SENESCENCE

Edited by **Tetsuji Nagata**

Senescence
Edited by Tetsuji Nagata

Published by InTech
Janeza Trdine 9, 51000 Rijeka, Croatia

Publishing Process Manager Iva Simcic

Technical Editor Teodora Smiljanic

Cover Designer InTech Design Team

Additional hard copies can be obtained from orders@intechopen.com

Senescence, Edited by Tetsuji Nagata
p. cm.
ISBN 978-953-51-0144-4

Meet the editor

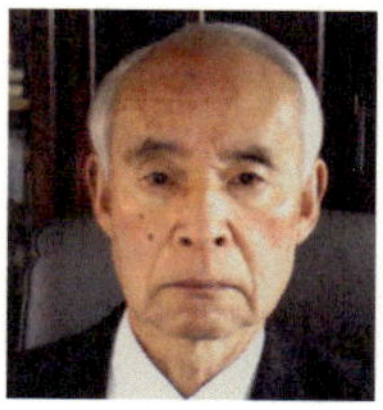

Tetsuji Nagata, M.D, Ph.D, Professor Emeritus (Department of Anatomy and Cell Biology, Shinshu University School of Medicine, Matsumoto, and Department of Anatomy, Shinshu Institute of Alternative Medicine and Welfare, Nagano) was Born in Nagano, Japan, February 5, 1931. After high school he finished premedical course at Shinshu University College of Liberal Arts and Sciences; medical education at Shinshu University School of Medicine, Matsumoto, Japan, 1951-1955. He received his PhD in Anatomy 1961., also at Shinshu University Graduate School of Medicine, Matsumoto, Japan. Dr. Nagata received several awards and honors. He is author of 10 single-authored books and 112 co-authored books, 586 original and review papers, 713 contributed papers at national and international conferences in Asian-Pacific, European and American countries.

Contents

Preface

This book is aimed to describe all the phenomena related to aging and senescence of all forms of life on Earth, i.e. plants, animals and the human beings. The book is comprised of 36 chapters written by diverse authors, including botanists, zoologists and physicians who study the aging and senescence of plants, animals and humans from structural and functional viewpoints.

Aging is the time frame during which a person, animal or a plant has lived, or a thing has existed. On the contrary, senescence are the signs of old age that a person, animal or a plant shows once they get old. This book aims to describe all the phenomena appearing in plants, animals and humans after they got old and became senescent.

The book contains 36 carefully reviewed chapters written by different authors, aiming to describe the aging and senescent changes of living creatures, i.e. plants and animals.

In each section, the chapters are arranged from lower plants or animals to higher creatures, as well as from the organ of movement to cardiovascular, visceral and neuro-sensory systems, according to the order of anatomy and histology. Thus, the readers will be able to carry each volume easily.

The Editor hopes that this book will have an interactive role in various fields of biology and medicine necessary to conduct further studies on aging and senescence. It should recount the background and current status of our knowledge in this field as well.

Finally, the Editor would like to express sincere gratitude to all the contributing authors and the staff of InTech – Open Access Publisher, especially Ms. Iva Simcic who regularly communicated with the editor and the respective authors, for their expertise and cooperation in the publication of this book.

Dr. Tetsuji Nagata
Shinshu University School of Medicine
Japan

Part 1

Plant

1

Photo- and Free Radical-Mediated Oxidation of Lipid Components During the Senescence of Phototrophic Organisms

Jean-François Rontani
Laboratory of Microbiology, Geochemistry and Marine Ecology (UMR 6117), Center of Oceanology of Marseille, Aix-Marseille University, Campus of Luminy, Marseille, France

1. Introduction

Recently, the role played by photochemical and free radical-mediated processes in the degradation of lipid components during the senescence of phototrophic organisms was investigated. The present paper reviews the results obtained in the course of these studies.

In a first part, visible and UV light-induced photooxidation of the main lipid cell components (chlorophylls, carotenoids, sterols, unsaturated fatty acids, highly branched isoprenoid and linear alkenes, alkenones, cuticular waxes ...) in senescent phototrophic organisms (phytoplankton, cyanobacteria, higher plants, purple sulfur bacteria and aerobic anoxygenic phototrophic bacteria) is examined. Probably due to its long lifetime in hydrophobic micro-environments and thus in senescent cells, singlet oxygen plays a key role in the photodegradation of most of the lipid components.

The second part of this paper describes the free radical oxidation (autoxidation) of lipid components during the senescence of phototrophic organisms, which have been virtually ignored until now in the literature. In senescent phototrophic organisms, the mechanism of initiation of free-radical oxidation seems to be the homolytic cleavage (catalyzed by some metal ions) of photochemically produced hydroperoxides. It was also demonstrated recently that viral infection and autocatalytic programmed cell death could also lead to elevated production of reactive oxygen species (ROS) able to induce the degradation of cell components.

2. Photodegradation processes in phototrophic organisms

Several works suggested photo-oxidation as an important sink of organic matter in the photic layer of oceans (Zafiriou, 1977; Zafiriou et al., 1984). However, due to the lack of suitable markers this phenomenon has never been fully addressed. Owing to the problem of stratospheric ozone depletion, some studies have recently examined the degradative effects of enhanced UV-B doses on phytoplanktonic lipids (He and Häder, 2002). However, photochemical damages in phytoplanktonic cells are not a monopoly of UV radiation. In fact, due to the presence of chlorophylls (which are very efficient photosensitizers (Foote, 1976; Knox and Dodge, 1985)), numerous organic components of phytoplankton are susceptible to being photodegraded during senescence by photosynthetically active radiation (PAR).

2.1 Photodegradation of the main lipidic components of phytoplankton during senescence

When a chlorophyll molecule absorbs a quantum of light energy, an excited singlet state (^{1}Chl) is formed which, in healthy cells, leads predominantly to the characteristic fast reactions of photosynthesis (Foote, 1976). However, a small proportion (<0.1%) undergoes intersystem crossing (ISC) to form the longer lived triplet state (^{3}Chl; Knox and Dodge, 1985). ^{3}Chl is not only itself potentially damaging in type I reactions (hydrogen atom or electron abstraction) (Knox and Dodge, 1985), but can also generate highly reactive oxygen species (ROS) and, in particular, singlet oxygen ($^1O_2$), by reaction with ground state oxygen ($^3O_2$) via Type II processes. In order to avoid oxidative damage, there are many antioxidant protective mechanisms in chloroplasts. Carotenoids quench ^{3}Chl and $^1O_2$ by energy transfer mechanisms at very high rates (Foote, 1976) and tocopherols can remove $^1O_2$, $O_2^{\bullet-}$, $HOO^\bullet$ and $HO^\bullet$ by acting as sacrificial scavengers (Halliwell, 1987). Superoxide dismutase enzyme (SOD) and ascorbic acid may also scavenge $O_2^{\bullet-}$ (Halliwell, 1987), while catalase activity decreases H_2O_2 levels.

In senescent phototrophic organisms, the fast reactions of photosynthesis clearly do not operate, so an accelerated rate of formation of ^{3}Chl and $^1O_2$ would be expected (Nelson, 1993). The rate of formation of these potentially damaging species can then exceed the quenching capacity of the photoprotective system and photodegradation can occur (photodynamic effect; Merzlyak and Hendry, 1994). In phytodetritus, when the ordered structure of the thylakoid membranes has been disrupted, pigments tend to remain associated with other hydrophobic cellular components such as membrane lipids (Nelson, 1993). As a result, the photooxidative effect of chlorophyll sensitization might be strongly amplified within such a hydrophobic micro-environment. Moreover, the lifetime of $^1O_2$ produced from sensitizers in a lipid-rich hydrophobic environment could be longer, and its potential diffusive distance greater, than its behaviour in aqueous solution (Suwa et al., 1977). It is not surprising, therefore, that photodegradation processes act on the majority of unsaturated lipid components of senescent phytoplankton.

2.1.1 Chlorophylls

Irradiation of dead phytoplankton cells by PAR and UVR radiations results in rapid degradation of chlorophylls (Nelson, 1993; Rontani et al., 1995; Christodoulou et al., 2010). Photodegradation of chlorophyll-*a* and -*c* in killed cells of *E. huxleyi* appeared to be induced by both PAR and UVR (Christodoulou et al., 2010). The photochemical degradation of chlorophylls has so far been studied almost exclusively with respect to the macrocycle moiety of the molecule, which is the more reactive. Despite some progress regarding intermediary photoproducts (Engel et al., 1991; Iturraspe et al., 1994), no stable and specific markers for the chlorophyll macrocycle photodegradation have been characterised.

The isoprenoid phytyl side-chain of chlorophylls is also sensitive to photochemical processes. In fact, in phytodetritus, the photodegradation rates were only 3 to 5 times higher for the chlorophyll tetrapyrrolic structure than for the phytyl side-chain (Cuny et al., 1999; Christodoulou et al., 2010). Analysis of isoprenoid photoproducts of chlorophylls after irradiation of different dead phytoplanktonic cells by visible light clearly established that the photodegradation of the chlorophyll phytyl side-chain in phytodetritus involved mainly

$^1O_2$. The type II (i.e. involving $^1O_2$) photosensitized oxidation of the phytol moiety of chlorophylls leads to the production of photoproducts of structures **a** and **b** (Fig. 1), quantifiable after $NaBH_4$-reduction and alkaline hydrolysis respectively in the form of 6,10,14-trimethylpentadecan-2-one (**1**) (phytone) and 3-methylidene-7,11,15-trimethyl-hexadecan-1,2-diol (phytyldiol) (**2**) (Fig. 1) (Rontani et al., 1994).

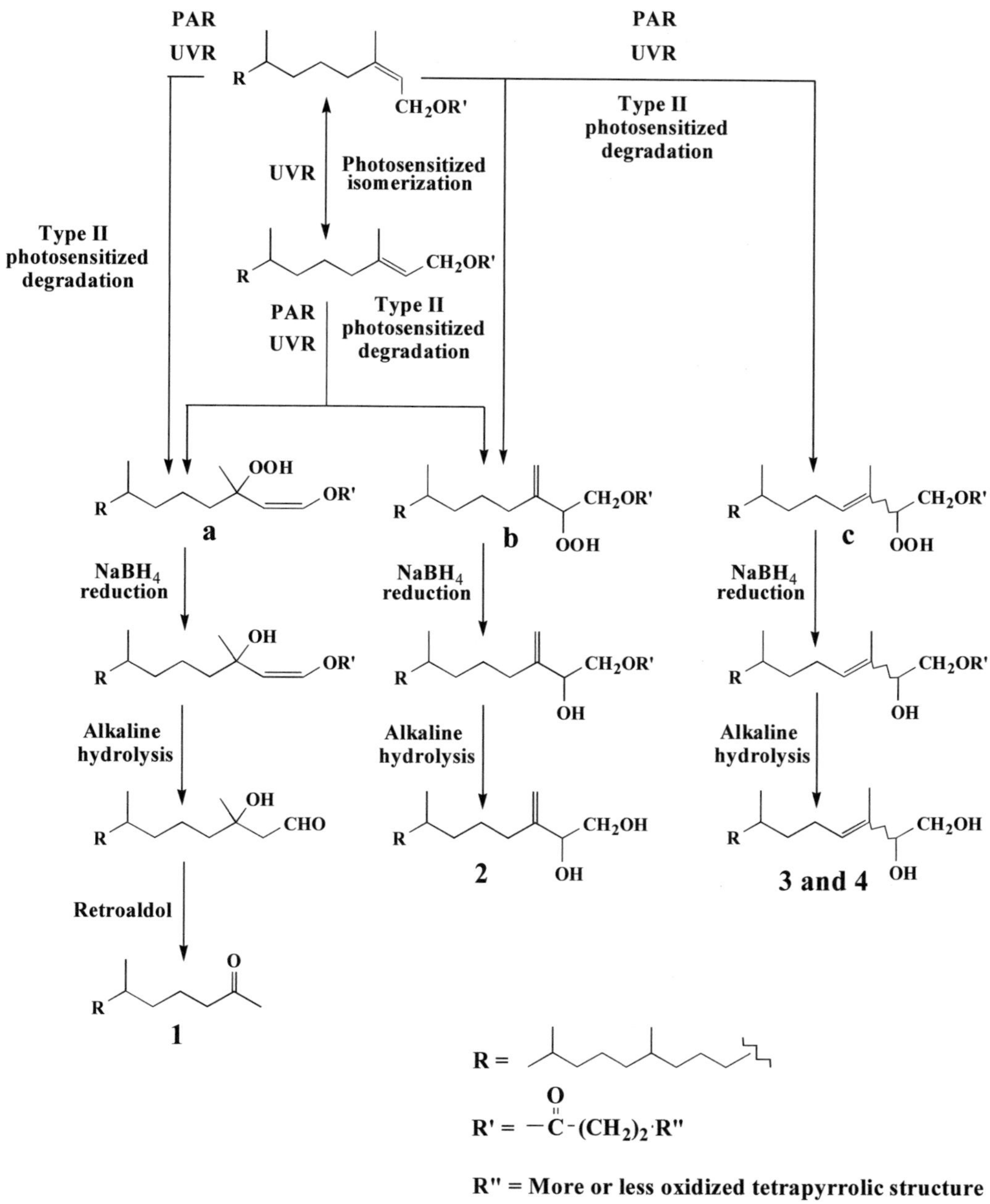

Fig. 1. Photooxidation of chlorophyll phytyl side-chain and reactions of oxidation products during alkaline hydrolysis.

Irradiation with UVR resulted in the additional production of small amounts of Z-phytol and Z and E-3,7,11,15-tetramethylhexadec-3-en-1,2-diols (**3,4**) (Christodoulou et al., 2010). The detection of Z-phytol allowed to demonstrate the induction of *cis-trans* photosensitized isomerization by UVR. These reactions probably involve triplet states of ketones as sensitizers. Type II photosensitized oxidation of the Z configuration of phytol, which should lead to the production of photoproducts of structures **a**, **b** and **c** (Fig. 1) (Schulte-Elte et al., 1979), explains the detection of small amounts of Z and E-3,7,11,15-tetramethylhexadec-3-en-1,2-diols (**3,4**) after irradiation with UVR. Irradiation with UVR also resulted in a faster degradation of chlorophyll phytyl side-chain oxidation products (Christodoulou et al., 2010). This higher reactivity was attributed to UVR-induced homolysis of the peroxyl group of photoproducts of structures **a**, **b** and **c** (Fig. 1).

Phytyldiol (**2**) is ubiquitous in the marine environment and has been proposed as tracer for photodegradation of chlorophyll's phytyl side chain (Rontani et al. 1994; 1996a; Cuny and Rontani 1999). Further, the molar ratio phytyldiol:phytol (Chlorophyll Phytyl side-chain Photodegradation Index, CPPI) was employed to estimate the extent of chlorophyll photodegraded in natural marine samples by the empirical equation: chlorophyll photodegradation % = $(1-(\text{CPPI} + 1)^{-18.5}) \times 100$ (Cuny et al. 2002).

2.1.2 Carotenoids

In phytodetritus, chlorophylls and carotenoids remain in a close molecular-scale association at relatively high localized concentrations, even though the structure of the thylakoid membrane has been disrupted (Nelson, 1993). Thus, the sensitized photooxidation of carotenoids is enhanced. The photosensitized oxidation (involving $^1O_2$) of carotenoids in solvents has been studied (Iseo et al., 1972) and loliolide (**5**), *iso*-loliolide (**6**) and dihydroactinidiolide (**7**) (Fig. 2) were identified as major photoproducts, depending on the functionality of carotenoids at C-3. Loliolide (**5**) and *iso*-loliolide (**6**) have been detected in killed cells of *Dunaliella* sp. irradiated by visible light (Rontani et al., 1998). However, due to their apparent production by anaerobic bacteria (Repeta, 1989) and during dark incubations of killed phytoplanktonic cells (Rontani et al., 1998), these compounds cannot constitute unequivocal indicators of photooxidative processes.

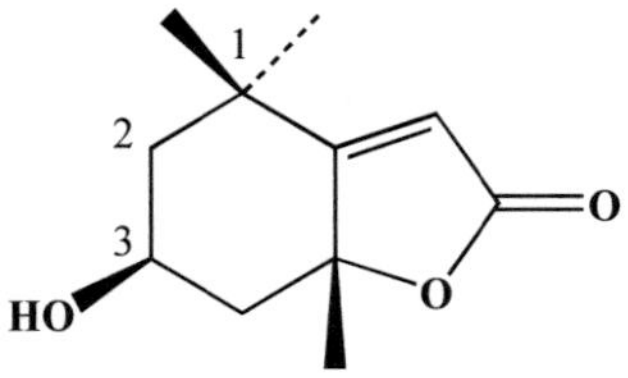

5

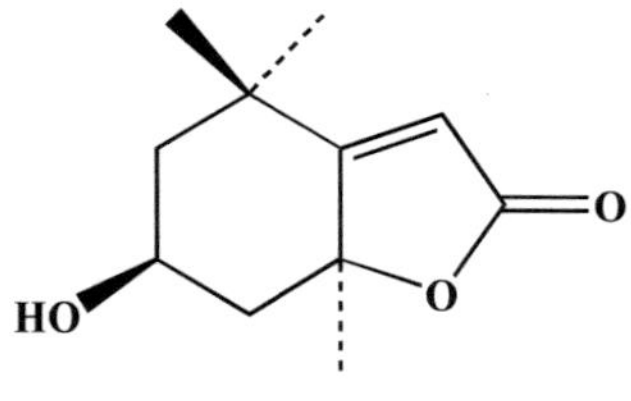

6

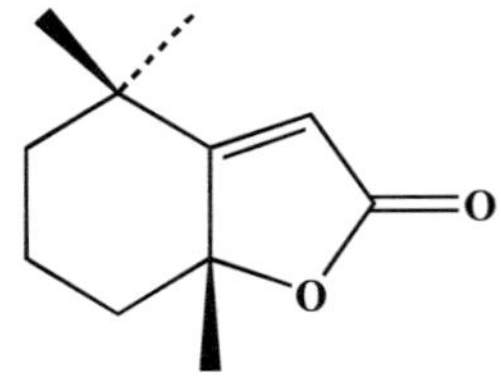

7

Fig. 2. Structure of the main carotenoid oxidation products.

2.1.3 Δ^5-sterols

As important unsaturated components of biological membranes, Δ^5-sterols are highly susceptible to photooxidative degradation during the senescence of phytoplankton. Irradiation by visible light of killed cells of *Skeletonema costatum*, *Dunaliella* sp.,

Phaeodactylum tricornutum and *Emiliania huxleyi* (Rontani et al., 1997a; 1997b; 1998) resulted in a quick photodegradation of the sterol components of these algae. The results obtained clearly established that the photooxidation of sterols in senescent cells of phytoplankton involves type II photoprocesses. These processes mainly produce Δ^6-5α-hydroperoxides (**8**) and to a lesser extent Δ^4-6α/6β-hydroperoxides (**9** and **10**) (Fig. 3) (Nickon and Bagli, 1961; Kulig and Smith, 1973). Δ^6-5α-hydroperoxysterols (**8**) are relatively unstable and may undergo allylic rearrangement to Δ^5-7α-hydroperoxysterols (**11**), which in turn epimerize to the corresponding 7β-hydroperoxides (**12**) (Fig. 3) (Smith, 1981). It was previously demonstrated that during singlet oxygen-mediated photooxidation of sterols in biological membranes (Korytowski *et al.*, 1992) and senescent phytoplanktonic cells (Rontani *et al.*, 1997a) the photogeneration of Δ^4-6α/6β-hydroperoxides (**9** and **10**) was more favourable than in homogeneous solution (ratio Δ^4-6α/6β-hydroperoxides/Δ^6-5α-hydroperoxysterols ranging from 0.30 to 0.35 instead of 0.1).

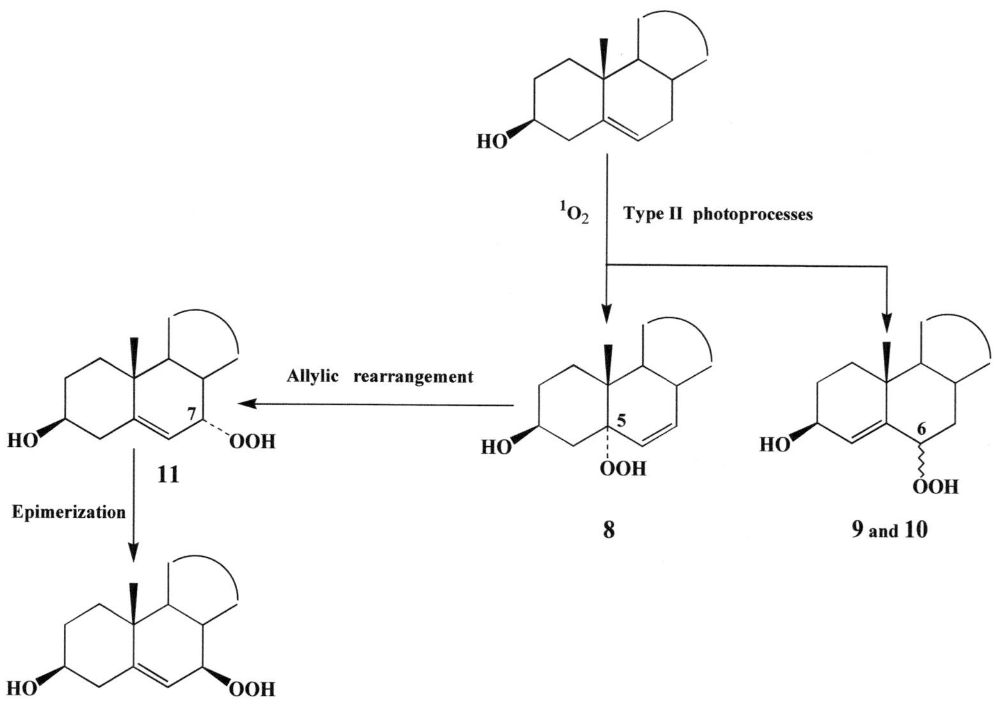

Fig. 3. Type II photosensitized oxidation of Δ^5 sterols.

Allylic rearrangement of Δ^6-5α-hydroperoxides (**8**) appeared to take place very weakly in senescent phytoplanktonic cells (Rontani et al., 1997a; 1997b; 1998). This surprising stability was attributed by Korytowski et al. (1992) either to hydrogen bonding between the unsaturated fatty acyl chain of phospholipids and Δ^6-5α-hydroperoxides (**8**) which could hinder the allylic rearrangement, or to differences of polarity in the carbon 7-10 zone of the fatty acyl chain (where sterols tend to localize in phospholipid/sterol bilayers (MacIntosch, 1978)). It is also interesting to note that the reduction of hydroperoxysterols to the corresponding diols weakly operates in killed phytoplanktonic cells (Rontani et al., 1997a).

Δ^6-5α-Hydroperoxysterols (**8**) are potential type II photodegradation markers, not only because they are the major products of singlet oxygen attack on the steroidal Δ^5-3β- system, but also because biological functionalization of steroids at C-5 is rare. Unfortunately, if these compounds are particularly stable in phytodetritus, they decay slowly in the sediment to their corresponding Δ^5-7α/β-derivatives (**11** and **12**) (Rontani and Marchand, 2000), which are not selective markers (see chapter 3.3). Moreover, according to the stability of the alkyl radicals formed during β-scission of the corresponding alkoxyl radicals, the following order of stability was proposed: Δ^4-6-hydroperoxysterols (**9** and **10**) > Δ^5-7-hydroperoxysterols (**11** and **12**) > Δ^6-5-hydroperoxy-sterols (**8**) (Christodoulou et al., 2009). Consequently, Δ^4-6α/β-hydroperoxysterols (**9** and **10**) (or their degradative products Δ^4-6α/β-hydroxysterols and Δ^4-6α/β-oxosterols) may be considered as more reliable *in situ* markers of type II photodegradation processes than Δ^6-5α-hydroperoxides (**8**).

2.1.4 Unsaturated fatty acids

Chloroplast membrane components are particularly susceptible to type II photooxidation (Heath and Packer, 1968). This is the case notably for unsaturated fatty acids, which generally predominate in algal lipids, particularly in the photosynthetic membranes (Woods, 1974). In killed phytoplanktonic cells, the photodegradation rates of unsaturated fatty acids logically increase with their unsaturation degree (Rontani et al., 1998). Singlet oxygen-mediated photooxidation of monounsaturated fatty acids involves a direct reaction of $^1O_2$ with the carbon–carbon double bond by a concerted 'ene' addition (Frimer 1979) and leads to formation of hydroperoxides at each carbon of the original double bond. Thus, photooxidation of oleic acid produces a mixture of 9- and 10-hydroperoxides with an allylic *trans*-double bond (Frankel et al. 1979; Frankel, 1998), which can subsequently undergo stereoselective radical allylic rearrangement to 11-*trans* and 8-*trans* hydroperoxides, respectively (Porter et al. 1995) (Fig. 4).

The free radical nature of the allylic hydroperoxide rearrangement is supported by the observation that the rearrangement is catalysed by free radical initiators or light and inhibited by phenolic antioxidants (Porter et al., 1995). This allylic rearrangement weakly intervenes in most of the killed phytoplanktonic cells examined (Rontani et al., 1998). This was attributed to the relatively high localized fatty acid concentrations present in phytodetritus (Nelson, 1993), which favoured the dimerisation of hydroperoxides. Hydrogen atom abstraction to form allylperoxyl radicals does indeed occur readily from hydroperoxide monomers but not from hydroperoxide dimers (Porter et al., 1995).

During early diagenesis, isomeric hydroperoxyacids undergo heterolytic cleavage to aldehydes and ω-oxocarboxylic acids (Frimer, 1979) or homolytic cleavage and subsequent transformation to the corresponding alcohols or ketones (Fig. 5).

Taking into account the high amounts of photoproducts of mono-unsaturated fatty acids detected in the particulate matter samples (Marchand and Rontani, 2001; Christodoulou et al., 2009; Rontani et al., 2011a), and the well known increasing photooxidation rates of fatty acids with their degree of unsaturation (Frankel., 1998), it can be concluded that considerable amounts of poly-unsaturated fatty acids must be photooxidized during the senescence of phytoplankton in the marine environment. However, at this time photooxidation products of this kind of fatty acids could not be detected in natural samples.

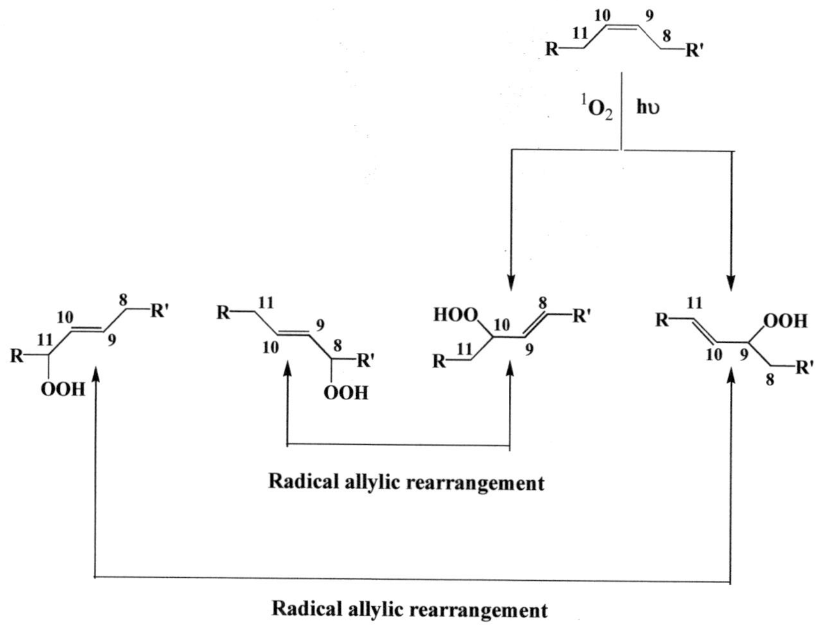

R = $-(CH_2)_6-CH_3$

R' = $-(CH_2)_6-COOH$

Fig. 4. Type II photosensitized oxidation of oleic acid.

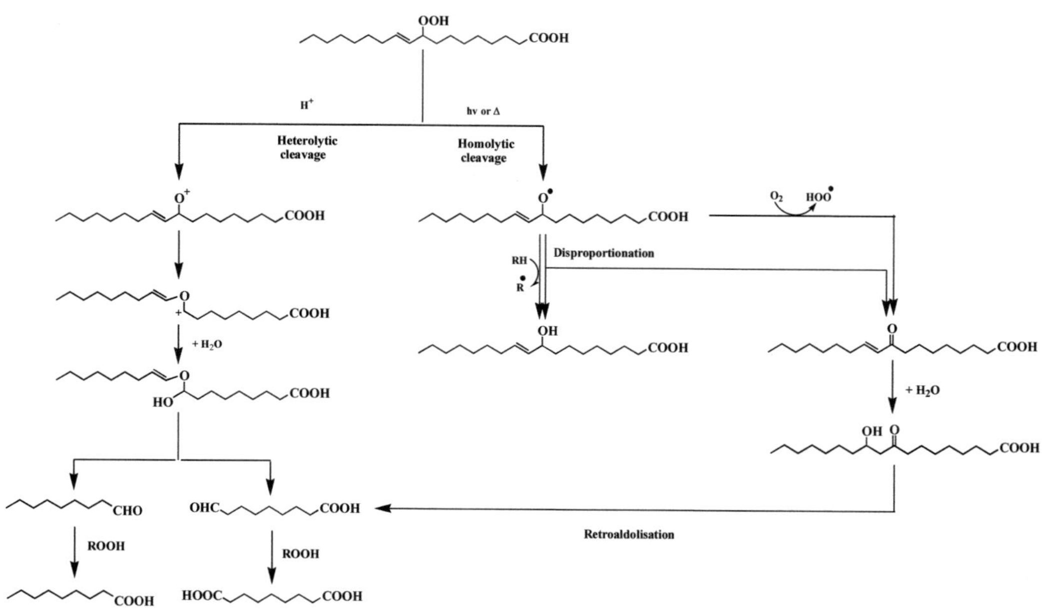

Fig. 5. Degradation of allylic hydroperoxides resulting from Type II photosensitized oxidation of monounsaturated fatty acids (the example given is this of 9-hydroperoxyoctadec-10-enoic acid) (RH = hydrogen donors, e.g. lipids or reduced sensitizers).

This is possibly due to: (i) the instability of the hydroperoxides formed, or (ii) the involvement of cross-linking reactions leading to the formation of macromolecular structures (Neff et al., 1988) non-amenable by gas chromatography.

2.1.5 Alkenones

Alkenones are a class of mono-, di-, tri-, tetra- and penta-unsaturated C_{35}-C_{40} methyl and ethyl ketones (Boon et al., 1978; Volkman et al., 1980; de Leeuw et al., 1980; Marlowe et al., 1984; Prahl et al., 2006; Jaraula et al., 2010), which are produced by certain marine haptophytes. *Emiliania huxleyi* and *Gephyrocapsa oceanica* are the major sources of alkenones in the open ocean (Volkman et al., 1980; 1995; Conte et al., 1994). The unsaturation ratio of C_{37} alkenones, defined as $U_{37}^{K'} = [C_{37:2}] / ([C_{37:2}] + [C_{37:3}])$ where $[C_{37:2}]$ and $[C_{37:3}]$ are the concentrations of di- and tri-unsaturated C_{37} alkenones respectively, varies positively with the growth temperature of the alga (Prahl and Wakeham, 1987; Prahl et al., 1988). The $U_{37}^{K'}$- growth temperature relationship in haptophyte algae and transferred to sinking marine particulate matter leads to a linear relationship between sedimentary C_{37} alkenone composition and mean annual SST records throughout the oceans (Rosell-Melé et al., 1995; Müller et al., 1998). The $U_{37}^{K'}$ index is now routinely used for paleotemperature reconstruction.

For alkenones to be useful as measures of sea surface temperature in the geological record, it is essential that any effects of degradation in the water column and in sediments either do not affect the temperature signal established during their initial biosynthesis by the alga (Harvey, 2000; Grimalt et al., 2000), or if there is a change its extent can be reasonably estimated.

Visible light-induced photodegradation of these compounds was thus previously investigated in order to determine if photochemical processes could appreciably modify $U_{37}^{K'}$ ratios during algal senescence (Rontani et al., 1997b; Mouzdahir et al., 2001; Christodoulou et al., 2010). Though potentially selective, photochemical degradation of alkenones is not fast enough in killed cells of *E. huxleyi* to induce strong modifications of the $U_{37}^{K'}$ ratio before the photodestruction of the photosensitizing substances (Rontani et al., 1997b; Mouzdahir et al., 2001). UVR also appeared to be inefficient to alter the $U_{37}^{K'}$ ratio (Christodoulou et al., 2010).

This stability was attributed to the *trans* configuration of alkenone double bonds (Rechka and Maxwell, 1988) that is 7 to 10 times less sensitive against singlet oxygen-mediated oxidation than the classical *cis* configuration of fatty acids (Hurst et al., 1985). This may explain the difference of photoreactivity observed between the alkenones and fatty acids with the same number of unsaturations. We also previously attributed the poor photoreactivity of alkenones to a localisation of these compounds elsewhere than in cell membranes (Rontani et al., 1997b; Mouzdahir et al., 2001), which could significantly decrease the likelihood of interaction between singlet oxygen and alkenones. Although this hypothesis is well supported by the recent results of Eltgroth et al. (2005), who demonstrated that alkenones are mainly localized into cytoplasmic vesicles, the migration of singlet oxygen from phytodetritus to attached heterotrophic bacteria previously observed (Rontani et al., 2003a; Christodoulou et al., 2010) strongly suggests a diffusion of this excited form of oxygen also in these cytoplasmic vesicles.

2.1.6 n-Alkenes

The visible light-induced degradation of *n*-alkenes was previously investigated in killed cells of the Prymnesiophycea *E. huxleyi* and the Eustigmatophycea *Nannochloropsis salina* (Mouzdahir et al., 2001).

In *E. huxleyi* killed cells, minor C_{31} and C_{33} *n*-alkenes were strongly photodegraded, while the major C_{37} and C_{38} *n*-alkenes appeared particularly recalcitrant towards photochemical processes. These strong differences of photoreactivity imply distinct biological syntheses and/or functions for these two groups of hydrocarbons in *E. huxleyi* cells. Interestingly, the stereochemistry of the internal double bonds in C_{31} and C_{33} n-alkenes has been established to be *cis*, while C_{37} and C_{38} alkenes internal double bonds exhibit a *trans* geometry (Rieley et al., 1998; Grossi et al., 2000). The photochemical recalcitrance of C_{37} and C_{38} n-alkenes could thus be partly attributed to the *trans* geometry of their internal double bonds.

Irradiation of dead cells of *N. salina* resulted in a strong modification of the hydrocarbon fraction. It did not provide evidence of a significant light-dependent degradation of monounsaturated hydrocarbons; this result was attributed to the terminal position of the double bond in these compounds (Gelin et al., 1997), which is poorly reactive towards singlet oxygen (Hurst et al., 1985). In contrast, di-, tri-, and tetraenes were strongly photodegraded during irradiation. The visible light-dependent degradation of phytoplanktonic *n*-alkenes showed apparent second-order kinetics with respect to light exposure and the half-life doses obtained logically decrease with increasing number of double bonds in these compounds (Mouzdahir et al., 2001).

2.1.7 Highly branched isoprenoid (HBI) alkenes

HBI alkenes are widely distributed in aquatic environments (Rowland and Robson, 1990; Sinninghe-Damsté et al., 2004), although they appear to originate from a relatively small number of diatomaceous algae including *Haslea* spp., *Rhizosolenia* spp., *Pleurosigma* spp. and *Navicula* spp. (Volkman et al., 1994; Sinninghe-Damsté et al., 2004; Belt et al., 2000, 2001; Allard et al., 2001; Grossi et al., 2004). Despite this, they have been commonly reported in marine sediments worldwide and provide some insight into the deposition of organic matter from the water column. One HBI alkene, a mono-unsaturated isomer termed IP_{25}, has been used as a proxy for the occurrence of spring sea ice in the Arctic (e.g. Belt et al., 2007, 2010; Massé et al., 2008).

Examination of the photoreactivity of several mono-, di-, tri- and tetra-unsaturated HBI alkenes in the presence of a photosensitizer solution and in dead cells of *H. ostrearia* allowed to show that HBI alkenes possessing at least one tri-substituted double bond may be photo-oxidized at similar or higher rates compared to other highly reactive lipids (e.g. PUFAs, vitamin E and chlorophyll *a*) during the senescence of diatom cells (Rontani et al., 2011b). As a consequence, it is proposed that HBI alkenes possessing trisubstituted double bonds are likely to be susceptible to photodegradation within the euphotic zone. In contrast, HBIs containing only mono- and di-substituted double bonds were found to be significantly less reactive towards $^1O_2$ and should, therefore, be relatively preserved during sedimentation through the water column (Rontani et al., 2011b). The kinetic experiments are supported by product analysis, which revealed that the main reaction with $^1O_2$ primarily occurs with the trisubstituted double bonds of HBI alkenes affording tertiary and secondary allylic hydroperoxides (Fig. 6). In contrast, the extremely low photoreactivity of the HBI monoene

IP_{25}, can be attributed to its containing only the least photochemically reactive double bond. This lack of reactivity supports (in part) the good preservation of IP_{25} generally observed in sediments (Belt et al., 2007, 2010; Massé et al., 2008).

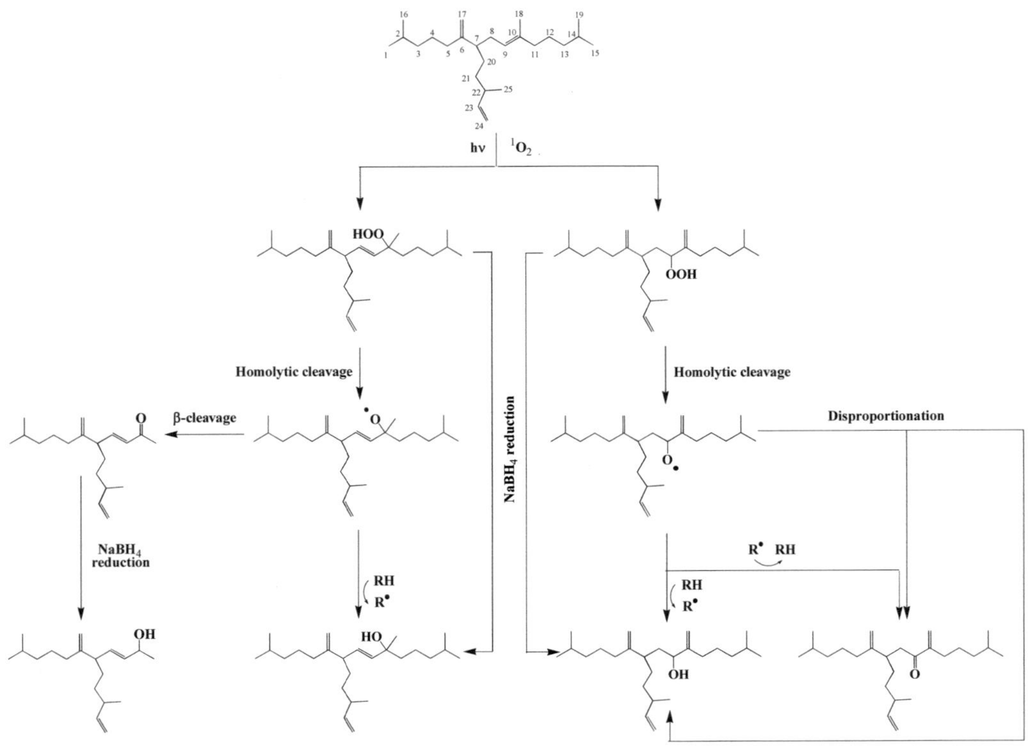

Fig. 6. Type II photosensitized oxidation of HBI alkenes (RH = hydrogen donors)

2.2 Photodegradation processes in other phototrophic organisms

Visible light-dependent degradation processes have been also studied in senescent cells of two purple sulfur bacteria (*Thiohalocapsa halophila* and *Halochromatium salexigens*) isolated from microbial mats from Camargue (France) (Marchand and Rontani, 2003). These reactions act intensively on the phytyl side chain of bacteriochlorophyll-*a* and lead to the production of phytone (**1**) and phytyldiol (**2**) as in the case of chlorophylls (Fig. 1). Palmitoleic and *cis*-vaccenic acids also undergo strong photodegradation, affording mainly isomeric allylic oxo-, hydroxy- and hydroperoxyacids.

These processes were also investigated in aerobic anoxygenic phototrophic bacteria (AAPs) (Rontani et al., 2003a). These organisms constitute a relatively recently discovered bacterial group (Yurkov and Beatty, 1998) and seem to be widespread in the open ocean (Kolber et al., 2000). They perform photoheterotrophic metabolism, requiring organic carbon for growth, but they are capable to use photosynthesis as an auxiliary source of energy (Kolber et al., 2001). Though sensitive to photochemical processes in senescent purple sulfur bacteria (Marchand and Rontani., 2003), the isoprenoid phytyl side-chain of bacteriochlorophyll -*a* is not significantly photodegraded in senescent cells of AAPs (Rontani et al., 2003a). In contrast, significant amounts of allylic hydroxyacids arising from the photo-oxidation of the major unsaturated fatty acid of these organisms (*cis*-vaccenic acid) could be detected after irradiation (Rontani et al., 2003a).

As in the case of phytoplankton and cyanobacteria, visible light-dependent degradation processes act significantly on the chlorophyll phytyl side-chain (Rontani et al., 1996b), unsaturated fatty acids and sterols (Rontani, Unpublished results) during terrestrial higher plant senescence affording similar photoproducts. 9-Hydroperoxy-18-hydroxyoctadec-10(*trans*)-enoic (**13**) and 10-hydroperoxy-18-hydroxyoctadec-8(*trans*)-enoic (**14**) acids deriving from type II photooxidation of 18-hydroxyoleic acid (**15**) (Fig. 7) were detected after visible light-induced senescence experiments carried out with *Petroselinum sativum* and subsequent cutin depolymerisation (Rontani et al., 2005a).

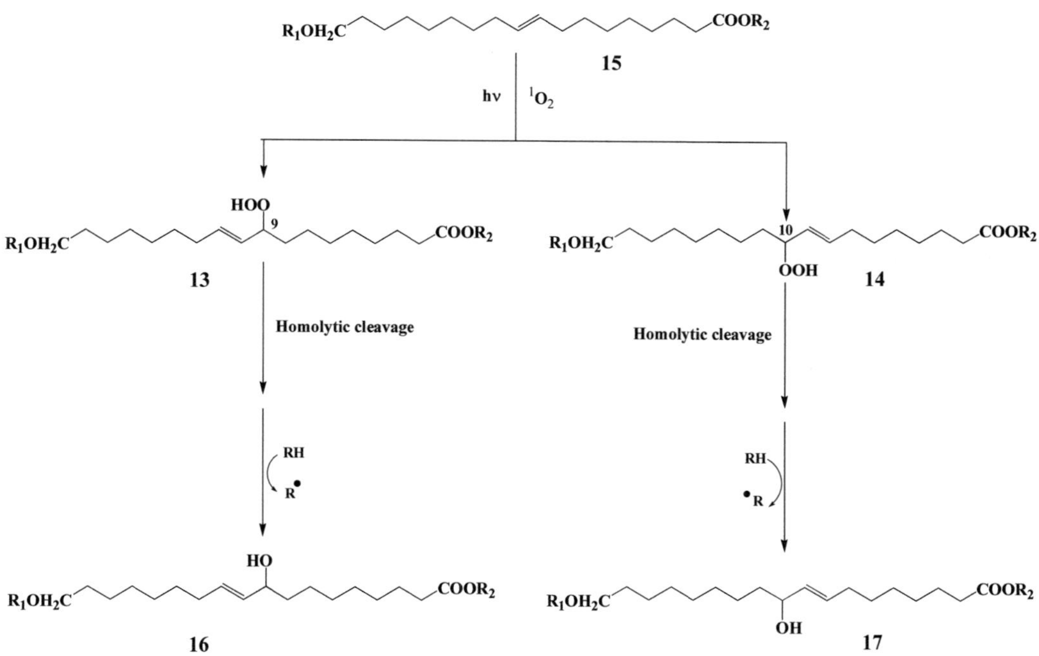

Fig. 7. Type II photosensitized oxidation of 18-hydroxyoleic acid in cutin polymers.

These results showed that in senescent plants, where the $^1O_2$ formation rate exceeds the quenching capacity of the photoprotective system, $^1O_2$ can migrate outside the chloroplasts and affect the unsaturated components of cutins. Significant amounts of 9,18-dihydroxyoctadec-10(*trans*)-enoic (**16**) and 10,18-dihydroxyoctadec-8(*trans*)-enoic (**17**) acids resulting from the reduction of these photoproducts of 18-hydroxyoleic acid were also detected in different natural samples (Rontani et al., 2005a). These results well support the significance of the photooxidation of the unsaturated components of higher plant cutins in the natural environment.

3. Free radical degradation (autoxidation) processes in phototrophic organisms

Autoxidation is the direct reaction of molecular oxygen with organic compounds under mild conditions. The autoxidation of organic compounds (in particular, lipids) involves free radical reaction chains and thus includes an initiation, a propagation and a termination phase. Mechanisms of initiation for the free radical processes have been the subject of many studies. In senescent phytoplanktonic cells, initiation seems to result from the decomposition of hydroperoxides produced during photodegradation of cellular organic matter (Rontani et al., 2003b). Until now, autoxidative degradation in the marine environment has been largely ignored. Specific markers of these reactions have been highlighted by *in vitro* studies (Frankel, 1998; Rontani et al., 2003b; Rontani and Aubert, 2005). Using these markers, it was demonstrated *in situ* that autoxidation plays a very significant role in the degradation of particulate organic matter (Marchand et al., 2005; Rontani et al., 2006; Christodoulou et al., 2009; Rontani et al., 2011a).

Although the occurrence of autoxidation processes was clearly demonstrated *in situ*, it is not easy to induce these processes in laboratory cultures. Indeed, the mechanism of initiation of lipid radical oxidation, which has been debated for many years, seems to be the homolytic cleavage of photochemically produced hydroperoxides in phytodetritus (Rontani et al., 2003b). Redox-active metal ions are generally considered as the initiators of perhaps greatest importance for lipid oxidation in biological systems (Pokorny, 1987; Schaich, 1992). They may direct the cleavage of hydroperoxides either through alkoxyl or peroxyl radicals. In classical culture media (such as f/2) the metal chelator EDTA, which is present in high amounts, tightly binds free catalytic metal ions and thus renders them unavailable. EDTA thus acts in the culture media as an antioxidant and strongly limits radical oxidation processes.

Recently, autoxidative damages in cells of *E. huxleyi* strain CS-57 could be induced after incubation of this strain under an atmosphere of air + 0.5% CO_2 (Rontani et al., 2007a). The presence of additional CO_2 allowed: (i) to induce a stress that favoured oxidative damage and (ii) to decrease the pH of the culture medium releasing metal ions from EDTA complexes, which can act as catalysts of hydroperoxide homolysis.

It was also demonstrated recently that viral infection (Evans et al., 2006) and autocatalytic programmed cell death (Bidle and Falkowski, 2004) of phytoplanktonic cells could also lead to elevated production of reactive oxygen species (ROS) able to induce the degradation of cell components.

3.1 Chlorophyll phytyl side-chain

Autoxidation of the esterified chlorophyll phytyl chain involves either addition of peroxyl radicals to the double bond or hydrogen abstraction at the allylic carbon 4 (Rontani and Aubert, 1994; Rontani and Aubert, 2005). Classical addition of peroxyl radical to the double bond gives a tertiary radical (Fig. 8). This radical can then: (i) lead to *Z* and *E* epoxides (**18** and **19**) by fast intramolecular homolytic substitution (Fossey et al., 1995), or (ii) react with molecular oxygen affording (after hydrogen abstraction on another molecule of substrate) a diperoxide (**20**) (Fig. 8). Subsequent $NaBH_4$-reduction and alkaline hydrolysis of these compounds gives 3,7,11,15-tetramethylhexadecan-1,2,3-triol (**21**) (Fig. 8). In contrast, abstraction (by photochemically-produced peroxyl radicals) of a hydrogen atom at the allylic carbon 4 of the phytyl chain and subsequent oxidation of the allylic radicals thus formed affords (after $NaBH_4$-reduction and alkaline hydrolysis) *Z* and *E* 3,7,11,15-tetramethylhexadec-3-en-1,2-diols (**3** and **4**) and *Z* and *E* 3,7,11,15-tetramethyl-hexadec-2-en-1,4-diols (**22** and **23**) (Fig. 8). Compounds **22 and 23** (which are well specific markers of free radical oxidation) could be detected in particulate matter samples (Marchand et al., 2005) and *E. huxleyi* cells (Rontani et al., 2007a) attesting to the involvement of such processes in senescent phytoplanktonic cells.

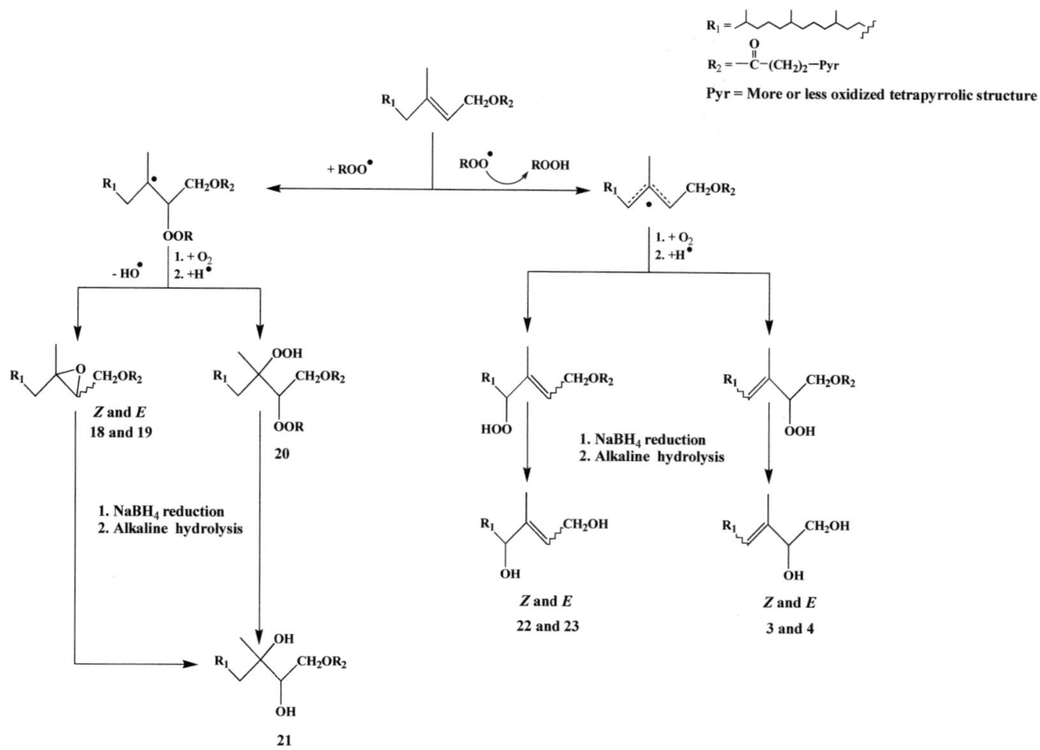

Fig. 8. Free radical-mediated oxidation of chlorophyll phytyl side-chain.

Free radical oxidation of chlorophyll phytyl chain appeared to be different in senescent cells of *S. costatum* (Rontani et al., 2003b). The differences observed were attributed to the well documented high chlorophyllase activity of this strain (Jeffrey and Hallegraeff, 1987) catalysing the hydrolysis of chlorophyll to free phytol and chlorophyllide. Indeed, in the case of free allylic alcohols hydrogen abstraction at carbon 1 is strongly favoured to the detriment of addition reactions (Huyser and Johnson, 1968).

3.2 Unsaturated fatty acids

Free radical oxidation of isolated classical 1,2-disubstituted double bonds generally involved mainly allylic hydrogen abstraction. Addition of peroxyl or alkoxyl radicals to the double bond becomes competitive only in the case of conjugated, terminal, or trisubstituted double bonds (Schaich, 2005). Effectively, autoxidation of mono-unsaturated fatty acids appears to mainly involve allylic hydrogen abstraction and subsequent oxidation of the allylic radical thus formed. For example, autoxidation of oleic acid mainly results in the formation of 9-hydroperoxyoctadec-*trans*-10-enoic (**24**), 10-hydroperoxyoctadec-*trans*-8-enoic (**25**), 11-hydroperoxyoctadec-*trans*-9-enoic (**26**), 11-hydroperoxyoctadec-*cis*-9-enoic (**27**), 8-hydroperoxyoctadec-*trans*-9-enoic (**28**) and 8-hydroperoxyoctadec-*cis*-9-enoic (**29**) acids (Fig. 9) (Frankel, 1998).

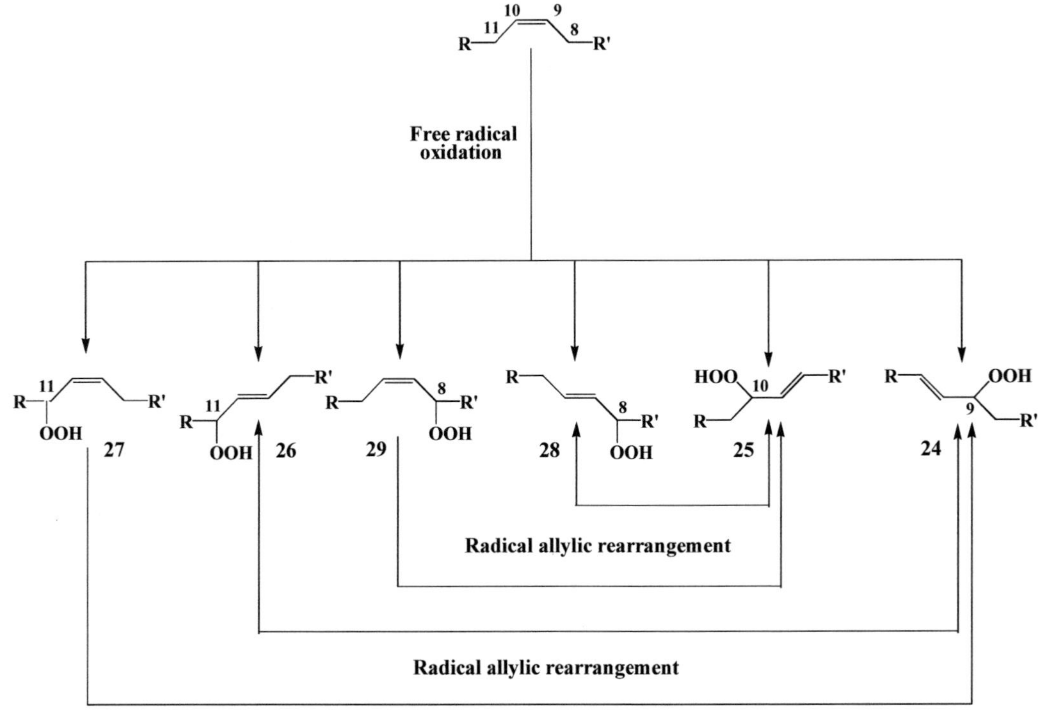

R = $-(CH_2)_6-CH_3$

R' = $-(CH_2)_6-COOH$

Fig. 9. Free radical-mediated oxidation of oleic acid.

Free radical oxidative processes can be easily characterised based on the presence of *cis* allylic hydroperoxyacids, which cannot be produced photochemically (see Fig. 4) and are specific products of these degradation processes (Porter et al., 1995; Frankel, 1998).

Large amounts of oxidation products of oleic acid could be detected in cells of *E. huxleyi* grown under an atmosphere of air + 0.5% CO_2 for 10 days (Rontani et al., 2007a). The presence (after $NaBH_4$-reduction) of a high proportion of 11-hydroxyoctadec-*cis*-9-enoic (**27**) and 8-hydroxyoctadec-*cis*-9-enoic (**29**) acids (Fig. 10) showed that under these conditions the degradation of oleic acid mainly involved free radical oxidation processes.

3.3 Δ^5-sterols

Free radical autoxidation of Δ^5-stenols yields mainly 7*α*- and 7*β*-hydroperoxides and, to a lesser extent, 5*α*/*β*,6*α*/*β*-epoxysterols and 3*β*,5*α*,6*β*-trihydroxysterols (Smith, 1981; Morrissey and Kiely, 2006) (Fig. 11).

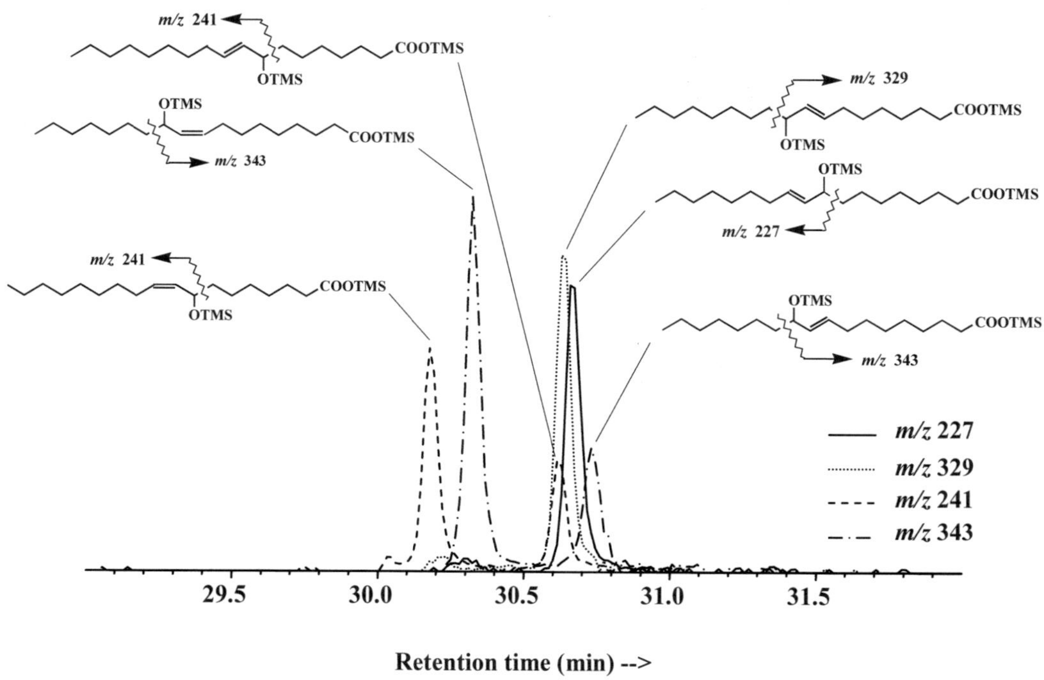

Fig. 10. Partial mass chromatogram of *m/z* 227, 329, 241 and 343 revealing the presence of oxidation products of oleic acid in the saponified fraction of *E. huxleyi* strain CS-57 grown under an atmosphere of air + 0.5% CO_2.

Owing to: their lack of specificity (possible formation by allylic rearrangement of photochemically-produced 5-hydroperoxides (see chapter 2.1.3), 7-hydroperoxides cannot be employed as tracers of autoxidation processes in phytodetritus. In contrast, it is generally considered that 5*α*/*β*,6*α*/*β*-epoxysterols arise mainly from peroxidation processes (Breuer and Björkhem, 1995; Giuffrida et al., 2004). Unfortunately, these compounds are not very stable and may be easily hydrolysed to the corresponding triol in seawater and during the treatment of the samples. 5*α*/*β*,6*α*/*β*-Epoxysterols and the corresponding 3*β*,5*α*,6*β*-trihydroxysterols were thus finally selected as tracers of sterol autoxidation..

5*α*/*β*,6*α*/*β*-Epoxysterols and 3*β*,5*α*,6*β*-trihydroxysterols corresponding to sitosterol, stigmasterol and campesterol were previously detected in young and old cell cultures of *Chenopodium rubrum* (Meyer and Spiteller, 1997). The results showed that the increase of these oxidation products well correlated with the age of the culture.

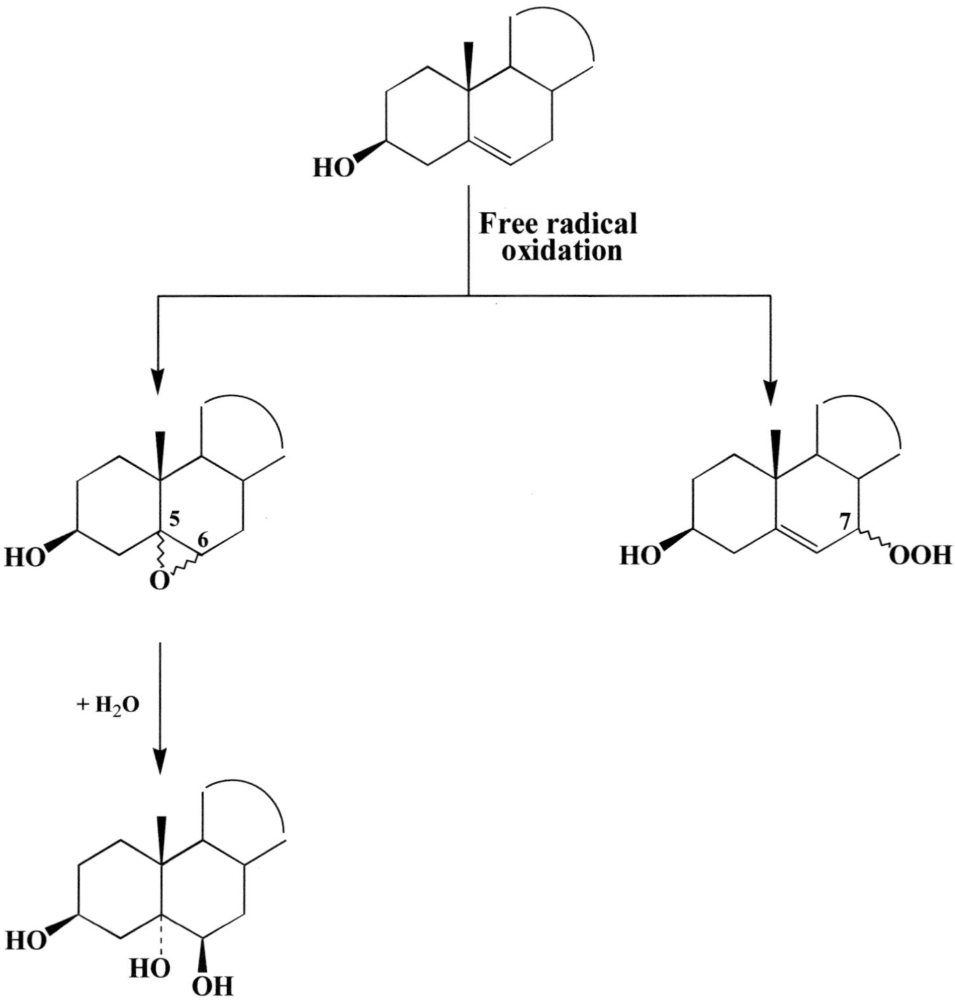

Fig. 11. Free radical-mediated oxidation of Δ^5 sterols.

3.4 Vitamin E

Vitamin E is relatively abundant in most photosynthetic organisms, such as higher plants (Rise et al., 1988; Schultz, 1990), cyanobacteria (Dasilva and Jensen, 1971), microalgae (Brown et al., 1999) and macroalgae (Sanchez-Machado et al., 2002), where it plays an essential role in the removal of toxic forms of oxygen (singlet oxygen, superoxide anion, hydroxyl and peroxyl radicals), by acting as sacrificial chemical scavenger (Halliwell, 1987); the process results in the irreversible oxidation of the tocopherol molecule. Vitamin E reacts rapidly with peroxyl radicals, affording small amounts of phytone (**1**), 4,8,12,16-tetramethylheptadecan-4-olide, α-tocopherylquinone and epoxy-α-tocopherylquinones, and dimers and trimers as major oxidation products (Liebler, 1994; Frankel, 1998; Rontani et al., 2007b) (Fig. 12).

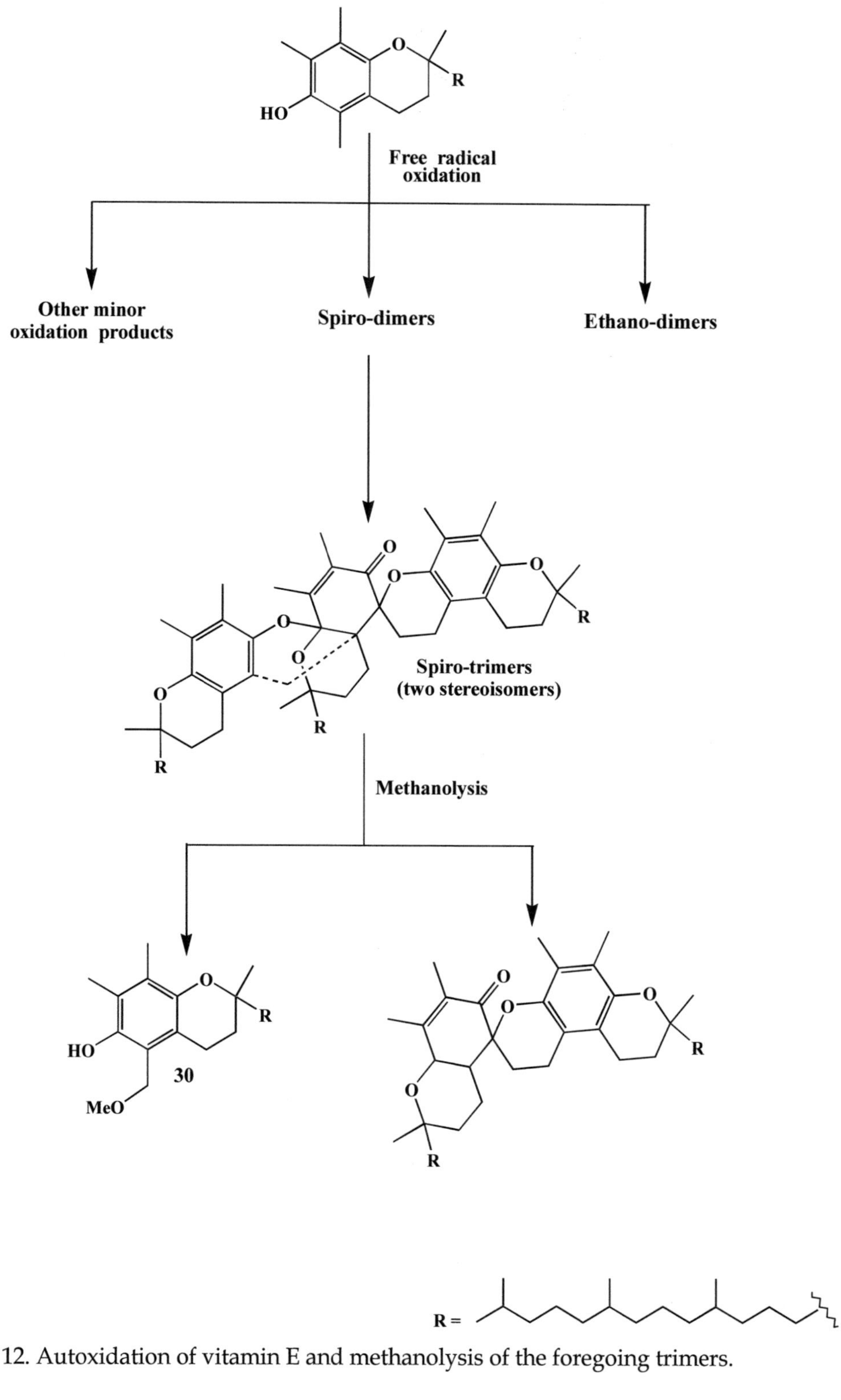

Fig. 12. Autoxidation of vitamin E and methanolysis of the foregoing trimers.

Isomeric trimers have been previously observed as products in numerous oxidations of vitamin E (e.g. Suarna et al., 1988; Krol et al., 2001). Such compounds cannot be easily detected since they are too heavy to be amenable by gas chromatography. However, methanolysis of the residues obtained resulted to the formation of high amounts of 5a-methoxytocopherol (**30**) arising from the methanolysis of the ketal group of trimers (Fig. 12) (Yamauchi et al., 1988). ESI-TOF MS analyses of oxidation products were also carried out in order to confirm the presence of high proportions of trimers (Nassiry et al., 2009).

Despite the intensive study of vitamin E oxidation since several decades, trimeric oxidation products could be detected in plants only very recently by Row et al. (2007). These authors detected these trimers in seeds of *Euryale ferox* containing extraordinarily high content of tocopherols. It is interesting to note that trimers were previously obtained as the major reaction products of vitamin E autoxidized under mild conditions in solution (1%) in methyl linoleate (Yamauchi et al., 1988). In plastoglobules, which are lipid monolayer subcompartments of the thylakoid membranes of chloroplasts (Maeda and Dellapenna, 2007), the concentration of tocopherols can reach 10% of the total fatty acids (Vidi et al., 2006). At such a concentration, the formation of a high proportion of trimers during photodynamic damages is thus very likely. In order to check this hypothesis, we searched for the presence of 5a-methoxytocopherol (**30**) after methanolysis of $NaBH_4$-reduced and non-reduced lipid extracts obtained from cells of *Emiliania huxleyi* strain TWP1 and *Chrysotila lamellosa* strain HAP17. The detection of significant amounts of this methanolysis product of trimers (Yamauchi et al., 1988) in these extracts (Nassiry et al., 2009) well supported the presence of such trimeric oxidation products of vitamin E in these algae.

3.5 Alkenones

The autoxidative reactivity of alkenones was studied in the laboratory in the presence of a radical initiator (di-*tert*-butyl nitroxide) and a radical enhancer (*tert*-butyl hydroperoxide) (Rontani et al., 2006). Alkenones appeared to be more sensitive towards oxidative free radical processes than analogues of other common marine lipids such as phytyl acetate, methyl oleate and cholesteryl acetate, and their oxidation rates increase in proportion with their number of double bonds. As the result of this increasing reactivity with degree of unsaturation, the $U_{37}^{K'}$ ratio increased significantly (up to 0.20) during the incubation.

Autoxidation of alkenones appears to mainly involve allylic hydrogen abstraction and subsequent oxidation of the allylic radical thus formed (Fig. 13). According to these processes, oxidation of each double bond of alkenones and subsequent $NaBH_4$ reduction affords four positional isomeric alkenediols. These compounds could be very useful indicators of autoxidation of alkenones but, unfortunately, they did not accumulate during the incubation. Indeed, due to the presence of additional reactive double bonds, hydroperoxyalkenones may undergo subsequent oxidation reactions affording, di-, tri- and tetrahydroperoxyalkenones according to the degree of unsaturation of the starting alkenone. In seawater, these different hydroperoxides may undergo two main degradative processes: (i) homolysis of the O-O bond leading to carbonyl (dehydration), alcoholic (reduction) and fragmentation (β-scission) products (Rontani et al., 2007c) and (ii) heterolysis of the O-O bond leading to the formation of two carbonyl fragments (Hock cleavage), this proton-catalysed cleavage being initiated by migration of groups to positive oxygen (Frimer, 1979). Dimeric and oligomeric compounds cross-linked through either peroxide or ether linkages (Frankel, 1998) may also be formed during autoxidation of alkenones.

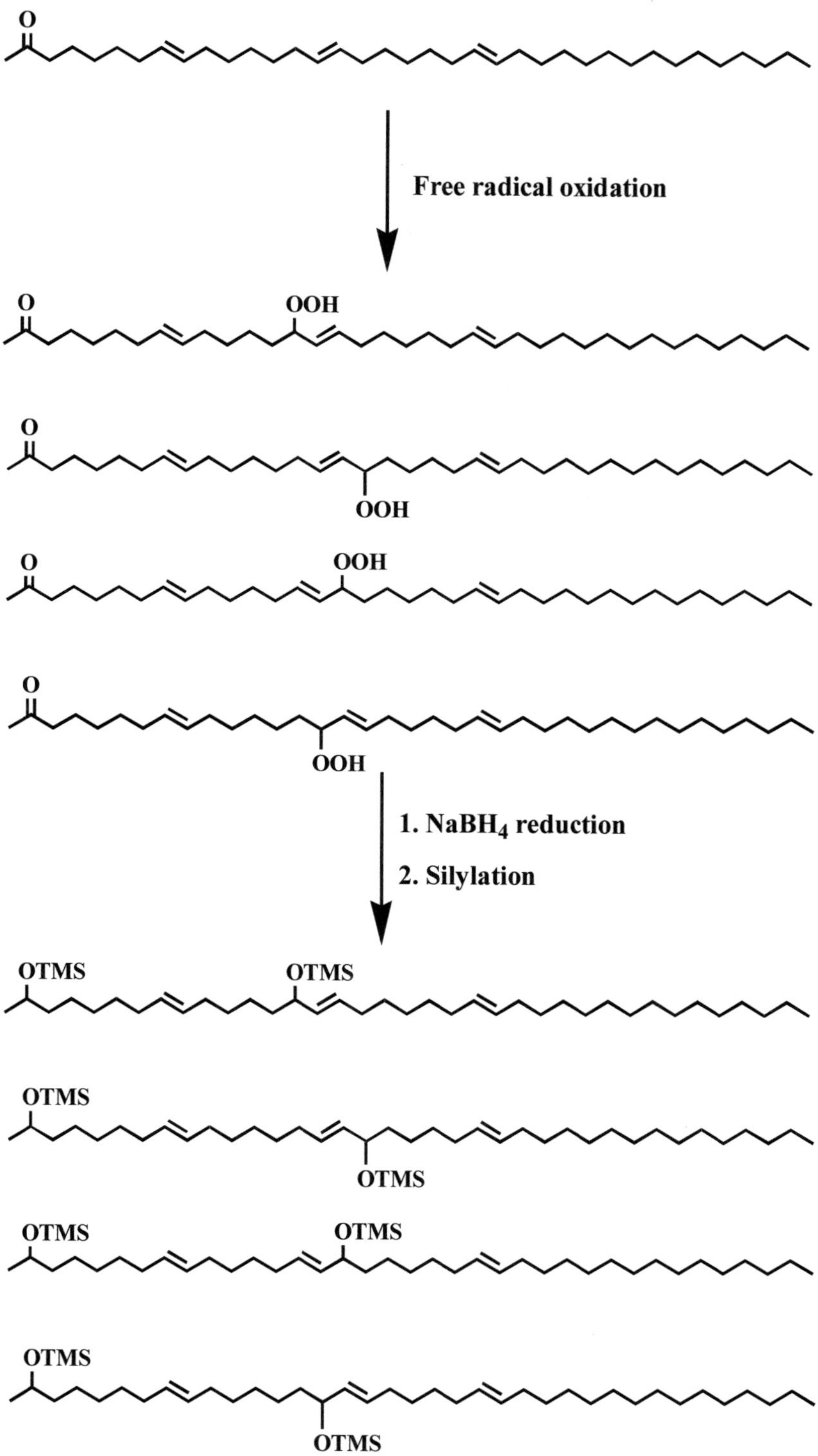

Fig. 13. Characterization of oxidation products derived from the autoxidation of the ω22 double bond of the $C_{37:3}$ alkenone (TMS = trimethylsilyl).

These results were corroborated by the further finding of significant amounts of alkenediols arising from $NaBH_4$-reduction of the corresponding hydroperoxyalkenones in cultures of *E. huxleyi* strain CS-57 grown under an atmosphere of air + 0.5% CO_2 (Rontani et al., 2007a) and more recently after incubation of a culture of the strain *E. huxleyi* TWP1 under darkness (Rontani, Unpublished results) (Fig. 14) both exhibiting an anomalously high unsaturation ratio It seems thus that autoxidation processes have the potential to affect alkenone distributions leading to a warm bias in estimates of palaeotemperatures derived from alkenone ratios in sediments.

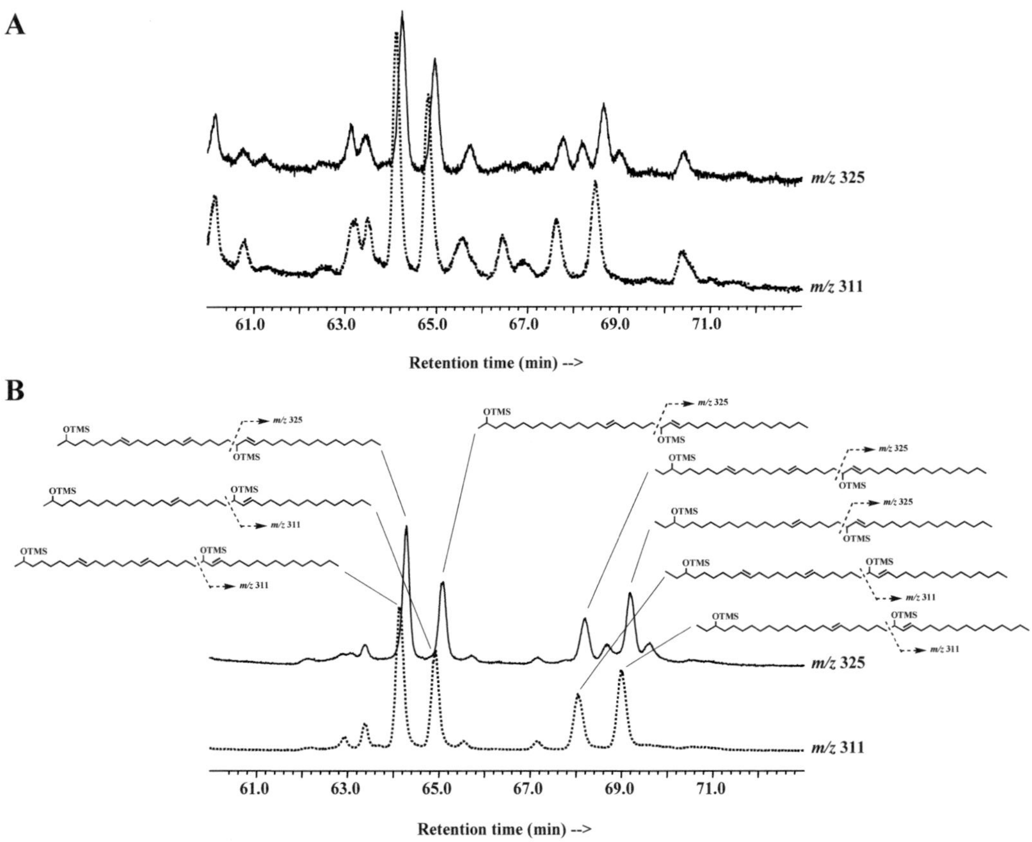

Fig. 14. Partial mass fragmentograms of *m/z* 311 and 325 revealing the presence of silylated C_{37} and C_{38} alkenediols after $NaBH_4$-reduction and silylation of the total lipid extract of *E. huxleyi* cells incubated under darkness (A) and standard autoxidation products of alkenones (B).

4. Conclusions

Due to the lack of adequate tracers, the role played by light-induced photochemical and free radical-mediated (autoxidative) processes during the degradation of lipid components of phototrophic organisms has been virtually ignored until now.

It was recently demonstrated that most of the unsaturated lipid components of these organisms (chlorophylls, carotenoids, unsaturated fatty acids, sterols, *n*-alkenes and HBI alkenes) could be photodegraded by visible and UV radiations during the senescence. This degradation mainly involves type II (i.e. involving $^1O_2$) photoprocesses. Singlet oxygen appeared to be sufficiently stable in this hydrophobic micro-environment to migrate outside the chloroplasts and affect the unsaturated components of cutins of higher plants.

Free radical-mediated oxidation (autoxidation) processes also intervene intensively during the senescence of phototrophic organisms. Induction of these processes seems to mainly result from the homolytic cleavage (catalyzed by some metal ions) of photochemically produced hydroperoxides. Unsaturated fatty acids, chlorophyll phytyl side-chain, vitamin E, sterols and alkenones appeared to be strongly affected by these degradative processes. In the case of alkenones, it is very important to note that autoxidative degradation processes may alter significantly their unsaturation ratio and thus constitute a potential source of biases during paleotemperature reconstruction.

5. Acknowledgements

Financial support over many years from the Centre National de la Recherche Scientifique (CNRS) and the Université de la Méditerranée is gratefully acknowledged.

6. References

Allard, W. G., Belt, S.T., Massé, G., Naumann, R., Robert, J.-M. & Rowland, S.J. (2001). Tetra-unsaturated sesterterpenoids (Haslenes) from *Haslea ostrearia* and related species. *Phytochemistry* 56, 795-800.

Belt, S.T., Allard, W.G., Massé, G., Robert, J.-M. & Rowland, S.J. (2000). Highly branched isoprenoids (HBIs): Identification of the most common and abundant sedimentary isomers. *Geochimica & Cosmochimica Acta* 64, 3839-3851.

Belt, S.T., Massé, G., Rowland, S.J., Poulin, M., Michel, C. & Leblanc, B. (2007). A novel chemical fossil of palaeo sea ice : IP_{25}. *Organic Geochemistry* 38, 16-27.

Belt, S.T., Vare, L.L., Massé, G., Manners, H., Price, J., MacLachlan, S., Andrews, J.T. & Schmidt, S. (2010). Striking similarities in temporal changes to seasonal sea ice conditions across the central Canadian Arctic Archipelago during the last 7,000 years. *Quaternary Science Reviews* 29, 3489-3504.

Bidle, K.D. & Falkowski, P.G. (2004). Cell death in planktonic, photosynthetic microorganisms. *Nature Review 2*, 643-655.

Boon, J.J., van der Meer, F.W., Schuyl, P.J., De Leeuw, J.W., Schenck, P.A. & Burlingame, A.L. (1978). Organic geochemical analyses of core samples from site 362 Walvis Ridge. DSDP Leg 40, *Initial Reports. DSDP* Leg 38, 39, 40 and 41, Suppl., pp. 627-637.

Breuer, O. & Blörkhem, I. (1995). Use of $^{18}O_2$ inhalation technique and mass isotopomer distribution analysis to study oxygenation of cholesterol in rat: evidence for in vitro formation of 7-oxo-, 7b-hydroxy-, and 25-hydroxycholesterol. *Journal of Biological Chemistry* 270, 20278-20284.

Brown, M.R., Mular, M., Miller, I., Farmer, C. & Trenerry, C. (1999). The vitamin content of microalgae used in aquaculture. *Journal of Applied Phycology* 11, 247-255.

Christodoulou S., Marty J.-C., Miquel J.-C., Volkman J.K. & Rontani J.-F. (2009). Use of lipids and their degradation products as biomarkers for carbon cycling in the northwestern Mediterranean Sea. *Marine Chemistry* 113, 25-40.

Christodoulou S., Joux F., Marty J.-C., Sempéré R. & Rontani J.-F. (2010). Comparative study of UV and visible light induced degradation of lipids in non-axenic senescent cells of *Emiliania huxleyi*. *Marine Chemistry* 119, 139-152.

Conte, M.H., Volkman, J.K. & Eglinton, G. (1994). Lipid biomarkers of the Haptophyta. In:Green, J.C., Leadbeater, B.S.C. (Eds.), *The Haptophyte Algae. Systematics Association* Special Volume No. 51, Clarendon Press, Oxford, pp. 351-377.

Cuny, P. & Rontani, J.-F. (1999). On the widespread occurrence of 3-methylidene-7,11,15-trimethylhexadecan-1,2-diol in the marine environment: a specific isoprenoid marker of chlorophyll photodegradation. *Marine Chemistry* 65, 155-165.

Cuny, P., Romano, J.-C., Beker, B. & Rontani, J.-F. (1999). Comparison of the photodegradation rates of chlorophyll chlorin ring and phytol side chain in phytodetritus: is the phytyldiol versus phytol ratio (CPPI) a new biogeochemical index? *Journal of Experimental Marine Biology and Ecology* 237, 271-290.

Cuny, P., Marty, J.-C., Chiaverini, J., Vescovali, I., Raphel, D. & Rontani, J.-F. (2002). One-year seasonal survey of the chlorophyll photodegradation process in the Northwestern Mediterranean Sea. *Deep Sea Research II* 49, 1987-2005.

DaSilva, E.J. & Jensen, A. (1971). Content of α-tocopherol in some blue-green algae. *Biochimica et Biophysica Acta* 239, 345-347.

De Leeuw, J.W., van der Meer, J.W., Rijpstra, W.I.C. & Schenck, P.A. (1980). On the occurrence and structural identification of long chain ketones and hydrocarbons in sediments. In: Douglas, A.G., Maxwell, J.R. (Eds.), *Advances in Organic Geochemistry 1979*. Pergamon Press, Oxford, pp. 211-7.

Eltgroth, M.L., Watwood, R.L. & Wolfe, G.V. (2005). Production and cellular localization of neutral long-chain lipids in the Haptophyte algae *Isochrysis galbana* and *Emiliania huxleyi*. *Journal of Phycology* 41, 1000–1009.

Engel, N., Jenny, T. A., Mooser, V. & Gossauer, A. (1991). Chlorophyll catabolism in *Chlorella protothecoides*. Isolation and structure elucidation of a red biline derivative. *FEBS Letters* 293, 131-133.

Evans, C., Malin, G. & Mills, G.P. (2006). Viral infection of *Emilinia huxleyi* (Prymnesiophyceae) leads to elevated production of reactive oxygen species. *Journal of Phycology* 42, 1040-1047.

Foote, C.S. (1976). Photosensitized oxidation and singlet oxygen: consequences in biological systems. In: Pryor, W.A. (Ed.), *Free Radicals in Biology*. Academic Press, New York, pp. 85-133.

Fossey, J., Lefort, D. & Sorba, J. (1995). *Free radicals in organic chemistry*. Masson. Paris, pp 1-307.

Frankel, E.N., Neff, W.E. & Bessler, T.R. (1979). Analysis of autoxidized fats by gas chromatography-mass spectrometry: V. photosensitized oxidation. *Lipids* 14, 961–967.

Frankel, E.N. (1998). *Lipid Oxidation*. The Oily Press, Dundee.

Frimer, A.A. (1983). Singlet oxygen in peroxide chemistry. In: Patai, S. (Ed.), *The Chemistry of Functional Groups, Peroxides*. John Wiley & sons Ltd., pp. 202-229.

Gelin, F., Boogers, I., Noordeloos, A. A. M., Sinninghe Damsté, J. S., Riegman, R. & de Leeuw, J. W. (1997). Resistant biomacromolecules in marine microalgae of the classes Eustigmatophyceae and chlorophyceae: Geochemical implications. *Organic Geochemistry* 26, 659-675.

Giuffrida, F., Destaillats, F., Robert, F., Skibsted, L.H. & Dionisi F. (2004) Formation and hydrolysis of triacylclycerol and sterol epoxides : role of unsaturated triacylglycerol peroxyl radicals. *Free Radical Biology & medicine* 37, 104-114.

Grimalt, J.O., Rullkötter, J., Sicre, M.-A., Summons, R., Farrington, J., Harvey, H.R., Goñi, M. & Sawada, K. (2000). Modifications of the C_{37} alkenone and alkenoate composition in the water column and sediment: possible implications for sea surface temperature estimates in paleoceanography. *Geochemistry Geophysics and Geosystems* 1, doi: 10.1029/2000G000053.

Grossi, V., Raphel, D., Aubert, C. & Rontani, J.-F. (2000). The effect of growth temperature on the long-chain alkene composition in the marine coccolithophorid *Emiliania huxleyi*. *Phytochemistry* 54, 393-399.

Grossi, V., Beker, B., Geenevasen, J.A.J., Schouten, S., Raphel, D., Fontaine, M.-F. & Sinninghe-Damsté, J.S. (2004). C_{25} highly branched isoprenoid alkenes from the marine benthic diatom *Pleurosigma strigosum*. *Phytochemistry* 65, 3049-3055.

Halliwell, B. (1987). Oxidative damage, lipid peroxidation and antioxidant protection in chloroplasts. *Chemistry and Physics of lipids* 44, 327-340.

Harvey, H.R. (2000). Alteration processes of alkenones and related lipids in water columns and sediments. *Geochemistry Geophysics and Geosystems* 1, doi: 2000GC000054.

He, Y.Y. & Häder, D.P. (2002) Reactive oxygen species and UV-B effect on cyanobacteria. *Photochemical and Photobiological Sciences* 1, 729-736.

Heath, R.L. & Packer, L. (1968). Photoperoxidation in isolated chloroplasts. II. Role of electron transfer. *Archives of Biochemistry and Biophysics 125*, 850-857.

Hurst, J.R., Wilson, S.L. & Schuster, G.B. (1985). The ene reaction of singlet oxygen: kinetic and product evidence in support of a perepoxide intermediate. *Tetrahedron* 41, 2191-2197.

Huyser, E.S. & Johnson, K.L. (1968). Concerning the nature of the polar effect in hydrogen atom abstractions from alcohols, ethers and esters. *Journal of Organic Chemistry 33*, 3972-3974.

Iseo, S., Hyeon, S.B., Katsumura, S. & Sakan, T. (1972). Photooxygenation of carotenoids. II- The absolute configuration of loliolide and dihydroactinidiolide. *Tetrahedron Letters 25*, 2517-2520.

Iturraspe, J., Engel, N. & Gossauer, A. (1994). Chlorophyll catabolism. Isolation and structure elucidation of chlorophyll b catabolites in *Chlorella protothecoides*. *Phytochemistry* 35, 1387-1390.

Jaraula, C.M.B., Brassell, S.C, Morgan-Kiss, R, Doran, P.T. & Kenig, F. (2010) Origin and distribution of tri to pentaunsaturated alkenones in Lake Fryxell, East Antarctica. *Organic Geochemistry* 41, 386-397.

Jeffrey, S.W. & Hallegraeff, G.M. (1987). Chlorophyllase distribution in ten classes of phytoplankton: a problem for chlorophyll analysis. *Marine Ecology Progress Series* 35, 293-304.

Knox, J.P. & Dodge, A.D. (1985). Singlet oxygen and plants. *Phytochemistry* 24, 889-896.

Kolber, Z.S., Van Dover, C.L., Niederman, R.A. & Falkowski, P.G. (2000) Bacterial photosynthesis in surface waters of the open ocean. *Nature 407*, 177-179.

Kolber, Z.S., Plumley, F.G., Lang, A.S., Beatty, J.T., Blankenship, R.E., VanDover, C.L., Vetriani, C., Koblizek, M., Rathgeber, C. & Falkowski, P.G. (2001) Contribution of aerobic photoheterotrophic bacteria to the carbon cycle in the ocean. *Science 292*, 2492-2495.

Korytowski, W., Bachowski, G.J. & Girotti, A.W. (1992). Photoperoxidation of cholesterol in homogeneous solution, isolated membranes, and cells: comparison of the 5α- and 6β-hydroperoxides as indicators of singlet oxygen intermediacy. *Photochemistry and Photobiology* 56, 1-8.

Krol, E.S., Escalante, D.D.J. & Liebler, D.C. (2001). Mechanisms of dimer and trimer formation from ultraviolet-irradiated α-tocopherol. *Lipids* 36, 49-55.

Kulig, M.J. & Smith, L.L. (1973). Sterol metabolism. XXV. Cholesterol oxidation by singlet molecular oxygen. *Journal of Organic Chemistry* 38, 3639-3642.

Liebler, D.C. (1994). Tocopherone and epoxytocopherone products of vitamin E oxidation. *Methods in Enzymology* 234, 310-316.

MacIntosh, T.J. (1978). The effect of cholesterol on the structure of phosphatidylcholine bilayers. *Biochimica et Biophysica Acta 513*, 43-58.

Maeda, H. & DellaPenna, D. (2007). Tocopherol functions in photosynthetic organisms. *Current Opinion in Plant Biology* 10, 260-265.

Marchand, D. & Rontani, J.-F. (2001). Characterization of photooxidation and autoxidation products of phytoplanktonic monounsaturated fatty acids in marine particulate matter and recent sediments. *Organic Geochemistry* 32, 287-304.

Marchand, D. & Rontani, J.-F. (2003). Visible light-induced oxidation of lipid components of purple sulphur bacteria: A significant process in microbial mats, *Organic Geochemistry* 34, 61-79.

Marchand, D., Marty, J.-C., Miquel, J.-C. & Rontani, J.-F. (2005). Lipids and their oxidation products as biomarkers for carbon cycling in the northwestern Mediterranean Sea: results from a sediment trap study. *Marine Chemistry* 95, 129-147.

Marlowe, I.T., Green, J.C., Neal, A.C., Brassell, S.C., Eglinton, G. & Course, P.A. (1984). Long chain (n-C_{37}–C_{39}) alkenones in the Prymnesiophyceae. Distribution of alkenones and other lipids and their taxonomic significance. *British Phycology Journal* 19, 203-216.

Massé, G., Rowland, S.J., Sicre, M.-A., Jacob, J., Jansen, E. & Belt, S.T. (2008). Abrupt climate changes for Iceland during the last millennium: Evidence from high resolution sea ice reconstructions. *Earth and Planetary Science Letters* 269, 565-569.

Merzlyak, M.N. & Hendry, G.A.F. (1994). Free radical metabolism, pigment degradation and lipid peroxidation in leaves during senescence. *Proceedings of the Royal Society of Edinburgh* 102B, 459-471.

Meyer, W. & Spiteler, G. (1997). Oxidized phytosterols increase by ageing in photoautotrophic cell cultures of *Chenopodium rubrum*. *Phytochemistry* 45, 297-302.

Morrissey, P. A. & Kiely, M. (2006). Oxysterols: formation and biological function. In. *Advanced Dairy Chemistry 3rd edition*, Vol. 2 Lipids, Fox. P.F. & McSweeney, P.L.H., eds., Spinger, New-York, pp. 641-674.

Mouzdahir A., Grossi, V., Bakkas, S. & Rontani, J.-F. (2001). Photodegradation of long-chain alkenes in senescent cells of *Emiliania huxleyi* and *Nannochloropsis salina. Phytochemistry* 56, 677-684.

Müller, P.J., Kirst, G., Ruhland, G., von Storch, I. & Rosell-Melé, A. (1998). Calibration of the alkenone paleotemperature index $U_{37}^{K'}$ based on core-tops from the eastern South Atlantic and global ocean (60°N-60°S). *Geochimica & Cosmochimica Acta* 62, 1757-1772.

Nassiry, M., Aubert, C., Mouzdahir, A. & Rontani, J.-F. (2009) Generation of isoprenoid compounds and notably of prist-1-ene through photo- and autoxidative degradation of vitamin E. *Organic Geochemistry* 40, 38-50.

Neff, W.E., Frankel, E.N. & Fujimoto, K. (1988). Autoxidative dimerization of methyl linolenate and its monohydroperoxides, hydroperoxy epidioxides and dihydroperoxides. *Journal of the American Oil Chemical Society* 65, 616-623.

Nelson, J.R. (1993). Rates and possible mechanism of light-dependent degradation of pigments in detritus derived from phytoplankton. *Journal of Marine Research* 51, 155- 179.

Nickon, A. & Bagli, J.F. (1961). Reactivity and geochemistry in allylic systems. I. Stereochemistry of photosensitized oxygenation of monoolefins. *Journal of the American Chemical Society* 83, 1498-1508.

Pokorny, J. (1987). Major factors affecting the autoxidation of lipids. In: Chan, H.W.-S. (Ed.), *Autoxidation of Unsaturated Lipids*. Academic Press, London, pp. 141–206.

Porter, N.A., Caldwell, S.E. & Mills, K.A. (1995). Mechanisms of free radical oxidation of unsaturated lipids. *Lipids* 30, 277-290.

Prahl, F.G. & Wakeham, S.G. (1987). Calibration of unsaturation patterns in long-chain ketone compositions for palaeotemperature assessment. *Nature* 330, 367-369.

Prahl, F.G., Muehlhausen, L.A. & Zahnle, D.L. (1988). Further evaluation of long-chain alkenones as indicators of paleoceanographic conditions. *Geochimica & Cosmochimica Acta* 52, 2303-2310.

Prahl F. G., Rontani J.-F., Volkman J. K., Sparrow M. A. & Royer I. M. (2006). Unusual C_{35} and C_{36} alkenones in a paleoceanographic benchmark strain of *Emiliania huxleyi. Geochimica & Cosmochimica Acta* 70, 2856-2867.

Rechka, J.A. & Maxwell, J.R. (1988). Unusual long chain ketones of algal origin. *Tetrahedron Leters*. 29, 2599-600.

Repeta, D.J. (1989). Carotenoid diagenesis in recent marine sediments. II- Degradation of fucoxanthin to loliolide. *Geochimica & Cosmochimica Acta 53*, 699-707.

Rieley, G., Teece, M. A., Peakman, T. M., Raven, A. M., Greene, K. J., Clarke, T. P., Murray, M., Leftley, J. W., Campbell, C. N., Harris, R. P., Parkes, R. J. & Maxwell, J. R. (1998). Long-chain alkenes of the Haptophytes *Isochrysis galbana* and *Emiliania huxleyi. Lipids* 33, 617-625.

Rise, M., Cojocaru, M., Gottlieb, H.E. & Goldschmidt, E.E. (1988). Accumulation of α-tocopherol in senescing organs as related to chlorophyll degradation. *Plant Physiology* 89, 1028-1030.

Rontani, J.-F. & Aubert, C. (1994) Effect of oxy-free radicals upon the phytyl chain during chlorophyll-*a* photodegradation. *Journal of Photochemistry and Photobiology*, A79, 167-172.

Rontani, J.-F., Grossi, V., Faure, R. & Aubert, C. (1994). "Bound" 3-methylidene-7,11,15-trimethylhexadecan-1,2-diol: a new isoprenoid marker for the photodegradation of chlorophyll-a in seawater. *Organic Geochemistry* 21, 135-142.

Rontani, J.-F., Beker, B., Raphel, D. & Baillet, G. (1995). Photodegradation of chlorophyll phytyl chain in dead phytoplanktonic cells. *Journal of Photochemistry and Photobiology* 85A, 137-142.

Rontani, J.-F., Raphel, D. & Cuny, P. (1996a). Early diagenesis of the intact and photooxidized chlorophyll phytyl chain in a recent temperate sediment. *Organic Geochemistry* 24, 825-832.

Rontani, J.-F., Cuny, P. & Grossi, V. (1996b). Photodegradation of chlorophyll phytyl chain in senescent leaves of higher plants. *Phytochemistry* 42, 347-351.

Rontani, J.-F., Cuny, P. & Aubert, C. (1997a). Rates and mechanism of light-dependent degradation of sterols in senescing cells of phytoplankton. *Journal of Photochemistry and Photobiology* 111A, 139-144.

Rontani, J.-F., Cuny, P., Grossi, V. & Beker, B. (1997b). Stability of long-chain alkenones in senescing cells of *Emiliania huxleyi*: effect of photochemical and aerobic microbial degradation on the alkenone unsaturation ratio ($U_{37}^{K'}$). *Organic Geochemistry* 26, 503-509.

Rontani, J.-F., Cuny, P. & Grossi, V. (1998). Identification of a pool of lipid photoproducts in senescent phytoplanktonic cells. *Organic Geochemistry* 29, 1215-1225.

Rontani, J.-F. & Marchand, D. (2000) Δ^5-Stenol photoproducts of phytoplanktonic origin: a potential source of hydroperoxides in marine sediments? *Organic Geochemistry* 31, 169-180.

Rontani J.-F., Koblizek M., Beker B., Bonin P. & Kolber Z. (2003a). On the origin of *cis*-vaccenic photodegradation products in the marine environment. *Lipids* 38, 1085-1092.

Rontani, J.-F., Rabourdin, A., Marchand, D. & Aubert, C. (2003b). Photochemical oxidation and autoxidation of chlorophyll phytyl side chain in senescent phytoplanktonic cells: potential sources of several acyclic isoprenoid compounds in the marine environment. *Lipids* 38, 241-253.

Rontani, J.-F. & Aubert, C. (2005). Characterization of isomeric allylic diols resulting from chlorophyll phytyl side-chain photo- and autoxidation by electron ionization gas chromatography/mass spectrometry. *Rapid Communications in Mass Spectrometry* 19, 637-646.

Rontani, J.-F., Rabourdin, A., Pinot, F., Kandel, S. & Aubert, C. (2005) Visible light-induced oxidation of unsaturated components of cutins: a significant process during the senescence of higher plants. *Phytochemistry* 66, 313-321.

Rontani, J.-F., Marty, J.-C., Miquel, J.-C. & Volkman, J.K. (2006). Free radical oxidation (autoxidation) of alkenones and other microalgal lipids in seawater. *Organic Geochemistry* 37, 354-368.

Rontani, J.-F., Jameson, I., Christodoulou, S. & Volkman, J.K. (2007a). Free radical oxidation (autoxidation) of alkenones and other lipids in cells of *Emiliania huxleyi*. *Phytochemistry* 68, 913-924.

Rontani, J.-F., Nassiry, M. & Mouzdahir, A. (2007b). Free radical oxidation (autoxidation) of α-tocopherol (vitamin E): A potential source of 4,8,12,16-tetramethylheptadecan-4-olide in the environment. *Organic Geochemistry* 38, 37-47.

Rontani, J;-F., Harji, R. & Volkman, J.K. (2007c) Biomarkers derived from heterolytic and homolytic cleavage of allylic hydroperoxides resulting from alkenone autoxidation. *Marine Chemistry* 107, 230-243.

Rontani, J.-F., Zabeti, N. & Wakeham, S.G. (2011a) Degradation of particulate organic matter in the equatorial Pacific Ocean: biotic or abiotic? *Limnology and Oceanography* 56, 333-349.

Rontani, J.-F., Belt, S.T., Vaultier, F. & Brown, T.A. (2011b) Visible light-induced photo-oxidation of highly branched isoprenoid (HBI) alkenes: a significant dependence on the number and nature of the double bonds. *Organic Geochemistry* 42, 812-822

Rosell-Melé, A., Carter, J.F., Parry, A.T. & Eglinton, G. (1995). Determination of the $U_{37}^{K'}$ index in geological samples. *Analytical Chemistry* 67, 1283-1289.

Row, L.-C., Ho, J.-C. & Chen, C.-M. (2007). Cerebrosides and tocopherol trimers from the seeds of *Euryale ferox*. *Journal of Natural products* 70, 1214-1217.

Rowland, S.J. & Robson, J.N. (1990). The widespread occurrence of highly branched isoprenoid acyclic C_{20}, C_{25} and C_{30} hydrocarbons in recent sediments and biota.- a review. *Marine Environmental Research* 30, 191-216.

Sanchez-Machado, D.I., Lopez-Hernandez, J. & Paseiro-Losada, P. (2002). High-performance liquid chromatographic determination of α-tocopherol in macroalgae. *Journal of Chromatography* 976A, 277-284.

Schaich, K.M. (1992). Metals and lipid oxidation. Contemporary issues. *Lipids* 27, 209–218.

Schaich, K.M. (2005) Lipid oxidation: theoretical aspects. In: *Bailey's Industrial Oil and Fat Products*, Sixth edition, Shahidi, F. (Ed.), John Wiley & Sons, pp. 269-355.

Schulte-Elte, K.H., Muller, B.L. & Pamingle, H. (1979). Photooxygenation of 3,3-dialkylsubstituted allyl alcohols. Occurrence of syn preference in the ene addition of $^1O_2$ at *E/Z*-isomeric alcohols. *Helvetica Chimica Acta* 62, 816–828.

Schultz, G. (1990). Biosynthesis of α-tocopherol in chloroplasts of higher plants. *Fett Wissenschaft Technologie* 92, 86-91.

Sinninghe-Damté, J.S., Muyzer, G., Abbas, B., Rampen, S.W., Massé, G., Allard, W.G., Belt, S.T., Robert, J.-M., Rowland, S.J., Moldovan, J.M., Barbanti, S.M., Fago, F.J., Denisevich, P., Dahl, J., Trindade, L.A.F. & Schouten, S. (2004). The rise of the Rhizosolenoid diatoms. *Science* 304, 584-587.

Smith, L.L. (1981). *The Autoxidation of Cholesterol*. Plenum Press, New York.

Suarna, C., Craig, D.C., Cross, K.J. & Southwell-Keely, P.T. (1988). Oxidations of vitamin E (α-tocopherol) and its model compound 2,2,5,7,8-pentamethyl-6-hydroxychroman. A new dimer. *Journal of Organic Chemistry* 53, 1281-1284.

Suwa, K., Kimura, T. & Schaap, A.P. (1977). Reactivity of singlet molecular oxygen with cholesterol in a phospholipidic membrane matrix: a model for oxidative damage of membranes. *Biochemistry and Biophysical Research Communications 75*, 785-792.

Vidi, P.-A., Kanwischer, M., Bagninsky, S., Austin, J.R., Csucs, G., Dörmann, P., Kessler, F. & Bréhélin, C. (2006). Tocopherol cyclase (VTE1) localization and vitamin E accumulation in chloroplast plastoglobule lipoprotein particles. *Journal of Biological Chemistry* 281, 11225-11234.

Volkman, J.K., Eglinton, G., Corner, E.D.S. & Forsberg, T.E.V. (1980). Long chain alkenes and alkenones in the marine coccolithophorid *Emiliania huxleyi*. *Phytochemistry* 19, 2619–2622.

Volkman, J. K., Barrett, S. M. & Dunstan, G. A. (1994). C_{25} and C_{30} highly branched isoprenoid alkenes in laboratory cultures of two marine diatoms. *Organic Geochemistry* 21, 407-414.

Volkman, J.K., Barrett, S.M., Blackburn, S.I. & Sikes, E.L. (1995). Alkenones in *Gephyrocapsa oceanica* - implications for studies of paleoclimate. *Geochimica & Cosmochimica Acta* 59, 513–520.

Wood, B.J.B. (1974). Fatty acids and saponifiable lipids. In: Steward, W.D. (Ed.), *Algal Physiology and Biochemistry*. University of California Press, Berkeley, pp. 236-265.

Yamauchi, R., Kato, K. & Ueno, Y. (1988). Formation of trimers of α-tocopherol and its model compound, 2,2,5,7,8-pentamethylchroman-6-ol, in autoxidizing methyl linoleate. *Lipids* 23, 779-783.

Yurkov, V.V. & Beatty, J.T. (1998) Aerobic anoxygenic phototrophic bacteria, *Microbiology and Molecular Biology Review* 62, 695-724.

Zafiriou, O.C. (1977) Marine organic photochemistry previewed. *Marine Chemistry* 5, 497-522.

Zafiriou, O.C., Joussot-Dubien, J., Zepp, R.G. & Zika, R.G. (1984) Photochemistry in natural waters. *Environmental Science and Technology* 18, 358A-370A.

2

Role of Intracellular Hydrogen Peroxide as Signalling Molecule for Plant Senescence

Ulrike Zentgraf, Petra Zimmermann and Anja Smykowski
ZMBP, University of Tübingen
Germany

1. Introduction

All aerobic organisms use molecular oxygen as terminal oxidant during respiration. Oxygen is neither very reactive nor harmful, but it has the potential to be only partially reduced, leading to the formation of very reactive and therefore toxic intermediates, like singlet oxygen ($^1O_2$), superoxide radical ($O_2^{\cdot-}$), hydroperoxylradical ($HO_2^{\cdot-}$), hydrogen peroxide (H_2O_2) and hydroxylradical ($\cdot OH$). These forms are called "reactive oxygen species" (ROS). All ROS are extremely reactive and may oxidize biological molecules, such as DNA, proteins and lipids. However, these reactive molecules are unavoidable by-products of an aerobic metabolism. It is known that reactive oxygen species may have a dual role in plant stress response (Dat et al. 2000). Whereas high concentrations of hydrogen peroxide are toxic for the cell, low concentrations may act as signal which triggers the plant response upon a variety of biotic and abiotic stresses (Dat et al., 2000; Grant & Loake, 2000). It has been known for many years that common signal transduction molecules like MAPKs and calmodulin play an important role in some of these ROS signal transduction pathways.

Mitochondria are an important origin of ROS. During respiration, the ubiquinone pool is the main source for superoxide production. The alternative oxidase (AOX) could be identified in plants and protists, e.g. Trypanosoma, fungi, like *Neurospora crassa* and *Hansenula anomala* and in green algae, e.g. in Chlamydomonas (McIntosh, 1994). It acts as a quinoloxidase by transferring electrons from the reduced ubiquinone directly to molecular oxygen forming water (Siedow & Moore, 1993). AOX mediates an energy-wasteful form of respiration, but its physiological significance is still a matter of intense debate (Rasmusson et al., 2009; Vanlerberghe et al., 2009; Millar et al., 2011). The plant alternative oxidases form homodimers (Moore et al., 2002) and are encoded by a small gene family. In *Arabidopsis thaliana* five genes are known, *AOX1a, AOX1b, AOX1c, AOX1d* and *AOX2*, each exhibiting organ specific expression (Saisho et al., 1997; https:/www.genevestigator.com). Among these five *AOX* genes in *Arabidopsis thaliana, AOX1a* is the major isoform expressed in leaves (Clifton et al., 2006). One important function of the alternative oxidase is to prevent the formation of excess of reactive oxygen molecules (Maxwell et al., 1999). AOX ensures a low reduction status of the ubiquinone pool by oxidizing ubiquinol. Thus, the electron flow is guaranteed (Millenaar & Lambers, 2003). This reaction is necessary, if the cytochrome *c* dependent pathway is restricted by naturally occurring cyanide, NO, sulphide, high concentrations of CO_2, low temperatures or phosphorus deprivation (Millenaar & Lambers, 2003) as well as wounding, drought, osmotic stress, ripening and pathogen infection

(McIntosh, 1994; Moore et al., 2002). Photo-oxidative stress of chloroplasts is also involved in *AOX* up-regulation (Yoshida et al. 2008). Moreover, ascorbate biosynthesis in mitochondria is linked to the electron transport chain between complexes III and IV (Bartoli et al., 2000) and leaves of the *AOX*-overexpressing lines accumulate more ascorbic acid than wild-type leaves (Bartoli et al., 2006). A lack of AOX can lead to an up-regulation of transcripts of the antioxidant defense system at low temperature (Watanabe et al, 2008). Therefore, it is likely that AOX is an important component in antioxidant defense mechanisms.

In addition, it is proposed that AOX also has important functions outside the mitochondria (Arnholdt-Schmitt et al., 2006; Clifton et al., 2006; Van Aken et al., 2009). Furthermore, a beneficial role for AOX in illuminated leaves has been suggested and AOX-deficient *aox1a* mutant showed a lowered operating efficiency of photosystem II and an enhanced activity of cyclic electron transport around photosystem I (CET-PSI) at high irradiance (Yoshida et al., 2011). However, in most cases, transgenic plants with altered levels of AOX exhibited no obvious variation in plant growth phenotype (Vanlerberghe et al., 2009), implying that AOX does not severely affect photosynthetic carbon gain and biomass productivity. In addition, AOX also has an effect on the control of NO levels in plant cells (Wulff et al., 2009).

There is some evidence that alternative respiration is correlated with senescence and longevity. Aging potato slides showed a decline in the capacity of cytochrome *c* dependent respiration whereas the alternative respiration as well as the protein content of AOX increased (Hiser & McIntosh, 1990). Expression of *AOX1a* of Arabidopsis is highest in rosette leaves at the onset of senescence (https:/www.genevestigator.com). Interestingly, the inactivation of subunit V of the cytochrome *c* oxidase complex in the fungus *Podospora anserina* led to the exclusive use of the alternative respiration pathway and to a decline in ROS formation in these mutants. This inactivation of the cytochrome *c* oxidase resulted in an extraordinary longevity of this fungus (Dufour et al. 2000). There are several lines of evidence that beside mitochondria also chloroplasts and peroxisomes trigger leaf senescence. For peroxisomes a ROS-mediated function in leaf senescence has been described (del Río et al. 1998). Tobacco deficient in the thylacoid Ndh complex showed a delay in leaf senescence. It was discussed that the senescence delay was achieved by lower ROS production (Zapater et al., 2005).

In different Arabidopsis mutants a tight correlation between extended longevity and tolerance against oxidative stress has been observed (Kurepa et al., 1998). The most extended longevity mutant of this collection which also showed the highest tolerance against paraquat treatment was *gigantea3*. GIGANTEA acts in blue light signaling and has biochemically separable roles in circadian clock and flowering time regulation (Martin-Tryon et al., 2007). However, the link between this nuclear localized protein and resistance to oxidative stress is still unclear. CATALASE2 (CAT2) and CATALASE3 (CAT3) enzymes, which are expressed under the control of the circadian clock, might be good candidates. They exhibit a higher activity in the *gigantea3* mutant which might be responsible for the elevated oxidative stress tolerance (Zentgraf & Hemleben, 2007). In contrast, the delayed leaf senescence mutants of Arabidopsis *ore1, ore3,* and *ore9* also exhibit increased tolerance to various types of oxidative stress but the activities of antioxidant enzymes were similar or lower in the mutants, as compared to wild type providing evidence that oxidative stress tolerance is also genetically linked to control of leaf longevity in plants (Woo et al., 2004).

In addition, the expression of many SAGs is enhanced by increased levels of reactive oxygen species (Miller et al., 1999; Navabpour et al., 2003) indicating that elevated levels of ROS might be used as a signal to promote senescence. In Arabidopsis the coordinate regulation of the hydrogen peroxide scavenging enzymes catalase (CAT) and ascorbate peroxidase (APX) leads to a defined increase of hydrogen peroxide content during bolting time (Ye et al., 2000; Zimmermann et al., 2006). Removing the bolt and thereby delaying the decrease in APX activity led to a delay in chlorophyll degradation and senescence (Ye et al., 2000). Since APX enzyme activity appears to be regulated on the posttranscriptional level (Panchuk et al., 2005; Zimmermann et al., 2006) and appears to be inhibited by hydrogen peroxide itself in this developmental stage, the initial event to create the hydrogen peroxide peak during bolting time at the onset of senescence is the transcriptional down-regulation of *CAT2*. The transcription factor responsible for this down-regulation was isolated by a yeast-one hybrid screen and turned out to be a member of the bZIP transcription factor family, namely GBF1. If *GBF1* is knocked out by a T-DNA insertion, the down-regulation of *CAT2* during bolting time is abolished, the hydrogen peroxide peak during bolting time disappears and senescence is delayed (Smykowski et al., 2010). This hydrogen peroxide peak is discussed to trigger senescence induction by activating the systemic expression of the senescence-related transcription factors e.g. *WRKY53* (Miao et al., 2004).

In order to understand the correlation between mitochondrial ROS production and senescence in *Arabidopsis thaliana*, we treated cell cultures and whole Arabidopsis plants with antimycin A, an inhibitor of cytochrom *c* oxidase, and measured hydrogen peroxide production and senescence parameters. In addition, two different genes encoding the peroxisomal enzyme catalase have been knocked-out and the single knock-out plants *cat2* and *cat3* have been crossed to produce double knock-out plants *cat2/3*. In these plants also the consequences on hydrogen peroxide levels and leaf senescence were analysed.

2. Results and discussion

2.1 Changes in mitochondrial hydrogen peroxide production

Dufour and others (2000) characterized an almost immortal mutant of the fungus *Podospora anserina* carrying a mutation in the gene encoding subunit V of the cytochrom *c* oxidase complex. These mutants exclusively used the alternative respiration pathway thus clearly leading to a lower content of reactive oxygen species than in normal growing fungi. In Arabidopsis resistance to oxidative stress and longevity are also tightly correlated (Kurepa et al., 1998; Woo et al., 2004). Therefore, we wanted to analyse Arabidopsis plants and cells with increased alternative respiration for mitochondrial ROS production and a delay in senescence.

2.1.1 Antimycin A treatment of cell cultures and whole plants

The alternative respiration in plants can be induced by application of antimycin A (Vanlerberghe & McIntosh, 1992), which was isolated from *Streptomyces* sp. and inhibits specifically the electron transport between cytochrome *b* and c_1. To investigate the influence of antimycin A on the production of ROS, we analysed antimycin A treated *Arabidopsis thaliana* cell cultures for their hydrogen peroxide contents. Two hours after treatment with 5 µM antimycin A or 0.02 % ethanol as control the H_2O_2 concentration slightly increased, whereas further incubation clearly lowered H_2O_2 content in antimycin A treated cells in comparison to control cells (Fig. 1 A). The transient increase in H_2O_2 levels might be a result of the inhibition of cytochrome *c* oxidase as it was already shown by Maxwell and coworkers (1999) for tobacco cells. Here an initial hydrogen peroxide production after antimycin A treatment could be localized almost exclusively to the mitochondria using laser scanning microscopy of H_2DCF-DA and mitotracker double-labelled cells. Dot blot analyses of 10 µg total RNA isolated from Arabidopsis culture cells and subsequent hybridization revealed that alternative oxidase 1a (AOX 1a) was induced by antimycin A as well as by hydrogen peroxide treatment (Fig. 1 B). This was also observed in tobacco cells, where antimycin A led to a more efficient alternative respiration capacity (Maxwell et al., 2002) and subsequently to a reduced mitochondrial ROS formation (Maxwell et al., 1999).

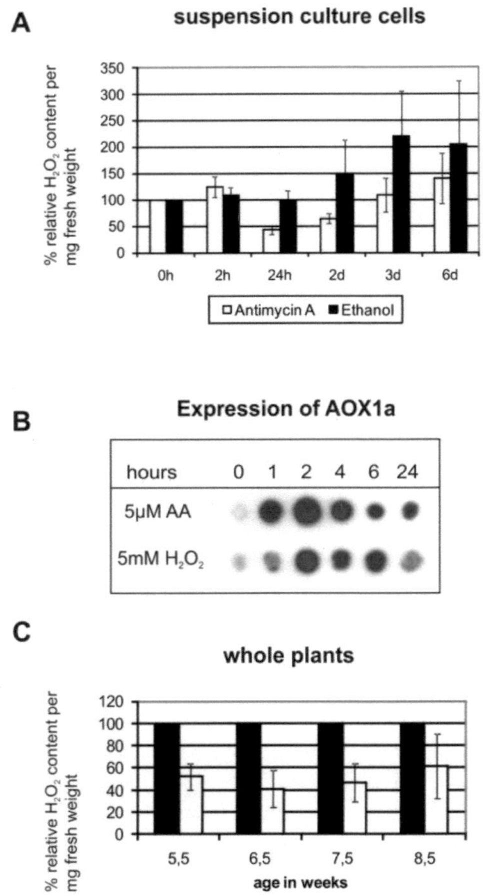

Fig. 1. *Short term treatment of cell cultures and whole plants with antimycin A.*
A) *Arabidopsis thaliana* cell cultures were treated with 5 µM antimycin A or 0.02 % ethanol as control and were analysed for their hydrogen peroxide content. The 0 h value was referred to as 100%. The error bars indicate the standard deviation of 4 independent experiments.
B) Hybridization of 10µg of total RNA isolated from antimycin A or H_2O_2 treated culture cells dotted on a nylon filter with an *AOX1a* specific probe. **C)** *Arabidopsis thaliana* plants of different developmental stages were watered with 10 ml of a 20 µmol antimycin A solution whereas control plants were treated with 0.8 % ethanol and were analysed for their hydrogen peroxide content after 24 hours. The values of ethanol treated plants were referred to as 100%. The error bars indicate the standard deviation of 4 independent experiments.

Since we were interested in analyzing the induction of senescence in whole Arabidopsis plants, we watered plants of different developmental stages with antimycin A and measured the hydrogen peroxide content 24 h after the treatment. In all developmental stages the hydrogen peroxide content was significantly lower in leaves of antimycin A treated plants (Fig. 1 C) indicating that in all developmental stages AOX and alternative respiration was induced to reduce mitochondrial ROS production.

2.1.2 Long term treatment of plants with antimycin A

In order to elucidate the long term effects of alternative respiration on plant development and senescence, soil grown Arabidopsis plants were watered over a time period of five weeks with 10 ml 20 µmol antimycin A solution every second day beginning with 5-week-old plants. Control plants were treated with 0.8 % ethanol in which antimycin A was dissolved. Since it was possible to reduce the hydrogen peroxide levels by the induction of the alternative pathways in all developmental stages, we assume that these plants grew under conditions favouring the alternative respiration from week 5 on. We have chosen this experimental design in order to guarantee that plant growth and development is not impaired in early stages by the lack of a functional cytochrome *c* pathway and the ATP it generates. Therefore, we did not use cytochrome *c* oxidase knock-out mutants, which appear to be impaired in growth and development from early on (data not shown).

The hydrogen peroxide content of antimycin A watered and control plants was measured weekly and the H_2O_2 level at the beginning of the experiment was set as 100 % (Fig. 2A). H_2O_2 concentrations of the control plants exhibit a peak in 7-week-old plants during the time of bolting and an increase in late stages of development as it was already shown before (Miao et al. 2004; Zimmermann et al. 2006).

In contrast, the antimycin A treated plants showed a slight decrease up to 8 weeks and recovered in older stages to the starting level (Fig. 2A). This coincides with the results of Dufour and coworkers (2000) for the fungus *Podospora anserine*, where long term activated alternative respiration led to lower hydrogen peroxide contents and strongly increased longevity. However, in Arabidopsis no obvious differences in the development and the progression of senescence could be detected phenotypically in antimycin A treated plants (Fig. 2B). In contrast, a transgenic Arabidopsis line overexpressing the senescence-associated transcription factor *WRKY53* exhibited an accelerated senescence phenotype (Fig. 2B; Miao et al., 2004). In accordance with the phenotype, chlorophyll and total protein content differed only slightly between antimycin A and ethanol treated plants, but were reduced earlier in 35S:*WRKY53* plants (Fig. 2C). Northern blot analyses revealed that the senescence-specific cystein protease gene *SAG12* was induced earlier and stronger in the antimycin A treated plants (Fig. 2D). This implies that even though less reactive oxygen species are produced in plants with favoured alternative respiration, development and senescence are not impaired or even slightly accelerated. Maxwell et al. (2002) presented evidence that, besides AOX, different senescence associated genes of tobacco (e.g. ACC, GST and Cystein protease precursor) can rapidly be induced by antimycin A treatment and this rapid induction can be prevented by ROS scavengers (Maxwell et al., 2002). In addition, overexpression of AOX in tobacco culture cells led to a decline in ROS concentration and a reduced expression of antioxidative enzymes, like superoxide dismutase or glutathione peroxidase (Maxwell et al., 1999).

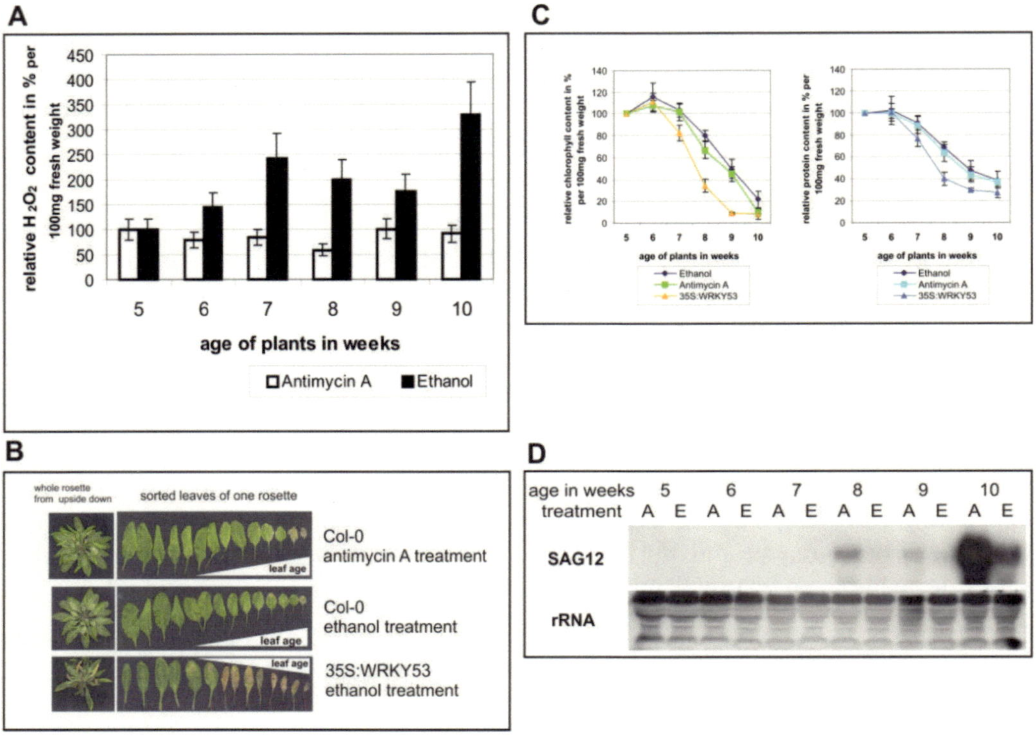

Fig. 2. *Long term treatment of whole plants with antimycin A.*
A) *Arabidopsis thaliana* plants were watered with 10 ml of a 20 µmol antimycin A solution every second day over a time period of five weeks beginning with 5-week-old plants. Control plants were treated with 0.8 % of ethanol. These plants were analysed for their hydrogen peroxide content every week. The values of the 5-week-old plants were referred to as 100%. The error bars indicate the standard deviation of 3 independent experiments.
B) Phenotypic analyses of antimycin A or ethanol treated 8-week-old wildtype plants and ethanol treated transgenic *WRKY53* overexpressing line (35S:*WRKY53*). Whole plants are shown upside down to visualize older leaves of the rosette. In addition, the leaves were sorted according to their age using a specific colour code. **C)** Chlorophyll (left) and total protein (right) were measured in ethanol treated wildtype plants (Col-0), antimycin A treated wildtype plants and ethanol treated *WRKY53* overexpessing plants (35S:*WRKY53*). The values of 5-week-old plants were referred to as 100%. The error bars indicate the standard deviation of 3 independent experiments. **D)** Northern blot analyses of 15 µg of total RNA isolated from antimycin A (A) or ethanol treated (E) plants. The nylon filters were hybridized with a *SAG12* specific probe. Rehybridization with a 25S rRNA probe was used as loading control.

Transgenic tobacco culture cells carrying an antisense construct for *AOX* show an increased ROS formation and an elevated transcript abundance of catalase (Maxwell et al., 1999). In contrast, Umbach and coworkers (2005) observed that in *AOX* overexpressing or *AOX* antisense transgenic Arabidopsis lines transcript levels of the antioxidative enzymes MnSOD, organellar APX, cytosolic and organellar glutathione reductase and peroxiredoxins were not altered. This indicates that in Arabidopsis the lower production of ROS does not lead to compensatory reduction of oxidative stress enzymes. A senescence phenotype was also not observed in these lines.

2.1.3 Transgenic plants overexpressing *AOX1a*

The analysis of transgenic plants is helpful to gain more information about the function of a gene. For this reason, plants expressing the genes *AOX1a* under the constitutive 35S promoter were generated. This isoform was selected since it is strongly expressed in leaves. Plants of the T2 generation of these overexpressing lines were tested for *AOX1a* expression and three lines were obtained which overexpressed the transgene about 20-fold. The H_2O_2 content of these lines was analysed and a clear reduction in the hydrogen peroxide content in the transgenic lines could be measured (Fig.3B). Again, no obvious senescence phenotype could be detected (Fig. 3A). If at all, a slight acceleration of leaf senescence can be observed in the 35S:*AOX1a* lines. Fiorani et al. (2005) could observe a phenotype in 35S:*AOX1a* lines under low temperature conditions (12°C) with increased leaf area and larger rosettes. This could not be observed in our 35S:*AOX1a* lines under normal growth conditions. However, the cytochrom *c* dependent respiration is still functional in these plants probably masking the effect of increased levels of AOX.

Millenaar and Lambers (2003) describe that there is no clear positive correlation between the concentration of AOX protein and its activity *in vivo*, since an increase in protein formation does not change pyruvate concentration and the reduction state of ubiquinone, which are necessary for the activation of the AOX protein. For example, tobacco leaves infected with tobacco mosaic virus showed an increased AOX protein level but no change in activity of the alternative respiration (Lennon et al., 1997). In the transgenic plants overexpressing AOX, the capacity of the alternative respiration pathway appears to be elevated, but this does not necessarily reflect its activation. In the same line of evidence neither overexpression nor inactivation of AOX caused a change in ROS formation in the fungus *Podospora anserina* (Lorin et al., 2001). There was no effect on lifespan or senescence in the transgenic fungi either. However, in our transgenic lines the ROS production is clearly reduced indicating an activation of the alternative respiration pathway but nevertheless no effect on senescence could be observed.

Overexpression of *AOX* in tobacco culture cells leads to a decline in ROS concentration and a reduced expression of other antioxidative enzymes, like superoxide dismutase or glutathione peroxidase (Maxwell et al., 1999) whereas transgenic tobacco culture cells carrying an antisense construct for *AOX* show an increased ROS formation and an elevated transcript abundance of catalase (Maxwell et al., 1999). This would suggest that the plants would be either more sensitive or more resistant to oxidative stress. In contrast, in transgenic Arabidopsis lines either overexpressing *AOX* or an *AOX* antisense construct transcript levels of the antioxidative enzymes MnSOD, organellar APX, cytosolic and organellar glutathione reductase and peroxiredoxins were not altered (Umbach et al., 2005). In consistence with these findings, no altered resistance against oxidative stress could be observed in the transgenic 35S:*AOX1a* transgenic plants, which we germinated on MS plates and applied oxidative stress by spraying the seedlings with hydrogen peroxide (Fig. 3C).

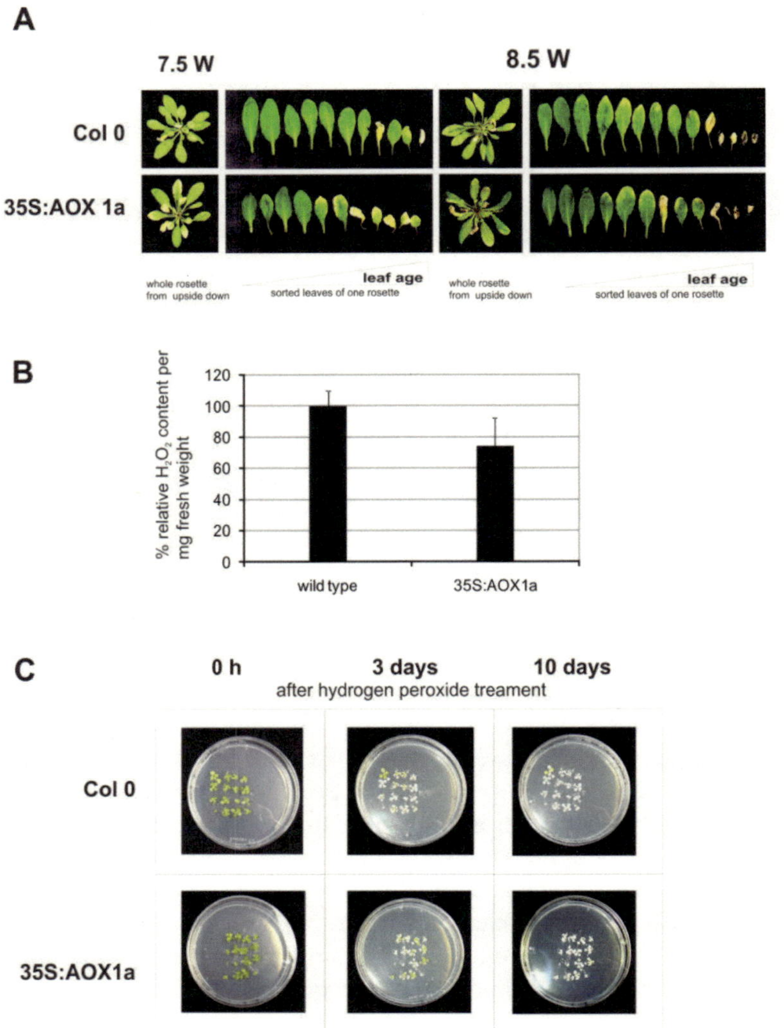

Fig. 3. *Transgenic plants overexperessing AOX1a*
A) Phenotypic analyses of wildtype (Col-0) and 35S:*AOX1a* transgenic plants. Whole plants are shown upside down to visualize older leaves of the rosette. In addition, the leaves were sorted according to their age using a specific colour code. **B)** 4-6 wildtype (Col-0) and 35S:*AOX1a* transgenic plants were pooled and analysed for their hydrogen peroxide content. The values of the wild type plants were referred to as 100%. The error bars indicate the standard deviation of 2 independently collected plant pools. **C)** Phenotypic analyses of hydrogen peroxide treated seedlings of wild type (Col-0) and 35S:*AOX1a* transgenic plants.

2.1.4 Senescence-associated and circadian expression of *AOX1a*

The family of alternative oxidases comprises five genes with an organ specific expression (Saisho et al., 1997; https://www.genevestigator.com). In general, *AOX* is expressed only at a very low level under normal conditions. By using leaf material of plants of different age harvested in the morning hours, a senescence dependent expression of *AOX1a* could be observed with the highest transcript abundance in old plants. In young, up to 7-week-old plants, no expression could be detected by Northern blot analyses (Fig. 4A). This coincides with genevestigator data and with the *AOX* expression in different stages of the leaf development in potatoes, where an increase in AOX protein from young to mature leaves could be observed (Svensson & Rasmusson, 2001; https:/www.genevestigator.com). Furthermore, there is a *de novo* synthesis of alternative oxidase in aging potato slides (Hiser & McIntosh, 1990). Our *in silico* analysis of about 1500 bp upstream the coding region of the *AOX1a* gene revealed, amongst others, several W-box core elements and one sequence for a circadian element. The W-boxes indicate a regulation by WRKY transcription factors which are involved in senescence or pathogen dependent regulation (Eulgem et al., 2000; Miao et al., 2004) whereas the circadian element points out a clock dependent regulation. Based on these results, we used 8.5-week-old plants to harvest leaf material every three hours over 27 h. A circadian regulation of *AOX1a* could be detected with the maximum of expression in the early morning hours with the beginning of illumination (Fig. 4B). This corresponds to the expression of *AOX* in tobacco (Dutilleul et al., 2003).

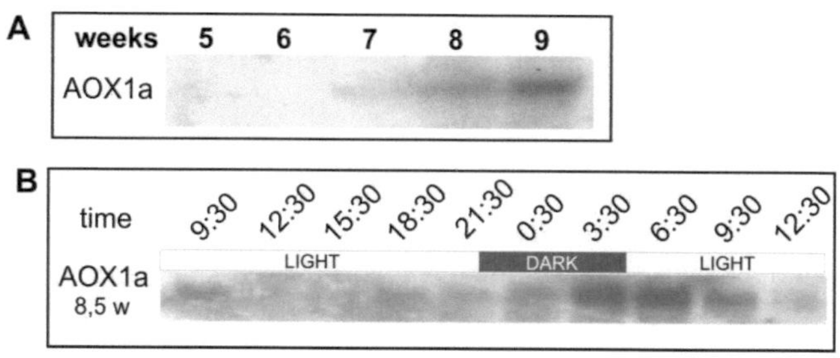

Fig. 4. *Senescence-associated expression of AOX1a*
Northern blot analyses of 15 µg of total RNA isolated from plants of **A)** 5-week-old to 9-week-old plants and **B)** 8-week-old plants at different day times. The nylon filters were hybridized with an *AOX1a* specific probe. Equal loading was controlled by Toluidin blue staining of the membranes.

2.2 Changes in peroxisomal hydrogen peroxide production

Peroxisomes are organelles encircled by only a single membrane layer embedding an extensive oxidative metabolism. These organelles are found in all eukaryotic organisms. In plants, peroxisomes participate in many physiological processes like seed germination, leaf senescence, fruit maturation, response to abiotic and biotic stress, photomorphogenesis, biosynthesis of the plant hormones jasmonic acid and auxin, and in cell signaling by reactive oxygen and nitrogen species. A specific feature of peroxisomes is their dynamic metabolism meaning that the enzymatic constitution of peroxisomes is adjusted to the organism, cell or tissue-type, and also to a variety of environmental conditions (Palma et al., 2009). One important source for ROS formation, especially for H_2O_2, is photorespiration. During CO_2 fixation, ribulose-1,5-bisphosphate-carboxylase (RubisCO) can use CO_2 to carboxylate ribulose-1,5-bisphosphate but also molecular oxygen to oxygenate ribulose-1,5-bisphosphate forming glycolate. The glycolate is then transported from the chloroplasts into the peroxisomes where it is oxidized generating H_2O_2 as a by-product. Peroxisomes and ROS generated in these organelles were shown to play a central role in natural and dark induced senescence in pea (del Rio et al., 1998) and appear to play an important role as a supplier of signal molecules like NO· (nitric oxide), $O_2^{\cdot -}$, H_2O_2 and possibly S-nitrosoglutathione (del Rio et al., 1998; 2002; 2003). These signaling molecules can trigger specific gene expression by so far largely unknown signal transduction pathways (Corpas et al., 2001; 2004; del Rio et al., 2002). However, the concentration of these molecules is tightly regulated by a sensitive balance between production and decomposition by different specific scavenging systems. Catalases are the most abundant enzymes in peroxisomes and convert hydrogen peroxide into water and oxygen without the consumption of reducing equivalents. Besides catalases all enzymes of the antioxidant ascorbate-glutathione cycle, also called Foyer-Halliwell-Asada cycle, are present in peroxisomes to detoxify H_2O_2 through the oxidation of ascorbate and glutathione in an NADPH-dependent manner, thus complementing the action of catalase in peroxisomes. If the mitochondrial and the peroxisomal ascorbate-glutathione cycles are compared during progression of senescence, it can be speculated that peroxisomes may participate longer in the cellular oxidative mechanism of leaf senescence than mitochondria, since mitochondria appear to be affected by oxidative damage earlier than peroxisomes (Jiménez et al. , 1998; del Rio et al., 2003).

Catalases are tetrameric heme containing enzymes and are present in all aerobic organisms. Due to a very high apparent Michaelis constant catalases are not easily saturated with substrate and can act over a wide range of H_2O_2 concentrations maintaining a controlled intracellular H_2O_2 concentration. Whereas animals have only one form of catalase, plants have evolved small gene families encoding catalases. The plant catalases can be grouped into three classes depending on their expression and physiological parameters. In *Arabidopsis*, the small catalase gene family has been characterized to consist of three members, the class III catalase *CAT1*, class I catalase *CAT2* and class II catalase *CAT3*. All three Arabidopsis catalases show a senescence-specific alteration in expression and activity (Zimmermann et al., 2006). *CAT2* expression and activity is down-regulated at an early time point when plants are bolting. Subsequently, expression and activity of *CAT3* is up-regulated during progression of senescence. In contrast to *CAT2* expression, which is predominantly located in mesophyll cells, *CAT3* expression is mainly expressed in vascular tissue indicating that the vascular system appears to be protected against oxidative stress during senescence to guarantee the transport of nutrients and minerals out of the senescing tissue into developing parts of the plant like e.g. the seeds (Zimmermann et al., 2006). CAT1 expression and activity is very low during plant development and only increases significantly during germination and in very late stages of senescence. Due to this expression pattern, its activity is discussed to be related to fatty acid degradation which takes place when peroxisomes are converted into glyoxisomes.

Especially the transcriptional down-regulation of *CAT2* appears to be involved in the regulation of the onset of senescence. This down-regulation is executed by the bZIP transcription factor GBF1. Insertion of a T-DNA into the *GBF1* gene revealed a loss of *CAT2* down-regulation and resulted in the loss of a hydrogen peroxide increase during bolting time. These *gbf1* mutant plants exhibit a delayed onset of senescence (Smykowski et al., 2010). Consequently, the idea suggests itself that *CAT2* knock-out plants also have a senescence phenotype. Taking into consideration that *CAT2* is expressed not only in leaves but also in roots, stems and flowers contributing substantially to the regulation of intracellular hydrogen peroxide contents and the protection of the cells against ROS in stress situations, the knock-out of this gene would have severe effects on the plants. The loss of such an important enzyme has to be compensated somehow during development but it would be expected that these knock-out plants are more sensitive against all stresses implying an increased ROS production and that they most likely show a senescence phenotype. The lack of peroxisomal catalase CTL-2 in *Caenorhabditis elegans* causes a progeric phenotype whereas the lack of the cytosolic catalase CTL-1 has no effect on nematode aging (Petriv & Rachubinski, 2004). In yeast, catalase T activity but not catalase A activity was necessary to assure longevity under repressing conditions on glucose media. However, under derepressing conditions, on ethanol media, both catalases were required for longevity assurance (Van Zandycke et al., 2002) indicating a correlation between CAT activity and longevity in animal systems.

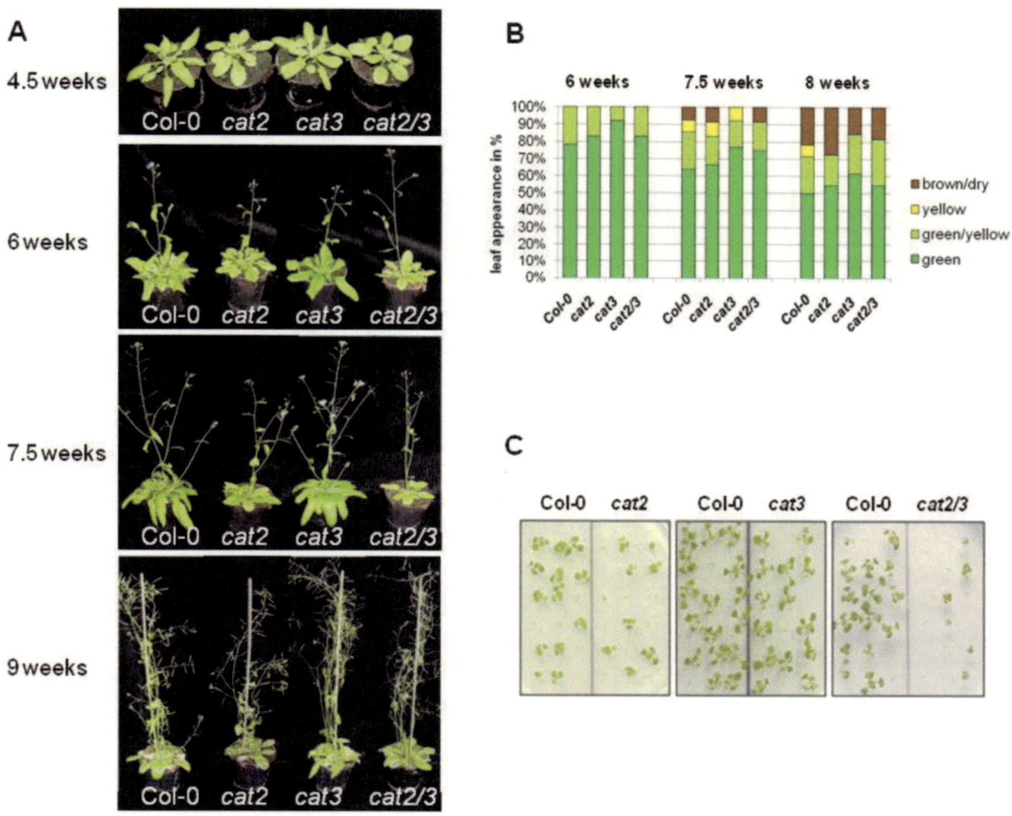

Fig. 5. *Phenotypic analyses of catalase mutants*
A) Plant development, **B)** Percantage of phenotypical appearance of the leaves of ten rosettes, **C)** Germination rate of wild type (Col-0), *cat2*, *cat3*, and *cat2/3* mutant plants.

Surprisingly, *cat2* knock-out plants appear to be more or less inconspicuous. They are slightly impaired in germination (Fig. 5C) but once germinated the plants developed relatively normaly (Queval et al., 2007; Fig. 5A). Photoperiod and CO_2 levels have a high impact on the phenotypic appearance of the plants and on the ascorbate and glutathione contents and their balances of the oxidized and reduced form, respectively. Under high CO_2

conditions no obvious phenotype could be observed whereas growth under ambient air, which favours photorespiration, led to a lower biomass production of the rosette and an altered leaf shape (Queval et al., 2007; Fig 5). We characterized SALK T-DNA insertion lines for *CAT2* and *CAT3* for homozygous insertion of the T-DNA and crossed the homozygous *cat2* and *cat3* mutants and selected the offsprings for a homozygous double knock-out line *cat2/3*. After separation of leaf protein extracts of these lines on native PAGEs, we could confirm that according to the gene knock-out the activity of the respective isoform disappeared (Fig. 6 A). When we analyzed plant development under long day conditions, leaf or plant senescence does not seem to be impaired (Fig. 5A, B); only leaf shape and biomass production were slightly altered in *cat2 and cat2/3* plants. However, the mutant plant populations did not senesce as homogenously as the wildtype populations. If the hydrogen peroxide content was measured, the profiles appeared to be not much different indicating that a very efficient compensation of the loss of CAT activity has been activated (Fig 6A).

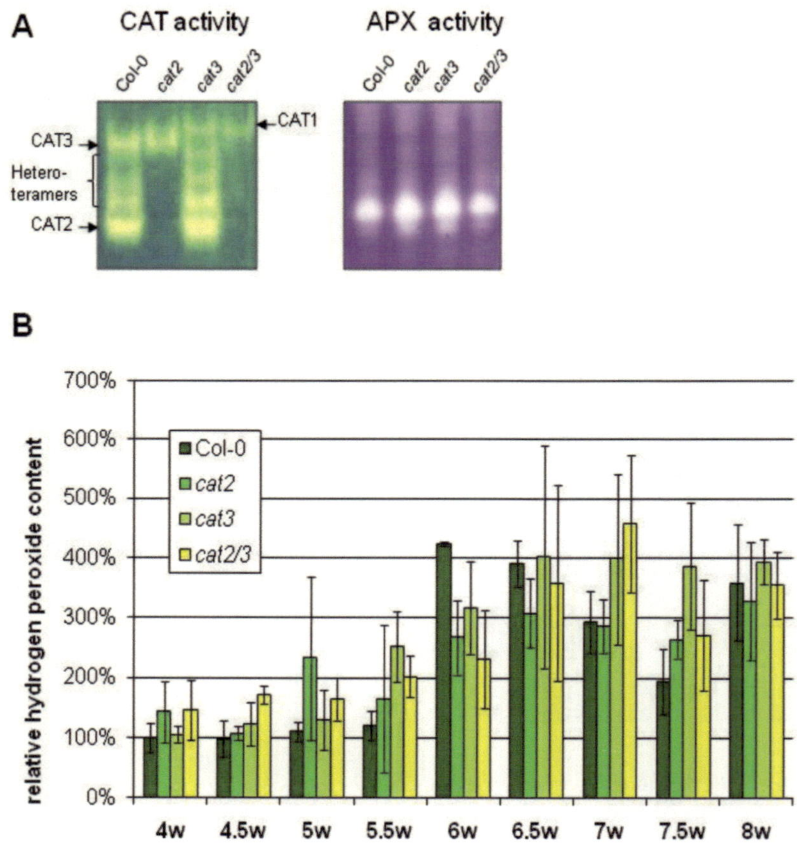

Fig. 6. *Physiological analyses of catalase mutants*
A) Catalase activity, **B)** Ascorbate peroxidase activity. **C)** Hydrogen peroxide content of wild type (Col-0), cat2, cat3, and cat2/3 mutant plants. The value of the 4-week-old wildtype plants was referred to as 100%. The error bars indicate the standard deviation of 4 independent experiments.

However, the hydrogen peroxide content between different leaves and plants varied remarkably so that the standard deviation was quite high in the measurements of the mutants. How the CAT2 or CAT3 activity losses were compensated is not yet clear but APX activity appeared to be not elevated (Fig 6B); in contrast, it appeared to be even slightly reduced in the double mutant. Hydrogen peroxide levels in these plants clearly indicated that the loss of the CAT activity must have been compensated. This is consistent with the finding of Rizhky and co-workers (2002), who claimed that there appears to be a sensitive balance between the antioxidant enzymes with compensating mechanisms, since they observed that double antisense plants for CAT or APX are more tolerant to oxidative stress than single antisense plants (Rizhsky et al., 2002). A slight activation of CAT1 can be observed in all our catalase mutants, especially in the *cat3* and *cat2/3* mutant plants. This is also indicated by the heterodimer formation between CAT2 and CAT1 in the *cat3* mutant. However, the activity of this isoform appears to be only low compared to the loss of catalase activity which would be present in wild type plants (Fig. 6B). Remarkably, glutathione levels are increased and shifted towards the more oxidized form in *cat2* plants under long day conditions (Queval et al., 2007). Taken together, the ROS levels appear to be very tightly regulated on many levels with the possibility of compensation if one detoxifying system fails.

3. Conclusion

Antimycin A treatment leads to the inhibition of the cytochrom *c* dependent electron transport lowering the production of hydrogen peroxide in mitochondria. Conversely, it is assumed that if stress occurs in a cellular compartment and increasing amounts of hydrogen peroxide are formed, these hydrogen peroxide molecules also can pass membranes and can be transported into the cytosol. This signal can then be transduced into the nucleus, where it induces the expression of many genes including *AOX*. As soon as the newly synthesized AOX protein is active, it minimizes the formation of ROS in the mitochondria by preventing the overreduction of the electron transport chain. Therefore, alternative oxidase might be regarded as mechanism to protect the plant from oxidative stress. Even though oxidative stress tolerance and longevity in Arabidopsis are tightly correlated (Kurepa et al. 1998, Woo et al., 2004) and hydrogen peroxide is discussed as signalling molecule to induce leaf senescence in Arabidopsis (Navabpour et al., 2003; Miao et al. 2004; Zimmermann et al., 2006), minimizing hydrogen peroxide production in the mitochondria by long-term antimycin A treatment did not delay senescence. In contrast, if down-regulation of *CAT2* expression and activity is abolished in *gbf1* mutants, the onset of senescence is delayed. On the other hand, if *CAT2* gene expression is prevented from early on in development in *cat2* T-DNA insertion lines, also no effect on senescence could be observed and hydrogen peroxide contents are not significantly altered. Therefore, we can assume that the intracellular origin but also the developmental time point of the hydrogen peroxide production might have an impact on its signalling function. In addition, the loss of one detoxifying system can be compensated by the cells and there seems to be a very sensitive balance between the different antioxidative protection systems. Remarkably, hydrogen peroxide plays a role in many different signal transduction pathways but how specificity is mediated is still an open question. Compartment-specific hydrogen peroxide fluorescent sensor molecules like roGFP or Hyper will help to clarify whether the intracellular origin of the hydrogen peroxide and changes during specific developmental time points might be important for its signalling function.

4. Experimental procedures

4.1 Plant material

Seeds from *Arabidopsis thaliana,* ecotype Columbia, were grown in a climatic chamber at 22°C under 16 h of illumination under low light conditions (60 µmol $s^{-1}m^{-2}$). Under these conditions plants developed flowers within 7 weeks, mature seeds could be harvested after 12 weeks. For long term treatment, plants were watered every second day with 5 ml of 40 µM antimycin A or 0.8 % ethanol as a control in addition to normal watering.

Suspension cells of *Arabidopsis thaliana,* ecotype Landsberg erecta, were grown under constant light on a rotary shaker (120 rpm) at 20°C and were subcultured every 7 days by 30-fold dilution in fresh growth medium (100 ml culture in 250 ml flasks). The Murashige and Skoog growth medium contains 3 % (w/v) sucrose, 0.5 mg/l α-naphthaleneacetic acid and 0.05 mg/l kinetin; pH was adjusted to 5.8 with KOH. Cell cultures with a density of about 100 mg/ml medium were treated with 5 µM antimycin A (Sigma) or 5 mM hydrogen peroxide.

The full length cDNA of AOX1a (At3g22370) was amplified by PCR form reverse transcripted poly A^+ RNA isolated from mature leaf material. The cDNA was cloned into the vector PY01 adjacent to a CaMV35S promoter. The construct was verified by sequencing. Arabidopsis transformation was performed by the vacuum infiltration procedure (Bechthold & Pelletier, 1998). The seeds of the transgenic plants were selected by spraying with 0.1% Basta. *WRKY53* overexpressing plants were constructed as described before (Miao et al., 2004)

T-DNA insertion lines in *CAT2* (SALK_057998) and *CAT3* (SALK_092911) were obtained from the Nottingham Arabidopsis Stock Centre (NASC). Homozygous lines were characterized by PCR using gene specific and T-DNA left border primers (LBb1 5'GCGTGG ACC GCT TGC TGC AAC T 3'; CAT2-LP2 5' TCG CAT GAC TGT GGT TGG TTC 3'; CAT2-RP2 5' ACC ACC AAC TCT GGT GCT CCT 3'; CAT3-LP 5' CAC CTG AGT AAT CAA ATC TAC ACG 3'; CAT3-RP 5' TCA GGG ATC CTC TCT CTG GTG AA 3'). Homozygous plants were crossed and homozygous double knock-out lines were selected by PCR screening using the same primers. Knock-out was verified by native PAGE and subsequent CAT activity staining. Since *CAT2* and *CAT3* are under circadian regulation, leaves were always harvested 3 h after the beginning of illumination. Leaves were pooled in all experiments.

4.2 RNA isolation and Northern and dot blot analyses

Total RNA was isolated from leaves according to the protocol of PURESCRIPT RNA isolation kit (Gentra). Total RNA was either denatured 15 min at 55°C and spotted on nylon membranes or separated on MOPS-formaldehyde (6.2 %) agarose gels (1.5 %) and transferred to nylon membranes using 10 x SSC as transfer buffer. The membranes were hybridized at 65°C, washed twice at room temperature for 20 min with 2 x SSPE, 0.1 % SDS and once at 65°C for 30 min with 0.2 x SSPE, 0.1 % SDS. A fragment of the 5′ UTR of the *AOX1a* gene or of the 3′UTR of the *SAG12* gene (At5g45890) was used as radioactive labeled hybridization probe.

4.3 Measurement and detection of hydrogen peroxide

Hydrogen peroxide was measured according to the method described by Kuźniak and others (1999). Ten leaf discs (diameter 1 cm) or pelleted suspension cells (approx. 100 mg) were incubated for 2 h in 2 ml reagent mixture containing 50 mM potassium phosphate buffer pH 7.0, 0.05 % guaiacol (Sigma) and horseradish peroxidase (2.5 u/ml, Serva) at room temperature in the dark. Four moles of hydrogen peroxide are required to form 1 mole of tetraguaiacol, which has an extinction coefficient of ε = 26.6 $cm^{-1}mM^{-1}$ at 470 nm. The absorbance in the reaction mixture was measured immediately at 470 nm.

4.4 Chlorophyll and total protein content

Leaf discs were homogenized in 0.2 ml 25 mM potassium phosphate buffer, pH 7.0, containing 2 mM EDTA. Subsequently, 0.8 ml acetone was added, and the samples were shaken vigorously for 1 h at room temperature. After centrifugation at 14000 g for 30 min at room temperature, the total chlorophyll content of the supernatant was measured and calculated following the method described by Arnon (1949). To determine total protein content, leaf discs were ground in 100 mM potassium phosphate buffer, pH 7.0, containing 1 mM EDTA at 4°C. After centrifugation at 14000 g for 30 min at 4°C, the supernatant was directly used for protein quantification according to the method of Bradford (1976) using BSA as standard.

4.5 CAT and APX acitivities

For analyses of APX isozymes, crude protein extracts were separated on 10% native polyacrylamide gels (0.375 M Tris-HCl, pH 8.8, as gel buffer) with a 5% stacking gel (0.125 M Tris-HCl, pH 6.8, as gel buffer) for 16 h (120V) at 4°C using 2 mM ascorbate, 250 mM glycine, and 25 mM Tris-HCl, pH 8.3, as electrophoresis buffer. After electrophoresis, the gels were soaked in 50 mM potassium phosphate buffer, pH 7.0, containing 2 mM ascorbate for 10 min (3x) and, subsequently, in 50 mM potassium phosphate buffer, pH 7.0, containing 4 mM ascorbate, and 1 mM H_2O_2 for 20 min. After rinsing in water, the gels were stained in 50 mM potassium phosphate buffer, pH 7.8, containing 14 mM TEMED (*N,N,N´,N´*-tetramethylethylenediamine) and 2.45 mM NBT (nitro blue tetrazolium) for 10-30 min. For the analyses of CAT isozymes the protein extracts were separated on 7.5% native polyacrylamide gels (0.375 M Tris-HCl, pH 8.8, as gel buffer) with a 3.5% stacking gel (0.125 M Tris-HCl, pH 6.8, as gel buffer) for 16 h (70-80V) at 18°C using 250 mM glycine and 25 mM Tris-HCl, pH 8.3, as electrophoresis buffer. Subsequently, the gels were stained for the activity of catalases as follows: The gels were soaked in 0.01% of hydrogen peroxide solution for 5 min, washed twice in water and incubated for 5 min in 1% $FeCl_3$ and 1% $K_3[Fe(CN)_6]$. After staining, the gels were washed once more in water.

5. Acknowledgment

We thank the Nottingham Arabidopsis Stock Centre (NASC) for providing seeds of the T-DNA insertion lines for *CAT2* (SALK_057998) and *CAT3* (SALK_092911). This work was supported by the Deutsche Forschungsgemeinschaft (SFB 446).

6. References

Arnholdt-Schmitt, B.; Costa, J.H. & de Melo, D.F. (2006). AOX- a functional marker for efficient cell reprogramming under stress? *Trends Plant Sciences* 11(6), pp. 281-287, ISSN 1360-1385

Arnon, D.I. (1949). Copper enzymes in isolated chloroplast. Polyphenoloxidase in *Beta vulgaris*. *Plant Physiology* 24, pp. 1-15, ISSN 0032-0889, online ISSN 1532-2548

Bartoli ,C.G.; Pastori ,G.M. & Foyer, C.H. (2000). Ascorbate biosynthesis in mitochondria is linked to the electron transport chain between complexes III and IV. *Plant Physology* 123, pp. 335–344, ISSN 0032-0889, online ISSN 1532-2548

Bartoli, C.G.; Yu, J.; Gómez, F.; Fernández, L.; McIntosh, L. & Foyer, C.H. (2006). Interrelationships between light and respiration in the control of ascorbic acid synthesis and accumulation in Arabidopsis thaliana leaves. *Journal of Experimental Botany* 57 (8), pp. 1621-1631, ISSN 0022-0957, online ISSN 1460-2431

Bechtold, N. & Pelletier, G. (1998). In planta Agrobacterium-mediated transformation of adult Arabidopsis thaliana plants by vacuum infiltration. *Methods in Molecular Biology* 82, pp. 259-266, ISSN 1064-3745

Bradford, M.M. (1976). A rapid and sensitive method for the quantification of microgram quantities of protein utilizing the principle of protein-dye binding. *Annals of Biochemistry* 72, pp. 248-254 , ISSN 0305-7364, online ISSN 1095-8290

Clifton, R.; Millar, A.H. & Whelan, J. (2006). Alternative oxidases in Arabidopsis: a comparative analysis of differential expression in the gene family provides new insights into function of non-phosphorylating bypasses. *Biochimica et Biophysica Acta (BBA)* 1757 (7), pp. 730-741, ISSN 0005-2728, online ISSN 1879-2650

Corpas, F.J.; Barroso, J.B. & del Río, L.A. (2001). Peroxisomes as a source of reactive oxygen species and nitric oxide signal molecules in plant cells. *Trends in Plant Science* 6 (4), pp. 145–150, ISSN 1360-1385

Dat, J.; Vandenabeele, S.; Vranová, E.; Van Montagu, M.; Inzé, D. & Van Breusegem, F. (2000). Dual action of the active oxygen species during plant stress responses. *Cellular and Molecular Life Sciences* 57 (5), pp. 779-795, ISSN 1420-682X, online ISSN 1420-9071

del Río, L.A.; Pastori, G.M.; Palma, J. M.; Sandalio, L.M.; Sevilla, F.; Corpas, F.J.; Jiménez A.; López-Huertas, E. & Hernández, J. A. (1998). The activated oxygen role of peroxisomes in senescence. *Plant Physiology* 116 (4), pp. 1195–1200, ISSN 0032-0889, online ISSN 1532-2548

del Río, L.A.; Corpas, F.J.; Sandalio, L.M. ; Palma, J.M. & Barroso J.B. (2003). Plant peroxisomes, reactive oxygen metabolism and nitric oxide. *IUBMB Life* 55(2), pp. 71-81, ISSN 1521-6543, online ISSN 1521-6551

del Río, L.A.; Corpas, F.J.; Sandalio, L.M.; Palma, J.M.; Gómez, M. & Barroso, B. (2002). Reactive oxygen species, antioxidant systems and nitric oxide in peroxisomes. *Journal of Experimental Botany* 53 (372), pp. 1255–1272, ISSN 0022-0957, online ISSN 1460-2431

Dufour, E.; Boulay, J.; Rincheval, V. & Sainsard-Chanet, A. (2000). A causal link betweeen respiration and senescence in *Podospora anserina*. *Proceedings of the National Academy of Sciences USA* 97 (8), pp. 4138-4143, ISSN 0027-8424, online ISSN 1091-6490

Dutilleul, C.; Garmier, M.; Noctor, G.; Mathieu, C.; Chétrit, P.; Foyer, C.H. & de Paepe, R. (2003). Leaf mitochondria modulate whole cell redox homeostasis, set antioxidant capacity, and determine stress resistance through altered signaling and diurnal regulation. *Plant Cell* 15 (5), pp. 1212-1226, ISSN 1040-4651, online ISSN 1532-298X

Eulgem, T.; Rushton, P. J.; Robatzek, S. & Somssich, I. E. (2000). The WRKY superfamily of plant transcription factors. *Trends in Plant Science* 5 (5), pp. 199-206, ISSN 1360-1385

Fiorani, F.; Umbach, A.L. & Siedow, J.N. (2005). The alternative oxidase of plant mitochondria is involved in the acclimation of shoot growth at low temperature. A study of Arabidopsis AOX1a transgenic plants. *Plant Physiology* 139 (4), pp. 1795-1805, ISSN 0032-0889, online ISSN 1532-2548

Grant, J.J. & Loake, G.J. (2000). Role of reactive oxygen intermediates and cognate redox signalling in disease resistance. *Plant Physiology* 124 (1), pp. 21-29, ISSN 0032-0889, online ISSN 1532-2548

Hiser, C. & McIntosh, L. (1990). Alternative oxidase of potato is an integral membrane protein synthesized de novo during aging of tuber slices. *Plant Physiology* 93 (1), pp. 312-318, ISSN 0032-0889, online ISSN 1532-2548

Jiménez, A.; Hernandez, J.A.; Pastori, G.; del Rio, L.A. & Sevilla, F. (1998). Role of the ascorbate-glutathione cycle of mitochondria and peroxisomes in the senescence of pea leaves. *Plant Physiology* 118 (4), pp. 1327-1335, ISSN 0032-0889, online 1532-2548

Kurepa, J.; Smalle, J.; Van Montagu, M. & Inzé, D. (1998). Oxidative stress tolerance and longevity in Arabidopsis: the late flowering mutant *gigantea* is tolerant to paraquat. *Plant Journal* 14 (6), pp. 759-764, Online ISSN: 1365-313X

Kuźniak, E.; Patykowski, J. & Urbanek, H. (1999). Involvement of the antioxidative system in tomato response to fusaric acid treatment. *Journal of Phytopathology* 147, pp. 385-390, ISSN 0931-1785, online 1439-0434

Lennon, A.M.; Neuenschwander, U.H.; Ribas-Carbo, M.; Giles, L.; Ryals, J.A. & Siedow, J. N. (1997). The effects of salicylic acid and tobacco mosaic virus infection on the alternative oxidase of tobacco. *Plant Physiology* 115 (2), pp. 783-791, ISSN 0032-0889, online ISSN 1532-2548

Lorin, S.; Dufour, E.; Boulay, J.; Begel, O.; Marsy, S. & Sainsard-Chanet, A. (2001). Overexpression of the alternative oxidase restores senescence and fertility in a long- lived respiration-deficient mutant of *Podospora anserina*. *Molecular Microbiology* 42 (5), pp. 1259-1267, ISSN 0950-382X, online ISSN 1365-2958

Martin-Tryon, E.L.; Kreps, J.A. & Harmer, S.L. (2007). GIGANTEA acts in blue light signaling and has biochemically separable roles in circadian clock and flowering time regulation. *Plant Physiology* 143 (1), pp. 473-486, ISSN 0032-0889, online 1532-2548

Maxwell, D.P.; Nickels, R. & McIntosh, L. (2002). Evidence of mitochondrial involvement in the transduction of signals required for the induction of genes associated with pathogen attack and senescence. *Plant Journal* 29 (3), pp. 269-279, online ISSN 1365-313X

Maxwell, D.P.; Wang, Y. & McIntosh, L. (1999). The alternative oxidase lowers mitochondrial reactive oxygen production in plant cells. *Proceedings of the National Academy of Sciences USA* 96 (14), pp. 8271-8276, ISSN 0027-8424, online ISSN 1091-6490

McIntosh, L. (1994). Molecular biology of the alternative oxidase. *Plant Physiology* 105 (3), pp. 781-786, ISSN 0032-0889, online ISSN 1532-2548

Miao, Y.; Laun, T.; Zimmermann, P. & Zentgraf, U. (2004). Targets of the WRKY53 transcription factor and its role during leaf senescence in *Arabidopsis thaliana*. *Plant Molecular Biology* 55 (6), pp. 853-867, ISSN 0167-4412, online ISSN: 1573-5028

Millar, A.H.; Whelan, J.; Soole, K.L. & Day, D.A. (2011). Organization and regulation of mitochondrial respiration in plants. *Annual Review of Plant Biology* 62, pp. 79–104, ISSN: 1543-5008

Millenaar, F.F. & Lambers, H. (2003). The Alternative Oxidase: *in vivo* Regulation and Function. *Plant Biology* 5 (1), pp. 2-15, ISSN 1435-8603, online ISSN 1438-8677

Miller, J.D.; Arteca, R. N. & Pell, E.J. (1999). Senescence-associated gene expression during ozone-induced leaf senescence in Arabidopsis. *Plant Physiology* 120 (4), pp. 1015-1024, ISSN 0032-0889, online 1532-2548

Moore, A.L.; Albury, M.S.; Crichton, P.G. & Affourtit, C. (2002). Function of the alternative oxidase: is it still a scavenger? *Trends in Plant Science* 7 (11), pp. 478-481, ISSN 1360-1385

Navabpour, S.; Morris, K.; Allen, R.; Harrison, E.; Mackerness, S.A.H. & Buchanan-Wollaston V. (2003). Expression of senescence-enhanced genes in response to oxidative stress. *Journal of Experimental Botany* 54 (391), pp. 2285-2292, ISSN 0022-0957, online 1460-2431

Palma, J.M. ; Copras, F.J. & del Rio, L.A. (2009). Proteome of plant peroxisomes: new perspectives on the role of these organelles in cell biology. *Proteomics* 9 (9), pp. 2301–2312, ISSN 1615-9853, online ISSN 1615-9861

Panchuk, I. I.; Zentgraf, U. & Volkov, R. A .(2005). Expression of the *Apx* gene family during leaf senescence of *Arabidopsis thaliana. Planta* 222 (5), pp. 926-932, ISSN 0032-0935, online ISSN 1432-2048

Petriv, O.I. & Rachubinski, R.A. (2004). Lack of peroxisomal catalase causes a progeric phenotype in Caenorhabditis elegans. *Journal of Biological Chemistry* 279 (19), pp. 19996-20001, ISSN 0021-9258, online ISSN 1083-351X

Queval, G.; Issakidis-Bourguet, E.; Hoeberichts, F.A.; Vandorpe, M.; Gakière, B.; Vanacker, H.; Miginiac-Maslow, M.; Van Breusegem, F. & Noctor, G. (2007). Conditional oxidative stress responses in the Arabidopsis photorespiratory mutant cat2 demonstrate that redox state is a key modulator of daylength-dependent gene expression, and define photoperiod as a crucial factor in the regulation of H_2O_2-induced cell death. *Plant Journal* 52 (4), pp. 640-657, Online ISSN: 1365-313X

Rasmusson, A.G.; Fernie, A.R. & van Dongen, J.T. (2009). Alternative oxidase: a defence against metabolic fluctuations? *Physiologia Plantarum* 137 (4), pp. 371–382, ISSN 0031-9317, online ISSN 1399-3054

Rizhsky, L.; Hallak-Herr, E.; Van Breusegem, F.; Rachmilevitch, S.; Barr, J.E.; Rodermel, S.; Inzé, D. & Mittler, R. (2002). Double antisense plants lacking ascorbate peroxidase and catalase are less sensitive to oxidative stress than single antisense plants lacking ascorbate peroxidase or catalase. *Plant Journal* 32 (3), pp. 329-342, Online ISSN: 1365-313X

Saisho, D.; Nambara, E.; Naito, S.; Tsutsumi, N.; Hirai, A. & Nakazono, M. (1997). Characterization of the gene family for alternative oxidase from *Arabidopsis thaliana. Plant Molecular Biology* 35 (5), pp. 585-596, ISSN 0167-4412, online ISSN: 1573-5028

Siedow, J. N. & Moore, A. L. (1993). A kinetic model for the regulation of electron transfer through the cyanide-resistant pathway in plant mitochondria. *Biochimica et Biophysica Acta - Bioenergetics* 1142 (1-2), pp. 165-174, ISSN 0006-3002

Smykowski, A.; Zimmermann, P. & Zentgraf, U. (2010). G-Box binding Factor1 reduces CATALASE2 expression and regulates the onset of leaf senescence in Arabidopsis. *Plant Physiology* 153 (3), pp. 1321-1331, ISSN 0032-0889, online 1532-2548

Svensson, A. S. & Rasmusson, A. G. (2001). Light-dependent gene expression for proteins in the respiratory chain of potato leaves. *Plant Journal* 28 (1), pp. 73-82, Online ISSN 1365-313X

Umbach, A.L.; Fiorani, F. & Siedow, J.N. (2005). Characterization of transformed Arabidopsis with altered alternative oxidase levels and analysis of effects on reactive oxygen species in tissue. *Plant Physiology* 139 (4), pp. 1806-1820, ISSN 0032-0889, online ISSN 1532-2548

Van Aken, O.; Zhang ,B.; Carrie, C.; Uggalla ,V.; Paynter, E.; Giraud, E. & Whelan, J. (2009). Defining the mitochondrial stress response in Arabidopsis thaliana. *Molecular Plant* 2 (6), pp. 1310–1324, ISSN 1674-2052, online ISSN 1752-9867

Van Zandycke, S.M.; Sohier, P.J. & Smart, K.A. (2002). The impact of catalase expression on the replicative lifespan of Saccharomyces cerevisiae. *Mechanisms of Ageing and Development* 123 (4), pp. 365-373, ISSN 0047-637

Vanlerberghe, G. C. & McIntosh, L. (1992). Coordinate regulation of cytochrome and alternative pathway respiration in tobacco. *Plant Physiology* 100 (4), pp. 1846-1851, ISSN 0032-0889, online ISSN 1532-2548

Vanlerberghe, G.C.; Cvetkovska, M. & Wang, J. (2009). Is the maintenance of homeostatic mitochondrial signaling during stress a physiological role for alternative oxidase? *Physiologia Plantarum* 137 (4), pp. 392–406, ISSN 0031-9317, online ISSN 1399-3054

Watanabe, C.K.; Hachiya, T.; Terashima, I. & Noguchi, K. (2008). The lack of alternative oxidase at low temperature leads to a disruption of the balance in carbon and nitrogen metabolism, and to an up-regulation of anti-oxidant defense systems in Arabidopsis thaliana leaves. *Plant, Cell & Environment* 31 (8), pp. 1190–1202, ISSN 0140-7791, online ISSN1365-3040

Woo, H.R.; Kim, J.H.; Nam, H.G. & Lim, P.O. (2004). The delayed leaf senescence mutants of Arabidopsis, ore1, ore3, and ore9 are tolerant to oxidative stress. *Plant & Cell Physiology* 45 (7), pp. 923-932, ISSN 0140-7791, online ISSN1365-3040

Wulff, A.; Oliveira, H.C.; Saviani, E.E.& Salgado, I. (2009). Nitrite reduction and superoxide-dependent nitric oxide degradation by Arabidopsis mitochondria: influence of external NAD(P)H dehydrogenases and alternative oxidase in the control of nitric oxide levels. *Nitric Oxide* 21(2), pp. 132-139, ISSN 1089-8603

Ye, Z.Z.; Rodriguez, R.; Tran, A.; Hoang, H.; de los Santos, D.; Brown, S. & Vellanoweth, R.L. (2000). The developmental transition to flowering represses ascorbate peroxidase activity and induces enzymatic lipid peroxidation in leaf tissue in *Arabidopsis thaliana*. *Plant Science* 158 (1-2), pp. 115-127, ISSN 0168-9452

Yoshida, K.; Watanabe, C. Kato, Y.; Sakamoto, W. & Noguchi, K. (2008). Influence of chloroplastic photo-oxidative stress on mitochondrial alternative oxidase capacity and respiratory properties: a case study with Arabidopsis yellow variegated 2. *Plant & Cell Physiology* 49 (4), pp. 592-603, ISSN 0032-0781, online ISSN 1471-9053

Yoshida, K.; Watanabe, C.K.; Terashima, I. & Noguchi, K. (2011). Physiological impact of mitochondrial alternative oxidase on photosynthesis and growth in Arabidopsis thaliana. *Plant Cell & Environment*, Jun 24. doi: 10.1111/j.1365-3040.2011.02384.x, ISSN 0140-7791, online ISSN1365-3040

Zapata, J.M.; Guera, A.; Esteban-Carrasco, A.; Martin, M. & Sabater, B. (2005). Chloroplasts regulate leaf senescence: delayed senescence in transgenic ndhF-defective tobacco. *Cell Death and Differentiation* 12 (10), pp. 1277-1284, ISSN 1350-9047

Zentgraf; U. & Hemleben, V. (2007). Molecular cell biology: Are reactive oxygen species regulators of leaf senescence? In: Lüttge, U.; Beyschlag, W. & Murata, J. (Eds), Progress in Botany, Vol. 69, Springer, Berlin, Heidelberg, New York, pp. 117-138, ISBN 978-3-540-72953-2, ISSN 0340-4773

Zimmermann, P.; Orendi, G.; Heinlein, C. & Zentgraf, U. (2006). Senescence specific regulation of catalases in *Arabidopsis thaliana* (L.) Heynh. *Plant Cell & Environment* 29 (6), pp. 1049-1060, ISSN 0140-7791, online ISSN1365-3040

3

Metabolic Regulation of Leaf Senescence in Sunflower (*Helianthus annuus* L.) Plants

Eloísa Agüera, Purificación Cabello,
Lourdes de la Mata, Estefanía Molina and Purificación de la Haba
Department of Botany, Ecology and Plant Physiology,
University of Córdoba
Spain

1. Introduction

The leaf is the main photosynthetic organ of plants and its development a complex process governed by a combination of environmental factors and intrinsic and genetically regulated signals (Van Lijsebettens & Clarke, 1998). Usually, leaf ontogeny includes an early phase of increasing photosynthetic rates while the leaf is actively expanding, a mature phase where such rates peak and a senescence phase where they decline (Gepstein, 1988; Miller et al., 2000). During early development, the leaf is a sink receiving nutrients from the rest of the plant; however, as soon as it reaches full photosynthetic capacity, it becomes the main source organ of the plant. After this productive period, the leaf enters the senescence phase, during which most compounds present in it are removed and reused (Hörtensteiner & Feller, 2002; Buchanan-Wollaston et al., 2003a). Leaf senescence, which is last stage in leaf development, is a highly regulated and programmed degeneration process governed by a variety of developmental and environmental signals (Lim et al., 2003). This important phase in the leaf lifespan period may last as long as leaf maturation and involves a shift from nutrient assimilation to nutrient remobilization and recycling (Guiboileau et al., 2010). In senescent leaf metabolism, carbon and nitrogen assimilation are replaced by catabolism of chlorophyll and macromolecules such as proteins, RNA and membrane lipids, the degradation of which marks the senescence phase. Unsurprisingly, senescence alters the expression of many genes. These senescence-associated genes include regulatory genes encoding transcription factors; genes involved in degradative processes that code for hydrolytic enzymes such as proteases, lipases and ribonucleases; and genes with secondary functions in senescence that code for proteins involved in nutrient remobilization (e.g. glutamine synthetase, which catalyses the conversion of ammonium into glutamine to enable nitrogen recycling in senescing cells) (Taiz & Zeiger, 2010). Environmental cues such as day length and temperature, and various biotic and abiotic sources of stress, can also affect the initiation and progress of such a high complex as leaf senescence.

During senescence, some metabolic pathways are triggered and others turned off. These dramatic metabolic changes result in orderly degradation of cellular structures, starting with chloroplasts (Wiedemuth et al., 2005), and also in the subsequent remobilization of the resulting materials. Chloroplasts play a dual role; thus, they are the main source of nitrogen and also the regulators of their own degradation during senescence (Zapata et al., 2005). Most of the protein in green cells is located in chloroplasts, which thus constitute their main reserves of organic nitrogen. Efficient recycling of nitrogen from the photosynthetic apparatus during early senescence requires the presence of intact mitochondrial, nuclear and cellular membranes (Gan & Amasino, 1997; Nam, 1997; Noodén et al., 1997; Hörtensteiner & Feller, 2002; Cabello et al., 2006). Leaf proteins (particularly photosynthetic proteins) are extensively degraded during senescence (Martínez et al., 2008), which confirms that one of the primary functions of leaf senescence is to recycle nutrients (especially through nitrogen remobilization) (Himelblau & Amasino, 2001). Protein breakdown starts early in senescence and proteolysis is believed to start within chloroplasts. Some proteins (e.g. chlorophyll-binding light-harvesting proteins LHCII) seem to be entirely degraded within chloroplasts, whereas Rubisco and other chloroplastic proteins may be broken down via a hybrid pathway involving both chloroplasts and extraplastidic compartments such as the central vacuole and small senescence-associated vacuoles (SAVs), which are absent from mature, non-senescing leaves but present in large numbers during senescence (Otegui et al., 2005; Martínez et al., 2008). Degradation of chloroplastic proteins releases potentially phototoxic chlorophylls that necessitate degradation. Therefore, leaf senescence is characterized by a decline in photosynthetic activity and chlorophyll content, and the rapid chlorophyll loss associated with chloroplast degeneration is frequently used as a biomarker for the start of senescence. Although chlorophyll degradation is an early senescence signal, leaf yellowing is not an appropriate marker of early senescence because it is observed when senescence has progressed to a great extent (Diaz et al., 2005). Nitrogen and carbon metabolism plays a crucial role in the senescence process, which is seemingly governed by both external and internal factors. Thus, leaf senescence induction involves the joint action of external (nitrogen availability, light) and internal signals (regulating metabolites, C/N ratio) (Wingler et al., 2006; Wingler & Roitsch, 2008).

Other important signals for induction or progression of senescence include the redox status of leaf cells and the production of reactive oxygen species (ROS) such as hydrogen peroxide and superoxide radical (Kukavica & Veljovic-Jovanovic, 2004; Zimmermann & Zentgraf, 2005). There are many sources of reactive oxygen species, which are produced during aerobic metabolism in chloroplasts, mitochondria and peroxisomes in both photosynthetically active and senescent cells. The toxicity of these reactive species is dictated by various enzymatic and non-enzymatic protective antioxidant defences. Superoxide dismutases, catalases, peroxidases and the ascorbate–glutathione cycle enzymes are the primary antioxidant enzymes. Plant ageing increases oxidative stress and the levels of reactive oxygen species, which may additionally diminish antioxidant protection (Buchanan-Wollaston et al., 2003b; Zimmermann & Zentgraf, 2005). Chloroplasts are probably the main target of age-associated oxidative stress in plants (Munné-Bosch & Alegre, 2002). Therefore, a plausible model for regulation of leaf senescence is a shifted balance between the production of reactive oxygen species and their removal by antioxidant systems.

In this chapter, we describe various aspects of leaf senescence in sunflower plants, with special emphasis on changes in the contents of some nitrogen and carbon metabolites potentially acting as regulators or markers of senescence during sunflower leaf development, and also on the role of oxidative stress in this process and the influence of external factors such nitrogen supply and irradiance exposition on it.

2. Growth-related parameters and photosynthetic activity during sunflower leaf senescence

We examined various markers widely used to monitor leaf development (viz. photosynthetic pigment level, protein content and CO_2 fixation rate) in primary leaves of sunflower plants grown for 42 days. The start of senescence in sunflower plants was associated with a considerable decrease in protein content and specific leaf masses referred as weight (Table 1).

Leaf age (days)	Soluble protein (mg g^{-1} DW)	Specific leaf mass (mg DW cm^{-2})
16	152.3 ± 9.4	2.2 ± 0.11
22	178.5 ± 7.7	3.1 ± 0.28
28	108.1 ± 4.6	3.0 ± 0.27
36	89.6 ± 1.9	2.5 ± 0.23
42	62.2 ± 1.4	2.2 ± 0.29

Table 1. Changes in soluble protein and specific leaf mass during sunflower primary leaf ageing. Data are means ± SD for duplicate determinations in three separated experiments.

These changes may reflect alterations in N and C compound distributions as a consequence of N remobilization, the efficiency of which is related to the ratio between biomass in the sink and source organs (Wiedemuth et al., 2005; Diaz et al., 2008). Since chloroplasts contain the largest amounts of protein in leaves, their breakdown releases most of the nitrogen that is reused by other plant organs. The mechanisms behind chloroplast degradation in senescing leaves are poorly understood (especially those for the degradation of Rubisco and chlorophyll-binding light-harvesting proteins, which are the most abundant chloroplastic proteins) (Martínez et al., 2008). Chloroplasts contain a large number of proteases, some of which are encoded by senescence-associated genes, which are up-regulated during senescence. Degradation of some thylakoid proteins such as LHCII seemingly occurs exclusively within chloroplasts and requires the prior release and breakdown of pigments (Hörtensteiner & Feller, 2002; Buchanan-Wollaston et al., 2003a). CND41 protease is believed to be involved in Rubisco degradation and in the translocation of nitrogen during senescence in tobacco leaves (Kato et al., 2004, 2005). However, the central vacuole and SAVs also play a role here, as they help complete the degradation of Rubisco and other stromal proteins (Martínez et al., 2008). The relative rates of degradation of some photosynthetic components may be altered by the environmental conditions. Thus, LHCII degradation in rice is delayed by low irradiances (Hidema et al., 1991). Also, the protein content in senescing sunflower leaves was found to drop earlier in nitrogen-deficient plants than in high-nitrogen plants (Agüera et al., 2010). Changes in photosynthetic pigment contents also indicate progress of leaf senescence (Yoo et al., 2003; Guo & Gan, 2005; Ougham et al., 2008). The chlorophyll breakdown pathways operating during leaf senescence are well-known and require pigment degradation and avoiding photodamage in order to maintain the ability to export released nutrients to other plant parts (Hörtensteiner,

2006; Ougham et al., 2008). Chlorophylls in sunflower plants are more susceptible to degradation than are carotenoids during leaf senescence, and both total chlorophyll and carotenoid contents are high in young and mature leaves, their levels peaking at 22 days and decreasing afterwards during senescence (Fig. 1). Carotenoid degradation is usually slower than chlorophyll breakdown and can be especially complex depending on the particular pigment species (Suzuki & Shioi, 2004).

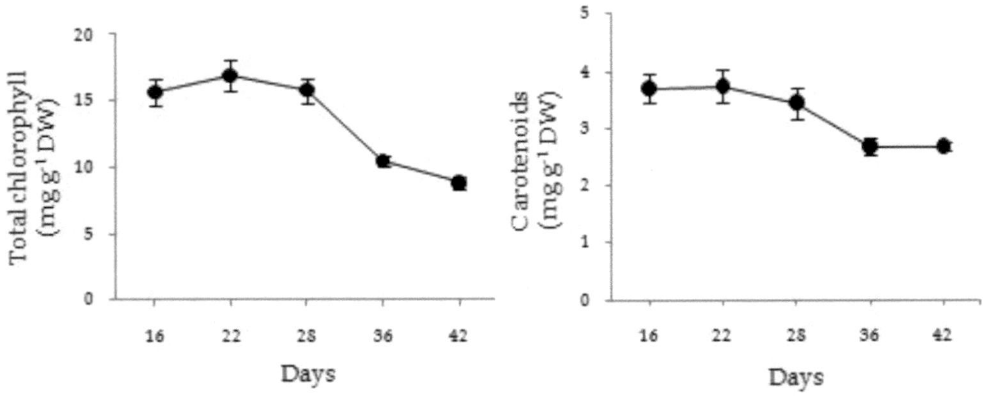

Fig. 1. Changes in pigment levels during ageing of sunflower primary leaves. Data are means ± SD for duplicate determinations in three separated experiments.

Chlorophyll loss in sunflower plants is also a typical phenomenon of leaf senescence of potential use as an indicator. The marked decrease in total chlorophyll observed after 28 days is mainly due to the loss of chlorophyll *a*, which is the form most strongly affected by leaf ageing as revealed by a significant decrease in Chl *a*/Chl *b* ratio in senescent leaves (Cabello et al., 2006). In radish cotyledons, however, the ratio of Chl *a* to Chl *b* increases slightly during senescence, which suggests that Chl *b* is degraded faster than is Chl *a* (Suzuki & Shioi, 2004).

Other typical changes observed during senescence are a rapid decline in photosynthetic activity, which may be a senescence-inducing signal (Bleecker & Patterson, 1997; Quirino et al., 2000), and a reduction in transpiration rate, which is probably due to an increase in abscisic acid levels inducing stomatal closure, although this is not a direct induction factor for senescence (Weaver & Amasino, 2001). A marked decrease in CO_2 fixation rate and transpiration in sunflower plants was observed during natural leaf senescence, a process that starts and develops in plants aged 28–42 days (Fig. 2).

Although natural senescence is the final stage of leaf development, it may start prematurely by effect of exposure to environmental stress or nutrient deprivation (Quirino et al., 2000; Lim et al., 2003, 2007, Wingler et al., 2009). In fact, poor nitrogen nutrition and exposure to high irradiance are known to lead to early senescence in sunflower leaves (Agüera et al., 2010). Thus, the decrease in chlorophyll content associated to leaf senescence starts earlier in sunflower plants grown with low nitrogen, which suggests that leaf senescence is accelerated under these conditions. In addition, the decline in photosynthetic activity is more apparent with nitrogen deficiency (Agüera et al., 2010). Similarly, the loss of photosynthetic activity is more marked in leaves of sunflower plants grown at high irradiance than in others grown at a low photon flux density, also indicating that an increased irradiance may accelerate leaf senescence.

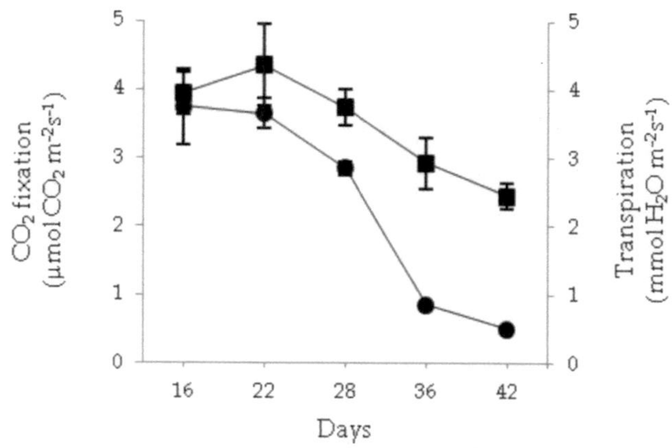

Fig. 2. Carbon dioxide fixation rates and transpiration in sunflower primary leaves of different age. Data are means ± SD of measured values on primary leaves of ten plants randomly selected for each age.

3. Carbon and nitrogen metabolites as regulators of leaf senescence in sunflower plants

The contents in soluble sugars of sunflower plants increase with leaf ageing, and the opposite holds for the starch content. Our results show that accumulation of soluble sugars in plants grown at high irradiance is not much greater than in plants grown at low irradiance, although a substantial increase in the monosaccharide-to-sucrose ratio is observed at the start of senescence (especially at high irradiance levels) (Fig. 3). The accumulation of soluble sugars is associated to leaf age but unrelated to photosynthetic activity because CO_2 fixation rates decrease during ageing; rather, it is due to starch hydrolysis. The increase in soluble sugars may also be ascribed to senescence causing a loss of functional and structural integrity in cell membranes, thereby boosting membrane lipid catabolism and hence sugar production by gluconeogenesis (Buchanan-Wollaston et al., 2003b; Lim et al., 2007). Leaf senescence is a plastic process triggered by a variety of external and internal factors (Weaver & Amasino, 2001; Buchanan-Wollaston et al., 2003a; Balibrea-Lara et al., 2004; Wingler et al., 2006). Senescence reduces photosynthetic carbon fixation, but is important for the recycling of nitrogen and other nutrients (Díaz et al., 2005; Wingler et al., 2005). By virtue of its lying at the crossroads of carbon and nitrogen metabolism, senescence is regulated by carbon and nitrogen signals. Increasing evidence suggests a role for hexose accumulation in ageing leaves as a signal for either senescence initiation or acceleration in annual plants (Masclaux et al., 2000; Moore et al., 2003; Díaz et al., 2005; Masclaux-Daubresse et al., 2005; Parrott et al., 2005; Pourtau et al., 2006; Wingler & Roitsch, 2008; Agüera et al., 2010). Recently, the role of sugar accumulation or starvation in leaf senescence was critically evaluated by van Doorn (2008), who pointed out that little is known about sugar concentrations and senescence regulation in different tissues and cells.

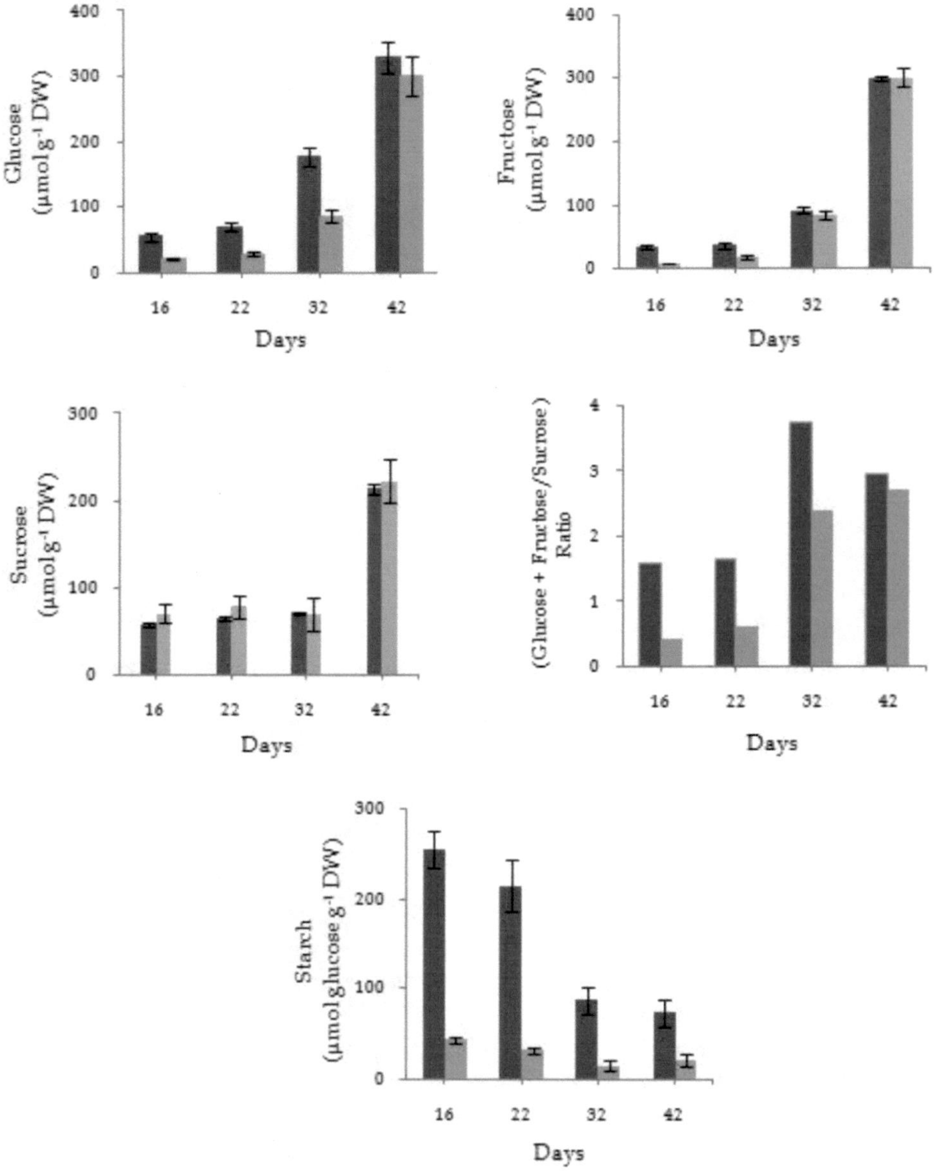

Fig. 3. Changes in glucose, fructose, sucrose and starch contents, and in hexoses-to-sucrose ratio, during development of sunflower primary leaves. Plants were grown at 125 µmol photons m^{-2} s^{-1} (grey bars) or 350 µmol photons m^{-2} s^{-1} (black bars). Data are means ± SD for duplicate determinations in three separate experiments.

Although sugars may not always be the direct cause of leaf senescence, there is enough evidence suggesting that sugar signalling plays a role in senescence regulation in a complex network involving a variety of other signals (Masclaux-Daubresse et al., 2007; Wingler & Roitsch, 2008; Wingler et al., 2009). Thus, cytokinin oxidase/dehydrogenase activity and senescence are positively correlated. The enzyme probably boosts senescence by destroying cytokinins and light is known to increase cytokinin oxidase/dehydrogenase activity during senescence of barley leaf segments (Schlüter et al., 2011).

Some results also suggest that leaf senescence is regulated by the carbon–nitrogen balance (Masclaux et al., 2000). However, in spite of the drastic changes in leaf metabolism occurring during senescence, carbon and nitrogen metabolite contents have scarcely been determined (Diaz et al., 2005). Cabello et al. (2006) found sunflower leaf senescence to be associated with significant changes in the contents of carbon and nitrogen metabolites. The highest ammonium concentrations were found in young and senescent leaves, as reported in tobacco (Masclaux et al., 2000). Our results indicate that sunflower plants exhibit their peak ammonium contents in young and late senescing leaves (Table 2). The high ammonium contents of young leaves are probably a result of strong photosynthetic nitrate reduction activity and photorespiration. In addition, young leaves have low contents in soluble carbohydrates, and sugar availability is known to be a limiting factor for ammonium assimilation (Morcuende et al., 1998). The high ammonium contents of senescent leaves are mainly due to protein degradation, amino acid deamination and nucleic acid catabolism, but also to photorespiration.

Senescent leaves contain low levels of free amino acids, probably because their remobilization is essential with a view to supplying developing organs in the plant (Buchanan-Wollaston, 1997). The concentrations of glutamate (a precursor of other amino acids) and aspartate (a direct product of glutamate transamination) decrease in the final stages of senescence in *Arabidopsis*. Glutamine and asparagine, the major amino acids translocated in the phloem sap, are mobilized more efficiently during late senescence (Diaz et al., 2005). As suggested by a genome array study (Lin & Wu, 2004), the synthesis of asparagine for nitrogen remobilization during dark-induced leaf senescence in *Arabidopsis* seems to occur via a novel biochemical pathway. Cabello et al. (2006) found glutamate to be the most abundant free amino acid in sunflower leaves as previously also found in rice (Kamachi et al., 1991), tobacco (Masclaux et al., 2000; Tercé-Laforgue et al., 2004) and *Arabidopsis* (Diaz et al., 2005). The ratio (Glu + Asp)/(Gln + Asn) peaked in sunflower leaves of 22 days, but decreased gradually in leaves of 28, 36 and 42 days (Table 2), which suggests that N-rich amino acids (specially Asn, which has a lower C to N ratio) are produced for efficient export from leaves in late senescence, as proposed for *Arabidopsis* (Diaz et al., 2005).

Leaf age (days)	Ammonium (μmol g^{-1} DW)	(Glu + Asp/Gln + Asn) Ratio
16	11.40 ± 1.0	2.11
22	8.57 ± 0.9	2.29
28	7.29 ± 0.7	1.77
36	8.94 ± 0.5	1.51
42	10.91 ± 0.7	1.44

Table 2. Changes in ammonium content and glutamate + aspartate /glutamine + asparagine ratio during sunflower primary leaf ageing. Data are means ± SD for duplicate determinations in three separated experiments

We examined changes in glutamine synthetase (GS) expression and activity during leaf development (Cabello et al., 2006). GS, which is the key enzyme in ammonia assimilation, is present as chloroplastic (GS2) and cytosolic (GS1) isoforms in sunflower leaves (Cabello et al., 1991). In order to confirm whether these isoforms are differently affected by senescence in sunflower leaves, we determined their specific activity during plant development. As shown in Figure 4, total GS activity decreased with the leaf age. The decrease was consequence of a strong decline in chloroplastic GS2 activity. On the other hand, cytosolic GS1 activity increased with ageing. It should be noted that GS1 was the predominant isoform in senescent leaves of 42 days, but accounted for only 7 % of total GS activity in young leaves (16 days). As a result, the GS2/GS1 ratio decreased from 13.3 in young leaves (16 days) to 0.9 in senescent leaves (42 days) (Fig. 4). These results indicate that leaf senescence has an adverse effect on the activity of chloroplastic GS2 (the main glutamine synthetase isoform) and reduces total GS activity despite its boosting GS1 activity.

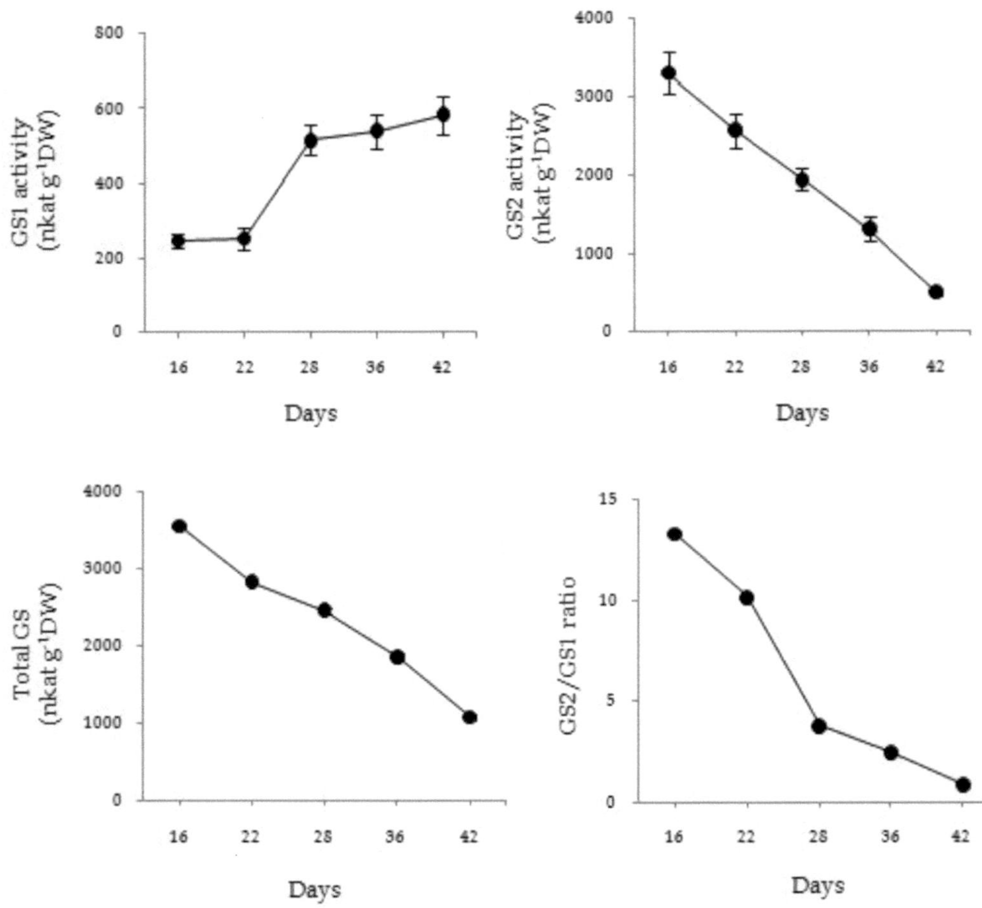

Fig. 4. Effect of ageing on total GS activity and on the activities of GS1 and GS2 isoforms in sunflower leaves. Data are means ± SD of duplicate determinations from three separated experiments.

Ageing affects glutamine synthetase activity but plays a direct role in the regulation of GS gene expression (Cabello et al., 2006). A Northern blot test using a probe corresponding to an internal fragment from *Helianthus annuus* GS2 cDNA revealed that the levels of GS2 transcripts decreased during leaf development and were very low in the late stage of senescence (42 days) (Fig. 5). Glutamine synthetase activity has been found to decrease during natural leaf senescence in a wide variety of plants including cereals, tomato and tobacco (Streit & Feller, 1983; Kamachi et al., 1991; Pérez-Rodríguez & Valpuesta, 1996; Masclaux et al., 2000). This loss of activity is mainly due to a gradual decrease in the major plastidial GS2 isoform since the cytosolic GS1 isoform remains constant or increases during leaf ageing (Pérez-Rodríguez & Valpuesta, 1996; Masclaux et al., 2000).

Northern blots and immunological analyses indicate that both GS transcripts and polypeptides are affected (Pérez-Rodríguez & Valpuesta 1996). GS1 plays a major role in the synthesis of glutamine for transport and remobilization of leaf organic nitrogen (Tercé-Laforgue et al., 2004), whereas GS2 takes part in the reassimilation of ammonium from photorespiration in photosynthetic tissues (Kamachi et al., 1992). The stimulation of the cytosolic GS1 isoform during senescence can be ascribed to the need for toxic ammonium to be reassimilated in order to produce glutamine for export to sink organs; this has led some authors to assume a shift in ammonia assimilation from the chloroplast to the cytosol of leaf cells during senescence (Brugière et al., 2000). Total GS activity was found to drop by a effect of a strong decrease in GS2 activity was found during sunflower leaf ageing despite the simultaneous increase in GS1 activity. GS2 transcript levels also diminished during ageing. Our results (Figs. 4 and 5) are therefore consistent with others previously reported for tomato and tobacco.

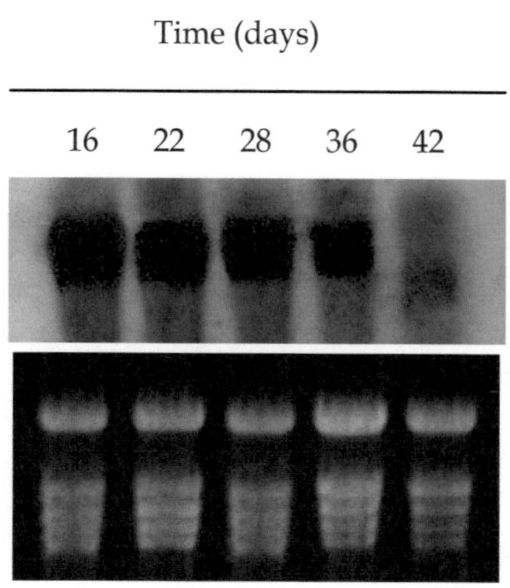

Fig. 5. Effect of ageing on GS2 mRNA accumulation in sunflower leaves.

Amino acids and other metabolites related to N metabolism deficit may act as signals to induce senescence in combination with hexose accumulation. Thus, leaf senescence in sunflower plants is induced by high sugar levels and accelerated by a low nitrogen supply, which supports the view that high sugar/low nitrogen conditions trigger senescence and facilitate its development (Wingler et al., 2009). Our results suggest that leaf senescence in sunflower plants is accelerated by nitrogen deficiency and high irradiance, and also that some factors such the levels of soluble sugars and amino acids may interact in a complex network to promote this process.

4. Oxidative stress in sunflower plants

Leaf senescence is an oxidative process that involves degradation of cellular and subcellular structures and macromolecules, and mobilization of the degradation products to other parts of the plants (Vanacker et al., 2006). Oxidative stress during senescence may be caused or increased by a loss of antioxidant enzymatic activities (Zimmermann & Zentgraf, 2005; Zimmermann et al., 2006; Procházkova & Wilhelmova, 2007). Senescence is also accompanied by an increase in ROS, one of the origins of which is an imbalance between the production and consumption of electrons in the photosynthetic electron transport chain caused by preferential inhibition of stromal reactions in contrast with photosystem II photochemistry (Špundová et al., 2003). The inhibition of stromal reactions increases the electron flow to molecular oxygen and causes ROS to accumulate and chloroplast components to be damaged as a result (Špundová et al., 2005; Couée et al., 2006). Chloroplasts are the main source of ROS in plants (Zimmermann & Zentgraf, 2005) and also the major target of oxidative damage (Munné-Bosch & Alegre, 2002). Stromal protein degradation during leaf senescence may be initiated by oxidative processes associated with the generation of free radicals and reactive species (Procházkova et al., 2001). Like Rubisco and other chloroplastic proteins, GS2 is susceptible to degradation initiated by reactive oxygen species (Ishida et al., 2002). The chloroplastic GS2 isoform is one of the first targets of oxidative damage at high irradiation levels (Palatnik et al., 1999). Oxidized GS becomes more susceptible to proteolysis (Ortega et al., 1999); under photo-oxidative stress, GS2 cleavage occurs preferentially around the catalytic site (Ishida et al., 2002). Senescence may therefore have a direct impact on GS2 activity through enzyme degradation initiated by reactive oxygen species as reported in Rubisco (Ishida et al., 1997; Roulin & Feller, 1998). Our results indicate that the decrease in GS2/GS1 ratio during sunflower leaf ageing may be partly due to a different sensitivity to oxidative stress of the two isoforms; in fact, chloroplastic GS2 is much more sensitive to oxidative modification *in vitro* than is cytosolic GS1 (Cabello et al., 2006). Therefore, ageing induces oxidative stress in sunflower leaves and can thus have an adverse effect on chloroplastic GS2, as well as on photosynthetic pigments. Antioxidant enzyme activities in sunflower leaves were found to decline during late senescence (42 days). Similar results have been reported for tobacco (Dhindsa et al., 1981), *Arabidopsis* (Ye et al., 2000), pea (Olsson, 1995) and maize (Procházkova et al., 2001). Oxidative stress during late senescence may be caused or increased by the loss of antioxidant enzymatic activities (Zimmermann & Zentgraf, 2005). Also, the decline in antioxidant activities is believed to be a consequence rather than the origin of senescence (Dertinger et al., 2003).

Susceptibility to oxidative stress depends on the overall balance between production of oxidants and cell antioxidant capability. In sunflower plants, considerable oxidative stress has been observed *in vivo* during leaf senescence, as revealed by lipid peroxidation, H_2O_2 accumulation and a decrease in the levels of antioxidant enzymes such as catalase, ascorbate peroxidase and superoxide dismutase (Table 3). Lipid peroxidation only occurs during the late stage of senescence (Berger et al., 2001; Jongebloed et al., 2004; Wingler et al., 2005). High irradiance causes reversible photoinhibition of photosynthesis in pea chloroplasts and increases ROS potentially regulating the accumulation of mRNA encoding antioxidant enzymes (Hernández et al., 2006).

Age (days)	H_2O_2 (μmol g^{-1} DW)	Catalase	Ascorbate peroxidase (U g^{-1} DW)	Superoxide dismutase	Lipid peroxidation (nmol MDA g^{-1} DW)
16	1.22 ± 0.15	1.12 ± 0.10	17.21 ± 1.22	336.4 ± 28	87.6 ± 8.2
22	1.38 ± 0.14	1.70 ± 0.12	17.99 ± 2.12	356.2 ± 39	85.6 ± 7.4
28	3.84 ± 0.42	2.25 ± 0.26	28.22 ± 3.22	538.5 ± 42	155.5 ± 12.3
36	4.76 ± 0.30	1.94 ± 0.17	21.34 ± 2.19	1450.5 ± 112	171.5 ±14.5
42	5.28 ± 0.51	1.24 ± 0.15	14.53 ± 1.17	985.2 ± 92	188.4 ± 12.8

Table 3. Hydrogen peroxide accumulation, catalase, ascorbate peroxidase and superoxide dismutase activities, and lipid peroxidation levels during sunflower primary leaf development. Data are means ± SD for duplicate determinations in three separated experiments.

The activity and expression of antioxidant enzymes are seemingly sensitive to high irradiance stress (Yoshimura et al., 2000; Hernández et al., 2004).

We found H_2O_2 accumulation in senescent sunflower to be slightly more marked in plants grown under a nitrogen deficiency; the differences, however, were not large enough to assume that H_2O_2 is a major factor regulating the induction of leaf senescence in N-deficient plants (Table 3). Interestingly, catalase and ascorbate peroxidase activity decreased steadily in plants grown with low nitrogen, but increased during early leaf development and then declined during senescence in plants grown with high nitrogen (Agüera et al., 2010). Production of ROS during leaf senescence is essentially governed by chloroplasts, which have a strong photooxidative potential (Zapata et al., 2005). A simultaneous increase in lipid peroxidation was observed. Mutations in the *Arabidopsis CPR5/OLD1* gene may cause early senescence through deregulation of the cellular redox balance (Jing et al., 2008). Also, there is evidence suggesting that inadequate oxidant and carbonyl group production are intrinsically related to plant ageing, and that low mitochondrial, superoxide dismutase and ascorbate peroxidase activities may contribute to extensive protein carbonylation (Vanacker et al., 2006; Srivalli & Khanna-Chopra, 2009).

In conclusion, during sunflower leaf development some coordinated metabolic and physiological changes are produced, and the senescence process induces significant alterations in the levels of carbon and nitrogen metabolites. Glutamine synthetase of sunflower leaves is regulated both at transcriptional and enzyme levels during leaf ontogeny. Post-translational regulation of the GS2 isoform could be due, at least partially, to oxidative processes. GS activity may be used as a biochemical marker of leaf ageing, since the beginning of senescence at about 28 days is accompanied by a drastic drop in the GS2/GS1 ratio due to the increase of the cytosolic GS1 activity and the decline of the chloroplastic GS2 activity. Our results suggest that both high irradiance and nitrogen deficiency accelerates senescence of the primary leaf, probably for maintaining the functionality of the young leaves, and that one of the reasons for this accelerated senescence may be the high cellular oxidation and oxidative damage caused by the earlier decline of the activity of the antioxidant enzymes in these plants (Pompelli et al., 2010).

5. Acknowledgment

This work was supported by Junta de Andalucía (grant P07-CVI-02627 and PAI group BIO-0159) and DGICYT (AGL2009-11290).

6. References

Agüera, E., Cabello, P., & de la Haba, P. (2010). Induction of leaf senescence by low nitrogen nutrition in sunflower (*Helianthus annuus* L.) plants. *Physiologia Plantarum,* Vol.138, pp. 256-267, ISSN 0031-9317

Balibrea-Lara, M.E., González-García, M.C., Fatima, T., Ehneß, R., Lee, T.K., Proels, R., Tanner, W., & Roitsch, T. (2004). Extracellular invertase is an essential component of cytokinin-mediated delay of senescence. *Plant Cell,* Vol.16, pp. 1276-1287, ISSN 1040-4651

Berger, S., Weichert, H., Porzel, A., Wasternack, C., Kühn, H., & Feussner, I. (2001). Enzymatic and non-enzymatic lipid peroxidation in leaf development. *Biochimica et Biophysica Acta,* Vol.1533, pp. 266-276, ISSN 0304-4165

Bleecker, A.P., & Patterson, S.E. (1997). Last exit: Senescence, abscission, and meristem arrest in *Arabidopsis. Plant Cell,* Vol.9, pp. 1169-1179, ISSN 1040-4651

Buchanan-Wollaston, V. (1997). The molecular biology of leaf senescence. *Journal of Experimental Botany,* Vol.48, pp. 181-199, ISSN 0022-0957

Buchanan-Wollaston, V., Earl, S., Harrison, E., Mathas, E., Navabpour, S., Page, T., & Pink, D. (2003a). The molecular analysis of leaf senescence- a genomics approach. *Plant Biotechnology Journal,* Vol.1, pp. 3-22, ISSN 1467-7644

Buchanan-Wollaston, V., Wellesbourne, H.R.I., & Warwick, U.K. (2003b). Senescence, leaves, In: *Encyclopedia of Applied Plant Sciences,* Elsevier Academic Press, 808-816

Brugière, N., Dubois, F., Masclaux, C., Sangwan, R.S., & Hirel, B. (2000) Immunolocalization of glutamine synthetase in senescing tobacco (*Nicotiana tabacum* L.) leaves suggests that ammonia assimilation is progressively shifted to the mesophyll cytosol. *Planta,* Vol. 211, pp. 519-527, ISSN 0032-0935

Cabello, P., de la Haba, P., & Maldonado, J.M. (1991). Isoforms of glutamine synthetase in cotyledons, leaves and roots of sunflower plants. *Journal of Plant Physiology,* Vol.137, pp. 378-380, ISSN 0176-1617

Cabello, P., Agüera, E., & de la Haba, P. (2006). Metabolic changes during natural ageing in sunflower (*Helianthus annuus*) leaves: expression and activity of glutamine synthetase isoforms are regulated differently during senescence. *Physiologia Plantarum,* Vol.128, pp. 175-185, ISSN 0031-9317

Couée, I., Sulmon, C., Gouesbet, G., & El-Amrani, A. (2006). Involvement of soluble sugars in reactive oxygen species balance and responses to oxidative stress in plants. *Journal of Experimental Botany,* Vol.3, pp. 449-459, ISSN 0022-0957

Dertinger, U., Schaz, U., & Schulze, E.D. (2003). Age-dependence of the antioxidative system in tobacco with enhanced glutathione reductase activity or senescence-induced production of cytokinins. *Physiologia Plantarum,* Vol.119, pp. 19-29, ISSN 0031-9317

Dhindsa, R.A., Plumb-Dhindsa, P., & Thorpe, T.A. (1981). Leaf senescence: correlated with increased permeability and lipid peroxidation, and decreased levels of superoxide dismutase and catalase. *Journal of Experimental Botany*, Vol.126, pp. 93-101, ISSN 0022-0957

Diaz, C., Purdy, S., Christ, A., Morot-Gaudry, J.F., Wingler, A., & Masclaux-Daubresse, C. (2005). Characterization of markers to determine the extent and variability of leaf senescence in Arabidopsis. A metabolic profiling approach. *Plant Physiology*, Vol.138, pp. 898-908, ISSN 0032-0889

Diaz, C., Lemaître, T., Christ, A., Azzopardi, M., Kato, Y., Sato, F., Morot-Gaudry, J.F., Le Dily, F., & Masclaux-Daubresse, C. (2008). Nitrogen recycling and remobilization are differentially controlled by leaf senescence and development stage in *Arabidopsis* under low nitrogen nutrition. *Plant Physiology*, Vol.147, pp. 1437-1449, ISSN 0032-0889

Gan, S., & Amasino, R.M. (1997). Making sense of senescence. *Plant Physiology*, Vol.113, pp. 313-319, ISSN 0032-0889

Gepstein, S. (1988). Photosynthesis, In: *Senescence and Aging in Plants*, L.D. Noodén & A.C. Leopold, (Eds.), 85-109, Academic Press Publishers, San Diego, USA

Guiboileau, A., Sormani, R., Meyer, C., & Masclaux-Daubresse, C. (2010). Senescence and death of plant organs: nutrient recycling and developmental regulation. *Comptes Rendus Biologies*, Vol.333, pp. 382-391 ISSN 1631-0691

Guo, I., & Gan, S. (2005). Leaf senescence: signals, execution, and regulation. *Current Topics in Developmental Biology*, Vol.71, pp. 83-112, ISSN 0070-2153

Hernández, J.A., Escobar, C., Creissen, G., & Mullineaux, P.M. (2004). Role of hydrogen peroxide and the redox state of ascorbate in the induction of antioxidant enzymes in pea leaves under excess light stress. *Functional Plant Biology*, Vol.31, pp. 359-368, ISSN 1445-4408

Hernández, J.A., Escobar, C., Creissen, G., & Mullineaux, P.M. (2006). Antioxidant enzyme in pea plants under high irradiance. *Biologia Plantarum*, Vol.50, pp. 395-399, ISSN 0006-3134

Hidema, J., Makino, A., Mae, T., & Ojima, T. (1991). Photosynthetic characteristics of rice leaves aged under different irradiances from full expansion through senescence. *Plant Physiology*, Vol.97, pp.1287-1293, ISSN 0032-0889

Himelblau, E., & Amasino, R.M. (2001). Nutrients mobilized from leaves of *Arabidopsis thaliana* during senescence. *Journal of Plant Physiology*, Vol.158, pp. 1317-1323, ISSN 0176-1617

Hörtensteiner, S. (2006). Chlorophyll degradation during senescence. *Annual Review of Plant Biology*, Vol.57, pp. 55-77, ISSN 1543-5008

Hörtensteiner, S., & Feller, U. (2002). Nitrogen metabolism and remobilization during senescence. *Journal of Experimental Botany*, Vol.53, pp. 927-937, ISSN 0022-0957

Ishida, H., Nishimori, Y., Sugisawa, M., Makino, A., & Mae, T. (1997). The large subunit of ribulose-1,5-bisphosphate carboxilase/oxygenase is fragmented into 37 kDa and 16 kDa polypeptides by active oxygen in the lysates of chloroplasts from primary leaves of wheat. *Plant and Cell Physiology*, Vol. 38, pp. 471-479, ISSN 0032-0781

Ishida, H., Anzawa, D., Kokubun, N., Makino, A., & Mae, T. (2002). Direct evidence for non-enzymatic fragmentation of chloroplastic glutamine synthetase by a reactive oxygen species. *Plant Cell and Environment*, Vol.25, pp. 625-631, ISSN 0140-7791

Jing, H.C., Hebeler, R., Oeljeklaus, S., Sitek, B., Stühler, K., Meyer, H.E., Sturre, M.J., Hille, J., Warscheid, B., & Dijkwell, P.P. (2008). Early leaf senescence is associated with an altered cellular redox balance in *Arabidopsis* cpr5/old1 mutants. *Plant Biology*, Vol.1, pp. 85-98, ISSN 1435-8603

Jongebloed, U., Szederkényi, J., Hartig, K., Schobert, C., & Komor, E. (2004). Sequence of morphological and physiological events during natural ageing and senescence of a castor bean leaf: sieve tube occlusion and carbohydrate back-up precede chlorophyll degradation. *Physiologia Plantarum*, Vol.120, pp. 338-346, ISSN 0031-9317

Kamachi, K., Yamaya, T., Mae, T., & Ojiva, K. (1991). A role for glutamine synthetase in the remobilization of leaf nitrogen during natural senescence in rice leaves. *Plant Physiology*, Vol.96, pp. 411-417, ISSN 0032-0889

Kamachi, K., Yamaya, T., Hayakawa, T., Mae, T., & Ojima, K. (1992). Changes in cytosolic glutamine synthetase polypeptide and its mRNA in a leaf blade of rice plants during natural senescence. *Plant Physiology*, Vol.98, pp. 1323-1329, ISSN 0032-0889

Kato, Y., Murakami, S., Yamamoto, Y., Chatani, H., Kondo, Y., Nakano, T., Yokota, A., & Sato, F. (2004). The DNA-binding protease, CND41, and the degradation of ribulose-1,5-bisphosphate carboxylase/oxygenase in senescent leaves of tobacco. *Planta*, Vol.220, pp. 97-104, ISSN 0032-0935

Kato, Y., Yamamoto, Y., Murakami, S., Sato, F. (2005). Post-translational regulation of CND41 protease activity in senescent tobacco leaves. *Planta*, Vol.222, pp. 643-651, ISSN 0032-0935

Kukavica, B., & Veljovic-Jovanovic, S. (2004). Senescence-related changes in the antioxidant status of ginkgo and birch leaves during autumn yellowing. *Physiologia Plantarum*, Vol.122, pp. 321-327, ISSN 0031-9317

Lim, P.O., Woo, H.R., & Nam, H.G. (2003). Molecular genetics of leaf senescence in *Arabidopsis. Trends in Plant Science*, Vol.8, pp. 272-278, ISSN 1360-1385

Lim, P.O., Kim, H.J., & Nam, H.G. (2007). Leaf senescence. Annual Review of Plant Biology, Vol.58, pp. 115-136, ISSN 1543-5008

Lin, J.F., & Wu, S.H. (2004). Molecular events in senescing *Arabidopsis* leaves. *Plant Journal*, Vol.39, pp. 612-628, ISSN 0960-7412

Martínez, D.E., Costa, M.L., & Guiamet, J.J. (2008). Senescence-associated degradation of chloroplast proteins inside and outside the organelle. *Plant Biology*, Vol.1, pp.15-22, ISSN 1435-8603

Masclaux, C., Valadier, M.H., Brugière, N., Morot-Gaudry, J.F., & Hirel, B. (2000). Characterization of the sink/source transition in tobacco (*Nicotiana tabacum* L.) shoots in relation to nitrogen management and leaf senescence. *Planta*, Vol.211, pp. 510-518, ISSN 0032-0935

Masclaux-Daubresse, C., Carrayol, E., & Valadier, M.H. (2005). The two nitrogen mobilization- and senescence-associated GS1 and GDH genes are controlled by C and N metabolites. *Planta*, Vol.221, pp. 580–588, ISSN 0032-0935

Masclaux-Daubresse, C., Purdy, S., Lemaître, T., Pourtau, N., Naconnat, L., Renou, J.P., & Wingler, A. (2007). Genetic variations suggest interaction between cold acclimation and metabolic regulation of leaf senescence. *Plant Physiology*, Vol.143, pp. 434-446, ISSN 0032-0889

Miller, A., Schlagnhaufer, C., Spalding, M., & Rodermel, S. (2000). Carbohydrate regulation of leaf development: prolongation of leaf senescence in Rubisco antisense mutants of tobacco. *Photosynthesis Research*, Vol.63, pp. 1-8, ISSN 0166-8595

Moore, B., Zhou, L., Rollanf, F., Hall, Q., Cheng, W.H., Líu, Y.X., Hwang, I., Jones, T., & Sheen, J. (2003). Role of the *Arabidopsis* glucose sensor HXK1 in nutrient, light and hormonal signalling. *Science*, Vol.300, pp. 332-336, ISSN 0036-8075

Morcuende, R., Krapp, A., Hurry, V., & Stitt, M. (1998). Sucrose-feeding leads to increased rates of nitrate assimilation, increased rates of α-oxoglutarate synthesis, and increased synthesis of a wide spectrum of amino acids in tobacco leaves. *Planta*, Vol.206, pp. 394-409, ISSN 0032-0935

Munné-Bosch, S., & Alegre, L. (2002). Plant aging increases oxidative stress in chloroplasts. *Planta*, Vol.214, pp. 608-615, ISSN 0032-0935

Nam, H.G. (1997). The molecular genetic analysis of leaf senescence. *Current Opinion in Biotechnology*, Vol.8, pp. 200-207, ISSN 0958-1669

Noodén, L.D., Guiamét, J.J., & John, I. (1997). Senescence mechanisms. *Physiologia Plantarum*, Vol.101, pp. 746-753, ISSN 0031-9317

Olsson, M. (1995). Alteration in lipid composition and antioxidative protection during senescence in drought stressed plants and non-drought stressed plants of *Pisum sativum*. *Plant Physiology and Biochemistry*, Vol.33, pp. 547-553, ISSN 0981-9428

Ortega, J.L., Roche, D., & Sengupta-Gopalan, C. (1999). Oxidative turnover of soybean root glutamine synthetase. In vitro and in vivo studies. *Plant Physiology*, Vol.119, pp. 1483-1495, ISSN 0032-0889

Otegui, M., Noh, Y.S., Martínez, D.E., Vila-Petroff, M., Staehelin, A., Amasino, R., & Guiamet, J.J. (2005). Senescence-associated vacuoles with intense proteolytic activity develop in senescing leaves of *Arabidopsis* and soybean. *Plant Journal*, Vol.41, pp. 831-844, ISSN 0960-7412

Ougham, H., Hörtensteiner, S., Armstead, I., Donnison, I., King, I., Thomas, H., & Mur, L. (2008). The control of chlorophyll catabolism and the status of yellowing as a biomarker of leaf senescence. *Plant Biology*, Vol.10, pp. 4-14, ISSN 1435-8603

Palatnik, J.F., Carrillo, N., & Valle, E.M. (1999). The role of photosynthetic electron transport in the oxidative degradation of chloroplastic glutamine synthetase. *Plant Physiology*, Vol.121, pp. 471-478, ISSN 0032-0889

Parrott, D., Yang, L., Shama, L., & Fischer, A.M. (2005). Senecence is accelerated, and several proteases are induced by carbon "feast" conditions in barley (*Hordeum vulgare* L.) leaves. *Planta*, Vol.222, pp. 989-1000, ISSN 0032-0935

Pérez-Rodríguez, J., & Valpuesta, V. (1996). Expression of glutamine synthetase genes during natural senescence of tomato leaves. *Physiologia Plantarum*, Vol.97, pp. 576-582, ISSN 0031-9317

Pompelli, M.F., Martins, S., Antunes, W.C., Chaves, A., & DaMatta, F.M. (2010). Photosynthesis and photoprotection in coffee leaves is affected by nitrogen and light availabilities in winter conditions. *Journal of Plant Physiology*, Vol.167, pp. 1052-1060, ISSN 0176-1617

Pourtau, N., Jennings, R., Pelzer, E., Pallas, J., & Wingler, A. (2006). Effect of sugar-induced senescence on gene expression and implications for the regulation of senescence in *Arabidopsis*. *Planta*, Vol.224, pp. 556-568, ISSN 0032-0935

Prochazkova, D., Sairam, R.K., Srivastava, G.C., & Singh, D.V. (2001). Oxidative stress and antioxidant activity as the basis of senescence in maize leaves. *Plant Science*, Vol.161, pp. 765-771, ISSN 0168-9452

Procházkova, D., & Wilhelmova, N. (2007). Leaf senescence and activities of the antioxidant enzymes. *Biologia Plantarum*, Vol.51, pp. 401-406, ISNN 0006-3134

Quirino, B.F., Noh, Y.S., Himelblau, E., & Amasino, R.M. (2000). Molecular aspects of leaf senescence. *Trends in Plant Science*, Vol.5, pp. 278-282, ISSN 1360-1385

Roulin, S., & Feller, U. (1998). Dithiothreitol triggers photo-oxidative stress and fragmentation of the large subunit of ribulose-1,5-bisphosphate carboxylase/oxygenase in intact pea chloroplasts. *Plant Physiology and Biochemistry*, Vol.36, pp. 849-856, ISSN 0981-9428

Schlüter, T., Leide, J., & Conrad, K. (2011). Light promotes an increase of cytokinin oxidase/dehydrogenase activity during senescence of barley leaf segments. *Journal of Plant Physiology*, Vol.168, pp. 694-698, ISSN 0176-1617

Špundová, M., Popelková, H., Ilík, P., Skotnica, J., Novotný, R., & Nauš, J. (2003). Ultra-structural and functional changes in the chloroplasts of detached barley leaves senescing under dark and light conditions. *Journal of Plant Physiology*, Vol.160, pp. 1051-1058, ISSN 0176-1617

Špundová, M., Sloukova, K., Hunková, M., & Nauš, J. (2005). Plant shading increases lipid peroxidation and intensifies senescence-induced changes in photosynthesis and activities of ascorbate peroxidase and glutathione reductase in wheat. *Photosynthetica*, Vol.43, pp. 403-409, ISSN 0300-3604

Srivalli, S., & Khanna-Chopra, R. (2009). Delayed wheat flat leaf senescence due to removal of spikelets is associated with increased activities of leaf antioxidant enzymes, reduced glutathione/oxidized glutathione ratio and oxidative damage to mitochondrial proteins. *Plant Physiology and Biochemistry*, Vol.47, pp. 663-670, ISSN 0981-9428

Streit, L., & Feller, U. (1983). Changing activities and different resistance to proteolytic activity of two forms of glutamine synthetase in wheat leaves during senescence. *Physiologie Végétale*, Vol.21, pp. 103-108, ISSN 0031-9368

Suzuki, Y., & Shioi, Y. (2004). Changes in chlorophyll and carotenoid contents in radish (*Raphanus sativus*) cotyledons show different time courses during senescence. *Physiologia Plantarum*, Vol.122, pp. 291-296, ISSN 0031-9317

Taiz, L., & Zeiger, E. (2010). *Plant Physiology* (5th edition). Sinauer Associates Inc., ISBN 978-0-87893-866-7, Sunderland, Massachusetts USA

Tercé-Laforgue, T., Mäck, G., & Hirel, B. (2004). New insights towards the function of glutamate dehydrogenase revealed during source-sink transition of tobacco (*Nicotiana tabacum*) plants grown under different nitrogen regimes. *Physiologia Plantarum*, Vol.120, pp. 220-228, ISSN 0031-9317

Van Doorn, V.G. (2008). Is the onset of senescence in leaf cells of intact plants due to low or high sugars level? *Journal of Experimental Botany*, Vol.59, pp. 1963-1972, ISSN 0022-0957

Van Lijsebettens, M., & Clarke, J. (1998). Leaf development in *Arabidopsis*. *Plant Physiology and Biochemistry*, Vol.36, pp. 47-60, ISSN 0981-9428

Vanacker, H., Sandalio, L.M., Jiménez, A., Palma, J.M., Corpas, F.J., Meseguer, V., Gómez, M., Sevilla, F., Leterrier, M., Foyer, C.H., & del Río, L.A. (2006). Roles for redox regulation in leaf senescence of pea plants grown on different sources of nitrogen nutrition. *Journal of Experimental Botany*, Vol.57, pp. 1735-1745, ISSN 0022-0957

Weaver, L.M., & Amasino, R.M. (2001). Senescence is induced in individually darkened *Arabidopsis* leaves, but inhibited in whole darkened plants. *Plant Physiology*, Vol.127, pp. 876-886, ISSN 0032-0889

Wiedemuth, K., Müller, J., Kahlau, A., Amme, S., Mock, H.-P., Grzam, A., Hell, R., Egle, K., Beschow, H., & Humbeck, K. (2005). Successive maduration and senescence of individual leaves during barley whole plant ontogeny reveals temporal and spatial regulation of photosynthetic function in conjunction with C and N metabolism. *Journal of Plant Physiology*, Vol.162, pp. 1226-1236, ISSN 0176-1617

Wingler, A., & Roitsch, T. (2008). Metabolic regulation of leaf senescence: interactions of sugar signalling with biotic and abiotic stress response. *Plant Biology*, Vol.10, pp. 50-62, ISSN 1435-8603

Wingler, A., Bownhill, E., & Pourtau, N. (2005). Mechanisms of light-dependent induction of cell death in tobacco plants with delayed senescence. *Journal of Experimental Botany*, Vol.56, pp. 2897-2905, ISSN 0022-0957

Wingler, A., Purdy, S., Maclean, J.A., & Pourtau, N. (2006). The role of sugars in integrating environmental signals during the regulation of leaf senescence. *Journal of Experimental Botany*, Vol.57, pp. 391-399, ISSN 0022-0957

Wingler, A., Maxclaux-Daubresse, C., & Fischer, A.M. (2009). Sugars, senescence, and ageing in plants and heterotrophic organisms. *Journal of Experimental Botany*, Vol.60, pp. 1063-1066, ISSN 0022-0957

Ye, Z., Rodríguez, R., Tran, A., Hoang, H., de los Santos, D., Brown, S., & Vellanoweth, R.L. (2000). The development transition to flowering repress ascorbate peroxidase activity and induces enzymatic lipid peroxidation in leaf tissue in *Arabidopsis thaliana*. *Plant Science*, Vol.158, pp. 115-127, ISSN 0168-9452

Yoo, S.D., Greer, D.H., Laing, W.A., & McManus, M.T. (2003). Changes in photosynthetic efficiency and carotenoid composition in leaves of white clover at different developmental stages. *Plant Physiology and Biochemistry*, Vol.4, pp. 887-893, ISSN 0981-9428

Yoshimura, K., Yabuta, Y., Ishikawa, T., & Shigeoka, S. (2000). Expression of spinach ascorbate peroxidase isoenzymes in response to oxidative stress. *Plant Physiology*, Vol.123, pp. 223-233, ISSN 0032-0889

Zapata, J.M., Guéra, A., Esteban-Carrasco, A., Martin, M., & Sabater, B. (2005). Chloroplasts regulate leaf senescence: delayed senescence in transgenic *ndh*F-defective tobacco. Cell Death and Differentiation, Vol.12, pp. 1277-1284, ISSN 1350-9047

Zimmermann, P., & Zentgraf, U. (2005). The correlation between oxidative stress and leaf senescence during plant development. *Cellular & Molecular Biology Letters*, Vol.10, pp. 515-534, ISSN 1425-8153

Zimmermann, P., Heinlein, C., Orendi, G., & Zentgraf, U. (2006). Senescence-specific regulation of catalases in *Arabidopsis thaliana* (L.) Heynh. *Plant Cell and Environment*, Vol.29, pp. 1049-1060, ISSN 0140-7791

4

Functional Approaches to Study Leaf Senescence in Sunflower

Paula Fernandez, Sebastián Moschen, Norma Paniego and Ruth A. Heinz
Biotechnology Institute - CICVyA- INTA Castelar
Argentina

1. Introduction

Senescence is an age-dependent process at the cellular, tissue, organ or organism level, leading to death at the end of the life span (Noodén 1988). Annual plants as grain and oil crops undergo a visual process towards the end of the reproductive stage that is accompanied by nutrient remobilization from leaf to developing seeds (Buchanan-Wollaston et al. 2003). The final stage of this process is leaf death but this is actively delayed until all nutrients have been removed and recycle through the process of developmental senescence. It have been documented that a delay in leaf senescence has an important impact on grain yield trough the maintenance of the photosynthetic leaf area during the reproductive stage in different crops (Ewing & Claverie 2000), including sunflower (Sadras et al. 2000; De la Vega et al. 2011). The potential yields of sunflower crop are far from the real ones in all Argentina productive regions. In Balcarce, for example, while the potential yields are estimated in 5,000 $kg.ha^{-1}$, those obtained by the best producers only reach 3,000 kg.ha-1, and the average in the region ranges in 1,800 $kg.ha^{-1}$ (Dosio & Aguirrezábal 2004). These differences could possibly be due to the inability of current hybrids to keep their green leaf area for long periods, which would allow greater use of the incident radiation during the grain filling period which plays an important role in determining the yield and oil concentration in sunflower (Dosio et al. 2000; Aguirrezábal et al. 2003).

Besides autonomous (internal) factors as age, reproductive stage and phytohormone levels, leaf senescence is hardly affected by environmental factors. Among these environmental factors, including extreme temperature, drought, shading, nutrient deficient and pathogen infection, the most limiting ones are water and nutrient availability (Gan & Amasino 1997; Sadras et al. 2000; Sadras et al. 2000; Dosio et al. 2003; Lim et al. 2003; Aguera et al. 2010).

During leaf senescence, critical and dramatic changes occurred in a highly regulated manner following a genetically programmed process of high complexity. Chlorophyll degradation, nutrient recycling and remobilization are preceded or paralleled by RNA and protein degradation. Even though leaf senescence has been widely recognized and accepted as a type of Programmed Cell Death (PCD) (Noodén & Leopold 1987), the onset and progression of senescence is accompanied by global changes in gene expression. Thus, deep extensive efforts have been achieved to reveal relevant molecular process by identifying and analysing

Senescence Associated Genes (SAGs) as prior tags to disclosure the core of this complex process (Kim et al. 2007). SAGs genes have been extensively studied in model plant species (Audic & Claverie 1997; Gepstein et al. 2003; Balazadeh et al. 2008; Hu et al. 2010) and in some agronomical relevant crops (Andersen et al. 2004; Conesa et al. 2005; Espinoza et al. 2007). Yet, although senescence and ageing might be considered synonyms, a distinct reference was previously discussed because the former comprises all those degenerative changes and cellular degradation occurring with little or non-reference to death, whereas the latter is considered the final developmental stage culminating in death (Nooden & Leopold 1988; Shahri 2011). In the last year, considering this limitation, many efforts are being achieved to disclosure and obtain genomic information for this oil crop (Kane et al. 2011) but complete sequence information are still no available.

Sunflower (*Helianthus annuus L.*) is one of the most relevant crops as source of edible oil and many efforts have been achieved to build up useful functional genomics tools for cultivated sunflower involving transcriptional and metabolic profiles (Fernandez et al. 2003; Cabello et al. 2006; Paniego et al. 2007; Fernandez et al. 2008; Peluffo et al. 2010). Although, molecular studies focused on the onset of the senescence process in sunflower leaf are scarce (Fernandez et al. 2003; Dezar et al. 2005; Manavella et al. 2006; Jobit et al. 2007; Paniego et al. 2007; Fernandez et al. 2008; Manavella et al. 2008; Peluffo et al. 2010; Fernandez et al. 2011). Thus, two different approaches are envisage for studying molecular events occurring during leaf senescence: the first strategy relays on the identification of sunflower SAGs based on a candidate gene approach while the second approach involves concerted gene expression studies based on high density oligonucleotide microarrays, whole transcriptome shotgun sequencing and microRNA detection by RNA-seq (Buermans et al. 2010; Dhahbi et al. 2011).

Leaf senescence is a complex and highly coordinated process (Noodén et al. 1997). Although symptoms have been explored, the involved processes and the mechanisms that control it have not been characterized yet (Buchanan-Wollaston et al. 2003). The distinctive symptom of leaf senescence is the breakdown of chloroplasts, therefore the decrease in chlorophyll content becomes a key indicator of the process (Hörtensteiner 2006). Both, the beginning and the rate of senescence may be affected by autonomous and environmental signals.

Environmental factors such as light (Weaver & Amasino 2001), nutrient availability, concentration of CO_2, abiotic and biotic stresses caused by disease (Sadras et al. 2000) may affect the rate of senescence. A previous work (Pic et al. 2002) showed that the sequence of certain events at macroscopic, biochemical and molecular level in pea leaf senescence were not modified in leaves of different age, or under conditions of moderate water stress. Since some of the environmental conditions that affect senescence have important effects on carbon metabolism, previous works assigned to sugar content in leaves an integrating role of environmental signals, regulating leaf senescence (Wingler et al. 2006). Reproductive growth is mentioned as a factor that usually impacts on leaf senescence, and particularly in sunflower, the lack of sinks delays the onset of senescence (Sadras et al. 2000). Control of senescence by growth of reproductive structures was not observed in *Arabidopsis thaliana* (Noodén & Penny 2001). Moreover, determining the onset of senescence is complex because there is no a "symptom" indicating this moment. Visual parameters are often used to assess these processes, but both the variation in chlorophyll content and yellowing or necrosis of leaves, are detectable long after the signalling cascade of senescence process is activated.

Senescence studies are generally based on the accumulation of messenger RNA coding for enzymes involved in degradation of structures, however, this process has a high degree of interaction between endogenous and environmental signals, involving different genes whose expression is induced or inhibited in different stages of the process (Gan & Amasino 1997). On the other hand, there are relevant studies that inversely correlate senescence with a high level of nitrogen in soil. According to these evidences a high nutritional nitrogen performance along soil profile should lead to a delay leaf senescence in sunflower, avoiding the pronounced symptoms occurred for chlorophyll content (Aguera et al. 2010).

2. Candidate gene approach to identify SAGs in sunflower

Senescence Associated Genes (SAGs) refer to genes whose expression level is up-regulated during senescence, in contrast with Senescence Down-regulated Genes (SDGs). These genes could be classified into two classes depending on their expression patterns: Class I genes are those whose expression is only activated during senescence (senescence-specific) whereas class II are those that maintain a basal level of expression during early leaf development, but this level increases when senescence begins (Gan & Amasino 1997). The expression patterns of these genes may change in response to different conditions of plant growth. Many of these genes can be shared by different regulatory pathways whereas others may belong to a particular pathway. Thus, the inactivation or overexpression of many SAGs may not exhibits significant effect, suggesting a complex regulatory network in leaf senescence process. SAGs can be grouped into several categories based on their predictive function, including macromolecular degradation and recycling, amino acid transport, metabolism, detoxification, regulatory genes, among others (Gepstein et al. 2003).

The main objective in sunflower to open new insights into the early leaf senescence process focuses in the identification and characterization of genetic sequences and metabolic pathways involved in the onset and evolution of the leaf senescence process. This aim involved the analysis of transcriptional and metabolic profiles in leaves from plants growing under different conditions that may alter the senescence rate, concomitant with studies of physiological and biochemical aspects. The specific items involved in this work include:

1. Study of the evolution of leaf area, chlorophyll and sugar content in leaf of different ages in a traditional sunflower hybrid subjected to treatments that alter the senescence under both field and greenhouse conditions.
2. Identification in public sunflower databases of gene sequences orthologous to Senescence Associated Genes (SAG) or Senescence Down-regulated Genes (SDG).
3. Identification of new candidate genes through a sunflower microarray expression analysis.
4. Verification and quantification of the expression profiles of these genes under conditions that accelerate or delay the senescence process.
5. Study of metabolic changes that occurred during the senescence process.
6. Integration of metabolic and transcriptional profile analysis and physiological variables for the detection of useful biomarkers for application in sunflower breeding.

Following a candidate genes strategy, a preliminary assay to detect putative SAGs in sunflower was achieved by selecting few candidates previously described for *Arabidopsis thaliana*, due to the fact that this was the very first model plant for which a large-scale SAG transcriptome was available (Gepstein et al. 2003). For this purpose six candidate SAGs were selected from this plant model (Moschen 2009) to search for orthologous genes in the sunflower EST database using the tblastx algorithm (Altschul et al. 1990), employing bioinformatics tools locally installed and developed. Sequences showing significant similarity parameters were selected and confirmed. Specific oligonucleotides were designed to amplify fragments of approximately 150 bp for further evaluation by quantitative PCR. In a previous study, we have reported the evaluation and identification of a panel of eight reference genes for their application to transcriptional analysis of the leaf senescence process, thus enabling the use of genuine reference genes in ongoing expression studies (Fernandez et al. 2011). Exploratory studies of senescence by qPCR comparing two treatments which affect the rate of leaf senescence were performed: water stress and head excision, relative to a control condition. Samples were taken from two leaves of different ages, leaf 15 and 25 in order to identify functional markers for this process. Two of the selected genes, a gamma vacuolar processing enzyme (AN At5g60360) (D3 gene) involved in the maturation and activation of vacuolar proteins and an aleurain protease AALP, (AN At1g18210) (D4 gene), belonging to the cystein-protease family are classified in the group of macromolecular degradation and recycling; the third gene, a calcium binding protein (AN At4g32940) (R2 gene) belongs to the group of regulatory genes (Gepstein et al. 2003). Furthermore two reference genes were evaluated against these conditions for relative expression studies, Elongation Factor 1-α (AN) and α-Tubuline, selected from a previous study of the performance of different reference genes against these experimental conditions in sunflower (Fernandez et al. 2011). Alfa tubuline (α-Tubuline) showed the most stable behavior; therefore, it was selected as internal control in further analysis of expression of these SAGs (Figure 1).

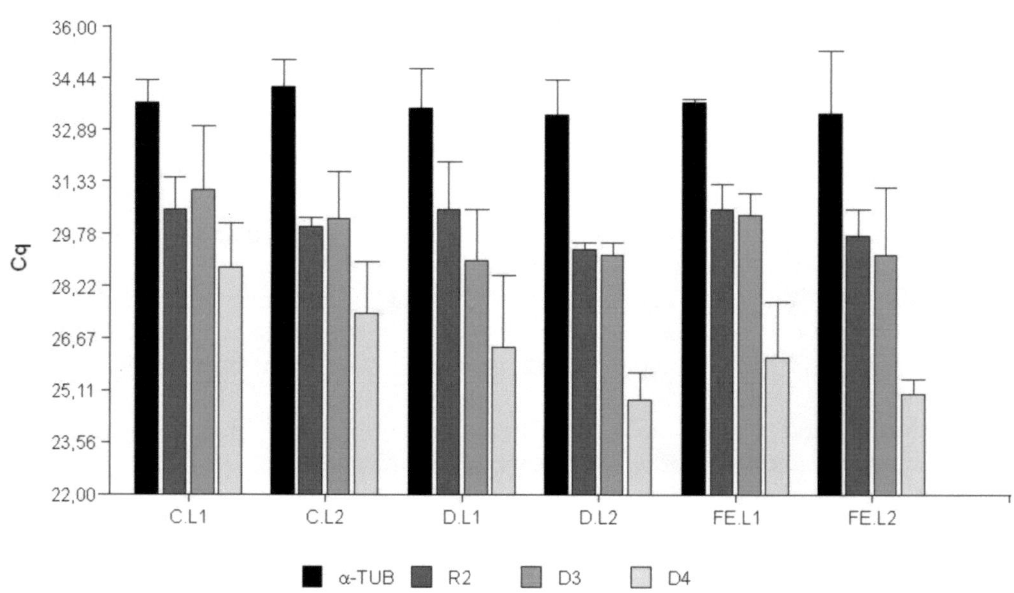

Fig. 1. Average Cq of analyzed SAGs genes normalizing against a-TUB as RG. Error bars show standard deviation (Fernandez et al. 2011).

The three selected genes did not show significant differences between the evaluated conditions at the sampling times tested (63 days post-emergence) (Table 1). It is worth noting that the target genes showed high expression levels even in controls plants with values close to the water stressed samples. Thus, these genes were probably induced by internal plant factors at an early time point, prior to the tested time in that assay. On the other hand, sampling for the incidence of head excision assessment on senescence could be consistent with an early stage of bud development in which there would be no evident differences between the two conditions (Zavaleta-Mancera et al. 1999a; Zavaleta-Mancera et al. 1999b; Thomas & Donnisson 2000).

		SAGs genes (Gepstein et al. 2003)						RGs genes (Fernandez et al. 2011)			
		R2 (AN At4g32940)		D3 (AN At5g60360)		D4 (AN At1g18210)		α-TUB (AN AF401481.1)		EF-1α (AN CAA37212.1)	
Treatment	Samples	Cq	CV	Cq	CV	Cq	CV	Cq	CV	Cq	CV
C.L1	3	30.49	2.5	31.06	5.0	28.74	3.9	33.69	1.7	30.08	2.6
C.L2	3	30.00	0.8	30.19	3.8	27.42	4.5	34.20	1.9	25.57	7.2
FE.L1	3	30.46	3.9	28.96	4.3	26.42	6.6	33.52	2.9	27.16	1.7
FE.L2	3	29.28	0.6	29.13	1.1	24.84	2.7	33.32	2.6	26.73	12.9
D.L1	3	30.45	2.1	30.31	1.7	26.10	5.1	33.67	0.2	27.80	6.7
D.L2	3	29.75	2.0	29.12	5.5	24.98	1.5	33.38	4.5	30.07	5.7

Table 1. Average Cq and CV value for R2, D3 and D4 genes and the two best ranked RGs for three biological replicates per treatment (Fernandez et al. 2011).

As a result from these analyses, the adjustment of the sampling time and frequency turns out as a highly critical point in studying gene expression profiling of candidate genes, according to the treatments on evaluation. Earlier samplings are necessary to detect the trigger moment of different candidate genes for leaf senescence process in sunflower. Considering Table 1, it is worth mentioning that relative quantification of a putative SAG would be overestimated if EF-1α (AN CAA37212.1) would have been used as a single reference gene, which reinforces the importance of normalizing against two or more experimentally validated RG when quantifying transcripts (Fernandez et al. 2011). In order to reach a wider search of new candidate genes, an additional set of new published genes were considered and their predicted functionality was evaluated with the aim to give new insights into this process. For a preliminary detection of potential SAGs, classical macromolecular degradation SAGs were discarded of our analysis because they are probably not associated with early leaf senescence, but with induced changes later in the time course of the process. In this sense, Chlorophyll-Binding Proteins (CBP) were first isolated in soybean (Guiamet et al. 1991) whereas SAGs N4 and SAG12 were detected by differential screen of *Arabidopsis* leaf senescence cDNA libraries (Gan & Amasino 1995; Park et al. 1998). They encode an apparent cysteine proteinase and their expression is highly senescence specific (Lohman et al. 1994; Gan & Amasino 1995; Martinez et al. 2007) mainly localized in small senescence associated vacuoles (Saeed et al. 2003; Otegui et al. 2005). However, neither SAG12 nor SEN4 match any full sequence in sunflower with a high identity score level. For this reason, a second set of candidate SAGs (OsNAC5, WRKY6, ORS1 YUCCA6, among others) (Ülker & Somssich 2004; Balazadeh et al. 2011; Kim et al. 2011; Song et al. 2011) was compared against *Helianthus annuus* unigene collection but a low score level to *Helianthus annuus* sequences was detected. Therefore, other candidate genes were added to be functionally tested for early leaf senescence in sunflower. The special case of transcription factors (TFs) as crucial regulators of gene expression by binding to distinct cis-elements, generally located in the 5' upstream regulatory regions of target genes, were specially considered to detect early senescence leaf makers (Balazadeh et al. 2008). NAC transcription factors related to senescence have been recently identified in model species and they play a relevant role in the regulation of development of leaf senescence related to programmed cell death (Olsen et al. 2005; Kim et al. 2009; Balazadeh et al. 2010; Hu et al. 2010; Nuruzzaman et al. 2010; Balazadeh et al. 2011). A single one NAC gene (AtNAP), also called NAC2 or ANAC029 (Guo & Gan 2006), has been the main one identified to control leaf senescence, although approximately 20 NAC genes in *Arabidopsis* shown high expression in senescing leaves (Guo et al. 2004; Lin & Wu 2004). ROS reagents acting as senescence stimulus were also reported within a narrow cross talk involving hormones and TFs both in natural and stress-related senescence (Rivero et al. 2007; Khanna-Chopra 2011), indicating that elevated ROS levels might be detected as a potential signal of senescence induction. Under this assumption *ORE1*, a NAC transcription factor that has been extensively studied in recent years, has been described as strongly related to leaf senescence, probably coevolving genes with ORS1 (Ooka et al. 2003). This TF can be considered a new further positive regulator of senescence in conjunction with AtNAP (Balazadeh et al. 2011), controlling leaf senescence in *Brassicaceae*. In *Arabidopsis*, *ORE1* mutants show a delay in leaf senescence whereas overexpression through an inductive promoter, accelerates senescence in relation to wild type plants (Balazadeh et al. 2010) and the forest tree *Populus trichocarpa* in which approximately 2,900 TFs were reported (Hu et al. 2010) and will be soon tested for sunflower candidate SAG detection. Microarray studies showed that 46% of up regulated genes in *Arabidopsis ORE1* overexpression lines, are known as senescence-associated genes, including many genes previously reported as senescence regulated, suggesting an important role in the development of the senescence process (Balazadeh et al. 2010). In wheat, it was reported that NAC TFs not only accelerate senescence but also improve nutrient remobilization by increasing protein, iron and zinc content (Uauy et al. 2006). ORE1 expression is under control of the ethylene signaling pathway and is subjected to regulation by miRNA164, being negatively regulated. When the leaf is young, miR164 transcripts remain at high levels regulating the expression of ORE1 but during the leaf aging process, its expression gradually decreases, thus increasing the expression of ORE1 (Kim et al. 2009).

In sunflower, a sequence similar ORE1 has been detected in the *Helianthus annuus* unigene collection developed at INTA (ATGC Sunflower Database: http://bioinformatica.inta.gov.ar/ATGC) with a Blast score of 96 and E-value of e-10 (Altschul et al. 1990). Expression profiles studies at different sunflower developmental stages showed a significant increase of putative ORE1 transcripts in samples close to anthesis stage, prior to the start of the first symptoms of senescence, when the critical period of grain filling has already begun (Figure 2). These results are consistent with those observed in *Arabidopsis*, and turn this gene a potential functional marker of the progress of senescence, representing an important tool for future implications in the sunflower crop improvement (Moschen et al. 2010). In order to confirm *in-situ* the functionality of this putative ORE1 gene in sunflower, a comparative bioinformatics analysis has been performed using the Blastx algorithm (Altschul et al. 1990), searching for proteins in the database at the National Center for Biotechnology Information NCBI (http://www.ncbi.nlm.nih.gov/), using as query the nucleotide sequence of putative sunflower ORE1. These results showed a high similarity with ORE *Arabidopsis* protein (GI 15241819) suggesting a possible role of this gene as NAC transcription factor. Moreover, searches for functional protein domains in Pfam (http://pfam.sanger.ac.uk/) revealed that main protein domain in sunflower ORE1-like gene sequence corresponds to the family of NAM transcription factors (No Apical Meristem) (pfam02365), as well as the *Arabidopsis ORE1 sequence* pfam02365. Figure 3 shows *Arabidopsis* alignments and putative sunflower ORE1 proteins against Pfam NAC domain. Others relevant *in-silico* candidates for a putative sunflower SAG are: RAV1 gene, a transcription factor whose expression is closely associated with leaf maturation and senescence (Woo et al. 2010), which has been detected with a high score level and statistically low E-value, and CAT2, a member of a small gene H_2O_2 detoxifying enzyme family, widely characterized in *Arabidopsis* (Gergoff et al. 2010; Smykowski et al. 2010), although not yet tested in sunflower.

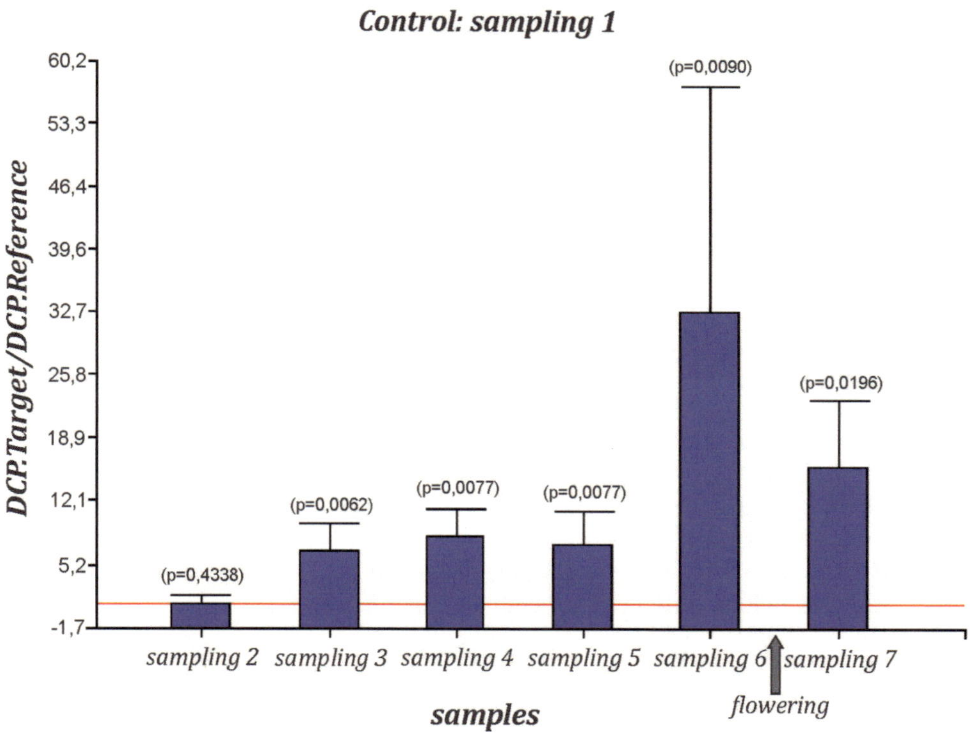

Fig. 2. Differential expression of putative sunflower *ORE1* gene in subsequent samplings, taking as control condition sampling number 1 and referred to α-TUB expression level (Moschen et al. 2010).

```
                           10        20        30        40        50        60        70        80
                   ....*....|....*....|....*....|....*....|....*....|....*....|....*....|....*....|
gi 15241819     20 LPPGFRFHPTDEELITHYLKPKVF-NTFFSATAIGEVDLNKIEPWDLPW-KAKMGEKEWYFFCVRDRKYPTGLRTNRATE 97
Cdd:pfam02365    1 LPPGFRFHPTDEELVVYYLKRKVLgKPLPLLEVIPEVDIYKFEPWDLPDgKAKGGDREWYFFSPRDRKYPNGSRTNRATG 80
Sunflower ORE1   1 MPPGFRFHPTDEELITHYLSNKVV-DNNFVAKAIAEVDMNKIEPWELPK-LAKLGGKEWYFFCVNDKKYPTGLRTNRATA 78

                           90       100       110       120       130
                   ....*....|....*....|....*....|....*....|....*....|
gi 15241819     98 AGYWKATGKDKEIF-KGKSLVGMKKTLVFYKGRAPKGVKTNWVMHEYRLE 146
Cdd:pfam02365   81 SGYWKATGKDKPILsKGGEVVGMKKTLVFYKGRAPKGEKTDWVMHEYRLE 130
Sunflower ORE1  79 AGYWKATGKDKEIS-RGKLLVGMKXTLVFYMGRAPKGEKTNWVIHEYRLE 128
```

Fig. 3. *Arabidopsis* NAM domain and putative *sunflower* ORE1 protein alignment (pfam02365) (http://www.ncbi.nlm.nih.gov/cdd/).

As mentioned above, the execution of the senescence process consists of multiple interconnecting pathways which regulate and/or modulate this series of orderly steps; therefore different transcription factors play an important role as regulators of these pathways. Recently, a list of transcription factors that regulate leaf senescence in *Arabidopsis* has been published (Balazadeh et al. 2008). The search for tentative orthologous genes in the *Helianthus annuus* unigene collection, using Blast algorithm, led to the identification of 42 genes with a significant score value to transcription factors like NAC, MYB, WRKY, ARP among others, some of these genes are being studied their expression patterns by qPCR.

3. Concerted gene expression studies to elucidate sunflower senescence process

Although microarray technology started a new era of high-throughput transcriptomic analysis approximately ten years ago, starting with 8,000 printed genes by Affymetrix in *Arabidopsis thaliana* (Zhu & Wang 2000) and later on scaling up to 45,000 printed genes in rice (Jung et al. 2008) and 90,000 in *Brassica* (Trick et al. 2009), next generation sequencing (NGS) technologies are nowadays opening a new era of even deeper understanding of genomics and transcriptomics in different species . However, for the foreseeable future both technologies will coexist each focusing on different tasks, or by complementing biological and value information (Fenart et al. 2010) or by designing dedicated oligonucleotide arrays to support functional studies on a specified pathway/developmental stage (Kusnierczyk et al. 2008; Cosio & Dunand 2010; Ott et al. 2010). One obvious application of microarray technology is the transcriptional profiling in species that have neither their own genome sequenced nor a reference genome from a closely related species. For some of these species a commercial microarray based on an existing own-design are available (Agilent, Affimetrix, Nimblegen, etc) (Close et al. 2004; Li et al. 2008; Martinez-Godoy et al. 2008; Mascarrell-Creus et al. 2009; Trick et al. 2009; Booman et al. 2010; Curtiss et al. 2011). Sunflower is a species that fits into this framework, even though a genome sequence initiative is in progress (Kane et al. 2011), there is no reference genome available. In this case, the only source of functional information is limited to ESTs databases, which in the case of cultivated sunflower is rather extensive, more than 133,000 ESTs are publicly available (http://ncbi.nlm.nih.gov/dbEST/dbEST_summary.html) covering libraries prepared from several lines and cultivars (Table2). However, it should also be noted that ESTs libraries tend to be significantly contaminated with vector sequences and chimeras, and have relatively low quality DNA information derived from the library sequencing strategy which prioritizes obtaining a large number of single pass sequences, being necessary to standardize a set of bioinformatics routines in order to clean and decontaminate public raw sequences (Figure 4).

Microarrays using ESTs and full length gene sequences allowed SAGs identification during leaf senescence at the genome-wide scale in *Arabidopsis* and other plants (Lim et al. 2007). In parallel, other high-throughput system has been assayed in other species: cDNA macro and microarray were developed for sunflower to study sunflower seed development (Hewezi et al. 2006) and the response to biotic (Alignan et al. 2006), and abiotic stresses (Hewezi et al. 2006; Roche et al. 2007; Fernandez et al. 2008). This last work reported for the first time, a concerted study on gene expression in early responses to chilling and salinity using a fluorescence microarray assay based on organ-specific unigenes in sunflower. These two strategies, although useful, are limited to the analysis of a limited set of genes. Currently, the shortage of candidate genes underlying agronomically important traits represents one of the main drawbacks in sunflower molecular breeding. In this context, functional tools which allow concerted transcriptional studies, as high density oligonucleotide microarray, strongly support the discovery and characterization of novel genes. Oligonucleotide-based chips not only allow the analysis for a whole transcriptome but they are also considered more accurate than cDNA-based chips due to the reduction of manipulation steps (Larkin et al. 2005; Lai et al. 2006). The possibility to implement this technology on any custom array system like Agilent, Nimblegen, and others, has the potential to create a very useful tool for gene discovery in orphan crops (Nazar et al. 2010; Ophir et al. 2010). In addition, the use of longer probe format represents a major advantage of Agilent oligonucleotide microarrays over others technologies based on a higher stability in the presence of sequence mismatches, being consequently, more suitable for the analysis of highly polymorphic regions (Hardiman 2004).

In general, the analysis of complex biological processes based on a gene by gene approach seldom leads to limited or erroneous conclusions requiring an alternative approach based on systemic association studies. Under this assumption, new insights into molecular senescence events might be cleared up by high-resolution microarray data, for example, considering different points of leaf development (Breeze et al. 2011) or predicting putative SAGs by tissue and functional categories (Thomas et al. 2009). In our lab, a public and proprietary datasets of *H. annuus L.* ESTs have been used to create a comprehensive sunflower unigene collection. This dataset comprises 34 cDNAs libraries available from different cultivars, various tissues and anatomical parts, from plants grown at different physiological conditions.

Figure 4 describes the routines applied for the *H. annuus L* unigene collection design.

A Digital Gene Expression Profile (Audic & Claverie 1997) was assayed with the EST public data in order to detect any bias that would be pseudo-enriching the gene index by full representation of one library over another considering full public ESTs derived from public collections (Table 2). This analysis ("digi-Northern") detected that ESTs were equally represented among differential cDNA libraries, showing that the *H. annuus* unigene collection generated would be fully represented by different transcripts, lacking of a potential enrichment or overestimation among organ-specific ESTs libraries. This unigene collection was used to design the first custom sunflower oligonucleotide-based microarray based on Agilent technology as a main goal for functional genomics approaches, generated within the frame of a collaborative project involving Argentinean research sunflower groups (Sunflower PAE Consortium), Facultad de Agronomía (UBA) and the Bioinformatics facility at the Principe Felipe Institute, Valencia , España. A Chado-based database (Mungall et al.

2007) and a visualization tool call ATGC (Clavijo et al., unpublished) was developed to integrate and browse sunflower transcriptome information. Figure 5 shows the output of the ATGC interface for one functional annotated sunflower unigene.

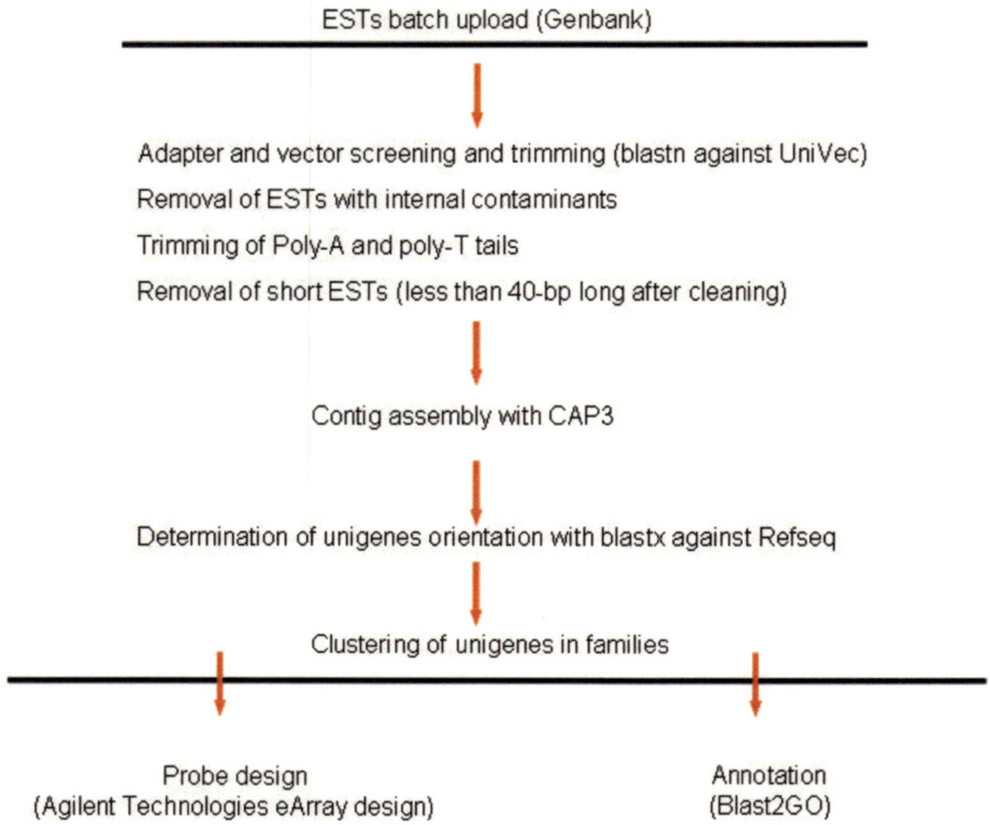

Fig. 4. Bioinformatics routines applied to design *Helianthus annuus* unigene collection (http://bionformatica.inta.gov.ar/ATGC/).

Sunflower gene expression chip probes were designed using eArray® web application (Agilent Technologies). For this instance, two probe sets were designed: one including non-control specific probes for the sequences of sunflower unigene collection and a second control probe set consisting in 74 probes derived from 80 differentially expressed sunflower genes identified in a previously work (Fernandez et al. 2008). The latest group was used as 'Replicate Controls' with 10 replicates each. To utilize the full capacity of the microarray, probes were randomly selected to be represented in duplicate in the final design, which also included Agilent Technologies' standard panel of quality control and spike-in probes. This design was then used to manufacture microarrays using Agilent SurePrint™ Technology in the 4 x 44 format. Agilent's microarrays include the Spike-In Kit that consists of a set of 10 positive control transcripts optimized to anneal to complementary probes on the microarray, minimizing self-hybridization or cross-hybridization. This work contemplates the microarray validation through diverse differential expression analysis in order to analyze early senescence in sunflower through a classical approach and a pipeline-based methodology. Differential gene expression was also carried out using the limma package (Smyth 2004). Multiple testing adjustments of p-values was done according to Benjamini and Hochberg methodology (Benjamini & Hochberg 1995). Gene set analysis was carried out according to the Gene Ontology terms using FatiScan (Al-Shahrour et al. 2007) integrated in Babelomics suite (Al-Shahrour et al. 2005).

Library ID	Developmental stage
HaSSH	Molecular characterization of phosphorus-responsive genes in sunflower
CCF (STU)	EST sequences from several different strains/cultivars
QH-RHA 280/QH_ABCDI sunflower RHA801	shoots/hulls/flowers environmental stress/chemical induction
CHA(XYZ) common wild sunflower	girasol silvestre (wild sunflower)
HaHeaS	heart-shaped embryo vs cotyledonary embryo
HaHeaR	heart-shaped embryo
HaCotR	cotyledonary embryo
HaGlbR	globular embryo
HaDevS1	4 days after self-pollination embryo
HaDevS2	7 days after self-pollination embryo
HaDevR1	leaves
HaDevR2	terminal bud
HaDevR3	stem
HaDevR6	embryo
HaDevR5	4 days after self-pollination embryo
HaDevR8	15 days after self-pollination embryo
HaDis	unknown/cotyledons/ (Genoplante)
HaSemS4	hypocotyl
HaDpsR1	hypocotyl
HaDplR2	hypocotyl 1-5 days
HaDplR	protoplast
HaERF	embryo
HaERS	embryo
HaR	INTA: organ-specific cDNA libraries (root)
HaT	INTA: organ-specific cDNA libraries (stem)
HaEF	INTA: organ-specific cDNA libraries (early flower)
HaF	INTA: organ-specific cDNA libraries (flower)
HaH	INTA: organ-specific cDNA libraries (leaf)

Table 2. Public cDNA libraries deposited in GenBank for which *H. annuus* unigene collection was designed.

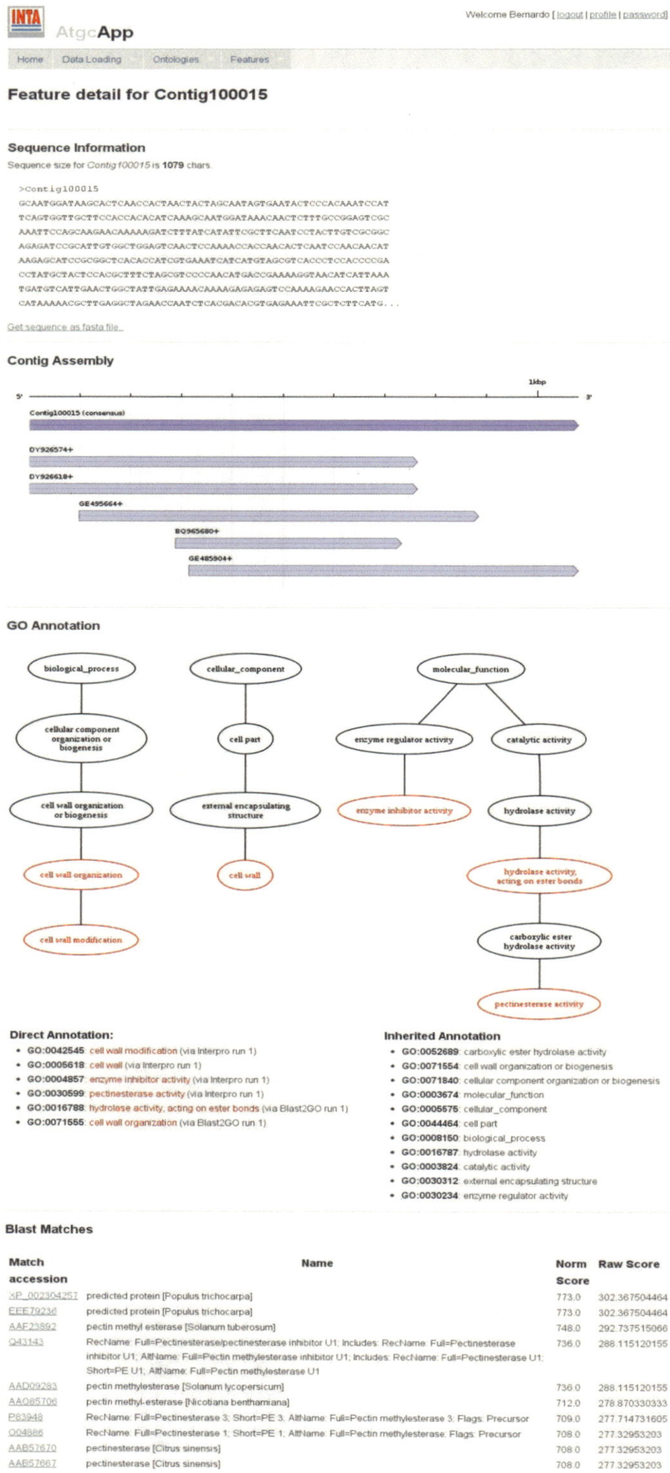

Fig. 5. ATGC view for an annotated sunflower unigene.

4. Conclusions and perspectives

Knowing the time of onset the the cascade of events that trigger senescence could determine the causes of this process and generate molecular tools to facilitate future interventions on it, useful for application in assisted breeding of this crop with major growing oil impact in the world.

The sunflower chip, designed within a PAE Consortium made up of six laboratories and one private company working in different areas of research and development, was validated by means of the analysis of global changes in gene expression profiles in response to water deficit as a physiological event which induces senescence, taken as a model experiment, for which reference genes have also been previously identified (Fernandez et al. 2011). This high-throughput transcriptome tool will allow the discovery, identification and analysis of a new set of putative SAGs for sunflower which would bring novel insights for this process. The integrated analysis of transcriptional and metabolic profiles will allow the identification of concerted regulation of distinct metabolic pathways facilitating the discovery of robust candidate genes and key metabolic pathways involved in the outbreak of the early senescence process in sunflower leaves. We expect that the integration of the information generated by this project will allow the construction of the quantitative predictive model of senescence in sunflower, under field and greenhouse conditions, which is required to interpret the regulation of the underlying complex biological processes. There will also be practical applications in directed gene discovery for other important agronomic traits involving plant responses to biotic and abiotic stresses. Finally, this project will have impact based in the establishment of microarray technologies and metabolic analysis, as well as on the knowledge of appropriated statistical and bioinformatics procedures supporting functional genomics ranging from the transcriptome to the metabolome.

5. Acknowledgment

This research was supported by CONICET PIP 5788, ANPCyT/FONCYT, Préstamo BID PICT 15-32905 and PICT 0960, INTA-PE AEBIO 241001and 245001, INTA-PE AEBIO 245732, INTA-AEBI0 243532, INTA PN CER 1336 and UNMdP, AGR212, AGR260. Lic. Sebastián Moschen holds a fellowship from ANPCyT to support his PhD studies whereas Dr. PdCF, Dr. RAH, Dr. NBP are career members of the Consejo Nacional de Investigaciones Científicas y Técnicas (CONICET, Argentina) and INTA researchers.

6. References

Aguera, E., P. Cabello and P. de la Haba (2010). "Induction of leaf senescence by low nitrogen nutrition in sunflower (*Helianthus annuus*) plants." *Physiol Plant* 138(3): 256-267.

Aguirrezábal, L. A. N. A., Y. Lavaud, G. A. A. Dosio, N. Izquierdo, F. Andrade and L. González (2003). "Intercepted solar radiation during seed filling determines sunflower weight per seed and oil concentration." *Crop Science* 43: 152-161.

Al-Shahrour, F., L. Arbiza, H. Dopazo, J. Huerta-Cepas, P. Minguez, D. Montaner and J. Dopazo (2007). "From genes to functional classes in the study of biological systems." *BMC Bioinformatics* 8(1): 114.

Al-Shahrour, F., P. Minguez, J. M. Vaquerizas, L. Conde and J. Dopazo (2005). "BABELOMICS: a suite of web tools for functional annotation and analysis of groups of genes in high-throughput experiments." *Nucleic Acids Res* 33(Web Server issue): W460-464.

Alignan, M., T. Hewezi, M. Petitprez, G. Dechamp-Guillaume and L. Gentzbittel (2006). "A cDNA microarray approach to decipher sunflower (*Helianthus annuus*) responses to the necrotrophic fungus *Phoma macdonaldii*." *New Phytol* 170(3): 523-536.

Altschul, S., W. Gish, W. Miller, E. Myers and D. Lipman (1990). "Basic local alignment search tool." *Journal of Molecular Biology* 215: 403-410.

Andersen, C., J. Jensen and T. Orntoft (2004). "Normalization of real-time quantitative reverse transcription–PCR data: a model-based variance estimation approach to identify genes suited for normalization, applied to bladder and colon cancer data sets." *Cancer Res* 64: 5245–5250.

Audic, S. and J. M. Claverie (1997). "The significance of digital gene expression profiles." *Genome Research* 7(10): 986-995.

Balazadeh, S., M. Kwasniewski, C. Caldana, M. Mehrnia, M. I. Zanor, G. P. Xue and B. Mueller-Roeber (2011). "ORS1, an HO-responsive NAC transcription factor, controls senescence in Arabidopsis thaliana." *Mol Plant* 4(2): 346-360.

Balazadeh, S., D. M. Riaño-Pachón and B. Mueller-Roeber (2008). "Transcription factors regulating leaf senescence in *Arabidopsis thaliana*." *Plant Biology* 10((Suppl. 1)): 63-75.

Balazadeh, S., H. Siddiqui, A. D. Allu, L. P. Matallana-Ramirez, C. Caldana, M. Mehrnia, M.-I. Zanor, B. Köhler and B. Mueller-Roeber (2010). "A gene regulatory network controlled by the NAC transcription factor ANAC092/AtNAC2/ORE1 during salt-promoted senescence." *The Plant Journal* doi: 10.1111/j.1365-313X.2010.04151.x.

Balazadeh, S., H. Siddiqui, A. D. Allu, L. P. Matallana-Ramirez, C. Caldana, M. Mehrnia, M. I. Zanor, B. Kohler and B. Mueller-Roeber (2010). "A gene regulatory network controlled by the NAC transcription factor ANAC092/AtNAC2/ORE1 during salt-promoted senescence." *Plant J* 62(2): 250-264.

Balazadeh, S., A. Wu and B. Mueller-Roeber (2010). "Salt-triggered expression of the ANAC092-dependent senescence regulon in Arabidopsis thaliana." *Plant Signal Behav* 5(6): 733-735.

Benjamini, Y. and Y. Hochberg (1995). "Controlling the False Discovery Rate: A Practical and Powerful Approach to Multiple Testing." *Journal of the Royal Statistical Society* 57(1): 289-300.

Booman, M., T. Borza, C. Y. Feng, T. S. Hori, B. Higgins, A. Culf, D. Leger, I. C. Chute, A. Belkaid, M. Rise, A. Kurt Gamperl, S. Hubert, J. Kimball, R. J. Ouelelette, S. C. Johnson, S. Bowman and M. L. Rise (2010). "Development and Experimental Validation of a 20K Atlantic Cod (*Gadus morhua*) Oligonucleotide Microarray Based on a Collection of over 150,000 ESTs." *Mar Biotechnol* DOI: 10.1007/s10126-010-9335-6.

Breeze, E., E. Harrison, S. McHattie, L. Hughes, R. Hickman, C. Hill, S. Kiddle, Y.-s. Kim, C. A. Penfold, D. Jenkins, C. Zhang, K. Morris, C. Jenner, S. Jackson, B. Thomas, A. Tabrett, R. Legaie, J. D. Moore, D. L. Wild, S. Ott, D. Rand, J. Beynon, K. Denby, A. Mead and V. Buchanan-Wollaston (2011). "High-Resolution Temporal Profiling of Transcripts during Arabidopsis Leaf Senescence Reveals a Distinct Chronology of Processes and Regulation." *The Plant Cell Online* 23(3): 873-894.

Buchanan-Wollaston, V., S. Earl, E. Harrison, E. Mathas, S. Navabpour, T. Page and D. Pink (2003). "The molecular analysis of leaf senescence -a genomic approach." *Plant Biotechnology Journal* 1: 3-22.

Buermans, H., Y. Ariyurek, G. van Ommen, J. den Dunnen and P. 't Hoen (2010). "New methods for next generation sequencing based microRNA expression profiling." *BMC Genomics* 11(1): 716.

Cabello, P., E. Agüera and P. De la Haba (2006). "Metabolic changes during natural ageing in sunflower (*Helianthus annuus*) leaves: expression and activity of glutamine synthetase isoforms are regulated differently during senescence." *Physiol Plant* 128: 175-185.

Close, T. J., S. I. Wanamaker, R. A. Caldo, S. M. Turner, D. A. Ashlock, J. A. Dickerson, R. A. Wing, G. J. Muehlbauer, A. Kleinhofs and R. P. Wise (2004). "A New Resource for Cereal Genomics: 22K Barley GeneChip Comes of Age." *Plant Physiology* 134: 960-968.

Conesa, A., S. Gotz, J. M. Garcia-Gomez, J. Terol, M. Talon and M. Robles (2005). "Blast2GO: a universal tool for annotation, visualization and analysis in functional genomics research." *Bioinformatics* 21(18): 3674-3676.

Cosio, C. and C. Dunand (2010). "Transcriptome analysis of various flower and silique development stages indicates a set of class III peroxidase genes potentially involved in pod shattering in Arabidopsis thaliana." *BMC Genomics* 11(1): 528.

Curtiss, J., L. Rodriguez-Uribe, J. M. Stewart and J. Zhang (2011). "Identification of differentially expressed genes associated with semigamy in Pima cotton (Gossypium barbadense L.) through comparative microarray analysis." *BMC Plant Biol* 11: 49.

De la Vega, A., M. A. Cantore, N. N. Sposaro, N. Trapani, M. Lopez Pereira and A. J. Hall (2011). "Canopty stay green and yield in non stressed sunflower." *Fields Crop Researchs* 121: 175-185.

Dezar, C. A., G. M. Gago, D. H. Gonzalez and R. L. Chan (2005). "Hahb-4, a sunflower homeobox-leucine zipper gene, is a developmental regulator and confers drought tolerance to *Arabidopsis thaliana* plants." *Transgenic Res* 14(4): 429-440.

Dhahbi, J. M., H. Atamna, D. Boffelli, W. Magis, S. R. Spindler and D. I. K. Martin (2011). "Deep Sequencing Reveals Novel MicroRNAs and Regulation of MicroRNA Expression during Cell Senescence." *PLoS ONE* 6(5): e20509.

Dosio, G. A., H. Rey, J. Lecoeur, N. G. Izquierdo, L. A. Aguirrezabal, F. Tardieu and O. Turc (2003). "A whole-plant analysis of the dynamics of expansion of individual leaves of two sunflower hybrids." *J Exp Bot* 54(392): 2541-2552.

Dosio, G. A. A. and L. A. N. Aguirrezábal (2004). Variaciones del rendimiento en girasol. Identificando las causas. *Revista Agromercado,* Cuadernillo de girasol. 90: 7-10.

Dosio, G. A. A., L. A. N. A. Aguirrezábal, F. H. Andrade and P. V. R. (2000). "Solar radiation intercepted during seed filling and oil production in two sunflower hybrids." *Crop Science* 40(1637-1644).

Espinoza, C., C. Medina, S. Somerville and P. Arce-Johnson (2007). "Senescence-associated genes induced during compatible viral interactions with grapevine and *Arabidopsis*." *Journal of Experimental Botany* 58(12): 3197-3212.

Ewing, R. M. and J. M. Claverie (2000). "EST databases as multi-conditional gene expression datasets." *Pac Symp Biocomput*: 430-442.

Fenart, S., Y.-P. Assoumou Ndong, J. Duarte, N. Rivière, J. Wilmer, O. van Wuytswinkel, A. Lucau, E. Cariou, G. Neutelings, L. Gutierrez, B. Chabbert, X. Guillot, R. Tavernier, S. Hawkins and B. Thomasset (2010). "Development and validation of a flax (*Linum usitatissimum L.*) gene expression oligo microarray." *BMC Genomics* 11(592).

Fernandez, P., J. Di Rienzo, L. Fernandez, H. Hopp, N. Paniego and H. R.A. (2008). "Transcriptomic identification of candidate genes involved in sunflower responses to chilling and salt stresses based on cDNA microarray analysis." *BMC Plant Biology* 8(11).

Fernandez, P., J. Di Rienzo, S. Moschen, D. GAA, L. Aguirrezabal, H. Hopp, N. Paniego and H. R.A. (2011). "Comparison of predictive methods and biological validation for qPCR reference genes in sunflower leaf senescence transcript analysis." *Plant Cell Report* 30(1): 63-74.

Fernandez, P., N. Paniego, S. Lew, H. E. Hopp and R. A. Heinz (2003). "Differential representation of sunflower ESTs in enriched organ-specific cDNA libraries in a small scale sequencing project." *BMC Genomics* 4(1): 40.

Gan, S. and R. M. Amasino (1995). "Inhibition of leaf senescence by autoregulated production of cytokinin." *Science* 270(5244): 1986-1988.

Gan, S. and R. M. Amasino (1997). "Making sense of senescence." *Plant Physiology* 113: 313-319.

Gepstein, S., G. Sabehi, M.-J. Carp, T. Hajouj, M. F. O. Nesher, I. Yariv, C. Dor and M. Bassani (2003). "Large-scale identification of leaf senescence-associated genes." *The Plant Journal* 36: 629-642.

Gergoff, G., A. Chaves and C. G. Bartoli (2010). "Ethylene regulates ascorbic acid content during dark-induced leaf senescence." *Plant Science* 178: 207-212.

Guiamet, J. J., E. Schwartz, E. Pichersky and L. D. Nooden (1991). "Characterization of Cytoplasmic and Nuclear Mutations Affecting Chlorophyll and Chlorophyll-Binding Proteins during Senescence in Soybean." *Plant Physiol* 96(1): 227-231.

Guo, Y., Z. Cai and S. Gan (2004). "Transcriptome of Arabidopsis leaf senescence." *Plant, Cell and Environment* 27: 521-549.

Guo, Y. and S. Gan (2006). "AtNAP, a NAC family transcription factor, has an important role in leaf senescence." *The Plant Journal* 46(4): 601-612.

Hardiman, G. (2004). "Microarray platforms--comparisons and contrasts." *Pharmacogenomics* 5(5): 487-502.

Hewezi, T., M. Leger, W. El Kayal and L. Gentzbittel (2006). "Transcriptional profiling of sunflower plants growing under low temperatures reveals an extensive down-regulation of gene expression associated with chilling sensitivity." *J Exp Bot* 57(12): 3109-3122.

Hewezi, T., M. Petitprez and L. Gentzbittel (2006). "Primary metabolic pathways and signal transduction in sunflower (*Helianthus annuus L.*): comparison of transcriptional profiling in leaves and immature embryos using cDNA microarrays." *Planta* 223(5): 948-964.

Hörtensteiner, S. (2006). "Chlorophyll degradation during senescence." *The Annual Review of Plant Biology* 57: 55-77.

Hu, R., G. Qi, Y. Kong, D. Kong, Q. Gao and G. Zhou (2010). "Comprehensive Analysis of NAC Domain Transcription Factor Gene Family in *Populus trichocarpa*." *BMC Plant Biology* 10(145).

Jobit, C., A. Boisson, E. Gout, C. Rascle, M. Feyre, P. Cotton and R. Bligny (2007). "Metabolic processes and carbon nutrient exchanges between host and pathogen sustain the disease development during sunflower infection by *Sclerotinia sclerotiorum*." *Planta* 226: 251-265.

Jung, K. H., C. Dardick, L. E. Bartley, P. Cao, J. Phetsom, P. Canlas, Y. S. Seo, M. Shultz, S. Ouyang, Q. Yuan, B. C. Frank, E. Ly, L. Zheng, Y. Jia, A. P. Hsia, K. An, H. H. Chou, D. Rocke, G. C. Lee, P. S. Schnable, G. An, C. R. Buell and P. C. Ronald (2008). "Refinement of light-responsive transcript lists using rice oligonucleotide arrays: evaluation of gene-redundancy." *PLoS ONE* 3(10): e3337.

Kane, N. C., N. Gill, M. J. King, J. E. Bowers, H. Berges, J. Gouzy, E. Bachlava, N. B. Langlade, Z. Lai, M. Stewart, J. M. Burke, P. Vincourt, S. J. Knapp and L. H. Rieserberg (2011). "Progress towards a reference genome for sunflower." *Botany* 89: 429-437.

Khanna-Chopra, R. (2011). "Leaf senescence and abiotic stresses share reactive oxygen species-mediated chloroplast degradation." *Protoplasma.*

Kim, J. H., P. O. Lim and H. G. Nam (2007). Molecular regulation of leaf senescence. "*Senescence Process in Plants*". S. Gan. Ithaca, Blackwell Publishing.

Kim, J. H., H. R. Woo, J. Kim, P. Ok Lim, I. C. Lee, S. H. Choi, D. E. Hwang and H. Gil Nam (2009). "Trifurcate Feed-Forward Regulation of Age-Dependent Cell Death Involving miR164 in Arabidopsis." *Science* 323(5917): 1053-1057.

Kim, J. I., A. S. Murphy, D. Baek, S. W. Lee, D. J. Yun, R. A. Bressan and M. L. Narasimhan (2011). "YUCCA6 over-expression demonstrates auxin function in delaying leaf senescence in Arabidopsis thaliana." *J Exp Bot* 62(11): 3981-3992.

Kusnierczyk, A., P. Winge, T. S. Jorstad, J. Troczynska, J. T. Rossiter and A. M. Bones (2008). "Towards global understanding of plant defence against aphids--timing and dynamics of early Arabidopsis defence responses to cabbage aphid (Brevicoryne brassicae) attack." *Plant Cell Environ* 31(8): 1097-1115.

Lai, Z., B. L. Gross, Y. Zou, J. Andrews and L. H. Rieseberg (2006). "Microarray analysis reveals differential gene expression in hybrid sunflower species." *Mol Ecol* 15(5): 1213-1227.

Larkin, J. E., B. C. Franc, H. Gavras, R. Sultana and J. Quackenbush (2005). "Independence and reproducibility across microarray platforms." *Nat. Methods* 2(5): 337-344.

Li, X., H.-I. Chiang, J. Zhu, S. E. Dowd and H. Zhou (2008). "Characterization of a newly developed chicken 44K Agilent microarray." *BMC Genomics* 9:60.

Lim, P., H. Kim and H. Nam (2007). "Leaf Senescence." *Annual Rev. Plant Biol.* 58: 115-136.

Lim, P. O., H. R. Woo and H. G. Nam (2003). "Molecular genetics of leaf senescence in *Arabidopsis*." *Trends in Plant Science* 8: 272-278.

Lin, J.-F. and S.-H. Wu (2004). "Molecular events in senescing Arabidopsis leaves." *The Plant Journal* 39(4): 612-628.

Lohman, K. N., S. Gan, M. C. John and R. M. Amasino (1994). "Molecular analysis of natural leaf senescence in Arabidopsis thaliana." *Physiol Plant* 92(2): 322-328.

Manavella, P. A., A. L. Arce, C. A. Dezar, F. Bitton, J. P. Renou, M. Crespi and R. L. Chan (2006). "Cross-talk between ethylene and drought signalling pathways is mediated by the sunflower Hahb-4 transcription factor." *Plant J* 48(1): 125-137.

Manavella, P. A., C. A. Dezar, G. Bonaventure, I. T. Baldwin and R. L. Chan (2008). "HAHB4, a sunflower HD-Zip protein, integrates signals from the jasmonic acid and ethylene pathways during wounding and biotic stress responses." *The Plant Journal* 56(3): 376-388.

Martinez-Godoy, M. A., N. Mauri, J. Juarez, M. Carmen Marques, J. Santiago, J. Forment and J. Gadea (2008). "A genome-wide 20K citrus microarray for gene expression analysis." *BMC Genomics* 9(318).

Martinez, D. E., C. G. Bartoli, V. Grbic and J. J. Guiamet (2007). "Vacuolar cysteine proteases of wheat (*Triticum aestivum L.*) are common to leaf senescence induced by different factors." *J Exp Bot* 58(5): 1099-1107.

Mascarrell-Creus, A., J. Cañizares, J. Vilarrasa-Blasi, S. Mora-Garcia, J. Blanca, D. Gonzalez-Ibeas, M. Saladié, C. Roig, W. Deleu, B. Picó-Silvent, N. López-Bigas, M. A. Aranda, J. Garcia-Mas, F. Nuez, P. Puigdomènech and A. Caño-Delgado (2009). "An oligo-based microarray offers novel transcriptomic approaches for the analysis of pathogen resistance and fruit quality traits in melon (*Cucumis melo L.*)." *BMC Genomics* 10(467).

Moschen, S. (2009). "Identificación y caracterización de genes asociados a la senescencia tempana en girasol". Tesis de Grado. Lic. en Genética.

Moschen, S., P. Fernandez, N. Paniego and R. A. Heinz (2010). ""Análisis de los perfiles de expresión de factores de transcripción NAC asociados a la senescencia foliar en girasol (*Helianthus annuus L.*)"." *Reunión Argentina de Fisiología Vegetal.*

Mungall, C. J., D. B. Emmert and T. F. Consortium (2007). "A Chado case study: an ontology-based modular schema for representing genome-associated biological information." *Bioinformatics* 23(13): i337-i346.

"National Center for Biotechnology Information (NCBI)." *http://www.ncbi.nlm.nih.gov/.*

Nazar, N. R., P. Chen, D. Dean and J. Robb (2010). "DNA Chip Analysis in Diverse Organisms with Unsequenced Genomes." *Mol. Biotechnol* 44: 8-13.

Noodén, L. and J. Penny (2001). "Correlative controls of senescence and plant death in *Arabidopsis thaliana* (Brassicaceae)." *J. Exp. Bot.* 52: 2151-2159.

Noodén, L. D. (1988). The phenomena of senescence and aging. . *Senescence and Aging in Plants.* A. C. L. L.D. Noodén. San Diego, Academic: 1-50.

Noodén, L. D., J. J. Guiamet and J. Isaac (1997). "Senescence mechanisms." *Physiologia plantarum* 101: 746-753.

Noodén, L. D. and A. C. Leopold (1987). "Phytohormones and the endogenous regulation of senescence and abscission". *"Phytohormones and related compounds: A comprehensive treatise"*. Amsterdam, Elsevier: 329-370.

Nooden, L. D. and Z. C. Leopold (1988). "The phenomena of senescence and aging. In "Senescence and aging in plants"." *Academic Press.* San Diego CA, USA: 1-50.

Nuruzzaman, M., R. Manimekalai, A. M. Sharoni, K. Satoh, H. Kondoh, H. Ooka and S. Kikuchi (2010). "Genome-wide analysis of NAC transcription factor family in rice." *Gene* 465(1-2): 30-44.

Olsen, A. N., H. A. Ernst, L. L. Leggio and K. Skriver (2005). "NAC transcription factors: structurally distinct, functionally diverse." *Trends Plant Sci* 10(2): 79-87.

Ooka, H., K. Satoh, K. Doi, T. Nagata, Y. Otomo, K. Murakami, K. Matsubara, N. Osato, J. Kawai, P. Carninci, Y. Hayashizaki, K. Suzuki, K. Kojima, Y. Takahara, K. Yamamoto and S. Kikuchi (2003). "Comprehensive analysis of NAC family genes in Oryza sativa and Arabidopsis thaliana." *DNA Res* 10(6): 239-247.

Ophir, R., R. Eshed, R. Harel-Beja, G. Tzuri, V. Portnoy, Y. Burger, S. Uliel, N. Katzir and A. Sherman (2010). "High-throughput marker discovery in melon using a self-designed oligo microarray." *BMC Genomics* 11: 269.

Otegui, M. S., Y. S. Noh, D. E. Martinez, M. G. Vila Petroff, L. A. Staehelin, R. M. Amasino and J. J. Guiamet (2005). "Senescence-associated vacuoles with intense proteolytic activity develop in leaves of Arabidopsis and soybean." *Plant J* 41(6): 831-844.

Ott, H., C. Schroder, M. Raulf-Heimsoth, V. Mahler, C. Ocklenburg, H. F. Merk and J. M. Baron (2010). "Microarrays of recombinant Hevea brasiliensis proteins: a novel tool for the component-resolved diagnosis of natural rubber latex allergy." *J Investig Allergol Clin Immunol* 20(2): 129-138.

Paniego, N., R. Heinz, P. Fernandez, P. Talia, V. Nishinakamasu and H. Hopp (2007). Sunflower. *Genome Mapping and Molecular Breeding in Plants.* C. Kole. Berlin Heidelberg, Springer-Verlag. 2: 153-177.

Park, J. H., S. A. Oh, Y. H. Kim, H. R. Woo and H. G. Nam (1998). "Differential expression of senescence-associated mRNAs during leaf senescence induced by different senescence-inducing factors in Arabidopsis." *Plant Mol Biol* 37(3): 445-454.

Peluffo, L., V. Lia, C. Troglia, C. Maringolo, N. Paniego, R. A. Heinz and F. Carrari (2010). "Metabolic profiles of sunflower genotypes with contrasting response to *Sclerotinia sclerotiorum* infection." *Phytochemistry.*

Pic, E., B. Teyssandier de la Serve, F. Tardieu and O. Turc (2002). "Leaf senescence induced by mild water deficit follows the same sequence of macroscopic, biochemical, and molecular events as monocarpic senescence in pea." *Plant Physiology* 128: 236-246.

Rivero, R. M., M. Kojima, A. Gepstein, H. Sakakibara, R. Mittler, S. Gepstein and E. Blumwald (2007). "Delayed leaf senescence induces extreme drought tolerance in a flowering plant." *Proc Natl Acad Sci U S A* 104(49): 19631-19636.

Roche, J., T. Hewezi, A. Bouniols and L. Gentzbittel (2007). "Transcriptional profiles of primary metabolism and signal transduction-related genes in response to water stress in field-grown sunflower genotypes using a thematic cDNA microarray." *Planta* DOI 10.1007/s00425-007-0508-0.

Sadras, V. O., L. Echarte and A. F. H. (2000). "Profiles of Leaf Senescence During Reproductive Growth of Sunflower and Maize." *Annals of Botany* 85(2): 187-195.

Sadras, V. O., M. Ferreiro, F. Gutheim and A. G. Kantolic (2000). Desarrollo fenológico y su respuesta a temperatura y fotoperíodo. *Bases para el manejo del maíz, el girasol y la soja.* I. B. F. d. C. A. UNMP: 29-60.

Sadras, V. O., F. Quiroz, L. Echarte, E. A. and P. V. R. (2000). "Effect of *Verticillium dahliae* on Photosynthesis, Leaf Expansion and Senescence of Field-grown Sunflower." *Annals of Botany* 86: 1007-1015.

Saeed, A., V. Sharov, J. White, J. Li, W. Liang, N. Bhagabati, J. Braisted, M. Klapa, T. Currier, M. Thiagarajan, A. Sturn, M. Snuffin, A. Rezantsev, D. Popov, A. Ryltsov, E. Kostukovich, I. Borisovsky, Z. Liu, A. Vinsavich, V. Trush and J. Quackenbush (2003). "TM4: a free, open-source system for microarray data management and analysis." *Biotechniques* 34(2): 374-378.

Shahri, W. (2011). "Senescence: Concepts and Symptoms." *Asian Journal of Plant Sciences* 10(1): 24-28.

Smykowski, A., P. Zimmermann and U. Zentgraf (2010). "G-Box Binding Factor1 Reduces CATALASE2 Expression and Regulates the Onset of Leaf Senescence in Arabidopsis." *Plant Physiol* 153(3): 1321-1331.

Smyth, G. (2004). "Linear models and empirical bayes methods for assessing differential expression in microarray experiments." *Stat Appl Genet Mol Biol* 3: Article3.

Song, S.-Y., Y. Chen, J. Chen, X.-Y. Dai and W.-H. Zhang (2011). "Physiological mechanisms underlying OsNAC5-dependent tolerance of rice plants to abiotic stress." *Planta* 234(2): 331-345.

Thomas, H. and I. Donnisson (2000). "Back from the brink: plant senescence and its reversibility." *Symp Soc Exp Biol.* 52: 149-162.

Thomas, H., L. Huang, M. Young and H. Ougham (2009). "Evolution of plant senescence." *BMC Evol Biol* 9: 163.

Trick, M., F. Cheung, N. Drou, F. Fraser, E. K. Lobenhofer, P. Hurban, A. Magusin, C. D. Town and I. Bancroft (2009). "A newly-developed community microarray resource for transcriptome profiling in *Brassica* species enables the confirmation of *Brassica*-specific expressed sequences." *BMC Plant Biology* 9(50).

Uauy, C., A. Distelfeld, T. Fahima, A. Blechl and J. Dubcovsky (2006). "A NAC Gene regulating senescence improves grain protein, zinc, and iron content in wheat." *Science* 314(5803): 1298-1301.

Ülker, B. and E. I. Somssich (2004). "WRKY transcription factors: from DNA binding towards biological function." *Current Opinion in Plant Biology* 7: 491-498.

Weaver, M. and R. Amasino (2001). "Senescence is induced in individually darkened *Arabidopsis* leaves, but inhibited in whole darkened plants." *Plant Physiology* 127: 876-886.

Wingler, A., S. Purdy, J. A. MacLean and N. Pourtau (2006). "The role of sugars in integrating environmental signals during the regulation of leaf senescence." *Journal of Experimental Botany* 57(2): 391-399.

Woo, H. R., J. H. Kim, J. Kim, U. Lee, I. J. Song, H. Y. Lee, H. G. Nam and P. O. Lim (2010). "The RAV1 transcription factor positively regulates leaf senescence in Arabidopsis." *J Exp Bot* 61(14): 3947-3957.

Zavaleta-Mancera, H. A., B. J. Thomas, H. Thomas and I. M. Scott (1999a). "Regreening of senescent Nicotiana leaves: II Redifferentiation of plastids." *Journal of Experimental Botany* 50(340): 1683-1689.

Zavaleta-Mancera, H. A., B. J. Thomas, H. Thomas and I. M. Scott (1999b). "Regreening of senescent Nicotiana leaves: I Reappearance of NADPH-protochlorophyllide oxidoreductase and light-harvesting chlorophyll a/b-binding protein." *Journal of Experimental Botany* 50(340): 1677-1682.

Zhu, T. and X. Wang (2000). "Large-scale profiling of the Arabidopsis transcriptome." *Plant Physiol* 124(4): 1472-1476.

5

Plant Ageing, a Counteracting Agent to Xenobiotic Stress

David Delmail[1,2] and Pascal Labrousse[2]
[1]*University of Rennes 1, Lab. of Pharmacognosy & Mycology, UMR CNRS 6226 SCR/PNSCM, Rennes*
[2]*University of Limoges, Lab. of Botany & Cryptogamy, GRESE EA 4330, Limoges*
France

1. Introduction

A xenobiotic can be defined as any chemical or other substance that is not normally found in the ecosystems or that is present at concentrations harmful to all biological organisms. This general definition could be applied to anthropogenic and naturally occurring constituents. Organic contaminants can include pesticides, solvents and petroleum products. Inorganic xenobiotics include heavy metals, nonmetals, metalloids, radionuclides and simple soluble salts (Schwab, 2005).

Indeed, after absorption in plant cell, these toxics induce a broad range of disturbances like competition between elements. But the main effect remains the oxidative stress which disrupts many physiological pathways. Reactive oxygen species which initiate the oxidation are produced through several mechanisms in all cell compartments (Delmail et al., 2009; Thompson et al., 1987). Some reactive oxygen species are less deleterious to the plant cell than others but they can act as initiator of the production of more toxic compounds (Delmail et al., 2011c, 2011d).

To prevent from the production of reactive oxygen species, plants can use the senescence process to eliminate the xenobiotics from their organisms. Toxic compounds like radionuclides can be sequestrated by metallothioneins preferentially in vacuoles of specific organs like trichomes and old leaves. Indeed, morphological structures as non-glandular trichomes which are not implied in any physiological process, could store many xenobiotics. Moreover, potentially abscised organs as mature leaves are used to eliminate toxics from the living parts to protect the young organs from any disturbance of the photosynthetic pathways (Delmail et al., 2011c, 2011d).

This chapter will focus on xenobiotics having anthropogenic origins and will address organic and inorganic xenobiotics. Moreover, the origin of the oxidative stress induced by the xenobiotic assimilation, its consequence on the ageing of morphological, physiological and cellular patterns, as well as the functioning of antioxidant pathways, the implication of scavengers and the role of the senescence in reducing the oxidative disturbance, will be discussed in this chapter.

2. The xenobiotics

A xenobiotic (from the Greek *xenos* "stranger" and *biotic* "related to living beings") is a biological (Qiu et al., 2002), physical (Sacco et al., 2004) or chemical disturbance which above a certain degree, and in certain environmental conditions, could lead to toxic effects on a part or the whole ecosystem. It implies that a xenobiotic acts as a pollutant or a contaminant of one or several compartments of the natural environments (atmosphere, lithosphere and hydrosphere) and of biological organisms among the biosphere. This compound disrupts the ecosystem functioning above the limit of tolerance.

The pollution introduced directly or indirectly by humans in all natural compartments, could have prejudicial consequences on its own species and others, on biological resources, on climates and on infrastructures (Delmail, 2007). This impact depends on the type of pollution as it could be distinguished the pollution of proximity and the regional/global pollution (Delmail et al., 2011a; Ritter et al., 2002). The first one is constituted by factory smokes, fumes, sewer gas, etc. and it is directly produced by an anthropogenic source. The second one results from more complex and diverse physicochemical phenomenon (e.g. ozone synthesis in troposphere, acid rains, greenhouse effect).

The xenobiotics could be classified according to their nature (solid, liquid, gas, mineral, organic), their radiation (X, ultraviolet, infrared, radioactivity) and their origin (natural, synecological, autoecological, chemical, industrial) (Fig. 1). They may be also distinguished depending on their environmental targets (air, soil, and water), their biological targets (e.g. plants, fungi, mammals, invertebrates) and their cytotoxicity (e.g. cell types, organites). Their mode of action brings also information as some xenobiotics have an acute (death) or chronic toxicity (e.g. carcinogenesis, mutagenesis), or synergistic effect on organisms. They could be toxic at infinitesimal concentrations (micropollutants) or at a more concentrated range (macropollutants) (Delmail et al., 2010; Delmail et al., 2011b). Moreover, their effects have different duration of action: they could be degradable or persistent, or have a half-life like radioelements from several microseconds to many thousands of years.

Ecological exposure to environmental stressors occurs when a xenobiotic in a form that is bioavailable, reaches an organism. In order to be bioavailable, a xenobiotic must reach a location on or in an organism where it can cause an effect. The notion of phytoavailability defines the fraction of a bioavailable compound which could be absorbed by roots (Hinsinger et al., 2005).

The phytoavailability of xenobiotics is strongly correlated to the concentrations of contaminant species that occurred in the natural environments (Kabata-Pendias & Pendias, 2000). It is also linked to the physicochemical properties of the environment, the plant taxon and the xenobiotic considered. Thus, the phytoavailability is dependent from several parameters allowing the transfer from aerial, solid or aqueous phase to the plant: the availability (or chemical mobility), the accessibility (or physical mobility) and the assimilation (or biological mobility) (Hinsinger et al., 2005).

The xenobiotics could be observed under free forms depending on environmental conditions, but in many cases they may interact with different elements from the environments which will have an influence on its behavior. They could be included in primary minerals originated from the rock crystallization, or in secondary minerals developed from primary ones after oxidation and hydrolysis processes. Moreover, they may be adsorbed on the organic matter in soils and waters, or on microorganisms (which could also absorb and accumulate them). Associations between colloids and xenobiotics could be observed in all natural compartments as a colloidal system may be solid, liquid or gaseous.

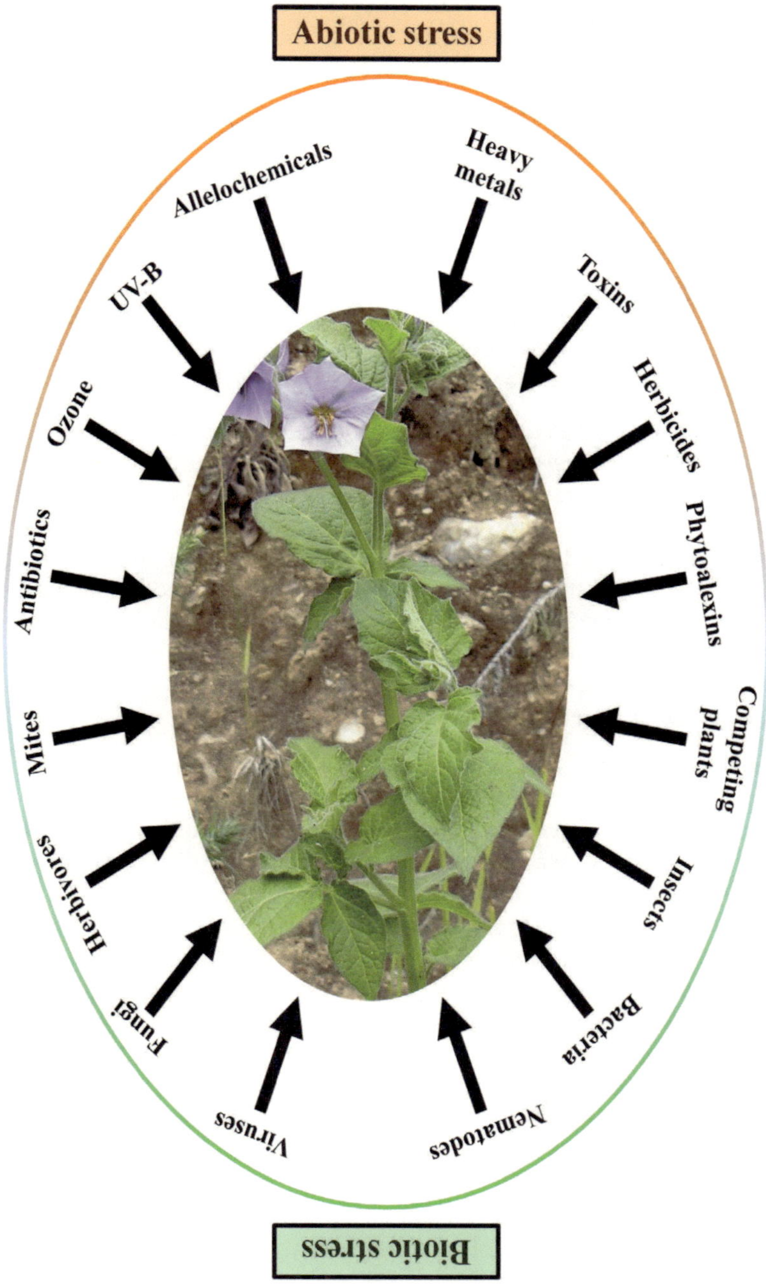

Fig. 1. Overview of selective environmental stress factors which could threaten plants. Biotic and abiotic environmental selective factors are considered.

3. The reactive oxygen species

All plants use the dioxygen as a source of energy for their development. However, this aerobic process could lead to the production of reactive oxygen species which are diversified chemically reactive molecules containing oxygen. Reactive oxygen species are a natural byproduct of the metabolism and play important roles in homeostasis and cell signaling. However, under environmental stress, their levels can increase dramatically which lead to disruptions and damages in cell compartments.

3.1 Diversity and toxicity

An uncompleted reduction of the dioxygen through cytochroms from the respiratory chain implies the production of reactive oxygen species as singlet oxygen ($^1O_2$) and superoxide radical ($O_2^{\bullet -}$) which leads to the synthesis of hydroxyl radical ($^\bullet OH$), hydroperoxyl radical ($^\bullet O_2H$) and hydrogen peroxide (H_2O_2) (Fig. 2). The radicals alkoxyl ($RO^\bullet$) and peroxyl ($RO_2^\bullet$) are the consequence of the peroxidation of membrane phospholipids (or lipoperoxidation) by the previous reactive oxygen species (Fig. 3) (Edreva, 2005; Lagadic et al., 1997; Li et al., 1994; Thompson et al., 1987).

At the same time, the photosynthetic electron transport chains could product high concentrations of reactive oxygen species. Indeed, the electrons tetravalently reduce the intracellular oxygen to water. But, some electrons could leak from many sites along the electron transport chain, resulting in a univalent reduction of dioxygen to form the extremely reactive superoxide radical which can dismutate to form hydrogen peroxide (Alscher et al., 2002). This last reaction is spontaneous or catalyzed by one of the superoxide dismutases (Fig. 2) depending on the cell compartment where the reaction occurs: manganese-superoxide dismutase (mitochondria, peroxisome), iron-superoxide dismutase (chloroplast) or copper/zinc-superoxide dismutase (chloroplast, cytosol) (Fornazier et al., 2002; Gill & Tuteja, 2010; Pereira et al., 2002).

The hydrogen peroxide is not a free radical due to all its matched electrons. However, it has a strong toxicity potential: it has a long lifespan and a high diffusibility far from its synthesis site. Indeed, it could pass through biological membranes via aquaporins as it presents a chemical structure close to water (Bienert et al., 2006, 2007; Parent et al., 2008). The concentration of this oxidative compound is regulated by antioxidant enzymes like the ascorbate peroxidase, the catalase or the glutathione peroxidase (Fig. 2). These proteins use the nicotinamide adenine dinucleotide phosphate (NADPH) produced during the photosynthesis in chloroplasts for their functioning (Fig. 2). However, the reactive oxygen species could disrupt the photosynthetic electron transport chains in thylakoid membranes and some electrons are deflected. Without a normal synthesis of NADPH, plants use a cytosolic secondary catabolism pathway to produce it, the pentose phosphate pathway (Fig. 4) (Delmail, 2011; Kruger & von Schaewen, 2003). The hydrogen peroxide could be also produced through the bivalent reduction of the oxygen in presence of oxidases like the peroxisomal glycolate oxidase or the amine oxidase (Parent et al., 2008). The toxicity of hydrogen peroxide is also linked to its implication in the synthesis of the hydroxyl and hydroperoxyl radicals through the Haber-Weiss and Fenton reactions (Fig. 2). Like their reactive-oxygen-species mother, these short-lifespan radicals are very diffusive through biological membranes and they could disturb and affect all organites and cell compartments. They are also mainly implied in the lipoperoxidation (Fig. 3) (Edreva, 2005 ; Lagadic et al.,

1997). The produced fatty-acid radical then reacts with molecular oxygen, thereby creating a peroxyl fatty acid radical. This last one reacts with another phospholipid, producing a new radical and a lipid peroxide, or a cyclic peroxide if it reacts with itself. This cycle continues as a chain reaction mechanism (Schaich, 2005). This process ends up when two radicals react and produce a non-radical compound. It happens when the concentrations of radicals is high enough. Living organisms have evolved different molecules that speed up termination by catching the reactive oxygen species (Paramesha et al., 2011). Among such antioxidants, the most important are the scavengers mainly constituted with α-tocopherol (or vitamin E) and carotenoids (β-caroten, xantophylls) (Figs. 2 and 3) (Delmail et al., 2011c, 2011d).

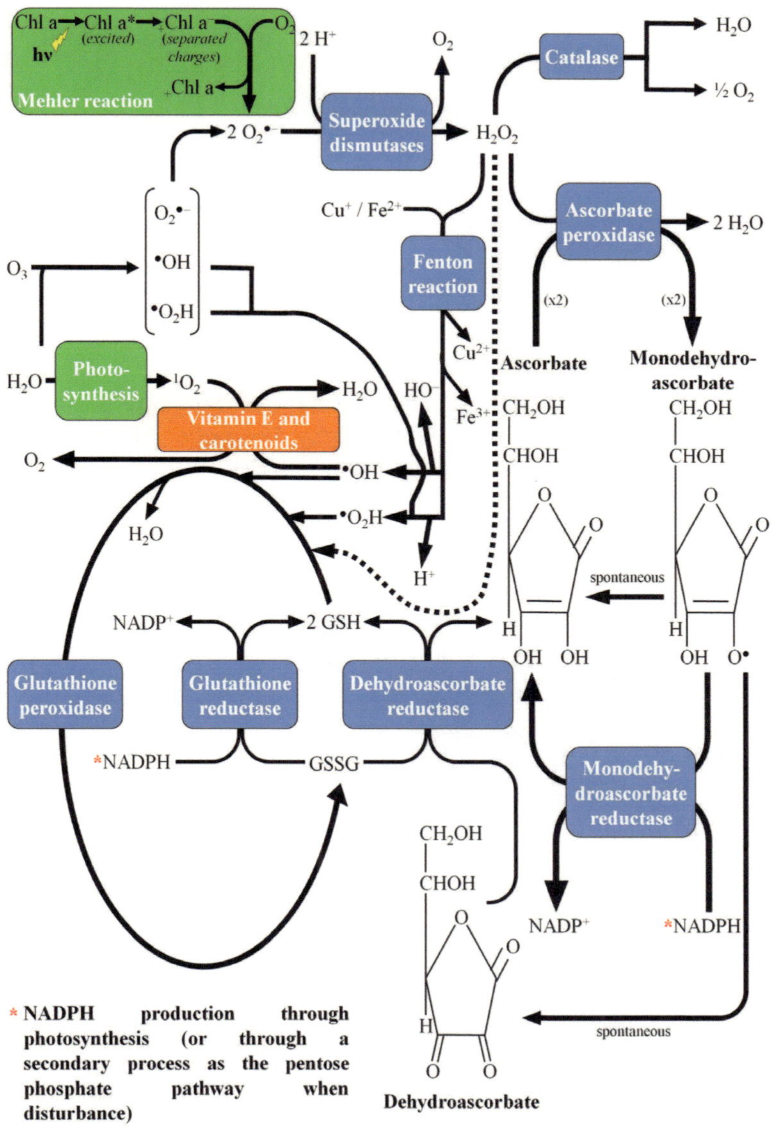

Fig. 2. Main plant antioxidant pathways including enzymes and scavengers (based on Delmail (2011)).

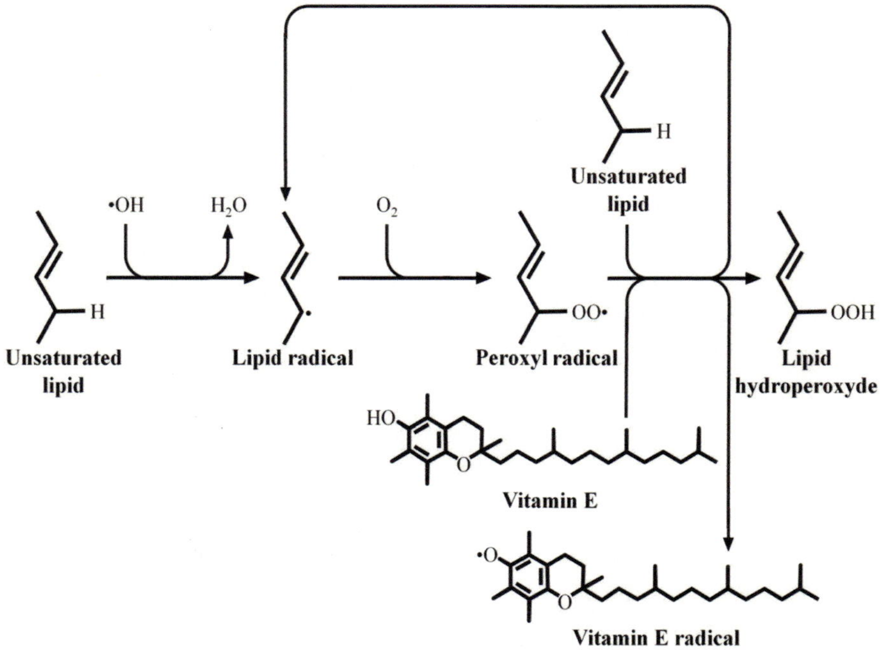

Fig. 3. Mechanisms of lipid peroxidation in biological membranes. The produced peroxyl radicals could react either with another lipid to supply the lipoperoxidative chain reaction mechanism or with a scavenger like the vitamin E which disrupts and stops the oxidative process.

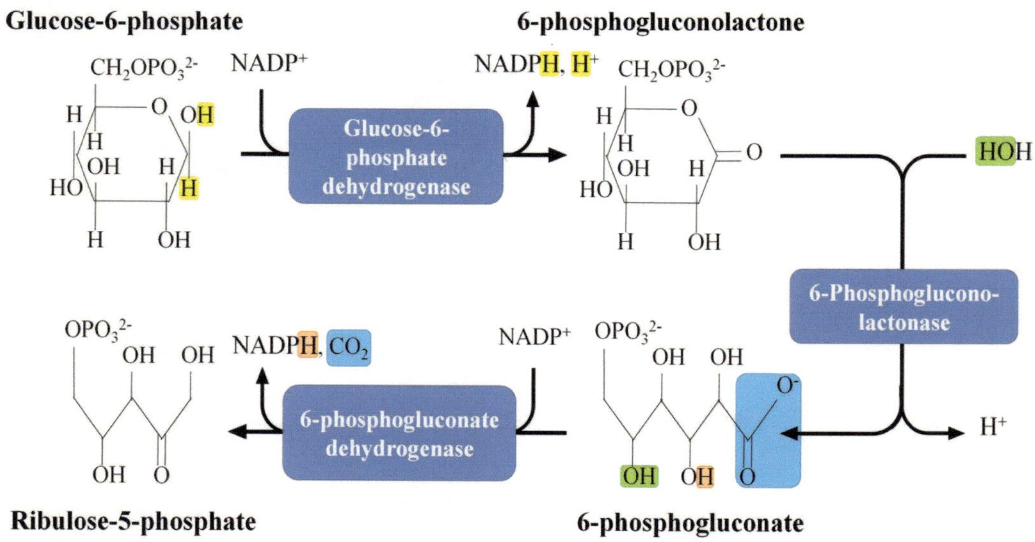

Fig. 4. Reactions of NADPH synthesis through the oxidative phase of the pentose phosphate pathway of plants (based on Delmail (2011)).

Considering all these elements, the reactive oxygen species are considered as phytotoxic compounds. However, it is currently admitted that their synthesis, in relation to the respiratory and photosynthetic metabolisms, plays an essential role in the life and the death of plant cells. Indeed, they could play an alternative role and act as cell signalization molecules to establish some defense mechanisms towards a xenobiotic stress (Parent et al., 2008).

3.2 Role in cell death and protection of living parts

The reactive oxygen species are known for their importance in the plant responses towards environmental disturbances. Several symptoms like necrosis (Fig. 5), are the consequences of a high oxidative-compound accumulation and a disturbance of cell homeostasis.

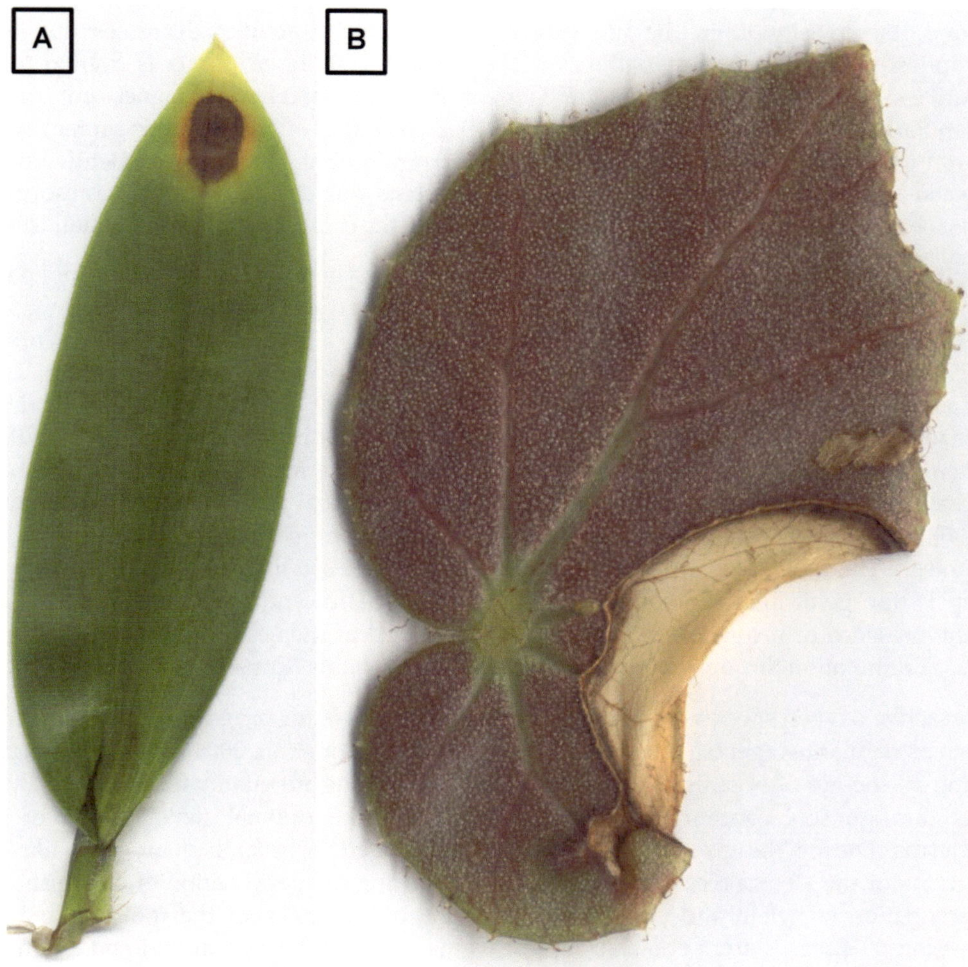

Fig. 5. Leaf of *Tradescantia sp.* (A) and *Begonia sp.* (B) with symptoms of photosynthetic-pigment oxidation and cell necrosis.

This phenomenon is due to an oxidation of photosynthetic pigments in chlorophyllian organs and to the death of isolated cells or groups of cells in many plant tissues. Despite that reactive oxygen species could be produced in normal conditions, the increase of their concentrations in plants is often linked to xenobiotics (Parent et al., 2008). For example, an increase of hydrogen peroxide is observed in peroxisomes of the aquatic macrophyte *Myriophyllum alterniflorum* after an exposition to cadmium chloride from 0.5 to 10 $\mu g.l^{-1}$ (Delmail, 2011). Moreover, the oxidative stress generated by this reactive oxygen species is all the more important during the 2-3 weeks of contamination that the heavy-metal concentration is high. Indeed, the activity of the catalase is higher during a longer period when the toxicity increases (Delmail, 2011).

It could be also noted that many of the symptoms due to the xenobiotics stress are amplified by the presence of reactive oxygen species. In the same species, when *M. alterniflorum* is contaminated with copper sulphate from 5 to 100 $\mu g.l^{-1}$, an increase of the catalase activity is observed up to 25 $\mu g.l^{-1}$ to reduce this reactive oxygen species into water (Delmail, 2011). Beyond this toxicity limit, the intensity of the enzymatic activity decreases due to a disruption of the antioxidant pathways. The catalase activity of plants is known to be sensitive to oxidative stress when a lack of iron (or sometimes magnesium) occurs (Esfandiari et al., 2010; Iturbe-Ormaetxe et al., 1995; Tewari et al., 2005) as this protein needs an iron ion in its constitutive heme (Arménia Carrondo et al., 2007). A competitive effect between the excess of copper and the other elements during the adsorption/absorption (Bernal et al., 2007) could lead to a disturbance during the catalase synthesis (Delmail, 2011).

Despite of their extremely toxic nature, the reactive oxygen species are also implied in cascades of signalization which induce the expression and the regulation of many genes. These genes could be involved in the defense mechanisms, like the phytochelatine synthase which allows the synthesis of heavy-metal binding peptides, the phytochelatins. These compounds play important roles in the detoxification of toxic heavy metals and the regulation of intracellular concentrations of essential metals in plants (Hirata et al., 2005). The primary structure of phytochelatins generally have the form $(\gamma\text{-glutamate-cysteine})_n$-glycine and these peptides could form complexes with heavy metals such as cadmium (Fig. 6), copper, zinc, mercury, silver and arsenic, which are stored as inactive in the cell vacuoles. The expression of phytochelatin synthase in *Populus tremula x tremuloides* cv. Etrepole transgenic lines expressing the wheat phytochelatin synthase TaPCS1 is stimulated by the presence of heavy metal and this protein aimed at increasing metal tolerance and metal accumulation through overproduction of phytochelatins (Couselo et al., 2010).

The reactive oxygen species are also implied in the apoptosis (or programmed cell death) of plants as regulating agents (Dat et al., 2003; Van Breusegem et al., 2006). This event occurs during all the life of organisms and selected cells or organs are eliminated from the living parts through senescence or abscission to maintain the optimal development of the organisms. During the growth, the apoptosis is involved in several phenomena like the triggering of the aleurone cells to release amylase during the germination of caryopsis, the differentiation of xylem and phloem elements, the development of the root cap and the abscission of leaves (Parent et al., 2008). But plants may use this apoptosis to adapt and to resist towards environmental stress like pathogens. For example, the infection of *Nicotiana obtusifolia* by the downy mildew pathogen *Peronospora tabacina* resulted in a compatible interaction, in which *P. tabacina* penetrated and colonized host leaf tissue (Heist et al., 2004).

This interaction becomes incompatible several days later and it leads to an oxidative burst, with the appearance of necrotic lesions due to reactive oxygen species, which isolates the pathogen from the living parts. This conducts to the inhibition of the pathogen growth. These necrotic lesions are due to hypersensitive cell death in the host and the resistance phenotype was due to the action of a gene known to confer a hypersensitive response, Rpt1 (Heist et al., 2004).

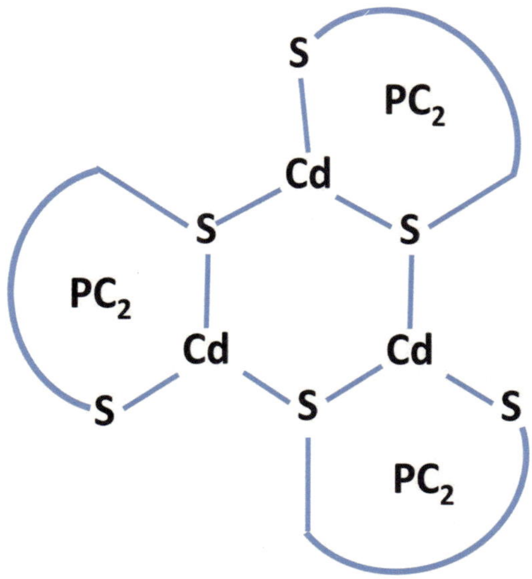

Fig. 6. Schematic structure and organization of phytochelatins implied in the sequestration mechanism of cadmium (Cd) through thiol function (SH) and constituted each of 2 γ-glutamylcysteine parts (PC_2) (based on Delmail (2011)).

4. Senescence and abscission

Leaf senescence is a highly regulated process particularly well studied in crop plants and *Arabidopsis* (Balazadeh et al., 2008). Nowadays it is conspicuous that environmental stresses can induce precocious senescence (Balazadeh et al., 2008) as hypothesized since 1997 by Ouzounidou et al. during the observation of the effect of cadmium on wheat; but the effect of heavy metal ions on this phenomenon is still poorly documented. However, it was demonstrated that protein functioning as metal chelator like metallothionein may be needed to protect normal cell functions from the toxic effects of metal ions released during senescence. In that sense, metallothioneins may be involved in chaperoning released metal ions to avoid metal toxicity or metal induced-oxidative stress in plant cell during the senescence process. Guo et al. (2003) indicated that all the *Arabidopsis* metallothionein genes expressed in vegetative tissues were upregulated in senescing leaves thus protecting cells from metal ions toxicity during senescence. A similar observation of the implication of some metallothioneins in leaf senescence and in heavy metal stress was done in barley by Heise et al. (2007).

Another important molecule involved during senescence is the yellow stripe-like transporter family (YSL). Curie et al. (2009) indicated that five out the eight Arabidopsis YSL genes are most strongly expressed in senescent leaves. Indeed, the expression of AtYSL1 and

AtYSL3 is increased during senescence and although the leave of the double ysl1ysl3 mutant loses only 10% of copper content between the 4th and the 5th week of growth, the wild type *Arabidopsis* loses almost 60%. More recently Xiao & Chye (2011) evidenced new roles for acyl-CoA-binding proteins (ACPBs). Indeed, in *Arabidopsis* the expression of AtACPB3 was upregulated during senescence and AtACPB3-KOs *Arabidopsis* displayed delayed leaf senescence whereas AtACPB3-overexpressors *Arabidopsis* present an accelerated leaf senescence phenotype. On the other hand these authors indicated that *Arabidopsis* AtACPB2-overexpressors were more tolerant to cadmium in the growing media.

Among the different mechanisms adopted by plants to cope with metallic stress (phenological escape, exclusion, amelioration and tolerance), the amelioration one implies that the ion must be removed from the circulation or tolerated within the cytoplasm. These amelioration processes include excretion either actively - through glands on aerial part or by roots - or passively by accumulation in old leaves followed by abscission (Adams & Lamoureux, 2005). The simplest form of excretion is the loss of an organ which has accumulated the toxic compounds. This is generally true for the old leaves that present higher content of toxics than the young leaves and buds. For example, Yasar et al. (2006) noticed that the toxic sodium ion was stored in old leaves of the salt-tolerant Gevas Sirik 57 (GS57) green bean genotype acting as a protection mechanism from the detrimental effect of sodium for young leaves. In the same way, Szarek-Lukaszewska et al. (2004) indicated that an *Armeria maritima* population from metalliferous soil directed to the oldest leaves a part of the metal transported to aboveground plant organs. For these authors the ability to accumulate metals in withering leaves characterizes plants growing under strong environmental pressure from metal contamination. Detoxification mechanism by leaf fall was a strategy previously suggested by Dahmani-Mueller et al. (2000) in *Armeria maritima spp. halleri* where metal content (cadmium, copper, lead and zinc) in ageing leaves (brown leaves) were 3-8 times higher than in green leaves. A similar observation was done by Monni et al. (2001) on a shrub (*Empetrum nigrum*) which accumulates metals (cadmium, copper, iron, lead, nickel and zinc) in older tissues, mainly leaves and bark, by both accumulation and surface contamination. For tree species, Pahalawattaarachchi et al. (2009) shown that in *Rhizophora mucronata* chromium, cadmium and lead were accumulated in leaves before abscission and thus eliminated. A major disadvantage of the excretion strategy for plant is that they are stationary so the excreted substance will remain in the root zone and may eventually lead to a build-up of the xenobiotic (Adams & Lamoureux, 2005).

Only few data were available on aquatic macrophyte, a case where this major disadvantage did not apply. For example in *Spirodela polyrrhiza*, the excess of iron and copper induces plant necrosis, colony disintegration and root abscission (Xing et al., 2010). It should be noted that in another aquatic macrophyte, *Lemna minor*, the frond abscission could be used to test water toxicity induced by metal and other compounds (Henke et al., 2011). Our previous data (Delmail et al., 2011d) suggest that as in terrestrial plants a similar excretion strategy could occur in aquatic plants. Indeed, *Myriophyllum alterniflorum* old leaves are much more affected by heavy-metal pollution than younger ones. Previous study of Jana & Chouduri (1982) on three submerged aquatic macrophytes (*Potamogeton pectinatus, Vallisneria spiralis* and *Hydrilla verticillata*) demonstrated that all the heavy metals tested (cadmium, copper, lead and mercury) hastened the senescence process. These authors evidenced the role of the plant growth regulator kinetin in the reduction of the senescence induced by heavy metals.

The role of plant growth regulator in senescence and in heavy-metal resistance is quite complex but cytokinins for their senescence delaying action (for a review see Werner & Schmulling, 2009) and brassinosteroids for their role in responses to various environmental stress (for a review see Bajguz & Hayat, 2009) appeared as major candidates for further studies to understand the heavy-metal induced senescence processes. Indeed, Arora et al. (2010) demonstrated that the brassinosteroid 24-epibrassinolide present stress-ameliorative properties in *Brassica juncea* plant during chromium stress as an improved growth and antioxidant enzymes activities. Similar conclusion was highlighted by Anuradha & Rao (2007) on *Raphanus sativus* plant were brassinosteroids supplementation alleviated the toxic effect of cadmium. More recently, Bajguz (2011) noted on *Chlorella vulgaris* that the brassinosteroid application to the culture prevents chlorophyll, sugar and protein loss and increases phytochelatin synthesis during heavy metal stress (cadmium, copper and lead). These reactions call to mind the delayed senescence process observed previously in aquatic macrophytes when treated with cytokinins during a heavy-metal stress. In the same way, brassinosteroid treatment improves sunflower (genotype 2603) and turnip (var. rave du Limousin) resistance to cadmium stress in terms of photosynthesis activities (Figs. 7 and 8, Delmail et al. unpublished data).

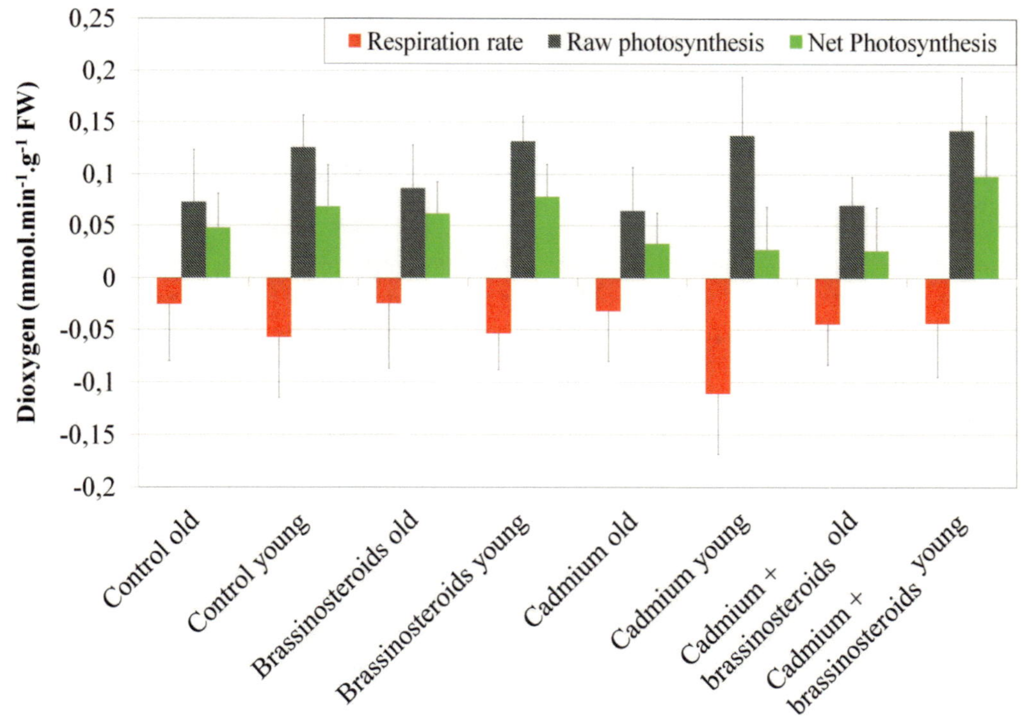

Fig. 7. Photosynthetic activities and respiration rate of one-month old sunflower specimens after 48h of cadmium exposure (1 mM) combined or not with 3 μM 24-epibrassinolid (Delmail et al. unpublished data). FW, fresh weight.

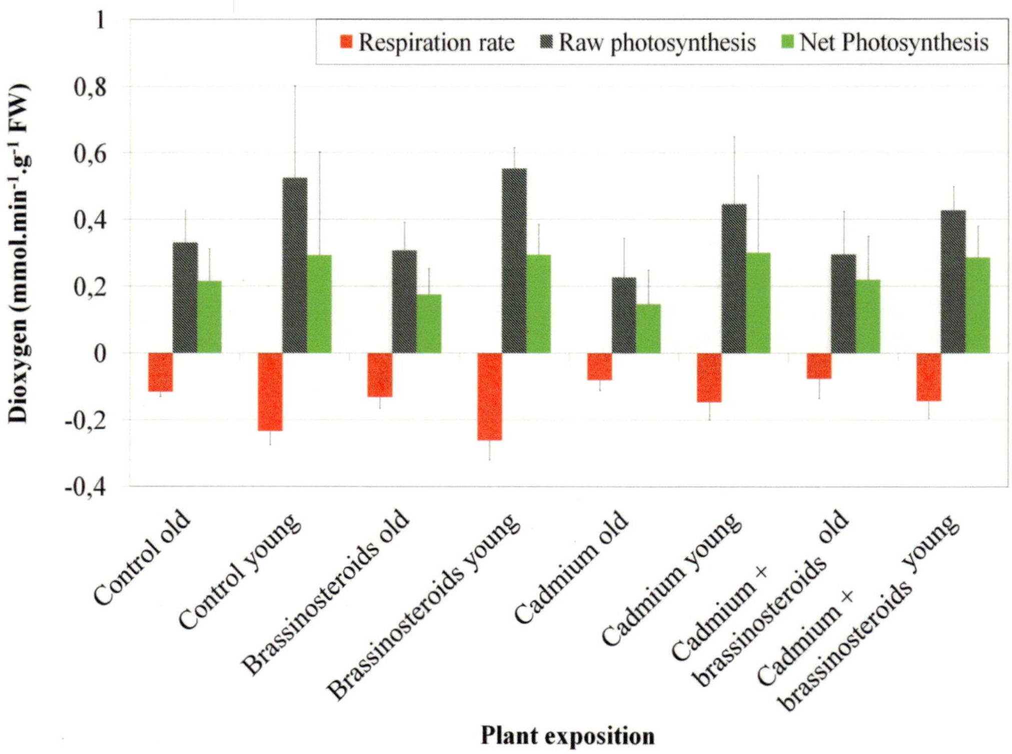

Fig. 8. Photosynthetic activities and respiration rate of one-month old turnip specimens after 72h of cadmium exposure (1 mM) combined or not with 3 µM 24-epibrassinolid (Delmail et al. unpublished data). FW, fresh weight.

Moreover, the effect of brassinosteroids on antioxidant enzymatic activities during cadmium stress could be similar in young and old leaves as shown in Fig. 9 for a decrease in catalase activity of sunflower plants treated with phytohormons during a heavy-metal stress. On the other hand, as demonstrated in turnip (Fig. 10) a differential effect between old and young leaves could appear with an increase in superoxide-dismutase activity in young leaves and a decrease in old leaves (Delmail et al. unpublished data). In these two plants, brassinosteroid application clearly has a protective effect on the raw photosynthesis activity, probably indicating a delayed heavy-metal senescence. These protective actions probably also occur on the enzymatic antioxidant system even if the complexity of the involved cascade reactions lead to a more unclear landscape inducing pattern variations between studied enzymes, age of plant parts and plant species. It appears clearly that much more studies are needed to understand the complex interwoven relationship existing between plant physiology under heavy-metal stress, senescence and plant growth regulators.

Concerning the organic xenobiotics effect on plant senescence even much less data are available. For example, Cape et al. (2003) noted that in *Lotus corniculatus* exposes to a mixture of six volatile organic compounds (acetone, acetonitrile, dichloromethane, ethanol, methyl t-butyl ether and toluene), a premature senescence occurs but in this case a premature senescence refers to advanced timing of seed pot production. Another example concerns the die-back symptom of *Phragmites communis* where the premature senescence of shoot appears to result at least in part from phytotoxin action (acetic, propionic, n- and iso-butyric and n-caproic acids and sulphide) (Armstrong & Armstrong, 2001).

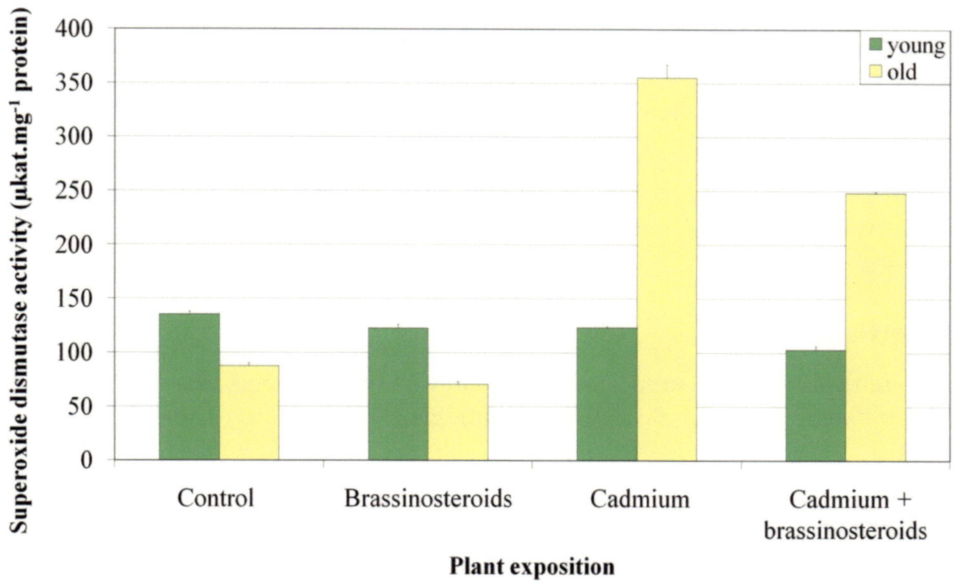

Fig. 9. Superoxide dismutase activity of one-month old sunflower specimens after 48h of cadmium exposure (1 mM) combined or not with 3 µM 24-epibrassinolid (Delmail et al. unpublished data).

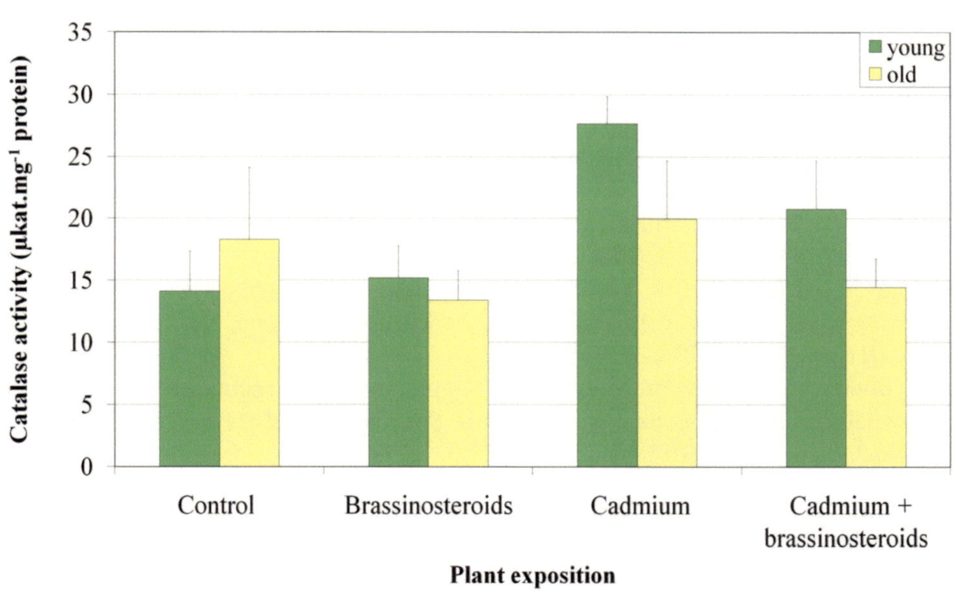

Fig. 10. Catalase activity of one-month old turnip specimens after 72h of cadmium exposure (1 mM) combined or not with 3 µM 24-epibrassinolid (Delmail et al. unpublished data).

5. Conclusion

Senescence implies a succession of physiological events integrated with developmental program which lead to the loss of several organs from the plant. This biological process constitutes an integral part of the normal plant developmental cycle which can be observed at different organization levels (cell, tissue and organ). The senescence is the final event in the life of many plant tissues and it is a highly regulated process that involves structural, biochemical and molecular changes.

Organic and inorganic xenobiotics could hasten the senescence processes and they may lead to a premature death of the plants. At the opposite, the senescence occurring in the plant organs could isolate the stressors and/or eliminate the toxics from the living parts through induced abscission.

6. Acknowledgment

This research was partially supported by the University of Limoges, the GRESE (Research Group on Water, Soil and the Environment) EA 4330, and the Conseil Régional du Limousin.

7. References

Adams, P.W., Lamoureux, S. (2005). Resistance to toxicity, In: *A literature review of the use of native Northern plants for the re-vegetation of Arctic mine tailings and mine waste*, 31.08.2011, Available from http://www.enr.gov.nt.ca/_live/documents/content/WKSS_Northern_Plants_Re-vegetation-2005.pdf

Alscher, R.G., Erturk, N., Heath, L.S. (2002). Role of superoxide dismutases (SODs) in controlling oxidative stress in plants. *Journal of Experimental Botany*, Vol.53, No.372, (May 2002), pp. 1331-1341, ISSN 0022-0957

Anuradha, A., Rao, S.S.R. (2007). The effect of brassinosteroids on radish (*Raphanus sativus* L.) seedlings growing under cadmium stress. *Plant, Soil and Environment*, Vol.53, No.11, (November 2007), pp. 465-472, ISSN 1214-1178

Arménia Carrondo, M., Bento, I., Matias, P.M., Lindley, P.F. (2007). Crystallographic evidence for dioxygen interactions with iron proteins. *Journal of Biological Inorganic Chemistry*, Vol.12,No.4, (May 2007), pp. 429-442, ISSN 0949-8257

Armstrong, J., Armstrong, W. (2001). An overview of the effects of phytotoxins on *Phragmites australis* in relation to die-back. *Aquatic Botany*, Vol.69, No.2-4, (April 2001), pp. 251-268, ISSN 0304-3770

Arora, P., Bhardwaj, R., Kanwar, M.K. (2010). 24-epibrassinolide regulated diminution of Cr metal toxicity in *Brassica juncea* L. plants. *Brazilian Journal of Plant Physiology*, Vol.22, No.3, (September 2010), pp. 159-165, ISSN 1677-0420

Bajguz, A. (2011). Suppression of *Chlorella vulgaris* growth by cadmium, lead, and copper stress and its restoration by endogenous brassinolide. *Archives of Environmental Contamination and Toxicology*, Vol.60, No.3, (April 2011), pp. 406-416, ISSN 0090-4341

Bajguz, A., Hayat, S. (2009). Effects of brassinosteroids on the plant responses to environmental stresses. *Plant Physiology and Biochemistry*, Vol.47, No.1, (January 2009), pp. 1-8, ISSN 0981-9428

Balazadeh, S., Riaño-Pachón, D.M., Mueller-Roeber, B. (2008). Transcription factors regulating leaf senescence in Arabidopsis thaliana. *Plant Biology*, Vol.10, No.SUPPL.1, (September 2008), pp. 63-75, ISSN, 1435-8603

Bernal, M., Cases, R., Picorel, R., Yruela, I. (2007). Foliar and root Cu supply affect differently Fe-and Zn-uptake and photosynthetic activity in soybean plants. *Environmental and Experimental Botany*, Vol.60, No., (2), pp. 145-150, ISSN 0098-8472

Bienert, G.P., Schjoerring, J.K., Jahn, T.P. (2006). Membrane transport of hydrogen peroxide. *Biochimica et Biophysica Acta – Biomembranes*, Vol.1758, No.8, (August 2006), pp. 994-1003, ISSN 0005-2736

Bienert, G.P., Møller, A.L.B., Kristiansen, K.A., Schulz, A., Møller, I.M., Schjoerring, J.K., Jahn, T.P. (2007). Specific aquaporins facilitate the diffusion of hydrogen peroxide across membranes. *The Journal of Biological Chemistry*, Vol.282, No.2, (January 2007), pp. 1183-1192, ISSN 0021-9258

Cape, J.N., Leith, I.D., Binnie, J., Content, J., Donkin, M., Skewes, M., Price, D.N., Brown, A.R., Sharpe, A.D. (2003). Effects of VOCs on herbaceous plants in an open-top chamber experiment. *Environmental Pollution*, Vol.124, No.2, (July 2003), pp. 341-353, ISSN 0269-7491

Couselo, J.L., Navarro-Avĩnó, J., Ballester, A. (2010). Expression of the phytochelatin synthase TaPCS1 in transgenic aspen, insight into the problems and qualities in phytoremediation of Pb. *International Journal of Phytoremediation*, Vol.12, No.4, (April 2010), pp. 358-370, ISSN 1522-6514

Curie, C., Cassin, G., Couch, D., Divol, F., Higuchi, K. , Le Jean, M. , Misson, J. , Schikora, A. , Czernic, P., Mari, S. (2009). Metal movement within the plant: Contribution of nicotianamine and yellow stripe 1-like transporters. *Annals of Botany*, Vol.103, No.1, (January 2009), pp. 1-11, ISSN 0305-7364

Dahmani-Muller, H., Van Oort, F., Gélie, B., Balabane, M. (2000). Strategies of heavy metal uptake by three plant species growing near a metal smelter. *Environmental Pollution*, Vol.109, No.2, (August 2000), pp. 231-238, ISSN 0269-7491

Dat, J.F., Pellinen, R., Beeckman, T., Van De Cotte, B., Langebartels, C., Kangasjarvi, J., Inze, D., Van Breusegem, F. (2003). Changes in hydrogen peroxide homeostasis trigger an active cell death process in tobacco. *The Plant Journal*, Vol.33, No.4, (February 2003), pp. 621-632, ISSN 0960-7412

Delmail, D. (2007). Ecologie florale bretonne. *La Garance Voyageuse*, Vol.79, No.1, (September 2007), pp. 14-17, ISSN 0988-3444

Delmail, D. (2011). *Contribution de Myriophyllum alterniflorum et de son périphyton à la biosurveillance de la qualité des eaux face aux métaux lourds*, Université de Limoges, Limoges, France

Delmail, D., Labrousse, P., Buzier, R., Botineau, M. (2009). Importance of *Myriophyllum alterniflorum* D.C., an aquatic macrophyte, in biomonitoring of trace metal pollution in running freshwater, *Proceedings of EMEC10 10th European Meeting on Environmental Chemistry*, pp. 66, Limoges, France, December 2-5, 2009

Delmail, D., Labrousse, P., Hourdin, P., Botineau, M. (2010). Use of *Myriophyllum alterniflorum* (Haloragaceae) for restoration of heavy-metal-polluted freshwater environments: preliminary results, *Proceedings of 7th SER European Conference on Ecological restoration and sustainable development,* pp. 103, Avignon, France, August 23-27, 2010

Delmail, D., Labrousse, P., Crassous, P., Hourdin, P., Guri, M., Botineau, M. (2011a). Simulating the dynamics of epiphytic diatom metacommunity in stream environments contaminated with heavy metals, *Proceedings of ECEM 2011 7th European Conference on Ecological hierarchy from the genes to the biosphere,* pp. 112, Riva del Garda, Italy, May 30-June 2, 2011

Delmail, D., Labrousse, P., Hourdin, P., Botineau, M. (2011b). Evidence of copper impact on freshwater environments using *Myriophyllum alterniflorum*: restoration, biomonitoring and management, *Proceedings of IAVS 2011 54th International Symposium on Vegetation in and around water: patterns, processes and threats,* pp. 157, ISBN 978-2-9539515-1-6, Lyon, France, June 20-24, 2011

Delmail, D., Labrousse, P., Hourdin, P., Larcher, L., Moesch, C., Botineau, M. (2011c). Differential responses of *Myriophyllum alterniflorum* DC (Haloragaceae) organs to copper: physiological and developmental approaches. *Hydrobiologia,* Vol.664, No.1, (April 2011), pp. 95-105, ISSN 0018-8158

Delmail, D., Labrousse, P., Hourdin, P., Larcher, L., Moesch, C., Botineau, M. (2011d). Physiological, anatomical and phenotypical effects of a cadmium stress in different-aged chlorophyllian organs of *Myriophyllum alterniflorum* DC (Haloragaceae). *Environmental and Experimental Botany,* Vol.72, No.2, (September 2011), pp. 174-181, ISSN 0098-8472

Edreva, A. (2005). Generation and scavenging of reactive oxygen species in chloroplasts: a submolecular approach. *Agriculture, Ecosystems and Environment,* Vol.106, No.2-3, (April 2005), pp. 119-133, ISSN 0167-8809

Esfandiari, E., Shokrpour, M., Alavi-Kia, S. (2010). Effect of Mg deficiency on antioxydant enzymes activities and lipid peroxidation. *Journal of Agricultal Science,* Vol.2, No.3, (September 2010), pp. 131-136, ISSN 1916-9752

Fornazier, R.F., Ferreira, R.R., Vitória, A.P., Molina, S.M.G., Lea, P.J., Azevedo, R.A. (2002). Effects of cadmium on antioxidant enzyme activities in sugar cane. *Biologia Plantarum,* Vol.45, No.1, (January 2002), pp. 91-97, ISSN 0006-3134

Gill, S.S., Tuteja, N. (2010). Reactive oxygen species and antioxidant machinery in abiotic stress tolerance in crop plants. *Plant Physiology and Biochemistry,* Vol.48, No.12, (December 2010), pp. 909-930, ISSN 0981-9428

Guo, W.-J., Bundithya, W., Goldsbrough, P.B. (2003). Characterization of the *Arabidopsis* metallothionein gene family: Tissue-specific expression and induction during senescence and in response to copper. *New Phytologist,* Vol.159, No.2, (August 2003), pp. 369-381, ISSN 0028-646X

Heise, J., Krejci, S., Miersch, J., Krauss, G.-J., Humbeck, K. (2007). Gene expression of metallothioneins in barley during senescence and heavy metal treatment. *Crop Science,* Vol.47, No.3, (May 2007), pp. 1111-1118, ISSN 0011-183X

Heist, E.P., Zaitlin, D., Funnell, D.L., Nesmith, W.C., Schardl, C.L. (2004). Necrotic lesion resistance induced by *Peronospora tabacina* on leaves of *Nicotiana obtusifolia. Phytopathology,* Vol.94, No.11, (November 2004), pp. 1178-1188, ISSN 0031-949X

Henke, R., Eberius, M., Appenroth, K.-J. (2011). Induction of frond abscission by metals and other toxic compounds in *Lemna minor*. *Aquatic Toxicology*, Vol.101, No.1, (January 2011), pp. 261-265, ISSN 0166-445X

Hinsinger, P., Schneider, A., Dufey J.E. (2005). Le sol : ressource en nutriments et biodisponibilité, In : *Sols et Environnement*, M.-C. Girard, C. Walter, J.-C. Rémy, J. Berthelin, J.-L. Morel (Eds.), 285-305, Dunod, ISBN 978-2-1005-1695-7, Paris, France

Hirata, K., Tsuji, N., Miyamoto, K. (2005). Biosynthetic regulation of phytochelatins, heavy-metal-binding peptides. *Journal of Bioscience and Bioengineering*, Vol.100, No.6, (December 2005), pp. 593-599, ISSN 1389-1723

Iturbe-Ormaetxe, I., Moran, J.F., Arrese-Igor, C., Gogorcena, Y., Klucas, R.V., Becana, M. (1995). Activated oxygen and antioxidant defences in iron-deficient pea plants. *Plant, Cell and Environment*, Vol.18, No.4, (April 1995), pp. 421-429, ISSN 0140-7791

Jana, S., Choudhuri, M.A. (1982). Senescence in submerged aquatic angiosperms: Effects of heavy metals. *New Phytologist*, Vol.90, No.3, (), pp. 477-484, ISSN 0028-646X

Kabata-Pendias, A., Pendias, H. (2000). *Trace elements in soils and plants*, CRC Press, ISBN 978-0-8493-1575-6, Boca Raton, Florida, USA

Kruger, N.J., von Schaewen, A. (2003). The oxidative pentose phosphate pathway: structure and organisation. *Current Opinion in Plant Biology*, Vol.6, No.3, (June 2003), pp. 236-246, ISSN 1369-5266

Lagadic, L. , Caquet, T., Amiard J.-C. (1997). Biomarqueurs en écotoxicologie : principes et définitions, In: *Biomarqueurs en écotoxicologie*, L. Lagadic, T. Caquet, J.C. Amiard, (Eds.), 1-10, Masson Press, ISBN 2-225-83053-3, Paris, France

Li, Y., Trush, M.A., Yager, J.D. (1994). DNA damage caused by reactive oxygen species originating from a copper-dependent oxidation of the 2-hydroxy catechol of estradiol. *Carcinogenesis*, Vol.15, No.7, (July 1994), pp. 1421-1427, ISSN 0143-3334

Monni, S., Uhlig, C., Junttila, O., Hansen, E., Hynynen, J. (2001). Chemical composition and ecophysiological responses of *Empetrum nigrum* to aboveground element application. *Environmental Pollution*, Vol.112, No.3, (May 2001), pp. 417-426, ISSN 0269-7491

Ouzounidou, G., Moustakas, M., Eleftheriou, E.P. (1997). Physiological and ultrastructural effects of cadmium on wheat (*Triticum aestivum* L.) leaves. *Archives of Environmental Contamination and Toxicology*, Vol.32, No.2, (February 1997), pp. 154-160, ISSN 0090-4341

Pahalawattaarachchi, V., Purushothaman, C.S., Vennila, A. (2009). Metal phytoremédiation potential of Rhizophora mucronata (Lam.). *Indian Journal of Marine Sciences*, Vol.38, No.2, (June 2009), pp. 178-183, ISSN 0379-5136

Parent, C., Capelli, N., Dat, J. (2008). Formes réactives de l'oxygène, stress et mort cellulaire chez les plantes. *Comptes Rendus Biologies*, Vol.331, No.4, (April 2008), pp. 255-261, ISSN 1631-0691

Paramesha, S., Vijay, R., Bekal, M., Kumari, S., Pushpalatha, K.C. (2011). A study on lipid peroxidation and total antioxidant status in diabetes with and without hypertension. *Research Journal of Pharmaceutical, Biological and Chemical Sciences*, Vol.2, No.1, (January-March 2011), pp. 329-334, ISSN 0975-8585

Pereira, G.J.G., Molina, S.M.G., Lea, P.J., Azevedo, R.A. (2002). Activity of antioxidant enzymes in response to cadmium in *Crotalaria juncea*. Plant and Soil, Vol.239, No.1, (January 2002), pp. 123-132, ISSN 0032-079X

Qiu, J., Zhu, K., Zhang, J., Zhang, Z. (2002). Diversity of the microorganisms degrading aromatic hydrocarbons. *Chinese Journal of Applied Ecology*, Vol.13, No.12, (December 2002), pp. 1713-1715, ISSN 1001-9332

Ritter, L., Solomon, K., Sibley, P., Hall, K., Keen, P., Mattu, G., Linton, B. (2002). Sources, pathways, and relative risks of contaminants in surface water and groundwater: A perspective prepared for the Walkerton inquiry. *Journal of Toxicology and Environmental Health - Part A*, Vol.65, No.1, (January 2002), pp. 1-142, ISSN 1528-7394

Sacco, M.G., Amicone, L., Catò, EM., Filippini, D., Vezzoni, P., Tripodi, M. (2004). Cell-based assay for the detection of chemically induced cellular stress by immortalized untransformed transgenic hepatocytes. *BMC Biotechnology*, Vol.4, No.5, (March 2004), pp. 1-7, ISSN 1472-6750

Schwab, A.P. (2005). Pollutants: Organic and Inorganic, In: *Encyclopedia of Soil Science*, L. Rattan, (Ed.), 1334-1337, CRC Press, ISBN 978-0-8493-3830-4

Schaich, K.M. (2005). Lipid oxidation: theoretical aspects, In: *Bailey's Industrial Oil and Fat Products*, F. Shahidi, (Ed.), 269-355, Wiley J., Sons Publishers, ISBN 978-0-471-38460-1

Szarek-Łukaszewska, G., Słysz, A., Wierzbicka, M. (2004). Response of *Armeria maritima* (Mill.) Willd. to Cd, Zn and Pb. *Acta Biologica Cracoviensia Series Botanica*, Vol.46, No.1, (December 2004), pp. 19-24, ISSN 0001-5296

Tewari, R., Kumar, P., Sharma, P. (2005). Signs of oxidative stress in the chlorotic leaves of iron starved plants. *Plant Science*, Vol.169, No.6, (December 2005), pp. 1037-1045, ISSN 0168-9452

Thompson, J.E., Legge, R.L., Barber, R.F. (1987). The role of free radicals in senescence and wounding. *New Phytologist*, Vol.105, No.3, (March 1987), pp. 317-344, ISSN 0028-646X

Van Breusegem, F., Dat, J.F. (2006). Reactive oxygen species in plant cell death. *Plant Physiology*, Vol.141, No.2, (June 2006), pp. 384-390, ISSN 0032-0889

Werner, T., Schmülling, T. (2009). Cytokinin action in plant development. *Current Opinion in Plant Biology*, Vol.12, No.5, (October 2009), pp. 527-538, ISSN 1369-5266

Xiao, S., Chye, M.-L. (2011). New roles for acyl-CoA-binding proteins (ACBPs) in plant development, stress responses and lipid metabolism. *Progress in Lipid Research*, Vol.50, No.2, (April 2011), pp. 141-151, ISSN 0163-7827

Xing, W., Huang, W., Liu, G. (2010). Effect of excess iron and copper on physiology of aquatic plant *Spirodela polyrrhiza* (L.) schleid. *Environmental Toxicology*, Vol.25, No.2, (April 2010), pp. 103-112, ISSN 1520-4081

Yasar, F., Uzal, O., Tufenkci, S., Yildiz, K. (2006). Ion accumulation in different organs of green bean genotypes grown under salt stress. *Plant, Soil and Environment*, Vol.52, No. 10, (October 2006), pp. 476-480, ISSN 1214-1178

6

Some Aspects of Leaf Senescence

Hafsi Miloud and Guendouz Ali
Laboratory of Improvement and Development of Livestock and Crop Production, Department of Agronomy, Faculty of Natural Sciences and Life, Ferhat ABBAS University, Setif Algeria

1. Introduction

The word *senescence* derives from two Latin words: *senex* and *senescere*. *Senex* means 'old'; this Latin root is shared by 'senile', 'senior', and even 'senate'. In ancient Rome the 'Senatus' was a 'council of elders' that was composed of the heads of patrician families. *Senescere* means 'to grow old'. The Merriam-Webster online dictionary defines *senescence* as 'the state of being old or the process of becoming old'. Aging is also the process of getting older. Therefore, aging has been regarded as a synonym of senescence, and the two words have often been used interchangeably, which, in some cases, is fine but in some other cases causes confusion. This paper will first briefly discuss the terminology of senescence, and then will review the literature related to mitotic senescence, a topic that has not been well discussed in the plant senescence research area and discuss some results relating to nutrient remobilization during leaf senescence.

2. Terminology and types of senescence

Senescence is a universal phenomenon in living organisms, and the word *senescence* has been used by scientists working on a variety of systems, such as yeast, fruit fly, worm, human being and plants. However, the meaning of the word *senescence* to scientists working on different organisms can be different, and the difference can be subtle in some cases and very obvious in some other cases.

3. Plants exhibit mitotic senescence, post mitotic senescence and cell quiescence

Plants exhibit both types of senescence. An example of mitotic senescence in plants is the arrest of apical meristem; the meristem consists of non differentiated, germ line-like cells that can divide finite times to produce cells that will be then differentiated to form new organs such as leaves and flowers. The arrest of apical meristem is also called proliferative senescence in plant literature .This is similar to replicative senescence in yeast and animal cells in culture. Another example of mitotic senescence is the arrest of mitotic cell division at early stages of fruit development. Fruit size is a function of cell number, cell size and intercellular space, and cell number is the major factor.

Cell number is determined at the very early stage of fruit development and remains unchanged thereafter. Post mitotic senescence occurs in some plant organs, such as leaves and floral petals. Once formed, cells in these organs rarely undergo cell division; their growth is mainly contributed by cell expansion; thus, their senescence, unlike mitotic senescence, is not due to an inability to divide. This type of senescence involving predominantly somatic tissues is very similar to that.

4. Physiological regulation

Reproductive development appears to play an important role in regulating proliferative senescence in plants, which is especially true in many monocarpic plants. Hensel *et al.* (1994) found that meristems of all inflorescence branches in the wild-type *Arabidopsis* ecotype Landsberg *erecta* (L*er*) ceased to produce flowers coordinately, but such a coordinated proliferative arrest did not occur in the wild-type L*er* plants with their fruits surgically removed. Similarly, meristem arrest was not observed in a male-sterile line that never sets seeds. This result suggests that the arrest of inflorescence meristems is regulated by developing fruits/seeds (Hensel *et al.*, 1994). Hensel *et al.* further proposed two models to explain the effect of developing fruits on the mitotic activity of meristems. One model is that a factor necessary for sustaining mitotic activity at the SAM is gradually taken and eventually depleted by developing fruits, resulting in arrest. The other model is that developing fruits produce a negative regulator of mitotic activities and that the negative regulator is transferred to and accumulated in the SAM to a threshold level so that the SAM is arrested. The factor, either positive or negative, is unknown.

5. Nutrient remobilization during leaf senescence

Senescence is the last stage in the development of leaves and other plant organs. While many plants are perennial (barring adverse conditions leading to premature death), and some species even very long-lived (at least from a human perspective), senescence and death of organs such as leaves is often an annual event. Due to its importance for agriculture, the senescence of annual crops (e.g. corn, rice, wheat, barley and some legumes) has been most intensely studied (Feller & Fischer, 1994; Hayati *et al.*, 1995; Crafts-Brandner *et al.*, 1998; Yang *et al.*, 2003; Robson *et al.*, 2004; Parrott *et al.*, 2005;Weng *et al.*, 2005). Additionally, as in other areas of plant science research,*Arabidopsis* has emerged as an important model system (Diaz *et al.*, 2005; Levey & Wingler, 2005; Otegui *et al.*, 2005). These plants show monocarpic senescence, i.e. fruit set and maturation are directly associated with whole-plant senescence and death. Other types of senescence, such as top senescence (in species with bulbs, tubers, tap roots or rhizomes), deciduous senescence (in some trees and shrubs of temperate climate zones) and progressive senescence (e.g. in evergreen trees) have received less attention. In contrast to annuals, leaf (or whole-shoot) senescence is often not directly associated with seed filling in perennial plants (Feller & Fischer 1994; Nood´en *et al.*, 2004). However, nutrient remobilization from senescing plant parts to surviving structures is a hallmark of the 'execution' of the senescence process in both annual plants, in which nutrients are retranslocated to the seeds, and perennial species, in which nutrients are transported to surviving structures such as bulbs and roots.

Plants need a number of elements in higher quantities or concentrations to complete their life cycle (macronutrients, including C, O, H, N, P, S, K, Mg and Ca), while a number of additional elements (micronutrients, including Fe, Mn, Zn, Cu, B, Mo, Cl and Ni) are needed in comparatively small quantities (Marschner, 1995). Some elements are essential only for specific taxonomic groups (e.g. Na, Si) and/or are considered beneficial (Marschner, 1995).

5.1 Nitrogen remobilization

Quantitatively, nitrogen is the most important mineral nutrient in plants (Marschner, 1995). It is often a limiting factor for plant growth, yield and/or quality (Gastal & Lemaire, 2002; Good *et al.*, 2004). Additionally, as for carbon, the principal form in which many plants acquire nitrogen from the environment (nitrate) is more oxidized than the form in which it can be integrated into metabolites and macro molecules, demanding substantial energy input for the synthesis of nitrogen compounds. Although the biochemistry involved is different, the establishment and maintenance of a symbiosis with N2-fixing microorganisms (e.g. in legumes) is also costly (Crawford *et al.*, 2000; Lodwig & Poole, 2003). For these reasons, efficient N remobilization increases the competitiveness of wild plants. Additionally, due to the economic and ecological (N runoff from agricultural soils) cost of N fertilization, this trait is of considerable importance to farmers.

In most plant tissues, the largest fraction of organic nitrogen, which is potentially available for remobilization during senescence, is contained in proteins. In photosynthetically active tissues of C3 species, over 50% of this nitrogen is found in soluble (Calvin cycle) and insoluble (thylakoid) chloroplast proteins (Peoples and Dalling, 1988; Feller and Fischer, 1994). Intriguingly, ribulose-1,5-bisphosphate carboxylase/ oxygenase (Rubisco) alone represents 50% of the total plastidial nitrogen.

All other cellular nitrogen fractions, including cytosolic and other proteins, nucleic acids, chlorophylls and free amino acids, while not negligible, represent relatively minor stores of organic nitrogen. Efforts at understanding nitrogen remobilization during leaf senescence have therefore focused on the biochemistry of plastidial protein degradation. Mae *et al.* (1983), using elegant 15 N-labeling techniques, have demonstrated that the synthesis and degradation phases of Rubisco are surprisingly clearly separated during leaf development. High rates of synthesis were observed until full leaf expansion; after this point, synthesis was minimal, but degradation rates started to increase. In this context, it is well known that the photosynthetic capacity of a leaf declines early during leaf senescence, while mitochondrial integrity and respiration are maintained longer (Gepstein, 1988; Feller and Fischer, 1994). That efficient N remobilization is associated with (early) loss of CO2 assimilation represents a formidable problem in annual crops. In this context, agronomists are well aware of the negative correlation between seed protein and yield.

5.2 Macro- and micronutrient remobilization

Developing (young) leaves constitute significant net importers ('sinks') for all nutrients, which are utilized to build the organ's cellular and molecular components. After the so-called sink–source transition (Ishimaru *et al.*, 2004; Jeong *et al.*, 2004), leaves become net exporters ('sources') of carbohydrates from photosynthesis, while import (through the xylem) and export (through the phloem) of phloem-mobile nutrients are (roughly) at an equilibrium in mature leaves (Marschner, 1995). The onset of leaf senescence is associated with a transition to net export of 'mobile' (see below) compounds, i.e. total (per leaf) content of some nutrients starts to decrease (Marschner, 1995). The literature often refers to this situation as 'redistribution', 'retranslocation', 'resorption' or 'remobilization' (Marschner, 1995; Killingbeck, 2004).

The main transport route from senescing leaves to nutrient sinks is the phloem (Atkins, 2000; Tilsner *et al.*, 2005). Using various approaches, including sampling and analysis of phloem sap and (radioactive) tracer studies, it has been established that macronutrients with the exception of calcium (i.e. N, P, S, K and Mg) are generally highly mobile in the phloem, while micronutrients with the exception of manganese (i.e. Fe, Zn, Cu, B, Mo, Cl and Ni) show at least moderate mobility (Marschner, 1995). As a consequence, while some mobile nutrients decrease during leaf senescence, this is not true for calcium, which continues to accumulate throughout a leaf's life span. The molecular form, in which nutrients fulfill their biological functions, determines the biochemical steps necessary to make them phloem mobile. A certain percentage of many nutrients is biochemically inert, and cannot be remobilized (Marschner, 1995; Killingbeck, 2004). Cell wall components are a good example, and explain why fully senesced (dead) leaves are usually rich in carbon as compared to nitrogen. Some macronutrients, including carbon, nitrogen, phosphorus and sulfur, are covalently bound in myriads of both low-molecular-weight metabolites and macromolecules. Proteins and nucleic acids are important stores of nitrogen, phosphorus (nucleic acids) and sulfur (proteins); these macromolecules have to be degraded by specific hydrolases prior to phloem loading and transport. Metals (both macro- and micronutrients) can also be tightly bound, mostly by macromolecules, e.g. cell wall compounds or proteins. Their release is therefore often linked with the degradation of the functional complexes/macromolecules, to which they belong.

5.3 Carbon

Because it is taken up in gaseous form and a large amount of energy is needed for its reduction prior to its incorporation into metabolites, carbon occupies a special position in plant metabolism. Additionally, as discussed obove, degradation of the photosynthetic apparatus is an early event during leaf senescence, leading to a decrease of photoassimilate production and export to sinks, and to an increasing dependence of senescing tissues on respiratory metabolism (Gepstein, 1988; Feller & Fischer, 1994). Metabolization and, to some degree, remobilization of reduced carbon are therefore important for senescing leaves. In this context, Gut and Matile (1988, 1989) observed an induction of key enzymes of the glyoxylate cycle, isocitrate lyase and malate synthase, in senescent barley leaves. Based on these data, and based on low respiratory quotients (0.6), these authors suggested a reutilization of plastidial (thylakoid) lipids via *β*-oxidation, glyoxylate cycle and gluconeogenesis, allowing export of at least some of the carbon 'stored' in plastidial lipids from the senescing leaf. These observations have since been confirmed and extended (Pistelli *et al.*, 1991; Graham *et al.*, 1992; McLaughlin & Smith, 1994). He and Gan (2002) have shown an essential role for an *Arabidopsis* lipase in leaf senescence; however, it is not yet clear if this or other lipases are involved in preparing substrates (free fatty acids) for *β*-oxidation and gluconeogenesis. Roulin *et al.* (2002) have found an induction of (1→3, 1→4)-*β*-d-glucan hydrolases during dark-induced senescence of barley seedlings, suggesting a remobilization of cell wall glucans under these conditions.

Using radioactive labeling studies,Yang *et al.* (2003) demonstrated considerable remobilization of pre-fixed 14C from vegetative tissues to grains in senescent wheat plants. Interestingly, this process was enhanced under drought conditions, when leaf photosynthetic rates declined faster. Together, these data suggest that while C remobilization during leaf senescence has received less attention than N remobilization, it probably makes important contributions to seed development, at least in annual crops.

5.4 Sulfur

Besides carbon and nitrogen, sulfur is the third nutrient, which (relative to its main form of uptake, sulfate) is reduced by plants prior to its incorporation into certain metabolites and macromolecules. It is noteworthy, however, that plants also contain oxidized ('sulfated') sulfur metabolites (Crawford et al., 2000). Identically to carbon and nitrogen, sulfur is an essential element of both low-molecular weight compounds (including the protein amino acids cysteine and methionine) and macromolecules (proteins). Glutathione (γ -glutamyl-cysteinyl-glycine) represents the quantitatively most important reduced sulfur metabolite; it can reach millimolar concentrations in chloroplasts (Rennenberg and Lamoureux, 1990). Sulfur remobilization from older leaves has been shown; however, the extent of its retranslocation appears to depend on the nitrogen status, at least in some systems (Marschner, 1995). Sunarpi & Anderson (1997) demonstrated the remobilization of both soluble (non protein) and insoluble (protein) sulfur from senescing leaves. This study also indicated that homoglutathione (containing β-alanine instead of glycine) is the principal export form of metabolized protein sulfur from senescing soybean leaves.

5.5 Potassium

Next to nitrogen, potassium is the mineral nutrient required in the largest amount by plants. It is highly mobile within individual cells, within tissues and in long-distance transport via the xylem and phloem (Marschner, 1995). In contrast to the nutrients discussed above, potassium is not metabolized, and it forms only weak complexes, in which it is easily exchangeable. Next to the transport of carbohydrates and nitrogen compounds, potassium transport has been studied most intensely, using both physiological and molecular approaches (Kochian, 2000). Many plant genes encoding K+ transporters have been identified, and some of them have been studied in detail in heterologous systems, such as K+-transport-deficient yeast mutants. Similarly to the situation discussed for nitrogen transport, analysis of K+ transport is complicated by the fact that these transporters are organized in multigene families with (partially?) redundant functions (Kochian, 2000). Potassium was repeatedly reported to be remobilized in significant quantities from senescing tissues (Hill *et al.*, 1979; Scott *et al.*, 1992; Tyler, 2005). However, it has to be considered that this element easily leaches from tissues, especially senescing tissues (Tukey, 1970; Debrunner & Feller, 1995). Therefore, actually remobilized potassium quantities may be smaller than those reported in the literature.

5.6 Phosphorus

Unlike carbon dioxide, nitrate and sulfate, phosphate (main form of P uptake) is not reduced, but utilized in its oxidized form by plants (Marschner, 1995), both in lowmolecular- weight metabolites and in macromolecules (nucleic acids). Studies on P remobilization from senescing leaves are scarce. Snapp and Lynch (1996) concluded that in maturing common bean plants, leaf P remobilization supplied more than half of the pod plus seed phosphorus. In contrast, Crafts-Brandner (1992) observed no net leaf P remobilization during reproductive growth of soybeans cultivated at three different P regimes. Therefore, while P is a mobile nutrient, its remobilization may be influenced by a number of exogenous and endogenous/genetic factors, making generalizations on the importance of its remobilization difficult. Nucleic acids (especially RNA) constitute a major phosphorus store but, depending on the species and growth condition investigated, considerable P amounts are also present in lipids, in esterified (organic) form, and as inorganic phosphate (Hart & Jessop, 1984; Valenzuela *et al.*, 1996). Similarly to the situation with nitrogen 'bound' in proteins, release of phosphorus from nucleic acids depends on the activities of hydrolytic enzymes. A decrease in nucleic acid levels is typical for senescing tissues, and increases in nuclease activities have also been observed (Feller and Fischer, 1994; Lers *et al.*, 2001), indicating that if P is remobilized from senescing tissues, at least part of it is derived from the degradation of RNA and DNA.

5.7 Magnesium, calcium and micronutrients

Magnesium has not often been considered in studies on nutrient remobilization. However, despite the fact that this element is considered phloem mobile (Marschner, 1995), available results indicate a tendency of continued accumulation during leaf senescence (Killingbeck, 2004). Unsurprisingly, calcium, which is the least mobile of all macronutrients (Marschner, 1995), has repeatedly been found to increase in senescing leaves (Killingbeck, 2004).

Information on remobilization of micronutrients does not allow a generalized picture. For several of them, including Fe, Cu, Mn (which is the least phloem mobile among the micronutrients) and Zn, both remobilization from and accumulation in senescing leaves have been reported (Killingbeck, 2004, and references cited therein). Tyler (2005) gives a broad overview of the fate of numerous elements (including the micronutrients Fe, B, Mn, Zn, Cu, Mo and Ni) during senescence and decomposition of *Fagus sylvatica* leaves; however, in view of the results cited above, it is probably not possible to generalize conclusions from this study, e.g. with regard to the situation in annual crops.

6. Conclusions

This paper discussed some results relating to nutrient remobilization during leaf senescence.Complex regulatory network controlling senescence in plants may be the result of selection pressure driven by different environmental stresses for the development of senescence.Focus on limited number of model plant systems studied by plant senescence scientists may be required for more efficient research, and is likely to be highly relevant to agriculture as well as to our basic understanding of the senescence process in plants.

7. References

[1] Crafts-Brandner, S.J. (1992).Phosphorus nutrition influence on leaf senescence in soybean. Plant Physiol 98, 1128–1132.

[2] Crafts-Brandner, S.J., Holzer, R. & Feller, U. (1998).Influence of nitrogen deficiency on senescence and the amounts of RNA and proteins in wheat leaves. Physiol Plantarum 102,192–200.

[3] Crawford, N.M., Kahn, M.L., Leustek, T. & Long, S.R. (2000). Nitrogen and sulfur in Biochemistry and Molecular Biology of Plants (Eds Buchanan, B., Gruissem, W.and Jones, R.).American Society of Plant Physiologists, Rockville, MD, pp.786–849.

[4] Diaz, C., Purdy, S., Christ, A., Morot-Gaudry, J.-F., Wingler, A. & Masclaux Daubresse, C. (2005). Characterization of markers to determine the extent and variability of leaf senescence in Arabidopsis. A metabolic profiling approach. Plant Physiol 138,898–908.

[5] Debrunner, N. & Feller, U. (1995).Solute leakage from detached plant parts of winter wheat: Influence of maturation stage and incubation temperature. J Plant Physiol 145,257–260.

[6] Feller, U. & Fischer, A. (1994). Nitrogen metabolism in senescing leaves. Crit Rev Plant Sci 13(3), 241–273.

[7] Gastal, F. & Lemaire, G.(2002). N uptake and distribution in crops: an agronomical and ecophysio- Logical perspective. J Exp Bot 53(370), 789–799.

[8] Gepstein, S. (1988).Photosynthesis. In: Senescence and Aging in Plants (edsNood´ en, L.D.and Leopold, A.C.).Academic Press, SanDiego, CA, pp.85–109.

[9] Good, A.G., Shrawat, A. K. & Muench, D.G. (2004).Can less yield more? Is reducing nutrient in put into the environment compatible with maintaining crop production? Trends Plant Sci 9 (12), 597–605.

[10] Graham, I.A., Leaver, C.J. & Smiths. (1992).Induction of malate synthase gene expression in Senescent and detached organs of cucumber. Plant Cell 4,349-357.

[11] Gut, H. & Matile, P. (1989).Break down of galactolipids in senescent barley leaves. Bot Acta 102, 31–36.

[12] Gut, H.& Matile, P. (1988). Apparent induction of key enzymes of the glyoxylic acid cycle in senescent barley leaves. Planta 176,548–550.

[13] Hart, A. L. & Jessop, D.(1984).Leaf phosphorus fractionation and growth responses to phosphorus of the forage legumes *Trifolium repens, T.dubium* and *Lotus pedunculatus*. Physiol Plant 61, 435–440.

[14] Hayati, R., Egli, D.B. & Crafts-Brandner, S.J. (1995).Carbon and nitrogen supply during seed filling and leaf senescence in soybean. Crop Sci 35, 1063–1069.

[15] He, Y. & Gan, S. (2002).Agene encoding anacyl hydrolase is involved in leaf senescence in Arabidopsis. Plant Cell 14,805–815.

[16] Hensel, L.L., Nelson, M.A., Richmond, T.A. & Bleecker, A.B. (1994). The fate of inflorescence meristems is controlled by developing fruits in Arabidopsis. Plant Physiol 106,863–876.

[17] Hill, J., Robson, A.D.and Loneragan, J.F. (1979) .The effect of copper supply on the senescence and the retranslocation of nutrients of the oldest leaf of wheat. Ann Bot 44,279–287.

[18] Ishimaru, K., Kosone, M.,Sasaki, H.and Kashiwagi,T.(2004).Leaf contents differ depending on the position in a rice leaf sheath during sink-source transition. Plant Physiol Biochem 42,855- 860.

[19] Jeong,M.L.,Jiang,H.,Chen,H.-S.,Tsai,C.-J.andHarding,S.A.(2004)Metabolic profiling of the sink-to-source transition in developing leaves of quaking aspen. Plant Physiol 136, 3364–3375.

[20] Kilian, A., Stiff, C. & Kleinhofs,A.(1995) . Barley telomerees shorten during differentiation but grow in callus culture. Proc Natl Acad Sci U SA 92, 9555–9559.

[21] Killing beck, K.T. (2004) .Nutrient resorption.In: Plant Cell Death Processes (ed.Nood´ en, L.D.). Elsevier Academic Press, Amsterdam, pp.215–226.

[22] Kochian, L.V. (2000) .Molecular physiology of mineral nutrient acquisition, transport, and utilization. In: Biochemistry and Molecular Biology of Plants (Eds Buchanan, B., Gruissem, W. & Jones, R.).American Society of Plant Physiologists, Rockville, MD, pp.1204–1249.

[23] Lers, A., Lomaniec, E., Burd, S.& Khalchitski,A.(2001).The characterization of LeNUC1,a Nuclease associated with leaf senescence of tomato. Physiol Plantarum, 112,176–182.

[24] Levey, S. & Wingler, A. (2005).Natural variation in the regulation of leaf senescence and relation to other traits in Arabidopsis. Plant Cell Environ 28,223–231.

[25] Lodwig , E.& Poole, P. (2003) Metabolism of Rhizobium bacteroids. Crit Rev Plant Sci 22, 37–78.

[26] Mae, T., Makino, A. & Ohira, K. (1983). Changes in the amounts of ribulose bisphosphate carboxylase synthesized and degraded during the life spanofrice leaf (Oryzasativa L.). Plant Cell Physiol 24(6), 1079–1086.

[27] Marschner, H.(1995) Mineral Nutrition of Higher Plants. Academic Press, London.

[28] Mc Laughlin, J.C. & Smith, S. M.(1994)Metabolic regulation of glyoxylate-cycle enzyme synthesis in detached cucumber cotyledons and protoplasts. Planta 195, 22–28.

[29] Nood´ en, L .D. Guiam, J.L. & John, I. (2004) .Whole plant senescence. In: Plant Cell Death Processes (Ed .Nood´ en, L.D.).Elsevier Academic Press, Amsterdam, pp .227–244.

[30] Otegui, M.S., Noh, Y.S., Martinez, D.E., et al. (2005)Senescence-associated vacuoles within tense Proteolytic activity develop in leaves of Arabidopsis and soybean. Plant J 41(6), 831–844.

[31] Parrott, D., Yang, L., Shama, L. & Fischer, A.M. (2005) .Senescence is accelerated, and several proteases are induced by carbon 'feast' conditions in barley (*Hordeum vulgare* L.) Leaves. Planta 222,989–1000.

[32] Peoples, M.B. & Dalling, M.J. (1988).The interplay between proteolysis and amino acid metabolism during senescence and nitrogen reallocation. In: Senescence and Aging in Plants (Eds Nooden, L.D. & Leopold, A.C.).Academic Press, San Diego, CA, pp.181–217.

[33] Pistelli, L., DeBellis, L. & Alpi, A. (1991) Peroxisomal enzyme activities in attached senescing leaves. Planta 184,151–153.

[34] Rennenberg, H. & Lamoureux, G.L. (1990). Physiological processes that modulate the concentration of glutathione in plant cells. In: Sulfur Nutrition and Sulfur Assimilation in Higher Plants (ed. Rennenberg, H.). XPB Academic PublishersB.V., The Hague, pp.53–65.

[35] Robson, P.R.H., Donnison, I.S. & Wang., et al. (2004).Leaf senescence is delayed in maize expressing the Agrobacterium IPT gene under the control of a novel maize senescence-enhanced promoter. Plant Biotechnol J 2,101–112.

[35] Roulin, S., Buchala, A.J.and Fincher, G.B. (2002). Induction of (1→3, 1→4)-β-D-glucan hydrolases in leave sofdark-incubated barley seedlings. Planta 215, 51–59.

[36] Scott, D.A., Proctor. & Thompson. (1992). Ecological studies on a low land ever green rainforest on Maraca island, Brazil.II: Litter and nutrient recycling. J Ecol 80,705–717.

[37] Snapp, S.S. & Lynch, J.P. (1996). Phosphorus distribution and remobilization in bean plants as influenced by phosphorus nutrition. Crop Sci 36,929–935.

[38] Sunarpi and Anderson, J.W. (1997) .Effect of nitrogen nutrition on remobilization of protein sulfur in the leaves of vegetative soybean and associated changes insoluble sulfur metabolites. Plant Physiol 115, 1671–1680.

[39] Tukey, H.B. (1970). The leaching of substances from plants. Annu Rev Plant Physiol 21,305–324.

[40] Tyler, G.(2005) . Changes in the concentrations of major, minor and rare-earth elements during leaf Senescence and decomposition in a *Fagus sylvatica* forest. Forest Ecol Manage 206,167–177.

[41] Yang,J.C.,Zhang,J.H.,Wang,Z.Q.,Zhu,Q.S.& Liu,L.J.(2003). Involvement of abscisic acid and Cytokinins in the senescence and remobilization of carbon reserves in wheat subjected to water Stress during grain filling. Plant Cell Environ 26,1621–1631.

[42] Valenzuela, J.L., Ruız, J.M., Belakbir, A. & Romero, L. (1996). Effects of nitrogen, phosphorus and potassium treatments on phosphorus fractions in melon plants. Commun Soil Sci Plant Anal 27(5–8), 1417–1425.

[43] Weng, X.-Y., Xu, H.-X. & Jiang, D.-A. (2005). Characteristics of gas exchange, chlorophyll fluorescence and expression of key enzymes in photosynthesis during leaf senescence in rice plants. J Integr Plant Biol 47(5), 560–566.

7

Advances in Plant Senescence

Kieron D. Edwards,
Matt Humphry and Juan Pablo Sanchez-Tamburrino
Advanced Technologies (Cambridge) Ltd.
UK

1. Introduction

Senescence is an integral component of a plant's lifecycle, which refers to changes that take place as the plant matures. A general distinction between plant senescence and animal senescence is the events observed in the animal kingdom typically steer growth while plant senescence orchestrates a massive shutdown or coordinated cell death in response to various stimuli designed to facilitate survival of the plant itself or the plant species.

In order to assist in the survival of the plant species, a sequence of tightly regulated genetic events efficiently governs a plant's death. These events are observable in a variety of plant models and in the different plant parts such as leaves, petals, reproductive organs (stamens and style), root cap, cortex and germinating seed. Leaf senescence will be the primary focus of this chapter.

A popular aspect of leaf senescence is the bright hues that can be observed on trees and plants during Autumn. The brilliant burst of colour that precedes the browning of leaves is an indication of active metabolic changes that result in the recycling or redistribution of nutrients to other parts of the plant. Evidence indicates the primary purpose of senescence in plants is for mobilization and recycling, a phenomenon that has tremendous implications for crop growth and food production.

Senescence marks the final phase of a leaf's development thereby launching degradation processes integral to the recycling and redistribution of the leaf's nutrients. Plant growth regulators, reproduction, cellular differentiation and hormone levels are internal factors that influence senescence (Thomas and Stoddart 1980; Smart 1994). Environmental stress also influences growth and can promote premature senescence. Certain parts of the plant may be sacrificed to enhance the chances of survival for the rest of the plant. Environmental cues include stress factors that adversely affect plant development and productivity; such as: drought, waterlogging, high or low solar radiation, extreme temperatures, ozone and other air pollutants, excessive soil salinity and inadequate mineral nutrition in the soil (Thomas and Stoddart 1980; Smart 1994). These environmental cues may accelerate leaf senescence by affecting the endogenous factors previously mentioned (Alegre and Munné-Bosch, 2004). Regardless of the trigger, the endogenous and exogenous signals that induce senescence appear to be coordinated through a common signalling network (Hopkins, 2007) involving the signalling molecules ethylene, jasmonic acid (JA), salicylic acid (SA) and Abscisic Acid (ABA) (Smart, 1994; Buchanan-Wollaston et al., 2005; van der Graaff et al., 2006)

2. Progress of senescence in plants

The general purpose of a leaf is to gather and generate nutrients for the plant. As a green leaf grows and develops, it creates an organ packed with nutrients. When the plant no longer requires the leaf, the senescence process is induced and recycling of all the nutrients that can be remobilized occurs. Leaf death is the final stage in the process; however, death is actively delayed until all nutrients have been removed.

The dismantling of the leaf begins with the chloroplasts, the energy-generating, photosynthetic powerhouse of the plant. Not unlike another energy generating organelle (ie, the mitochondria), chloroplasts are semiautonomous and they possess their own genome with its inherent transcriptional and translational machinery. Gradually the chloroplasts shrink and transform into gerontoplasts, an artefact characterised by the disintegration of the thylakoid membranes and accumulation of the plastoglobulin (Friedrich and Huffaker, 1980; Mae et al., 1984). The process of breaking down the chlorophyll is so pronounced that chlorophyll loss and the associated yellowing of the leaves are commonly used as indicators of plant senescence (Noodén et al., 1997). Control of the process is so tightly regulated that experiments demonstrating the reversibility of senescence have shown that the chloroplasts can recover structural features, re-synthesize chloroplast proteins and re-commence photosynthesis (Thomas and Donnison, 2000; Zavaleta-Mancera et al., 1999).

Degradation and remobilization of the chloroplast proteins and RNA contribute nitrogen and other nutrients for seed growth (Wittenbach, 1978). The mechanisms governing degradation of the chloroplast are not completely understood and there are competing theories about where proteins are degraded; for example they may be degraded locally within the chloroplast or in a centralized vacuole for degradation (Hortensteiner and Feller, 2002). Findings that support the possibility that the photosynthetic machinery is degraded *in situ* by the chloroplast include the presence of chloroplast enzymes, which are localized hydrolases that catalyze the initial steps of chlorophyll breakdown. (Hortensteiner, 2006). Proteases of the Clp, FtsH and DegP families are also expressed in chloroplasts and representative genes for these proteases are up-regulated in senescing leaves (Sokolenko et al., 1998; Nakabayashi et al., 1999; Itzhaki et al., 1998; Haussühl et al., 2001). Despite this observation, chloroplastic proteases are unlikely to account for the degradation of most photosynthetic proteins (eg, Rubisco) during senescence. Senescence-associated vacuoles, with strong proteolytic activity, have been identified in senescing tissue and likely also contribute towards the degradation of soluble photosynthetic proteins (Hensell et al., 1993; Comai et al., 1989).

Chloroplast degradation is followed by lipid, protein and nucleic acid degradation. Membrane integrity and cellular compartmentalisation are maintained until the latter stages of leaf senescence (Lohman et al., 1994; Smart, 1994; Pruzinska et al., 2005). A decline in photosynthesis during senescence may result in sugar starvation leading to the activation of conversion of lipids to sugars. Thylakoid breakdown leads to release of lipids, which are known to be converted to sugars through the glycoxylate cycle (Buchanan-Wollaston and Ainsworth, 1997; Kim and Smith, 1994). The sugars produced by conversion of large amounts of lipids may be in excess to that required for respiration of the senescing leaves and this excess may be exported to other growing and demanding parts of the plant. It appears that the expression of genes for the enzymes participating in the process of gluconeogenesis for production of sucrose play an important role during senescence as the genes responsible for synthesis of the enzymes involved in gluconeogenesis are reported to be significantly expressed during this time (Buchanan-Wollaston and Ainsworth 1997; Kim and Smith, 1994).

Leaf senescence also results in the breakdown of nucleic acids to purines and pyrimidines, which ultimately degrade to small and transportable carbon and nitrogenous compounds that are transported to growing parts of the plant (Buchanan-Wollaston and Ainsworth, 1997). In addition to mobilization of carbon and nitrogen, other nutrients like sulphur and metallic ions are also known to be transported from senescing leaves. Sugar content can also be modified at the onset of senescence. Generally crops under a limited nitrogen nutrition and high light regimen undergo early senescence and this is usually accompanied by an incremental rise of sugar levels in the leaves. Sugar has been suggested to trigger a senescence response based on gain or loss function experiments with hexokinase genes, principal regulators of a glucose signalling pathway (van Doorn, 2008).

3. Regulation of senescence and potential for biotechnology

Before the advent of modern biotechnology, which enabled scientists to commence deciphering the relationship between genes and life, senescence was perceived as an uncoordinated collection of events resulting in the metabolic and physiological changes to plant organs described above. The study of plant genetics, genomics, proteomics and more recently metabolomics have altered this perception and demonstrated that the process is dynamic and well organised. Below, a few examples are provided to emphasize the importance of a better understanding of plant senescence and the consequent potential of applications derived from that understanding.

Several techniques and different plant models have been employed in the pursuit of understanding the genetic mechanisms underlying the changes in gene expression associated with senescence. The process of senescence is initiated in source tissues prompting dramatic changes in gene expression, during which genes involved in basic metabolism, including photosynthesis and protein biosynthesis, are down-regulated while those involved in programmed cell death and stress response and/or encoding various hydrolytic enzymes are up-regulated (Hopkins et al., 2007; Lim et al., 2007). Not surprisingly the initial discoveries involving Senescence Associated Genes (SAGs) were made in the model plant Arabidopsis (*Arabidopsis thaliana*) by methods including differential display (Lohman et al. 1994), senescence-specific enhancer trap line screening using a range of senescence promoting factors (He et al., 2001), subtractive hybridization (Gepstein et al., 2003) and microarray experiments (Andersson et al., 2004). Many of the genes expressed during senescence of tissues encode hydrolytic enzymes that are capable of disassembling the ultra-structure of the cell and the breakdown of macromolecules (Smart, 1994; Griffith et al., 1997; Watanabe et al., 1994). In addition, a large number of transcription factors, as well as genes encoding carbohydrate and nitrogen-mobilising enzymes, nucleases and stress-responsive proteins, have been found to exhibit increased expression in senescing leaves (Buchanan-Wollaston and Ainsworth, 1997; Comai et al., 1989; Kim and Smith, 1994). The gene expression changes and biological processes that are up- and down-regulated during senescence as indicated by such studies, have been reviewed elsewhere (Guo and Gan, 2005), so will only be touched on in this review. What is more in the scope of this review are the potential implications that senescence has for plant biotechnological applications.

In addition to the conventional use of crops as food sources, innovations continue to expand the role of crop species in society. With these changes, the importance of understanding senescence becomes even more significant. Crops and trees are being developed as an alternative fuel source. Plants are also being integrated into the production of pharmaceutical ingredients and complex protein therapies such as vaccines (Lossl and Waheed, 2011). These and other innovative uses for plants make obtaining a greater understanding of senescence a necessary step for harnessing the influence of senescence on the plant lifecycle and reducing the impact this has on product yields and stability. The SAGs found through Arabidopsis investigations have provided a reference point for studies in other plant species, providing the potential to translate fundamental understanding into applied tools. Delaying the onset of senescence could increase the production of the desired plant product. This may be of particular interest in plastid expression systems (reviewed in Day and Goldschmidt., 2010), given that the chloroplast degradation occurs at a relatively early stage of senescence.

3.1 *Populus tremula* and bio fuel

As suggested above, crops are being developed for alternative applications including bio fuels and paper production. The deciduous Aspen tree species *Populus tremula* is one such plant being developed for alternative fuel production. By comparing expressed sequence tag (EST) libraries generated from young fully-expanded leaves to leaves harvested immediately prior to visible signs of senescence, Bhalerao et al., (2003) identified *P. tremula* homologs for many known Arabidopsis SAGs. Altering the expression of these SAGs may have an effect on dormancy in this species with possible implications on the wood yield from these trees.

The onset of growth cessation and dormancy represents a critical ecological and evolutionary trade-off between survival and growth in most forest trees. Without this dormant stage nutrients stored in green leaves would be lost to frost, which would impact growth in the spring. Tight regulation over the timing of senescence is thus important. Latitudinal clines influence the critical photoperiod for onset of bud set (dormancy) and leaf senescence in Aspen (Fracheboud et al., 2009). This cline in dormancy was associated with multiple alleles of *PHYTOCHROME B2* (*PHYB2*), a photoreceptor that is related to light perception and light input to the circadian clock (the internal timing mechanism of the plant). The circadian clock enables the plant to co-ordinate its endogenous activities with the external environment to maximise the effectiveness of its activity. These activities occur on a daily basis, such as the timing of photosynthetic gene expression (Harmer et al., 2000, Edwards et al., 2006), and on an annual basis when measuring photoperiod and co-ordinating activities such as transitions to flowering, senescence or dormancy (reviewed in Jackson, 2009). Indeed, previous experiments suggest more accurate timing by the clock in relation to the external environmental cycles also has the potential to improve crop yields (Dodd et al., 2005). Such regulation governing the timing of critical events is relevant to all crop species grown in temperate climates. In the case of senescence, utilising regulatory mechanisms such as the circadian clock has the potential to alter the timing of this process with benefits to both wood production (reduced loss of nutrients to frost) as well as, for example, increasing the length of the grain filling period in other crops.

3.2 Impact on yield

During whole plant senescence, fixed carbon and nitrogen are mobilized to reproductive or storage organs, which are harvested for human consumption (Vierstra, 1996; Hopkins et al., 2007; Lim et al., 2007). The process of senescence impacts all crop species and so the increased understanding of the tight regulatory mechanisms that control the process could potentially have an immeasurable impact on the world's agricultural production. Whole plant senescence plays a key role in remobilizing and transferring nutrients into the vegetative tissue and eventually to grain. The grain filling period is a critical period because many processes can influence the final grain yield (Yang and Zhang, 2006). For example, delaying whole plant senescence can be achieved by heavy use of fertilizer or development of a stay-green phenotype produced using a genetic or transgenic strategy. Extending or delaying senescence is believed to augment the grain filling stage thereby increasing grain yield. Contrarily, stresses, such as drought, induce early senescence, prompting the reduction of photosynthesis and shortening the grain filling period (Gregerson et al., 2008) and thus having the opposite affect on yield. Ectopic expression of SAG101, a protein with acyl hydrolase activity, has been shown to cause precocious senescence in both attached and detached leaves of transgenic Arabidopsis plants (He and Gan, 2002). Antisense expression of the gene, resulting in repression of the endogenous genes expression, was shown to cause a delay in the onset of senescence (He and Gan, 2002). Utilising genes such as SAG 101 to induce a stay-green/delayed senescence phenotype could potentially be employed in biotechnological strategies to increase yields in crops such as wheat.

Effective recycling of nutrients could have a massive impact on crop yields. Recycling of carbon and nitrogen during senescence involves the sequestering of cytoplasm and organelles into special autophagic vesicles. These vesicles deliver their contents to the vacuole (or lysosome) for breakdown by localized hydrolases (Thompson and Vierstra, 2005; Bassham, 2007). The breakdown products are either consumed by the host cell or transported to other tissues and organs. Under normal growth conditions, autophagy takes place at a basal level. The process ramps up in response to nutritional demand, biotic or abiotic stresses, and senescence. Autophagy plays an important role in the proper recycling of nutrients especially as a plant scavenges available nutrients from storage tissues and older senescing leaves.

When a pathway has been highly conserved evolutionarily, other organisms can provide the reference point for understanding a system in plants. The genes associated with autophagy discovered in yeast, enabled investigators to identify homologous genes in Arabidopsis and, subsequently, in rice and maize. Genome searches of Arabidopsis identified a collection of proteins structurally and functionally related to many of the ATG components present in yeast (Thompson and Vierstra, 2005; Bassham, 2007). In an effort to determine the importance of autophagy to crop plants, investigators at the University of Wisconsin, using the Arabidopsis as a reference, described a collection of components that participate in the ATG8/12 conjugation cascades in both rice (*Oryza sativa*) and maize (*Zea mays*). Remarkably, all components required for ATG8/12 conjugation in yeast and Arabidopsis (Ohsumi, 2001; Thompson and Vierstra, 2005) were identified in both rice and maize suggesting that the pathway is highly conserved. The group went on to greater characterize the expression of the maize ATG genes (Chung et al., 2009). The investigators observed an increase in ATG transcripts during leaf senescence and under nitrogen and fixed-carbon limiting conditions. The results indicate that the highly conserved process of autophagy plays a key role in nutrient remobilization with some variations unique to maize. The description of the maize ATG system provides a set of molecular and biochemical tools to study autophagy in this crop under field conditions (Chung et al., 2009). The same is true for rice (Ohsumi, 2001; Thompson and Vierstra, 2005). This type of knowledge may help to reveal important control points in autophagy that could be manipulated in both food and bio fuel crops to enhance nutrient use efficiency or to better allocate carbon and nitrogen to specific organs for improved yield.

In addition to highly conserved genes, specific genes or gene families that can also be employed to influence grain quality and yield. Uauy et. al., (2006) cloned a Quantitative Trait Locus (QTL) associated with increased grain protein, zinc, and iron content known as Gpc-B1. The ancestral wild wheat allele encodes a functional NAC transcription factor (NAM-B1) that accelerates senescence and increases nutrient remobilization from leaves to developing grains. In contrast, modern wheat varieties carry a non-functional NAM-B1 allele. Reduction in RNA levels of the multiple NAM homologues by RNA interference delayed senescence by more than three weeks and reduced wheat grain protein, zinc, and iron content by more than 30%. Other examples of specific genes having an effect in senescence include the cytokinin synthesis gene IPT, which has been shown to delay leaf senescence (Gan and Amasino, 1995), thereby providing the potential to increase seed setting time and yield, but the affect this has on nutritional value must also be considered.

3.3 Ripening

Although the main focus of this review relates to leaf senescence, fruit ripening is an aspect of plant senescence that is also of global significance. The timing of ripening is a key consideration when harvesting and transporting fruit to market. Successful efforts to control fruit ripening are based on either reducing the biosynthesis of the plant hormone ethylene or slowing down the rate of fruit softening by targeting the genes involved in cell wall modification (Causier et al., 2002). The Flavr Savr tomato is an example of an early attempt to slow ripening using the latter strategy. Researchers at Calgene hoped to slow the ripening process of the tomato by engineering in an antisense gene to interfere with production of the enzyme polygalacturonase (Weasel, 2009). The enzyme normally degrades pectin in the cell walls and results in softening.

More recently, investigators have attempted to characterize the N-glycan processing enzymes and their role in during non-climacteric fruit softening. The plant hormone ethylene does not influence ripening of non climacteric fruits and different genes need to be targeted for the different categories of fruits (Causier et al., 2002). Two ripening-specific N-glycan processing enzymes, α-mannosidase (α-Man) and β-D-N-acetylhexosaminidase were identified in the fruit capsicum (*Capsicum annuum*, Ghosh et al., 2010). Using RNA interference to suppress production of such enzymes has the potential to improve the shelf life of fruits, with obvious implications for improved food stability/storage.

4. A view on tobacco biotechnology and senescence

Tobacco is different from many of the crops discussed above because the organ harvested for human use is the leaf rather than reproductive organs (i.e. seed and fruit). The smoke generated during the burning of tobacco is a complex mixture of thousands of chemicals (Rodgman and Perfetti, 2008). Research to identify and characterise the harmful components present in tobacco smoke is ongoing, with lists such as the 44 Hoffmann analytes, being produced by researchers and public health organisations (Hoffmann and Wynder 1967; Baker, 1999; Norman, 1999; Borgerding and Klus, 2005). A major focus of tobacco research is related to lowering the levels of these chemicals from smoke in an effort to reduce the harmful effects associated with tobacco use (for an overview of such research the scientific website of British American Tobacco [BAT] n.d.). Understanding the regulation and effect of senescence on tobacco leaf chemistry could be of particular importance to these traits since it is following the onset of senescence that 'ripe' tobacco leaves are harvested.

4.1 Gene expression changes in senescing tobacco leaves

The availability of microarrays has considerably increased the extent to which differentially expressed genes can be identified and this line of research provides valuable insights into the identification of senescence related genes. High throughput analysis makes it possible to monitor changes in gene expression throughout the lifecycle of a plant. Researchers from Advanced Technologies (Cambridge) have recently described the generation of a tobacco (*Nicotiana tabacum*) custom expression array (Edwards et al., 2010). This array was used to develop the Tobacco Expression Atlas (TobEA), a map of gene expression from multiple tissues sampled throughout the life cycle of the tobacco plant which can be used as a reference data set for plant researchers. The expression data is freely available via the Solanaceae Genomics Network (SGN), a web based genomic resource for plants of the Solanaceae family (Mueller et al., 2005). Studying the changes in gene expression has the potential to identify targets that enable modifications or changes to leaf constituents in tobacco using transgenic or non-transgenic (e.g. molecular breeding) approaches.

Included in the TobEA study was a set of leaves from different positions that were categorised into either green (sink) or four distinct senescent (source) leaves, based on the average amount of yellowing and chlorosis across the leaf (Figure 1A; data not shown). Analysis of the gene expression changes in the tobacco leaf series suggested that tobacco showed similar changes during the progression of senescence as Arabidopsis leaves. For example the defence-associated phytohormone SA is known to play a role in developmental leaf senescence in Arabidopsis, with mutants and transgenic lines defective in the SA-mediated signalling pathway exhibiting delayed senescence (Buchanan-Wollaston et al., 2005; Morris et al., 2000). A significant over-representation of genes associated with systemic acquired resistance and the SA-mediated signalling pathway was observed in the up-regulated genes in the TobEA dataset, including presumptive orthologues of *ENHANCED SUSCEPTIBILITY 1* (*EDS1*) and *PHYTOALEXIN DEFICIENT 4* (*PAD4*), central regulators of SA-mediated defence (Figures 1H and I; Feys et al., 2005; Morris et al., 2000).

There was also significant over-representation of Gene Ontology categories associated with defence against fungal pathogens as well as cell death and innate immune responses in leaves at more advanced stages of senescence. These included a homologue of the Arabidopsis basic chitinase *PR3* (Verburg and Huynh 1991) in addition to other components of plant immunity/defence. This supports the growing evidence that pathogen defence and senescence share common components (Quirino et al., 1999; Feys et al., 2005), presumably largely via the use of similar signalling pathways leading to accumulation of reactive oxygen species and cell death (Yoshida, 2003).

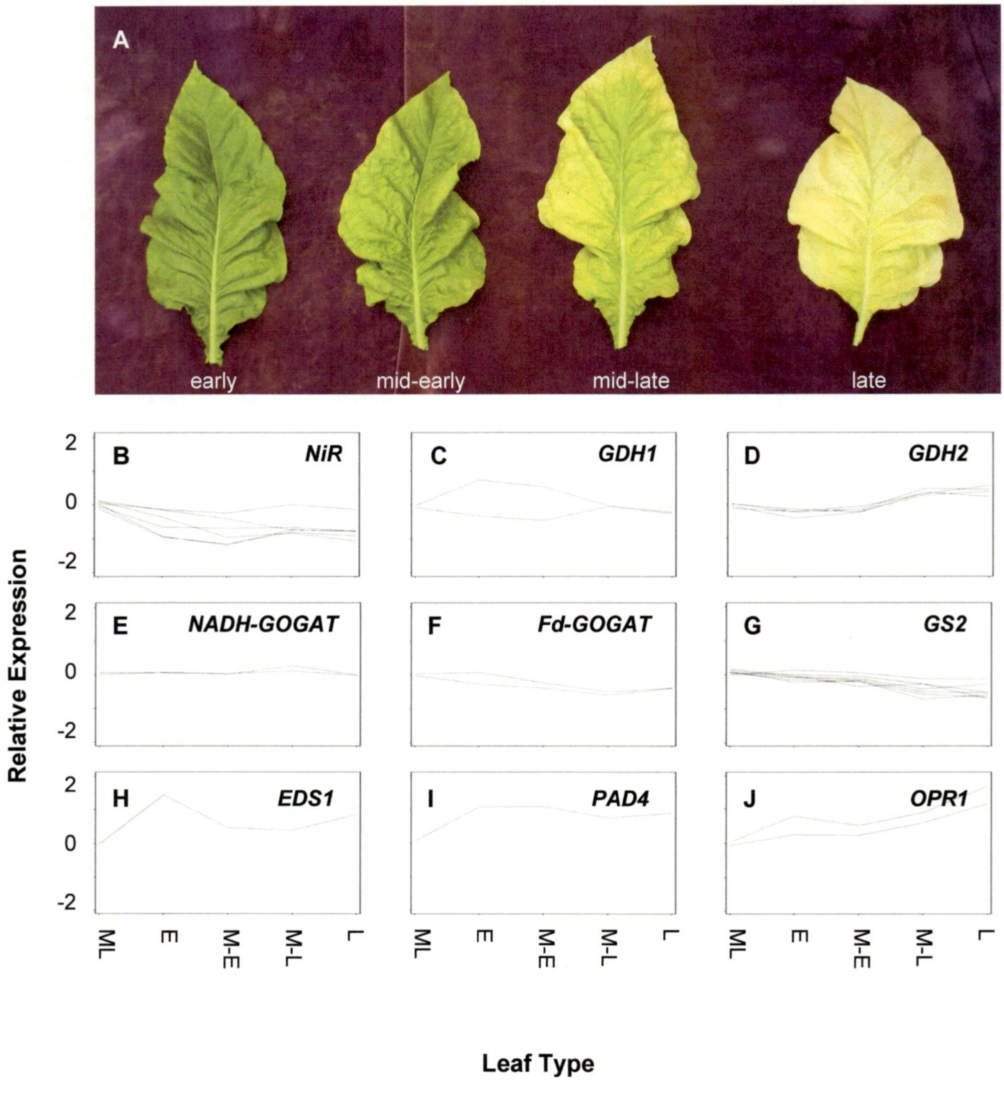

Fig. 1. Gene expression changes in tobacco source and sink leaves
(A) A sink to source series of leaves harvested from different positions on tobacco plants included in the Tobacco Expression Atlas and categorised as early- (E), mid-early- (M-E), mid-late- (M-L) and late- (L) senescent leaves based on level of Chlorosis (TobEA; Edwards et al., 2010). (B-J) Log expression data for selected transcripts associated with Nitrogen metabolism and plant hormone responses shown (See top right of each plot for transcript identification). Expression data was pre-processed with RMA and normalised against mature leaf (ML) samples showing no visible signs of senescence (also included in the TobEA data set). Differentially expressed genes from the sink-source series versus the mature leaf control were identified by one-way analysis of variance with Tukey HSD post hoc testing in GeneSpring GX 10 ($P < 0.05$). Gene ontology analysis of the up- and down-regulated genes in each condition (described in main text) were analysed by a custom script as described previously (Edwards et. al., 2010).

In addition to SA, several other hormone pathways were identified as being over-represented in the TobEA leaf senescence dataset including Jasmonic acid (JA). JA is known to have a role in developmental senescence, with both levels of JA itself and a number of JA biosynthetic genes found to increase during senescence (He et al., 2002). A similar response was observed in the developmental senescence dataset, with *12-OXOPHYTODIENOATE REDUCTASE* (*OPR*) family members being induced and an overall over-representation of genes involved in JA-meditated induced systemic resistance (Figure 1J; data not shown).

Ethylene is also known to play a role in promoting the onset of senescence (Grbic and Bleecker, 1995). Interestingly however, ethylene-mediated responses were not significantly over-represented in the TobEA data, suggesting that either ethylene is not as important in senescence of tobacco or that changes in this pathway are occurring post-transcriptionally. Stress can induce a senescence response in plants and one of the principal mediators of the stress response is the phyto-hormone Abscisic Acid or ABA (Smart 1994). ABA is a participant in drought (water) and cold stress responses (Wingler and Roitsch, 2008) and directly influences the sugar accumulation in response to stress. Interestingly, ABA will induce senescence during drought stress whereas it will delay senescence during cold stress (Xue -Xuan et al., 2010). In the TobEA data the ABA metabolic processes were significantly reduced late in senescence, the reason for which is unknown (data not shown).

Cytokinin levels in senescing leaves are though to play a key role in developmental leaf senescence, with both external and endogenous application resulting in delayed senescence (Smart 1994). This is largely reflected in the transcriptional responses to developmental senescence in Arabidopsis (Buchanan-Wollaston et al., 2005), as well as in the TobEA data, where cytokinin response processes were significantly down-regulated compared to controls.

Interestingly, phenylpropanoid biosynthesis was identified as a significantly down-regulated process the TobEA data. It would be expected that increased production of photo-protective phenylpropanoids, flavonoids in particular, would be observed during developmental leaf senescence, due to increased light stress during the degradation of chlorophyll (Buchanan-Wollaston 2005). Indeed, Buchanan-Wollaston et al., (2005) found a number of flavonoid biosynthesis genes had increased expression during developmental senescence.

Consistent with the phenotypic observations of the leaves themselves (Figure 1A), there was an enrichment of genes associated with photosynthesis being down-regulated in the TobEA data. This was accompanied by significant number of down-regulated genes associated with chloroplast components as well as responses to red, far-red and ultraviolet light stimuli. Over all the data suggest that similar processes occur during leaf senescence in Tobacco as in Arabidopsis and highlights the potential to translate findings in model species to biotechnological applications in other crops including Tobacco.

4.2 Nitrogen metabolism and harm reduction

Environmental and economic issues combined have increased the need to better understand the role and fate of nitrogen in crop production systems. Nitrogen is one of the most important nutrients recycled by the plant during senescence, with up to 90% recovered from the leaf during this process (reviewed in Liu et al., 2008). Adding nitrogen to the soil increases crop yields and delays senescence, whereas a reduced fertilizer regimen generally triggers early whole plant senescence in crops due to low nitrogen. A strong coordination of nitrogen-uptake, assimilation and remobilization is required for a beneficial grain filling stage (Hortensteiner and Feller 2002). The period that follows flowering can be critical in this process. Some crops, such as maize (C4 photosynthesis), use Nitrogen sourced both from the root's uptake and assimilation of NO_3- as well as nitrogen remobilized during leaf senescence. Other crops, such as oil seed rape, primarily rely on the remobilization of nitrogen from leaves, making these crops more dependent on the senescence process (Coque et. al., 2008). When nitrogen inputs to the soil system exceed crop needs, there is a possibility that excessive amounts of nitrate (NO_3^-) may enter either ground or surface water causing a detrimental effect on the environment.

In the case of tobacco, a greater understanding of the metabolism of nitrogen could also be applicable in an attempt to reduce the harmful constituents contained in cigarettes. One class of chemicals likely to feature in any future legislation of the tobacco industry is the Tobacco Specific Nitrosamines (TSNAs); 4-(N-methlynitrosamino)-1-(3-pyridyl)-1-butanone (NNK), N-nitrosonornicotine (NNN), N-nitrosoanabasine (NAB) and N-nitrosoanatabine (NAT).

TSNAs are principally formed by the nitrosation of tobacco alkaloids during the curing (drying) of tobacco leaf (Burton et al., 1989; Burton et al., 1994; Hoffmann et al., 1994; Spiegelhalder and Bartsch, 1996). Several studies have demonstrated a significant correlation between nitrite (formed by the microbial reduction of nitrate during curing) and TSNA levels in tobacco leaf, leading to the proposal of nitrite as the key nitrosating agent for TSNA formation (Burton et al., 1989; Fischer et al., 1989; Burton et al., 1994; Spiegelhalder and Bartsch, 1996; Wu et al., 2005). Curing conditions (including airflow, temperature and humidity) and their affect on microbial activity have been shown to affect the levels of TSNAs formed (Burton et al., 1989; Burton et al., 1994). Further understanding the nitrogen metabolism of tobacco could aid in reducing the potential for accumulating nitrosating agents during the curing process helping to limit the formation of TSNAs, and potentially reducing the levels of these toxicants in tobacco smoke.

Figure 2 shows a summary of the nitrogen assimilation pathway in plants. Plant nitrogen assimilation primarily occurs in mesophyll cells and involves the reduction of nitrate (taken up by the root) into ammonia by the enzymes—Nitrate Reductase (NR) and Nitrite Reductase (NiR; Figure 2). The ammonia is subsequently assimilated into the amino acids glutamine (gln) and glutamate (glu) via the cyclic action of Glutamine Synthetase (GS) and Glutamine-2-oxoglutarate aminotransferase (GOGAT; Figure 2; Lea and Miflin 1974).

Nitrogen assimilation is regulated by many factors, including the availability of sugars and other metabolites and also shows significant variation over the diurnal cycle (reviewed in Stitt et. al., 2002). The expression and activity of genes involved in nitrogen reduction and assimilation have previously been shown to be down-regulated in tobacco leaves at more advanced stages of senescence (Mascluax et. al., 2000). Masclaux et. al, compared leaves from different positions on mature tobacco plants and showed that there was a switch between nitrogen assimilation and nitrogen recycling from sink to source leaves at more advanced stages of senescence. The leaf series included in the TobEA microarray data set described above is similar to the leaf series tested by Masclaux et. al (Masclaux et. al 2000). Expression of nitrogen metabolism genes in the TobEA leaves compared with fully expanded mature leaves showing no visible signs of senescence (also included in the TobEA data), demonstrated consistent results with Masclaux et al., (2000; Figure 1).

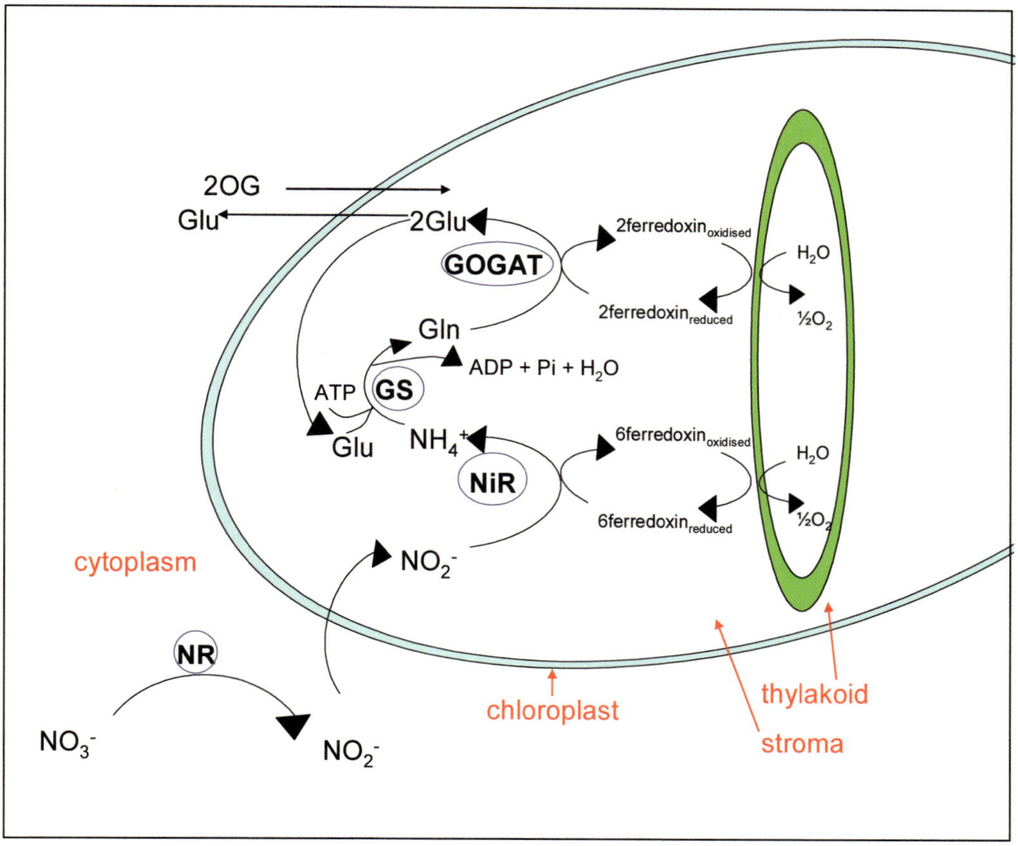

Fig. 2. Primary nitrogen assimilation in plants.
Representation of the primary nitrogen assimilation pathway in a mesophyll cell (modified from Mohr and Schopfer, 1994), showing reduction of Nitrate to Nitrite and then Ammonia by NR and NiR respectively and subsequent incorporation of nitrogen into gln and glu by the cyclic activity of the enzymes GS and GOGAT.

No probe sets for NR could be identified on the tobacco array, so the reduction in expression of this gene shown by Masclaux et al., (2000) could not be confirmed in the TobEA data. However, a decrease in NiR expression over the leaf series was shown, supporting a reduction in nitrogen fixation activity in the older leaves (Figure 1B). The ammonia generated by NR and NiR activity is incorporated into amino acids by the GS-GOGAT cycle. Plants have two types of GOGAT; ferredoxin dependent (Fd-GOGAT) and NADH dependent (NADH-GOGAT). Similarly *GS* genes can be subdivided into cytosolic and plastidic forms (*GS1* and *GS2* respectively). Fd-GOGAT functions in concert with GS2 and NADH-GOGAT is associated with GS1. In previous studies (Buchanan Wollaston 2005, Lin and Wu 2004), GS1 and NADH-GOGAT have demonstrated a co-ordinated increase in expression in Arabidopsis. *GS1* expression was previously shown to be induced in tobacco source leaves, whereas *GS2* transcripts were shown to be down regulated (Masclaux et al., 2000). No tobacco orthologues for *GS1* were identified on the tobacco microarray and transcripts for *NADH-GOGAT* did not demonstrate changes in expression over the TobEA dataset (Figure 1D). However, consistent with previous results, *GS2* transcripts were down regulated over the series of leaves (Figure 1C). A similar pattern of expression was also shown by tobacco *Fd-GOGAT* transcripts, supporting the proposed coordinated regulation and activity for these genes and a reduction of chloroplastic nitrogen assimilation in source leaves (Figures 1C and E).

Glutamate dehydrogenase (GDH) catalyses a reversible reaction adding or removing amino groups from glutamate. It has been proposed that the principal role of GDH is the deamination of glutamate in order to maintain a homeostatic balance of this amino acid that is thought to play a key role in the cross talk between the carbon and nitrogen assimilation pathways (Labboun et al., 2009). It has also been suggested that GDH amination may play a role in replacing glutamine synthetase (GS) activity in nitrogen assimilation within source leaves, which is lost during senescence (Masclaux et al., 2000). Previous studies have shown an increase in *GDH* expression in source leaves (Masclaux et al., 2000). Consistent with this, tobacco *GDH2* orthologs did show an increase in expression over the series; however, little change was shown by *GDH1* (Figures 1F and G).

Changes in the expression of genes involved in nitrogen assimilation shown by the leaves suggested that nitrogen metabolism was altered in source leaves towards remobilisation of the nitrogen resources to sink leaves. Consistent with this, gene ontology analysis of clusters of genes showing up-regulation in leaves demonstrating more advanced senescence revealed over representation of genes with functions related to proteolysis, the proteosome and endoplasmic reticulum associated protein catabolism. Increased understanding of the regulation of senescence in tobacco leaves could potentially help to limit the content of nitrate (and other nitrosonating agents) in harvested leaves prior to curing. This may augment efforts to reduce the levels of TSNAs in tobacco smoke; however, the study of senescence also provides other tools to facilitate TSNA reduction.

The main focus of agricultural research has been towards increased yield along with other agronomic traits. It is apparent in some crops that this has led towards an ignorance of flavour and texture components (as well as the associated nutritional value). Research is currently ongoing to understand and ultimately adjust the metabolic content of crops, such as those found in tomato, that contribute towards flavour and nutrition. This orientation toward flavour highlights the realisation that a perceived consumer benefit and consumer acceptance is becoming a more important driver in the development of new crops (Klee 2010). As indicated above, tobacco crops can be cured by multiple methods and the resulting leaf, or grades are blended together to produce the constituents of a cigarette. Dependent on the design, air cured tobacco typically only constitutes up to 30% of the blend in a cigarette, the rest being mainly made up of flue cured leaf (see Davis and Nielsen 1999 for a description of tobacco agronomy and chemistry). The conditions during air curing can lead to the formation of high levels of TSNAs. Thus, removing such grades from the blend could have beneficial affect on the overall level of TSNAs in the product. However, air cured grades make a significant contribution to the overall flavour of the cigarette, so the resulting product may not be consumer relevant and thus have no impact on harm reduction efforts. Replacing air cured grades with other grades that replace the flavour characteristics of these grades, but without the inherent higher levels of TSNAs provides one potential solution.

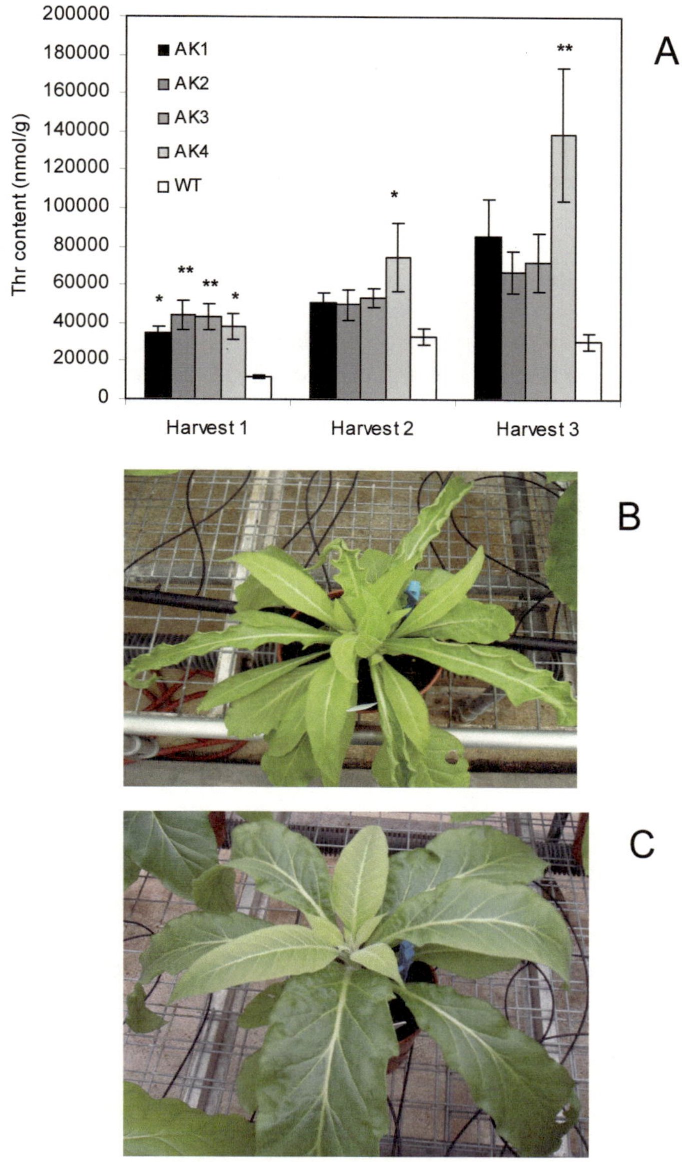

Fig. 3. Increased threonine production in tobacco leaves
Levels of threonine (nano moles per gram of cured leaf) for wild type tobacco and four independent transgenic tobacco lines expressing a mutated form of the Arabidopsis Aspartate Kinase AK:HSD (See inset key for line identification). Bars show mean threonine levels and error bars represent Standard Error of the mean. Leaves were taken from three harvest positions from the bottom to the top of the plant (Harvest 1 - 3). Asterisks represent significant difference between transgenic lines and WT for each harvest position based on one way analysis of variance with Tukey HSD post hoc testing (* $P < 0.005$, ** $P < 0.001$). Constitutive expression of the same gene results in increased threonine levels in tobacco leaves (data not shown), but results in reduced growth and altered morphology in (B) transgenic plants compared to (C) wild type plants.

Amongst other differences, air cured tobaccos tend to have lower levels of sugars and an altered balance of free amino acids compared to flue cured tobacco leaf (Davis and Nielsen 1999). Threonine (thr) is one of the amino acids observed in higher levels in air cured leaf compared to flue cured, indicating it may contribute towards the flavour and aroma of the tobacco. Within the leaf, the biosynthetic pathway leading to production of thr is tightly regulated by a negative feedback control loop. In the case of feedback inhibition the end-product, in this case thr, competitively inhibits the activity of the bifunctional enzyme ASPARTATE KINASE (AK) (EC 2.7.2.4) -HOMOSEREINE DESATURATE (HSD) (EC 1.1.1.3)– and consequently blocks the enzymatic processes leading to its own synthesis (Shaul and Galili,1993). Disabling the enzyme that switches off thr production would prompt a greater accumulation of the compound, but, if the accumulation takes place too early in the plant's life cycle, the fitness of the plant is severely compromised (Fig 3A: data not shown). To overcome this obstacle, the promoter of the senescence associated gene SAG12, identified in Arabidopsis (Lohman 1984), was used to drive expression of mutated forms of AK:HSD gene from Arabidopsis in tobacco. Elevated leaf thr levels were achieved in the modified plants without compromising the plant's fitness (Fig 3 B and C). If the increase in thr results in an increase of the air cured 'flavour' in the tobacco, then such an approach could provide the potential to reduce the amount of this tobacco in the blend resulting in an associated reduction in the TSNA levels.

Optimising the timing and absolute level of expression by selecting other senescence associated promoters from tobacco could help to increase the yield of thr present in harvested leaves. Such promoters, could also be used to up, or down regulate the synthesis of other target flavour or toxicant precursors at the correct stage in the plant's life cycle to maximise the target phenotype, with limited effect on the growth of the plant.

5. The translational nature of innovation

Nature has long been an infinite resource for the purpose of scientific discovery. Consequently, the study of plant senescence possesses immeasurable potential for increasing the understanding of the plant kingdom and the technological application of that knowledge. Genomics and the subsequent disciplines of proteomics and metabolomics have provided a complete reorientation toward the ways in which plants are designed to facilitate preservation of their own species. Thousands of genes that increase expression during leaf senescence have been isolated from a number of crop varieties; such as: Arabidopsis, wheat, tomato, maize, rice, and tobacco; these are just the tip of the iceberg.

Many of the recent advances in the understanding of plants (and organisms in general) can be attributed to the exponential increase in the sequencing and bioinformatics capacity of the world's research communities, coupled with numerous initiatives being driven by governments, academics and the private sector. Advances in gene sequencing techniques have made it possible to decipher entire genomes and high throughput microarray analysis and other techniques make it possible to monitor changes in a plant over time. By comparing what genes are switched on and off as a plant senesces, a collection of SAGs have already been discovered. Tracing the homology of conserved sequences through the evolutionary line, not only has facilitated the discovery of more SAGs, it has helped to elucidate the dynamics of an entire senescence-associated biosynthetic pathways such as ATG8/12. Comparative studies between species not only reveal similarities, researchers inevitably find unique differences specific to the plant variety and species contributing even more information to the pool.

Alternatively, Biotechnological tools (i.e. gene vectors) and progressive strategies, such as molecular breeding, make it possible to apply research findings to addressing modern challenges. For example, an understanding of the tight regulation of senescence can be applied to modify the grain filling stage in an appropriate plant organism in order to increase the grain yield (harvest index). Altering the senescence stage to enhance remobilization or delay senescence through stay-green strategies (the most successful approaches being enhancing endogenous cytokine pathways and reducing ethylene production or perception) has become a routine approach to increasing productivity (Gan and Amasino 1995). Similarly senescence promoters and pathways have already been used to augment the flavour and deter the spoilage of products such as tomatoes and augment the nutrition of wheat.

Development of transcriptional data-sets such as the one we describe in tobacco will continue to facilitate discovery and drive innovation. Understanding how plants use nitrogen could potentially lead to improving nitrogen strategies that increase productivity of the plant and enhance the sustainability of farming. In the case of tobacco, knowledge of senescence and nitrogen metabolism is being applied to altering the leaf to decrease the level of target chemicals found in tobacco smoke. The extent to which plant genome initiatives are being undertaken by governments, academics and industrial partners will serve to ensure that genomics and the related branches of research will continue to contribute new tools, including genes and pathways that can regulate senescence and applications that promise to have an impact on modern society.

6. Acknowledgement

We would like to acknowledge Susie Davenport and Gwendoline Leach for the provision of data and Barbara Nasto for assistance with the writing/editing of this manuscript.

7. References

Alegre, H., & Munné-Bosch S. (2004). Drought-induced changes in flavonoids and other low molecular weight antioxidants in *Cistus clusii* grown under Mediterranean field conditions, *Tree Physiology,* 24(11) pp 1303-1311

Andersson, A., Keskitalo, J., Sjödin, A., Bhalerao, R., Sterky, F., Wissel, K., Tandre, K., Aspeborg, H., Moyle, R., Ohmiya, Y., Bhalerao, R., Brunner, A., Gustafsson, P., Karlsson, J., Lundeberg, J., Nilsson, O., Sandberg, G., Strauss, S., Sundberg, B., Uhlen, M., Jansson, S., & Nilsson, P. (2004) A transcriptional timetable of autumn senescence, *Genome Biology,* 5: R24

Baker, R. R. (1999) Smoke chemistry, In: *Tobacco Producton, Chemistry and Technology,* Davis D L & Nielsen M. T., pp. 398-439, Blackwell Science Ltd., ISBN 0-632-04791-7, Oxford

Bassham, D. C. (2007) Plant autophagy--more than a starvation response, *Current Opinion in Plant Biology,* 10(6) pp 587-593

Borgerding, M., & Klus, H. (2005) Analysis of complex mixtures--cigarette smoke. *Exp Toxicol Pathol,* 57(1) pp 43-73.

Bhalerao, R., Keskitalo, J., Sterky, F., Erlandsson, R., Björkbacka, H., Birve, S. J., Karlsson, J., Gardeström, P., Gustafsson, P., Lundeberg, J. & Jansson, S. (2003) Gene expression in autumn leaves. *Plant Physiology,* 131(2) pp 430-442.

British American Tobacco (n.d.) Available from www.BAT-science.com

Buchanan-Wollaston, V. & Ainsworth, C. (1997) Leaf senescence in *Brassica napus*: cloning of senescence related genes by subtractive hybridisation. *Plant Molecular Biology,* 33(5) pp 821-834

Buchanan-Wollaston, V., Page, T., Harrison, E., Breeze, E., Lim, P. O., Nam, H. G., Lin, J. F., Wu, S. H., Swidzinski, J., Ishizaki, K. & Leaver, C. J. (2005) Comparative transcriptome analysis reveals significant differences in gene expression and signalling pathways between developmental and dark/starvation-induced senescence in Arabidopsis, *Plant Journal,* 42 pp 567-585

Burton, H. R., Bush, L. P. & Djordjevic, M. V., (1989) Influence of temperature and humidity on the accumulation of tobacco-specific nitrosamines in stored burley tobacco. *Journal of Agriculture Food Chemistry* 37, pp 1372-1377

Burton, H. R., Dye, N. K. & Bush, L. P., (1994) Relationship between Tobacco-Specific Nitrosamines and Nitrite from Different Air-Cured Tobacco Varieties. *Journal of Agriculture Food Chemistry* 42 (9), pp 2007–2011

Causier, B., Kieffer, M., Davies, B. (2002) Plant biology. MADS-box genes reach maturity, *Science,* 296(5566) pp275-276.

Comai, L., Dietrich, R. A., Maslyar, D. J., Baden, F. S. & Harada, J. J., Coordinate expression of transcriptionally regulated isocitrate lyase and malate synthase genes in Brassica napus L., *Plant Cell,* 1989, 1(3) pp 293–300

Coque, M., Martin, A., Veyrieras, J. B., Hirel, B. & Gallais, A. (2008) Genetic variation for N-remobilization and postsilking N-uptake in a set of maize recombinant inbred lines. 3. QTL detection and coincidences, *Theoretical and Applied Genetics,* 117(5) pp 729-747

Chung, T., Suttangkakul, A. & Vierstra, R. D. (2009) The ATG autophagic conjugation system in maize: ATG transcripts and abundance of the ATG8-lipid adduct are regulated by development and nutrient availability, *Plant Physiology* 149, pp220–234

Day, A. & Goldschmidt-Clermont, M. (2011) The chloroplast transformation toolbox: selectable markers and marker removal *Plant Biotechnology Journal* 9 (5) pp 540-553

Dodd, A., Salathia, N., Hall, A., Kévei, E., Tóth, R., Nagy, F., Hibberd, J. M., Millar, A. J. & Webb, A. A. R. (2005), Plant Circadian Clocks Increase Photosynthesis, Growth, Survival, and Competitive Advantage. *Science* 309(5734) pp 630-633

Davis, L. D. & Neilsen, M (1999) Tobacco Production Chemistry Technology, Blackwell Science Ltd., ISBN 0-632-04791-7, Oxford

Edwards K. D., Bombarely, A., Story, G. W., Allen, F., Mueller, L. A., Coates, S. A., Jones, L. (2010) TobEA: an atlas of tobacco gene expression from seed to senescence, *BMC Genomics,* 11:142.

Edwards, K., Anderson, P., Hall, A., Salathia, N., Locke, J., Lynn, J., Straume, M., Smith, J. & Millar, A. (2006) FLOWERING LOCUS C Mediates Natural Variation in the High-Temperature Response of the Arabidopsis Circadian Clock, *Plant Cell,* 18 pp 639–650

Feys B.J., Wiermer, M., Bhat, R. A., Moisan, L. J., Medina-Escobar, N., Neu, C., Cabral, A. & Parker, J. E. (2005) Arabidopsis SENESCENCE-ASSOCIATED GENE101 stabilizes and signals within an ENHANCED DISEASE SUSCEPTIBILITY1 complex in plant innate immunity. *Plant Cell,* 17(9) pp 2601-2613

Fischer, S., Spiegelhalder, B. & Preussmann, R. (1989) Preformed tobacco-specific nitrosamines in tobacco - role of nitrate and influence of tobacco type, *Carcinogenesis*, 10 pp1511-1517

Fracheboud, Y., Luquez, V., Björkén, L., Sjödin, A., Tuominen, H. & Jansson S. (2009) The control of autumn senescence in European aspen, *Plant Physiology*, 149(4) pp 1982-1891

Friedrich, J. W. & Huffaker, R. C. (1980) Photosynthesis, leaf resistances, and ribulose-1,5-bisphosphate carboxylase degradation in senescing barley leaves, *Plant Physiology*, 65(6) pp 1103-1107

Gan, S. & Amasino, R. M., (1995) Inhibition of Leaf Senescence by Autoregulated Production of Cytokinin, *Science* 270(5244) pp 1986-1988

Ghosh, S., Meli, V., Kumar, S., Thakur, A., Chakraborty, N., Chakraborty, S. & Datta, A. (2011) The N-glycan processing enzymes α-mannosidase and β-D-N-acetylhexosaminidase are involved in ripening-associated softening in the non-climacteric fruits of capsicum, *Journal of Experimetal Botany* 62(2) pp 571–582

Grbic, V. & Bleecker, A. (1995) Ethylene regulates the timing of leaf senescence in Aradopsis. *The Plant Journal*, 8(4) pp 595-602

Gepstein, S., Sabehi, G., Carp, M. J. T. H., Falah, M., Nesher, O., Yariv, I., Dor, C. & Bassani, M. (2003) Large-scale identification of leaf senescence-associated genes. *The Plant Journal* 36 pp 629-642

Gregersen, P. L. & Holm, P. B. (2007) Transcriptome analysis of senescence in the flag leaf of wheat (*Triticum aestivum L.*), *Plant Biotechnology Journal* 5(1) pp 192-206.

Gregersen, P. L., Holm, P. B. & Krupinska, K. (2008) Leaf senescence and nutrient remobilisation in barley and Wheat, *Plant Biology*, 10 pp 37-49

Griffith, C. M., Hosken, S. E., Oliver, D., Chojecki, J. & Thomas, H. (1997) Leaf senescence: Physiology and molecular biology, *Plant Molecular Biology*, 34 pp 815–821

Guo, Y. & Gan, S. (2005) Leaf Senescence: Signals, Execution, and Regulation *Current Topics in Developmental Biology*. 71 pp 83-112

Guo, Y., Cai, Z. & Gan, S. (2004) Transcriptome of Arabidopsis leaf senescence. *Plant Cell & Environment* 27 pp 521-549

Harmer, S. L., Hogenesch, J. B., Straume, M., Chang, H. S., Han, B., Zhu, T., Wang, X., Kreps, J. A. & Kay, S, A. (2000) Orchestrated transcription of key pathways in Arabidopsis by the circadian clock. *Science* 290(5499) pp 2110-2113

Harrington, G. & Bush, D. (2003) The Bifunctional Role of Hexokinase in Metabolism and Glucose Signaling, *Plant Cell*, 15(11) pp 2493–2496

Haussühl, K., Andersson, B. & Adamska, I. (2001) A chloroplast DegP2 protease performs the primary cleavage of the photodamaged D1 protein in plant photosystem II. *EMBO Journal* 20 pp 713–722

He, Y. & Gan, S. (2002) A gene encoding an acyl hydrolase is involved in leaf senescence in Arabidopsis, *Plant Cell*, 14(4) pp 805-815

He, Y., Tangm, W., Swain, J. D., Green, A. L., Jack, T. P. & Gan, S. (2001) Networking Senescence-Regulating Pathways by Using Arabidopsis Enhancer Trap Lines, *Plant Physiology*, 126 pp 707-716

Hensel, L. L., Garbic, V., Baumgarten, D. A. & Bleecker, A. B., (1993) Leaf senescence: Physiology and molecular biology. *Plant Cell*, 5 pp 553–564.

Hoffmann, D. & Wynder, E. L. (1967) The reduction of the tumorigenicity of cigarette smoke condensate by addition of sodium nitrate to tobacco, *Cancer Research,* 27(1) pp 172-174

Hopkins, M., Taylor, C., Liu, Z., Ma, F., McNamara, L., Wang, T. W. & Thompson, J. E. (2007) Regulation and execution of molecular disassembly and catabolism during senescence. *New Phytologist.* 175 pp 201-214

Hörtensteiner, S. (2006) Chlorophyll degradation during senescence. *Annual Reviews in Plant Biology* 57 pp 55-77

Hörtensteiner, S. & Feller, U. (2002) Nitrogen metabolism and remobilization during senescence, *Journal of Experimental Botany* 53(370) pp 927-37

Jackson, S. D. (2009) Plant responses to photoperiod, *New Phytologist,* 181(3) pp 517-531

Klee, H. J. (2010) Improving Flavor of Fresh Fruits: Genomics biochemistry and biotechnology *New Phytologist,* 187(1) pp 44-56

Kim, D. J. & Smith, S. M. (1994) Molecular cloning of cucumber phosphoenolpyruvate carboxykinase and developmental regulation of gene expression, *Plant Molecular Biology,* 26 pp 423–434

Labboun, S., Tercé-Laforgue, T., Roscher, A., Bedu, M., Restivo, F. M., Velanis, C. N., Skopelitis, D. S., Moschou, P. N., Roubelakis-Angelakis, K. A., Suzuki, A. & Hirel, B. (2009) Resolving the role of plant glutamate dehydrogenase. I. In vivo real time nuclear magnetic resonance spectroscopy experiments. *Plant Cell Physiology,* 50(10) pp 1761-1773

Lea, P. J. & Miflin, B. J., (1974) Alternative route for nitrogen assimilation in higher plants. *Nature.* 251(5476) pp 614-616

Lim, P. O., Kim, H. J. & Nam, H. G. (2007) Leaf senescence. *Annual Review of Plant Biology.* 58 pp 115-136

Lin, J. F. & Wu, S. H. (2004) Molecular events in senescing Arabidopsis leaves, *Plant Journal,* 39(4) pp612-628

Lohman, K., Gan, S., John, M. & Amasino, R. M. (1994) Molecular analysis of natural leaf senescence in *Arabidopsis thaliana, Physiologia Plantarum,* 92 pp 322-328

Lossl, A. & Waheed, M. (2011) Chloroplast-derived vaccines against human diseases: achievements, challenges and scopes, *Plant Biotechnology Journal,* 9 pp 527–539

Mae, T., Kai, N., Makino, A. & Ohira, K. (1984) Relation between ribulose bisphosphate carboxylase content and chloroplast number in naturally senescing primary leaves of wheat. *Plant Cell & Physiology,* 25 pp 333–336

Masclaux, C., Valadier, M. H., Brugière, N., Morot-Gaudry, J. F. & Hirel, B. (2000) Characterization of the sink/source transition in tobacco (Nicotiana tabacum L.) shoots in relation to nitrogen management and leaf senescence, *Planta,* 211(4) pp 510-518

Morris, K., MacKerness, S. A., Page, T., John, C. F., Murphy, A. M., Carr, J. P. & Buchanan-Wollaston, V. (2000) Salicylic acid has a role in regulating gene expression during leaf senescence, *Plant Journal,* 23(5) pp 677-685

Mueller, L. A., Solow, T. H., Taylor, N., Skwarecki, B., Buels, R., Binns, J., Lin, C., Wright, M. H., Ahrens, R., Wang, Y., Herbst, E. V., Keyder, E. R., Menda, N., Zamir, D. & Tanksley, S. D. (2005) The SOL Genomics Network. A Comparative Resource for Solanaceae Biology and Beyond. *Plant Physiol.* 138(3) pp 1310–1317.

Noodén, L. D., Guiamét, J. J. & John, I. (1997) Senescence mechanisms, *Physiologia Plantarum,* 101 pp 746-753

Otegui, M. S., Noh, Y. S., Martínez, D. E., Vila Petroff, M. G., Staehelin, L. A., Amasino & R. M., Guiamet, J. J. (2005) Senescence-associated vacuoles with intense proteolytic activity develop in leaves of Arabidopsis and soybean. *Plant Journal,* 41(6) pp 831-844

Norman, A. (1999). Cigarette Design and Materials. In: *Tobacco Producton, Chemistry and Technology,* Davis D L & Nielsen M. T., pp. 353-387, Blackwell Science Ltd., ISBN 0-632-04791-7, Oxford

Ohsumi, Y. (2001) Molecular mechanism of bulk protein degradation in lysosome/vacuole, *Tanpakushitsu Kakusan Koso,* 46(11) pp 1710-1716

Pruzinska, A., Tanner, G., Aubry, S., Anders, I., Moser, S., Muller, T., Ongania, K. H., Krautler, B., Youn, J. Y., Liljegren, S. J. & Hortensteiner, S. (2005) Chlorophyll Breakdown in Senescent Arabidopsis Leaves. Characterization of Chlorophyll Catabolites and of Chlorophyll Catabolic Enzymes Involved in the Degreening Reaction. *Plant Physiology,* 139 pp 52-63

Quirino, B. F., Normanly, J. & Amasino, R. M. (1999) Diverse range of gene activity during Arabidopsis thaliana leaf senescence includes pathogen-independent induction of defense-related genes. *Plant Molecular Biology,* 40(2) pp 267-278.

Rodgman, A. & Perfetti, T. A. (2009) The chemical components of tobacco and tobacco smoke. CRC press, Florida, USA. pp 1259. ISBN 978-1-4200-7883-1.

Shaul, O. & Galili, G. (1993) Concerted regulation of lysine and threonine synthesis in tobacco plants expressing bacterial feedback-insensitive aspartate kinase and dihydrodipicolinate synthase. *Plant Molecular Biology,* 23(4) pp 759-768.

Smart, C. M. (1994) Gene expression during leaf senescence. *New Phytologist* 126 pp 419-448

Sokolenko, A., Lerbs-Mache, S., Altschmied, L., Herrmann, R. G. (1998) Clp protease complexes and their diversity in chloroplasts. *Planta,* 207 pp 286–295

Spiegelhalder, B., Bartsch, H.(1996) Tobacco-specific nitrosamines, *European Journal of Cancer Prevention,* 5 pp 33-38

Stitt, M., Müller, C., Matt, P., Gibon, Y., Carillo, P., Morcuende, R., Scheible, W. R. & Krapp, A. (2002) Steps towards an integrated view of nitrogen metabolism, *Journal of Experimental Botany* 53(370) pp 959-70

Thomas, H. & Donnison, I. (2000) Back from the brink: plant senescence and its reversibility, *Symposium Society of Experimental Biology,* 52 pp 149-162

Thomas, H. & Stoddart, J. L. (1980). Leaf senescence, *Annual Review of Plant Physiology,* 31 pp 83–111

Thompson, A. R. & Vierstra, R. D. (2005) Autophagic recycling: lessons from yeast help define the process in plants, *Current Opinions in Plant Biology,* 8(2) pp 165-173

Tollenaar, M. & Wu, J. (1999). Yield improvement in temperate maize is attributable to greater stress Tolerance, *Crop Science,* 39 pp 1597–1604

Uauy, C., Distelfeld, A., Fahima, T., Blechl, A. & Dubcovsky J (2006) A NAC Gene regulating senescence improves grain protein, zinc, and iron content in wheat *Science,* 314(5803) pp 1298-1301

Van der Graaff, E., Schwacke, R., Schneider, A., Desimone, M., Flugge, U. I. & Kunze, R. (2006) Transcription Analysis of Arabidopsis Membrane Transporters and Hormone Pathways during Developmental and Induced Leaf Senescence, *Plant Physiology,* 141 pp 776-792

Van Doorn, W. G. (2008) Is the onset of senescence in leaf cells of intact plants due to low or high sugar levels? *Experimental Botany* 59(8) pp 1963-1972

Vierstra, R. D. (1996) Proteolysis in plants: mechanisms and functions. *Plant Molecular Biology*, 32(1-2) pp 275-302

Verburg, J. G., Huynh, Q.K. (1991) Purification and Characterization of an Antifungal Chitinase from Arabidopsis thaliana, *Plant Physiology*, 95(2) pp 450-455

Watanabe, A., Hamada, K., Yokoi, H. & Watanabe, A., (1994) Biophysical and differential expression of cytosolic glutamine synthetase genes of radish during seed germination and senescence of cotyledons, *Plant Molecular Biology*, 26 pp 1807–1817

Weasel, L. H. (2009) *Food Fray: Inside the Controversy over Genetically Modified Food*, Amacom, ISBN-13: 978-0814401644, New York

Wingler, A. & Roitsch, T. (2008) Metabolic regulation of leaf senescence: interactions of sugar signalling with biotic and abiotic stress responses, *Plant Biology*, 10 pp 50-62.

Wittenbach, V. A. (1978) Breakdown of Ribulose Bisphosphate Carboxylase and Change in Proteolytic Activity during Dark-induced Senescence of Wheat Seedlings, *Plant Physiology*, 62(4) pp 604-608

Wu, W., Zhang, L., Jain, R. B., Ashley, D. L. & Watson, C. H. (2005) Determination of carcinogenic tobacco-specific nitrosamines in mainstream smoke from U.S.-brand and non-U.S.-brand cigarettes from 14 countries, *Nicotine Tobacco Research*, 7(3) pp 443-451

Xue-Xuan, X., Hong-Bo, S., Yuan-Yuan, M., Gang, X., Jun-Na, S., Dong-Gang, G. & Cheng-Jiang, R. (2010) Biotechnological implications from abscisic acid (ABA) roles in cold stress and leaf senescence as an important signal for improving plant sustainable survival under abiotic-stressed conditions, *Critical Reviews in Biotechnology*, 30(3) pp 222-230

Yang, J. & Zhang, J. (2006) Grain filling of cereals under soil drying, *New Phytologist* 169(2) pp 223-236

Yoshida, S. (2003) Molecular regulation of leaf senescence, *Current opinion in plant biology*, 6 pp 79-84

Zavaleta-Mancera, H. A., Thomas, B. J., Thomas, H. & Scott, I. M. (1999) Regreening of senescent Nicotiana leaves, *Journal of Experimental Botany*, 50(340) pp 1683–1689

8

The Legume Root Nodule: From Symbiotic Nitrogen Fixation to Senescence

Laurence Dupont, Geneviève Alloing, Olivier Pierre, Sarra El Msehli, Julie Hopkins, Didier Hérouart and Pierre Frendo

[1]*UMR "Biotic Interactions and Plant Health" INRA 1301-CNRS 6243 University of Nice-Sophia Antipolis, F-06903 Sophia-Antipolis Cedex,*
[2]*Laboratory of Plant Physiology, Science University, Tunis,*
[1]*France*
[2]*Tunisia*

1. Introduction

Biological nitrogen fixation (BNF) is the biological process by which the atmospheric nitrogen (N_2) is converted to ammonia by an enzyme called nitrogenase. It is the major source of the biosphere nitrogen and as such has an important ecological and agronomical role, accounting for 65 % of the nitrogen used in agriculture worldwide. The most important source of fixed nitrogen is the symbiotic association between rhizobia and legumes. The nitrogen fixation is achieved by bacteria inside the cells of *de novo* formed organs, the nodules, which usually develop on roots, and more occasionally on stems. This mutualistic relationship is beneficial for both partners, the plant supplying dicarboxylic acids as a carbon source to bacteria and receiving, in return, ammonium. Legume symbioses have an important role in environment-friendly agriculture. They allow plants to grow on nitrogen poor soils and reduce the need for nitrogen inputs for leguminous crops, and thus soil pollution. Nitrogen-fixing legumes also contribute to nitrogen enrichment of the soil and have been used from Antiquity as crop-rotation species to improve soil fertility. They produce high protein-containing leaves and seeds, and legumes such as soybeans, groundnuts, peas, beans, lentils, alfalfa and clover are a major source of protein for human and animal consumption. Most research concentrates on the two legume-rhizobium model systems *Lotus-Mesorhizobium loti* and *Medicago-Sinorhizobium meliloti,* with another focus on the economically-important *Glycine max* (soybean) *-Bradyrhizobium japonicum* association. The legume genetic models *Medicago truncatula* and *Lotus japonicus* have a small genome size of *ca.* 450 Mbp while *Glycine max* has a genome size of 1,115 Mbp, and all are currently targets of large-scale *genome sequencing* projects (He et al., 2009; Sato et al., 2008; Schmutz et al., 2010). The complete genome sequence of their bacterial partners has been established (Galibert et al., 2001; Kaneko et al., 2000; Kaneko et al., 2002; Schneiker-Bekel et al., 2011).

1.1 Early interaction and nodule development

Symbiotic interaction begins with the infection process, which is initiated by a reciprocal exchange of signals between plant and the compatible bacteria. Aromatic compounds -

mostly flavonoids - are secreted by the plants into the rhizosphere and activate the bacterial NodD proteins that are members of the LysR family of transcriptional activators, which in turn induce the expression of the *nod* genes (Long, 2001). This results in the secretion by the bacteria of lipo-chitin oligosaccharide molecules called Nod factors, which are recognized by epidermal cells via specific receptor kinases containing extracellular LysM domains. The spectrum of flavonoids exuded by a legume, as well as the strain-specific chemical structures of the Nod factors, are primary determinants of host specificity (Broughton et al., 2000). Additional bacterial components such as exopolysaccharides, type III and type IV secretion systems are also required for an effective infection (Perret et al., 2000; Saeki, 2011).

Nod factor perception initiates a complex signalling pathway essential for bacterial invasion of the host plant and formation of the nodule. Nod factor signal transduction requires a calcium signalling pathway, which includes the activation of a calcium and calmodulin dependent protein kinase in response to nuclear calcium oscillations. The ensuing induction of gene expression results in rearrangements of the root hair cytoskeleton and initiation of bacterial infection at the epidermis. The root hairs curl and trap the rhizobia which enter the root hair through tubular structures called infection threads. Simultaneously Nod factors induce root cortex cells dedifferentiation and division, leading to the formation of nodule primordia which then differentiate into N_2-fixing nodules (Crespi & Frugier, 2008; Oldroyd et al. 2011). The growing infection threads traverse the root epidermis and cortex, penetrate primordial cells, and then invading bacteria are released into the host cells by an endocytosis-like mechanism (Ivanov et al., 2010). Each bacterium is surrounded by a plant cell membrane, the peribacteroid membrane (PBM), the whole forming an organelle-like structure called the symbiosome where bacteria differentiate into nitrogen-fixing bacteroids. These symbiosomes ultimately completely fill the cytoplasm of infected cells. As the bacteria differentiate, infected cells undergo enlargement coupled to repeated endoreduplication cycles - genomic DNA replication without mitosis or cytokinesis - and become large polyploid cells housing thousands of bacteroids (Jones et al., 2007; Kondorosi et al., 2000). Mature nodules actively fix nitrogen until they enter senescence upon aging or stress.

Nodule organogenesis is accompanied by major changes in plant gene expression. Several hundred of genes were found to be strongly and specifically up- or -down regulated during the nodulation process (Benedito et al., 2008; El Yahyaoui et al., 2004). In *M. truncatula*, two distinct waves of gene expression reprogramming accompany the differentiation of both the plant infected cell and bacteroids (Maunoury et al., 2010). Genes exclusively expressed or strongly up-regulated in nodules have been termed "nodulins". The early nodulins are involved in signal transduction and nodule development and the late nodulins are induced when N_2 fixation begins. Different expression profiling tools relying on genome and high-throughput EST-sequencing have been developed to identify nodulin genes on a large scale (Kuster et al., 2007; Schauser et al., 2008).

Nodules can be classified into two main groups according to their mode of development (Franssen et al., 1992; Maunoury et al., 2008) (Figure 1). Legumes such as *Phaseolus vulgaris* (bean), *Lotus japonicus* or *Glycine max* (soybean) form determinate nodules that have no permanent meristem and adopt a globular shape. The mature nodules contain a homogenous central tissue composed of infected cells fully packed with nitrogen-fixing bacteroids and some uninfected cells. Senescence in these nodules occurs radially, beginning at the center and extending to the periphery. Decaying nodules release bacteroids most of which are able to revert to a free-living lifestyle. Conversely, legumes such as *Medicago truncatula, Pisum sativum* (pea) or *Trifolium* (clover) form indeterminate nodules that possess a permanent meristem and elongate, to become cylindrical. In mature nodule of this type, several histological zones of consecutive developmental states can be distinguished (Vasse et al., 1990). The apical meristem, free of bacteria, is the zone I. Zone II is the infection zone in which post-mitotic cells enter the nodule differentiation programme and where infection threads penetrate the plant cells and release rhizobia. In zone III, the bacteroids are able to fix N_2. A root proximal senescence zone (zone IV) can be observed in older nodules, where the bacteroids, together with the plant cells, are degraded. Upon aging this zone gradually extends to reach the apical part and the nodule degenerates. Proximal to the zone IV is a region (zone V) containing undifferentiated bacteria, which appear to proliferate in the decaying plant tissue (Timmers et al., 2000). In contrast to bacteroids housed in determinate nodules, those from undeterminate nodules have lost their capacity to reproduce. Thus at the end of symbiosis, essentially bacteria that are released from infection threads can return to a free-living lifestyle and recolonize the rhizosphere (Mergaert et al., 2006).

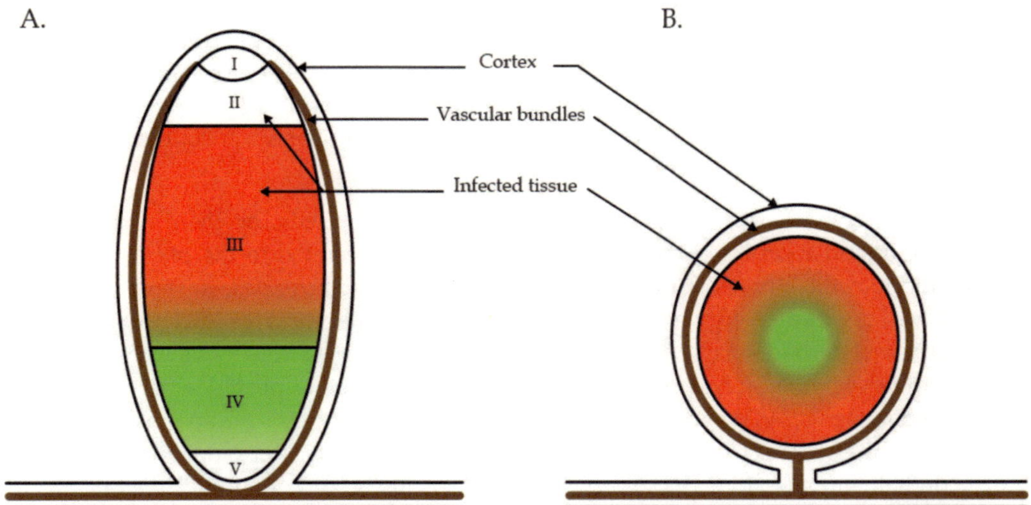

Fig. 1. Schematic representation of indeterminate (A) and determinate mature nodules (B) I, meristemic zone ; II, infection zone ; III, nitrogen fixing zone ; IV, senescence zone ; V, saprophytic zone.

Nitrogen fixing bacteroids in determinate and indeterminate nodules originate from distinct differentiation processes. Bacteroids in legume species forming determinate type nodules present the same cell size, genomic DNA content and reproductive capacity as the free-living bacteria. Conversely, differentiation of bacteroids in indeterminate nodules is linked to drastic morphological and cytological changes, such as cell elongation coupled to genome amplification, membrane permeabilisation and loss of reproductive capacity (Mergaert et al., 2006). This terminal differentiation is mediated by plant-host factors identified as the nodule-specific cysteine-rich (NCR) peptides (Kereszt et al., 2011; Van de Velde et al., 2010). In *M. truncatula* the NCR gene family encodes more than 300 different peptides, which resemble defensine-type antimicrobial peptides (AMPs) (Mergaert et al., 2003).

1.2 Nodule functioning

Bacteria that have completed the bacteroid differentiation program express the enzymes of the nitrogenase complex and begin to fix nitrogen. The reduction by nitrogenase of 1 molecule of N_2 to 2 molecules of NH_4^+ requires 16 molecules of ATP and 8 electrons (Jones et al., 2007). Thus, bacteroids require high rate flux of O_2 to enable high rates of ATP synthesis, but this must be achieved whilst maintaining a very low concentration of free O_2 to avoid inactivation of O_2-labile nitrogenase. These conditions exist due to the presence of an O_2 diffusion barrier and the synthesis of nodule-specific leghemoglobins, which accumulate to millimolar concentrations in the cytoplasm of infected cells prior to nitrogen fixation and buffer the free O_2 concentration at around 7-11 nM, while maintaining high O_2 flux for respiration (Appleby, 1984; Downie, 2005; Ott et al., 2005). The unique low-O_2 environment provided for the bacteroid is a key signal in bacteroid metabolism, inducing a regulatory cascade controlling gene expression of the nitrogenase complex and the microaerobic respiratory enzymes of the bacteroid. The O_2-sensing two-component regulatory system FixL-FixJ activates the transcription of the two intermediate regulators *nifA* and *fixK* genes, which induce the expression of *nif* and *fix* genes involved in nitrogen fixation and respiration (Reyrat et al., 1993). More generally, bacteroid differentiation is accompanied by a global change in gene expression compared with free-living bacteria. There is down-regulation of many genes such as most housekeeping genes and genes involved in synthesis of membrane proteins and peptidoglycan in favour of symbiosis specific processes (Becker et al., 2004; Bobik et al., 2006; Capela et al., 2006; Karunakaran et al., 2009; Pessi et al., 2007).

The reduction of N_2 to ammonium is accompanied, in bacteroids, by the switching-off of ammonium assimilation into amino acids. Ammonium is secreted to the plant cytosol, for assimilation into the amides glutamine and asparagine or into ureides. In return, the plant provides carbon and energy sources to bacteroids in the form of dicarboxylic acids, particularly malate and succinate, which are produced from sucrose via sucrose synthase and glycolytic enzymes. Their metabolization by the TCA cycle provides bacteroids with reducing equivalents, ATP and metabolites for amino acid synthesis and other biosynthetic pathways (White et al., 2007; Lodwig & Poole, 2003). Pea bacteroids also depend on plant for branched-chain amino-acid (LIV) supply, as the bacteroids become symbiotic auxotrophs for these amino-acids (Prell et al., 2009).

The nodule functioning has many peculiarities, involving a plant-microbe crosstalk associated to a metabolism which needs a high energy level under micro-oxic conditions. Nodule development and senescence also have specific features. Whereas multiple review articles have described the early steps of nodule formation and functioning, the rupture of the interaction has not been reviewed recently. In this context, this review focuses on the different characteristics of root nodule senescence.

2. Developmental senescence

For many years, the majority of the research concerning N-fixing symbioses focused on understanding the mechanisms leading to the establishment of this symbiotic relationship, from the invasion of plant cells to the N-fixing bacteroid state. In all nodule types, the N_2-fixation period is optimal between 4 and 5 weeks after infection. Beyond this period, first reductions of N_2-fixing bacteroid capacity are detectable and a senescence process occurs in the N -fixing nodule zone. This phenomena is related to the onset of pod filling in grain legumes like soybean, pea and common bean (Bethlenfalvay & Phillips, 1977; Lawn & Brun, 1977). Thus, the lifespan of the rhizobia-plant symbiotic relationship is relatively short and the disruption of this symbiosis affects the yield of the culture.

2.1 Structural analysis of developmental senescence

The spatial dynamics of the senescence process in nodules is nodule type dependent. The pink N_2-fixing tissues of the zone III become green in color in zone IV due to leghemoglobin breakdown (Lehtovaara & Perttila, 1978). In determinate nodules, histological analyses of cross-sections using this simple visible change revealed that senescence develops radially, starting from the center and gradually spreading toward the outside (Puppo et al., 2005). In contrast, in undeterminate nodules, histological analyses of longitudinal sections of nodules based on pink-to-green color changes or based on the expression pattern of bacteroid genes involved in the N_2-fixing process using promoter-lacZ fusions (i.e. NifH) have led many authors to consider the front of senescence as a planar structure (Puppo et al., 2005). Recently, using toluidine blue staining to discriminate senescent from healthy cells and studying the gene expression pattern of a small family of plant cysteine proteases as early markers of nodule senescence on serial transversal sections of *M. truncatula* nodules, Pérez Guerra and collaborators proposed a conical organization of the developmental senescence zone: the earliest signs of senescence in a few infected cells in the center of the N-fixing zone occurred similar to determined nodules, and this phenomena progressively extended toward the nodule periphery in subsequent proximal cell layers of the nodule (Pérez Guerra et al., 2010).

Comparison between N_2-fixing and senescent cells in soybean nodule showed a decrease of density of plant cytoplasm, the apparition of vesicles associated with the deterioration of symbiosomes and modifications in organelles like peroxisomes, mitochondria and plastids (Lucas et al., 1998; Puppo et al., 2005). Ultrastructural analysis of *M. truncatula* mature nodule cells has revealed at least two stages during the developmental senescence of N_2-fixing cells: first, a disintegration of bacteroids and symbiosomes revealed by the presence of numerous membranes in the plant cytoplasm associated with the formation of lytic symbiosome compartments probably involved in reabsorption processes and second, the decay of plant infected cells associated with collapse phenomena and that of the plant uninfected cells (Perez Guerra et al., 2010; Timmers et al., 2000; Van de Velde et al., 2006; Vasse et al., 1990). The fusion of symbiosomes to form lytic compartments resembles vacuole formation. Analysis of the relation between the symbiosome formation and the endocytic pathway showed that the lifespan of bacteria in individual symbiosomes compartments during the N_2-fixing stage is achieved by delaying the acquisition of vacuolar identity such as vacuolar SYP22 and VTI11 SNAREs (Limpens et al., 2009). The acquisition of vacuolar identity by symbiosomes upon senescence likely allows the delivery of newly formed proteases to facilitate nutrient remobilization and a sink-to-source transition. Indeed, nodule senescence is accompanied by increased plant proteolytic activities that might cause large-scale protein degradation in soybean (Malik et al., 1981), French bean (Pladys et al., 1991) and alfalfa (Pladys & Vance, 1993).

2.2 Physiological and biochemical modifications during developmental senescence

Developmental nodule senescence is a complex and programmed process which induces a decrease of N_2-fixing activity and leghemoglobin content, modifications in the nodule redox state components and an increase of proteolytic activity, ultimately leading to the death of infected cells.

Leghemoglobin (Lb), which has a fundamental role in nodule functioning, is an important physiological marker for following the progression of nodule senescence (Figure 2). Lb content progressively decreases with the onset of senescence. This diminution of Lb impacts not only general metabolism of nodule by decreasing the O_2 availability to bacteroids with a low free O_2 content but also by potentially releasing free iron to produce reactive oxygen species (ROS) via the Fenton reaction. Indeed, the auto-oxidation of the active form of Lb, ferro-Lb-O_2 (Lb-Fe^{2+}-O_2), is associated with superoxide anion ($O_2^{\cdot-}$) production (Fridovich, 1986; Puppo et al., 1981) and the degradation of the heme group of Lb by H_2O_2 likely allows the release of the catalytic Fe which enhances the production of OH• through the Fenton and the Haberweiss reactions (Becana & Klucas, 1992; Puppo & Halliwell, 1988). The importance of Lb in nodule ROS production has been shown in a transgenic *Lotus japonicus* line in which diminution of the Lb content is correlated with diminution of the H_2O_2 production (Gunther et al., 2007).

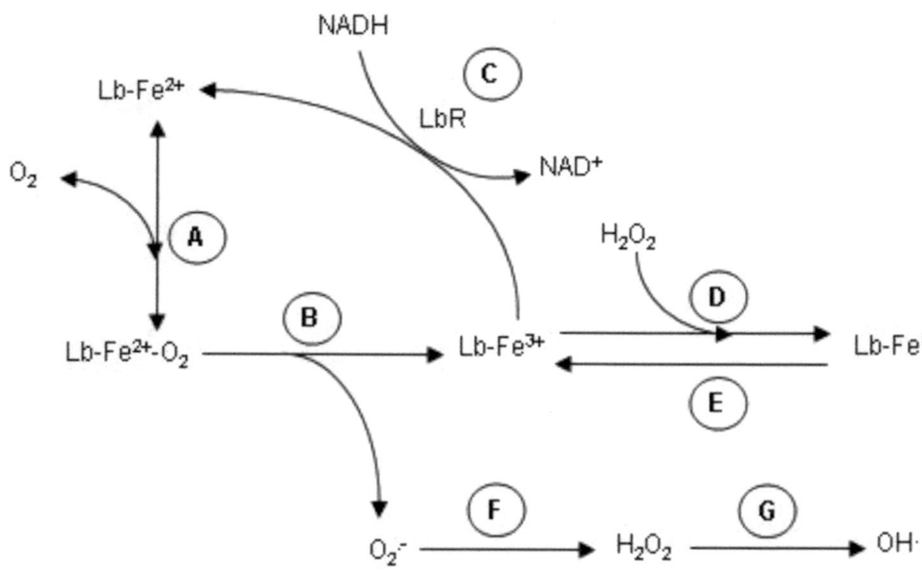

Fig. 2. Metabolic pathways involving Lb and formation of ROS.
A, Reversible oxygenation of Lb-Fe^{2+}; B, Autoxidation of Lb-Fe^{2+}-O_2 to Lb-Fe^{3+} with release of $O_2^{\cdot-}$; C, Lb-Fe^{3+} reduction by ferric Lb reductase (LbR); D, H_2O_2 reaction with Lb-Fe^{3+} to generate the inactive Lb-Fe^{IV} (ferryl) form; E, Lb-Fe^{IV} reduction to Lb-Fe^{3+} by ascorbate or thiols; other ROS can also be generated from $O_2^{\cdot-}$, by its dismutation to H_2O_2; F, and by H_2O_2 reduction to OH · through Fenton reaction (G).

Large modifications of the redox balance occur upon natural nodule senescence. Redox balance is defined by the equilibrium between the production of ROS and their degradation by the antioxidant defence system (Apel & Hirt, 2004). Ascorbate (Asc), homoglutathione (hGSH) and glutathione (GSH) are major antioxidants and redox buffers in plant nodule cells (Becana et al., 2010). The regulation of Asc and hGSH biosynthesis has been studied in common bean (*Phaseolus vulgaris*) nodules during aging (Loscos et al., 2008). The expression of five genes of the major Asc biosynthetic pathway was analyzed in nodules, and evidence was found that L-galactono-1,4-lactone dehydrogenase (GalLDH) , the last committed step of the pathway, is post-transcriptionally regulated. Large differences of Asc concentrations and redox states were observed in *P. vulgaris* nodules at different senescence stages suggesting that the lifespan of nodules is in part controlled by endogenous factors like Asc. Biochemical assays on alfalfa dissected nodules revealed that the senescent zone had lower GalLDH activity and ascorbate concentration compared to the infected zone (Matamoros et al., 2006). A strong positive correlation between N_2-fixing activity and nodule Asc and GSH contents was also observed during pea nodule development and senescence (Groten et al., 2005). Peroxiredoxins (Prx) have also been described in N_2-fixing nodules (Groten et al., 2006). Pea nodules contain at least two isoforms of Prx, located potentially in the cytosol (PrxIIB / C) and mitochondria (PrxIIF). The levels of PrxIIB /C declined with nodule senescence, but those of PrxIIF remained unaffected (Groten et al., 2006). The progressive decrease of antioxidant content during pea nodule senescence is not accompanied by an increase in ROS such as $O_2^{\cdot-}$ and H_2O_2 (Groten et al., 2005). In contrast, in aging soybean nodules, an oxidative stress has been detected including an increase of ROS, oxidized hGSH, catalytic Fe and oxidatively modified proteins and DNA bases, but no changes in Asc or tocopherol (Evans et al., 1999). The imbalance in redox state leading to oxidative stress induces the oxidation of lipids and proteins and the degradation of membranes. Lipid peroxidation was found to be elevated in senescent nodules of pigeon pea (*Cajanus cajan*) and bean (Loscos et al., 2008; Swaraj et al., 1995). In senescent soybean nodules, the presence of large amounts of H_2O_2 in the cytoplasmic and apoplastic compartments of the central infected tissue was detected and associated with a widespread expression of a cysteine protease gene (Alesandrini et al., 2003), suggesting a link between oxidative stress and proteolitic activities detected upon nodule senescence.

Various proteases, including those of the acid, serine, aspartic and cysteine types, have been isolated from senescing nodule tissue of soybean, alfalfa, French bean, and pea (Kardailsky & Brewin, 1996; Malik et al., 1981; Pfeiffer et al., 1983; Pladys & Vance, 1993; Pladys & Rigaud, 1985). The induction of cysteine protease genes during nodule senescence has been shown in soybean (Alesandrini et al., 2003), Chinese milk vetch (Naito et al., 2000), pea (Kardailsky & Brewin, 1996) and *M. truncatula* (Fedorova et al., 2002). The general transcriptomic analysis of senescent nodules in *M. truncatula* using cDNA-AFLP (Van de Velde et al., 2006) confirmed the predominant presence of genes encoding representatives of cysteine proteases that are highly homologous to one of the prominent markers of leaf senescence, *Sag12* (Lohman et al., 1994), indicating that these proteinases play an important role in the regulation of developmental nodule senescence. This hypothesis was confirmed in *Astragalus sinicus* since the silencing by RNA interference of the Asnodf32 gene, encoding a nodule-specific cysteine proteinase delayed root nodule senescence with a significant extention of the period of bacteroid active nitrogen fixation. Interestingly, elongated nodules were also observed on Asnodf32-silenced hairy roots (Li et al., 2008).

2.3 Transcriptomic analysis of developmental senescence

The onset of senescence involves the expression of genes whose products are required to carry out senescence-related processes (Gepstein, 2004). In order to isolate genes up- or down-regulated during nodule senescence, several genetic analyses including cDNA libraries and differential screening, mRNA differential display or cDNA-AFLP, have been performed in soybean (Alesandrini et al., 2003; Webb et al., 2008), and *M. truncatula* (Fedorova et al., 2002; Van de Velde et al., 2006). Using a mixture of effective nodules from 7 week-old plants, the first database specific to *M. truncatula* nodule senescence was obtained by isolating 140 000 Expressed Sequence Tags which are available in the J. Craig Venter Institute (http://www.jcvi.org/cms/research/groups/plant-genomics/resources/). To enrich plant material in senescent tissue, recent analyses in *M. truncatula* were performed from cross sections of nodules of 5 and 9 weeks by isolating the zones I, II and III from zones IV and V based on pink-to-green color changes (Van de Velde et al., 2006). This analysis using a modified cDNA-AFLP protocol has resulted in a collection of 508 gene tags that were expressed differentially. Functional clustering of these data has revealed a clear transition from carbon sink to nutriment source for the nodule by up-regulation of genes representative of several different proteases, genes involved in proteasome pathway and degradation of nucleic acids, membrane-derived lipids, and sugars. Moreover, this analysis suggests that three major hormones, ethylene, jasmonic acid and gibberellin, play an important role in nodule senescence (Van de Velde et al., 2006). From a more general point of view, it was been found that a significant overlap exists between genes expressed during leaf senescence in *Arabidopsis thaliana* and nodule senescence in *M. truncatula* (Van de Velde et al., 2006). However, more recent transcriptomic analysis of *M. truncatula* leaf senescence showed that only a minority of common genes are regulated during leaf and nodule senescence (De Michele et al., 2009).

2.4 Hormonal regulation of developmental senescence

Abscisic acid has been proposed to be an important signal in nodule senescence (Puppo et al., 2005), but no direct abscisic acid-responsive genes were present in the cDNA-AFLP dataset from *M. truncatula* nodules (Van de Velde et al., 2006). This analysis revealed that ethylene and jasmonic acid may play a positive role in nodule senescence, just as they do in the senescence of other plant tissues. The positive role of ethylene is illustrated by the up-regulation of ERF transcription factors and ethylene biosynthetic genes, such as S-adenosyl-Met (SAM) synthetase and 1-aminocyclopropane-1-carboxylate oxidase. Involvement of jasmonic acid is suggested by the induction of lipoxygenase genes during different stages of nodule senescence. Moreover, a strong induction of a gene coding for the GA 2-oxidase, that converts active gibberellins to inactive forms (Thomas et al., 1999), was observed in senescent nodule suggesting that gibberellins might repress the senescence process. Finally, the induction of genes encoding a SAM synthase and a spermidine synthethase suggests the involvement of polyamine biosynthetic pathways in nodule senescence. Concerning the potential implication of the two major hormones, auxin and cytokinin, in nodule senescence, only a small amount of data is available. In lupin (*Lupinus albus*), an elevated accumulation of the LaHK1 transcripts, encoding a cytokinin receptor homologue, was detected during nodule developmental senescence suggesting a putative role for this cytokinin receptor homologue in nodule senescence (Coba de la Pena et al., 2008).

3. Stress-induced senescence in legume root nodule

Legume BNF is particularly sensitive and perturbed by environmental stress conditions such as drought, salt stress, defoliation, continuous darkness and cold stress. Adverse environmental conditions affect nodule structure, impair nodule functioning and induce drastic metabolic and molecular modifications leading ultimately to a stress-induced senescence (SIS).

3.1 Stress induced senescence has typical features when compared to developmental senescence

As stated earlier, developmental induced senescence occurs typically in 5 to 11 week old nodules with a slow diminution of BNF during this time period (Evans et al., 1999; Puppo et al., 2005). In contrast, BNF declines drastically and quickly under environmental stress conditions. In less than a week, drought (Gonzalez et al., 1995; Larrainzar et al., 2007; Serraj et al., 1999), salt stress (Soussi et al., 1998; Swaraj and Bishnoi, 1999), dark stress (Matamoros et al., 1999; Gogorcena et al., 1997) and cold stress (van Heerden et al., 2008) decrease dramatically BNF. Thus, SIS is a much faster process than developmental senescence. Moreover, whereas developmental senescence is associated with the establishment of the nodule senescent zone which increases over time, SIS induces the degeneration of the whole nodule in a short time period (Matamoros et al., 1999; Perez Guerra et al., 2010; Vauclare et al., 2010). At the structural level, microscopic analyses also show that developmental senescence and dark stress-induced senescence present different features in *M. truncatula*. Dark-induced senescence leads to the condensation of the bacteroid content whereas the PBM remains intact even though most of the bacteroid content had disappeared (Perez Guerra et al., 2010). In contrast, developmental senescence induces a pronounced vesicle mobilisation in the host cytoplasm which is correlated with the degeneration of the PBM and the mixing of the symbiosome content with the cytoplasm (Perez Guerra et al., 2010; Van de Velde et al., 2006). However, structural analyses of the SIS have not been extensively performed on different nodule types for all the different environmental stress. Thus, it is possible that the different SIS do not develop similarly. Moreover, as for developmental senescence, SIS may process differently in determinate and indeterminate nodules. Indeed, nitrate induced senescence has been shown to induce bacteroid degradation in pea (indeterminate nodule) after two days of treatment in contrast to bean (determinate nodule), in which nitrate has little effect on the shape of bacteroids even after four days of 10mM nitrate treatment (Matamoros et al., 1999).

3.2 Stress induced senescence is characterized by modifications in nodule carbon metabolism and respiration

SIS is characterized by multiple early modifications of nodule physiology (Figure 2). Amongst them, modifications in carbon metabolism play a major role. As stated before, BNF is a highly energetic process which requires a constant energy supply. Modification of nodule sucrose content has been observed during drought stress (Galvez et al., 2005; Gordon et al., 1997), salt stress (Gordon et al., 1997; Lopez et al., 2008; Sanchez et al., 2011; Lopez et al., 2009; Ben Salah et al., 2009), dark stress (Gogorcena et al., 1997; Matamoros et al., 1999; Vauclare et al., 2010) and cold stress (Walsh & Layzell, 1986; van Heerden et al., 2008). However, whereas dark stress induces a diminution of sucrose concentration, drought stress, salt stress and cold stress lead in general to its accumulation in nodules. The diminution of sucrose concentration linked to a shortage in photosynthate feeding result in a deficiency in energy production. In contrast, the accumulation of sucrose during stress suggests that nodule glycolytic enzymes are affected. Sucrose synthase, which is involved in the degradation of sucrose into glucose and fructose in the root nodule, is inhibited during drought stress and salt stress (Ben Salah et al., 2009; Gordon et al., 1997) and malate content, which is one of the preferred substrates for bacteroid respiration (Prell and Poole, 2006), decreases under these two stress conditions (Marino et al., 2007; Galvez et al., 2005; Ben Salah et al., 2009). A fine-tuning of O_2 concentration is also important for nodule functioning, since a good supply of O_2 is determinant for nodule respiration and energy requirement while a low O_2 pressure must be maintained in the nitrogen fixing zone to prevent nitrogenase inhibition. The availability of O_2 through the nodule diffusion barrier and the rate of nodule respiration are thus important parameters of the nodule fitness and they have been shown to be modified during various SIS such as drought stress (Del Castillo et al., 1994; Guerin et al., 1990; Naya et al., 2007; Serraj & Sinclair, 1996; Vessey et al., 1988), salt stress (Bekki et al., 1987; Serraj et al., 1994; Aydi et al., 2004; L'Taief et al., 2007), dark stress (Gogorcena et al., 1997) and cold stress (van Heerden et al., 2008; Kuzma et al., 1995).

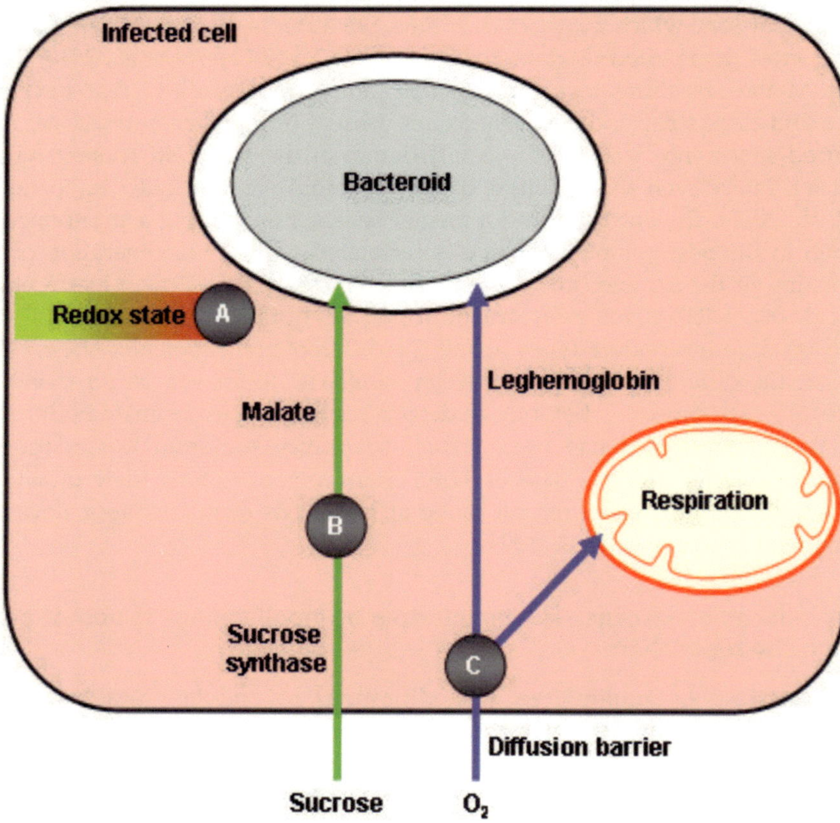

Fig. 3. Scheme showing the major processes modified during stress induced senescence. A, modification of the redox balance; B, alteration of the bacteroid nutrition; C, alteration of O_2 homeostasis.

However, nodule O_2 metabolic modifications are not always similar. Some types of stress decrease nodule permeability to O_2, lowering the O_2 availability to bacteroids, which in turn inhibits nitrogenase activity through a lower nodule respiration rate and lower energetic supply. In this context, a nitrate-nitric oxide respiration process has been identified in nodule which may play a role in the maintenance of energetic status under low oxygen conditions (Horchani et al., 2011). In contrast to stress which reduces oxygen availability, some stress increase nodule O_2 concentration (increased nodule permeability and/or lower respiration rate) which inhibits nitrogenase activity through a direct O_2-induced inactivation.

Leghemoglobin (Lb) is also a general physiological marker of SIS. As mentioned before, Lb has a crucial role in nodule functioning (Ott et al., 2009; Ott et al., 2005). Decrease of Lb content has been shown during drought stress (Gogorcena et al., 1995; Gordon et al., 1997; Guerin et al., 1990), salt stress (Gordon et al., 1997; Mhadhbi et al., 2011) and dark stress (Gogorcena et al., 1997; Matamoros et al., 1999). This diminution of Lb will impact the general metabolism of nodule by decreasing the O_2 availability to bacteroid and by potentially releasing free iron which may be a co-factor of the Fenton reaction to produce reactive oxygen species.

In conclusion, the general production of the high energy level needed for the efficient nitrogen fixation is generally altered at the onset of SIS.

3.3 Stress induced senescence is characterized by modifications in the nodule redox state components

As during developmental senescence, modifications of the redox balance are involved in nodule SIS. As discussed above, the high respiration rates, the important Lb concentration and the release of the catalytic Fe may be major ROS production systems. The accumulation of catalytic Fe has been detected during dark stress (Gogorcena et al., 1997; Becana & Klucas, 1992) and drought stress (Gogorcena et al., 1995) and participates in $OH^{\bullet}$ production during dark stress (Becana & Klucas, 1992). The modification of iron metabolism during SIS is also noticeable through the up regulation of ferritin and metallothionein during drought stress (Clement et al., 2008) and dark stress (Perez Guerra et al., 2010). These proteins sequester free Fe to decrease the Fenton reaction and protect the cellular primary components.

ROS accumulation is also regulated by antioxidant defence which participates in their degradation (Figure 4). Nodule antioxidant defence and the importance of the regulation of the redox balance has been extensively studied in root nodule (for review: Becana et al., 2010; Chang et al., 2009; Marino et al., 2009). Modifications of the antioxidant defence parameters have been used extensively as a marker for nodule SIS. Content and redox state of GSH and Asc, two antioxidant molecules, are modified during drought stress (Gogorcena et al., 1995; Marino et al., 2007), salt stress (Swaraj and Bishnoi, 1999) and dark stress (Matamoros et al., 1999; Gogorcena et al., 1997). Superoxide dismutase and catalase, two enzyme families involved in ROS degradation, are down regulated during dark stress (Matamoros et al., 1999; Gogorcena et al., 1997), salt stress (Jebara et al., 2005) and drought stress (Gogorcena et al., 1995; Rubio et al., 2002). Similarly, enzymes of the Asc-GSH cycle are modulated during nodule SIS (Gogorcena et al., 1995; Jebara et al., 2005; Matamoros et al., 1999; Mhadhbi et al., 2011). Nevertheless, whereas the majority of the reports suggest that SIS is associated with a decrease of the antioxidant defence, other articles have shown that some elements of the antioxidant defence are stable or even up regulated during stress. This discrepancy may be linked to the stress intensity, the plant adaptation to the treatment and to the growth conditions which modify the responses of plant to stress.

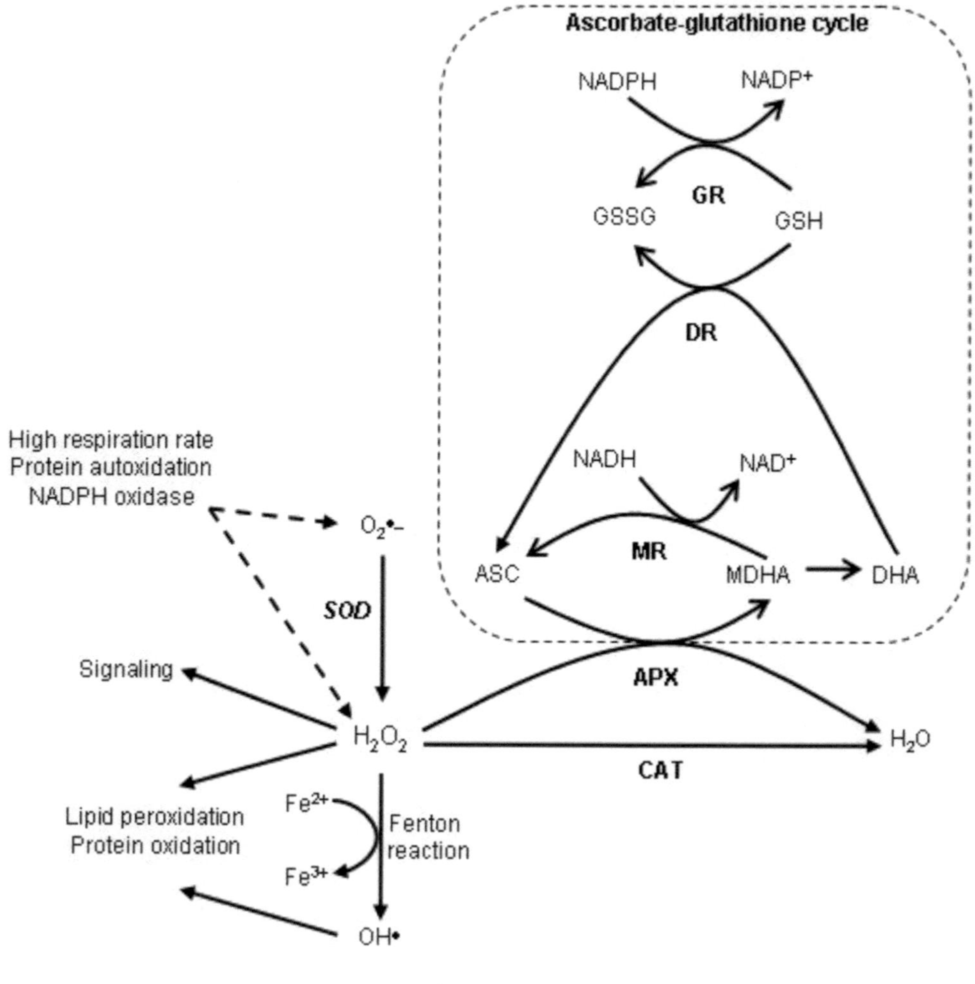

Fig. 4. Scheme showing processes for production and removal of Reactive Oxygen Species. CAT, catalase; SOD, superoxide dismutase; APX, ascorbate peroxidase; MR, monodehydroascorbate reductase; DR, dihydroascorbate reductase; GR, glutathione reductase; GSH, reduced glutathione; GSSG, oxidized glutathione; ASC, reduced ascorbate; MDHA, monodehydroascorbate; DHA, dehydroascorbate.

The imbalance in redox state leading to oxidative stress is characterized by the oxidation of major cellular components such as lipids and proteins. One of the major targets is the membrane. Lipid peroxidation, measured as the reaction of thiobarbituric acid with malondialdehyde, is significantly attenuated during dark stress (Matamoros et al., 1999; Gogorcena et al., 1997) in contrast to drought stress and salt stress during which lipid peroxidation increases (Gogorcena et al., 1995; Mhadhbi et al., 2011). Protein oxidation is increased during dark stress (Matamoros et al., 1999; Gogorcena et al., 1997) and drought stress (Gogorcena et al., 1995). The differential regulation in lipid peroxidation suggests that different degradation mechanisms may partially occur during SIS. This raises the question of SIS regulation and the specificity of the plant response to the different stress.

3.4 Nodule senescence induced by nitrate

One of the specificities of root nodule is the rapid onset of senescence occurring under nitrate treatment. Nitrate concentrations above 2 to 3 mM have strong detrimental effects on the NFS as there is inhibition of several developmental steps ranging from the infection process to the nitrogen fixation in mature nodule (Mortier et al., 2011; Streeter & Wong, 1988). As for other SIS, the inhibition of nitrogenase is correlated with an increase in O_2 diffusion and supply (Escuredo et al., 1996; Matamoros et al., 1999; Minchin et al., 1986; Minchin et al., 1989). Nitrate application also reduces carbon supply from leaves to nodules as measured by plant treatment with ^{11}C and ^{14}C-labelled CO_2 (Fujikake et al., 2003). This reduction in carbon supply is sometimes correlated with the diminution of the sucrose pool (Matamoros et al., 1999) and the down expression of sucrose synthase (Gordon et al., 2002). Nitrate treatment also decreases the antioxidant defence of the nodule with a diminution of the ascorbate pool and of the activities of ascorbate peroxidases and catalases (Escuredo et al., 1996; Matamoros et al., 1999). At the ultrastructural level, the symbiosome membrane seems to be affected by the senescence process before the bacteroid (Matamoros et al., 1999).

Nitrate effect results in both local and systemic regulation of the nodulation process (Jeudy et al., 2009). Systemic regulation has been described in numerous leguminous plants. Indeed, shoot-determined supernodulators with a nitrate-tolerant nodulation process have been described in soybean (Searle et al., 2003), pea (Duc & Messager, 1989), *L. japonicus* (Krusell et al., 2002) and *M. truncatula* (Penmetsa et al., 2003). Gene analyses have led to the identification of orthologous Leucine Rich Repeat-Receptor Like Kinases (LRR-RLKs) which play a crucial role in the autoregulation of nodulation. The systemic regulation may occur via the induction of specific CLV3/ESR (CLE) peptides produced after nitrate treatment (Okamoto et al., 2009; Reid et al., 2011). In this context, NOD3 is involved in the production or in the transport of the root signal molecule involved in the systemic regulation (Novak, 2010).

Finally, nitrogen limitation regulates nodule growth and stimulates BNF activity via a LRR-RLKs independent response suggesting that a local nodule adaptation may also be involved in the nitrate regulation of the BNF (Jeudy et al., 2009).

3.5 Molecular modifications occurring during stress induced senescence

The last review analyzing root nodule senescence presented oxidative stress and hormones as potential key players of the senescence process (Puppo et al., 2005). The concentration of abscissic acid (ABA), a hormone involved in plant response to abiotic and biotic stress (Cutler et al., 2010; Raghavendra et al., 2010), is strongly increased in soybean nodules under drought stress (Clement et al., 2008). The five-fold accumulation of ABA in stressed nodules compared to stressed roots shows that ABA accumulation is much higher in nodules than in roots. The effect of ABA on nodule functioning has been shown by exogenous treatment of pea nodules (Gonzalez et al., 2001). ABA treatment decreases the BNF and Lb content declines in parallel with the BNF. However, sucrose synthase activity, another parameter of drought stress effect, is not affected by this treatment suggesting that ABA is not the only player of nodule response to stress. Jasmonic acid (JA), another hormone involved in plant stress response (Reinbothe et al., 2009), has also been shown to be involved in the regulation of nodule functioning (Hause & Schaarschmidt, 2009). Exogenous JA treatment induces an accumulation of lipid peroxides and modifies ascorbate metabolism suggesting that JA could influence nodule senescence (Loscos et al., 2008).

Redox state modifications seem to be a regulatory element of the nodule SIS (Marino et al., 2006). Exogenous treatment with paraquat, which generates ROS, induces the alteration of the GSH and ASC pools toward a more oxidized state. This alteration of the redox state is associated with a diminution of BNF and decrease in Lb content. Moreover, an early decrease in sucrose synthase activity is also detected during the treatment. These results suggest that oxidative stress is involved in the signalling pathway leading to nodule SIS. Interestingly, sucrose synthase seems to be regulated at both the transcriptional and post-translational levels by oxidizing agents such as paraquat (Marino et al., 2008). Finally, genetic modifications allowing decrease and increase of GSH content in the nitrogen fixing zone has shown that BNF and Lb expression level are correlated with GSH content (El Msehli et al., 2011). These results strengthen the idea that cellular redox state plays a crucial role in the regulation of nodule functioning.

Developmental senescence and SIS present different structural and temporal features. At the transcriptomic level, analysis of the expression of 58 genes up regulated during developmental senescence has been performed during dark stress (Perez Guerra et al., 2010). 21 genes are induced during both types of senescence. Amongst these genes, some serine/threonine kinase and some genes involved in metal metabolism (metal transporters and metallothionein) have similar profiles of induction. Nine are up-regulated during both senescence types with different induction levels or transient induction during dark stress. Amongst these genes, cysteine and aspartic proteases are well represented. Finally, 28 genes are up regulated during developmental senescence and not by dark stress. Amongst these genes, proteins associated to proteasome function and vesicular trafficking are not induced during dark stress suggesting partial different regulatory processes between the two types of senescence. In soybean, a screen for genes involved in root nodule senescence has led to the isolation of the senescence-associated nodulin 1 (SAN1) multigene family showing a high homology with plant 2-oxoglutarate-dependent dioxygenases and including two functional genes *SAN1A* and *SAN1B* and a pseudogene *SAN1C* (Webb et al., 2008). Analyses of the steady-state mRNA levels of *SAN1A* and *SAN1B* during developmental senescence showed no significant differences for both genes. In contrast, during induced senescence by treatment with nitrate or darkness, *SAN1A* is down-regulated and *SAN1B* is up-regulated by both treatments.

Nevertheless, dark stress, drought stress and salt stress may induce specific senescence cascades and transcriptomic analyses will have to be realized to define the similarities and the differences in gene expression patterns in nodules subjected to the different stress.

4. Bacterial mutants and nodule senescence

The microsymbiont, differentiated into bacteroids inside the symbiosome, is not only dependent on "senescent" signals coming from the cytosolic environment of its host plant.

Mutations in some bacteroid genes have an incidence on its lifespan *in planta* and thus on the nodule integrity. However, it is difficult to assess the role of bacteroid genes on nodule senescence due to a lack of genetic tools to investigate this question.

Gene affected	Species	Function	Symbiotic phenotype	Reference
nifH, fixA, fixJ and fixK	*S. meliloti*	Nitrogen fixation	fix^{-}, elongated differentiated bacteroids	Maunoury et al., (2010)
lspB	*S. meliloti*	Lipopolysaccharide biosynthesis		
rpoH1	*S. meliloti*	σ^{23}-like protein , bacterial protection against environmental stresses	fix^{-}, reduced number of intracellular bacteria, mixture of normal elongated and abnormal bacteroids	Mitsui, (2004)
gltA	*S. meliloti*	Citrate synthase	fix$^{+/-}$ (20%/WT)	Grzemski et al., (2005)
aap bra	*R. leguminosarum*	Branched-chain amino acids transporters	fix$^{+/-}$ (30%/WT), fewer smaller bacteroids with a lower DNA content	Prell et al., (2009)
relA	*R. etli*	Stringent response	fix$^{+/-}$ (25%/WT), abnormal bacteroids, with an increased size	Moris et al., (2005)
sitA	*S. meliloti*	Manganese uptake	fix$^{+/-}$ (25%/WT), mixture of white, slightly pink and pink nodules	Davies et al., (2007)
katA katC	*S. meliloti*	Catalases	fix$^{+/-}$ (30%/WT), differentiated bacteroids irregular in shape	Jamet et al., (2003)
gshB	*S. meliloti*	Glutathione synthetase	fix$^{+/-}$ (25%/WT), senescence before or after differentiation into bacteroid	Harrison et al., (2005)
gshB	*R. tropici*	Glutathione synthetase	fix$^{+/-}$	Muglia et al., (2008)
lsrB1	*S. meliloti*	LysR-type transcriptional regulator	fix$^{+/-}$ (30%/WT), mixture of pink and white nodules	Luo et al., (2005)
hfq	*S. meliloti*	RNA chaperone	fix$^{+/-}$ (50%/WT), mixture of pink and white nodules	Torres-Quesada et al., (2010)

Table 1. Bacterial genes in which mutations cause early nodule senescence

Until now, there is no global transcriptomic study which could give information on the bacteroid gene expression profile when nitrogen fixing bacteroids turn off to become senescent. Moreover, due to the difficulty in finding a reliable and efficient screen to isolate bacteroid senescent mutants *in planta*, a library of such mutants is still not available. The data described below mostly come from the analysis of the symbiotic phenotype of rhizobial strains affected in one specific gene. The characteristics associated to these analyses include: plant yield, nodule morphology, nitrogen fixation efficiency, and sometimes, ultrastructure of the nodule and of the bacteroid. More recently, some symbiotic phenotype studies also include bacterial genome endoreduplication and transcriptome analyses. This section will mainly focus on the impact of a mutation in the bacterial genome on early nodule senescence and on delayed nodule senescence (Table 1).

4.1 Bacterial mutants and early nodule senescence

The rhizobial mutants that present a symbiotic phenotype are divided into four groups: the nodule deficient mutants impaired in the first steps of infection (nod$^-$ fix$^-$), the bacterial mutants which induce nodules that present an early nodule senescence phenotype i) blocked in their bacteroid differentiation process (nod$^+$ fix$^-$), ii) fully differentiated but unable to reduce N_2 (nod$^+$ fix$^-$) and iii) differentiated into bacteroids less efficient in N_2 fixation compared to the wild-type strain (nod$^+$ fix$^{+/-}$). Bacterial mutants leading to nodule development abortion due to a defect in bacteroid differentiation such as *bacA* (Saeki, 2011) or *parA* (Liu et al., 2011) mutants will not be presented here. The rhizobial nod$^+$ fix$^-$ mutants that could differentiate into bacteroids and pass the two transcriptome switch-points encountered during the differentiation of the wild-type bacteroids have been described recently (Maunoury et al., 2010). They are affected in genes encoding for symbiotic function and nitrogen fixation machinery (*nifH, fixA, fixJ* and *fixK*) or in lipopolysaccharide biosynthesis (*lspB*). The *rpoH1* mutant of *S. meliloti*, impaired in the synthesis of the σ^{32}-like protein, involved in bacterial protection against environmental stresses has also a nod$^+$ fix$^-$ symbiotic phenotype in interaction with alfalfa (Mitsui et al., 2004). The bacterial *rpoH1* mutant is still able to elicit nodule formation, efficient plant cell invasion and differentiation into bacteroids. But, the degeneration of bacteroids rapidly occurred in the proximal zone, adjacent to the infection zone, leading to ineffective white nodules associated to an early nodule senescence phenotype. Only the latter group of early nodule senescence mutants (nod$^+$ fix$^{+/-}$) will be described below. The genes affected in these mutants fall mainly into two categories: genes encoding function involved in carbon and nitrogen metabolism, and genes important for stress adaptation. Genes with other function will also be presented.

4.1.1 Genes encoding function involved in carbon and nitrogen metabolism of the bacteroid and in the nutriment stress response

The host plant supplies bacteroids with metabolites, including dicarboxylic and amino acids, used by the bacteroids to support the reduction of N_2 into ammonia in amounts sufficient for plant growth. To better understand the role of the decarboxylating part of the *S. meliloti* TCA cycle in a nitrogen fixing nodule, Gremski and collaborators (2005) have used an elegant approach (Grzemski et al., 2005). In *S. meliloti*, a mutant in the TCA cycle *gltA* gene encoding citrate synthase forms empty nodules devoid of intracellular bacteria. The *gltA* mutants are clearly unsuitable for experiments to determine whether citrate synthase (CS) is essential during nitrogen fixation in a mature nodule because they have a defect in development that prevents them from forming normal bacteroids. So, the authors constructed temperature-sensitive (ts) mutants in the *S. meliloti* citrate synthase (*gltA*) gene. This allows the formation of nitrogen-fixing nodules at the permissive temperature but, once nodule development was complete, an elevation of root temperature prevents CS expression. When alfalfa plants infected with the ts mutants were transferred to 30°C, the nodules lost the ability to fix nitrogen. Microscopic examination of the nodules revealed the loss of bacteroids in infected cells and morphological changes that resembled changes seen during nodule senescence.

These experiments with CS ts mutants showed that CS activity is needed in mature nodules to maintain bacteroid integrity and that removing CS activity via a temperature shift converts an effective nodule into an empty nodule. This implies that CS is essential for nodule maintenance as well as in the early stages of plant cell invasion.

Another example of early nodule senescence associated to a nutrient defect in *Rhizobium* has been described recently. Prell and collaborators (2009) have shown that *Rhizobium leguminosarum*, the bacterial partner of peas and broad beans (biovar *viciae*), becomes symbiotic auxotroph for the branched-chain amino acids Leucine, Isoleucine, Valine (LIV) when differentiated into bacteroids in root nodules (Prell et al., 2009). While these bacteria are prototrophs for LIV amino acids as free-living bacteria, they become dependent on the plant as nitrogen-fixing bacteroids, due to a major reduction in gene expression and activity of LIV biosynthetic enzymes. Peas inoculated with bacterial mutants impaired in their capacity to transport LIV, have an early senescent phenotype (nod$^+$, fix$^{+/-}$). Peas are yellow, have small, pale pink nodules and a dry weight similar to un-inoculated plants. This is correlated with a 70% decrease of the nitrogen fixation capacity for plants inoculated with these mutants compared to the plants inoculated with the *R. leguminosarum* wild-type strain. Thus, plants not only provide a carbon source (dicarboxylic acids) to the bacteroid but also precursors of proteins. The authors have shown that a defect in bacteroid LIV nutrition leads to a reduction in its persistence in plant infected cells, which in turn induces senescence. This means that the plant cell might receive information from the bacteroid in order to sense the fitness of the microsymbiont to maintain or interrupt the symbiotic interaction.

Concerning nutriment stress perceived by the bacteria *in planta*, a mutation in the *relA* gene of *Rhizobium etli*, induces symbiotic defects at the intermediate and/or late stages of the interaction with *Phaseolus vulgaris* (Moris et al., 2005). RelA allows the production of the alarmone (p)ppGpp, which mediates the stringent response in bacteria. This response results in transcriptional down regulation of ribosomal and tRNA genes, upon conditions of amino acid starvation. Despite this role, RelA has been reported to be important for biofilm formation and for interaction of bacteria, pathogenic or beneficial, with their eukaryotic host. Interaction of a *relA* mutant with common bean plants strongly reduces the nitrogen fixation efficiency by 75% and the plant yield. Microscopic studies showed that bacteria differentiated into bacteroids in the symbiosomes were larger in size than the wild-type ones. Thus, in the *R. etli* bacteroids, *relA* plays a role in physiology adaptation and regulation of gene expression. However, the step impaired in the nitrogen fixation defect of a *relA* mutant has not been investigated.

4.1.2 Genes encoding function involved in oxidative stress response

It is generally accepted that symbiotic bacteria are submitted to an oxidative burst released by the host plant during the first steps of infection (Pauly et al., 2006). In addition to this role as a general plant defence mechanism against bacterial invasion, oxidative burst might also play a role in the lifespan of the bacteroid. The high rate of bacteroid respiration necessary to supply energy required for the nitrogen reduction process generates high levels of ROS in the nodule. In legume root nodules, a large amount of H_2O_2 surrounding disintegrating bacteroids in senescent zone IV is detected (Rubio et al, 2004). This reflects the close relationship between oxidative stress and nodule senescence. Indeed, most of the bacterial mutant strains that show a symbiotic nod$^+$ fix$^{+/-}$ phenotype (early senescence) are affected in their antioxidant defence. To escape the stress generated by H_2O_2 and $O_2^{\cdot -}$, bacteria encode a set of enzymes such as superoxide dismutases, catalases and alkylhydroperoxidases, and also antioxidant molecules such as GSH.

In *S. meliloti,* disruption of the *sitA* gene induces a decrease in Mn/Fe SodB activity and a higher sensitivity to ROS (Davies and Walker, 2007). The *sitA* gene encodes a periplasmic protein involved in manganese uptake. During alfalfa interaction, a *sitA* mutant is either affected in its infection efficiency leading to small white nodules or is possibly altered in the survival of the differentiated form leading to intermediate nodules, with a slight pink fixing zone, smaller in size than the wild-type nodules. As a consequence, the nitrogenase activity and the plant yield are greatly reduced in these mutant infected plants compared to the plants inoculated with the wild-type bacteria. It is difficult to assess the role of the other superoxide dismutase of *S. meliloti* (SodA) in the natural senescence process since a *sodA* mutant failed to differentiate into bacteroids after release into plant cells (Santos et al., 2000).

To cope with H_2O_2 production, *S. meliloti* possesses three catalases. In free living bacteria, KatA and KatC are encoded by genes mainly transcribed in oxidative stress conditions while the *katB* gene is constitutively expressed. In 6 week-old nodules of *Medicago sativa,* KatA is the predominant catalase present in the bacteroids. The *katB* gene is also expressed in the nitrogen fixation zone III while *katC* is only transcribed in the infection zone II (Jamet et al., 2003). Single mutant strains of *katA, katB* or *katC* genes have no significant impact on nitrogen fixation efficiency of alfalfa nodules containing these mutants compared to those infected with wild-type bacteria. However a *katA katC* double mutant presents a dramatic decrease of nitrogen fixation capacity (Sigaud et al., 1999), associated with an early senescence of the nodule. These nodules were devoid of a clear zone III, instead the senescent zone IV was adjacent to interzone II-III (Jamet et al., 2003). In most plant cells, bacteria were correctly released from infection threads and were able to differentiate into bacteroids. This shows that efficient detoxification of H_2O_2 by the microsymbiont is essential in the latter steps of bacteroid differentiation leading to nitrogen fixing bacteria.

The antioxidant GSH plays an important role during symbiosis and nodule senescence. This tripeptide is synthesized by a two-step process. In bacteria, GshA catalyses the conjugation of glutamate and cysteine to form γEC and, in a second enzymatic step, GshB completes GSH synthesis by addition of glycine. In *S. meliloti,* while a *gshA* mutant is unable to form nodules (nod$^-$ fix$^-$ phenotype), a *gshB* mutant has a nod$^+$ phenotype coupled to a 75% reduction in the nitrogen fixation capacity (Harrison et al., 2005). In these nodules, bacteria are correctly released from the infection thread into host plant cells and enter into early senescence after differentiation into bacteroids. These data show that, in *S. meliloti,* GSH is important to maintain bacteroid during symbiotic interaction with alfalfa. This is also true in some determinate-type nodules as the survival of the common bean (*P. vulgaris)* microsymbiont, *Rhizobium tropicii,* is dependent on GSH production (Muglia et al., 2008). A *gshB* mutant has an early senescent pattern associated with increased levels of superoxide accumulation. Expression of this gene in a wild-type background is enhanced at late stage of nodule development, suggesting its antioxidant role against ROS accumulation during nodule senescence. In these species, GSH is important to keep nodules functional over time. In contrast, this does not hold true for *Bradyrhizobium* sp. where disruption of the *gshA* gene does not affect the ability to form effective nodules (Sobrevals et al., 2006). In this latter case, it is possible that the defect in intracellular GSH was compensated for by other compounds acting as antioxidants.

4.1.3 Genes encoding bacterial function involved in the regulation of gene expression

Ninety putative genes encoding LysR-type transcriptional regulators were identified in the *S. meliloti* genome. These regulators are typically 300 amino acids long with an N-terminal DNA binding domain and a C-terminal sensing domain for signal molecules and function as activators or repressors. LysR regulated genes have promoters which contain at least one TN11A motif and are usually divergently transcribed from the LysR regulator (Schell, 1993). To determine the role of LysR regulators in symbiosis, a mutagenesis analysis of all 90 putative *lysR* genes was realized (Luo et al., 2005). This allowed the isolation of the *lsrB1* mutant that presents a symbiotic phenotype. An *lsrB1* mutant was deficient in symbiosis and elicited a mixture of pink (45%) and white (55%) nodules on alfalfa plants. These plants exhibited lower overall nitrogenase activity (30%) than plants inoculated with the wild-type strain. This is consistent with the fact that most of the alfalfa plants inoculated with the *lsrB1* mutant were short (50 to 80% shorter than the plants inoculated with the WT strain) and light green. Cells of the *lsrB1* mutant were recovered from both pink and white nodules, suggesting that *lsrB1* mutants could be blocked either early or late during nodulation. Similar numbers of bacterial cells were recovered from the pink nodules of plants inoculated with the wild-type strain Rm1021 and pink and white nodules from the plants inoculated with the mutants. These findings suggest that the *lsrB1* mutants were able to invade plant cells. The *lsrB* gene is located downstream from the *trxB* gene for thioredoxin reductase, which also participates in the bacterial antioxidant defence. The *trxB* gene is transcribed from its own promoter in the same direction as the *lsrB* gene. The *trxB* promoter contains a nearly perfect recognition site (TN11A) for a LysR regulator so it is possible that LsrB regulates the expression of both the *trxB* and *lsrB* genes. The authors suggest that the early senescence phenotype observed *in planta* could be linked to a defect in detoxification of ROS in *S. meliloti*. However, this has not been demonstrated.

It has been shown recently that the *S. meliloti* RNA chaperone Hfq plays a role in the survival of the microsymbiont within the alfalfa nodule cells (Torres-Quesada et al., 2010). Hfq is considered to act as a global post-transcriptional regulator of gene expression since it interacts with diverse RNA molecules and small non-coding RNAs (sRNA). In free living bacteria, an *hfq* mutant down-regulates 91 genes mostly involved in central carbon metabolism (uptake and utilization of carbon substrates) and up-regulates genes involved in the uptake and catabolism of diverse N compounds. During late interaction with alfalfa (30 days post-infection), plants inoculated with the *hfq* mutant strain are composed of 60% of white non fixing nodules and 40% of pink fixing nodules. Thus, the plant yield was 64% of that of the wild-type-inoculated plants. Histological analysis of the white nodules revealed that the bacteroid differentiation was efficient but the bacteroid-infected tissues were restricted to the interzone II-III since the zone III was replaced by a large senescent zone IV. Indeed, an Hfq impaired mutant showed a premature senescent phenotype. The authors proposed that this phenotype could be linked to a defect in intracellular survival under prolonged stress present in the plant cell environment.

4.2 Bacterial mutants and delayed senescence

The delayed senescent bacterial mutants might have a nod$^+$ phenotype associated with a fix$^+$ phenotype for a period longer than the natural fixing period associated with the wild type bacteria in interaction with its host plant. Thus, such mutants are obligate differentiated bacteroids.

Compared to the data connected with the consequences of bacterial gene inactivation on early nodule senescence, little information on the role of bacterial mutants on delayed nodule senescence are available. Knowing that most of the mutations that induce an acceleration of senescence affect genes involved in ROS detoxification, in bacterial fitness, in import and/or processing of carbon skeletons, amino acids and antioxidants, we might suspect that a delayed senescence bacterial mutant should have a gain of function rather than an invalidated one. In that sense, it is possible that an increase in synthesis and/or activity of molecules involved in stress resistance, especially to ROS, should improve the bacteroid lifetime in the symbiosome and thus should enhance the nitrogen fixing period. This aspect of the role of bacterial genes in the functional life of symbiotic fixing nodules remains to be explored. However, one encouraging study sustains this postulate (Redondo et al., 2009). In fact, the authors of this work have overexpressed a cyanobacteria *Anabaena variabilis* gene encoding flavodoxin in *S. meliloti*. Knowing that natural senescence-inducing signals from the plant leads to a decrease in antioxidant content and thus an increase in ROS accumulation in an irreversible manner, they analyse the consequences of the over-expression of this flavodoxin protein involved in the response to oxidative stress. They have shown that the decline of nitrogenase activity was delayed and that the structural and ultrastructural modifications associated with nodule senescence had a later onset in flavodoxin-expressing nodules. Lipid peroxidation, a marker of senescence, was significantly reduced and the oxidative balance was improved in comparison to the control nodules. In conclusion, flavodoxin over-expression had an impact on bacteroid antioxidant metabolism, leading to delayed senescence.

In conclusion, we can propose that bacteroids inside the nodule infected cells are not only tributary from the plant to initiate nodule senescence. Genes encoding proteins implicated in bacterial nutrition and stress response are also essential since mutations in these genes alter the fitness of the differentiated bacteroids. In turn, this leads to the death of the microsymbiont followed by the senescence of the plant cells and nodule. Future aspects on the role of bacteroid genes on senescence should include the development of bacteroid genetic tools. The over-expression of pertinent genes specifically in the bacteroid or the conditional invalidation of rhizobial genes after bacteroid differentiation will be important to define senescence-related genes.

5. Perspectives

The data summarized in this review indicate that one of the general physiological features of nodule senescence is the decrease in nitrogen fixation efficiency. This diminution may be related to plant and/or bacterial-dependent factors. However whereas this diminution of the nitrogen fixation efficiency is observed during both developmental and stress induced-nodule senescence, the progression of senescence symptoms seems to be differentially controlled. Indeed, even if common general features have been described during nodule senescence, the few available microscopic and transcriptomic analyses show that nodule senescence may occur differently in developmental senescence and SIS. Moreover, the senescence occurring under different environmental stress conditions such as dark stress, drought stress or nitrate treatment may also involve different genetic and physiological programs. In this context, more detailed spatiotemporal analysis of the multiple senescence processes will have to be performed to determine the similarities and the differences between the various senescence processes. Microarray analysis or "Whole Transcriptome Shotgun Sequencing" will be valuable tools to analyse the transcriptome modifications occurring under the different senescence processes (Lister et al., 2009). In conditions in which the senescence process does not appear to be a homogenous process such as in developmental senescence, laser capture microdissection (Barcala et al., 2009) will allow the analysis of transcriptomic patterns of senescent infected cells. The development of two legume model systems, *M. truncatula* (http://www.medicago.org/) and *L. japonicus* (http://www.lotusjaponicus.org/) will facilitate an efficient analysis of the senescence process by developing tools dedicated to cell biology, genetic and transcriptomic analyses.

The role of the bacterial partner needs also to be clarified. Indeed, whereas senescence phenotypes are observed in nodules obtained with bacterial mutants affected in their nitrogen fixation efficiency, the regulation of this bacterial-induced senescence has not yet been studied. The abortion of nodule development when using such bacterial mutants suggests that the interaction may switch from a compatible to an incompatible interaction. In this context, the molecular events which trigger this switch still need to be defined. Nevertheless, the work with the flavodoxin overexpressing-bacterial strain showed that the symbiotic interaction may also be improved to resist to the various endogenous and environmental stress conditions. The construction of plant and bacteria with higher resistance to environmental stress (Zurbriggen et al., 2008) may be an interesting opportunity to increase the benefit from an efficient BNF in agronomy.

6. References

Alesandrini, F., Mathis, R., Van de Sype, G., Herouart, D. & Puppo, A. (2003). Possible roles for a cysteine protease and hydrogen peroxide in soybean nodule development and senescence. *New Phytol*, Vol. 158, No. 1, pp. 131-138

Apel, K. & Hirt, H. (2004). Reactive oxygen species: metabolism, oxidative stress, and signal transduction. *Annu Rev Plant Biol*, Vol. 55, pp. 373-399

Appleby, C. A. (1984). Leghemoglobin and Rhizobium respiration. *Annu Rev Plant Physiol Plant Mol Biol.*, Vol. 35, pp. 443-478

Aydi, S., Drevon, J. J. & Abdelly, C. (2004). Effect of salinity on root-nodule conductance to the oxygen diffusion in the *Medicago truncatula-Sinorhizobium meliloti* symbiosis. *Plant Physiol Biochem*, Vol. 42, No. 10, pp. 833-840

Barcala, M., Garcia, A., Cabrera, J., Casson, S., Lindsey, K., Favery, B., Garcia-Casado, G., Solano, R., Fenoll, C. & Escobar, C. (2009). Early transcriptomic events in microdissected Arabidopsis nematode-induced giant cells. *Plant J*, Vol. 61, No. 4, pp. 698-712

Becana, M. & Klucas, R. V. (1992). Transition metals in legume root nodules: iron-dependent free radical production increases during nodule senescence. *Proc Natl Acad Sci U S A*, Vol. 89, No. 19, pp. 8958-8962

Becana, M., Matamoros, M. A., Udvardi, M. & Dalton, D. A. (2010). Recent insights into antioxidant defenses of legume root nodules. *New Phytol*, Vol. 188, No. 4, pp. 960-976

Becker, A., Berges, H., Krol, E., Bruand, C., Ruberg, S., Capela, D., Lauber, E., Meilhoc, E., Ampe, F., de Bruijn, F. J., Fourment, J., Francez-Charlot, A., Kahn, D., Kuster, H., Liebe, C., Puhler, A., Weidner, S. & Batut, J. (2004). Global changes in gene expression in Sinorhizobium meliloti 1021 under microoxic and symbiotic conditions. *Mol Plant Microbe Interact*, Vol. 17, No. 3, pp. 292-303

Bekki, A., Trinchant, J.-C. & Rigaud, J. (1987). Nitrogen fixation (C_2H_2 reduction) by Medicago nodules and bacteroids under sodium chloride stress. *Physiologia Plantarum*, Vol. 71, No. 1, pp. 61-67

Ben Salah, I., Albacete, A., Martinez Andujar, C., Haouala, R., Labidi, N., Zribi, F., Martinez, V., Perez-Alfocea, F. & Abdelly, C. (2009). Response of nitrogen fixation in relation to nodule carbohydrate metabolism in Medicago ciliaris lines subjected to salt stress. *J Plant Physiol*, Vol. 166, No. 5, pp. 477-488

Benedito, V. A., Torres-Jerez, I., Murray, J. D., Andriankaja, A., Allen, S., Kakar, K., Wandrey, M., Verdier, J., Zuber, H., Ott, T., Moreau, S., Niebel, A., Frickey, T., Weiller, G., He, J., Dai, X., Zhao, P. X., Tang, Y. & Udvardi, M. K. (2008). A gene expression atlas of the model legume Medicago truncatula. *Plant J*, Vol. 55, No. 3, pp. 504-513

Bethlenfalvay, G. J. & Phillips, D. A. (1977). Ontogenetic Interactions between Photosynthesis and Symbiotic Nitrogen Fixation in Legumes. *Plant Physiol*, Vol. 60, No. 3, pp. 419-421

Bobik, C., Meilhoc, E. & Batut, J. (2006). FixJ: a major regulator of the oxygen limitation response and late symbiotic functions of Sinorhizobium meliloti. *J Bacteriol*, Vol. 188, No. 13, pp. 4890-4902

Broughton, W. J., Jabbouri, S. & Perret, X. (2000). Keys to symbiotic harmony. *J Bacteriol* Vol. 182, No. 20, pp. 5641-5652

Capela, D., Filipe, C., Bobik, C., Batut, J. & Bruand, C. (2006). Sinorhizobium meliloti differentiation during symbiosis with alfalfa: a transcriptomic dissection. *Mol Plant Microbe Interact*, Vol. 19, No. 4, pp. 363-372

Chang, C., Damiani, I., Puppo, A. & Frendo, P. (2009). Redox changes during the legume-rhizobium symbiosis. *Mol Plant*, Vol. 2, No. 3, pp. 370-377

Clement, M., Lambert, A., Herouart, D. & Boncompagni, E. (2008). Identification of new up-regulated genes under drought stress in soybean nodules. *Gene*, Vol. 426, No. 1, pp. 15-22

Coba de la Pena, T., Carcamo, C. B., Almonacid, L., Zaballos, A., Lucas, M. M., Balomenos, D. & Pueyo, J. J. (2008). A cytokinin receptor homologue is induced during root nodule organogenesis and senescence in Lupinus albus L. *Plant Physiol Biochem*, Vol. 46, No. 2, pp. 219-225

Crespi, M. & Frugier, F. (2008). De novo organ formation from differentiated cells: root nodule organogenesis. *Sci Signal*, Vol. 1, No. 49, pp. re11

Cutler, S. R., Rodriguez, P. L., Finkelstein, R. R. & Abrams, S. R. (2010). Abscisic acid: emergence of a core signaling network. *Annu Rev Plant Biol,* Vol. 61, pp. 651-679

Davies, B. W. & Walker, G. C. (2007). Disruption of sitA compromises Sinorhizobium meliloti for manganese uptake required for protection against oxidative stress. *J Bacteriol,* Vol. 189, No. 5, pp. 2101-2109

De Michele, R., Formentin, E., Todesco, M., Toppo, S., Carimi, F., Zottini, M., Barizza, E., Ferrarini, A., Delledonne, M., Fontana, P. & Lo Schiavo, F. (2009). Transcriptome analysis of Medicago truncatula leaf senescence: similarities and differences in metabolic and transcriptional regulations as compared with Arabidopsis, nodule senescence and nitric oxide signalling. *New Phytol,* Vol. 181, No. 3, pp. 563-575

Del Castillo, L. D., Hunt, S. & Layzell, D. B. (1994). The role of oxygen in the regulation of nitrogenase activity in drought-stressed soybean nodules. *Plant Physiol,* Vol. 106, No. 3, pp. 949-955

Downie, J. A. (2005). Legume haemoglobins: symbiotic nitrogen fixation needs bloody nodules. *Curr Biol,* Vol. 15, No. 6, pp. R196-198

Duc, G. & Messager, A. (1989). Mutagenesis of pea (Pisum sativum L.) and the isolation of mutants for nodulation and nitrogen fixation. *Plant Science,* Vol. 60, No. 2, pp. 207-213

El Msehli, S., Lambert, A., Baldacci-Cresp, F., Hopkins, J., Boncompagni, E., Smiti, S. A., Herouart, D. & Frendo, P. (2011). Crucial role of (homo)glutathione in nitrogen fixation in Medicago truncatula nodules. *New Phytol,* in press

El Yahyaoui, F., Kuster, H., Ben Amor, B., Hohnjec, N., Puhler, A., Becker, A., Gouzy, J., Vernie, T., Gough, C., Niebel, A., Godiard, L. & Gamas, P. (2004). Expression profiling in Medicago truncatula identifies more than 750 genes differentially expressed during nodulation, including many potential regulators of the symbiotic program. *Plant Physiol,* Vol. 136, No. 2, pp. 3159-3176

Escuredo, P. R., Minchin, F. R., Gogorcena, Y., Iturbe-Ormaetxe, I., Klucas, R. V. & Becana, M. (1996). Involvement of Activated Oxygen in Nitrate-Induced Senescence of Pea Root Nodules. *Plant Physiol,* Vol. 110, No. 4, pp. 1187-1195

Evans, P. J., Gallesi, D., Mathieu, C., Hernandez, M. J., de Felipe, M., Halliwell, B. & Puppo, A. (1999). Oxidative stress occurs during soybean nodule senescence. *Planta,* Vol. 208, No.1, pp. 73-79

Fedorova, M., van de Mortel, J., Matsumoto, P. A., Cho, J., Town, C. D., VandenBosch, K. A., Gantt, J. S. & Vance, C. P. (2002). Genome-wide identification of nodule-specific transcripts in the model legume Medicago truncatula. *Plant Physiol,* Vol. 130, No. 2, pp. 519-537

Franssen, H. J., Vijn, I., Yang, W. C. & Bisseling, T. (1992). Developmental aspects of the Rhizobium-legume symbiosis. *Plant Mol Biol,* Vol. 19, No. 1, pp. 89-107

Fridovich, I. (1986). Biological effects of the superoxide radical. *Arch Biochem Biophys,* Vol. 247, No. 1, pp. 1-11

Fujikake, H. - Yamazaki, A., Ohtake, N., Sueyoshi, K., Matsuhashi, S., Ito, T., Mizuniwa, C., Kume, T., Hashimoto, S., Ishioka, N.-S., Watanabe, S., Osa, A., Sekine, T., Uchida, H., Tsuji, A. & Ohyama, T. (2003). Quick and reversible inhibition of soybean root nodule growth by nitrate involves a decrease in sucrose supply to nodules. *J Exp Bot,* Vol. 54, No. 386, pp. 1379-1388

Galibert, F., Finan, T. M., Long, S. R., Puhler, A., Abola, P., Ampe, F., Barloy-Hubler, F., Barnett, M. J., Becker, A., Boistard, P., Bothe, G., Boutry, M., Bowser, L., Buhrmester, J., Cadieu, E., Capela, D., Chain, P., Cowie, A., Davis, R. W., Dreano, S., Federspiel, N. A., Fisher, R. F., Gloux, S., Godrie, T., Goffeau, A., Golding, B., Gouzy, J., Gurjal, M., Hernandez-Lucas, I., Hong, A., Huizar, L., Hyman, R. W., Jones, T., Kahn, D., Kahn, M. L., Kalman, S., Keating, D. H., Kiss, E., Komp, C., Lelaure, V., Masuy, D., Palm, C., Peck, M. C., Pohl, T. M., Portetelle, D., Purnelle, B., Ramsperger, U., Surzycki, R., Thebault, P., Vandenbol, M., Vorholter, F. J., Weidner, S., Wells, D. H., Wong, K., Yeh, K. C. & Batut, J. (2001). The composite genome of the legume symbiont Sinorhizobium meliloti. *Science,* Vol. 293, No. 5530, pp. 668-672

Galvez, L., Gonzalez, E. M. & Arrese-Igor, C. (2005). Evidence for carbon flux shortage and strong carbon/nitrogen interactions in pea nodules at early stages of water stress. *J Exp Bot,* Vol. 56, No. 419, pp. 2551-2561

Gepstein, S. (2004). Leaf senescence--not just a 'wear and tear' phenomenon. *Genome Biol,* Vol. 5, No. 3, pp. 212

Gogorcena, Y., Iturbe-Ormaetxe, I., Escuredo, P. R. & Becana, M. (1995). Antioxidant defenses against activated oxygen in pea nodules subjected to water stress. *Plant Physiol,* Vol. 108, No. 2, pp. 753-759

Gogorcena, Y., Gordon, A. J., Escuredo, P. R., Minchin, F. R., Witty, J. F., Moran, J. F. & Becana, M. (1997). N_2 fixation, carbon metabolism and oxidative damage in nodules of dark stressed Common Bean plants. *Plant Physiol,* Vol. 113, No.4, pp. 1193-1201

Gonzalez, E. M., Gordon, A. J., James, C. L. & Arrese-lgor, C. (1995). The role of sucrose synthase in the response of soybean nodules to drought. *J Ex Bot,* Vol. 46, No. 10, pp. 1515-1523

Gonzalez, E. M., Galvez, L. & Arrese-Igor, C. (2001). Abscisic acid induces a decline in nitrogen fixation that involves leghaemoglobin, but is independent of sucrose synthase activity. *J Exp Bot,* Vol. 52, No. 355, pp. 285-293

Gordon, A. J., Minchin, F. R., Skot, L. & James, C. L. (1997). Stress-induced declines in soybean N_2 fixation are related to nodule sucrose synthase activity. *Plant Physiol,* Vol. 114, No. 3, pp. 937-946

Gordon, A. J., Skot, L., James, C. L. & Minchin, F. R. (2002). Short-term metabolic responses of soybean root nodules to nitrate. *J Exp Bot,* Vol. 53, No. 368, pp. 423-428

Groten, K., Vanacker, H., Dutilleul, C., Bastian, F., Bernard, S., Carzaniga, R. & Foyer, C. H. (2005). The roles of redox processes in pea nodule development and senescence. *Plant, Cell & Environment,* Vol. 28, No. 10, pp. 1293-1304

Groten, K., Dutilleul, C., van Heerden, P. D., Vanacker, H., Bernard, S., Finkemeier, I., Dietz, K. J. & Foyer, C. H. (2006). Redox regulation of peroxiredoxin and proteinases by ascorbate and thiols during pea root nodule senescence. *FEBS Lett,* Vol. 580, No. 5, pp. 1269-1276

Grzemski, W., Akowski, J. P. & Kahn, M. L. (2005). Probing the Sinorhizobium meliloti-alfalfa symbiosis using temperature-sensitive and impaired-function citrate synthase mutants. *Mol Plant Microbe Interact,* Vol. 18, No. 2, pp. 134-141

Guerin, V., Trinchant, J. C. & Rigaud, J. (1990). Nitrogen Fixation (C(2)H(2) Reduction) by Broad Bean (Vicia faba L.) Nodules and Bacteroids under Water-Restricted Conditions. *Plant Physiol,* Vol. 92, No. 3, pp. 595-601

Gunther, C., Schlereth, A., Udvardi, M. & Ott, T. (2007). Metabolism of reactive oxygen species is attenuated in leghemoglobin-deficient nodules of Lotus japonicus. *Mol Plant Microbe Interact,* Vol. 20, No. 12, pp. 1596-1603

Harrison, J., Jamet, A., Muglia, C. I., Van de Sype, G., Aguilar, O. M., Puppo, A. & Frendo, P. (2005). Glutathione plays a fundamental role in growth and symbiotic capacity of Sinorhizobium meliloti. *J Bacteriol,* Vol. 187, No. 1, pp. 168-174

Hause, B. & Schaarschmidt, S. (2009). The role of jasmonates in mutualistic symbioses between plants and soil-born microorganisms. *Phytochemistry,* Vol. 70, No. 13-14, pp. 1589-1599

He, J., Benedito, V. A., Wang, M., Murray, J. D., Zhao, P. X., Tang, Y. & Udvardi, M. K. (2009). The Medicago truncatula gene expression atlas web server. *BMC Bioinformatics,* Vol. 10, pp. 441

Horchani, F., Prevot, M., Boscari, A., Evangelisti, E., Meilhoc, E., Bruand, C., Raymond, P., Boncompagni, E., Aschi-Smiti, S., Puppo, A. & Brouquisse, R. (2011). Both plant and bacterial nitrate reductases contribute to nitric oxide production in Medicago truncatula nitrogen-fixing nodules. *Plant Physiol,* Vol. 155, No. 2, pp. 1023-1036

Ivanov, S., Fedorova, E. & Bisseling, T. (2010). Intracellular plant microbe associations: secretory pathways and the formation of perimicrobial compartments. *Curr Opin Plant Biol,* Vol. 13, No. 4, pp. 372-377

Jamet, A., Sigaud, S., Van de Sype, G., Puppo, A. & Herouart, D. (2003). Expression of the bacterial catalase genes during Sinorhizobium meliloti-Medicago sativa symbiosis and their crucial role during the infection process. *Mol Plant Microbe Interact,* Vol. 16, No. 3, pp. 217-225

Jebara, S., Jebara, M., Limam, F. & Aouani, M. E. (2005). Changes in ascorbate peroxidase, catalase, guaiacol peroxidase and superoxide dismutase activities in common bean (*Phaseolus vulgaris*) nodules under salt stress. *J Plant Physiol,* Vol. 162, No. 8, pp. 929-936

Jeudy, C., Ruffel, S., Freixes, S., Tillard, P., Santoni, A. L., Morel, S., Journet, E. P., Duc, G., Gojon, A., Lepetit, M. & Salon, C. (2009). Adaptation of Medicago truncatula to nitrogen limitation is modulated via local and systemic nodule developmental responses. *New Phytol,* Vol. 185, No. 3, pp. 817-828

Jones, K. M., Kobayashi, H., Davies, B. W., Taga, M. E. & Walker, G. C. (2007). How rhizobial symbionts invade plants: the Sinorhizobium-Medicago model. *Nat Rev Microbiol,* Vol. 5, No. 8, pp. 619-633

Kaneko, T., Nakamura, Y., Sato, S., Asamizu, E., Kato, T., Sasamoto, S., Watanabe, A., Idesawa, K., Ishikawa, A., Kawashima, K., Kimura, T., Kishida, Y., Kiyokawa, C., Kohara, M., Matsumoto, M., Matsuno, A., Mochizuki, Y., Nakayama, S., Nakazaki, N., Shimpo, S., Sugimoto, M., Takeuchi, C., Yamada, M. & Tabata, S. (2000). Complete genome structure of the nitrogen-fixing symbiotic bacterium Mesorhizobium loti. *DNA Res,* Vol. 7, No. 6, pp. 331-338

Kaneko, T., Nakamura, Y., Sato, S., Minamisawa, K., Uchiumi, T., Sasamoto, S., Watanabe, A., Idesawa, K., Iriguchi, M., Kawashima, K., Kohara, M., Matsumoto, M., Shimpo, S., Tsuruoka, H., Wada, T., Yamada, M. & Tabata, S. (2002). Complete genomic sequence of nitrogen-fixing symbiotic bacterium Bradyrhizobium japonicum USDA110. *DNA Res,* Vol. 9, No. 6, pp. 189-197

Kardailsky, I. V. & Brewin, N. J. (1996). Expression of cysteine protease genes in pea nodule development and senescence. *Mol Plant Microbe Interact,* Vol. 9, No. 8, pp. 689-695

Karunakaran, R., Ramachandran, V. K., Seaman, J. C., East, A. K., Mouhsine, B., Mauchline, T. H., Prell, J., Skeffington, A. & Poole, P. S. (2009). Transcriptomic analysis of Rhizobium leguminosarum biovar viciae in symbiosis with host plants Pisum sativum and Vicia cracca. *J Bacteriol,* Vol. 191, No. 12, pp. 4002-4014

Kereszt, A., Mergaert, P., Maroti, G. & Kondorosi, E. (2011). Innate immunity effectors and virulence factors in symbiosis. *Current opinion in microbiology,* Vol. 14, No. 1, pp. 76-81

Kondorosi, E., Roudier, F. & Gendreau, E. (2000). Plant cell-size control: growing by ploidy? *Curr Opin Plant Biol,* Vol. 3, No. 6, pp. 488-492

Krusell, L., Madsen, L. H., Sato, S., Aubert, G., Genua, A., Szczyglowski, K., Duc, G., Kaneko, T., Tabata, S., de Bruijn, F., Pajuelo, E., Sandal, N. & Stougaard, J. (2002). Shoot control of root development and nodulation is mediated by a receptor-like kinase. *Nature,* Vol. 420, No. 6914, pp. 422-426

Kuster, H., Vieweg, M. F., Manthey, K., Baier, M. C., Hohnjec, N. & Perlick, A. M. (2007). Identification and expression regulation of symbiotically activated legume genes. *Phytochemistry,* Vol. 68, No. 1, pp. 8-18

Kuzma, M. M., Topunov, A. F. & Layzell, D. B. (1995). Effects of Temperature on Infected Cell O2 Concentration and Adenylate Levels in Attached Soybean Nodules. *Plant Physiol,* Vol. 107, No. 4, pp. 1209-1216

Larrainzar, E., Wienkoop, S., Weckwerth, W., Ladrera, R., Arrese-Igor, C. & Gonzalez, E. M. (2007). *Medicago truncatula* root nodule proteome analysis reveals differential plant and bacteroid responses to drought stress. *Plant Physiol,* Vol. 144, No. 3, pp. 1495-1507

Lawn, R. J. & Brun, W. A. (1977). Symbiotic Nitrogen Fixation in Soybeans. I. Effect of Photosynthetic Source-Sink Manipulations1. *Crop Sci.,* Vol. 14, No. 1, pp. 11

Lehtovaara, P. & Perttila, U. (1978). Bile-pigment formation from different leghaemoglobins. Methine-bridge specificity of coupled oxidation. *Biochem J,* Vol. 176, No. 2, pp. 359-364

Li, Y., Zhou, L., Li, Y., Chen, D., Tan, X., Lei, L. & Zhou, J. (2008). A nodule-specific plant cysteine proteinase, AsNODF32, is involved in nodule senescence and nitrogen fixation activity of the green manure legume Astragalus sinicus. *New Phytol,* Vol. 180, No. 1, pp. 185-192

Limpens, E., Ivanov, S., van Esse, W., Voets, G., Fedorova, E. & Bisseling, T. (2009). Medicago N2-fixing symbiosomes acquire the endocytic identity marker Rab7 but delay the acquisition of vacuolar identity. *Plant Cell,* Vol. 21, No. 9, pp. 2811-2828

Lister, R., Gregory, B. D. & Ecker, J. R. (2009). Next is now: new technologies for sequencing of genomes, transcriptomes, and beyond. *Curr Opin Plant Biol,* Vol. 12, No. 2, pp. 107-118

Liu, C. T., Lee, K. B., Wang, Y. S., Peng, M. H., Lee, K. T., Suzuki, S., Suzuki, T. & Oyaizu, H. (2011). Involvement of the azorhizobial chromosome partition gene (parA) in the onset of bacteroid differentiation during Sesbania rostrata stem nodule development. *Applied and environmental microbiology,* Vol. 77, No. 13, pp. 4371-4382

Lodwig, E. & Poole, P. S. (2003). Metabolism of Rhizobium bacteroids. *Crit Rev Plant Sci,* Vol. 22, No.1, pp. 37-78

Lohman, K. N., Gan, S., John, M. C. & Amasino, R. M. (1994). Molecular analysis of natural leaf senescence in Arabidopsis thaliana. *Physiologia Plantarum,* Vol. 92, No. 2, pp. 322

Long, S. R. (2001). Genes and signals in the rhizobium-legume symbiosis. *Plant Physiol,* Vol. 125, No. 1, pp. 69-72

Lopez, M., Herrera-Cervera, J. A., Iribarne, C., Tejera, N. A. & Lluch, C. (2008). Growth and nitrogen fixation in *Lotus japonicus* and *Medicago truncatula* under NaCl stress: Nodule carbon metabolism. *J Plant Physiol,* Vol. 165, No. 6, pp. 641-650

Lopez, M., Tejera, N. A. & Lluch, C. (2009). Validamycin A improves the response of Medicago truncatula plants to salt stress by inducing trehalose accumulation in the root nodules. *J Plant Physiol,* Vol. 166, No. 11, pp. 1218-1222

Loscos, J., Matamoros, M. A. & Becana, M. (2008). Ascorbate and homoglutathione metabolism in common bean nodules under stress conditions and during natural senescence. *Plant Physiol,* Vol. 146, No. 3, pp. 1282-1292

Lucas, M. M., Van de Sype, G., Hérouart, D., Hernandez, M. J., Puppo, A. & de Felipe, M. R. (1998). Immunolocalization of ferritin in determinate and indeterminate legume root nodules. *Protoplasma,* Vol. 204, No. 1, pp. 61-70

Luo, L., Yao, S. Y., Becker, A., Ruberg, S., Yu, G. Q., Zhu, J. B. & Cheng, H. P. (2005). Two new Sinorhizobium meliloti LysR-type transcriptional regulators required for nodulation. *J Bacteriol,* Vol. 187, No. 13, pp. 4562-4572

L'Taief, B., Sifi, B., Zaman-Allah, M., Drevon, J. J. & Lachaal, M. (2007). Effect of salinity on root-nodule conductance to the oxygen diffusion in the *Cicer arietinum-Mesorhizobium ciceri* symbiosis. *J Plant Physiol,* Vol. 164, No. 8, pp. 1028-1036

Malik, N. S., Pfeiffer, N. E., Williams, D. R. & Wagner, F. W. (1981). Peptidohydrolases of Soybean Root Nodules: Identification, separation and partial characterisation of enzymes from bacteroid-free extracts. *Plant Physiol,* Vol. 68, No. 2, pp. 386-392

Marino, D., Gonzalez, E. M. & Arrese-Igor, C. (2006). Drought effects on carbon and nitrogen metabolism of pea nodules can be mimicked by paraquat: evidence for the occurrence of two regulation pathways under oxidative stresses. *J Exp Bot,* Vol. 57, No. 3, pp. 665-673

Marino, D., Frendo, P., Ladrera, R., Zabalza, A., Puppo, A., Arrese-Igor, C. & Gonzalez, E. M. (2007). Nitrogen fixation control under drought stress. Localized or systemic? *Plant Physiol,* Vol. 143, No. 4, pp. 1968-1974

Marino, D., Hohnjec, N., Kuster, H., Moran, J. F., Gonzalez, E. M. & Arrese-Igor, C. (2008). Evidence for transcriptional and post-translational regulation of sucrose synthase in pea nodules by the cellular redox state. *Mol Plant Microbe Interact,* Vol. 21, No. 5, pp. 622-630

Marino, D., Pucciariello, C., Puppo, A. & Frendo, P. (2009).The Redox State, a Referee of the Legume-Rhizobia Symbiotic Game. In *Advances in Botanical Research: Oxidative Stress and Redox Regulation in Plants,* J. P. Jacquot, pp. 115-151, Burlington: Academic Press

Matamoros, M. A., Baird, L. M., Escuredo, P. R., Dalton, D. A., Minchin, F. R., Iturbe-Ormaetxe, I., Rubio, M. C., Moran, J. F., Gordon, A. J. & Becana, M. (1999). Stress induced legume root nodule senescence. Physiological, biochemical and structural alterations. *Plant Physiol,* Vol. 121, No.1, pp. 97-112

Maunoury, N., Kondorosi, A., Kondorosi, E. & Mergaert, P. (2008).Cell biology of nodule infection and development. In *Nitrogen-fixing Leguminous Symbioses* E. K. James, J. I. Sprent, W. E. Dilworth and N. W.E., pp. 153–189, Springer, the Netherlands

Maunoury, N., Redondo-Nieto, M., Bourcy, M., Van de Velde, W., Alunni, B., Laporte, P., Durand, P., Agier, N., Marisa, L., Vaubert, D., Delacroix, H., Duc, G., Ratet, P., Aggerbeck, L., Kondorosi, E. & Mergaert, P. (2010). Differentiation of symbiotic cells and endosymbionts in Medicago truncatula nodulation are coupled to two transcriptome-switches. *PLoS One,* Vol. 5, No. 3, pp. e9519

Mergaert, P., Nikovics, K., Kelemen, Z., Maunoury, N., Vaubert, D., Kondorosi, A. & Kondorosi, E. (2003). A novel family in Medicago truncatula consisting of more than 300 nodule-specific genes coding for small, secreted polypeptides with conserved cysteine motifs. *Plant Physiol,* Vol. 132, No. 1, pp. 161-173

Mergaert, P., Uchiumi, T., Alunni, B., Evanno, G., Cheron, A., Catrice, O., Mausset, A. E., Barloy-Hubler, F., Galibert, F., Kondorosi, A. & Kondorosi, E. (2006). Eukaryotic control on bacterial cell cycle and differentiation in the Rhizobium-legume symbiosis. *Proc Natl Acad Sci U S A,* Vol. 103, No. 13, pp. 5230-5235

Mhadhbi, H., Fotopoulos, V., Mylona, P. V., Jebara, M., Elarbi Aouani, M. & Polidoros, A. N. (2011). Antioxidant gene-enzyme responses in Medicago truncatula genotypes with different degree of sensitivity to salinity. *Physiol Plant,* Vol. 141, No. 3, pp. 201-214

Minchin, F. R., Minguez, M. I., Sheehy, J. E., Witty, J. F. & SkÃ˜T, L. (1986). Relationships Between Nitrate and Oxygen Supply in Symbiotic Nitrogen Fixation by White Clover. *J Ex Bot,* Vol. 37, No. 8, pp. 1103-1113

Minchin, F. R., Becana, M. & Sprent, J. I. (1989). Short-term inhibition of legume N_2 fixation by nitrate. II. Nitrate effects on nodule oxygen diffusion. *Planta,* Vol. 180, No.1, pp. 46-52

Mitsui, H., Sato, T., Sato, Y., Ito, N. & Minamisawa, K. (2004). Sinorhizobium meliloti RpoH1 is required for effective nitrogen-fixing symbiosis with alfalfa. *Mol Genet Genomics,* Vol. 271, No. 4, pp. 416-425

Moris, M., Braeken, K., Schoeters, E., Verreth, C., Beullens, S., Vanderleyden, J. & Michiels, J. (2005). Effective symbiosis between Rhizobium etli and Phaseolus vulgaris requires the alarmone ppGpp. *J Bacteriol,* Vol. 187, No. 15, pp. 5460-5469

Mortier, V., Holsters, M. & Goormachtig, S. (2011). Never too many? How legumes control nodule numbers. *Plant Cell Environ,* in press

Muglia, C., Comai, G., Spegazzini, E., Riccillo, P. M. & Aguilar, O. M. (2008). Glutathione produced by Rhizobium tropici is important to prevent early senescence in common bean nodules. *FEMS microbiology letters,* Vol. 286, No. 2, pp. 191-198

Naito, Y., Fujie, M., Usami, S., Murooka, Y. & Yamada, T. (2000). The involvement of a cysteine proteinase in the nodule development in Chinese milk vetch infected with Mesorhizobium huakuii subsp. rengei. *Plant Physiol,* Vol. 124, No. 3, pp. 1087-1096

Naya, L., Ladrera, R., Ramos, J., Gonzalez, E. M., Arrese-Igor, C., Minchin, F. R. & Becana, M. (2007). The response of carbon metabolism and antioxidant defenses of alfalfa nodules to drought stress and to the subsequent recovery of plants. *Plant Physiol,* Vol. 144, No. 2, pp. 1104-1114

Novak, K. (2010). Early action of pea symbiotic gene NOD3 is confirmed by adventitious root phenotype. *Plant Sci,* Vol. 179, No. 5, pp. 472-478

Oldroyd, G. E., Murray, J. D., Poole, P. S. & Downie, J. A. (2011). The Rules of Engagement in the Legume-Rhizobial Symbiosis. *Annu Rev Genet,* Vol.45, in press

Ott, T., van Dongen, J. T., Gunther, C., Krusell, L., Desbrosses, G., Vigeolas, H., Bock, V., Czechowski, T., Geigenberger, P. & Udvardi, M. K. (2005). Symbiotic leghemoglobins are crucial for nitrogen fixation in legume root nodules but not for general plant growth and development. *Curr Biol,*Vol. 15, No. 6, pp. 531-535

Ott, T., Sullivan, J., James, E. K., Flemetakis, E., Gunther, C., Gibon, Y., Ronson, C. & Udvardi, M. (2009). Absence of symbiotic leghemoglobins alters bacteroid and plant cell differentiation during development of Lotus japonicus root nodules. *Mol Plant Microbe Interact,* Vol. 22, No. 7, pp. 800-808

Pauly, N., Pucciariello, C., Mandon, K., Innocenti, G., Jamet, A., Baudouin, E., Herouart, D., Frendo, P. & Puppo, A. (2006). Reactive oxygen and nitrogen species and glutathione: key players in the legume-Rhizobium symbiosis. *J Exp Bot,* Vol. 57, No. 8, pp. 1769-1776

Penmetsa, R. V., Frugoli, J. A., Smith, L. S., Long, S. R. & Cook, D. R. (2003). Dual genetic pathways controlling nodule number in Medicago truncatula. *Plant Physiol,* Vol. 131, No. 3, pp. 998-1008

Perez Guerra, J. C., Coussens, G., De Keyser, A., De Rycke, R., De Bodt, S., Van De Velde, W., Goormachtig, S. & Holsters, M. (2010). Comparison of developmental and stress-induced nodule senescence in Medicago truncatula. *Plant Physiol,* Vol. 152, No. 3, pp. 1574-1584

Perret, X., Staehelin, C. & Broughton, W. J. (2000). Molecular basis of symbiotic promiscuity. *Microbiol Mol Biol Rev,* Vol. 64, No. 1, pp. 180-201

Pessi, G., Ahrens, C. H., Rehrauer, H., Lindemann, A., Hauser, F., Fischer, H. M. & Hennecke, H. (2007). Genome-wide transcript analysis of Bradyrhizobium japonicum bacteroids in soybean root nodules. *Mol Plant Microbe Interact,* Vol. 20, No. 11, pp. 1353-1363

Pfeiffer, N. E., Torres, C. M. & Wagner, F. W. (1983). Proteolytic Activity in Soybean Root Nodules : Activity in Host Cell Cytosol and Bacteroids throughout Physiological Development and Senescence. *Plant Physiol,* Vol. 71, No. 4, pp. 797-802

Pladys, D. & Rigaud, J. (1985). Senescence in French-bean nodules: Occurrence of different proteolytic activities. *Physiologia Plantarum,* Vol. 63, No. 1, pp. 43

Pladys, D., Dimitrijevic, L. & Rigaud, J. (1991). Localization of a protease in protoplast preparations in infected cells of French bean nodules. *Plant Physiol,* Vol. 97, No. 3, pp. 1174-1180

Pladys, D. & Vance, C. P. (1993). Proteolysis during Development and Senescence of Effective and Plant Gene-Controlled Ineffective Alfalfa Nodules. *Plant Physiol,* Vol. 103, No. 2, pp. 379-384

Prell, J. & Poole, P. (2006). Metabolic changes of rhizobia in legume nodules. *Trends Microbiol* Vol. 14, No. 4, pp. 161-168

Prell, J., White, J. P., Bourdes, A., Bunnewell, S., Bongaerts, R. J. & Poole, P. S. (2009). Legumes regulate Rhizobium bacteroid development and persistence by the supply of branched-chain amino acids. *Proc Natl Acad Sci USA,*Vol. 106, No. 30, pp. 12477-12482

Puppo, A., Rigaud, J. & Job, D. (1981). Role of superoxide anion in leghemoglobin autoxidation. *Plant Science Letters,* Vol. 22, No. 4, pp. 353

Puppo, A. & Halliwell, B. (1988). Formation of hydroxyl radicals from hydrogen peroxide in the presence of iron. Is haemoglobin a biological Fenton reagent? *Biochem J,* Vol. 249, No. 1, pp. 185-190

Puppo, A., Groten, K., Bastian, F., Carzaniga, R., Soussi, M., Lucas, M. M., de Felipe, M. R., Harrison, J., Vanacker, H. & Foyer, C. H. (2005). Legume nodule senescence: roles for redox and hormone signalling in the orchestration of the natural aging process. *New Phytol,* Vol. 165, No. 3, pp. 683-701

Raghavendra, A. S., Gonugunta, V. K., Christmann, A. & Grill, E. (2010). ABA perception and signalling. *Trends Plant Sci,* Vol. 15, No. 7, pp. 395-401

Redondo, F. J., de la Pena, T. C., Morcillo, C. N., Lucas, M. M. & Pueyo, J. J. (2009). Overexpression of flavodoxin in bacteroids induces changes in antioxidant metabolism leading to delayed senescence and starch accumulation in alfalfa root nodules. *Plant Physiol,*Vol. 149, No. 2, pp. 1166-1178

Reinbothe, C., Springer, A., Samol, I. & Reinbothe, S. (2009). Plant oxylipins: role of jasmonic acid during programmed cell death, defence and leaf senescence. *Febs J,* Vol. 276, No. 17, pp. 4666-4681

Reyrat, J. M., David, M., Blonski, C., Boistard, P. & Batut, J. (1993). Oxygen-regulated in vitro transcription of Rhizobium meliloti nifA and fixK genes. *J Bacteriol,* Vol. 175, No. 21, pp. 6867-6872

Rubio, M. C., Gonzalez, E. M., Minchin, F. R., Webb, K. J., Arrese-Igor, C., Ramos, J. & Becana, M. (2002). Effects of water stress on antioxidant enzymes of leaves and nodules of transgenic alfalfa overexpressing superoxide dismutases. *Physiol Plant,* Vol. 115, No. 4, pp. 531-540

Saeki, K. (2011). Rhizobial measures to evade host defense strategies and endogenous threats to persistent symbiotic nitrogen fixation: a focus on two legume-rhizobium model systems. *Cell Mol Life Sci,* Vol. 68, No. 8, pp. 1327-1339

Sanchez, D. H., Pieckenstain, F. L., Escaray, F., Erban, A., Kraemer, U., Udvardi, M. K. & Kopka, J. (2011). Comparative ionomics and metabolomics in extremophile and glycophytic Lotus species under salt stress challenge the metabolic pre-adaptation hypothesis. *Plant Cell Environ,* Vol. 34, No. 4, pp. 605-617

Santos, R., Herouart, D., Puppo, A. & Touati, D. (2000). Critical protective role of bacterial superoxide dismutase in rhizobium-legume symbiosis. *Molecular microbiology,* Vol. 38, No. 4, pp. 750-759

Sato, S., Nakamura, Y., Kaneko, T., Asamizu, E., Kato, T., Nakao, M., Sasamoto, S., Watanabe, A., Ono, A., Kawashima, K., Fujishiro, T., Katoh, M., Kohara, M., Kishida, Y., Minami, C., Nakayama, S., Nakazaki, N., Shimizu, Y., Shinpo, S., Takahashi, C., Wada, T., Yamada, M., Ohmido, N., Hayashi, M., Fukui, K., Baba, T., Nakamichi, T., Mori, H. & Tabata, S. (2008). Genome structure of the legume, Lotus japonicus. *DNA Res,*Vol. 15, No. 4, pp. 227-239

Schauser, L., Udvardi, M., Tabata, S. & Stougaard, J. (2008).Legume genomics relevant to N_2 fixation. In *Nitrogen-fixing Leguminous Symbioses,* S. J. James EK, Dilworth WE, Newton WE, pp. 211–233, Springer, the Netherlands

Schell, M. A. (1993). Molecular biology of the LysR family of transcriptional regulators. *Annu Rev Microbiol,* Vol. 47, pp. 597-626

Schmutz, J., Cannon, S. B., Schlueter, J., Ma, J., Mitros, T., Nelson, W., Hyten, D. L., Song, Q., Thelen, J. J., Cheng, J., Xu, D., Hellsten, U., May, G. D., Yu, Y., Sakurai, T.,

Umezawa, T., Bhattacharyya, M. K., Sandhu, D., Valliyodan, B., Lindquist, E., Peto, M., Grant, D., Shu, S., Goodstein, D., Barry, K., Futrell-Griggs, M., Abernathy, B., Du, J., Tian, Z., Zhu, L., Gill, N., Joshi, T., Libault, M., Sethuraman, A., Zhang, X. C., Shinozaki, K., Nguyen, H. T., Wing, R. A., Cregan, P., Specht, J., Grimwood, J., Rokhsar, D., Stacey, G., Shoemaker, R. C. & Jackson, S. A. (2010). Genome sequence of the palaeopolyploid soybean. *Nature,* Vol. 463, No. 7278, pp. 178-183

Schneiker-Bekel, S., Wibberg, D., Bekel, T., Blom, J., Linke, B., Neuweger, H., Stiens, M., Vorholter, F. J., Weidner, S., Goesmann, A., Puhler, A. & Schluter, A. (2011). The complete genome sequence of the dominant Sinorhizobium meliloti field isolate SM11 extends the S. meliloti pan-genome. *J Biotechnol,* Vol. 155, No. 1, pp. 20-33

Searle, I. R., Men, A. E., Laniya, T. S., Buzas, D. M., Iturbe-Ormaetxe, I., Carroll, B. J. & Gresshoff, P. M. (2003). Long-distance signaling in nodulation directed by a CLAVATA1-like receptor kinase. *Science,* Vol. 299, No. 5603, pp. 109-112

Serraj, R. & Sinclair, T. R. (1996). Inhibition of nitrogenase activity and oxygen permeability by water deficit. *J Exp Bot,* Vol. 47, No., pp. 1067-1073

Serraj, R., Vadez, V. V., Denison, R. F. & Sinclair, T. R. (1999). Involvement of ureides in nitrogen fixation inhibition in soybean. *Plant Physiol,* Vol. 119, No. 1, pp. 289-296

Sigaud, S., Becquet, V., Frendo, P., Puppo, A. & Herouart, D. (1999). Differential regulation of two divergent Sinorhizobium meliloti genes for HPII-like catalases during free-living growth and protective role of both catalases during symbiosis. *J Bacteriol,* Vol. 181, No. 8, pp. 2634-2639

Sobrevals, L., Muller, P., Fabra, A. & Castro, S. (2006). Role of glutathione in the growth of Bradyrhizobium sp. (peanut microsymbiont) under different environmental stresses and in symbiosis with the host plant. *Canadian journal of microbiology,* Vol. 52, No. 7, pp. 609-616

Soussi, M., Ocana, A. & Lluch, C. (1998). Effects of salt stress on growth, photosynthesis and nitrogen fixation in chick-pea (Cicer arietinum L.). *J Ex Bot,* Vol. 49, No. 325, pp. 1329-1337

Streeter, J. & Wong, P. P. (1988). Inhibition of legume nodule formation and N2 fixation by nitrate. *Critical Reviews in Plant Sciences,* Vol. 7, No. 1, pp. 1-23

Swaraj, K., Dhandi, S. & Sheokand, S. (1995). Relationship between defense mechanism against activated oxygen species and nodule functioning with progress in plant and nodule development in Cajanus cajan L. Millsp. *Plant Sci,* Vol. 112, No. 1, pp. 65

Swaraj, K. & Bishnoi, N. R. (1999). Effect of salt stress on nodulation and nitrogen fixation in legumes. *Indian J Exp Biol,* Vol. 37, No. 9, pp. 843-848

Thomas, S. G., Phillips, A. L. & Hedden, P. (1999). Molecular cloning and functional expression of gibberellin 2- oxidases, multifunctional enzymes involved in gibberellin deactivation. *Proc Natl Acad Sci U S A,*Vol. 96, No. 8, pp. 4698-4703

Timmers, A. C., Soupene, E., Auriac, M. C., de Billy, F., Vasse, J., Boistard, P. & Truchet, G. (2000). Saprophytic intracellular rhizobia in alfalfa nodules. *Mol Plant Microbe Interact,* Vol. 13, No. 11, pp. 1204-1213

Torres-Quesada, O., Oruezabal, R. I., Peregrina, A., Jofre, E., Lloret, J., Rivilla, R., Toro, N. & Jimenez-Zurdo, J. I. (2010). The Sinorhizobium meliloti RNA chaperone Hfq influences central carbon metabolism and the symbiotic interaction with alfalfa. *BMC microbiology,* Vol. 10, pp. 71

Van de Velde, W., Guerra, J. C., De Keyser, A., De Rycke, R., Rombauts, S., Maunoury, N., Mergaert, P., Kondorosi, E., Holsters, M. & Goormachtig, S. (2006). Aging in legume symbiosis. A molecular view on nodule senescence in Medicago truncatula. *Plant Physiol,* Vol. 141, No. 2, pp. 711-720

Van de Velde, W., Zehirov, G., Szatmari, A., Debreczeny, M., Ishihara, H., Kevei, Z., Farkas, A., Mikulass, K., Nagy, A., Tiricz, H., Satiat-Jeunemaitre, B., Alunni, B., Bourge, M., Kucho, K., Abe, M., Kereszt, A., Maroti, G., Uchiumi, T., Kondorosi, E. & Mergaert, P. (2010). Plant peptides govern terminal differentiation of bacteria in symbiosis. *Science,* Vol. 327, No. 5969, pp. 1122-1126

van Heerden, P. D., Kiddle, G., Pellny, T. K., Mokwala, P. W., Jordaan, A., Strauss, A. J., de Beer, M., Schluter, U., Kunert, K. J. & Foyer, C. H. (2008). Roles for the regulation of respiration and the oxygen diffusion barrier in soybean in the protection of symbiotic nitrogen fixation from chilling -induced inhibition and shoots from premature senescence. *Plant Physiol,* Vol. 148, No. 1, pp. 316-327

Vasse, J., de Billy, F., Camut, S. & Truchet, G. (1990). Correlation between ultrastructural differentiation of bacteroids and nitrogen fixation in alfalfa nodules. *J Bacteriol,* Vol. 172, No. 8, pp. 4295-4306

Vauclare, P., Bligny, R., Gout, E., De Meuron, V. & Widmer, F. (2010). Metabolic and structural rearrangement during dark-induced autophagy in soybean (Glycine max L.) nodules: an electron microscopy and 31P and 13C nuclear magnetic resonance study. *Planta,* Vol. 231, No. 6, pp. 1495-1504

Vessey, J. K., Walsh, K. B. & Layzell, D. B. (1988). Oxygen limitation of nitrogen fixation in stem-girdled and nitrate-treated soybean. *Physiol Plant,* Vol. 73, No., pp. 113-121

Walsh, K. B. & Layzell, D. B. (1986). Carbon and nitrogen assimilation and partitioning in soybeans exposed to low root temperatures. *Plant Physiol,* Vol. 80, No. 1, pp. 249-255

Webb, C. J., Chan-Weiher, C. & Johnson, D. A. (2008). Isolation of a novel family of genes related to 2-oxoglutarate-dependent dioxygenases from soybean and analysis of their expression during root nodule senescence. *J Plant Physiol,* Vol. 165, No. 16, pp. 1736-1744

White, J., Prell, J., James, E. K. & Poole, P. (2007). Nutrient sharing between symbionts. *Plant Physiol,* Vol. 144, No. 2, pp. 604-614

Zurbriggen, M. D., Tognetti, V. B., Fillat, M. F., Hajirezaei, M. R., Valle, E. M. & Carrillo, N. (2008). Combating stress with flavodoxin: a promising route for crop improvement. *Trends Biotechnol,* Vol. 26, No. 10, pp. 531-537

Part 2

Animal

9

The Nucleolus and Ribosomal Genes in Aging and Senescence

Nadine Hein[1,*], Elaine Sanij[1,2,*], Jaclyn Quin[1,3], Katherine M. Hannan[1], Austen Ganley[4,#] and Ross D. Hannan[1,3,5,6,#]

[1]*Division of Cancer Research, Peter MacCallum Cancer Centre, Melbourne,*
[2]*Department of Pathology, University of Melbourne, Melbourne,*
[3]*Department of Biochemistry and Molecular Biology, University of Melbourne, Melbourne,*
[4]*Institute of Natural Sciences, Massey University, Auckland,*
[5]*Department of Biochemistry and Molecular Biology, Monash University, Melbourne,*
[6]*School of Biomedical Sciences, The University of Queensland, Melbourne,*
[1,2,3,5,6]*Australia*
[4]*New Zealand*

1. Introduction

The nucleolus forms around the tandem repeats of the ribosomal RNA (rRNA) genes (rDNA) that are transcribed by RNA polymerase I (Pol I), giving rise to the production of rRNAs. These represent the nucleic acid backbone of the functional ribosomes in the cytoplasm, and as such rDNA transcription dictates the cells' protein translational capacity. More recently it has become apparent that the epigenetic status of these rDNA repeats and the integrity of the nucleolus can modulate cellular homeostasis beyond ribosome biogenesis. Such roles include mediating the titration of tumor suppressors and oncogenes, modulating the heterochromatic state of many RNA Polymerase II (Pol II) transcribed genes, and importantly, regulating the process of aging and senescence. This chapter will focus on the molecular and cellular evidence that the nucleolus and the rDNA repeats play critical roles in the control of aging and cellular senescence in yeast and mammals.

2. Introduction to rDNA transcription and the nucleolus

This section will provide a brief overview of the regulation of rDNA transcription, however, for more details refer to (Tschochner & Hurt, 2003; McStay & Grummt, 2008).

---

* These authors contributed equally to this work.
\# Corresponding Authors

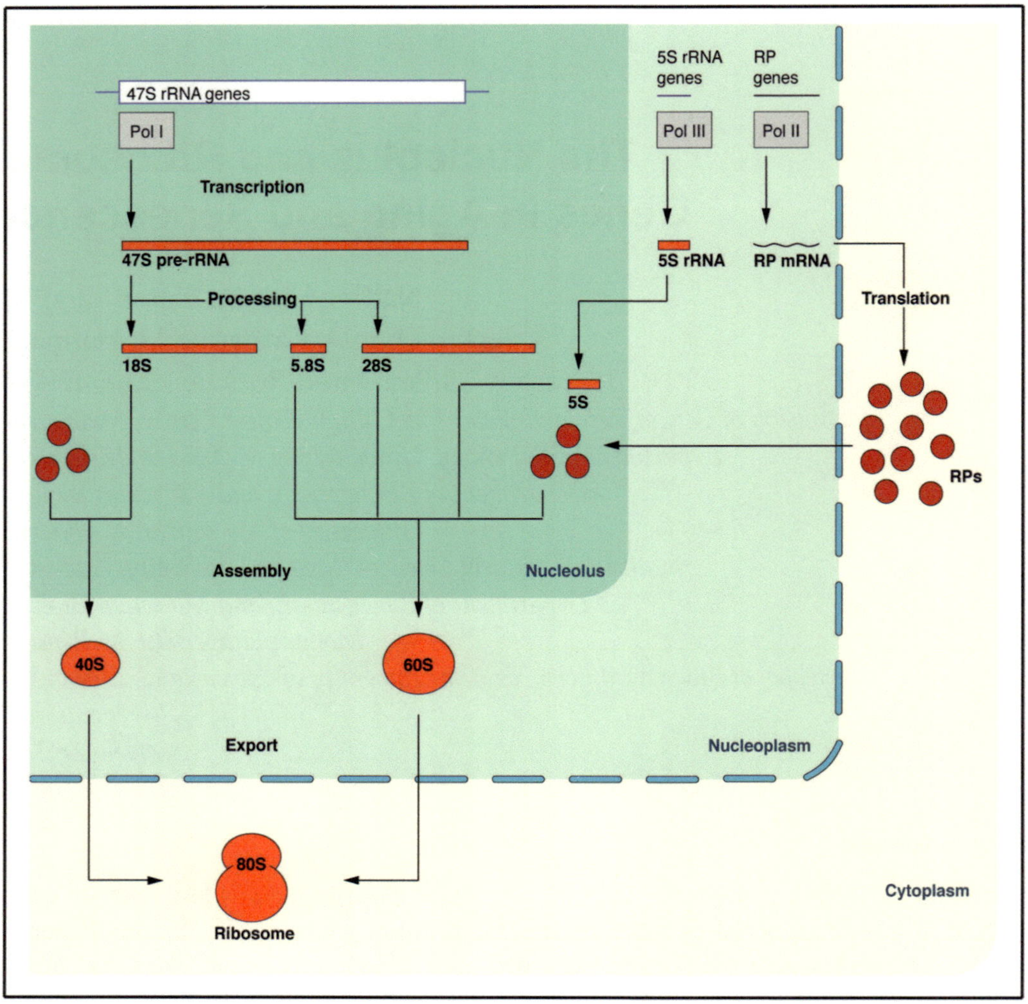

Fig. 1. Overview of ribosome biogenesis in mammalian cells.

2.1 Ribosome biogenesis

Ribosome biogenesis dictates the capacity of a cell to grow and proliferate, and is one of the most energy consuming processes in eukaryotic cells (Grummt & Pikaard, 2003). The synthesis of a ribosome is a highly complex, yet exquisitely coordinated process, which utilizes all three DNA-dependent RNA polymerases (Pol I, Pol II and Pol III) to produce approximately equimolar amounts of numerous ribosomal proteins (RP) and four rRNA (Fig. 1). Transcription of the Pol I-transcribed rRNA genes (the rDNA) has traditionally been considered the major rate-limiting step in ribosome biogenesis. Consistent with this dogma, any perturbations in the cellular environment, such as nutrient withdrawal, altered growth factor signaling, cell cycle cues and stress, are directly accompanied by modulation of the rate of rDNA transcription. However, in addition to the two key components of the ribosome (rRNAs and RPs) a multitude of non-ribosomal proteins and non-coding RNAs have been identified as essential for various steps in the generation of new ribosomes. These steps not only include Pol I transcription of the pre-RNA precursor but its subsequent processing and modifications, the nuclear import of RP's, and the final assembly of the large and small ribosomal subunits followed by their export to the cytoplasm (Grummt & Pikaard, 2003; Moss et al., 2007). The process of ribosome biogenesis is fundamental to cellular life and consequently is highly conserved, and this is illustrated by the numerous similarities between yeast and mammals.

In budding yeast (*Saccharomyces cerevisiae)* and mammals the rRNA gene is transcribed exclusively by Pol I in the nucleolus. While in yeast this generates a 35S rRNA precursor which is processed into the mature 18S, 5.8S and 26S rRNAs (Fig. 2a), in mammals a 47S rRNA precursor is generated and processed to give 18S, 5.8S and 28S rRNAs (Fig. 2b). There are also numerous similarities in the other component of the ribosome, the RPs, which in both cases are transcribed by Pol II in the nucleoplasm. In growing yeast it has been established that ~40 nascent ribosomes leave the nucleolus every second, 80% of the total RNA is rRNA, and ~50% of total protein consists of RPs (Tschochner & Hurt, 2003). Overall the process of ribosome biogenesis consumes between 60-80% of the cells total energy both in yeast and mammals (Moss & Stefanovsky, 2002). Thus for both systems, even minor perturbations to ribosome biogenesis are likely to have major repercussions for the cell.

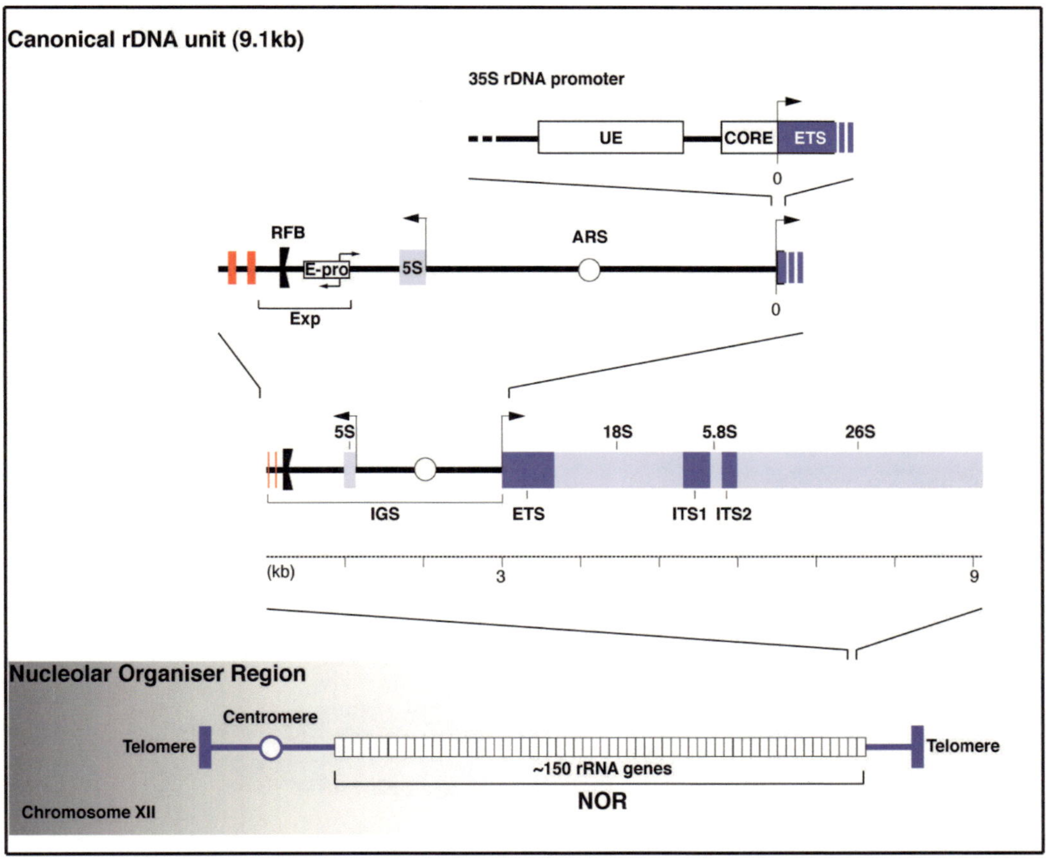

Fig. 2a. Organization of ribosomal RNA genes in yeast.

2.2 Organization of eukaryotic ribosomal RNA genes

The number of rDNA units per cell varies among eukaryotes, from 40 to ~19,000 in animals and from 150 to 26,000 in plants and correlates positively with genome size (Richard et al., 2008). In human cells there are up to 200 hundred copies of the ribosomal genes per haploid genome which are arranged in a head to tail orientation in clusters of tandem repeats. In yeast a single cluster consisting of ~150 copies of rRNA genes termed the nucleolar organizer region (NOR) is located on chromosome XII (Fig. 2a) and comprises over 10% of the whole genome (Kobayashi, 2011). During interphase a single nucleolus forms around this cluster. Two transcriptional regulatory DNA elements have been identified (Kulkens et al., 1991; Musters et al., 1989): the upstream element (UE), which is the binding site for the upstream activating factor (UAF); and the core promoter (CORE), which recruits the core factor (CF) (Elion & Warner, 1984). In addition to these regulatory DNA elements several non-coding regions have been identified within the gene and the IGS, including an origin of replication, called the ribosomal autonomous replicating sequence (ARS), and an expansion sequence containing a replication fork barrier (RFB) plus a bidirectional promoter (E-pro) that is required for rDNA amplification (Fig. 2a) (Brewer et al., 1992; Kobayashi et al., 1992).

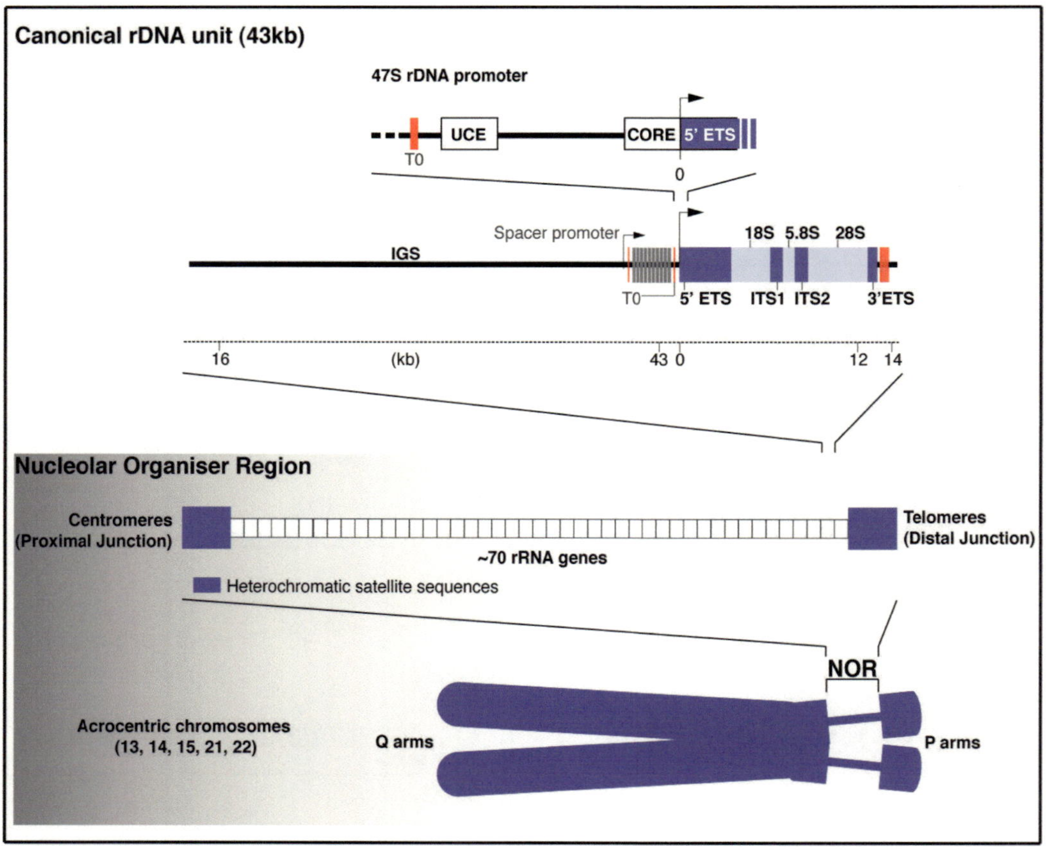

Fig. 2b. Organization of ribosomal RNA genes in mammalian cells.

In contrast to yeast, the rDNA repeats of higher eukaryotes are located in multiple NORs (Fig. 2b). For example, humans have five NORs located on the short arms of the acrocentric chromosomes (chromosomes 13, 14, 15, 21 and 22) that contain ~70 copies of the rRNA genes (Sakai et al., 1995). During interphase two or more NORs coalesce to form multiple nucleoli in exponentially growing cells (McStay & Grummt, 2008).

A single rDNA unit, containing a transcribed region followed by intergenic spacer (IGS) is referred to as a canonical rDNA unit. However, non-canonical units, which form a palindromic structure are present and arranged as a mosaic with the canonical units in human NORs (Caburet et al., 2005). These non-canonical units are likely to be non-functional and it is believed that they are silenced since their transcription would result in antisense transcripts that could use the RNAi machinery to degrade the 47S precursor rRNA. However, this has not been formally tested.

The rDNA repeats were not sequenced during the human genome project due to their repetitive nature and high copy number, thus the full sequence of only two repeats have been reported (Kuo et al., 1996). A canonical human rDNA repeat (43 kb) consists of a 13 kb coding region that encodes the 47S pre-rRNA, which is rapidly processed at the external transcribed spacer (ETS) and internal transcribed spacer (ITS) regions and ~30 kb of IGS (Fig. 2b). The IGS harbors several DNA regulatory elements, including the 47S rDNA promoter. The rDNA promoter has a bipartite architecture composed of a CORE and an upstream control element (UCE) located 100 bp upstream (McStay & Grummt, 2008). One or more terminator elements are located at the 5` and 3` ends of each mammalian rDNA repeat. Intriguingly, the IGS also contains one or more regions that are almost identical to the 47S rDNA promoter, and these are termed spacer promoters. Recent studies demonstrated that non-coding IGS transcripts play a role in the epigenetic control of rRNA gene silencing through modulation of the activity of the nucleolar remodeling complex (NoRC), the rDNA silencing complex (Mayer et al., 2006) (see below for more detail).

2.3 Epigenetic regulation of Pol I transcription

It is well established that even in exponentially growing cells only a subset of rRNA genes are active. In yeast, active and inactive rRNA genes are randomly distributed in the single NOR (French et al., 2003). However in higher eukaryotes it is thought that active and silent rRNA genes are clustered, thus generating active and silent NORs. Silent NORs are condensed and do not contribute to the formation of nucleoli during interphase. It is likely that active NORs may contain a mosaic of active and inactive units however this remains a matter for discussion (McStay & Grummt, 2008).

2.3.1 Epigenetic silencing of rDNA

While the precise mechanism controlling the silencing of rRNA genes is yet to be fully elucidated, there appears to be a marked difference between yeast and higher organisms in this process. For example, *S. cerevisiae* lacks the two major repressive methylation marks (CpG dinucleotide and H3K9 methylation) that are associated with the silencing of higher eukaryotic genes. Indeed, little is known about what regulates the number of active/inactive repeat units in yeast, although the histone deacetylase, Rpd3, is thought to play a role (Sandmeier et al, 2003), and TOR signaling regulates Pol I transcription and alters nucleolar compaction (Tsang et al, 2007). Instead, the majority of studies looking at rDNA silencing in yeast have looked at the silencing of Pol II genes in the rDNA, and it is this form of silencing that is most strongly linked to senescence and aging, particularly through the Pol II-dependent E-pro promoter in the rDNA (Kobayashi & Ganley, 2005).

Silencing of E-pro is regulated by Sir2p, a member of the Sirtuin family of NAD+ dependent protein deacetylases. Sir2p also regulates the silencing of the telomeres and the mating loci (Guarente, 1999). The Sir2p analog in mammals SIRT1 is a key component of the energy-dependent nucleolar silencing complex (eNoSC), which has been reported to repress rRNA gene transcription in response to altered intracellular energy status (Murayama et al., 2008). Sir2p together with Net1 and Cdc14 are part of a well-known epigenetic regulator of the yeast rDNA locus, the regulator of nucleolar silencing and telophase exit (RENT) complex (Huang & Moazed, 2003). In addition, Sir2p in a complex with accessory proteins such as condensin or cohesin can repress recombination events within the rDNA repeats (Huang et al., 2006; Machin et al., 2004). More recently it has become clear that the stability of the rDNA repeats and their accurate replication depends on the proportion of the epigenetically silenced rRNA genes (Kobayashi, 2011).

In higher eukaryotes methylation of CpG dinucleotides is a common modification associated with establishing stable transcriptional repression. This covalent modification is catalyzed by the DNA methyltransferases DNMT1, DNMT3a and DNMT3b, and is maintained during cell division (Klose & Bird, 2006). Stanchev et al (1979) demonstrated that CpG dinucleotide methylation marks are predominantly present in the promoter and enhancer regions of inactive rRNA genes (Fig. 3). In murine cells, methylation of a single CpG dinucleotide within the UCE (position -133 relative to the start of transcription) impairs the association of the Pol I transcription factor, upstream binding factor (UBF), to the rDNA and thus inhibits the assembly of the preinitiation complex (PIC) at the promoter (McStay & Grummt, 2008). In contrast, the human rDNA promoter contains ~25 CpG islands none of which are completely methylated or non-methylated. This suggests that the overall level of methylation rather than a binary on/off switch, dictates the transcriptional status of the rDNA. NoRC is the major complex involved in CpG methylation silencing of rDNA repeats (Santoro et al., 2002) (Fig. 3). The evolutionary logic underlying the additional complexity of rDNA silencing in higher eukaryotes compared to yeast is not clear but it potentially relates to regulation of cell differentiation and multicellular development.

2.3.2 Active rDNA repeats and activation of Pol I transcription

Regulation of rDNA transcription can occur at multiple levels, through regulatory elements defined by the primary DNA sequence as described above and also via the structure of the chromatin, which determines the accessibility of the DNA. Similar to regulation of Pol II and Pol III transcription, post-translational modification of the histones, such as acetylation, methylation, phosphorylation and ubiquitination, represent a key mechanism for the regulation of transcription by Pol I of active rDNA (Fig. 3).

In yeast it has been shown that the chromatin of actively transcribed rRNA genes is largely devoid of histone molecules, and instead is associated with the high-mobility group protein Hmo1, which interacts with the Pol I subunit Rpa49, binds across the entire 35S rDNA sequence and stabilize open rRNA gene chromatin (Hall et al., 2006; Merz et al., 2008).

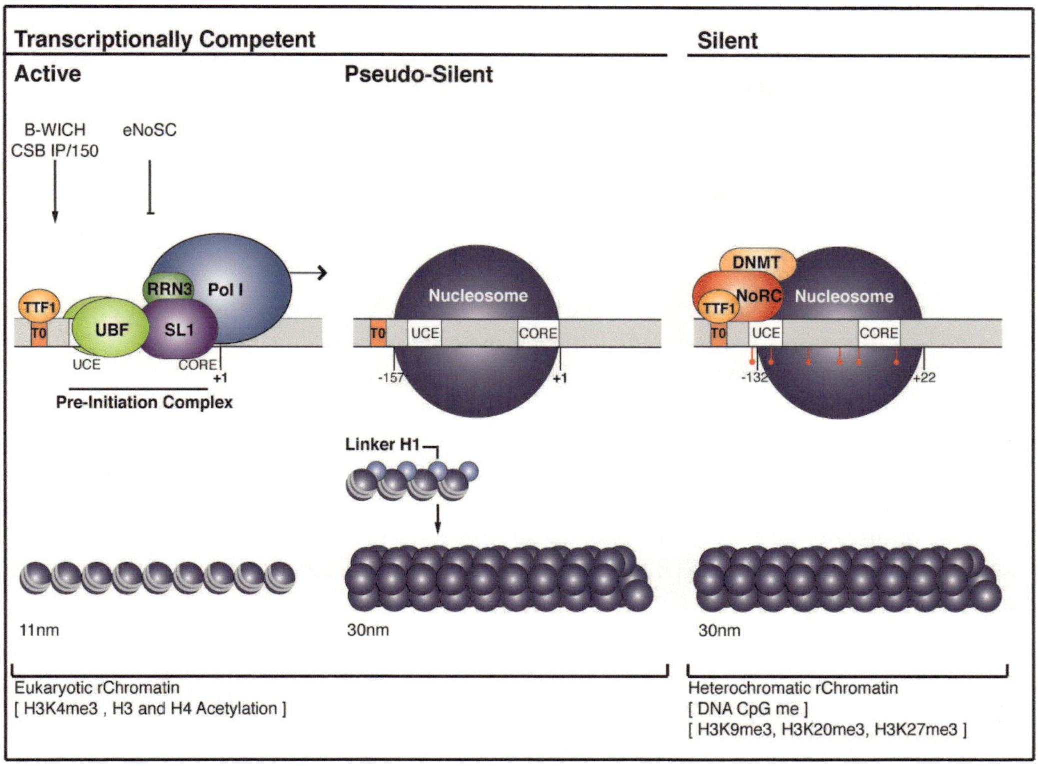

Fig. 3. Regulation of Pol I transcription in mammalian cells.

In mammals transcriptionally active rRNA genes lack repressive histone modifications such as H3K9, H3K20 and H3K27 methylation and CpG DNA methylation (Conconi et al., 1989). Furthermore, they are associated with markers for active genes including H3K4 methylation and acetylation of histone H3 and H4 (Fig. 3). Importantly, transcriptionally active mammalian rDNA are characterized by the presence of UBF, which is enriched at the promoter and the transcribed regions of the repeat, and to a lesser extent at the IGS (Fig. 3) (Sanij et al., 2008; Wright et al., 2006). UBF seems to play multiple roles at the rDNA including transcriptional initiation, promoter escape and elongation control (Stefanovsky et al., 2006). Most likely these functions relate to the essential role UBF plays in maintaining active genes in an open, uncondensed configuration, which is achieved, in part, through the ability of UBF to outcompete histone linker H1, thus preventing the formation of higher order chromatin (Sanij & Hannan, 2009; Sanij et al., 2008). Of note, active rRNA genes are around tenfold less condensed then adjacent DNA and remain uncondensed during mitosis (Heliot et al., 1997). This is undoubtedly due to the continual association of UBF and a subset of the Pol I transcription machinery with the rDNA repeats, which maintains them in an under-condensed configuration to allow the rapid resumption of rDNA transcription as cells re-enter the cell cycle (Prieto & McStay, 2007; Roussel et al., 1996).

One complex that has been described to promote the formation of an active chromatin environment for Pol I transcription is the chromatin remodeling complex B-WICH, which is composed of the William syndrome transcription factor (WSTF), SNF2h and nuclear myosin (NM1) has been described to promote the formation of an active chromatin environment for Pol I transcription (Vintermist et al., 2011) (Fig. 3). The remodeling activity of the B-WICH complex is restricted to a specific 200 bp region around the promoter, which includes the UCE, CORE and transcriptional start site (Vintermist et al., 2011). An ATP-dependent chromatin remodeling complex (CSB IP/150) also promotes transcription of active rRNA genes. CSB IP/150 consists of the Crockayne syndrome protein B (CSB), TFIIH and TIF1B (Bradsher et al., 2002) (Fig. 3).

A key similarity between yeast and mammals is that the rate of rRNA transcription is regulated in response to stress signals and the availability of nutrients as sensed by the TOR pathway. In mammals the Pol I transcription factors, UBF and Pol I-specific transcription initiation factor 1A (TIF-1A)/RRN3 (Hannan et al., 2003; Mayer et al., 2004) have been reported to be activated by TOR kinase. Similar finding have been made in yeast for Hmo1 and Rrn3p. Specifically binding of Hmo1 to the rDNA is TORC1 dependent, and nutrient starvation or rapamycin (inhibitor of mTOR) treatment prevents this association (Berger et al., 2007). In the absence of Hmo1 the histone H4 deacetylase, Rpd3, can associate with the rDNA, resulting in rDNA condensation and a reduction of nucleolar size (Tsang et al., 2003).

The basal Pol I transcription machinery in yeast involves two multiprotein complexes, the UAF consisting of Rrn5, Rrn9, and Rrn10 and UAF30 (Keys et al., 1996; Siddiqi et al., 2001) and the CF, consisting of Rrn7p, Rrn11p, and Rrn6p (Steffan et al., 1996). Both complexes interact with the TATA-box-binding protein TBP. Binding of UAF to the promoter is essential for the recruitment of CF, once the UAF-CF is established active Pol I is recruited to initiate transcription. Initiation in yeast and mammals requires the essential Pol I-associated factor Rrn3p. Rrn3p is only found associated with a small fraction of Pol I, and in yeast this association requires Pol I phosphorylation. Upon initiation of transcription Pol I enters into the elongation phase of transcription and Rrn3p is released.

As with yeast, in mammals the initiation of transcription of active rRNA genes requires the assembly of a PIC at the promoter, although some of the components are species specific (Grummt, 2003; Moss et al., 2007). In the mammalian system the PIC (Fig. 3) contains the selectivity factor I (SL1), a complex itself of 4 or more TATA association factors (TAFs) unique to Pol I transcription plus the TBP that is utilized by all three Pol's (Learned et al., 1985; Zomerdijk et al., 1994). Our current understanding is that SL1 is recruited to the promoter by UBF, and consequently stabilizes UBF interaction with the rDNA promoter. Upon formation of a stable UBF/SL1 complex, active Pol I (defined by its association with RRN3 (Hempel et al., 1996; Yuan et al., 2002) is then recruited to complete the PIC. Following Pol I transcription mediated initiation and promoter clearance, RRN3 is thought to be released to be recycled for another round of transcription. Various steps in transcription including initiation or elongation, are also regulated in response to extracellular signals such as nutrients, amino acids, ATP, stress, which is mediated by signaling pathways, including the PI3K/AKT/mTOR, RAS/RAF/ERK and JNK pathways (Chan et al., 2011; Hannan et al., 2003; Mayer et al., 2005; Stefanovsky et al., 2001). More recently the transcription termination factor (TTF1), which was originally identified for its role in the termination of Pol I transcription, has been implicated in modulating DNA looping at the rDNA repeat thus facilitating a specific interaction between the promoter and terminator elements of actively transcribed rDNA repeats (Sander & Grummt, 1997). Thus by creating an rDNA loop, TTF1 is thought to promote efficient re-initiation of the Pol I complex at the rDNA promoter (Grummt et al., 1985; Henderson & Sollner-Webb, 1986).

2.3.3 Pseudo-silenced rDNA repeats in higher eukaryotes

Interestingly, in mammals not all the transcriptionally active rRNA genes of interphasic nucleoli are transcribed at any one time (Sanij & Hannan, 2009). Transcriptionally competent genes can be subdivided into two categories; active genes and pseudo-silent genes (Fig. 3). Active genes are undermethylated, bound by the cytoarchitectural chromatin remodeling factor UBF and are highly transcribed, whereas pseudo-silent rRNA genes are undermethylated and bound by linker-histone H1, but not by UBF, and thus are not transcriptionally active. This pseudo-silenced conformation of rDNA repeats, when induced by RNA inference mediated knock down of UBF, is stably propagated throughout the cell cycle of many generations in the absence of changes in CpG methylation and can be reversed by restoration of UBF to wild-type level (Sanij et al., 2008). Importantly, pseudo-silencing seems to be a physiologically relevant phenomenon. For example, terminal differentiation of various cell types is associated with decreased UBF expression and a concomitant increase in the number of pseudo-silent rRNA genes (Poortinga et al., 2004; Poortinga et al., 2011; Sanij & Hannan, 2009). Moreover, the transition from a pre-malignant to malignant state is also associated with a decrease in the proportion of pseudo-silenced rRNA genes (Hannan RD and Bywater M, unpublished observation).

3. rDNA stability and aging in yeast

S. cerevisiae and its unique genetic and biochemical attributes have proven to be an outstanding model organism to analyze many aspects of eukaryotic ribosome biogenesis. This is evident as much of our current understanding of the link between the nucleolus/rDNA transcription with aging and senescence comes from studies utilizing the experimental advantages of budding yeast.

3.1 Maintenance of rDNA copy number in yeast

The highly repetitive nature of eukaryotic rDNA makes it one of the most fragile and dynamic regions of the genome, as recombination events within these repeats can cause either loss or gain of rDNA copies. Typically, such recombination events are highly regulated and are essential for maintenance of the rDNA copy number and the evolutionary stability of the rDNA repeats (Hawley & Marcus, 1989). Two mechanisms have been shown to be utilized for the repair of DNA double strand breaks (DSB) in the rDNA: homologous recombination (HR) and the single strand annealing (SSA) (Fishman-Lobell et al., 1992). Both these repair pathways can cause loss of rDNA copies, however the HR pathway can also result in a gain of copies. Despite the fluctuation resulting from the loss or gain of rDNA copies, an rDNA maintenance system provides a mechanism for the cell to keep copy number at a uniform level and ensure genomic stability (Fig. 4) (Kobayashi, 2006). Part of this maintenance system utilizes amplification of the rDNA, which rectifies the loss of rDNA copies (Kobayashi et al., 2004). Interestingly two of the key players in the regulation of rDNA copy number are also known as "aging associated genes", Fob1p and Sir2p (Fig. 4).

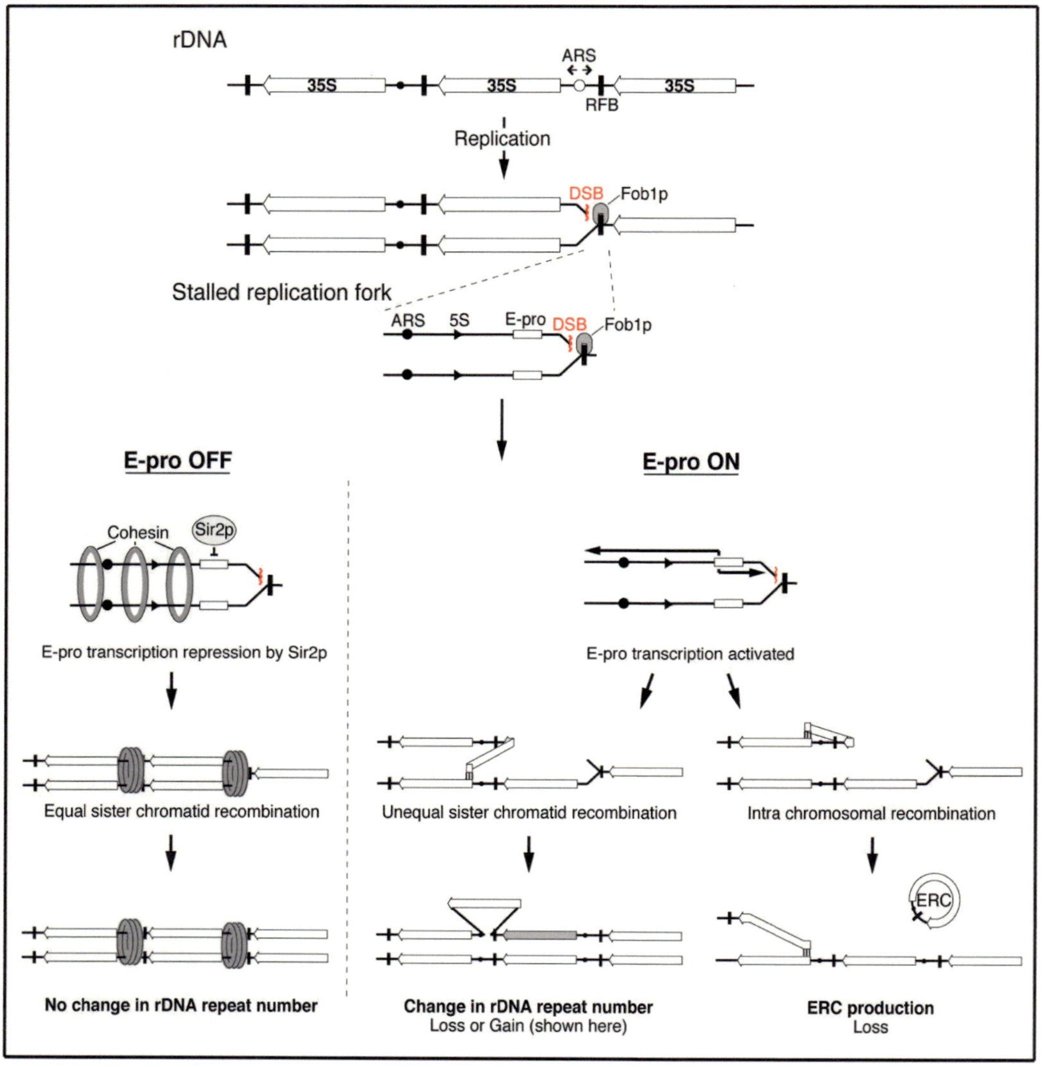

Fig. 4. Maintenance of rDNA copy number in yeast. Following initiation of replication from an ARS, Fob1p binding at the RFB inhibits replication fork progression. The outcome of the repair of these DSBs is dependent on the copy number of the rDNA. "E-pro OFF" illustrates cells containing wild-type copy number with no change in rDNA copy number. "E-pro ON" illustrates cells where rDNA copy number is altered, resulting in the production of an ERC.

During S-phase, initiation of DNA replication occurs at the origins of a subset of rDNA repeats (Pasero et al., 2002). The protein Fob1p binds in a sequence-specific manner to the rDNA at the RFB site, stalling the replication fork in one direction (Kobayashi, 2003). DNA

DSB can occur at these paused replication forks, and they are repaired using HR. The outcome of this repair is dependent on the copy number of the rDNA (Kobayashi & Ganley, 2005). In cells containing wild-type copy number, Sir2p represses noncoding Pol II-dependent transcription at the bidirectional promoter located in the IGS (Fig. 4: E-pro OFF), enabling the association of cohesin with the IGS. Cohesin is a chromosome-associated multisubunit complex that connects sister chromatids and plays an essential role in the correct segregation of chromosomes during cell division and post-replicative DNA repair (Merkenschlager, 2010). Cohesin complex association with the IGS prevents the broken end from using a non-cognate repeat as the template for HR, thereby ensuring repair through equal sister chromatid recombination, with no rDNA copy number change. If the number of rDNA copies is reduced, however, a transcription-dependent rDNA amplification mechanism is activated whereby Sir2p repression is lifted, thus activating bidirectional E-pro transcription (Fig. 4: E-pro ON). This non-coding transcription promotes the dissociation of cohesin from the IGS, allowing the broken end to use an unequal repeat as the repair template, resulting in a change of copy number. Copy number can either increase or decrease depending on whether the repeat used as the template for repair is upstream or downstream of the broken repeat (Ganley et al., 2005; Kobayashi & Ganley, 2005; Santangelo et al., 1988). If the template for repair is the same sister chromatid, a circular pop-out molecule, called an extra-chromosomal ribosomal circle (ERC) is formed. When rDNA copy number reaches wild-type levels E-pro transcription is silenced by Sir2p again, and rDNA amplification is inhibited. Sir2p mutant yeast cells can accumulate up to 300 copies due to non-restricted rDNA amplification (Kobayashi et al., 2004). Fob1p also meditates recombination events that are important for sequence homogenization of rDNA repeats and thus maintenance of the rRNA genes with identical or similar sequences (Ganley & Kobayashi, 2007). Whilst the mechanism by which cells monitor their rDNA copy number remains to be determined, it is clear that the maintenance of numerous copies of the rDNA is very important for genomic stability.

3.2 Silenced rDNA copies and DNA damage

A recent landmark study (Ide et al., 2010) demonstrated that the number of silenced rDNA copies determines the cells sensitivity to DNA damage inducing agents such as ultraviolet (UV) radiation and methyl methanesulfonate (MMS) (Fig. 5). By using low-rDNA copy number strains (20 copies), the ratio of actively transcribed rRNA genes increased, and these strains were deficient in their ability to repair DNA damage during S-phase. Low copy number strains mutated in the Pol I subunit Rpa135p or Rrn3p were not impaired in their DNA repair capacity and consequently do not exhibit a higher sensitivity to DNA damaging agents. These findings suggest that rDNA transcription determines the sensitivity to DNA damage by inhibiting DNA repair (Ide et al., 2010). The authors also reported that this transcription-dependent sensitivity resulted from the inability of the multi subunit complex condensin, that is important for establishing and maintaining chromosome condensation, to associate with actively-transcribing rDNA units. This results in premature sister-chromatid separation, which impairs accurate sister-chromatid recombination required for DNA repair. Strikingly the major site of condensin complex occupation in the genome is the NOR. Consistent with this, the binding of mitotic condensin to the rDNA was shown to be reduced when Pol I transcription was elevated, and this impaired proper DNA repair and chromatid cohesion, thus resulting in increased rDNA instability (Wang et al., 2006).

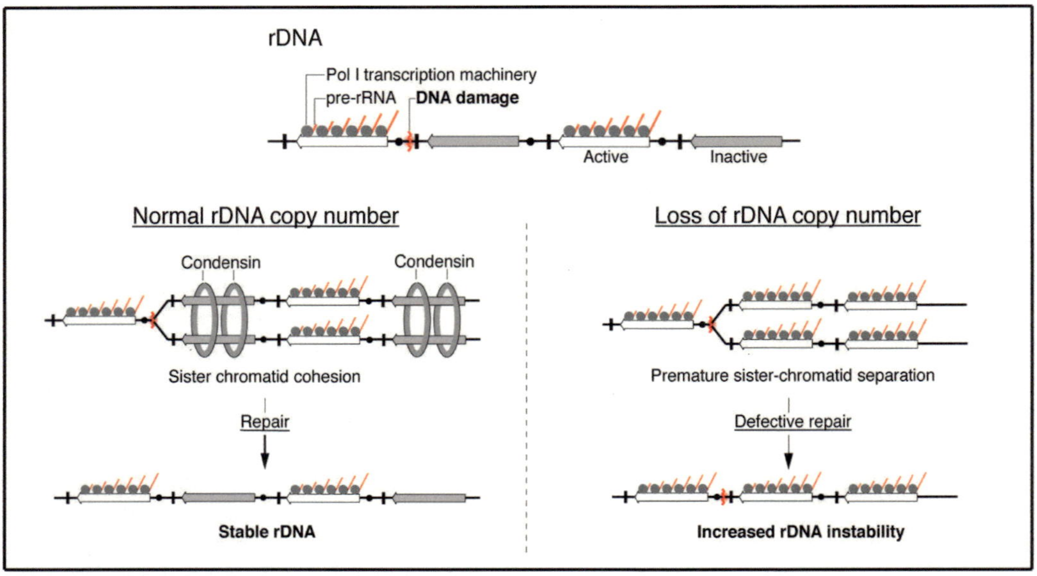

Fig. 5. Silenced rDNA copies and DNA damage in yeast. In cells with normal rDNA copy number, a proportion of genes are transcriptionally silent. Following DNA damage, condensin binds to untranscribed rDNA copies and facilitates sister chromatid cohesion, allowing repair of the rDNA by HR between sister chromatids at the stalled replication fork. Loss of rDNA copy number results in increased rates of transcription from the remaining rDNA repeats. Pol I transcription hinders the association of condensin with the rDNA, resulting in premature sister chromatid separation and preventing repair of the rDNA.

3.3 Aging in budding yeast

Aging can generically be defined as a progressive functional decline, or a gradual deterioration of physiological function and loss of viability (Partridge & Mangel, 1999). In *S. cerevisiae* an aged phenotype becomes apparent when the mother cell gets beyond ~10 asymmetric cell divisions, and this includes enlargement of the cell and vacuole, extension of the cell division cycle, and sterility. Furthermore aged wild-type cells display an extremely enlarged and often fragmented nucleolus (Shore, 1998). The average lifespan of wild-type yeast is ~ 20 buddings, after which time the mother cell dies (Jazwinski, 2001). In contrast, daughter cells are born with a full budding capacity independent of the age of the mother cell. Studies in the late 90`s implicated a role for the nucleolus in yeast aging (reviewed in Guarente, 1997). As mentioned above Sirtuins are a protein family of NAD+ dependent protein deacetylases, and they are linked to the process of yeast aging by acting as silencing factors at a site termed the *AGE* locus, prolonging life span. It has been shown that Sir3p relocalizes to the nucleolus with age and that deletion of Sir2, 3 and 4 can abbreviate yeast life span (Kennedy et al., 1997). Later studies revealed that Sir2p could repress recombination in the rDNA locus, maintain rDNA stability and promote yeast longevity (Kaeberlein et al., 1999), suggesting a role for rDNA stability in the regulation of life span. Intriguingly, extra copies of Sir2 orthologs are capable of extending the lifespan of both worms and flies (Bauer et al., 2009; Tissenbaum & Guarente, 2001), suggesting an evolutionary role for Sir2 in regulation of longevity. As discussed earlier in section 2, the mammalian Sir2p orthologue, SIRT1 is part of the eNoSC complex, which mediates epigenetic silencing of rDNA in response to varying intracellular energy status (Murayama et al., 2008). It has been proposed that the SIRT1-eNoSC complex and epigenetic regulation of rDNA may provide a novel regulatory pathway for mammalian aging, which is associated with lower metabolic rates (Salminen & Kaarniranta, 2009).

There is a clear prediction for aging factors in *S. cerevisiae,* as cell division is asymmetrical and the daughter cell receives a full lifespan, thus any aging factor must be preferentially sequestered in the mother cell and not passed on to the daughter. Indeed, Sinclair & Guarente (1997) demonstrated that aging wild-type yeast accumulated ERC, and these accumulated exclusively in mother cells. ERC accumulated even more rapidly in mutants (*sgs1*) that exhibit premature aging. In addition, accumulation of other extra-chromosomal genetic elements (i.e. plasmids) in the mother were shown to induce senescence. It was proposed that the accumulation of extra-chromosomal elements, including ERC and episomes, in the mother titrates genomic factors important for the maintenance of a young phenotype. A recent study suggested that it is not the ERC themselves that are the aging factor, but instead the rDNA recombination process that produces the ERC (Ganley et al., 2009). This study used strains with altered rDNA replication efficiencies. ERC exist in the cell effectively as plasmids because they harbour a replication origin. In the absence of selection, plasmid stability correlates with replication origin strength. Thus by altering rDNA replication strength, ERC production could be separated from their maintenance, and a strain with very little ERC accumulation was shown to age quickly when rDNA recombination was high. This study also reported that other episomes can induce genomic instability (Ganley et al., 2009), reconciling their results with those of Guarente and colleagues. ERCs have also been identified in *Drosophila* and humans (Gagnon-Kugler et al., 2009; Peng & Karpen, 2007) however its origin and role in aging is yet to be determined.

Other aging theories propose that senescence is caused by an accumulation of DNA damage or cytoplasmic senescence factors that remain within the mother cell due to asymmetrical segregation. These theories are supported by the observation showing that oxidized (damaged) proteins predominantly accumulate in mother rather than daughter cells (Erjavec et al., 2007). Nucleolar rDNA is proposed to be particularly sensitive to the presence of elevated levels of oxidized proteins, as this leads to an impaired protein turnover and defects in DNA repair. Furthermore, the asymmetrical segregation of oxidized proteins is Sir2p dependent (Erjavec et al., 2007), leads to rDNA instability and the accumulation of ERC in the mother cell, which then promotes cellular senescence (Kobayashi, 2008).

3.4 A specific role for rDNA in aging

The role of rDNA in aging is most clearly demonstrated in yeast with rDNA instability and cellular aging strongly correlating with rDNA copy number (Burkhalter & Sogo, 2004; Kobayashi et al., 2004). A recent review proposed the "rDNA theory" for aging. Specifically that dysfunction of DNA repair and the replication proteins, predominantly within the nucleolus of the mother cell, is a cause of increased rDNA instability. Because the nucleolus is the most sensitive cellular component to age-related DNA damage, the stability of the rDNA will in turn dictate the stability of the whole genome (Kobayashi,

2008). In both yeast and humans mutations within DNA repair genes result in a reduced lifespan (Park et al., 1999). In humans mutations associated with a premature aging phenotype (Werner and Bloom syndrome) are prominently found in RecQ homolog helicases, which are involved in rDNA repair (Ellis et al., 1995; Yu et al., 1996). In yeast, mutations in genes involved in rDNA transcription and elongation have been identified as modulators of rDNA stability and longevity (Heo et al., 1999; Hoopes et al., 2002; Merker & Klein, 2002). In conclusion whilst the findings in yeast clearly link the stability of rDNA, to aging and cellular senescence, relatively few studies in mammals investigating this link have been reported, predominantly due to the difficulties in studying this complicated part of the genome.

The idea that the rDNA has other, extra-coding functions has received increasing attention over the last few years (Kobayashi, 2011). In yeast, due to the fact that the rDNA cluster comprises ~10% of the genome, rDNA copy number and stability can influence the effective concentration of proteins and protein complexes located within the nucleus through titration. For example, studies investigating Sirtuins revealed that Sir2p is released from the nucleolus upon loss of rDNA copies. Sir2p, together with Sir3p, Sir4p and RAP1 can mediate silencing of telomeres and the mating-type loci. Intriguingly, depletion of ~50% of the rDNA repeats caused an increase in telomeric and mating-type gene silencing, suggesting that the effective concentration of Sir2p at different genomic loci plays a critical role in epigenetic regulation. The fact that mammalian rDNA comprises only ~0.3% of the genome raises the question of whether the association of genomic factors with the rDNA is sufficient to titrate silencing complexes to a similar extent to that reported in yeast. However, the mammalian nucleolus has been reported to influence various cellular functions via sequestering or releasing factors important for various cellular processes that regulate senescence and aging and this is described in more detail in section 4.

4. The nucleolus and senescence in mammals

Senescence is considered a manifestation of organismal aging at a cellular level, although this remains mechanistically unproven (Guarente, 1997; McCormick & Campisi, 1991). However, a number of studies have shown that senescent cells accumulate within mammalian tissues with increasing chronological age (Dimri et al., 1995; Y. Li et al., 1997; Pawelec et al., 1999). As discussed above, in yeast the rDNA locus, and hence the nucleolus, has been implicated in the regulation of longevity and senescence (Kobayashi, 2008). Consistent with this, a nontraditional role for the mammalian nucleolus is also now emerging that involves sequestration and release of tumor suppressors or oncogenes, cell cycle regulators and factors involved in modulating telomerase function (Olson et al., 2002; Olson, 2004; Olson & Dundr, 2005). Thus, similar to yeast, the mammalian nucleolus has been proposed to play an active role in senescence (Mehta et al., 2007; Olson et al., 2000).

Changes in nucleolar morphology are detected in aging cells (Mehta et al., 2007). While pre-senescent cells show a higher number of smaller nucleoli (Bemiller & Lee, 1978), senescent cells have a single prominent nucleolus. Cellular senescence however, does not always correlate with a concomitant decrease in rRNA gene transcription (Halle et al., 1997; Machwe et al., 2000). Even so, studies from many laboratories indicate that inhibition of rRNA synthesis and ribosome biogenesis and subsequent changes in nucleolar structure and function induce cell cycle arrest, implicating the nucleolus in regulation of cell survival and proliferation (Boisvert et al., 2007; Boulon et al., 2010). Indeed, a number of proteins regulated by their localization to the nucleolus, including the tumor suppressor protein ARF (alternative reading frame; p19ARF in mouse, p14ARF in human) and nucleophosmin (NPM), are involved in cellular senescence by mediating p53 stability (Colombo et al., 2002; Daniely et al., 2002). Therefore, it is likely that the nucleolus plays an active role in establishing and maintaining the senescent phenotype.

Senescent cells are growth arrested in the transition from G1 to S-phase of the cell cycle (Sherwood et al., 1988). The role of the G1-S and G2-M cell cycle checkpoints is to ensure that the cell accurately duplicates its genome and successfully divide into the two daughter cells. The tumor suppressor factors p53 and retinoblastoma protein (RB) regulate these cell cycle checkpoints, which upon activation induce cell cycle arrest, senescence or apoptosis. Correct cell division requires increased protein synthesis that, in turn, is achieved by upregulation of ribosome biogenesis, thus these processes are tightly linked and potentially regulated by common mechanisms (Montanaro, 2008). For example, rDNA transcription and subsequent assembly of the nucleoli during G1 have been shown to be prerequisites for G1-S progression (Pardee, 1989; Sirri et al., 2002). Conversely, decreases in rates of rDNA transcription and disassembly of the nucleoli are observed during mitosis (Grummt, 1999; Pyronnet et al., 2001; Sirri et al., 2002). In fact, the nucleolus can sense and respond to cellular stress by modifying its size and content throughout interphase (Nalabothula et al., 2010). Consequently, it is not surprising that the nucleolus has been recognized as a central regulatory link between ribosome biogenesis and cell cycle progression (Carmo-Fonseca et al., 2000). Certainly, an ever increasing number of nucleolar proteins have been reported to play multiple roles in regulating ribosome biogenesis and cell cycle progression (Boisvert et al., 2007). Although, the exact molecular mechanisms responsible for mediating this crosstalk remain largely unknown, the p53 pathway is prevailing as an important link between ribosome biogenesis and the cell cycle (Pestov et al., 2001).

Early evidence for p53 as a key mediator of the crosstalk between ribosome biogenesis and cell cycle progression came from studies showing that inhibition of Bop1 (block of proliferation), a factor involved in rRNA synthesis and assembly, led to a p53-dependent G1 checkpoint arrest (Pestov et al., 2001). This is consistent with the notion that ongoing ribosome synthesis acts as a checkpoint at the G1-S boundary. In support of this inhibition of rRNA synthesis by microinjecting antibodies to UBF, disruption of the *TIF-IA* gene by Cre-dependent HR, or low doses of actinomycin D (Act D), leads to perturbations in nucleolar structure and function, p53-dependent G1-S cell cycle arrest and apoptosis (Montanaro et al., 2007; Rubbi & Milner, 2003; Yuan et al., 2005).

We have previously shown that inhibition of Pol I transcription by CX-5461, a small molecule inhibitor of initiation of rRNA synthesis, induces senescence in solid tumor cell lines (Drygin et al., 2011). Moreover, CX-5461 treatment or low doses of Act D induces premature senescence in TERT immortalized primary human fibroblasts (BJ-TERT) (Fig. 6) (Hahn et al., 1999). Within 24 hours of treatment with Act D or CX-5461, the protein levels of p53 and its transcriptional target, p21, are upregulated and sustained for a further 24 hours (Fig. 6a). Inhibition of rRNA synthesis correlates with the appearance of single nucleoli, as visualized by fluorescence *in situ* hybridization (FISH) of rDNA (Fig. 6b), while in interphasic control cells the rDNA repeats are present as multiple nucleoli. The induction of p53 and nucleolar disorganization correlates with the subsequent appearance of γH2A.X foci indicative of DNA damage, which is associated with senescence (Gire et al., 2004). After 96 hours of Pol I transcription inhibition, BJ-TERT cells appear bigger in size with a flat cell morphology and display acidic β-galactosidase activity, characteristic phenotypic markers of senescence (Fig. 6c) (Dimri et al., 1995). UBF depletion in BJ-TERT cells is also associated with nucleolar disorganization and premature senescence, consistent with its role in establishing and maintaining nucleolar structure. Intriguingly, UBF depletion does not lead to decreased rates of rRNA synthesis, suggesting that the premature senescence may be a consequence of nucleolar disruption (Sanij E and Hannan RD, manuscript in preparation).

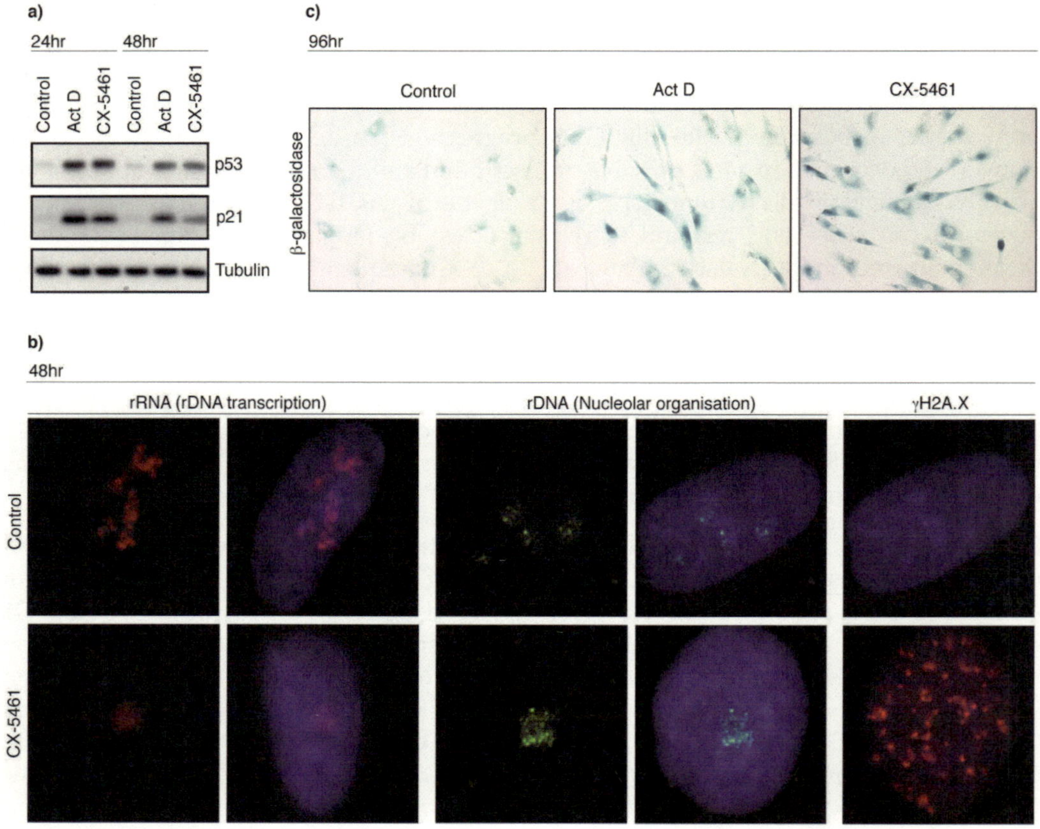

Fig. 6. Inhibition of Pol I transcription induces senescence. Following inhibition of Pol I transcription by treatment with either 5nM Act D or 1μM CX-5461, BJ-TERT fibroblasts display hallmarks of senescence. a) Western blot analysis of p53 and p21 after treatment with either Act D or CX-5461. b) Following 48hr CX-5461 treatment, from left to right: RNA FISH to the 5′ETS region of the 47S pre-rRNA (red); DNA FISH to the rDNA (green) combined with immunofluorescent analysis for γH2A.X (red). gDNA is visualized by DAPI (blue)
c) β-galactosidase staining of BJ-TERT cells after 96hr treatment with Act D or CX-5461.

Recent studies exploring the nucleolar proteome have revealed the involvement of the nucleolus in multiple biological processes including senescence, regulation of telomerase function, cell cycle regulation, and stress signaling (Boisvert et al., 2010; Boisvert et al., 2007). Furthermore, nucleolar structure and function are intimately linked with the regulation of p53 stabilization and activation of the p53 pathway, which firmly places the integrity of rDNA transcription and ribosome biogenesis at the centre of control of the cell cycle progression. In addition, over the last few years, significant advances have been made in understanding the higher order organization of nuclear structures, including the nucleolus, and their importance for the regulation of nuclear functions (Nemeth & Langst, 2011). Here, we address the impact of these recent results and discuss the molecular mechanisms underlying nucleolar function in the regulation of cell cycle progression and senescence.

4.1 The nucleolus in control of cell cycle regulation and senescence

An increasing number of nucleolar proteins have been reported to play multiple roles in regulating ribosome biogenesis and cell cycle progression. For instance, components of the DNA replication initiation machinery, origin of replication complex (ORC) and minichromosome maintenance (MCM) proteins, have been purified from human nucleoli (Boisvert et al., 2007; Couté et al., 2006) and were shown, in yeast, to associate with several 60S ribosomal synthesis factors that are required for pre-rRNA processing and are also essential for initiation of DNA replication by mediating the association of the ORC and MCM proteins at replication origins (Zhang et al., 2002). However, the most direct role for nucleoli in regulation of the cell cycle is via the sequestration or release of proteins directly involved in cell cycle progression.

The tumor suppressor protein RB is an important regulator of senescence (Campisi & di Fagagna, 2007). RB is generally active during senescence, indeed its enforced expression has been shown to induce senescence (Narita et al., 2003). RB was initially reported to accumulate in the nucleolus and to have a repressive role in Pol I transcription (Cavanaugh et al., 1995; Hannan et al., 2000). Subsequently, Nucleolin (NCL), a multifunctional nucleolar protein essential for rRNA processing (Mongelard & Bouvet, 2007) was reported to associate with hypophosphorylated (active) RB (pRB) during the G1 phase of the cell cycle (Grinstein et al., 2006). pRB mediates a cell cycle checkpoint between G_1 and S phase (Bartek et al., 1996) by targeting members of the E2F family of transcriptional activators (Chellappan et al., 1991) that are essential for cellular proliferation. While pRB has been reported to reside in the nucleoli in a cell type dependent manner (Angus et al., 2003) hyperphosphorylated RB (ppRB) is eliminated from the nucleolus until late S or G2 phase. Import of ppRB into the nucleolus in late S or G2 phase is mediated by its interaction with nucleolar NPM (Takemura et al., 2002). Although the functional significance of nucleolar retention and release of RB is currently unresolved, it has been proposed that its retention could represent a negative regulatory mechanism to sequester RB to prevent checkpoint activation during the cell cycle (Angus et al., 2003).

By far the most convincing studies linking the dynamic release of nucleolar proteins and cell cycle progression were performed in yeast. Cdc14p is a protein phosphatase that is crucial for promoting exit from mitosis into the G1 phase (Jin et al., 2008; Visintin et al., 1998; Zachariae et al., 1998). Cdc14p activation is also a prerequisite for successful chromosome segregation as it is necessary for condensin enrichment at the rDNA, which triggers rDNA segregation and ensures the completion of chromosome segregation (D'Amours et al., 2004). In G1 or during S phase, Cdc14p is sequestered to the nucleolus by its inhibitor Net1/Cfi1p, a component of the multifunctional protein complex RENT, where it remains inactive until the onset of anaphase, thereby preventing the premature onset of mitotic exit (Shou et al., 1999). The release of Cdc14p from the nucleolus is mediated through the sequential action of two regulatory networks: FEAR (CDC Fourteen Early Anaphase Release) and MEN (Mitotic Exit Network) that lead to Net1/Cfi1p phosphorylation reducing its affinity for Cdc14p and thus disassociation of the complex (Shou et al., 2002; Yoshida & Toh-e, 2002). The roles of the two human orthologs of Cdc14p (CDC14A and CDC14B) are not yet established. CDC14B has been shown to translocate from the nucleolus to the nucleoplasm following genotoxic stress in G2, leading to the activation of the APC/CDH1 complex and the establishment of a DNA damage induced G2 checkpoint (Bassermann et al., 2008). Nevertheless, a wider role in promoting mammalian cell cycle progression has been proposed for CDC14B including the governing of cell cycle re-entry after G2 block (De Wulf & Visintin, 2008).

Another example of nucleolar sequestration-mediated regulation of specific cellular activity during the cell cycle is the regulation of telomerase, the enzyme that adds telomeric repeats sequences to the ends of chromosomes (Fig. 7). Telomeres are composed of TTAGGG repeats that form a 3′ overhang of 100-400 nucleotides forming a T-loop structure that is stabilized by telomeric proteins (Griffith et al., 1999). Telomeres maintain chromosome integrity by protecting against end shortening and end-to-end fusions (de Lange, 2005; Sahin & Depinho, 2010). If telomere length is not maintained, the telomeres will reach a critically short length, triggering the cell to undergo replicative senescence (Harley et al., 1990; Stewart et al., 2003). Although the telomeres and the nucleolus are separate subnuclear domains, multiple telomeric components have been detected in the nucleolus suggesting an underling regulatory connection between the nucleolus and telomeres (Tsai, 2009).

The ribonucleoprotein (RNP) telomerase is composed of the telomerase RNA component (TERC) and the telomerase reverse transcriptase (TERT), which catalyzes *de novo* repeat addition by utilizing TERC as a template (Greider & Blackburn, 1989). Outside of S phase, TERC and TERT are localised within distinct nucleoplasmic foci separate from telomeres. In early S-phase, TERT moves to nucleoli while Cajal bodies containing TERC accumulate at the periphery of nucleoli (Fig. 7). Nucleolar transportation of TERC and TERT has been proposed as a prerequisite step in the process of telomerase RNP biogenesis (Etheridge et al., 2002; Narayanan et al., 1999; Yang et al., 2002) and/or the transport of active telomerase, which occurs during mid-S phase (Tomlinson et al., 2006). Nucleolar localization of telomerase has also been reported to be mediated by NCL, which interacts with the active telomerase complex and is involved either in the assembly or maturation of telomerase. Nucleolar NCL-telomerase complexes are exported and maintained in the nucleoplasm and delivered to the telomeres (Khurts et al., 2004). Cell-cycle dependent nucleolar localization of telomerase is lost in transformed cells or following DNA damage (Wong et al., 2002).

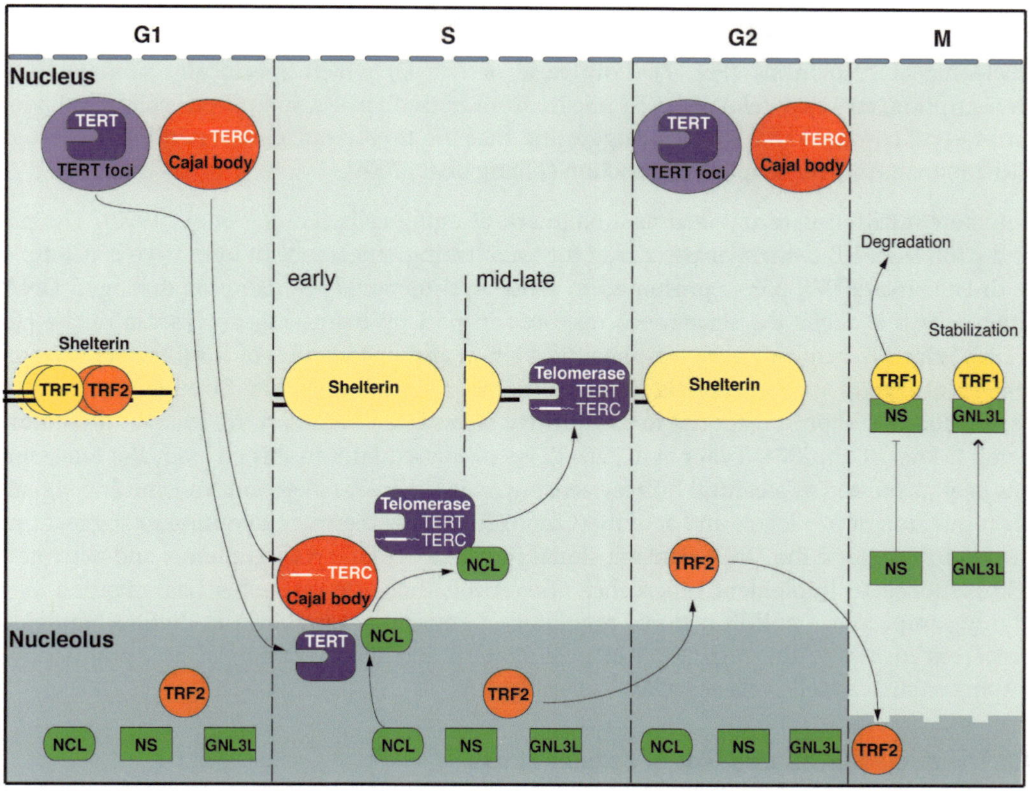

Fig. 7. Nucleolar regulation of telomere stability. Telomerase and the shelterin complex are regulated by the nucleolus through sequestration and release. In early S-phase, TERT moves to the nucleoli and Cajal bodies containing TERC accumulate at the periphery of the nucleoli. NCL-telomerase complexes are then exported to the telomeres during mid-S phase. TRF1 is regulated by NS and GNL3L in opposing manners. TRF2 is sequestered in the nucleolus during G1 and S phase, released to the nucleoplasm in G2, and returned to the nucleoli at cytokinesis.

In addition to telomerase, components of the shelterin telomere binding complex, including telomeric repeat binding factors 1 (TRF1) and TRF2 have been reported as regulated in part by localization to the nucleolus (Fig. 7) (Lin et al., 2008; Tsai, 2009; Wong et al., 2002; Zhang et al., 2004). TRF1, which is required for establishing 'closed' structures at the telomeres that are inaccessible to telomerase, has been shown to be regulated by a number of nucleolar proteins, including nucleostemin (NS) and guanine nucleotide binding protein-like 3-like (GNL3L). NS binding to TRF1 enhances its degradation, while GNL3L binding stabilizes TRF1 (Zhu et al., 2009). Since the majority of TRF1 resides in the nucleoplasm, nucleolar retention of NS and GNL3L renders them inactive in modulating TRF1 activity. However, their nucleoplasmic localization during mitosis or in response to nucleolar stress may allow modulation of TRF1 in regulating telomere capping (Tsai, 2009).

In addition, TRF2, the component of shelterin considered responsible for the formation of the protective telomeric T-loop structure required for protecting the telomeres, localizes to the nucleolus at G0 and S but diffuses into the nucleoplasm in G2 and returns to the nucleolus at cytokinesis (Fig. 7). Low dose of Act D, which specifically inhibits Pol I transcription, causes a delay in TRF2 release from nucleoli in G2 and mitotic cells displaying end-to-end chromosomal fusions, suggesting that the timely nucleolar retention/release of TRF2 regulates its nucleoplasmic function (Zhang et al., 2004).

Telomere attrition is recognized as a hallmark of aging cells (Harley et al., 1990). The p53 and p16INK4a-RB pathways are critical for establishing senescence in human cells (Campisi & di Fagagna, 2007). p53 is presumed to sense dysfunctional telomeres as damaged DNA, upon which it elicits the senescence response in part by increasing expression of the p21 CDKI, which in turn prevents the phosphorylation and inactivation of RB (Sherr & Roberts, 1999). In several mouse models, inappropriate p53 activity, either through deregulated expression of p53 or in response to constitutive stress like DNA damage, leads to premature aging (Maier et al., 2004; Tyner et al., 2002). As discussed later in this chapter, the nucleolus has been proposed as a central hub for sensing major cellular stress and transmitting signals for regulation of p53 levels and activity (Olson, 2004). It is therefore tempting to suggest that nucleoli may sense the DNA damage signal induced by damaged telomeres and activate a p53 response to implement senescence. Taken together, the nucleolus has emerged as a highly complex and multifunctional regulatory compartment involved in diverse biological processes including the regulation of proliferation and the execution of anti-proliferative responses such as cell cycle arrest and senescence.

4.2 The nucleolus as a sensor of cellular stress

One of the most intriguing roles proposed for the nucleolus is as a sensor of cellular stress and a means to couple cellular stress to the p53 pathway (Rubbi & Milner, 2003), a key regulator of senescence and longevity (Fig. 8) (Vigneron & Vousden, 2010) In this paradigm, under normal conditions, the nucleolus contributes to the maintenance of low p53 levels, while in response to cellular stress p53 levels and activity are dramatically elevated through the actions of select nucleolar proteins. Key to the nucleolar control of p53 is the oncogene MDM2 (mouse double minute 2; or HDM2 in humans). In proliferating cells, p53 activity is kept under surveillance by MDM2, via two complimentary mechanisms: (i) MDM2 acts as an E3 ubiquitin ligase directly transfering ubiquitin onto p53 thereby targeting it for 26S proteosomal degradation (Haupt et al., 1997; Kubbutat et al., 1997); and (ii) the direct binding of MDM2 to the N-terminal domain of p53 inhibits its transcriptional activity by abrogating its interaction with the basal Pol II transcription machinery (Momand et al., 1992; Oliner et al., 1993). The two best characterized mechanisms by which cellular stress modulates MDM2/p53 pathway in a nucleolar specific manner are in response to oncogenes (oncogenic stress) and to perturbations that alter ribosome biogenesis (nucleolar stress).

4.2.1 ARF and oncogenic / replicative stress

The *Ink4/Arf* locus encodes two tumor-suppressor proteins, p16INK4a and p19ARF, that govern the antiproliferative functions of RB and p53 proteins, respectively (Fig. 8). ARF binds to MDM2 and sequesters it into the nucleolus, thereby preventing negative-feedback regulation of p53 by MDM2, leading to the activation of p53 in the nucleoplasm (Honda & Yasuda, 1999; Palmero et al., 1998; Zindy et al., 1998). Under normal conditions, ARF is expressed at very low levels and is sequestered into to the nucleolus, due to its association with the nucleolar protein NPM (Gjerset & Bandyopadhyay, 2006; Korgaonkar et al., 2005). This prevents its interaction with MDM2. In contrast during replicative senescence of MEFs or stress induced by activation of oncogenes such as c-MYC and H-RAS, ARF rapidly accumulates to sufficient quantities and is able to bind and sequester MDM2 leading to p53 activation (Palmero et al., 1998; Sharpless et al., 2001; Weber et al., 1999). In addition ARF directly suppresses rRNA synthesis and processing to modulate ribosome biogenesis (Ayrault et al., 2006; Lessard et al., 2010; Sugimoto et al., 2003). Although, the importance of the later for modulation of p53 is unclear, a ribosome biogenesis-dependent-ARF pathway may complement ARF's function in modulating the p53 pathway.

4.2.2 Nucleolar stress

The protein content of the nucleolus has been shown to change dramatically under various stress conditions (Boulon et al., 2010). It is now clear that, the nucleolar proteome undergoes distinct spatial and temporal alterations in response to different stress insults, suggesting that the nucleolus responds to different stress stimuli in a unique and specific manner (Moore et al., 2011). The landmark study by Rubbi and Milner (2003) proposed that disruption of nucleolar structure and function and subsequent release of nucleolar components into the nucleoplasm as a common denominator in most or possibly all p53-inducing stresses (Reviewed in Olson, 2004). Consistent with this, it is now recognized that inactivation of rDNA transcription, RP synthesis, rRNA processing, and the assembly and nucleolar export of the 40S and 60S ribosomal subunits (Zhang & Lu, 2009) are established mechanisms for causing nucleolar disruption and activation of the p53 pathway. From these observations a model of nucleolar surveillance of ribosome biogenesis (also termed nucleolar stress) has been proposed to integrate a diverse array of metabolic irregularities and oncogenic stimuli whereby the rate or efficiency of ribosome production serves as a signal by which cells could regulate cell-cycle progression via controlling p53 levels (Fig. 8) (Boulon et al., 2010; Deisenroth & Zhang, 2010; Ruggero & Pandolfi, 2003; Shcherbik & Pestov, 2010). In addition, due to the repetitive nature of the rRNA genes as well as the high rate of transcription by Pol I complexes, the rDNA is considered unstable and has been proposed to act as a potential sensor for DNA damage (Boisvert & Lamond, 2010). Signals associated with stalled polymerases and/or reduced rRNA transcription could activate p53 and possibly other DNA damage response pathways (Boisvert & Lamond, 2010; Kobayashi, 2008) leading to cell cycle arrest or programmed cell death (Drygin et al., 2009). Under conditions of "nucleolar stress", p53 stabilization can be achieved via different mechanisms including posttranslational modifications, protein-protein interactions and increases in the translation rate of p53 mRNA. Of these mechanisms perhaps the best documented is the role of RPs which are able to interact directly with MDM2 leading to p53 stabilization in response to ribosomal stress. Interestingly, while the RPs are required for p53 response to ribosomal stress, ARF in this context is not required, suggesting that different cellular conditions, oncogenic stress or ribosomal stress modulate the binding of either ARF or RPs to MDM2 and subsequent activation of p53 (Pan et al., 2011).

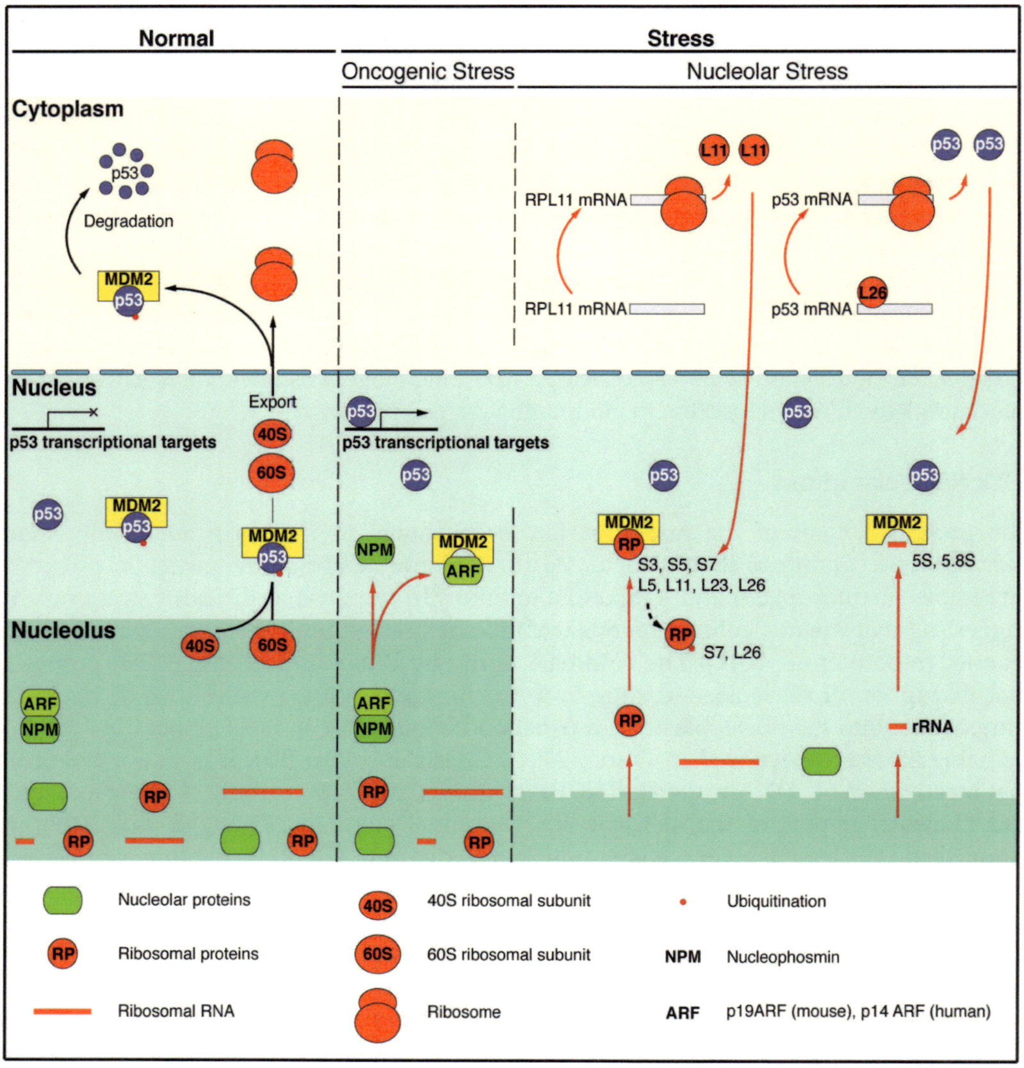

Fig. 8. The nucleolus as a sensor of cellular stress. Under normal conditions, p53 activity is maintained at low levels by MDM2, via two mechanisms: First, MDM2 ubiquitinates p53 thereby promoting its degradation; second, the binding of MDM2 to p53 abrogates its interaction with Pol II transcription machinery. Following oncogenic stress, ARF binds MDM2 and sequesters it in the nucleolus. Under nucleolar stress, p53 can be activated by the following mechanisms: (i). The co-transport of p53 and/or MDM2 with the ribosomal subunits to the cytoplasm is impaired; (ii). RPs interact directly with MDM2; (iii). 5.8S and 5S rRNA interact directly with MDM2; (iv). RPL26 binds p53mRNA and enhances its translation; (v). Increased RPL11 mRNA translation results in enhanced interaction between RPL11 and MDM2.

An increasing number of RPs (RPS3, RPS5, RPS7, RPL5, RPL11, RPL23, RPL26) as well as the 5.8S and 5S rRNAs are capable of interacting with MDM2 leading to p53 stabilization (Deisenroth & Zhang, 2010; Fontoura et al., 1992; Fumagalli et al., 2009; Ofir-Rosenfeld et al., 2008; Riley & Maher, 2007; Zhang & Lu, 2009). A number of different models have been proposed for how these various interactions might regulate p53 (Fig. 8). Under normal growth conditions, RPs are synthesized in equimolar amounts with the rRNAs and assembled with large and small ribosomal subunits in the nucleolus and transported to the cytoplasm to form functional ribosomes. In one model, so called "riding the ribosome", the interaction of p53 and/or MDM2 with the ribosomal subunits may facilitate p53/MDM2 transport from the nucleolus to the cytoplasm thus preventing p53 from interacting with its target genes in the nucleoplasm and/or promoting its ubiquitin-mediated degradation in the cytoplasm (Boulon et al., 2010). Conversely, stress signaling that impairs production and export of ribosome subunits, would be predicted to decrease p53/MDM2 transport to the cytoplasm, thus allowing p53 to activate transcription of its target genes in the nucleoplasm (Boulon et al., 2010). In a second and perhaps better described model, conditions that inhibit rRNA transcription or stall ribosome synthesis and assembly in the nucleolus are postulated to create a pool of free RPs (such as RPL5, RPL11 and RPL23) that are directly interact and sequester MDM2 resulting in suppression of p53 ubiquitination (Daniely et al., 2002; Deisenroth & Zhang, 2010; Lindstrom & Nister, 2010; Pestov et al., 2001; Warner & McIntosh, 2009; Zhang & Lu, 2009). However, Horn and Vousden (2008) observed a synergistic suppression of MDM2 activity through cooperation of RPL11 and RPL5, suggesting they have distinct roles in inhibiting MDM2 function. In addition, binding sites for ARF, RPL5, and RPL11 on MDM2 do not appear to overlap (Lindstrom et al., 2007; Zhang et al., 2003) suggesting that ARF and RPL5/L11 may respond to different stimuli and converge at the point of MDM2 inactivation (Shcherbik & Pestov, 2010).

RPL26 is so far unique in its ability to bind the 5`untranslated region of the p53 mRNA and enhance its translation. Its interaction with MDM2 triggers its own ubiquitination and degradation, which in turn causes downregulation of p53 mRNA translation (Ofir-Rosenfeld et al., 2008). The diverse roles of RPs in the regulation of the MDM2-p53 pathway is further supported by the finding that knockdown of RPS6 not only affects 40S ribosomal biogenesis but also enforces RPL11 mRNA translation. This leads to an enhanced interaction between RPL11 and MDM2 leading to the accumulation and activation of p53 (Fumagalli et al., 2009). Since multiple RPs have separate mechanisms for activating p53, it is plausible that they may have distinct roles in sensing different types of signals leading to activation of nucleolar stress response. In summary there is now a robust set of data demonstrating that the nucleolus and rDNA transcription indirectly play an important role in the regulation of tumor suppressors and oncogenes such as ARF, MDM2 and p53 and thus perturbation in the nucleolus are predicted to have profound effects on cellular functions that are controlled by these factors. In this manner the nucleolus can be considered as a sensitive cellular stress detector integrating various perturbations in homeostasis and converting them to appropriate responses such as cell cycle arrest and senescence.

4.3 Alterations in genome organization in and around the nucleolus are associated with senescence

The nucleus is compartmentalized into substructures that perform distinct nuclear activities (Lanctot et al., 2007). These nuclear structures include the nucleoli, nuclear envelope, nuclear bodies, nuclear matrix and chromosome territories (Cremer & Cremer, 2001). Organization and spatial location of chromosomes and their interactions with other nuclear substructures ensures that transcription is correctly regulated (Misteli, 2004). The periphery of the nucleolus consists of satellite DNA repeats, which are proposed to play a role in the formation of perinucleolar heterochromatin (Manuelidis, 1984), and its been suggested they serve as a distinct nuclear space with a primary function in maintaining repressive chromatin states (Nemeth & Langst, 2011; van Koningsbruggen et al., 2010). For example the inactive X chromosome (Xi) must continuously visit the perinucleolar compartment during S phase to maintain its epigenetic status (Zhang et al., 2007). Other conserved chromosomal regions have also been shown to interact with the nucleolus including a fraction of the human centromeres (Bridger & Bickmore, 1998; Leger et al., 1994; Park & De Boni, 1992). Furthermore, chromosome mobility studies demonstrated that nucleolar-associated chromatin is significantly less mobile then other genomic regions. Specifically disruption of the nucleolar structure enhanced chromatin mobility, thus implying the nucleoli plays an active role in constraining chromatin movement and maintaining the three-dimensional organization of the genome within the nucleus (Chubb et al., 2002). This is further supported by the identification of specific interactions between repetitive and non-repetitive loci within the yeast genome including specific repeated elements that interact with rRNA genes. Therefore, it has been proposed that genomic architecture is organized by restricting the mobility of these repeat elements relative to the nucleolar interaction point (O'Sullivan et al., 2009). Similar results have been obtained using live cell imaging, with frequent interactions observed between the nucleolar and non-nucleolar chromatin (Berger et al., 2008). Intriguingly, extensive disorganisation of nuclear architecture, at the level of whole chromosomes, is associated with the transition from proliferative to senescent states. The human non-rDNA bearing chromosome 18, for instance, exhibits altered spatial positioning, changing from the apical edge of the nucleus in proliferating cells to nucleoli in senescent cells (Bridger et al., 2000). It is plausible that the reorganisation of the genome as the cells enter senescence is responsible for extensive changes in the transcriptional status of the genome (Foster & Bridger, 2005). Consitent with this, we have recently found that reductions in UBF levels lead to disruptions in nucleolar structure and acrocentric chromosome organization and induces premature senescence in primary human fibroblasts (Huang S, Hannan RD, manuscript in preparation). Together, the data suggest a functional role for nucleoli in the organization of the genome and in the regulation of cellular senescence.

5. Conclusion

The nucleolus is a highly evolutionary conserved subnuclear compartment traditionally associated with rDNA transcription and ribosome-subunit production. However it is now apparent that the nucleolus is dynamic in nature and its organization, size and protein composition changes dramatically during the cell cycle and under different cellular conditions including stress. Consistent with this dynamic nature the nucleolus has now been implicated in regulating additional important cellular processes beyond ribosome-subunit synthesis, including cell-cycle control, stress responses, senescence and aging. The fundamental role the rDNA repeats play in aging of fission yeast is now overwhelming. Similarly, in higher eukaryotes, nucleolar function in coupling ribosome subunit biogenesis and cell-cycle progression, through the activity of the tumor suppressor protein p53, places the nucleolus at the centre of coordinating cellular stress response and determining cell fate such as survival and senescence. It is likely we have only begun to scratch the surface of the detail by which eukaryotes have evolved to utilise the unique subnuclear domain, the nucleolus, to control fundamental cellular process such as aging and senescence.

6. References

Angus, S.P., Solomon, D.A., Kuschel, L., Hennigan, R.F. & Knudsen, E.S. (2003). Retinoblastoma tumor suppressor: Analyses of dynamic behavior in living cells reveal multiple modes of regulation. Molecular and Cellular Biology *23*, 8172-8188.

Ayrault, O., Andrique, L., Fauvin, D., Eymin, B., Gazzeri, S. & Seite, P. (2006). Human tumor suppressor p14ARF negatively regulates rRNA transcription and inhibits UBF1 transcription factor phosphorylation. Oncogene *25*, 7577-7586.

Bartek, J., Bartkova, J. & Lukas, J. (1996). The retinoblastoma protein pathway and the restriction point. Current Opinion in Cell Biology *8*, 805-814.

Bassermann, F., Frescas, D., Guardavaccaro, D., Busino, L., Peschiaroli, A. & Pagano, M. (2008). The Cdc14B-Cdh1-Plk1 axis controls the G2 DNA-damage-response checkpoint. Cell *134*, 256-267.

Bauer, J.H., Morris, S.N., Chang, C., Flatt, T., Wood, J.G. & Helfand, S.L. (2009). dSir2 and Dmp53 interact to mediate aspects of CR-dependent lifespan extension in D. melanogaster. Aging (Albany NY) *1*, 38-48.

Bemiller, P.M. & Lee, L.H. (1978). Nucleolar changes in senescing WI-38 cells. Mech Ageing Dev *8*, 417-427.

Berger, A.B., Cabal, G.G., Fabre, E., Duong, T., Buc, H., Nehrbass, U., Olivo-Marin, J.C., Gadal, O. & Zimmer, C. (2008). High-resolution statistical mapping reveals gene territories in live yeast. Nat Methods *5*, 1031-1037.

Berger, A.B., Decourty, L., Badis, G., Nehrbass, U., Jacquier, A. & Gadal, O. (2007). Hmo1 is required for TOR-dependent regulation of ribosomal protein gene transcription. Mol Cell Biol *27*, 8015-8026.

Boisvert, F.M., Lam, Y.W., Lamont, D. & Lamond, A.I. (2010). A quantitative proteomics analysis of subcellular proteome localization and changes induced by DNA damage. Mol Cell Proteomics *9*, 457-470.

Boisvert, F.M. & Lamond, A.I. (2010). p53-Dependent subcellular proteome localization following DNA damage. Proteomics.

Boisvert, F.M., van Koningsbruggen, S., Navascues, J. & Lamond, A.I. (2007). The multifunctional nucleolus. Nat Rev Mol Cell Biol *8*, 574-585.

Boulon, S., Westman, B.J., Hutten, S., Boisvert, F.M. & Lamond, A.I. (2010). The nucleolus under stress. Mol Cell *40*, 216-227.

Bradsher, J., Auriol, J., Proietti de Santis, L., Iben, S., Vonesch, J.L., Grummt, I. & Egly, J.M. (2002). CSB is a component of RNA pol I transcription. Mol Cell *10*, 819-829.

Brewer, B.J., Lockshon, D. & Fangman, W.L. (1992). The arrest of replication forks in the rDNA of yeast occurs independently of transcription. Cell *71*, 267-276.

Bridger, J.M. & Bickmore, W.A. (1998). Putting the genome on the map. Trends Genet *14*, 403-409.

Bridger, J.M., Boyle, S., Kill, I.R. & Bickmore, W.A. (2000). Re-modelling of nuclear architecture in quiescent and senescent human fibroblasts. Curr Biol *10*, 149-152.

Burkhalter, M.D. & Sogo, J.M. (2004). rDNA enhancer affects replication initiation and mitotic recombination: Fob1 mediates nucleolytic processing independently of replication. Mol Cell *15*, 409-421.

Bystricky, K., Laroche, T., van Houwe, G., Blaszczyk, M. & Gasser, S.M. (2005). Chromosome looping in yeast: telomere pairing and coordinated movement reflect anchoring efficiency and territorial organization. J Cell Biol *168*, 375-387.

Caburet, S., Conti, C., Schurra, C., Lebofsky, R., Edelstein, S.J. & Bensimon, A. (2005). Human ribosomal RNA gene arrays display a broad range of palindromic structures. Genome Res *15*, 1079-1085.

Campisi, J. & di Fagagna, F.D. (2007). Cellular senescence: when bad things happen to good cells. Nat Rev Mol Cell Biol *8*, 729-740.

Carmo-Fonseca, M., Mendes-Soares, L. & Campos, I. (2000). To be or not to be in the nucleolus. Nat Cell Biol *2*, E107-112.

Cavanaugh, A.H., Hempel, W.M., Taylor, L.J., Rogalsky, V., Todorov, G. & Rothblum, L.I. (1995). Activity of RNA polymerase I transcription factor UBF blocked by Rb gene product. Nature *374*, 177-180.

Chan, J.C., Hannan, K.M., Riddell, K., Ng, P.Y., Peck, A., Lee, R.S., Hung, S., Astle, M.V., Bywater, M., Wall, M., Poortinga, G., Jastrzebski, K., Sheppard, K.E., Hemmings, B.A., Hall, M.N., Johnstone, R.W., McArthur, G.A., Hannan, R.D. & Pearson, R.B. (2011). AKT Promotes rRNA Synthesis and Cooperates with c-MYC to Stimulate Ribosome Biogenesis in Cancer. Sci Signal *4*, ra56.

Chellappan, S.P., Hiebert, S., Mudryj, M., Horowitz, J.M. & Nevins, J.R. (1991). The E2F transcription factor is a cellular target for the RB protein. Cell *65*, 1053-1061.

Chubb, J.R., Boyle, S., Perry, P. & Bickmore, W.A. (2002). Chromatin motion is constrained by association with nuclear compartments in human cells. Curr Biol *12*, 439-445.

Colombo, E., Marine, J.C., Danovi, D., Falini, B. & Pelicci, P.G. (2002). Nucleophosmin regulates the stability and transcriptional activity of p53. Nat Cell Biol *4*, 529-533.

Conconi, A., Widmer, R.M., Koller, T. & Sogo, J.M. (1989). Two different chromatin structures coexist in ribosomal RNA genes throughout the cell cycle. Cell *57*, 753-761.

Couté, Y., Burgess, J.A., Diaz, J.-J., Chichester, C., Lisacek, F., Greco, A. & Sanchez, J.-C. (2006). Deciphering the human nucleolar proteome. Mass Spectrometry Reviews *25*, 215-234.

Cremer, T. & Cremer, C. (2001). Chromosome territories, nuclear architecture and gene regulation in mammalian cells. Nat Rev Genet *2*, 292-301.

D'Amours, D., Stegmeier, F. & Amon, A. (2004). Cdc14 and condensin control the dissolution of cohesin-independent chromosome linkages at repeated DNA. Cell *117*, 455-469.

Daniely, Y., Dimitrova, D.D. & Borowiec, J.A. (2002). Stress-dependent nucleolin mobilization mediated by p53-nucleolin complex formation. Mol Cell Biol *22*, 6014-6022.

de Lange, T. (2005). Shelterin: the protein complex that shapes and safeguards human telomeres. Genes Dev *19*, 2100-2110.

De Wulf, P. & Visintin, R. (2008). Cdc14B and APC/C tackle DNA damage. Cell *134*, 210-212.

Deisenroth, C. & Zhang, Y. (2010). Ribosome biogenesis surveillance: probing the ribosomal protein-Mdm2-p53 pathway. Oncogene *29*, 4253-4260.

Dimri, G.P., Lee, X., Basile, G., Acosta, M., Scott, G., Roskelley, C., Medrano, E.E., Linskens, M., Rubelj, I., Pereira-Smith, O. & et al. (1995). A biomarker that identifies senescent human cells in culture and in aging skin in vivo. Proc Natl Acad Sci U S A *92*, 9363-9367.

Drygin, D., Lin, A., Bliesath, J., Ho, C.B., O'Brien, S.E., Proffitt, C., Omori, M., Haddach, M., Schwaebe, M.K., Siddiqui-Jain, A., Streiner, N., Quin, J.E., Sanij, E., Bywater, M.J., Hannan, R.D., Ryckman, D., Anderes, K. & Rice, W.G. (2011). Targeting RNA polymerase I with an oral small molecule CX-5461 inhibits ribosomal RNA synthesis and solid tumor growth. Cancer Res *71*, 1418-1430.

Drygin, D., Siddiqui-Jain, A., O'Brien, S., Schwaebe, M., Lin, A., Bliesath, J., Ho, C.B., Proffitt, C., Trent, K., Whitten, J.P., Lim, J.K., Von Hoff, D., Anderes, K. & Rice, W.G. (2009). Anticancer activity of CX-3543: a direct inhibitor of rRNA biogenesis. Cancer Res *69*, 7653-7661.

Elion, E.A. & Warner, J.R. (1984). The major promoter element of rRNA transcription in yeast lies 2 kb upstream. Cell *39*, 663-673.

Ellis, N.A., Groden, J., Ye, T.Z., Straughen, J., Lennon, D.J., Ciocci, S., Proytcheva, M. & German, J. (1995). The Bloom's syndrome gene product is homologous to RecQ helicases. Cell *83*, 655-666.

Erjavec, N., Larsson, L., Grantham, J. & Nystrom, T. (2007). Accelerated aging and failure to segregate damaged proteins in Sir2 mutants can be suppressed by overproducing the protein aggregation-remodeling factor Hsp104p. Genes Dev *21*, 2410-2421.

Etheridge, K.T., Banik, S.S., Armbruster, B.N., Zhu, Y., Terns, R.M., Terns, M.P. & Counter, C.M. (2002). The nucleolar localization domain of the catalytic subunit of human telomerase. J Biol Chem *277*, 24764-24770.

Fishman-Lobell, J., Rudin, N. & Haber, J.E. (1992). Two alternative pathways of double-strand break repair that are kinetically separable and independently modulated. Mol Cell Biol *12*, 1292-1303.

Fontoura, B.M., Sorokina, E.A., David, E. & Carroll, R.B. (1992). p53 is covalently linked to 5.8S rRNA. Mol Cell Biol *12*, 5145-5151.

Foster, H.A. & Bridger, J.M. (2005). The genome and the nucleus: a marriage made by evolution. Genome organisation and nuclear architecture. Chromosoma *114*, 212-9.

French, S.L., Osheim, Y.N., Cioci, F., Nomura, M. & Beyer, A.L. (2003). In exponentially growing Saccharomyces cerevisiae cells, rRNA synthesis is determined by the summed RNA polymerase I loading rate rather than by the number of active genes. Mol Cell Biol *23*, 1558-1568.

Fumagalli, S., Di Cara, A., Neb-Gulati, A., Natt, F., Schwemberger, S., Hall, J., Babcock, G.F., Bernardi, R., Pandolfi, P.P. & Thomas, G. (2009). Absence of nucleolar disruption after impairment of 40S ribosome biogenesis reveals an rpL11-translation-dependent mechanism of p53 induction. Nat Cell Biol *11*, 501-508.

Gagnon-Kugler, T., Langlois, F., Stefanovsky, V., Lessard, F. & Moss, T. (2009). Loss of human ribosomal gene CpG methylation enhances cryptic RNA polymerase II transcription and disrupts ribosomal RNA processing. Mol Cell *35*, 414-425.

Ganley, A.R., Hayashi, K., Horiuchi, T. & Kobayashi, T. (2005). Identifying gene-independent noncoding functional elements in the yeast ribosomal DNA by phylogenetic footprinting. Proc Natl Acad Sci U S A *102*, 11787-11792.

Ganley, A.R., Ide, S., Saka, K. & Kobayashi, T. (2009). The effect of replication initiation on gene amplification in the rDNA and its relationship to aging. Mol Cell *35*, 683-693.

Ganley, A.R. & Kobayashi, T. (2007). Highly efficient concerted evolution in the ribosomal DNA repeats: total rDNA repeat variation revealed by whole-genome shotgun sequence data. Genome Res *17*, 184-191.

Gire, V., Roux, P., Wynford-Thomas, D., Brondello, J.M. & Dulic, V. (2004). DNA damage checkpoint kinase Chk2 triggers replicative senescence. EMBO J *23*, 2554-2563.

Gjerset, R.A. & Bandyopadhyay, K. (2006). Regulation of p14ARF through subnuclear compartmentalization. Cell Cycle *5*, 686-690.

Greider, C.W. & Blackburn, E.H. (1989). A telomeric sequence in the RNA of Tetrahymena telomerase required for telomere repeat synthesis. Nature *337*, 331-337.

Griffith, J.D., Comeau, L., Rosenfield, S., Stansel, R.M., Bianchi, A., Moss, H. & de Lange, T. (1999). Mammalian telomeres end in a large duplex loop. Cell *97*, 503-514.

Grinstein, E., Shan, Y., Karawajew, L., Snijders, P.J., Meijer, C.J., Royer, H.D. & Wernet, P. (2006). Cell cycle-controlled interaction of nucleolin with the retinoblastoma protein and cancerous cell transformation. J Biol Chem *281*, 22223-22235.

Grummt, I. (1999). Regulation of mammalian ribosomal gene transcription by RNA polymerase I. Prog Nucleic Acid Res Mol Biol *62*, 109-154.

Grummt, I. (2003). Life on a planet of its own: regulation of RNA polymerase I transcription in the nucleolus. Genes Dev *17*, 1691-1702.

Grummt, I., Maier, U., Ohrlein, A., Hassouna, N. & Bachellerie, J.P. (1985). Transcription of mouse rDNA terminates downstream of the 3' end of 28S RNA and involves interaction of factors with repeated sequences in the 3' spacer. Cell *43*, 801-810.

Grummt, I. & Pikaard, C.S. (2003). Epigenetic silencing of RNA polymerase I transcription. Nat Rev Mol Cell Biol *4*, 641-649.

Guarente, L. (1997). Link between aging and the nucleolus. Genes Dev *11*, 2449-2455.

Hahn, W.C., Counter, C.M., Lundberg, A.S., Beijersbergen, R.L., Brooks, M.W. & Weinberg, R.A. (1999). Creation of human tumour cells with defined genetic elements. Nature *400*, 464-468.

Hall, D.B., Wade, J.T. & Struhl, K. (2006). An HMG protein, Hmo1, associates with promoters of many ribosomal protein genes and throughout the rRNA gene locus in Saccharomyces cerevisiae. Mol Cell Biol *26*, 3672-3679.

Halle, J.P., Muller, S., Simm, A. & Adam, G. (1997). Copy number, epigenetic state and expression of the rRNA genes in young and senescent rat embryo fibroblasts. Eur J Cell Biol *74*, 281-288.

Hannan, K.M., Brandenburger, Y., Jenkins, A., Sharkey, K., Cavanaugh, A., Rothblum, L., Moss, T., Poortinga, G., McArthur, G.A., Pearson, R.B. & Hannan, R.D. (2003). mTOR-dependent regulation of ribosomal gene transcription requires S6K1 and is mediated by phosphorylation of the carboxy-terminal activation domain of the nucleolar transcription factor UBF. Mol Cell Biol *23*, 8862-8877.

Hannan, K.M., Hannan, R.D., Smith, S.D., Jefferson, L.S., Lun, M. & Rothblum, L.I. (2000). Rb and p130 regulate RNA polymerase I transcription: Rb disrupts the interaction between UBF and SL-1. Oncogene *19*, 4988-4999.

Harley, C.B., Futcher, A.B. & Greider, C.W. (1990). Telomeres shorten during ageing of human fibroblasts. Nature *345*, 458-460.

Haupt, Y., Maya, R., Kazaz, A. & Oren, M. (1997). Mdm2 promotes the rapid degradation of p53. Nature *387*, 296-299.

Hawley, R.S. & Marcus, C.H. (1989). Recombinational controls of rDNA redundancy in Drosophila. Annu Rev Genet *23*, 87-120.

Heliot, L., Kaplan, H., Lucas, L., Klein, C., Beorchia, A., Doco-Fenzy, M., Menager, M., Thiry, M., O'Donohue, M.F. & Ploton, D. (1997). Electron tomography of metaphase nucleolar organizer regions: evidence for a twisted-loop organization. Mol Biol Cell *8*, 2199-2216.

Hempel, W.M., Cavanaugh, A.H., Hannan, R.D., Taylor, L. & Rothblum, L.I. (1996). The species-specific RNA polymerase I transcription factor SL-1 binds to upstream binding factor. Mol Cell Biol *16*, 557-563.

Henderson, S. & Sollner-Webb, B. (1986). A transcriptional terminator is a novel element of the promoter of the mouse ribosomal RNA gene. Cell *47*, 891-900.

Henras, A.K., Capeyrou, R., Henry, Y. & Caizergues-Ferrer, M. (2004). Cbf5p, the putative pseudouridine synthase of H/ACA-type snoRNPs, can form a complex with Gar1p and Nop10p in absence of Nhp2p and box H/ACA snoRNAs. RNA *10*, 1704-1712.

Heo, S.J., Tatebayashi, K., Ohsugi, I., Shimamoto, A., Furuichi, Y. & Ikeda, H. (1999). Bloom's syndrome gene suppresses premature ageing caused by Sgs1 deficiency in yeast. Genes Cells *4*, 619-625.

Honda, R. & Yasuda, H. (1999). Association of p19(ARF) with Mdm2 inhibits ubiquitin ligase activity of Mdm2 for tumor suppressor p53. EMBO J *18*, 22-27.

Hoopes, L.L., Budd, M., Choe, W., Weitao, T. & Campbell, J.L. (2002). Mutations in DNA replication genes reduce yeast life span. Mol Cell Biol *22*, 4136-4146.

Horn, H.F. & Vousden, K.H. (2008). Cooperation between the ribosomal proteins L5 and L11 in the p53 pathway. Oncogene *27*, 5774-5784.

Huang, J., Brito, I.L., Villen, J., Gygi, S.P., Amon, A. & Moazed, D. (2006). Inhibition of homologous recombination by a cohesin-associated clamp complex recruited to the rDNA recombination enhancer. Genes Dev *20*, 2887-2901.

Huang, J. & Moazed, D. (2003). Association of the RENT complex with nontranscribed and coding regions of rDNA and a regional requirement for the replication fork block protein Fob1 in rDNA silencing. Genes Dev *17*, 2162-2176.

Ide, S., Miyazaki, T., Maki, H. & Kobayashi, T. (2010). Abundance of ribosomal RNA gene copies maintains genome integrity. Science *327*, 693-696.

Jazwinski, S.M. (2001). New clues to old yeast. Mech Ageing Dev *122*, 865-882.

Jin, F., Liu, H., Liang, F., Rizkallah, R., Hurt, M.M. & Wang, Y. (2008). Temporal control of the dephosphorylation of Cdk substrates by mitotic exit pathways in budding yeast. Proc Natl Acad Sci U S A *105*, 16177-16182.

Kaeberlein, M., McVey, M. & Guarente, L. (1999). The SIR2/3/4 complex and SIR2 alone promote longevity in Saccharomyces cerevisiae by two different mechanisms. Genes Dev *13*, 2570-2580.

Kennedy, B.K., Gotta, M., Sinclair, D.A., Mills, K., McNabb, D.S., Murthy, M., Pak, S.M., Laroche, T., Gasser, S.M. & Guarente, L. (1997). Redistribution of silencing proteins from telomeres to the nucleolus is associated with extension of life span in S. cerevisiae. Cell *89*, 381-391.

Keys, D.A., Lee, B.S., Dodd, J.A., Nguyen, T.T., Vu, L., Fantino, E., Burson, L.M., Nogi, Y. & Nomura, M. (1996). Multiprotein transcription factor UAF interacts with the upstream element of the yeast RNA polymerase I promoter and forms a stable preinitiation complex. Genes Dev *10*, 887-903.

Khurts, S., Masutomi, K., Delgermaa, L., Arai, K., Oishi, N., Mizuno, H., Hayashi, N., Hahn, W.C. & Murakami, S. (2004). Nucleolin interacts with telomerase. Journal of Biological Chemistry *279*, 51508-51515.

Klose, R.J. & Bird, A.P. (2006). Genomic DNA methylation: the mark and its mediators. Trends Biochem Sci *31*, 89-97.

Kobayashi, T. (2003). The replication fork barrier site forms a unique structure with Fob1p and inhibits the replication fork. Mol Cell Biol *23*, 9178-9188.

Kobayashi, T. (2006). Strategies to maintain the stability of the ribosomal RNA gene repeats--collaboration of recombination, cohesion, and condensation. Genes Genet Syst *81*, 155-161.

Kobayashi, T. (2008). A new role of the rDNA and nucleolus in the nucleus--rDNA instability maintains genome integrity. Bioessays *30*, 267-272.

Kobayashi, T. (2011). Regulation of ribosomal RNA gene copy number and its role in modulating genome integrity and evolutionary adaptability in yeast. Cell Mol Life Sci *68*, 1395-1403.

Kobayashi, T. & Ganley, A.R. (2005). Recombination regulation by transcription-induced cohesin dissociation in rDNA repeats. Science *309*, 1581-1584.

Kobayashi, T., Hidaka, M., Nishizawa, M. & Horiuchi, T. (1992). Identification of a site required for DNA replication fork blocking activity in the rRNA gene cluster in Saccharomyces cerevisiae. Mol Gen Genet *233*, 355-362.

Kobayashi, T., Horiuchi, T., Tongaonkar, P., Vu, L. & Nomura, M. (2004). SIR2 regulates recombination between different rDNA repeats, but not recombination within individual rRNA genes in yeast. Cell *117*, 441-453.

Korgaonkar, C., Hagen, J., Tompkins, V., Frazier, A.A., Allamargot, C., Quelle, F.W. & Quelle, D.E. (2005). Nucleophosmin (B23) targets ARF to nucleoli and inhibits its function. Molecular and Cellular Biology *25*, 1258-1271.

Kubbutat, M.H., Jones, S.N. & Vousden, K.H. (1997). Regulation of p53 stability by Mdm2. Nature *387*, 299-303.

Kulkens, T., Riggs, D.L., Heck, J.D., Planta, R.J. & Nomura, M. (1991). The yeast RNA polymerase I promoter: ribosomal DNA sequences involved in transcription initiation and complex formation in vitro. Nucleic Acids Res *19*, 5363-5370.

Kuo, B.A., Gonzalez, I.L., Gillespie, D.A. & Sylvester, J.E. (1996). Human ribosomal RNA variants from a single individual and their expression in different tissues. Nucleic Acids Res *24*, 4817-4824.

Lam, Y.W., Lamond, A.I., Mann, M. & Andersen, J.S. (2007). Analysis of nucleolar protein dynamics reveals the nuclear degradation of ribosomal proteins. Curr Biol *17*, 749-760.

Lanctot, C., Cheutin, T., Cremer, M., Cavalli, G. & Cremer, T. (2007). Dynamic genome architecture in the nuclear space: regulation of gene expression in three dimensions. Nat Rev Genet *8*, 104-115.

Learned, R.M., Cordes, S. & Tjian, R. (1985). Purification and characterization of a transcription factor that confers promoter specificity to human RNA polymerase I. Mol Cell Biol *5*, 1358-1369.

Leger, I., Guillaud, M., Krief, B. & Brugal, G. (1994). Interactive computer-assisted analysis of chromosome 1 colocalization with nucleoli. Cytometry *16*, 313-323.

Lessard, F., Morin, F., Ivanchuk, S., Langlois, F., Stefanovsky, V., Rutka, J. & Moss, T. (2010). The ARF tumor suppressor controls ribosome biogenesis by regulating the RNA polymerase I transcription factor TTF-I. Mol Cell *38*, 539-550.

Li, Y., Yan, Q. & Wolf, N.S. (1997). Long-term caloric restriction delays age-related decline in proliferation capacity of murine lens epithelial cells in vitro and in vivo. Invest Ophthalmol Vis Sci *38*, 100-107.

Lin, J., Jin, R., Zhang, B., Chen, H., Bai, Y.X., Yang, P.X., Han, S.W., Xie, Y.H., Huang, P.T., Huang, C. & Huang, J.J. (2008). Nucleolar localization of TERT is unrelated to telomerase function in human cells. J Cell Sci *121*, 2169-2176.

Lindstrom, M.S., Jin, A., Deisenroth, C., White Wolf, G. & Zhang, Y. (2007). Cancer-associated mutations in the MDM2 zinc finger domain disrupt ribosomal protein interaction and attenuate MDM2-induced p53 degradation. Mol Cell Biol *27*, 1056-1068.

Lindstrom, M.S. & Nister, M. (2010). Silencing of ribosomal protein S9 elicits a multitude of cellular responses inhibiting the growth of cancer cells subsequent to p53 activation. PLoS One *5*, e9578.

Machin, F., Paschos, K., Jarmuz, A., Torres-Rosell, J., Pade, C. & Aragon, L. (2004). Condensin regulates rDNA silencing by modulating nucleolar Sir2p. Curr Biol *14*, 125-130.

Machwe, A., Orren, D.K. & Bohr, V.A. (2000). Accelerated methylation of ribosomal RNA genes during the cellular senescence of Werner syndrome fibroblasts. FASEB J *14*, 1715-1724.

Maier, B., Gluba, W., Bernier, B., Turner, T., Mohammad, K., Guise, T., Sutherland, A., Thorner, M. & Scrable, H. (2004). Modulation of mammalian life span by the short isoform of p53. Genes Dev *18*, 306-319.

Manuelidis, L. (1984). Different central nervous system cell types display distinct and nonrandom arrangements of satellite DNA sequences. Proc Natl Acad Sci U S A *81*, 3123-3127.

Mayer, C., Bierhoff, H. & Grummt, I. (2005). The nucleolus as a stress sensor: JNK2 inactivates the transcription factor TIF-IA and down-regulates rRNA synthesis. Genes Dev *19*, 933-941.

Mayer, C., Schmitz, K.M., Li, J., Grummt, I. & Santoro, R. (2006). Intergenic transcripts regulate the epigenetic state of rRNA genes. Mol Cell *22*, 351-361.

Mayer, C., Zhao, J., Yuan, X. & Grummt, I. (2004). mTOR-dependent activation of the transcription factor TIF-IA links rRNA synthesis to nutrient availability. Genes Dev *18*, 423-434.

McCormick, A. & Campisi, J. (1991). Cellular aging and senescence. Current Opinion in Cell Biology *3*, 230-234.

McStay, B. & Grummt, I. (2008). The epigenetics of rRNA genes: from molecular to chromosome biology. Annu Rev Cell Dev Biol *24*, 131-157.

Mehta, I.S., Figgitt, M., Clements, C.S., Kill, I.R. & Bridger, J.M. (2007). Alterations to nuclear architecture and genome behavior in senescent cells. In Biogerontology: Mechanisms and Interventions, pp. 250-263.

Merkenschlager, M. (2010). Cohesin: a global player in chromosome biology with local ties to gene regulation. Curr Opin Genet Dev *20*, 555-561.

Merker, R.J. & Klein, H.L. (2002). hpr1Delta affects ribosomal DNA recombination and cell life span in Saccharomyces cerevisiae. Mol Cell Biol *22*, 421-429.

Merz, K., Hondele, M., Goetze, H., Gmelch, K., Stoeckl, U. & Griesenbeck, J. (2008). Actively transcribed rRNA genes in S. cerevisiae are organized in a specialized chromatin associated with the high-mobility group protein Hmo1 and are largely devoid of histone molecules. Genes Dev *22*, 1190-1204.

Misteli, T. (2004). Spatial positioning; a new dimension in genome function. Cell *119*, 153-156.

Momand, J., Zambetti, G.P., Olson, D.C., George, D. & Levine, A.J. (1992). The mdm-2 oncogene product forms a complex with the p53 protein and inhibits p53-mediated transactivation. Cell *69*, 1237-1245.

Mongelard, F. & Bouvet, P. (2007). Nucleolin: a multiFACeTed protein. Trends Cell Biol *17*, 80-86.

Montanaro, L., Mazzini, G., Barbieri, S., Vici, M., Nardi-Pantoli, A., Govoni, M., Donati, G., Trere, D. & Derenzini, M. (2007). Different effects of ribosome biogenesis inhibition on cell proliferation in retinoblastoma protein- and p53-deficient and proficient human osteosarcoma cell lines. Cell Prolif *40*, 532-549.

Moore, H.M., Bai, B., Boisvert, F.M., Latonen, L., Rantanen, V., Simpson, J.C., Pepperkok, R., Lamond, A.I. & Laiho, M. (2011). Quantitative proteomics and dynamic imaging of the nucleolus reveals distinct responses to UV and ionizing radiation. Mol Cell Proteomics.

Moss, T., Langlois, F., Gagnon-Kugler, T. & Stefanovsky, V. (2007). A housekeeper with power of attorney: the rRNA genes in ribosome biogenesis. Cell Mol Life Sci *64*, 29-49.

Moss, T. & Stefanovsky, V.Y. (2002). At the center of eukaryotic life. Cell *109*, 545-548.

Murayama, A., Ohmori, K., Fujimura, A., Minami, H., Yasuzawa-Tanaka, K., Kuroda, T., Oie, S., Daitoku, H., Okuwaki, M., Nagata, K., Fukamizu, A., Kimura, K., Shimizu, T. & Yanagisawa, J. (2008). Epigenetic control of rDNA loci in response to intracellular energy status. Cell *133*, 627-639.

Musters, W., Knol, J., Maas, P., Dekker, A.F., van Heerikhuizen, H. & Planta, R.J. (1989). Linker scanning of the yeast RNA polymerase I promoter. Nucleic Acids Res *17*, 9661-9678.

Nalabothula, N., Indig, F.E. & Carrier, F. (2010). The Nucleolus Takes Control of Protein Trafficking Under Cellular Stress. Mol Cell Pharmacol 2, 203-212.

Narayanan, A., Lukowiak, A., Jady, B.E., Dragon, F., Kiss, T., Terns, R.M. & Terns, M.P. (1999). Nucleolar localization signals of box H/ACA small nucleolar RNAs. EMBO J *18*, 5120-5130.

Narita, M., Nunez, S., Heard, E., Lin, A.W., Hearn, S.A., Spector, D.L., Hannon, G.J. & Lowe, S.W. (2003). Rb-mediated heterochromatin formation and silencing of E2F target genes during cellular senescence. Cell *113*, 703-716.

Nemeth, A. & Langst, G. (2011). Genome organization in and around the nucleolus. Trends Genet *27*, 149-156.

O'Sullivan, A.C., Sullivan, G.J. & McStay, B. (2002). UBF binding in vivo is not restricted to regulatory sequences within the vertebrate ribosomal DNA repeat. Mol Cell Biol *22*, 657-668.

O'Sullivan, J.M., Sontam, D.M., Grierson, R. & Jones, B. (2009). Repeated elements coordinate the spatial organization of the yeast genome. Yeast *26*, 125-138.

Ofir-Rosenfeld, Y., Boggs, K., Michael, D., Kastan, M.B. & Oren, M. (2008). Mdm2 regulates p53 mRNA translation through inhibitory interactions with ribosomal protein L26. Mol Cell *32*, 180-189.

Oliner, J.D., Pietenpol, J.A., Thiagalingam, S., Gyuris, J., Kinzler, K.W. & Vogelstein, B. (1993). Oncoprotein MDM2 conceals the activation domain of tumour suppressor p53. Nature *362*, 857-860.

Olson, M.O., Dundr, M. & Szebeni, A. (2000). The nucleolus: an old factory with unexpected capabilities. Trends Cell Biol *10*, 189-196.

Olson, M.O., Hingorani, K. & Szebeni, A. (2002). Conventional and nonconventional roles of the nucleolus. Int Rev Cytol *219*, 199-266.

Olson, M.O.J. (2004). Sensing Cellular Stress: Another New Function for the Nucleolus? Sci STKE *2004*, pe10-.

Olson, M.O.J. & Dundr, M. (2005). The moving parts of the nucleolus. Histochem Cell Biol *123*, 203-216.

Palmero, I., Pantoja, C. & Serrano, M. (1998). p19ARF links the tumour suppressor p53 to Ras. Nature *395*, 125-126.

Pan, W., Issaq, S. & Zhang, Y. (2011). The in vivo role of the RP-Mdm2-p53 pathway in signaling oncogenic stress induced by pRb inactivation and Ras overexpression. PLoS One *6*, e21625.

Pardee, A.B. (1989). G1 events and regulation of cell proliferation. Science *246*, 603-608.

Park, P.C. & De Boni, U. (1992). Spatial rearrangement and enhanced clustering of kinetochores in interphase nuclei of dorsal root ganglion neurons in vitro: association with nucleolar fusion. Exp Cell Res *203*, 222-229.

Park, P.U., Defossez, P.A. & Guarente, L. (1999). Effects of mutations in DNA repair genes on formation of ribosomal DNA circles and life span in Saccharomyces cerevisiae. Mol Cell Biol *19*, 3848-3856.

Partridge, L. & Mangel, M. (1999). Messages from mortality: the evolution of death rates in the old. Trends Ecol Evol *14*, 438-442.

Pasero, P., Bensimon, A. & Schwob, E. (2002). Single-molecule analysis reveals clustering and epigenetic regulation of replication origins at the yeast rDNA locus. Genes Dev *16*, 2479-2484.

Pawelec, G., Wagner, W., Adibzadeh, M. & Engel, A. (1999). T cell immunosenescence in vitro and in vivo. Exp Gerontol *34*, 419-429.

Peng, J.C. & Karpen, G.H. (2007). H3K9 methylation and RNA interference regulate nucleolar organization and repeated DNA stability. Nat Cell Biol *9*, 25-35.

Pestov, D.G., Strezoska, Z. & Lau, L.F. (2001). Evidence of p53-dependent cross-talk between ribosome biogenesis and the cell cycle: effects of nucleolar protein Bop1 on G(1)/S transition. Mol Cell Biol *21*, 4246-4255.

Poortinga, G., Hannan, K.M., Snelling, H., Walkley, C.R., Jenkins, A., Sharkey, K., Wall, M., Brandenburger, Y., Palatsides, M., Pearson, R.B., McArthur, G.A. & Hannan, R.D. (2004). MAD1 and c-MYC regulate UBF and rDNA transcription during granulocyte differentiation. EMBO J *23*, 3325-3335.

Poortinga, G., Wall, M., Sanij, E., Siwicki, K., Ellul, J., Brown, D., Holloway, T.P., Hannan, R.D. & McArthur, G.A. (2011). c-MYC coordinately regulates ribosomal gene chromatin remodeling and Pol I availability during granulocyte differentiation. Nucleic Acids Res *39*, 3267-3281.

Prieto, J.L. & McStay, B. (2007). Recruitment of factors linking transcription and processing of pre-rRNA to NOR chromatin is UBF-dependent and occurs independent of transcription in human cells. Genes Dev *21*, 2041-2054.

Prieto, J.L. & McStay, B. (2008). Pseudo-NORs: a novel model for studying nucleoli. Biochim Biophys Acta *1783*, 2116-2123.

Pyronnet, S., Dostie, J. & Sonenberg, N. (2001). Suppression of cap-dependent translation in mitosis. Genes Dev *15*, 2083-2093.

Richard, G.F., Kerrest, A. & Dujon, B. (2008). Comparative genomics and molecular dynamics of DNA repeats in eukaryotes. Microbiol Mol Biol Rev *72*, 686-727.

Riley, K.J. & Maher, L.J., 3rd (2007). p53 RNA interactions: new clues in an old mystery. RNA *13*, 1825-1833.

Roussel, P., Andre, C., Comai, L. & Hernandez-Verdun, D. (1996). The rDNA transcription machinery is assembled during mitosis in active NORs and absent in inactive NORs. J Cell Biol *133*, 235-246.

Rubbi, C.P. & Milner, J. (2003). Disruption of the nucleolus mediates stabilization of p53 in response to DNA damage and other stresses. EMBO J *22*, 6068-6077.

Ruggero, D. & Pandolfi, P.P. (2003). Does the ribosome translate cancer? Nat Rev Cancer *3*, 179-192.

Sahin, E. & Depinho, R.A. (2010). Linking functional decline of telomeres, mitochondria and stem cells during ageing. Nature *464*, 520-528.

Sakai, K., Ohta, T., Minoshima, S., Kudoh, J., Wang, Y., de Jong, P.J. & Shimizu, N. (1995). Human ribosomal RNA gene cluster: identification of the proximal end containing a novel tandem repeat sequence. Genomics *26*, 521-526.

Salminen, A. & Kaarniranta, K. (2009). SIRT1 regulates the ribosomal DNA locus: Epigenetic candles twinkle longevity in the Christmas tree. Biochemical and Biophysical Research Communications *378*, 6-9.

Sander, E.E. & Grummt, I. (1997). Oligomerization of the transcription termination factor TTF-I: implications for the structural organization of ribosomal transcription units. Nucleic Acids Res *25*, 1142-1147.

Sanij, E. & Hannan, R.D. (2009). The role of UBF in regulating the structure and dynamics of transcriptionally active rDNA chromatin. Epigenetics *4*, 374-382.

Sanij, E., Poortinga, G., Sharkey, K., Hung, S., Holloway, T.P., Quin, J., Robb, E., Wong, L.H., Thomas, W.G., Stefanovsky, V., Moss, T., Rothblum, L., Hannan, K.M., McArthur, G.A., Pearson, R.B. & Hannan, R.D. (2008). UBF levels determine the number of active ribosomal RNA genes in mammals. J Cell Biol *183*, 1259-1274.

Santangelo, G.M., Tornow, J., McLaughlin, C.S. & Moldave, K. (1988). Properties of promoters cloned randomly from the Saccharomyces cerevisiae genome. Mol Cell Biol *8*, 4217-4224.

Santoro, R., Li, J. & Grummt, I. (2002). The nucleolar remodeling complex NoRC mediates heterochromatin formation and silencing of ribosomal gene transcription. Nat Genet *32*, 393-396.

Sharpless, N.E., Bardeesy, N., Lee, K.H., Carrasco, D., Castrillon, D.H., Aguirre, A.J., Wu, E.A., Horner, J.W. & DePinho, R.A. (2001). Loss of p16Ink4a with retention of p19Arf predisposes mice to tumorigenesis. Nature *413*, 86-91.

Shcherbik, N. & Pestov, D.G. (2010). Ubiquitin and ubiquitin-like proteins in the nucleolus: multitasking tools for a ribosome factory. Genes Cancer *1*, 681-689.

Sherr, C.J. & Roberts, J.M. (1999). CDK inhibitors: positive and negative regulators of G1-phase progression. Genes Dev *13*, 1501-1512.

Sherwood, S.W., Rush, D., Ellsworth, J.L. & Schimke, R.T. (1988). Defining cellular senescence in IMR-90 cells: a flow cytometric analysis. Proc Natl Acad Sci U S A *85*, 9086-9090.

Shore, D. (1998). Cellular senescence: lessons from yeast for human aging? Curr Biol *8*, R192-195.

Shou, W., Azzam, R., Chen, S.L., Huddleston, M.J., Baskerville, C., Charbonneau, H., Annan, R.S., Carr, S.A. & Deshaies, R.J. (2002). Cdc5 influences phosphorylation of Net1 and disassembly of the RENT complex. BMC Mol Biol *3*, 3.

Shou, W., Seol, J.H., Shevchenko, A., Baskerville, C., Moazed, D., Chen, Z.W., Jang, J., Charbonneau, H. & Deshaies, R.J. (1999). Exit from mitosis is triggered by Tem1-dependent release of the protein phosphatase Cdc14 from nucleolar RENT complex. Cell *97*, 233-244.

Siddiqi, I.N., Dodd, J.A., Vu, L., Eliason, K., Oakes, M.L., Keener, J., Moore, R., Young, M.K. & Nomura, M. (2001). Transcription of chromosomal rRNA genes by both RNA polymerase I and II in yeast uaf30 mutants lacking the 30 kDa subunit of transcription factor UAF. EMBO J *20*, 4512-4521.

Sinclair, D.A. & Guarente, L. (1997). Extrachromosomal rDNA circles--a cause of aging in yeast. Cell *91*, 1033-1042.

Sirri, V., Hernandez-Verdun, D. & Roussel, P. (2002). Cyclin-dependent kinases govern formation and maintenance of the nucleolus. Journal of Cell Biology *156*, 969-981.

Sirri, V., Urcuqui-Inchima, S., Roussel, P. & Hernandez-Verdun, D. (2008). Nucleolus: the fascinating nuclear body. Histochem Cell Biol *129*, 13-31.

Stancheva, I., Lucchini, R., Koller, T. & Sogo, J.M. (1997). Chromatin structure and methylation of rat rRNA genes studied by formaldehyde fixation and psoralen cross-linking. Nucleic Acids Res *25*, 1727-1735.

Stefanovsky, V., Langlois, F., Gagnon-Kugler, T., Rothblum, L.I. & Moss, T. (2006). Growth factor signaling regulates elongation of RNA polymerase I transcription in mammals via UBF phosphorylation and r-chromatin remodeling. Mol Cell *21*, 629-639.

Stefanovsky, V.Y., Pelletier, G., Hannan, R., Gagnon-Kugler, T., Rothblum, L.I. & Moss, T. (2001). An immediate response of ribosomal transcription to growth factor stimulation in mammals is mediated by ERK phosphorylation of UBF. Mol Cell *8*, 1063-1073.

Steffan, J.S., Keys, D.A., Dodd, J.A. & Nomura, M. (1996). The role of TBP in rDNA transcription by RNA polymerase I in Saccharomyces cerevisiae: TBP is required for upstream activation factor-dependent recruitment of core factor. Genes Dev *10*, 2551-2563.

Stewart, S.A., Ben-Porath, I., Carey, V.J., O'Connor, B.F., Hahn, W.C. & Weinberg, R.A. (2003). Erosion of the telomeric single-strand overhang at replicative senescence. Nat Genet *33*, 492-496.

Sugimoto, M., Kuo, M.L., Roussel, M.F. & Sherr, C.J. (2003). Nucleolar Arf tumor suppressor inhibits ribosomal RNA processing. Mol Cell *11*, 415-424.

Takemura, M., Ohoka, F., Perpelescu, M., Ogawa, M., Matsushita, H., Takaba, T., Akiyama, T., Umekawa, H., Furuichi, Y., Cook, P.R. & Yoshida, S. (2002). Phosphorylation-dependent migration of retinoblastoma protein into the nucleolus triggered by binding to nucleophosmin/B23. Exp Cell Res *276*, 233-241.

Tissenbaum, H.A. & Guarente, L. (2001). Increased dosage of a sir-2 gene extends lifespan in Caenorhabditis elegans. Nature *410*, 227-230.

Tomlinson, R.L., Ziegler, T.D., Supakorndej, T., Terns, R.M. & Terns, M.P. (2006). Cell cycle-regulated trafficking of human telomerase to telomeres. Molecular Biology of the Cell *17*, 955-965.

Trumtel, S., Leger-Silvestre, I., Gleizes, P.E., Teulieres, F. & Gas, N. (2000). Assembly and functional organization of the nucleolus: ultrastructural analysis of Saccharomyces cerevisiae mutants. Mol Biol Cell *11*, 2175-2189.

Tsai, R.Y.L. (2009). Nucleolar modulation of TRF1 A dynamic way to regulate telomere and cell cycle by nucleostemin and GNL3L. Cell Cycle *8*, 2912-2916.

Tsang, C.K., Bertram, P.G., Ai, W., Drenan, R. & Zheng, X.F. (2003). Chromatin-mediated regulation of nucleolar structure and RNA Pol I localization by TOR. EMBO J *22*, 6045-6056.

Tschochner, H. & Hurt, E. (2003). Pre-ribosomes on the road from the nucleolus to the cytoplasm. Trends Cell Biol *13*, 255-263.

Tyner, S.D., Venkatachalam, S., Choi, J., Jones, S., Ghebranious, N., Igelmann, H., Lu, X., Soron, G., Cooper, B., Brayton, C., Hee Park, S., Thompson, T., Karsenty, G., Bradley, A. & Donehower, L.A. (2002). p53 mutant mice that display early ageing-associated phenotypes. Nature *415*, 45-53.

van Koningsbruggen, S., Gierlinski, M., Schofield, P., Martin, D., Barton, G.J., Ariyurek, Y., den Dunnen, J.T. & Lamond, A.I. (2010). High-resolution whole-genome sequencing reveals that specific chromatin domains from most human chromosomes associate with nucleoli. Mol Biol Cell *21*, 3735-3748.

Vigneron, A. & Vousden, K.H. (2010). p53, ROS and senescence in the control of aging. Aging (Albany NY) *2*, 471-474.

Vintermist, A., Bohm, S., Sadeghifar, F., Louvet, E., Mansen, A., Percipalle, P. & Ostlund Farrants, A.K. (2011). The chromatin remodelling complex B-WICH changes the chromatin structure and recruits histone acetyl-transferases to active rRNA genes. PLoS One *6*, e19184.

Visintin, R., Craig, K., Hwang, E.S., Prinz, S., Tyers, M. & Amon, A. (1998). The phosphatase Cdc14 triggers mitotic exit by reversal of Cdk-dependent phosphorylation. Mol Cell *2*, 709-718.

Wang, B.D., Butylin, P. & Strunnikov, A. (2006). Condensin function in mitotic nucleolar segregation is regulated by rDNA transcription. Cell Cycle *5*, 2260-2267.

Warner, J.R. & McIntosh, K.B. (2009). How Common Are Extraribosomal Functions of Ribosomal Proteins? Molecular Cell *34*, 3-11.

Weber, J.D., Taylor, L.J., Roussel, M.F., Sherr, C.J. & Bar-Sagi, D. (1999). Nucleolar Arf sequesters Mdm2 and activates p53. Nat Cell Biol *1*, 20-26.

Wong, J.M.Y., Kusdra, L. & Collins, K. (2002). Subnuclear shuttling of human telomerase induced by transformation and DNA damage. Nat Cell Biol *4*, 731-U735.

Wright, J.E., Mais, C., Prieto, J.L. & McStay, B. (2006). A role for upstream binding factor in organizing ribosomal gene chromatin. Biochem Soc Symp, 77-84.

Yang, Y., Chen, Y., Zhang, C., Huang, H. & Weissman, S.M. (2002). Nucleolar localization of hTERT protein is associated with telomerase function. Exp Cell Res *277*, 201-209.

Yoshida, S. & Toh-e, A. (2002). Budding yeast Cdc5 phosphorylates Net1 and assists Cdc14 release from the nucleolus. Biochem Biophys Res Commun *294*, 687-691.

Yu, C.E., Oshima, J., Fu, Y.H., Wijsman, E.M., Hisama, F., Alisch, R., Matthews, S., Nakura, J., Miki, T., Ouais, S., Martin, G.M., Mulligan, J. & Schellenberg, G.D. (1996). Positional cloning of the Werner's syndrome gene. Science *272*, 258-262.

Yuan, X., Zhao, J., Zentgraf, H., Hoffmann-Rohrer, U. & Grummt, I. (2002). Multiple interactions between RNA polymerase I, TIF-IA and TAF(I) subunits regulate preinitiation complex assembly at the ribosomal gene promoter. EMBO Rep *3*, 1082-1087.

Yuan, X., Zhou, Y., Casanova, E., Chai, M., Kiss, E., Grone, H.J., Schutz, G. & Grummt, I. (2005). Genetic inactivation of the transcription factor TIF-IA leads to nucleolar disruption, cell cycle arrest, and p53-mediated apoptosis. Mol Cell *19*, 77-87.

Zachariae, W., Schwab, M., Nasmyth, K. & Seufert, W. (1998). Control of cyclin ubiquitination by CDK-regulated binding of Hct1 to the anaphase promoting complex. Science *282*, 1721-1724.

Zhang, L.F., Huynh, K.D. & Lee, J.T. (2007). Perinucleolar targeting of the inactive X during S phase: evidence for a role in the maintenance of silencing. Cell *129*, 693-706.

Zhang, S., Hemmerich, P. & Grosse, F. (2004). Nucleolar localization of the human telomeric repeat binding factor 2 (TRF2). J Cell Sci *117*, 3935-3945.

Zhang, Y. & Lu, H. (2009). Signaling to p53: ribosomal proteins find their way. Cancer Cell *16*, 369-377.

Zhang, Y., Yu, Z., Fu, X. & Liang, C. (2002). Noc3p, a bHLH protein, plays an integral role in the initiation of DNA replication in budding yeast. Cell *109*, 849-860.

Zhang, Y.P., Wolf, G.W., Bhat, K., Jin, A., Allio, T., Burkhart, W.A. & Xiong, Y. (2003). Ribosomal protein L11 negatively regulates oncoprotein MDM2 and mediates a p53-dependent ribosomal-stress checkpoint pathway. Molecular and Cellular Biology *23*, 8902-8912.

Zhu, Q., Meng, L., Hsu, J.K., Lin, T., Teishima, J. & Tsai, R.Y. (2009). GNL3L stabilizes the TRF1 complex and promotes mitotic transition. J Cell Biol *185*, 827-839.

Zindy, F., Eischen, C.M., Randle, D.H., Kamijo, T., Cleveland, J.L., Sherr, C.J. & Roussel, M.F. (1998). Myc signaling via the ARF tumor suppressor regulates p53-dependent apoptosis and immortalization. Genes Dev *12*, 2424-2433.

Zomerdijk, J.C., Beckmann, H., Comai, L. & Tjian, R. (1994). Assembly of transcriptionally active RNA polymerase I initiation factor SL1 from recombinant subunits. Science *266*, 2015-2018.

10

Senescence in Animals: Why Evolutionary Theories Matter

Thiago Monaco, Daniel Silvestre and Paulo S.P. Silveira
Department of Pathology, School of Medicine at the University of Sao Paulo, Sao Paulo Brazil

1. Introduction

Senescence, considered from the individual viewpoint can be characterized as a "progressive loss of fertility and increasing probability of death with increasing age"(Kirkwood & Austad, 2000). This phenomenon can also be considered from the populational perspective: senescent populations present increasingly higher death rates with increasing age (Masoro & Austad, 2006).

This is a clearly deleterious process, which seems difficult to conciliate with natural selection, which predicts evolution towards increasing fitness. Historically, the first evolutionary explanation able to conciliate these two processes is known as the mutation accumulation theory (Medawar, 1952). According to this theory, in age-structured populations the force of selection decreases with increasing age, allowing the accumulation of deleterious genes with age-specific effects on mortality rate (Hamilton, 1966). Under population genetics mechanisms, senescence is not necessarily deleterious: the original Medawar's proposition implies that the postponement of age-specific effects of harmful genes is equivalent to their elimination in such a way that they become effectively neutral. Hence, such postponement is beneficial and senescence can be regarded as a side effect of the process.

Medawar was convinced that these genes could only account for senescent manifestations encountered in protected populations after they reached ages not achievable in the wild and, therefore, that further explanation involving pleiotropy and linkage would be required to account for a gradual process of organic degeneration, but he did not elaborate on them. This was noted by Williams, who explained the maintenance of beneficial and deleterious traits together, giving rise to the antagonistic pleiotropy theory.

Essentially, the antagonistic pleiotropy theory relies on the existence of genes of a special kind, which are capable of increasing and decreasing fitness depending on the somatic environment and/or age. It is not necessary that the beneficial effects precede the deleterious effect as commonly believed e. g. (Futuyma, 1998; Masoro & Austad, 2006). Instead, Williams' original proposition only required an influx of pleiotropic alleles that may fixate in the population due to their overall beneficial effect. In this scenario, the observed senescence is understood as the composition of deleterious components from all present pleiotropic genes (Williams, 1957).

Instead of basing his arguments on genetics, a somewhat different view was offered by Kirkwood, elaborating on the error catastrophe of Orgel (Orgel, 1963). He approached senescence from an ecological argument in which energy resources may be allocated either to somatic cell maintenance or to reproduction, thus generating some sort of soma-germ conflict. Called disposable soma theory, it ultimately relies on the existence of specific genes controlling the accuracy of the transcription/translation machinery in an age-dependent manner. Kirkwood himself regards his theory as a specialization of the antagonistic pleiotropy of Williams (Kirkwood, 1977; Kirkwood & Holliday, 1975a;b; 1979). The difference is that Williams invokes the existence of genes responsible for beneficial and deleterious effects, but Kirkwood's theory, while not denying the existence of these genes, does not require them. The conflicting destination of energy either to body or reproduction maintenance would suffice for the evolution of senescence.

Senescence is a process that causes animals to become progressively less fertile (Medawar, 1946) and more vulnerable (Comfort, 1956) with age. It has long been noticed that senescence-associated frailty causes population death rates to rise exponentially with age (Gompertz, 1825).

Although a number of evidences have since been collected in support of each of these theories, in the last decades some phenomena have challenged all of them. This includes the effect of caloric restriction on longevity, the late-life mortality deceleration and the longevity pathways controlled by either a single or a few genes, such as the insulin pathway and the effect of sirtuins on longevity.

2. Measuring senescence

Although generally considered together, it is useful to take some time to consider the effects of senescence on individuals' survival and fertility (physiological senescence) or on populational survival curves (demographic senescence) separetly. By not doing so, the researcher may unwittingly take the risk of assuming demographic senescence to stem directly from physiological senescence. Although it might well be the case, there is no theoretical reason why it must be so.

The fact is that the genetic architecture of senescence, i.e., which genes are related to which measurable effects that we call senescence and how they relate to each other, will dictate the relationship between physiological and demographic senescence(s).

2.1 What is the genetic architecture of senescence?

Genetic architecture refers to the genetic basis of a phenotypic trait. Beyond comprehending the map of the genes linked to a given trait, genetic architecture considers all phenomena through which such genetic map produces the phenotype Masoro & Austad (2006).

The most common definition of the senescent phenotype combines individual effects (decrease in functional and reproductive abilities) with an effect which is measurable only in a population (age-dependent increase in mortality). This often leads us to conclude that it is exactly the same phenomenon that makes us individually more fragile and at greater risk of dying as we age.

Figure 1 shows that this is only one of the possible relationships between physiological senescence (progressive fall on functional capacity and fertility) and demographic senescence (increased mortality accompaining chronological aging) (Promislow et al., 2006).

While it is not necessarily clear what the relationship between the physiological and demographic components of senescence is, most "aging genes" described in the literature are simply genes whose variations influence the longevity of the studied species regardless of their physiological effect, and few genes were shown to affect the Mortality Rate Doubling Time (MRDT) of populations of mutants for such genes, and, therefore, to affect the speed of senescence (de Magalhães et al., 2005). Additionally, when strains carrying alleles for many of the so called *longevity genes* are mixed with wild populations, generally the "beneficial" mutation is lost over a few generations, indicating that although such variants increase longevity, they may exert a deleterious effect for fitness (Promislow et al., 2006).

For these reasons, the first decision before staring to seek for "aging genes" should be which model of senescence to assume. Otherwise, we might not know how to interpret the findings in a coherent way: suppose that human carriers of a given mutation have an increase of 5% in their annual mortality from 30 years of age – are them carriers of a genetic disease or of a deleterious mutation in a senescence pathway?

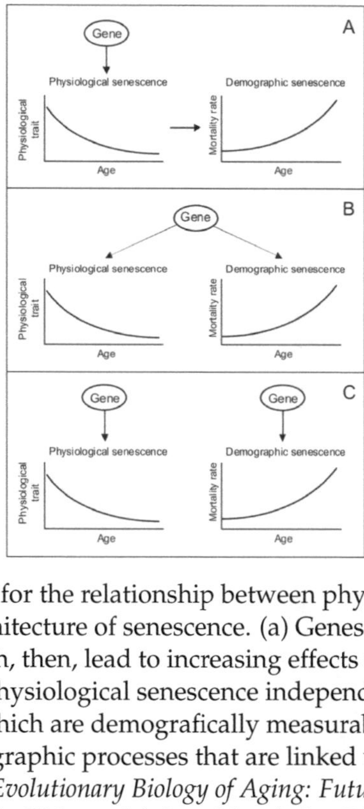

Fig. 1. Three different models for the relationship between physiological and demographic senescence on the genetic architecture of senescence. (a) Genes negatively influence physiological processes, which, then, lead to increasing effects on age-specific mortality. (b) The same genes that lead to physiological senescence independently lead to increasing age-dependent death rates, which are demograficaly measurable. (c) Different genes operate over physiological and demographic processes that are linked with senescence. Extracted from *Promislow, D. E. L. et al. Evolutionary Biology of Aging: Future Directions. In: Masoro EJ, Austad SN (Ed.). Handbook of the Biology of Aging. 6th. ed. San Diego: Academic Press, 2006. 217-242.*

If we suppose that senescence is a unique genetic phenomenon whose physiological effects lead to its demographic aspects (Figure 1 (a)), then "genes of senescence" should exert age-dependent deleterious effects in the physiology of organisms, and because more frail individuals are more prone to dye from a given insult, such genes would also increase mortality from their ages of onset.

On the other hand, genes that determine effects on demographic senescence may exert independent effects on the physiology of organisms. Such effects might not be linked to the demographic effects of the same genes (Figure 1 (b)).

Finally, physiological senescence could be genetically independent from demographic senescence, so that there would be a "genetic modularity" between the two phenomena, in which different groups of genes participate in each process (Figure 1 (c)).

This text assumes when necessary that genes linked to physiological senescence may impact probability of death (1 (a)). It does so relying on the fact that there is little evidence that there may be a genetic variability to the age-dependent physiological decline without its influencing on demographic senescence (Wessells et al., 2004).

Once delimited the senescent phenotype, we review some genetic phenomena that may have importance for the genetic architecture of senescence. Such phenomena include:

- Epistasis, when the expression of a gene negatively influences the expression of one another;
- Polygyny, where multiple genes contribute to a phenotypic trait;
- Pleiotropy, when multiple phenotypic characteristics are influenced by a single gene;
- Quasi-continuity, while a variation in a gene affects minimally a phenotype;
- Plasticity, when a single genotype can produce more than one distinct phenotype, such phenotypic diversity may occur among individuals of the same genotype, by action of different environmental influences on the same individual or *in the same individual at different ages*;
- Evolvability, when genotypic variations of a phenotype exist in a population and can lead to different degrees of adaptability, so that environmental changes will lead to readaptations.

Epistasis could function similarly to what is predicted on antagonistic pleiotropy theory: assuming two genes with positive effects for fitness, in which the first gene exerts a negative effect on the expression of the second gene, the first gene would have positive and negative effects on fitness The effect under selection, however, would be the average effect.

It is believed, since the formulation of the theory of mutation accumulation by Medawar, that senescence is a polygenic phenotype (Medawar, 1952). Indeed, recent decades have seen the description of "hundreds of aging genes" (Promislow et al., 2006). Summed to the fact that senescence is an early onset and gradually progressive phenotype in almost all of the species that has been described, it points to a polygenic inheritance with almost-continuity in organic response to genes that determine senescence.

3. The evolutionary theories of senescence

3.1 Introduction

It has always been difficult to conciliate senescence with natural selection, a biological mechanism generally expected to increase population fitness. Although acknowledged by Darwin (1872), the first tentative explanation for the evolution of senescence was offered by August Weismann in 1881. For Weismann, senescence had evolved for the good of species, in that the removal of older, weaker and less fertile individuals from a population would enhance the survival of younger individuals and overall reproduction of the species (Weismann, 1889).

Realizing his argument was circular (since it depended on older individuals being weaker and less fertile for senescence to evolve) Weismann withdrew his theory (Weismann, 1892).

More than half a century later, Medawar proposed the mutation accumulation theory of senescence (Medawar, 1952). He realized that even in an imaginary non senescent population, older individuals would be very rare simply because the cumulative incidence of death is necessarily dependent of age. This means that late acting mutations will affect population fitness only in the proportion of surviving individuals after such late ages. In other words, the force of natural selection decreases with age and deleterious mutations with effects that are late enough are in fact neutral mutations, which could randomly accumulate.

For Medawar, this would explain the existence of deleterious mutations fixed in ages to which individuals of a given species are not expected to survive in nature. Senescence evolved through such a process would only be observable in protected species, such as laboratory animals or our own species. Medawar, nonetheless, believed that animals did senesce in nature and, therefore felt the need for an early benefit to explain how a not so late acting deleterious mutation could evolve to fixation.

This was developed into the antagonistic pleiotropy theory (Williams, 1957). In short, Williams proposed that the fitness associated to mutations with more than one effect is the average fitness. Therefore, a mutation with earlier beneficial effects and later deleterious ones could be fixed by natural selection if the overall fitness be positive. Deleterious effects early enough to impact mortality in nature could be compensated by beneficial effects. Williams' theory depended on the existence of such special, pleiotropic genes, in numbers sufficient to explain the observed progressive increase in the effects of senescence.

In 1977, elaborating on the mechanistic error catastrophe theory of Orgel (1963), Kirkwood proposed an ecological argument for the evolution of senescence (Kirkwood, 1977). Since evolution is centered on reproduction and not directly in survival, the energetic and metabolic cost of maintenance and repair could affect reproduction negatively if taken to perfection. Therefore, the level of body maintenance and repair that can evolve is the minimum to assure reproduction. Any deleterious mutation that do not decrease reproduction can not only be neutral, but can enhance fitness if it results in more reproductive resources. This is the disposable soma theory of senescence.

These three theories are not mutually excluding, and can explain different aspects of the evolution of senescence (Kirkwood & Austad, 2000).

3.2 The mutation accumulation theory of senescence

According to Haldane, a deleterious mutation with effect only on later ages may escape natural selection, because either most individuals will be dead or will have reproduced at such ages. For Haldane, this implies in the fall of the force of natural selection with advancing ages (Haldane, 1941). Nevertheless, he failed to turn this observation into a theory of senescence.

It was Medawar who would do so. The gap between Haldane's observation of the falling force of natural selection and an evolutionary theory of senescence relies on the requirement of an age structure on populations for the fell in the force of selection. It is natural to suppose an age structure with many young individuals and rare older ones if senescence exists. In such a population, Haldane's explanation for Huntington's Disease works well, but such a model, which already pressuposes senescence, cannot acount for its evolutionary origins.

Medawar postulated that age-independent environmental hazards such as hunger, predation, accidents, etc. were a sufficient condition for the establishment of populational age structures. Older individuals, Medawar claimed, were rare because they have been exposed to such risks (termed extrinsic mortality) longer than young individuals. In other words, the existence of age structures in wild populations is a function of environmental hazards and not of senescence. Even a non senescent population would have an age structure (Medawar, 1952).

The importance of Medawar's reasoning is that older individuals in age structured populations, being necessarily rarer than younger ones, not only do not compete for environmental resources: they also don't contribute much offspring to newer generations. This is the key for Medawar's mutation accumulation theory of senescence – and also a basis for the next two hypotheses, antagonistic pleiotropy and disposable soma theories of senescence.

Figure 3 (age structured population)

Deleterious mutations, provided that it effects happen in sufficiently late ages, could accumulate in the genome According to mechanisms of population genetics, senescence is not necessarily harmful: Medawar's original proposition implies that the postponement of the effects of age-specific deleterious genes for late ages is equivalent to their elimination. Thus, these genes become effectively neutral (Medawar, 1952).

According to this theory, such evolutionary mechanism could only explain the manifestations found in senescent populations protected after individuals reach ages above those found in nature, since in nature, the age of accumulation would coincide with the maximum age of living individuals.

Medawar accepted that the effects of senescence also occurred at ages commonly found in nature. For this reason, he became convinced that another mechanism, involving either pleiotropy or linkage, would be necessary to explain the process of early and gradual degeneration which is charachteristic of senescence (Medawar, 1952). Medawar, however, didn't advance more details on this hypothesis.

3.3 The antagonistic pleiotropy theory

Although the accumulation of mutations justifies the existence of deleterious genes with late expression (and thus the already established senescent state), it didn't seem to explain the slow onset of senescence (Williams, 1957).

Seeking to understand how deleterious genetic effects expressed in relatively early ages could escape selection, Williams grounded his theory on four assumptions: the existence of a somatic cell line, i.e., non-transferable in whole or part by sexual or asexual reproduction, the natural selection of different alleles at a population, a decreasing probability of reproduction with increasing ages, the existence of pleiotropic genes with different effects on fitness at distinct ages (antagonistic pleiotropy). According to this idea, the evolutionary fundamental process to the establishment of senescence is a selective action on the inheritance of a gene with antagonistic effects on its carrier's fitness (Williams, 1957).

It is to note that the very existence of pleiotropic genes with antagonistic effects was not postulated by Williams. In a previous article, Sewall Wright describes an equation for calculating the impact of a pleiotropic gene on fitness:

$$W = (1 + S_1)(1 + S_2)...(1 + S_n) \,, \tag{1}$$

where W is the fitness of a gene and S_1, S_2 ... S_n are the separate selective coefficients for each age-specific effect of such gene on fitness (Wright, 1956).

Williams' merit was to note the implication of Wright's equation for the evolution of senescence in age structured populations. He applied to the Equation 1 the same reasoning applied by Medawar in relation to the age structure of populations: the magnitude of the effect of S_n of a gene may be reduced if it only starts at advanced ages. In a gene capable of expressing different effects on different ages, later effects will less be subject to natural selection than earlier effects.

By considering the effects of a given gene in distinct ages of expression, however, Williams proposed that the measure of the magnitude of each effect in question (advantages or disadvantages) is given by

$$S_n = m_n p_n \,, \tag{2}$$

where S_n is the effect under consideration, m_n its magnitude or impact on fitness and p_n is the proportion of a population's reproductive probability that is *relevant* to the age of manifestation of the effect S_n.

This allowed him to rewrite the Equation 1 considering the effect of age structure in the final selective coefficient of a pleiotropic gene:

$$W = (1 + m_1 p_1)(1 + m_2 p_2)...(1 + m_n p_n) \,. \tag{3}$$

From this equation we may extract the simplest case: the one of a pleiotropic gene with a late deleterious effect and a very early beneficial effect. To demonstrate the formula we need to know the values of p for each age.

Let us imagine a population (structured for simplicity on a human age-scale) with constant birth and death. This is necessary not to create an *ad hoc* argument, by starting with a previously non-senescent population and therefore with no age differences in mortality.

Let's say that this population has a constant mortality of 0.25 each 4 years, ie, 0.0625 per year, and that each 4-years extract is composed of 1000 individuals. This population age distribution is represented in Figure 2. The familiarity of this age distribution with any wild population is noticiable, as it is with any high-mortality human population (as an example, the Figure 3 represents the age distribution of the population of Afghanistan in 2008).

In this non-senescent population, organisms do not lose fertility with the progression of age and all individuals have the same reproductive probability. Therefore, p_x, i.e., the proportion of the reproductive probability associated with each age will be the proportion of remaining individuals with ages equal or superior to that in the population, since the effect of S remain after activated, i.e., be constant from its manifestation.

Williams could thus formulate an evolutionary hypothesis for the permanence (regardless of natural selection) of detrimental effects whose expression was sufficiently early to be influential in wild populations. It is important to notice that neither the equation nor any

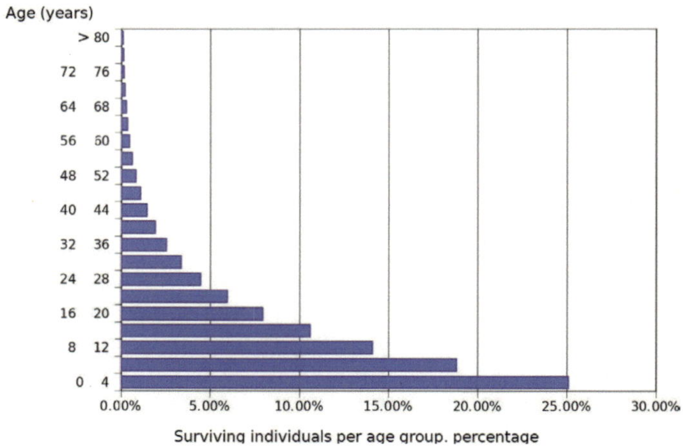

Fig. 2. Age distribution of an alleged non-senescent population exposed to a mortality of 6.25% per year.

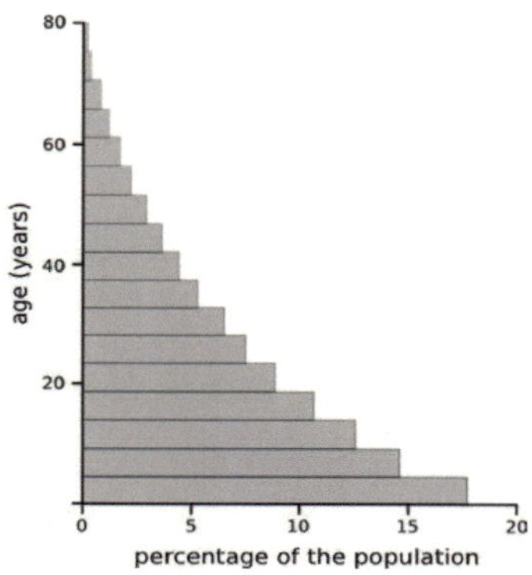

Fig. 3. Age distribution of the Afghan population in 2008 (data from U.S. Census, International Database, available at http://www.census.gov/).

comment on Williams' classic article (Williams, 1957) infer what the number of effects of a pleiotropic gene should be, nor which effect, beneficial or deleterious should happen earlier. While it is clear that the simplest case of antagonistic pleiotropy would be of a gene with an early beneficial effect and a late deleterious one, Equation 3 does not imply that this is the only possibility.

The literature, however, did not follow this conclusion. Williams' antagonistic pleiotropy came to be regarded precisely as the case in which a mutation with two actions, an early advantage and a later disadvantage, it is positively selected. It is worth quoting verbatim the concept of antagonistic pleiotropy found in the *Handbook of Biological Aging*, of 2006, in a chapter written by the editor of the book (Masoro, 2006):

"Another genetic mechanism, proposed by Williams (1957), is referred to as antagonistic pleiotropy. It proposes that those genes that increase evolutionary fitness in early life will be selected for, even if they have catastrophic deleterious effects in late life. Again, the deleterious effects of these genes will be evident only in subjects in protected environments that enable a long life. "

While Medawar discussed the age of onset of a characteristic deleterious and Williams called attention to the magnitude of genetic effects, no theory explicited discussed the influence of the magnitude of extrinsic mortality and random genetic drift on the selection of deleterious genes.

3.4 The disposable soma theory

From the 1970s, a new theory for the evolution of senescence was proposed by Thomas Kirkwood (Kirkwood & Holliday, 1975a;b), reasoning initially not about evolutionary mechanisms as maladaptive as Medawar or on pleiotropic genes as Williams, but on a strong ecological basis. Elaborating on the theory Orgell's "error catastrophe " (Orgel, 1963), Kirkwood gave us a somewhat different view from what had previously been formulated on the evolution of senescence.

Kirkwood addressed the issue of senescence under an ecological constraint in which energy resources available to individuals could be allocated either for maintenance somatic cells or for reproduction, generating a soma-germ conflict. Called disposable soma theory, this ultimately depends on the existence of specific genes that either influence or control the precision of the genetic replication / transcription and translation machineries in an age-dependent fashion; Kirkwood himself considered his theory as a specialization of the antagonistic pleiotropy theory of Williams (Kirkwood, 1977; Kirkwood & Holliday, 1979). The difference is that Williams posits the existence of genes for beneficial and deleterious effects, but the theory of Kirkwood, despite not denying the existence of these genes, do not need them. If, under Williams theory, natural selection would act on the average effects of a selected gene's mutant alleles, under Kirkwood's assumption a single genetic effect, determining the distribution of resources between reproduction and body maintenance would be sufficient for the evolution of senescence. Senescence would be the inevitable result of selection for an "'ideal" energy allocation between reproduction and body maintenance.

This is the first theory to propose that the evolution of organisms can optimize the allocation of metabolic resources between the maintenance of the somatic lineage (the individual itself) and the effort of reproduction (investment in next generation). Under it, the physiological mechanisms that postpone senescence consume metabolic resources, which become less available for reproduction, and vice versa. As reproduction of the species by natural selection is prioritized, the body is "disposable" after its reproductive function has been sufficiently fulfilled, and the aging process may appear, without sufficient opposition from natural selection.

There is some experimental support for this theory. When fruit flies are selected for a longer life expectancy, there is decrease in fertility. Conversely, exposure of females to earlier reproduction was correlated with a decline in their lifetimes as compared to virgin females (Sgro & Partridge, 1999).

The disposable soma theory changes the fundamental question about the evolution of senescence: instead of questioning why we senesce, we could wonder why we, humans, live as much as we do (Kirkwood & Rose, 1991).

4. The evolutionary theories of senescence today

4.1 Is there senescence in the wild indeed?

Does anyone die of old age? The existence of senescence in wild populations in their habitats, which, as mentioned, led Medawar and Williams to think of antagonistic pleiotropy, was harshly questioned in the literature by influential researchers like Hayflick and Comfort (Comfort, 1956; Hayflick, 2000).

In a large study, however, Promislow described significant evidence of senescence in 26 species of mammals *in natura* (Promislow, 1991). In fact, in recent years, several studies have demonstrated demographic senescence (Austad, 1993; Bronikowski et al., 2002; Ericsson et al., 2001; Orell & Belda, 2002) and reproductive senescence in mammals and birds in their habitats (Austad, 1993; Broussard et al., 2003; Ericsson et al., 2001; Reid et al., 2003; Saino et al., 2003).

Finally, a strong indication that senescence does exist in wild populations comes from our species: if the data collected by Gompertz and those who followed him can be extrapolated to primitive humans, then our mortality progresses under a Gompertzian regime from around 12 years of age. Senescence starting in such an early age certainly would have impacted on mortality of early human populations (Gompertz, 1825).

Evidence is thus, that death due to senescence is actually happening in the wild. We must change the question from someone dies of old to " someone dies because of senescence '?"And the answer, backed by extensive literature is a resounding yes (Carey & Judge, 2000).

4.2 Findings supporting each evolutionary theory

Evidence for the genetic basis of senescence accumulate in the literature. With respect to the specific theories on the evolution of senescence, experimental evidence supports each of the three theories mentioned above (Hughes & Reynolds, 2005).

In Drosophila, it is possible to obtain two distinct lineages in relation the speed of installation of its senescence by systematically separating over generations, the first (beginning of reproductive life) or the last oviposition (immediately prior to reproductive senescence). The flies of the the second group senesce more slowly and live up to 50% longer than the first group flies (Baret & Lints, 1993; Fukui et al., 1995; Luckinbill & Clare, 1985; Rose & Charlesworth, 1980; 1981).

According to Rose, while the flies in the control group focus their greater efficiency in the early reproductive life, the group submitted to selective pressure for older reproduction requires the of the opposite strategy. In both groups, according to the evolutionary concept of senescence, mutations of late manifestation accumulate and propagate to the new generations. These changes will not affect the flies of the first group, but the second group will largely benefit if such manifestations are delayed. Mutations that make deleterious effects to occur later will improve fitness of individuals in the second group, but not in the first group. This mechanism, over generations, makes the senescent manifestations in the second group to become even later, so that the flies of this group evolve longevity. Interestingly, even with the suspension of the selective pressure, the difference persists, and the strains of flies arising from these experiments remain more long-lived than wild flies (Rose, 1991).

Hughes and others have found evidence in favor of mutation accumulation in the experimental evolution of accelerated senescence (decrease in MRDT) in fruit flies as the predominant phenomenon (Hughes et al., 2002), argument which is sustained by Cortopassi in relation to human senescence (Cortopassi, 2002). Physiological senescence in our species, however, is easily noticeable between the fourth and fifth decades of life. This is not incompatible with Medawar's observation (Medawar, 1952) that the accumulation of mutations explain only senescence in artificially protected populations: modern man is an excellent example of a protected population.

Pleiotropic mechanisms have currently been described. The gene for the juvenile hormone (JH) found in specimens of wild Drosophila is expressed early in its life cycle, and takes to an increase in fertility, early sexual maturation and augmented vitellogenesis. On the other hand, it undermines resistance to stress factors, reduces immunity and the maximum life expectancy (Flatt et al., 2005). In geese, artificial selection for early sexual maturation causes, as adverse effects, a faster reproductive senescence; quantitative analysis revealed a genetic correlation between these two features (Charmantier et al., 2006). Finally, several programmed cell death mechanisms known in mammals also perform "important vital functions such as energy production, metabolism differentiation or the cell cycle" (Ameisen, 2004; 2005). It was recently suggested that Alzheimer's disease, which appears to be specific to humans, could be an example of antagonistic pleiotropy (Bufill & Blesa, 2006).

Holliday argues that the mammals' life cycle strongly illustrates the idea behind the disposable soma theory: there is in mammals an inverse relationship between maximum reproductive potential and maximum longevity; small mammals are very short-lived and fertile, the great mammals are less fertile and very long-lived (Holliday, 1997; 2005). This contrast between longevity and reproduction also appears in a historical cohort analysis of demographic data of the aristocracy of Britain in which with female longevity correlated with a lower number of children (Westendorp & Kirkwood, 1998).

It is noteworthy that the evolutionary theories of senescence (mutation accumulation, antagonistic pleiotropy, and disposable soma) are not mutually exclusive. Although the three currently accepted evolutionary processes for the evolution of senescence can coexist, a current problem of the evolutionary research on senescence is to know how much each of the processes have contributed to the emergence of this phenomenon (Gavrilov & Gavrilova, 2006).

4.3 The evolutionary theories of senescence and the increasing knowledge on evolution

Charlesworth's cumulative effect model (Charlesworth, 2001). The potential effect of genetic drift and natural selection on deleterious and pleiotropic mutations: effective population size on age-structured populations(Charlesworth, 1980; Felsenstein, 1971), infinite sites model of molecular mutation (Kimura & CROW, 1964), infinite alleles model of polymorphism and the neutral theory of evolution (Kimura and Ohta).

4.3.1 Randon genetic drift

A greater effect of random genetic drift is expected in populations with age structure (where the effective population size, N_e is smaller than the real population size, N), than in populations without age structure (and where $N_e \approx N$). Suppose that a genetic effect in a population is expressed at an advanced age (arbitrarily defined as significantly higher than the age of reproductive maturation of a species). We can use this to divide this population age into two subsets: that of individuals who have not expressed the genetic trait and those who have already expressed.

Let us consider what happens with the genetic trait in question under natural selection on these two subpopulations. Obviously, on the first subpopulation, the gene with the deleterious effect, not having expressed itself, is effectively neutral and therefore can evolve only by drift. In the second subpopulation, there is evolution by selection. Clearly, the effect of selection on the population as a whole will be less than what it would be if the mentioned gene was expressed at younger ages. This is just another way of saying that the force of selection falls with age.

Now let us consider the effect of genetic drift on the second subpopulation. Being it a fraction of the total population, its N_e will be considerably smaller than the the initial population's N_e. Thus, besides being subject to progressively smaller selection forces as a function of the age of onset, late onset of deleterious genes should be subject to progressively more intense phenomena of genetic drift. This point, not addressed in the current theories about the evolution senescence, might prove to be crucial.

This last aspect makes it fundamental to understand the roles of mutation, selection and drift as a whole in the evolution of senescence, since, at least in part, the force of selection declines with advancing ages precisely due to the decrease on the effective sizes of the subpopulations.

5. Conclusion

For decades, researchers in the field of senescence were divided between the proponents of proximal or mechanistic theories and the proponents of the distal or evolutionary theories of senescence (Masoro & Austad, 2006). Fortunately, recent decades have seen an excellent understanding of the importance of a joint reasoning between "mechanistic" and "evolutionary" thoughts: more and more studies focused on the evolution of senescence seek to understand its physiological mechanisms of onset and progression and researchers focusing on the mechanisms of senescence are increasingly seeking to understand the theoretical evolutionary basis of senescence (Masoro & Austad, 2006, Preface).

The evolutionary study of senescence seeks to explain why this phenomenon exists, providing researchers with mechanistic insights into what could be the proximal causes of senescence and how genetics produces the senescent phenotype (Kirkwood & Austad, 2000). By pointing to non-adaptive origins for senescence, the evolutionary theory may drive mechanistic researchers away from adaptive programs such as apoptosis as a plausible basis of senescence. After all, "nothing in biology makes sense except in the light of evolution" (Dobzhansky, 1973).

6. References

Ameisen, J. C. (2004). Looking for death at the core of life in the light of evolution., *Cell Death Differ* 11(1): 4–10.
URL: *http://www.ncbi.nlm.nih.gov/pubmed/14647240*

Ameisen, J.-C. (2005). [selective "death programs" or pleiotropic "life programs"? looking for programmed cell death in the light of evolution], *J Soc Biol* 199(3): 175–89.
URL: *http://www.ncbi.nlm.nih.gov/pubmed/16471257*

Austad, S. N. (1993). Retarded senescence in an insular population of virginia opossums (*didelphis virginiana*), *Journal of Zoology* 229(4): 695–708.

Baret, P. & Lints, F. A. (1993). Selection for increased longevity in *drosophila melanogaster*: a new interpretation., *Gerontology* 39(5): 252–9.
URL: *http://www.ncbi.nlm.nih.gov/pubmed/8314091*

Bronikowski, A. M., Alberts, S. C., Altmann, J., Packer, C., Carey, K. D. & Tatar, M. (2002). The aging baboon: comparative demography in a non-human primate., *Proc Natl Acad Sci U S A* 99(14): 9591–5.
URL: *http://www.ncbi.nlm.nih.gov/pubmed/12082185*

Broussard, D. R., Risch, T. S., Dobson, F. S. & Murie, J. O. (2003). Senescence and age-related reproduction of female columbian ground squirrels, *Journal of Animal Ecology* 72(2): 212–219.

Bufill, E. & Blesa, R. (2006). [Alzheimer's disease and brain evolution: is alzheimer's disease an example of antagonistic pleiotropy?], *Rev Neurol* 42(1): 25–33.
URL: *http://www.ncbi.nlm.nih.gov/pubmed/16402323*

Carey, J. & Judge, D. (eds) (2000). *Longevity records: life spans of mammals, birds, reptiles, amphibians and fish.*, Odense University Press.

Charlesworth, B. (1980). *Evolution in Age Structured Populations*, Cambridge University Press, Cambridge.

Charlesworth, B. (2001). Patterns of age-specific means and genetic variances of mortality rates predicted by the mutation-accumulation theory of ageing., *J Theor Biol* 210(1): 47–65.
URL: *http://www.ncbi.nlm.nih.gov/pubmed/11343430*

Charmantier, A., Perrins, C., McCleery, R. H. & Sheldon, B. C. (2006). Quantitative genetics of age at reproduction in wild swans: support for antagonistic pleiotropy models of senescence., *Proc Natl Acad Sci U S A* 103(17): 6587–92.
URL: *http://www.ncbi.nlm.nih.gov/pubmed/16618935*

Comfort, A. (1956). *The Biology of Senescence*, Rinehart & Company, Inc., New York.

Cortopassi, G. A. (2002). Fixation of deleterious alleles, evolution and human aging., *Mech Ageing Dev* 123(8): 851–5.
URL: *http://www.ncbi.nlm.nih.gov/pubmed/12044933*

Darwin, C. (1872). The origin of species by means of natural selection, or the preservation of favoured races in the struggle for life.
URL: *http://darwin-online.org.uk*

de Magalhães, J. P., Cabral, J. A. S. & Magalhaes, D. (2005). The influence of genes on the aging process of mice: a statistical assessment of the genetics of aging., *Genetics* 169(1): 265–74.
URL: *http://www.ncbi.nlm.nih.gov/pubmed/15466429*

Dobzhansky, T. (1973). Nothing in biology makes sense except in the light of evolution, *American Biology Teacher* 35: 125–129.

Ericsson, G., Wallin, K., Ball, J. P. & Broberg, M. (2001). Age-related reproductive effort and senescence in free-ranging moose, alces alces, *Ecology* (82): 1613–1620.

Felsenstein, J. (1971). Inbreeding and variance effective numbers in populations with overlapping generations., *Genetics* 68(4): 581–97.
URL: *http://www.ncbi.nlm.nih.gov/pubmed/5166069*

Flatt, T., Tu, M.-P. & Tatar, M. (2005). Hormonal pleiotropy and the juvenile hormone regulation of drosophila development and life history., *Bioessays* 27(10): 999–1010. URL: *http://www.ncbi.nlm.nih.gov/pubmed/16163709*

Fukui, H. H., Pletcher, S. D. & Curtsinger, J. W. (1995). Selection for increased longevity in drosophila melanogaster: a response to baret and lints., *Gerontology* 41(2): 65–8. URL: *http://www.ncbi.nlm.nih.gov/pubmed/7744268*

Futuyma, D. (1998). *Evolution*, Sinauer Associates, Sunderland, MA, U.S.A.

Gavrilov, L. A. & Gavrilova, N. S. (2006). Reliability theory of aging and longevity., *in* E. J. Masoro & S. N. Austad (eds), *Handbook of the Biology of Aging.*, 6th edn, Academic Press, San Diego, pp. 3–40.

Gompertz, B. (1825). On the nature of the function expressive of the law of human mortality and on a new mode of determining life contingencies., *Philos Trans Roy Soc London* (115): 513–85.

Haldane, J. B. S. (1941). *New Paths in Genetics*, Allen and Unwin, London.

Hamilton, W. D. (1966). The moulding of senescence by natural selection., *J Theor Biol* 12(1): 12–45.
URL: *http://www.ncbi.nlm.nih.gov/pubmed/6015424*

Hayflick, L. (2000). The future of ageing., *Nature* 408(6809): 267–9.
URL: *http://www.ncbi.nlm.nih.gov/pubmed/11089985*

Holliday, R. (1997). Understanding ageing., *Philos Trans R Soc Lond B Biol Sci* 352(1363): 1793–7.
URL: *http://www.ncbi.nlm.nih.gov/pubmed/9460062*

Holliday, R. (2005). Ageing and the extinction of large animals., *Biogerontology* 6(2): 151–6.
URL: *http://www.ncbi.nlm.nih.gov/pubmed/16034683*

Hughes, K. A., Alipaz, J. A., Drnevich, J. M. & Reynolds, R. M. (2002). A test of evolutionary theories of aging., *Proc Natl Acad Sci U S A* 99(22): 14286–91.
URL: *http://www.ncbi.nlm.nih.gov/pubmed/12386342*

Hughes, K. A. & Reynolds, R. M. (2005). Evolutionary and mechanistic theories of aging., *Annu Rev Entomol* 50: 421–45.
URL: *http://www.ncbi.nlm.nih.gov/pubmed/15355246*

Kimura, M. & CROW, J. F. (1964). The number of alleles that can be maintained in a finite population, *Genetics* 49: 725–38.
URL: *http://www.ncbi.nlm.nih.gov/pubmed/14156929*

Kirkwood, T. B. (1977). Evolution of ageing., *Nature* 270(5635): 301–4.
URL: *http://www.ncbi.nlm.nih.gov/pubmed/593350*

Kirkwood, T. B. & Austad, S. N. (2000). Why do we age?, *Nature* 408(6809): 233–8.
URL: *http://www.ncbi.nlm.nih.gov/pubmed/11089980*

Kirkwood, T. B. & Holliday, R. (1975a). Commitment to senescence: a model for the finite and infinite growth of diploid and transformed human fibroblasts in culture., *J Theor Biol* 53(2): 481–96.
URL: *http://www.ncbi.nlm.nih.gov/pubmed/1195775*

Kirkwood, T. B. & Holliday, R. (1975b). The stability of the translation apparatus., *J Mol Biol* 97(2): 257–65.
URL: *http://www.ncbi.nlm.nih.gov/pubmed/1177323*

Kirkwood, T. B. & Holliday, R. (1979). The evolution of ageing and longevity., *Proc R Soc Lond B Biol Sci* 205(1161): 531–46.
URL: *http://www.ncbi.nlm.nih.gov/pubmed/42059*

Kirkwood, T. B. & Rose, M. R. (1991). Evolution of senescence: late survival sacrificed for reproduction., *Philos Trans R Soc Lond B Biol Sci* 332(1262): 15–24.
URL: *http://www.ncbi.nlm.nih.gov/pubmed/1677205*

Luckinbill, L. S. & Clare, M. J. (1985). Selection for life span in drosophila melanogaster., *Heredity* 55 (Pt 1): 9–18.
URL: *http://www.ncbi.nlm.nih.gov/pubmed/3930429*

Masoro, E. J. (2006). Are age-associated diseases an integral part of aging?, *in* E. J. Masoro & S. N. Austad (eds), *Handbook of the Biology of Aging.*, 6th edn, Academic Press, London, UK, pp. 43–62.

Masoro, E. J. & Austad, S. N. (2006). *Handbook of the Biology of Aging*, sixth edition edn, Oxford Academic Press, London, UK.

Medawar, P. B. (1946). Old age and natural death, *Modern Quarterly* 1: 30–56.

Medawar, P. B. (1952). *An unsolved problem of biology*, H.K. Lewis and Co., Oxford, UK.

Orell, M. & Belda, E. J. (2002). Delayed cost of reproduction and senescence in the willow tit parus montanus, *Journal of Animal Ecology* 71(1): 55–64.

Orgel, L. E. (1963). The maintenance of the accuracy of protein synthesis and its relevance to ageing., *Proc Natl Acad Sci U S A* 49: 517–21.
URL: *http://www.ncbi.nlm.nih.gov/pubmed/13940312*

Promislow, D. E. L. (1991). Senescence in natural populations of mammals: A comparative study, *Evolution* 45(8): 1869–1887.

Promislow, D. E. L., Fedorka, K. M. & Burger, J. M. S. (2006). Evolutionary biology of aging: Future directions., *in* E. J. Masoro & S. N. Austad (eds), *Handbook of the Biology of Aging.*, 6th edn, Academic Press, London, UK, pp. 217–242.

Reid, J. M., Bignal, E. M., Bignal, S., McCracken, D. I. & Monaghan, P. (2003). Age-specific reproductive performance in red-billed choughs pyrrhocorax pyrrhocorax: patterns and processes in a natural population, *Journal of Animal Ecology* 72(5): 765–776.

Rose, M. & Charlesworth, B. (1980). A test of evolutionary theories of senescence., *Nature* 287(5778): 141–2.
URL: *http://www.ncbi.nlm.nih.gov/pubmed/6776406*

Rose, M. R. (1991). *Evolutionary biology of aging*, 1 edn, Oxford University Press, Oxford, UK.

Rose, M. R. & Charlesworth, B. (1981). Genetics of life history in drosophila melanogaster. i. sib analysis of adult females., *Genetics* 97(1): 173–86.
URL: *http://www.ncbi.nlm.nih.gov/pubmed/6790340*

Saino, N., Ferrari, R. P., Romano, M., Rubolini, D. & MÃÂ ÿller, A. P. (2003). Humoral immune response in relation to senescence, sex and sexual ornamentation in the barn swallow (hirundo rustica)., *J Evol Biol* 16(6): 1127–34.
URL: *http://www.ncbi.nlm.nih.gov/pubmed/14640404*

Sgro, C. M. & Partridge, L. (1999). A delayed wave of death from reproduction in drosophila., *Science* 286(5449): 2521–4.
URL: *http://www.ncbi.nlm.nih.gov/pubmed/10617470*

Weismann, A. (1889). *Essays upon heredity and kindred biological problems. I*, Vol. 1, 2n ed. edn, Oxford University Press Warehouse, Amen Corner, E. C.

Weismann, A. (1892). *Essays upon heredity and kindred biological problems. II*, Vol. II, 2n ed. edn, Oxford, Clarendon Press, Amen Corner, E. C.

Wessells, R. J., Fitzgerald, E., Cypser, J. R., Tatar, M. & Bodmer, R. (2004). Insulin regulation of heart function in aging fruit flies., *Nat Genet* 36(12): 1275–81.
URL: *http://www.ncbi.nlm.nih.gov/pubmed/15565107*

Westendorp, R. G. & Kirkwood, T. B. (1998). Human longevity at the cost of reproductive success., *Nature* 396(6713): 743–6.
URL: *http://www.ncbi.nlm.nih.gov/pubmed/9874369*

Williams, G. C. (1957). Pleiotropy, natural selection and the evolution of senescence, *Evolution* 11: 398–411.

Wright, S. (1956). Modes of selection, *The American Naturalist* 90(850): 5–24.

11

The Quest for Immortality in Triatomines: A Meta-Analysis of the Senescence Process in Hemimetabolous Hematophagous Insects

Paula Medone[1], Jorge Rabinovich[1], Eliana Nieves[1], Soledad Ceccarelli[1], Delmi Canale[2], Raúl L. Stariolo[2] and Frédéric Menu[3]
[1]Parasitological and Vector Studies Center (CEPAVE), National University of La Plata, La Plata,
[2]Vectors Reference Center, National Coordination of Vectors Control, Direction of Transmitted Vectors Diseases, National Ministry of Health, Córdoba,
[3]Laboratory of Biometry and Biology Evolutionary, CNRS, UMR 5558, Lyon University F-69000 Lyon, Claude Bernard University, Lyon 1 F-69622, Villeurbanne,
[1,2]Argentina
[3]France

1. Introduction

There are different views on senescence as a process. In its most general conception it represents the change in the biology of an organism as it ages. However this process may be viewed either at the physiological or at the demographic level. In the former sense senescence deals with changes affecting cells and tissues of the organism and their function and its effect on the organism as a whole (somatic senescence). In the demographic sense (actuarial senescence) the emphasis is in the population's survival decrease as a function of age (Promislow 1991, Tatar et al., 1993); this very general definition does not necessary imply somatic senescence (a physiological deterioration) because the organism may suffer an increased age-specific mortality rate because of an increased reproductive effort (Roff, 2002); the decrease in the reproductive performance with age may be termed reproductive senescence. Williams (1957), based on evolutionary arguments, claims that natural selection will frequently maximize vigor in youth at the expense of vigor later on and thereby he identifies senescence as a declination in vigor during adult life, using the term vigor as associated with a reproductive probability distribution. Here we are interested in this second approach to senescence, and we adhere to the definition of Rose (1991, cited in Roff 2002): "a persistent decline in the age-specific fitness components of an organism due to internal physiological deterioration".

According to Charlesworth & Partridge (1997) there are two main theories trying to explain the senescence process: (1) natural selection is less effective at reducing the frequency of later-acting mutations in populations, and so ageing is expected to evolve, and this is known as the "mutation accumulation" theory of ageing; (2) mutations that increase fitness at younger ages (perhaps because they increase fertility) but at the expense of decreasing fitness at later ages (perhaps because they increase the death rate) can be incorporated into a population because natural selection will act more strongly on the earlier, beneficial effect. This is the reasoning behind the "antagonistic pleiotropy" or "trade-off" theory of ageing (Williams, 1957).

Abrams & Ludwig (1995), based on an extension of the "disposable soma" model (Kirkwood & Holliday, 1979), provide an explicit realization of the trade-off idea which postulates a conflict between the allocation of resources to reproduction and to the repair of somatic damage. A reduction in damage repair at a given age is assumed to cause an elevated death rate at all subsequent ages. Given a functional relationship between repair allocation and reproductive rate at a given age, the age-specific pattern of allocation to repair versus reproduction that maximizes life-time reproductive success can be determined, yielding a prediction of the age-specific pattern of mortality for the optimal life history (Charlesworth & Partridge, 1997).

Longevity and senescence patterns in mammals and birds are very variable according to the life-history of these organisms (Gaillard et al., 2004), and variation within and between phyla can be expected. Despite phylogenetic similarity is reciprocal to taxonomic level of relatedness (Cheverud et al., 1985) it is also possible that species phylogenetically related show different senescence and/or longevity patterns. So a comparative approach focused on the frequency of senescence in closely related species may contribute to our knowledge of the senescence process. Comparative studies in insects are scarce as compared to mammals and birds; within the insects, demographic analyses of senescence have been carried out mainly for the Diptera (Styer et al., 2007; Curtsinger et al., 1992; Carey et al., 1992, 2005; Fukui et al., 1993), and the Coleoptera (Tatar et al., 1993), and very few studies have considered hemimetabolous species (Dingle, 1966, Chaves et al., 2004a,b, Rabinovich et al., 2010).

In this chapter we investigate the frequency of senescence in a closely related species group of insects: the Triatominae (Hemiptera: Reduviidae). We compiled from the bibliography and resorted to personal data to have phylogeny and life history traits of 27 species reared under laboratory controlled and comparable conditions, and analyzed mortality and fecundity through several death and reproductive parameters. In particular we investigated: (a) species patterns of mortality with respect to age (from cohort studies that followed all individuals from the egg stage until the death of the last individual), (b) the relationship between mortality and different life-history traits (size, reproductive allocation), and (c) the relationship between mortality and environmental factors. Being the 27 selected triatomine species close relatives (they belonged to only five different genera), for our comparative study we included in the analysis a correction for the possible effect of the degree of phylogenetic relatedness.

The advantage of working on laboratory data is that we can estimate intrinsic mortality and fecundity rates without confounding effects resulting from extrinsic factors acting on mortality and fecundity (predation, accidental deaths, starvation, etc.). Even if work with triatomines has the advantage that under natural conditions all life stages occur in a single type of environment and have similar biological requirements, there is always the disadvantage that laboratory data does not reflect natural condition: insects are fed *ad libitum*, and predators, parasites and pathogens are kept out, so that it does not constitute the best of conditions to detect trade-offs between reproductive effort and mortality. However, we think (in agreement with Mueller et al., 2005) that the identification of which aspects of the environment matter in the evolution of trade-offs can only be obtained by performing experiments in which these environmental variables are carefully manipulated; additionally, if even under such stable and near optimal conditions we are able to detect trade-offs, then our conclusions become much more robust.

Although life history traits such as fecundity, juvenile and adult survival, fasting capacity, developmental time, mortality patterns, and life span have been estimated under controlled conditions in the laboratory for a variety of triatomine species (about 500 scientific articles have been written on these aspects since 1910), very few studies have considered recent evolutionary ecology concepts (although see Menu et al., 2010) to shed some light on the trade-off aspects of life history traits. Understanding the mortality pattern in this group of insects is important both for academic and human health reasons. In the former sense we will provide elements to contribute to the theory of senescence and we discuss our results within of this theoretical background; in particular we will analyze the senescence pattern looking into the relationship between reproductive effort and mortality. In the latter sense, our analyses will provide information about a group of insects that are the vectors of Chagas disease, and represent a health threat estimated in 28 million people, living mostly in Latin America (see WHO, 2007).

2. Materials and methods

2.1 Demographic parameters

The basic information for the demographic parameters was obtained from a database compiled by one of us (JER). The original dataset comprised information on 534 case studies of triatomines representing 71 species; however, many of those cases had only partial information on demographic parameters and were not adequate for the present study. From the ones with complete information (55 cases) we selected 29 species that had relatively homogenous rearing conditions in the laboratory, to render them adequate for meta-analysis. The 29 species were later reduced to 27 species because two of them were not in the phylogenetic tree used for the application of the Phylogenetic Independent Contrast method (see section 2.4). The final list of species is shown in Table 1.

For each species we calculated basic life table parameters following Carey (2001): (i) age-specific survival or fraction alive at age x ($l_x = N_x / N_0$) (where N_x= number of individuals alive at age x), (ii) age-specific period survival or fraction alive at age x surviving to $x + 1$ ($p_x = l_{x+1} / l_x$), (iii) age-specific period mortality (probability of dying over the one-week interval used ($q_x = 1 - p_x$), and (iv) the force of mortality or instantaneous mortality rate ($\mu_x = -\ln(p_x)$). For more details on the definitions and formulae of the life table parameters see Rabinovich & Nieves (2011). The original values obtained from the laboratory (N_x, or number of individuals alive at age x, and M_x or total number of eggs laid by all females of the cohort aged x) were processed with a special program (called TriTV) developed by one of us (JER) that calculates the life table statistics and population growth rate parameters. As it is usual with laboratory cohorts, data of the last time-units of the cohorts are based on a very small number of individuals; thus the mortality rate estimated over the last living individual were excluded from the analysis, due to the unreliability of the mortality rate estimates (Carey et al., 1992). The TriTV software was programmed in Delphi language, and is available under request to the second author (the interested user should have an adequate command of the Spanish language).

We considered of interest the division of the female's adult life in two, three or four periods of equal length, to analyze possible lag effects between reproductive effort and mortality. For that purpose, the reproductive effort (m_x= number of female eggs per female per unit time) and the instantaneous mortality rates (μ_x) were averaged for each of the periods in which the female's adult life was divided. We also accumulated mortality from the egg to the last adult female ($\sum\mu_x$) and the female's *per capita* fecundity ($\sum m_x$) to look for a relationship of one with respect to the other along the female´s adult life (after scaling both between 0 and 1).

2.2 Mortality pattern models

For several reasons (see Rabinovich et al., 2010) we preferred the use of mortality analysis over survival analysis; in particular because we agree with Carey (2001) in that, despite mortality and survival are intimately related, death can be considered as an event whereas survival is a "non-event", that is, the absence of the mortality event. For the analysis of the age-specific mortality pattern of the 27 triatomine species selected for this study the following two mortality models were used with the formulation proposed by Carey (2001): the Gompertz model

$$\mu_x = a\, e^{bx}$$

and the Logistic model

$$\mu_x = (n\, x^{n-1})/(g^n + x^n)$$

We also used a third model based on reliability theory as proposed by Gavrilov & Gavrilova (2001), but simplified to two parameters, and which, for simplicity, will be called hereafter "Gavrilovs". Its formulation is given as:

$$\mu_x = n\, k^n\, x^{n-1}$$

In all models x is the age (in our case in weekly time-units), and for the interpretation of the model's parameters, one of them usually represents the "base" mortality rate, and the other the shape of the function (more directly related to the rate of increase of mortality with age, also called the ageing parameter in the case of the Gompertz model). The reason we selected these three models among about a dozen available models for the analysis of mortality patterns, is that Rabinovich et al. (2010), fitting seven models to the instantaneous mortality rate to another triatomine species (*R. neglectus*), found that these three models offered the best fit to the data.

2.3 Model fitting to the data

We used several tools and procedures to fit the three models to the age-specific instantaneous mortality data (μ_x): (i) the R language (R Development Core Team, 2007), (ii) the Kolmogorov-Zurbenko Adaptive smoothing package (kza) in R language (used with parameter q= 2) (Zurbenko et al., 1996), (iii) the Statistica software (StatSoft, 2009),

(iv) the "Online Curve Fitting and Surface Fitting Web Site" (accessible at http://ZunZun.com/) (Christopoulos & Lew, 2000), and (v) the Solver utility of the Excel 2007 program. The reason for the variety of procedures resorted to for fitting the data, is that -even after smoothing- the age-specific instantaneous mortality data was quite irregular, and frequently a given software was not able to succeed in fitting the data to the models while another did. This would happen even if the parameter starting values for fitting the data would have been successfully estimated with the Solver utility of the Excel 2007 program. All software products used, if successful in fitting the data, provided the standard deviation of each parameter and the probability for deciding on the significance of the parameters' estimates. When more than one model fitted the data of the same species, the sum of squares ($SSQ = \Sigma(\mu_{obs} - \mu_{mod})^2$) was calculated and the model with the smallest SSQ was selected. We did not use the Akaike model selection criterion (Akaike, 1974) because the three models tested had the same number of parameters, so the SSQ goodness of fit values would not be affected by any penalty due to the number of degrees of freedom of each model.

2.4 Phylogenetic Independent Contrasts

Comparative studies, either among life-history traits or between those traits and environmental variables, frequently imply resorting to statistical methods such as regressions, correlations and contingency tables, which assume that the data is drawn from a common and independent distribution. However, the comparison among species that are related among each other with different degrees of phylogenetic relatedness does not necessary comply with this assumption. Methods are available to correct for this violation of the assumption of independence. For such purpose we used the Phylogenetic Independent Contrast method (Paradis, 2006) that corrects this violation when derived from phylogeny. The application of this method requires the topology of the phylogenetic tree, and an estimate of the degree of relatedness, generally expressed by the length of the branches of the phylogenetic tree. Calculations were carried out in language R using package "ape".

The phylogenetic tree used for this purpose was the one provided by Silva de Paula et al. (2005), who analyzed the Reduviidae phylogeny by aligning groups of sequences using Clustal-X under gap opening/gap extension penalties, and treating the gaps as missing. For Cladistic analysis Silva de Paula et al. (2005) used the programs PAUP and MacClade to derive trees based both on maximum parsimony (MP) and on maximum likelihood (ML); parsimony bootstrap values were conducted with PAUP employing heuristic search with 100 bootstrap replicates. Decay index for the strict consensus trees (Bremer support) were retained using the decay commands performed by the MacClade software with the heuristic search command activated, and executed with PAUP. This phylogenetic tree covered 57 species of Triatominae, and included 27 species of the 29 species we had selected from the demographic dataset (see section 2.1); thus *Triatoma breyeri* and *Panstrongylus lignarius* were deleted from the analysis, which remained composed by 27 species (Table 1).

3. Results

The following are the main results obtained from our analyses.

3.1 Demographic parameters

Table 1, provides a list of the species analyzed and some of their main environmental information (average annual temperature and precipitation) and provides information about rearing conditions of each species analyzed. In the last column the initial number of eggs (both sexes) with which each cohort was initiated is given; as the sex ratio at the egg stage cannot be established, it was assumed to be 50% for each sex (see Rabinovich et al., 2010 for a justification of this procedure). Initial cohort size was between 35 and 500 eggs (mean: 167 eggs/cohort). Because the senescence analysis was based on female mortality, the initial number for each species was assumed to be one half of original total number of eggs. Feeding frequency of all cohorts was once a week.

Species	Country of origin	Area of distribution (km²)	Average annual temp. (°C)	Average precipitation (mm/year)	Laboratory rearing conditions			
					Temp. (°C)	R.H (%)	Feeding source	Initial Number of eggs
Dipetalogaster maximus	Mexico	36,074	22.2	198.42	28	70	pigeon	35
Eratyrus mucronatus	Venezuela	6,257,724	25.69	2340.64	26	60	chicken	200*
Panstrongylus geniculatus	Venezuela	12,040,606	24.45	1843.01	26	60	chicken	100
Panstrongylus herreri	Peru	354,387	21.46	1764.42	28	70	pigeon	105
Panstrongylus megistus	Brazil	3,739,358	22.55	1281.21	28	70	pigeon	96*
Rhodnius nasutus	Brazil	403,797	25.49	989.55	26	60	chicken	500*
Rhodnius neglectus [a]	Brazil	2,381,373	23.3	1318.39	26	60	chicken	500*
Rhodnius neivai	Venezuela	155,568	24.73	1347.3	26	60	chicken	100
Rhodnius prolixus	Colombia	5,281,236	25.46	2286.3	28	70	pigeon	102
Rhodnius robustus	Venezuela	3,133,393	25.68	2132.36	26	60	chicken	500*
Triatoma delpontei	Argentina	705,366	20.58	733.59	28	70	pigeon	108*
Triatoma dimidiata	Ecuador	2,176,134	24.26	1807.86	28	70	pigeon	45
Triatoma eratyrusiformis	Argentina	540,347	16.72	407.53	28	70	pigeon	112*
Triatoma garciabesi	Argentina	930,966	19.11	668.67	28	70	pigeon	132*
Triatoma guasayana	Argentina	1,412,079	19.38	747.88	28	70	pigeon	108*
Triatoma infestans [b]	Chile	5,198,083	19.26	957.3	26	60	chicken	500*
Triatoma maculata [c]	Venezuela	152,506	24.26	1421.51	26	60	chicken	50*
Triatoma matogrossensis	Argentina	205,258	22.3	815.29	28	70	pigeon	108
Triatoma mazzotti	Mexico	267,872	20.82	876.65	28	70	pigeon	56
Triatoma pallidipennis	Mexico	1,631,377	16.29	621.44	28	70	pigeon	138*
Triatoma patagonica	Argentina	53,047	20.5	915.06	28	65	pigeon	90
Triatoma platensis	Argentina	1,653,623	18.22	734	28	70	pigeon	126*
Triatoma protracta	USA	2,082,288	16.27	404.55	28	70	pigeon	68*
Triatoma pseudomaculata	Brazil	2,650,721	23.7	1198.89	28	70	pigeon	225*
Triatoma rubrovaria	Argentina	470,659	18.57	1472.36	28	70	pigeon	201*
Triatoma sordida	Brazil	4,408,479	22.25	1170.12	28	70	pigeon	120*
Triatoma vitticeps	Brazil	524,660	21.06	1352.76	28	70	pigeon	135*

Table 1. Natural environmental and laboratory rearing conditions of triatomine species selected for the analysis. R. H.=relative humidity. * Pool of several cohorts. Published sources: [a] Rabinovich & Nieves (2010), [b] Rabinovich (1972), [c] Feliciangeli & Rabinovich (1985); for *T. patagonica* original data from Dr. Elena Visciarelli; the rest of species: original data from this study.

Fig. 1 shows the instantaneous mortality and the fecundity rates of the 27 triatomine species analyzed. The senescence pattern is clear: instantaneous mortality rates stay at extremely low levels during most of the juvenile stages (except in the egg stage for some species) and during the first part of the adult stage, increasing greatly in the old ages (i.e., for old females). Most triatomine species seem to invest more in reproduction during the earlier and intermediate periods (but in general with lower effort) of the female's life. Only three species (*R. nasutus, R. neivai* and *D. maximus*) seem to invest more in the intermediate ages. However, six species (*T. eratyrusiformis, T. mazzotti, T. platensis, T. sordida, E. mucronatus,* and *P. geniculatus*) invest in reproduction during all periods of the reproductive life of the female. The difference in the reproductive effort pattern seem to be related to particular genera.

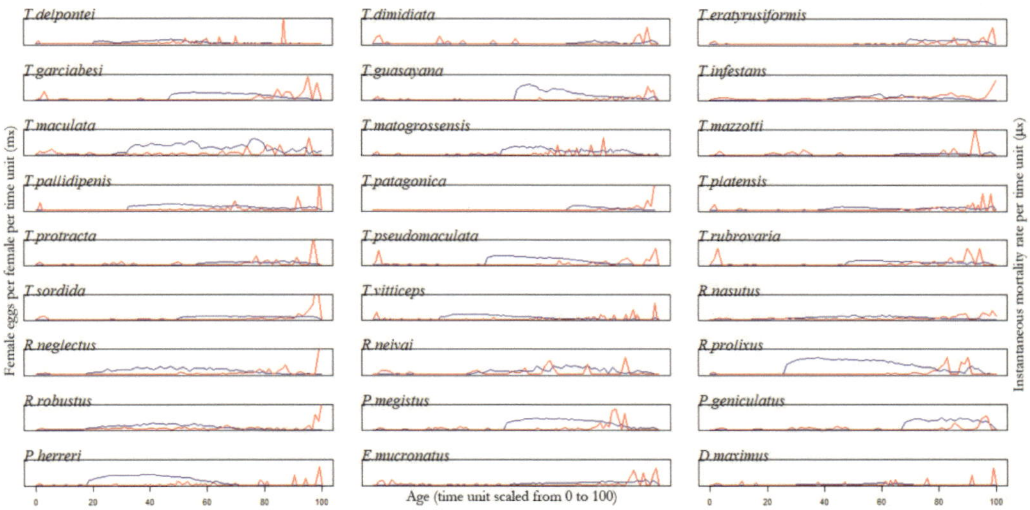

Fig. 1. Age-specific fecundity and instantaneous mortality rates for 27 triatomine species.

Age-specific fecundity (blue lines) and instantaneous mortality rates (red lines) for the 27 species analyzed. All species have a common scale for fecundity and mortality. Fecundity is represented in a scale from 0 to 25 ♀ eggs/♀/unit-time (not shown for better clarity); mortality is represented in a scale from 0 to 1 per unit-time; the x-axis is the age, originally in weeks, but scaled from 0 to 100 to have a common scale for all species.

3.2 Reproductive effort and mortality relationship

Fig. 2 shows the female adult accumulated mortality ($\sum\mu_x$) with respect the female adult accumulated fecundity ($\sum m_x$), both scaled from 0 to 1, in the form of a scatterplot ($\sum\mu_x$ vs $\sum m_x$); to facilitate interpretation of the different patterns, the scatterplots for all species were drawn in the same scale and with a 45° line to be used as a frame of reference. From those graphs we defined six groups with respect of the $\sum\mu_x$ vs $\sum m_x$ observed patterns. Despite the relationships differ among the species of the six groups, the species classed in the first five groups invest strongly in reproduction before a high mortality has been accumulated to a high degree (most of the curves stay below the 45° line) although with increased initial female adult mortality from Group 1 to Group 5; while Group 6 (R. neivai) has a different pattern with a curve that stays above this line during a long period, indicating no significant reproductive accumulation effort in relation to the accumulated mortality rate

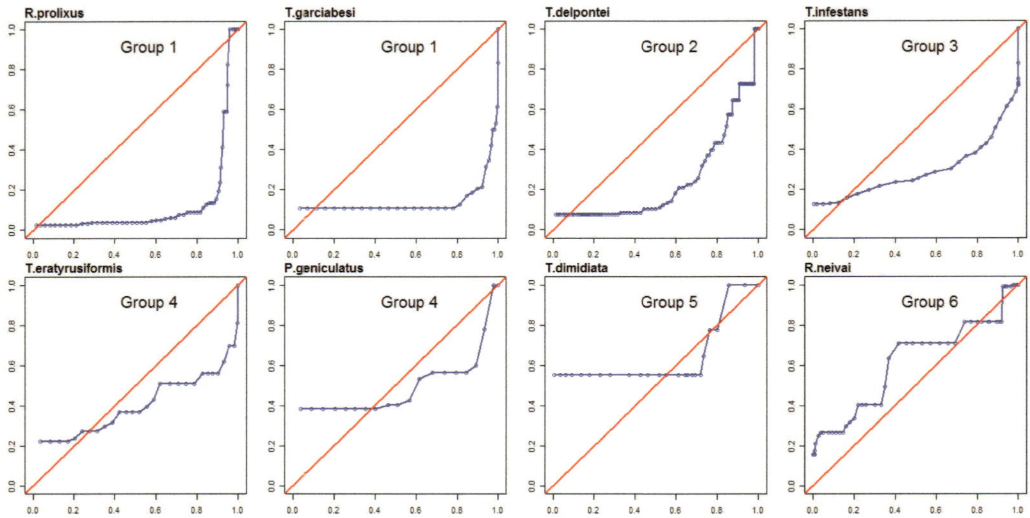

Fig. 2. Grouping of the accumulated mortality and accumulated fecundity relationship

Female adult accumulated instantaneous mortality rate ($\sum\mu_x$) (y- axis) with respect to the female adult accumulated fecundity ($\sum m_x$) (x- axis) (blue line), both scaled from 0 to 1. The 45° line was drawn as a reference (red line). Only selected species representative of each group are shown. For the criteria for grouping and description of the groups see text.

The species classed in first group (n=11) are: *T. garciabesi, T. guasayana, T. pallidipennis, T. vitticep, T. pseudomaculata, T. sordida, R. neglectus, R. prolixus, E. mucronatus, D. maximus* and *P. herreri;* in the second group (n=8): *T. delpontei, T. platensis, T. rubrovaria, T. pallidipennis, T. protracta, T. matogrossensis, T. mazzotti* and *P. megistus;* in the third group (n=4): *T. infestans, T. maculata, R. nasutus* and *R. robustus;* in fourth group (n=2): *T. eratyrusiformis* and *P. geniculatus;* in fifth group (n=1): *T. dimidiata,* and in last group (n=1): *R. neivai.*

3.3 Mortality pattern models

Table 2 shows the coefficients of the fit of the kza- smoothed instantaneous mortality rate (μ_x) to the three mortality models tested (Gavrilovs, Gompertz, and Logistic). Asterisks indicate a statistically significant coefficient with $p< 0.05$. The squared residuals (SSQ) are also shown. Certain mortality models could not be fitted to the instantaneous mortality rate data of some species; additionally, no single model fitted the mortality pattern of all species (Fig. 3, Table 2).

The fit is statistically significant for 14 out of 15 successful fits, for 10 out of 18 successful fits, and for 20 out of 21 successful fits, for the Gavrilovs, Gompertz, and Logistic models, respectively. From the results of the model fitting, Fig. 3 shows three main types of mortality patterns. A first group (Group I) shows a mortality pattern that we called "Late-spiky senescence" and is defined by a very long period in which the mortality rates are low and stable, with a high increase in the mortality rate at the end of the adult female life. In a second group, called "Gradual-medium senescence" (Group II), the increase in the mortality rate with age is more progressive than in the Group I and the mortality rate values stay at an intermediate level. In these two groups, no stabilization of mortality rate occurs at old age.

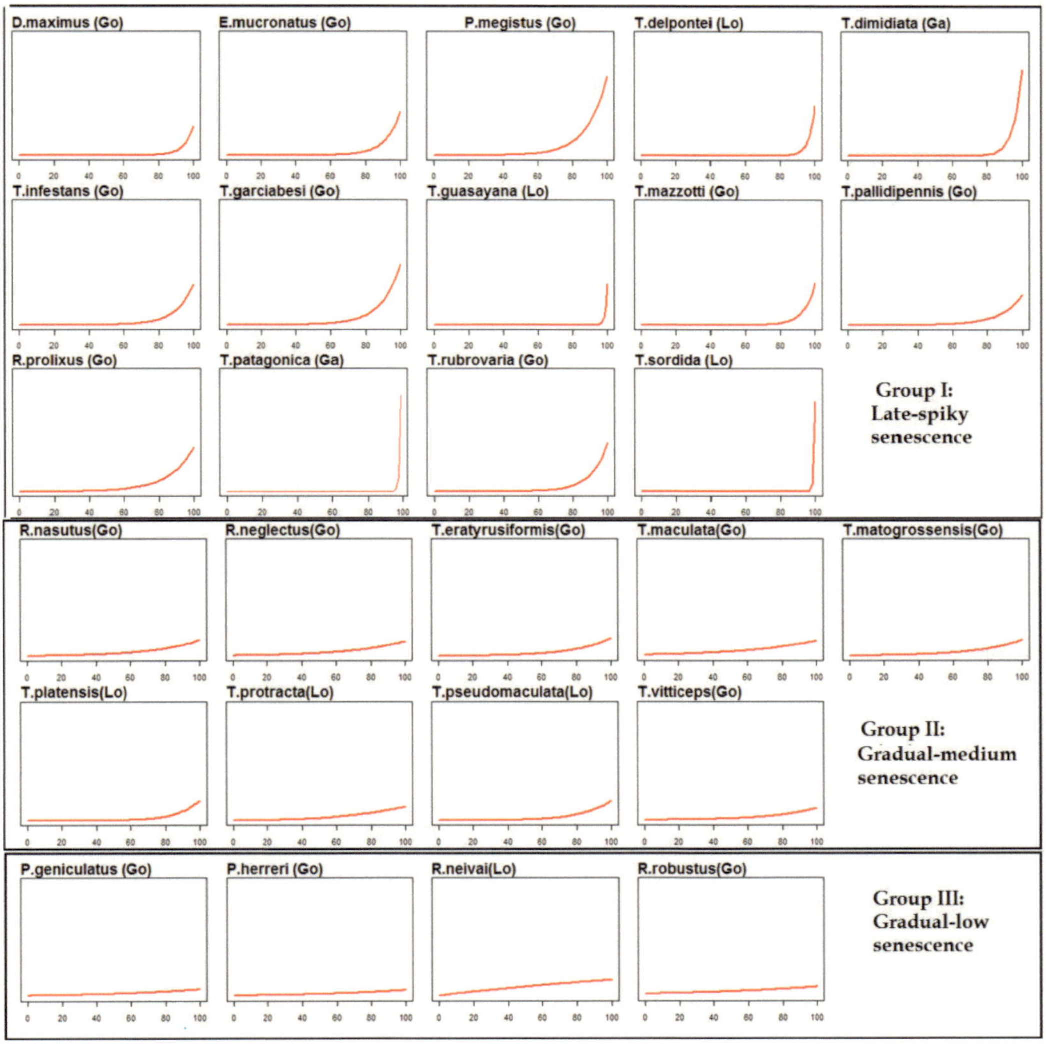

Fig. 3. Age specific mortality patterns of 27 species of triatomines.

The abbreviations in parenthesis indicate the best model that fitted the age-specific instantaneous mortality rate (Go= Gompertz, Lo= Logistic, and Ga= Gavrilovs). Axes have a common scale: from 0 to 1 in the ordinates (not shown) and from 0 to 100 in the abscissa; the latter covers from the egg stage to the last female adult alive.

	Gavrilovs model			Gompertz model			Logistic model		
Species	K	n	SSQ	a	b	SSQ	n	g	SSQ
D. maximus	6.7E-03*	18.78*	1.7E-01	1.5E-09*	1.6E-01*	1.7E-01	18.94*	149.8*	1.7E-01
E. mucronatus	-	-	-	1.6E-06*	1.4E-01*	1.8E-01	11.76*	115.3*	1.7E-01
P. geniculatus	6.7E-03*	18.78*	5.1E-02	1.1E-02*	9.3E+00*	4.8E-02	0.57	3310.3	5.0E-02
P. herreri	-	-	-	7.4E-03*	1.6E-02*	7.2E-02	-	-	-
P. megistus	1.1E-02*	8.18*	3.1E-01	7.9E-05*	1.4E-01*	3.3E-01	8.52*	85.7*	3.0E-01
R. nasutus	4.9E-03*	3.46*	9.4E-02	3.6E-03*	4.5E-02*	8.7E-02	3.56*	200.1*	9.4E-02
R. neglectus	-	-	-	5.0E-03*	3.9E-02*	7.6E-02	2.64*	260.3*	7.1E-02
R. neivai	2.0E-03	0.82	4.6E-01	-	-	-	0.93*	374.1*	4.6E-01
R. prolixus	8.5E-03*	6.32*	7.2E-02	2.6E-04	9.7E-02*	1.7E-01	6.49*	115.8*	1.6E-01
R. robustus	-	-	-	2.1E-02*	1.6E-02*	3.2E-01	-	-	-
T. delpontei	6.1E-03*	29.39*	3.2E-01	-	-	-	29.59*	162.7*	3.2E-01
T. dimidiata	1.2E-02*	28.09*	6.1E-01	-	-	-	-	-	-
T. eratyrusiformis	-	-	-	1.3E-03	5.1E-02*	1.3E-01	3.65*	225.2*	1.4E-01
T. garciabesi	1.2E-02*	8.49*	7.8E-02	4.1E-05	1.5E-01*	8.7E-02	8.72*	85.6*	7.6E-02
T. guasayana	8.9E-03*	88.89*	7.4E-02	-	-	-	89.28*	111.7*	7.4E-02
T. infestans	2.3E-02*	11.85*	5.8E-02	6.0E-06	3.3E-01*	5.4E-02	-	-	-
T. maculata	4.2E-03*	2.10*	1.3E-01	1.0E-02*	4.0E-02*	1.3E-01	2.18*	222.8*	1.3E-01
T. matogrossensis	-	-	-	2.6E-03*	4.1E-02*	7.7E-02	3.07*	270.4*	7.9E-02
T. mazzotti	-	-	-	2.8E-08	3.3E-01*	7.9E-02	15.69*	63.6*	7.7E-02
T. pallidipennis	-	-	-	5.8E-05	7.0E-02*	4.3E-01	-	-	-
T. patagonica	1.3E-02*	137.98*	2.0E-02	-	-	-	-	-	-
T. platensis	5.8E-03*	7.71*	7.9E-02	-	-	-	7.78*	172.5*	7.9E-02
T. protracta	-	-	-	-	-	-	2.96*	192.7*	1.5E-01
T. pseudomaculata	-	-	-	-	-	-	5.64*	163.4*	1.2E-01
T. rubrovaria	1.1E-02*	10.33*	1.8E-01	8.2E-06	1.7E-01*	1.8E-01	10.59*	86.6*	1.8E-01
T. sordida	-	-	-	-	-	-	146.65*	60.1*	4.3E-02
T. vitticeps	-	-	-	1.9E-03	2.8E-02*	2.0E-01	3.29*	406.0*	1.9E-01

Table 2. Fit to the Gavrilovs, Gompertz, and Logistic mortality models.

Parameter values of the mortality models fitted to the laboratory instantaneous mortality rates (μ_x). A "*" indicates a statistically significant coefficient of $p< 0.05$. $SSQ= \Sigma(\mu_{obs} - \mu_{mod})^2$. A "-" indicates that the model could not be fitted to the data.

The third group (Group III), which we called "Gradual-low senescence", is defined by a low and progressively increasing instantaneous mortality rate with age. In this group, particularly in *R. neivai*, the mortality rate seems to stabilize at old ages. The senescence pattern variation does not seem to be homogeneous for a given genus: all senescence pattern groups seem to occur in all genera, particularly in the dominant ones (*Triatoma, Rhodnius*).

3.4 Phylogenetic Independent Contrasts

The results of a series of phylogenetic independent contrasts among several dependent variables related to mortality and other variables related to the longevity and reproduction of the triatomines are shown in Tables 3-10. For a better illustration about the phylogenetic relationships we present (Fig. 4) the phylogenetic tree provided by Silva de Paula et al. (2005) but restricted to the 27 species used in our analysis. In Fig. 4 numbers close to the bifurcations identify each node of the phylogenetic tree. Numbers above the branches indicate the length of each branch, estimated by a branch length/decay index (Bremer support); it is proportional to the distance to ancestors. To the right of each species there is a label with a roman numeral corresponding to the Group into which each species has been classified as following a certain age-specific mortality pattern (Group I= "Late-spiky senescence"; Group II= "Gradual-medium senescence", and Group III= "Gradual-low senescence"; see Section 3.3 for definition of each group).

No significant relationship exists between the female's post reproductive period (FPRP) and the total length of adults or the age of first reproduction (non scaled, weeks) (Table 3). The relationship is statistically significant and positive between FPRP and the age of first reproduction scaled by total longevity. A statistically significant and negative correlation exists between FPRP and the female's reproductive period (scaled by longevity), the female reproductive life period (weeks, i.e., not scaled), and fecundity (expressed as ♀ eggs/♀/life).

Independent variables	Coefficient	Std Dev	t value	p
Female's reproductive period (longevity scaled)	-0.12288	0.05419	-2.26754	0.03226
Total length of adults (mm)	-0.00362	0.00192	-1.88994	0.07042
Female reproductive life period (weeks)	-0.00113	0.00043	-2.61769	0.01481
Fecundity (♀eggs/♀/life)	-0.00007	0.00002	-2.84123	0.00881
Age of first reproduction (weeks) (α)	0.00068	0.00107	0.64255	0.52636
α scaled by total longevity	0.11125	0.04857	2.29050	0.03070

Table 3. Female's post-reproductive period regressed on several independent variables

Simple lineal regression results, using the Phylogenetic Independent Contrast method, of the effect of several independent variables on the female's post-reproductive period (scaled in terms of lifespan) using 27 species of triatomines.

Therefore, the female's post reproductive period decreases with reproductive effort, which means that females live less after their last reproduction in those triatomine species in which the reproductive effort is high.

We show in Table 4 a statistically significant and negative correlation between the mean instantaneous mortality rate (called hereafter $\overline{\mu}_x$) and the average total female longevity since the egg stage, but no statistically significant relationship with the female's total length.

Independent variable	Coefficient	Std. Error	t value	p
Total average ♀ longevity (from the egg stage)	-0.00070	0.00014	-4.86	5.0E-05
Total length (mm)	-0.00076	0.00105	-0.73	0.4740

Table 4. Mean instantaneous mortality rate ($\overline{\mu}_x$) regressed on longevity and total length
Simple lineal regression results, using the Phylogenetic Independent Contrast method, of the effect of average female longevity and total body length as independent variables on the mean instantaneous mortality rate ($\overline{\mu}_x$).

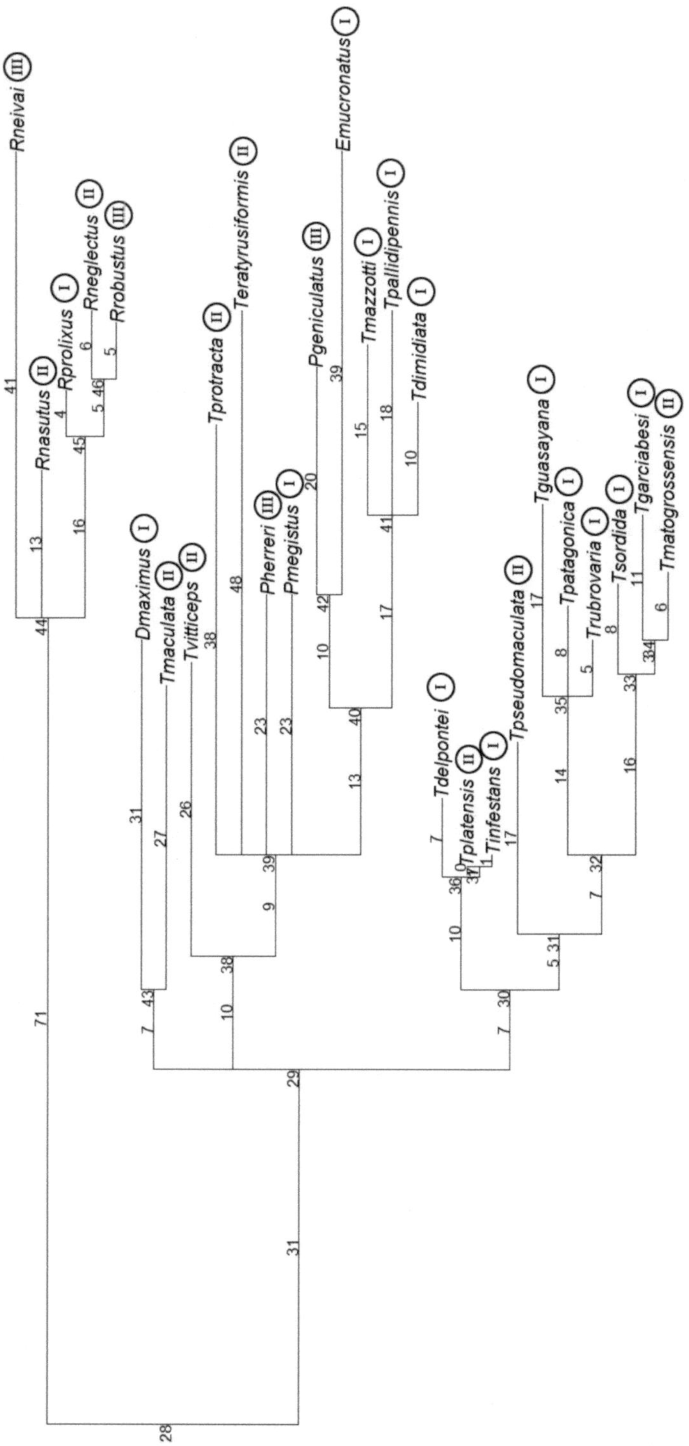

Fig. 4. Phylogenetic tree of the 27 triatomine species analyzed left from the original phylogenetic tree based on 72 species of Reduviidae proposed by Silva de Paula (2005)

Two indicators of mortality, total mean female mortality (1/e0) and the mean female mortality after the first reproduction ($1/e_{\alpha}$), are significantly correlated to two reproductive effort indicators (total eggs per female per life and reproductive weeks of females), decreasing with higher reproductive effort (Table 5). The mortality indicator $1/e_0$ is statistically significant and negatively correlated with both reproductive effort indicators used. Therefore, the total mean female mortality seems to decrease with the reproductive effort.

Dependent variables: total mean ♀ mortality (1/e0)				
Independent variable	**Coeff.**	**Std. Err.**	**T value**	**p**
Total eggs/♀/life	-2.7E-05	2.5E-06	-11.05	4.1E-11
Reproductive weeks of ♀	-0.00092	0.00012	-7.96	2.6E-08
Dependent variable: mean ♀ mortality after first reproduction ($1/e_{\alpha}$)				
Independent variable	**Coeff.**	**Std. Err.**	**T value**	**p**
Total eggs/♀/life	-3.0E-05	4.5E-06	-6.72	4.8E-07
Reproductive weeks of ♀	-0.00127	9.4E-05	-13.54	5.2E-13

Table 5. Two indicators of mortality rate regressed on two reproductive effort variables

Simple lineal regression results, using the Phylogenetic Independent Contrast method, of the effect of reproductive effort indicators as independent variables on two measures of mortality using 27 species of triatomines. The parameter e_0 is the expectation of life at birth (weeks).

Independent variable	**Coefficient**	**Std**	**t value**	**p**
Average ♀eggs/♀/week	-0.01099	0.07154	-0.15368	0.87979
Average ♀eggs/♀/life	0.00076	0.00133	0.56869	0.57746
α scaled by total longevity	-0.67365	0.89178	-0.75539	0.46099
α scaled by lifespan	-0.98590	0.87855	-1.12219	0.27834
Age of first reproduction (weeks) (α)	-0.01470	0.01375	-1.06885	0.30100
Total female longevity (weeks)	0.00478	0.00692	0.69122	0.49933
Total length (mm)	-0.03625	0.02683	-1.35086	0.19554

Table 6. The parameter *b* of the Gompertz model regressed on several independent variables

Simple lineal regression results, using the Phylogenetic Independent Contrast method, of the effect of several independent variables on the parameter *b* of the Gompertz mortality model. The phylogenetic tree used was reduced to the 18 species with $\bar{\mu}_x$ data that could be fitted to the Gompertz model. α represents the female's age (weeks) of first reproduction.

No statistically significant relationship was observed between the parameter *b* of the Gompertz mortality model (which is related to the shape of the mortality pattern) and the life history traits indicated in Table 6. Additionally, no statistically significant correlation was observed between the parameter *b* of the Gompertz mortality model and the geographic and/or climatic variables indicated in the table (Table 7).

Independent variable	Coefficient	Std Dev	t value	p
Surface area	-0.02572	0.02877	-0.89415	0.38449
Average annual precipitation (mm)	0.00027	0.00023	1.19358	0.25004
95% Lower precipitation (mm)	0.00029	0.00043	0.66386	0.51623
95% Upper precipitation (mm)	0.00021	0.00014	1.52282	0.14732
Colwell's precipitation index of predictability	2.40489	2.66950	0.90088	0.38101
Precipitation coefficient of variation (%)	0.03058	0.02010	1.52139	0.14768
NDVI coefficient of variation (%)	-0.11072	0.12554	-0.88195	0.39086
Maximum rain of the rainiest month (mm)	0.00405	0.00520	0.77925	0.44721
Minimum rain of the driest month (mm)	0.00204	0.00170	1.20070	0.24734

Table 7. The *b* Gompertz model parameter regressed on geographic/climatic variables

Simple lineal regression results, using the Phylogenetic Independent Contrast method, of the effect of several climatic variables used as independent variables on the parameter *b* of the Gompertz model. The phylogenetic tree was reduced to the 18 species with $\bar{\mu}_x$ that could be fitted to the Gompertz model. The NDVI is the Normalized Difference Vegetation Index.

Table 8 shows that from several geographic and/or climatic variables analyzed only the surface area and various precipitation indicators are correlated (negatively) with the mean mortality rate (defined here as $1/e_0$), while with the coefficient of variation (in %) of the Normalized Difference Vegetation Index (NDVI, a common indicator of live green vegetation obtained from satellite data) it was found to be positively correlated. In other words, species' geographical range size and some climatic factors, mainly the ones related to precipitation, seem to be related to mean mortality.

However, mortality ($1/e_0$) is probably not a good estimator of mean mortality because in our data the mortality rate varies greatly with age and this violates the hypothesis underlying this parameter as estimator of mean mortality rate. In consequence, we also used a more reliable estimator of the mean mortality rate from our data: the average for different time periods of the female's adult life ($\bar{\mu}_x$) (see Tables 9 and 10).

Independent variables	Coefficient	Std Err	t value	p
Surface area (km^2)	-0.00140	0.00022	-6.43226	9.8E-07
Modal latitude (degrees)	0.00034	0.00022	1.54316	0.13536
Modal longitude (degrees)	0.00025	0.00021	1.20700	0.23900
Average altitude (m)	1.1E-05	1.1E-05	1.05245	0.30266
Average annual temperature (°C)	-0.00060	0.00180	-0.33135	0.74315
Minimum annual temperature (°C)	0.00162	0.00137	1.18693	0.24641
Maximum annual temperature (°C)	0.00225	0.00210	1.07133	0.29425
Average annual precipitation (mm)	-1.5E-05	4.2E-06	-3.56725	0.00149
95% Lower precipitation (mm)	-2.6E-05	7.7E-06	-3.33849	0.00264
95% Upper precipitation (mm)	-9.3E-06	2.7E-06	-3.47074	0.00190
Colwell's rain index of predictability	-0.15913	0.04713	-3.37684	0.00240
Rain coefficient of variation (%)	0.00114	0.00044	2.61404	0.01494
Temperature amplitude (°C)	0.00047	0.00121	0.38703	0.70201
Temperature coefficient of variation (%)	0.00072	0.00055	1.30837	0.20265
Average annual NDVI	-0.05010	0.03350	-1.49561	0.14727
NDVI coefficient of variation (%)	0.00804	0.00263	3.06192	0.00520
Average AET (mm)	-0.00023	0.00015	-1.47877	0.15169
Minim temperature of coldest month (°C)	0.00088	0.00093	0.94976	0.35133
Maximum temperature of the warmest month (°C)	-9.8E-05	0.00272	-0.03617	0.97144
Maximum rain of the rainiest month (mm)	-0.00033	0.00008	-3.99956	0.00050
Minimum rain of the driest month (mm)	-0.00011	3.2E-05	-3.26415	0.00317
Number of dry months/year	0.00197	0.00108	1.83082	0.07907
Number of humid months/year	0.00214	0.00181	1.18209	0.24829
Number of super-humid months/year	-0.00200	0.00089	-2.25957	0.03282

Table 8. Average mortality ($1/e_0$) regressed on various geographic/climatic variables

Simple lineal regression results, using the Phylogenetic Independent Contrast method, of the effect of several climatic variables used as independent variables on the average mortality ($1/e_0$) using 27 species of triatomines.

The results obtained from the regressed of mean instantaneous mortality rate $\bar{\mu}_x$ were statistically non-significant with respect to the mean reproductive effort (first line in Table 9). However, if we divide the individual female adult life in two, three or four periods of equal length, some correlations between $\bar{\mu}_x$ for a given period and the mean reproductive effort for the same period are statistically significant and positive (Table 9 except the first line). Furthermore, we observe several significant positive correlations between $\bar{\mu}_x$ for a given period and the reproductive effort in the previous period(s) (Table 10). For instance, when divided in two periods, the $\bar{\mu}_x$ value in the second period is significantly and positively correlated to the reproductive effort during the first period (first line in Table

10) or during the first and second ones (second line in Table 10). Similarly, when divided in three periods, the $\bar{\mu}_x$ value of the third period is significantly and positively correlated to the reproductive effort during the all three periods (lines 4 and 6 in Table 10). Similarly for four periods.

Independent variable	Dependent variable	Coefficient	Std Err	t value	p
$\bar{m}_x$ 1/1	$\bar{\mu}_x$1/1	0.00021	0.001126	0.187	0.85354
$\bar{m}_x$ 1/2	$\bar{\mu}_x$1/2	-0.00556	0.00047	-11.96	7.7E-12
$\bar{m}_x$ 2/2	$\bar{\mu}_x$2/2	0.01840	0.00501	3.67	0.00115
$\bar{m}_x$ 1/3	$\bar{\mu}_x$1/3	-0.00266	0.00027	-9.75	5.3E-10
$\bar{m}_x$ 2/3	$\bar{\mu}_x$2/3	-0.00696	0.00212	-3.29	0.00300
$\bar{m}_x$ 3/3	$\bar{\mu}_x$3/3	0.02206	0.00813	2.71	0.01190
$\bar{m}_x$ 1/3	$\bar{\mu}_x$2/3	-0.00437	0.00062	-7.00	2.0E-07
$\bar{m}_x$ 2/3	$\bar{\mu}_x$3/3	0.01603	0.00327	4.91	4.7E-05
$\bar{m}_x$ 1/4	$\bar{\mu}_x$1/4	-0.00216	0.00022	-9.60	7.3E-10
$\bar{m}_x$ 2/4	$\bar{\mu}_x$2/4	-0.01076	0.00103	-10.41	1.4E-10
$\bar{m}_x$ 3/4	$\bar{\mu}_x$3/4	0.00910	0.00678	1.34	0.37520
$\bar{m}_x$ 4/4	$\bar{\mu}_x$4/4	0.02308	0.00877	2.63	0.01438
$\bar{m}_x$ 1/4	$\bar{\mu}_x$2/4	-0.00769	0.00066	-11.73	1.2E-11
$\bar{m}_x$ 2/4	$\bar{\mu}_x$3/4	0.01196	0.00148	8.07	2.0E-08
$\bar{m}_x$ 3/4	$\bar{\mu}_x$4/4	0.00822	0.00607	1.35	0.23480

Table 9. Average mortality and fecundity variables lagged by periods

Simple lineal regression results, using the Phylogenetic Independent Contrast method, of the effect of average fecundity ($\bar{m}_x$) on the average instantaneous mortality rates ($\bar{\mu}_x$) by periods of equal length (see text) using 27 species of triatomines.

Independent variable	Dependent variable	Coefficient	Std Err	t value	p
$\bar{m}_x$ 1/2	$\bar{\mu}_x$2/2	0.00528	0.00121	4.38	0.00019
$\bar{m}_x$ 1+2/2	$\bar{\mu}_x$2/2	0.01071	0.00197	5.45	1.2E-05
$\bar{m}_x$ 1+2/3	$\bar{\mu}_x$2/3	-0.00583	0.00102	-5.73	5.7E-06
$\bar{m}_x$ 1+2/3	$\bar{\mu}_x$3/3	0.00960	0.00203	4.73	7.5E-05
$\bar{m}_x$ 2+3/3	$\bar{\mu}_x$3/3	0.02390	0.00489	4.89	4.9E-05
$\bar{m}_x$ 1+2+3/3	$\bar{\mu}_x$3/3	0.01430	0.00276	5.18	2.3E-05
$\bar{m}_x$ 1+2/4	$\bar{\mu}_x$2/4	-0.00903	0.00079	-11.37	2.3E-11
$\bar{m}_x$ 1+2/4	$\bar{\mu}_x$3/4	0.00970	0.00128	7.56	6.5E-08
$\bar{m}_x$ 2+3/4	$\bar{\mu}_x$3/4	0.02099	0.00267	7.85	3.3E-08
$\bar{m}_x$ 2+3/4	$\bar{\mu}_x$4/4	0.00450	0.00436	1.03	0.21760
$\bar{m}_x$ 1+2+3/4	$\bar{\mu}_x$3/4	0.01455	0.00176	8.25	1.3E-08
$\bar{m}_x$ 1+2+3/4	$\bar{\mu}_x$4/4	0.00231	0.00301	0.77	0.47810
$\bar{m}_x$ 1+2+3+4/4	$\bar{\mu}_x$4/4	0.00374	0.00383	0.98	0.31270

Table 10. Accumulated average mortality and fecundity variables lagged by periods

Simple lineal regression results, using the Phylogenetic Independent Contrast method, of the effect of accumulated average fecundity on the accumulated average instantaneous mortality rates by periods of equal length (see text) using 27 species of triatomines.

4. Discussion

The following are our concepts on triatomine senescence in the light of evolutionary ecology.

4.1 Senescense in the triatomines

Since the first attempt to explain evolution of ageing was made by Weismann (1891, cited in Kirkwood & Holliday 1979) senescence has been a major topic of research in evolutionary ecology, both from an experimental and a theoretical approach. Being such a general area of investigation it is not surprising that it has relied strongly on the use of a comparative approach across a wide range of taxa. The phylogenetic variation in rates of senescence has been considered a consequence of a combination of factors that decrease the rate of decline in reproductive probability (and intensifying selection against senescence) and factors that increase this rate (relaxing selection against senescence). We applied a comparative meta-analyses approach within a single subfamily (Triatominae) correcting, for the first time in this group, the regression analyses by the phylogeny.

Williams (1957) has argued that the rate of senescence shown by any species will reflect the balance between a direct adverse selection of senescence as an unfavorable character, and an indirect, favorable selection through the age-related bias in the selection of pleiotropy genes. Thus positive variations in fecundity increase adult mortality rate, and affect other life-history traits (e.g., the shape of the distribution of reproductive effort with age) and thereby influence the evolution of senescence and phylogenetic variation. This theory predicts that (a) rapid morphogenesis should be associated with rapid senescence, (b) that senescence should always be a generalized deterioration of many organs and systems, and (c) that post-reproductive periods should be short and infrequent in any wild population. The latter prediction seems to have been confirmed in the case of triatomines (at least in the laboratory). This is another reason why, despite having selected for our study a relatively low taxonomic level (the species of only five genera, so we can expect a strong degree of phylogenetic relatedness), it is important to have the phylogeny included in these comparisons.

Our study shows that the 27 triatomine species analyzed present a senescence pattern that does not decrease at older ages. Mortality rate stays very low during most of the juvenile stages (except in the egg stage for some species) and during the first part of adult stage, and then increases greatly in the old ages in most species. This senescence pattern observed in triatomine species are in contrast with patterns reported for various Diptera: *Drosophila melanogaster* (Curtsinger et al., 1992; Pletcher & Curtsinger, 1998), *Ceratitis capitata* (Carey et al., 1992, 1998), *Anastrepha ludens* (Carey et al., 2005), and *Aedes aegypti* (Styer et al., 2007).

The mortality pattern of triatomines (Chaves et al., 2004a, Rabinovich et al 2010, and this study) seems to be more similar to that reported in *Oncopeltus fasciatus* (Dingle, 1966), *Dysdercus fasciatus* (Dingle, 1966), and *Callosobruchus maculatus* (Tatar et al., 1993) and is consistent with models of senescence based on the decline in physiological functions with age (known as the "disposable soma" theory for the evolution of senescence; Kirkwood & Holliday, 1979; Kirkwood & Rose, 1991; Kirkwood & Austad, 2000; Kirkwood, 2002), which can be considered a consequence of the equilibrium predictions of the antagonistic-pleiotropy and mutation accumulation hypotheses (Abrams & Ludwig, 1995).

In our comparative analysis we have used several measures of mortality. Although the use of the Gompertz model to describe the acceleration of mortality with age has been a matter of debate (Nusbaum et al., 1996), for a comparative study this model seems more sound than, e.g., maximum lifespan, particularly because of the sensitivity of maximum lifespan to the initial numbers of a cohort. Nusbaum et al. (1996) have analyzed the evolutionary relationships among several measures of mortality (Gompertz parameters, and average and maximum longevity) in 50 related populations of *D. melanogaster*; they included populations that had been selected for postponed aging and in their conclusions they give credit to a redundancy among these measures of aging, and consider that both the maximum lifespan and the Gompertz equation as adequate indices of aging in evolutionary research. This gives support to their use in our study.

4.2 High variation in senescence pattern

Our results show that the mortality pattern with age varies greatly among triatomine species (showing late-spiky, gradual-medium, and gradual-low senescence) despite our study was based on cohorts reared under very homogeneous environmental conditions; the present challenge is to understand which are the ultimate factors underlying such diversity of mortality patterns in triatomines (Fig. 3). These different patterns are observed in all the species we studied, even in the more phylogenetic related species within any given genus (Fig. 4). We do not dismiss the possibility that the small initial number of eggs of some cohorts may have played a role in the estimation of demographic parameters (e.g. threshold mortality) (Carey, 2001), and thus in the high degree of mortality patterns variability; however, we still think that the variability found is genuine and could reflects multiple underlying causes.

Despite most of the studied species show "late-spiky" (n= 14) or "gradual-medium" senescence (n= 9), the species in the “gradual-low" group (n= 4), particularly *R. neivai*, seem to show a weak late-life mortality plateau. Some demographic findings point to the existence of a late-life mortality plateau in a few dipteran insects (Mueller & Rose, 1996), with both antagonistic pleiotropy and mutation accumulation as driving population genetic mechanisms; this late-life attribute is a switch from accelerating mortality to a relatively stable mortality (Rauser et al., 2006); such plateaus seem to depend on the collection of high numbers of late-life data (Carey et al., 1992). One plausible explanation of the "plateau" behavior was introduced by Vaupel et al. (1979) assuming a life-long heterogeneity in the mortality rates: more robust subgroups survive to later ages, slowing the rate of decline in average survival probabilities at late ages among large cohorts. The older remaining individuals from the cohort are expected to be much more robust so that the mortality rate becomes a very shallow function of age, resembling a plateau. However this demographic heterogeneity model does not seem to be a reasonable explanation of demographic patterns and it has only a weak biological basis (Mueller et al., 2003).

With rare exceptions the Triatominae are exclusively hematophagous, and they also show strict hematophagy across all developmental stages. This may be a potential key to the explanation of the observed mortality pattern: hematophagy from vertebrate blood leads to the digestion of vertebrate hemoglobin resulting in the production of large amounts of heme, a potentially cytotoxic molecule that can exert biological damage (Graca-Souza et al., 2006). The evolution of hematophagy has resulted in many adaptations developed by blood-feeding insects and ticks to counteract those deleterious effects. Antioxidant enzymes and urates are known to play a major role in the protection of cells against free radical damage, and massive amounts of urates have been found in the haemolymph of *R. prolixus* (Souza et al., 1997). Given the strict hematophagy of triatomines these mechanisms that reduce the accumulation of oxidative substances associated with aging (Graca-Souzaet al., 2006) may be one of the basic mechanisms that may help explain the senescence patterns observed in the triatomines.

The relationships between average instantaneous mortality rates $\bar{\mu}_x$ and average fecundity by periods show a delay in the effect of the latter on the former, indicating an important reproductive investment before a high accumulated instantaneous mortality rate occurs. The negative relationship between the average instantaneous mortality rate $\bar{\mu}_x$ and average female longevity suggests that species with high longevity can invest in reproduction with a relatively low mean mortality and then a smaller senescence rate than the species with low longevity. This type of relationship between reproductive effort and the effects on age-specific mortality rate is similar to the one found in the beetle *C. maculatus* (Tatar et al., 1993) and confirms the observation of Sulbaran & Chaves (2006) in the kissing bug *R. prolixus*.

Additionally, the female's post reproductive period decreases with reproductive effort indicating that longevity after their last reproduction is shorter in species in which the reproductive effort is high. The above results suggest a trade-off between mortality rate and reproductive effort: a large investment in the reproduction during the first and/or intermediate part of the female adult life that seems to result in an increase in high mortality, and then a high senescence rate at the end of the adult life. Such trade-off could contribute to explain the variation between species in the mean mortality and in the post-reproductive period duration but probably not the difference in the senescence pattern since no significant relationship exists between the parameter *b* of the Gompertz model and other variables used as indicators of reproductive effort.

4.3 Triatominae senescence in the light of evolutionary ecology

The balance between extrinsic and intrinsic mortality rates is an important factor underlying the evolution and the diversity of senescence patterns. Williams (1957) proposed that organisms living in environments with high extrinsic mortality rate may evolve towards high senescence rates. Physiological senescence results from an optimal equilibrium between energy allocation in somatic maintenance and other competitive traits as reproduction (Kirkwood, 2005). In habitats in which life expectancy is short resulting from extrinsic factors (as high predation, starvation, etc.), the maintenance of costly mechanisms to guarantee the reparation of metabolic deterioration is not evolutionary stable.

Conversely, species living in habitats with low extrinsic mortality may increase energy allocation in somatic maintenance until old age and increase longevity by natural selection.

In triatomines no quantitative data exists concerning extrinsic mortality factors in the field. The levels of extrinsic mortality in relation to the habitat (domestic, peri-domestic and sylvatic), is still little known in triatomines. However, our results show a negative relationship between mortality rate and female longevity supporting Williams' (1957) prediction, contrary to other empirical observations that do not support this prediction (Promislow, 1991; Ricklefs, 1998; Reznicket et al., 2004), which has also been criticized on conceptual grounds due to the difficulty in separating extrinsic and intrinsic mortality rates (Williams & Day, 2003).

In a recent comparative analysis of mammal and bird survival senescence Jones et al. (2008) arrived to generalizations such as that mammals senesce faster than similarly sized birds. Furthermore, McCoy & Gillooly (2008) developed a model of natural mortality (relating body size and temperature to biological rate processes) and tested it with extensive field data from plants, invertebrates, fish, birds and mammals; their results indicate that much of the heterogeneity in natural mortality rates can be predicted, explicitly and quantitatively, despite the high diversity of extrinsic sources of mortality in natural systems, something that suggests that mortality rates may be governed by common rules.

We show that the geographical range size of species and some climatic factors, mainly the ones related to precipitation, seem to be related to total mean mortality ($1/e_0$). These results suggest that the influence of geographic and climatic factors on the senescence pattern deserves further investigation. However, can the potential senescence that is observed and measured in the laboratory be expressed in natural habitats where extrinsic mortality occurs? In the field, triatomines could die before intrinsic mortality and decreasing fecundity occurs, due to extrinsic factors such as predation, parasitism, extreme climatic conditions, etc. Recent studies in vertebrates (Adams, 1985; Gaillard et al., 1993; Reznick et al., 2002; Rebke et al., 2010) show that senescence is observed under natural conditions, but that kind of information is lacking for triatomines and needs to be investigated. Williams (1957) claimed that greater rates of extrinsic mortality (age- and condition-independent) favored more rapid senescence, but Abrams (1991) showed that the effects of the "extrinsic" mortality affect differentially the rate of senescence as a function of the degree of density-dependence. Abrams (1991) also showed that mortality patterns, contrary to Williams' (1957) predictions, are possible when density-dependence is present, and acts primarily on the survival or fertility of later ages, or when most of the variation in mortality rates is due to variation in non-extrinsic mortality.

There are few laboratory evaluations of the density-dependent processes in triatomines. Rodríguez & Rabinovich (1980) showed that in *R. prolixus* density had a significant effect on the development rate of second, third, and fourth instars, but not on the survivorship of either the first or fifth instars, or even of the adults, nor on the instantaneous population parameters, or the age-specific parameters. Influence of density-dependence on the senescence pattern in triatomines still needs more research.

How organisms distribute their "investment" in reproduction with respect to age is a major question in the senescence theory. It will be optimal for an organism to "invest" more in its reproduction when it becomes old-aged (Williams, 1966). An extension of William's (1966) theory is that old individuals may increase their reproductive effort during their last reproductive occasion(s) because it is their last chance to reproduce. This extension was called the "hypothesis of terminal investment" (Ricklef, 2000; Coulson & Fairweather, 2001; Ricklefs, 2008). Thus senescent individuals may invest more in reproduction than the non-senescent individuals. Our observations in the triatomines do not support these predictions. Indeed most of the reproductive effort (about 50 to 90%) occurs in the first and intermediate part of the adult life and before the high mortality that takes place at older ages. Furthermore, the duration of the post-reproductive period decreases with reproductive effort suggesting a trade-off between reproduction allocation and future survival. Recently William's (1966) prediction and the concept of terminal investment have been criticized because of scarce empirical support and for resorting to two hypotheses based on quite unrealistic assumptions: (i) organisms must have a fixed longevity, which implies that individual trajectories cannot influence longevity, and (ii) in order to increase their reproductive effort at the end of their life during their last reproductive occasion(s), individuals must be able to anticipate their future, i.e., they have to use cues indicating when their death may occur (Gadgil & Bossert, 1970).

Environmental heterogeneity, and particularly high environmental uncertainty (stochastic effects), affect circumstances that are very important in insects, such as encounter rates associated to suitable oviposition sites, food and refuge availability, physiological state (e.g., reserves for producing oocytes, egg maturation rate, and somatic maintenance costs), and expected reproductive success that can lead to different patterns of behavior and rates of mortality and reproduction (Partridge & Mangel, 1999). Environmental stochasticity and/or density-dependence processes can select bet-hedging dormancy including a development delay in insects (e.g., Menu et al., 2000; Gourbière & Menu, 2009; Rajon et al., 2009). Such a risk spreading strategy has been postulated to exist in triatomines (Menu et al., 2010) and we recommend that this approach be incorporated in future studies for understanding senescence in insects.

Mortality rates of triatomine vectors have epidemiological importance through the demography of its populations (Chaves et al., 2004a). Particularly, it has been shown in these insects that important changes in life-history traits take place when reared under laboratory conditions; for example, in *T. infestans*, *T. pseudomaculata*, *T. brasiliensis*, and *P. megistus* after only four years in the laboratory, the reduction in the number of eggs within the first month of oviposition and the average female life span was in average 37.5 and 45.9%, respectively (Perlowagora-Szumlewicz, 1976). Similar changes, including a reduction in life history traits and population growth parameters, during four successive and separate generations of *T. infestans* of Argentina (reared in the laboratory from a first generation from a sylvatic individual) have also been found (G. Martí, personal communication).

The adaptation to a domestic environment causes similar effects on triatomines as the adaptation to laboratory conditions (Forattini, 1980): indoor conditions of rural houses provide better chances of feeding, and are characterized by smaller predation risks, and smaller fluctuations of temperature and relative humidity that exclude potentially deleterious extreme values. In our study we did not analyze possible adaptations to the laboratory because the precise number of laboratory generations was known for only a few cohorts; however, it is recommended that, when estimating trade-offs, and in particular the senescence pattern, the influence of such changes should be taken into account.

Furthermore, as the data for our comparative analyses did not indicate the mean body length of the individuals used in the experiments we used the estimates provided by Galíndez Girón et al. (1998) based on the types and paratypes of triatomine measurements in museum collections. As the individual's body size distribution can vary with respect to each population, it is recommended that future cohort studies in the laboratory measure the body length of the individuals used. In consequence, we must take with some reservation the lack of a statistically significant correlation between life history traits and total length as obtained in this study and based on 27 triatomine species.

5. Conclusions

Most studies in triatomines have investigated physiology, population genetics, phylogeny (see Gourbière et al., 2011 for a review) and ecology of a given species (e.g., Dumonteil et al., 2002; Gourbière et al., 2008; Barbu et al., 2011) but very few studies have investigated the evolution of life history traits in the light of evolutionary ecology concepts (Menu et al., 2010). Our study is the first comparative analysis to the senescence pattern and its relationship with life history traits in triatomines.

Our results indicate that triatomines show both an actuarial and a reproductive senescence, with a high diversity of mortality patterns, even within a given genus. We believe that the relationship between life history traits, and particularly the trade-off between reproductive effort and future survival, is central to understand this diversity in mortality patterns. In order to identify ultimate and proximate factors underlying this diversity, we need longitudinal studies conducted in the field in order to estimate if the potential senescence observed in the laboratory can be expressed under natural (sylvatic and domestic) conditions. The analysis of senescence in relation to other life history traits in triatomines has not only academic value but also impinges in the areas of vector population management and epidemiology.

6. Acknowledgments

We are extremely grateful to the Vectors Reference Center of the National Ministry of Health, Córdoba, Argentina and to Dr. Elena Visciarelli for allowing the use of original data from 21 species of triatomines and from *T. patagonica,* respectively. We thank to Mr. Waldo Hasperué for his collaboration in the data processing with the computer program TriTV. This work has been supported by the French National Research Agency (grant reference «ANR-08-MIE-007»), the CNRS and the *Agencia Nacional de Promoción Científica y Tecnológica* of Argentina (grant PICT2008-0035).

7. References

Abrams P. A. & Ludwig, D. (1995). Optimality theory, Gompertz' law, & the disposable soma theory of senescence. *Evolution,* Vol.49, pp. 1055-1066

Abrams, P. A. (1991). Life History and the Relationship between Food Availability and Foraging Effort. *Ecology,* Vol.72, No.4, pp. 1242-1252

Adams, C. E. (1985). Reproductive senescence, In: *Reproduction in Mammals,* C. R. Austin & R. V. Short (Eds.), 210-233. Cambridge, Univ. Press

Akaike, H. (1974). A new look at statistical model identification. *IEEE Transactions on Automatic Control,* Vol.19, pp. 716-723

Barbu, C.; Dumonteil, E. & Gourbière, S. (2011). Evaluation of Spatially Targeted Strategies to Control Non-Domiciliated *Triatoma dimidiata* Vector of Chagas Disease. *PLoS Negl Trop Dis,* Vol.5, No.5, pp. e1045

Carey, J. R. (2001). Insect Biodemography. *Annual Review of Entomology,* Vol.46, pp. 79-110

Carey, J. R.; Liedo, P.; Müller, H.-G.; Wang, J.-L. & Vaupel, J. W. (1998). Dual Modes of Aging in Mediterranean Fruit Fly Females. *Science, New Series,* Vol.281, No.5379, pp. 996-998

Carey, J. R.; Liedo, P.; Muller, H-G.; Wang, J-L.; Senturke, D. & Harshman, L. (2005). Biodemography of a long-lived tephritid: Reproduction & longevity in a large cohort of female Mexican fruit flies, *Anastrepha ludens. Experimental Gerontology,* Vol.40, pp. 793-800

Carey, J. R.; Liedo, P.; Orozco, D. & Vaupel, J. W. (1992). Slowing of mortality rates at older ages in large medfly cohorts. *Science,* Vol. 258, pp. 457-461

Charlesworth, B. & Partridge, L. (1997). Ageing: Levelling of the Grim Reaper. *Current Biology,* Vol.7, pp. 440-442

Chaves, L. F.; Hernández, M. J.; Revilla, T. A.; Rodríguez, D. J. & Rabinovich, J. E. (2004a). Mortality profiles of *Rhodnius prolixus* (Heteroptera: Reduviidae), vector of Chagas disease. *Acta Tropica,* Vol.92, pp. 119-125

Chaves, L. F.; Zamora, E. & Aldana, E. (2004b). Mortality profile of female *Rhodnius robustus* (Heteroptera: Reduviidae). *Revista de Saúde Pública,* Vol.38, pp. 466-468

Cheverud, J. M.; Dow, M. M. & Leutenegger, W. (1985). The Quantitative Assessment of Phylogenetic Constraints in Comparative Analyses: Sexual Dimorphism in Body Weight Among Primates. *Evolution,* Vol.39, No.6, pp. 1335-1351

Christopoulos, A. & Lew, M. J. (2000). Beyond Eyeballing: Fitting Models to Experimental Data. Critical Reviews in *Biochemistry and Molecular Biology,* Vol.35, No.5, pp. 359-391

Coulson, J. C. & Fairweather, J. A. (2001). Reduced reproductive performance prior to death in the Black-legged Kittiwake: senescence or terminal illness? *Journal of Avian Biology,* Vol.32, pp. 146-152

Curtsinger, J. W.; Fukui, H. H.; Townsend, D. R. & Vaupel, J. W. (1992). Demography of genotypes: failure of the limited life-span paradigm in *Drosophila melanogaster. Science,* Vol.258, pp. 461-463

Dingle, H. (1966). The effect of population density on mortality & sex ratio in the milkweed bug, *Oncopeltus,* & the cotton stainer, *Dysdercus* (Heteroptera). *American Naturalist,* Vol.100, pp. 465-470

Dumonteil, E.; Gourbière, S.; Barrera-Perez, M.; Rodriguez-Félix, E.; Ruiz-Piña, H.; Banos-Lopez, O.; Ramirez-Siera, M. J.; Menu, F. & Rabinovich, J. E. (2002). Geographic distribution of *Triatoma dimidiata* and transmission dynamics of *Trypanosoma cruzi* in the Yucatan peninsula Mexico. *American Journal of Tropical Medicine and Hygiene,* Vol.67, pp. 176-183

Feliciangeli, M. D. & Rabinovich, J. E. (1985). Vital Statistics of Triatominae (Hemiptera: Reduviidae) under Laboratory Conditions. II. *Triatoma maculata. Journal of Medical Entomology,* Vol.22, pp. 43-48

Forattini, O. P. (1980). Biogeography, origin, and distribution of triatominae domiciliarity in Brazil. *Revista de Saúde Pública,* Vol.14, pp. 265-299.

Fukui, H. H.; Xiu, L. & Curtsinger, J. W. (1993). Slowing of age-specific mortality rates in *Drosophila melanogaster. Experimental Gerontology,* Vol.28, pp. 585-599

Gadgil, M. & Bossert, W. H. (1970). Life Historical Consequences of Natural Selection. *Am. Nat.,* Vol.104, No.935, pp. 1-24.

Gaillard, J.-M. ; Viallefont, A. ; Loison, A. & Festa-Bianchet, M. (2004). Assessing Senescence Patterns in Populations of Large Mammals. *Animal Biodiversity & Conservation,* Vol.27, No.1, pp. 47–58

Galíndez Girón, I.; Carcavallo, R. U.; Jurberg, J.; Galvao, C.; Lent, H.; Barata, J. M. S.; Pinto Serra, O. & Valderrama, A. (1998). Morfology and external anatomy. A: General, In: *Atlas of Chagas' Disease Vectors in the Americas,* R. U. Carcavallo, I. Galíndez Girón, J. Jurberg & H. Lent (Comps.), 53-73, FioCruz, Rio de Janeiro, Brazil

Gavrilov, L. A & Gavrilova, N. S. (2001) The reliability theory of aging and longevity. *Journal of Theoretical Biology,* Vol.213, No.4, pp. 527–545

Ghalambor, C. K.; Reznick, D. N. & Walker, J. A. (2004). Constraints on Adaptive Evolution: the Functional Trade-Off between Reproduction and Fast-Start Swimming Performance in the Trinidadian Guppy (*Poecilia reticulata*). *Am. Nat.,* Vol.164, No.1, pp. 38-50

Gourbière, S. & Menu, F. (2009). Adaptive dynamics of dormancy duration variability: evolutionary trade-off and priority effect lead to suboptimal adaptation. *Evolution,* Vol.63, No.7, pp. 1879-1892

Gourbière, S. ; Dumonteil, E. ; Rabinovich, J. E. ; Minkoue, R. & Menu, F. (2008). Demographic and Dispersal Constraints for Domestic Infestation by Non-Domicilated Chagas Disease Vectors in the Yucatan Peninsula Mexico. *American Journal of Tropical Medicine and Hygiene,* Vol78, pp. 133-139

Gourbière, S.; Dorn, P.; Tripet, F. & Dumonteil, E. (2011). Genetics and evolution of triatomines: from phylogeny to vector control. *Heredity,* pp. 1–13

Graca-Souza, A. V.; Maya-Monteiro, C.; Paiva-Silva, G. O.; Braz, G. R. C.; Paes, M. C.; Sorgine, M. H. F.; Oliveira, M. F. & Oliveira, P. L. (2006). Adaptations against heme toxicity in blood-feeding arthropods. *Insect Biochemistry and Molecular Biology,* Vol.36, pp. 322-335

Jones, O. R.; Gaillard, J.-M.; Tuljapurkar, S.; Alho, J. S.; Armitage, K. B.; Becker, P. H.; Bize, P.; Brommer, J.; Charmantier, A.; Charpentier, M.; Clutton-Brock, T.; Dobson, F. S.; Festa- Bianchet, M.; Gustafsson, L.; Jensen, H.; Jones, C. G. & Lillandt, B.-G. (2008). Senescence rates are determined by ranking on the fast-slow life-history continuum. *Ecology Letters,* Vol.11, pp. 664-673

Kirkwood, T. B. L. & Austad, S. N. (2000) Why do we age? *Nature* Vol.408, pp. 233-238

Kirkwood, T. B. L. & Holliday, R. (1979). The Evolution of Ageing & Longevity, *Proceedings of the Royal Society of London, Series B, Biological Sciences* Vol.205, No.1161, pp. 531-546

Kirkwood, T. B. L. & Rose, M. R. (1991). Evolution of senescence: late survival sacrificed for reproduction. *Transactions of the Royal Society, London B,* Vol.332, pp. 15–24

Kirkwood, T. B. L. (2002). Evolution of Ageing. *Mechanisms of Ageing & Development* Vol.123, pp. 737-745.

Kirkwood, T. B. L. (2005). Understanding the odd science of aging. *Cell* Vol.120, pp. 437-447

McCoy, M. W. & Gillooly, J. F. (2008). Predicting natural mortality rates of plants and animals. *Ecology Letters,* Vol.11, pp. 710-716

Menu F.; Roebuck, J. P. & Viala, M. (2000). Bet-hedging diapause strategies in stochastic environment. *The American Naturalist,* Vol.155, pp. 724-734

Menu, F.; Ginoux, M.; Rajon, E.; Lazzari, C. R. & Rabinovich, J. E. (2010). Adaptive Developmental Delay in Chagas Disease Vectors: An Evolutionary Ecology Approach. *PLoS Neglected Tropical Diseases,* Vol.4, No.5, pp. 1-10

Mueller, L. D. & Rose, M. R. (1996). Evolutionary theory predicts late-life mortality plateaus. *Proceedings of the National Academy of Sciences* Vol.93, pp. 15249-15253

Mueller, L. D.; Drapeau, M. D.; Adams, C. S.; Hammerle, C. W.; Doyal, K. M.; Jazayeri, A. J.; Ly, T.; Beguwala, S. A.; Mamidi, A. R. & Rose, M. R. (2003). Statistical Tests of Demographic Heterogeneity Theories. *Experimental Gerontology* Vol.38, pp. 373-386

Mueller, L. D.; Rauser, C. L. & Rose, M. R. (2005). Population Dynamics, Life History, & Demography: Lessons From *Drosophila*. *Advances in Ecological Research*, Vol.37, pp. 77-99

Nusbaum, T. J.; Mueller, L. D. & Rose, M. R. (1996). Evolutionary Patterns Among Measures of Aging. *Experimental Gerontology*, Vol.31, No.4, pp. 507-516

Paradis, E. (2006). *Analysis of Phylogenetics and Evolution with R*. Springer-Verlag, Heidelberg. ISBN 978-0-387-32914-7

Partridge, L. & Mangel, M. (1999). Messages from Mortality: the Evolution of Death Rates in the Old . *Trends in Ecology & Evolution*, Vol.14, No.11, pp. 438-442

Perlowagora-Szumlewicz, A. (1976). Laboratory Colonies of Triatominae, Biology, and Population Dynamics. *Proceedings of an International Symposium, New Approaches in American Trypanosomiasis Research*, pp. 63-82. Belo Horizonte, Minas Gerais, Brazil, March 18-21, 1975

Pletcher, S. D. & Curtsinger, J. W. (1998). Mortality Plateaus and the Evolution of Senescence: Why are Old-Age Mortality Rates so Low? *Evolution*, Vol.52, No.2, pp. 454-464

Promislow, D. E. L. (1991). Senescence in Natural Populations of Mammals: A Comparative Study. *Evolution*, Vol.45, No.8, pp. 1869-1887

R Development Core Team (2007) *R: A Language and Environment for Statistical Computing*. R Foundation for Statistical Computing, Vienna, Austria. Available from <http//www.R-project.org>

Rabinovich J. E. & Nieves, E. L. (2011). Vital Statistics of Triatominae (Hemiptera: Reduviidae) Under Laboratory Conditions III. *Rhodnius neglectus*. *Journal of Medical Entomology*, Vol.48, No.4, pp. 775-787

Rabinovich, J. E. (1972). Vital statistics of Triatominae (Hemiptera: Reduviidae) under laboratory conditions. I. *Triatoma infestans* Klug. *Journal of Medical Entomology*, Vol.9, No.4, pp. 351-370

Rabinovich, J. E.; Nieves, E. L. & Chaves, L. F. (2010). Age-specific mortality analysis of the dry forest kissing bug, *Rhodnius neglectus*. *Entomologia Experimentalis et Applicata*, Vol.135, No.3, pp. 252-262

Rajon, E.; Venner, S. & Menu, F. (2009). Spatially heterogeneous stochasticity and the adaptive diversification of dormancy. *Journal of Evolutionary Biology*, Vol.22, pp. 2094-2103

Rauser, C. L.; Mueller, L. D. & Rose, M. R. (2006). The Evolution of Late Life. *Ageing Research Reviews*, Vol.5, pp. 14-32

Rebke, M.; Coulson, T.; Becker, P. H. & Vaupel, J. W. (2010). Reproductive improvement and senescence in a longlived bird. *Proceedings of the National Academy of Sciences*, Vol.107, pp. 7841-7846

Reznick, D.; Bryant, M. J. & Bashey, F. (2002). r- and K- selection revisited: the role of population regulation in life history evolution. *Ecology*, Vol.83, No.6, pp. 1509-1520

Ricklefs, R. E. (1998). Evolutionary Theories of Aging: Confirmation of a Fundamental Prediction, with Implications for the Genetic Basis and Evolution of Life Span. *Am. Nat.*, Vol.152, No.1, pp. 24-44

Ricklefs, R. E. (2000). Intrinsic aging-related mortality in birds. *Journal of Avian Biology*, Vol.31, pp. 103-111

Ricklefs, R. E. (2008) The evolution of senescence from a comparative perspective. *Functional Ecology*, Vol.22, pp. 379-392

Rodríguez, D. & Rabinovich, J. E. (1980). The Effect of Density on some Population Parameters of *Rhodnius prolixus* (Hemiptera: Reduviidae) under Laboratory Conditions. *Journal of Medical Entomology*, Vol.17, No.2, pp. 165-171

Roff, D. A. (2002). *Life History Evolution. Sinauer Associates*, Inc. Sunderland, Massachusetts, USA.

Silva de Paula, A.; Diotaiuti, L. & Schofield, C. J. (2005). Testing the sister-group relationship of the Rhodniini and Triatomini (Insecta: Hemiptera: Reduviidae: Triatominae). *Molecular Phylogenetics and Evolution*, Vol.35, pp. 712-718

Souza, A. V. G.; Petretski, J. H.; Demasi, M.; Bechara, E. J. H.; Oliveira, P. L. (1997). Urate protects a blood-sucking insect against hemin induced oxidative stress. *Free Rad. Biol. Med.*, Vol.22, pp. 209–214

StatSoft (2009) STATISTICA (Data Analysis Software System), version 9.0. Statsoft, Tulsa, OK, USA.

Styer, L. M.; Carey, J. R.; Wang, J.-L. & Scott, T. W. (2007). Mosquitoes do senesce: departure from the paradigm of constant mortality. *American Journal of Tropical Medicine & Hygiene*, Vol.76, pp. 111–117

Sulbaran, J. E. & Chaves, L. F. (2006). Spatial complexity and the fitness of the kissing bug, *Rhodnius prolixus*. *Journal of Applied Entomology*, Vol.130, No.1, pp. 51-55

Tatar M.; Carey, J. R. & Vaupel, J. W. (1993). Long-term cost of reproduction with & without accelerated senescence in *Callosobruchus maculatus*: analysis of age-specific mortality. *Evolution*, Vol.47, pp. 1302-1312

Vaupel, J. W. Manton, K. G. & Stallard, E. (1979). The impact of heterogeneity in individual frailty on the dynamics of mortality. *Demography* Vol.16, No.3, pp. 439-454.

WHO (World Health Organization). 2007. Reporte sobre la enfermedad de Chagas. Grupo de trabajo científico 17–20 de abril de 2005, Buenos Aires, Argentina..

Williams, G. C. (1957). Pleiotropy, Natural Selection, & the Evolution of Senescence. *Evolution*, Vol.11, No.4, pp. 398-411

Williams, G. C. (1966). Natural Selection, the Costs of Reproduction, and a Refinement of Lack's Principle. *Am. Nat.*, Vol.100, No.916, pp. 687-690

Williams, P. D. & Day, T. (2003). Antagonistic Pleiotropy, Mortality Source Interactions, and the Evolutionary Theory of Senescence. *Evolution*, Vol. 57, No. 7 pp. 1478-1488

Zurbenko, I.; Porter, P. S.; Rao, S. T.; Ku, J. Y.; Gui, R.; Eskridge, R. E. (1996). Detecting Discontinuities in Time Series of Upper-air Data: Development and Demonstration of an Adaptive Filter Technique. *Journal of Climate*, Vol.9, No.12, pp. 3548-3560

12

Programming and Implementation of Age-Related Changes

Jaba Tkemaladze[1], Alexander Tavartkiladze[2] and Konstantin Chichinadze[3,4]

[1]Georgian Systemic Research Center, Tbilisi,
[2]Grigol Robakidze University's Oncology Department, Tbilisi,
[3]Life Science Research Center, Tbilisi,
[4]I. Javakhishvili Tbilisi State University, Tbilisi,
Georgia

1. Introduction

From the songs of my childhood I can remember one such song: " The cranes are flying far and they will never come back, the rumour is spread ... . " The author of the song text assumes that the cranes can not come back , but he/she can't bear the thought of losing lovely birds and adds: " it's a rumour !" However ,I am saying once more he lets the thought that maybe the cranes won't be back any more .... I loved this song and while listening sorrow used to enter my soul quietly. Although I knew that birds return from warm countries ... And still there was something ominous in those " never come back." Then , after so long in Dinara Kasradze's monograph ("Quantum satis ", 2005) I read the following: "Each species has it's own quantity of wing waving , after which the bird dies ." ..yhat's where that subconscious sorrow came from ... mine or of that song text author, as we mentioned above... Yes, it's so, the organism tissues , cells "get worn" while acting and get restored too; The only bad thing is that with age , damage of cells exceeds their reparation i. e. the mentioned fact becomes expressed with aging! Every creature turned to have its own strictly defined potential, after which the life expires. Then where is immortality? Only in fairy tales ? "The truth used to be written in fairy tails , the truth , written in a creative and "fairy" way " ,-"In fairy tales , many secrets of nature are explained in "fairy" language ,many things that are unsolved and not clear at all! "... Then where's immortality? The water or spring of immortality ? Maybe it is nearby , here next to us...

2. Hayflick's limit

With the age, damage of molecules exceeds its reparation i. e. the mentioned fact gets more expressed with aging. The question is : What are molecular reasons for wearing cells out. Hayflick's experiments are important in this way: in 1961 Leonard Hayflick demonstrated (at Wister Institute , Philadelphia) that the cells of normal human fetus managed to divide 40-60 times. The scientist in vitro observed human, normal, diploid fibroblast cultures and he saw that these cells have absolutely defined life expectancy - they stop multiplication and get older after 50 times division (doubling). On the contrary, fibroblasts of the patients , ill with Progeria or Verner syndrome (early aging) , used to double 10-12 times - instead of 40-60 . Adopted term , so acceptable nowadays, Hayflick's limit comes from the above . This limit i.e. border was fixed in the culture as for all differential (i.e. mature) cells, also for other multi cell organisms. Maximum number of divisions in one organism is different according to the type of the cell and difference is much more expressed in different organisms. For most of the cells Hayflick's Limit is 52 divisions. The history of Hayflick's experiments is also interesting. He worked together with Paul Moorhead . In one of the tests they mixed equal quantities of normal males' fibroblasts (that had been divided 40 times) and normal females' fibroblasts (that had been divided only 10 times) i.e. men's older cells were mixed with women's younger cells and they received mixed culture."Not mixed" culture (males') was used for control. When division in the controlling culture of the males cells stopped , in that very moment mixed culture was studied and it turned out that only women's cells were left there. This meant: The older cells "remembered" that they were old, even when they were surrounded by young cells.

Hayflick differed the following phases of cell division in the culture: At the beginning of the experiment, he called the "firstly" culture "phase one"; then the period when cells were multiplying was the "phase two". Division (doubling) period after numerous months was called "the third phase phenomenon" - when cell growth was reduced and stopped. The reason for replication aging is uncertain. It is supposed that genes of aging are activated. (They are located in the first and fourth chromosomes), the growth regulating genes are changed or lost (which at last causes growth inhibition in aging cells too. The genes, speeding (accelerating) aging process are revealed. For example, reducing signal transmission by means of Factor 1 , similar to insulin, causes Drosophila, also Nematode c. Elegans and increasing of life expectancy in mice. The reason for such difference in replication intensity is unknown. It can be caused by activating specific genes at an old age. For example, during reduction of replication Kinaza inhibitor genes (p21) are revealed. Replication aging is also induced by increased expression of p 161NK4a - the cell cycle inhibitor and DNA lesion.

3. The telomeres

The essence of genes' chromosome telomere shortening is interesting. The limited replication ability of the cell can be explained by the following: During each division, the chromosomal endings go through the unfinished replication (telomere shortening). After each division telomeres shorten, that ultimately causes stopping the cell division. Telomeres are important in stabilization of terminal parts of the chromosomes and also their fixing at the nucleus matrix. Telomeres gradually get shorter in later passages of the culture and also in older people's cell cultures. Telomeres are the longest in spermatozoids, they are longer in fetus than in an adult. As it seems, DNA loss in the terminal parts of chromosomes and telomere shortening causes deletion of important genes.

De novo synthesis of telomeres is regulated by means of enzym telomeraza. Correlation between the telomere length and telomeraza consistence is found. Hayflick's limit depends on telomere size reduction. Telomeres are DNA short repeated successions (TTAGGG) which are located at the end of chromosomes. If the cell doesn't have active telomeraza (as, for example, most of somatic cells), after each division the telomere size is reduced as DNA polymeraza can't replicate the ends of DNA molecule. In spite of this, taking this event into consideration , telomeres must shorten very slowly-- by 3-6 nucleotides after one cell cycle; According to the Hayflick's limit, after certain number of divisions telomeres shorten by 150-300 nucleotides.

Nowadays, epigenetic theory of aging is delivered by B.A. Galitski (2009),according to which telomere erosion is explained first of all by activation of cell recombinazas, which are activated in respond to the DNA lesion, which is mainly caused by age depression of genome mobile elements. When after certain number of divisions telomeres absolutely disappear, the cell remains at certain stage of the cell cycle or it turns apoptosis mechanism on. It is interesting that A.M. Olivnikov (who was the first to suppose existence of telomeres (1973,1996)) said: "Telomeres action is proved. However, it shouldn't have had direct link with aging".

In spite of theories or certain plurality of opinions, it is clear today that cell aging is caused by a number of factors. Not only endogenous molecular way of cell aging is important, but also harmful exogenous affects during the whole life, which is followed by, so called, cell "wearing". In the course of time lethal changes are gathered in the cell lesions, which lead the cells to death, as ability to respond to lesions is gradually reduced.

Certainly human cells division is not infinite, except embryonic, sex and cancer cells. The cells which have short telomeres, are often "not valid" as their chromosomes are no longer stable. The chromosomes become less protected against various damaging factors, as in norm , their defending telomeres i.e. their endings can't protect them.

During the experiment researchers (group- "Geron Corporation") could change the route of the aging process: They installed genes in the DNA. The genes were responsible for relomeraza synthesis. In these cells Hayflick's limit was doubled (100 divisions) and the life expectancy accordingly increased . According to these scientists' opinion, it is possible to change ordinary human cells that they will be able to divide infinitely. In January 1998 all the media sources informed the world that American scientists were able to force human normal cells to overcome Hayflick's limit: Instead of aging, the cells continued to multiply; and what is remarkable, they didn't transform into cancer cells. Brilliant! Bravo! If it was managed to overcome Hayflick's limit and increase life expectancy so, that cancer transformation didn't take place! And still we must point out that much care and attention is necessary in handling this process!

Telomeraza was discovered in 1984 by Carol W. Greider. For opening of the protecting mechanisms of chromosomes (terminal replication by the help of telomerazas) Elizabeth Blackburn , Carol Grider and Jack Szostak received Nobel Prizes. Human telomeraza's structure was explained by Scott Cohen and his group (Australia, Children's medicine Research Institute, 2007). Telomeraza consists of telomeraza reverse transcriptaza (TERT.), telomeraza RNM (hTR or TERC) and diskerin (two molecules of each substance). TERT, as we pointed out, is the ferment reverse-transcriptaza, which creates one-string DNA on the basis of template one-string RNA (i.e. telomeraza represents a reverse - transcriptaza and a special molecule of RNA is connected with it , which is used as a matrix for the reverse-transcriptaza during lengthening of the telomeres.) Two subunits of the ferment are encoded by two different genes. TERT has a glove shape, which allows it to fix at the chromosome and add to it one-string parts. It is considered that telomeraza is the key to the cell immortality. Thanks to this ferment, cells multiply fast and don't get older.

Telomeraza is the most intensively revealed in the embryonic cells , then-in Germinational cells, very slightly-in adult organism labile cells (cells, that must divide frequently, for example, intestinal epithelial cells), but their detection is difficult in the most of the somatic cells. (More correctly, it doesn't happen at all).

Telomeraza is used in the cosmetic production (The product TA-65 was received from the plant Astragal, which activates telomeraza). Michael Fossel supposed in one of the interviews (2006, int. by D, J Brown), that treatment by telomeraza could be used not only for struggle against cancer , but also for fight against aging i.e. for increasing life expectancy.

When cells come closer to the Hayflick's limit, it is possible to stop aging if deactivation of those genes will happen , which are responsible for creation of the albumin (p53 and pR6) , suppressing cancer . Sooner or later such , changed cells get to the condition , which is called "crisis" i.e. when big part of the cells (in the culture) die (However, sometimes the cell doesn't stop multiplication during the crisis period). As a rule, telomeres are absolutely destroyed at the time and condition of the chromosomes worsens after each division.

4. Cancer

The naked endings of the chromosomes mean splitting of the both DNA strings. Neutralization of such type of lesion happens by connecting split endings. Also endings of different chromosomes can make confluence as they are no longer protected by telomeres. This story as if temporarily relieves telomere absence. However, in the anaphase of the cell division, linked chromosomes come apart quite accidentally, which is followed by a lot of mutations and chromosomal anomaly development and with the process development the cell genome is more and more injured. Ultimately the moment comes when apoptosis is turned on (The gene substance is so much injured) or the mutation is added to the injured genome which activates telomeraza.

After activation of telomeraza some types of cells obtain immortality. Their chromosomes don't become less stable for the number of divisions and the death process doesn't start. Many cancer cells are considered to be immortal as the telomeraza gene is activated in them which allows these cells to divide infinitely and this is the reason for cancer growth.

Hela's cells are good example for cancer cells eternity, which were received in 1951 from Henrietta Lack's cervix cancer tissue. The name of the culture comes from the above. This culture is still used in studies today. Hela's cells are really immortal: They are produced daily in tons and they are descendants of the removed cancer cells from H. Lack's organism.

In spite of the fact, that cancer modeling in the cell culture is effective and it has already been used for years, it is still not exact. At first, it was unknown which was the influence, that causes cell multiplication in this model. Finding the answer became gradually possible: Different mutations were caused in the model cells (Which we meet in different cancer cells in human) which allowed the scientists to reveal several confluent mutations, that was sufficient for creating cancer cells from different types.

Mutations are confluent in different ways in different types of cells. However, in most of these confluences the following is fixed: 1.Activation of telomeraza 2.Cycle damage of the albumin p 53. 3. Activation of Ras , Myc and other protooncogenes . 4.Violation of PP2A phosphataza formation. These changes provide "turning off " the death mechanism by means of damaging chromosome destruction or apoptosis process. With this endless multiplication of the cell begins.

In cell cultures, this model of cancer clears up the telomeraza's role in cancer development. In 90 percent of cancers telomeraza's activation is observed.

In cancers without TERT activation in cells , they mainly used other mechanism of telomeres' protection , which is called ALT (alternative lengthening of telomeres). Details of this mechanism are unknown.

According to Elizabeth Blackburn's works (1985, 2001), telomeraza is also involved in regulation of 70 genes which participate (or probably participate) in cancer origin and development. Furthermore, telomeraza activates glycolysis, which allows cancer cells to use sugar in order to maintain growth and division rate. This speed is equal to the same process rate in embryo.

Fight with the cancer is difficult. If it was possible to receive such a medication, which would cause telomeraza's blockage in cancer cells, then telomere shortening would be renewed. Mutations would appear and cancer cells would die!

Working in this direction has started (Koreans have just created the preparation "Telovak", which in the opinion of creators, activates immune system, that ultimately is directed to suppress telomeraza. After trying it on volunteers, ill with cancer "Telovak" prolonged patients' life by merely one year. It also gifted three months of life to the patients who were on the last stage of cancer. The question is : Maybe not only in cancer cells is telomeraza suppressed? Subsequently, will it ultimately make life shorter?

5. Senescence

Cancer cell is divided infinitely, telomeraza's gene is expressed , " inserted " in it i.e. malignant cell looks like a sex or embryonic cell (Probably, these are the only cells and its product restores normal length of the telomere).

Hereby , we take the liberty of a small comment: Yes ! - Today, immortal cells of cancer are widely discussed , which is said to be the fault of telomerazas . However, it shouldn't be absolutely right. Not all multiplied cancer cells are divided, i.e. among them there are some cells that divide ,so there is the limit too. As regards the culture, it is possible to initiate growth in all the ways . Besides , in vivo , cancer cells gradually cannot divide . Ultimately, they don't have "strength " of even it and die (These are famous facts , pathology -anatomists like to point it out. I remember the talk with Omar Khardzeishvili about this very question) i.e. part of cancer cells die by themselves in the lifetime of the ill organism. (It is an axiom today too); However, the person dies before all the cancer cells die !

In human fibroblasts, Kamozin can increase Hayflicks's Limit by means of reduction of telomeres shortening quality. However, the scientists say , that vertebrates' cells have certain potential of replication. More importantly, A.Melk and his group (2003) saw that in vivo aging is possible without telomere shortening.

The surgeon, Nobeliant Alexsis Carrel said : "All the cells , that grow in the culture , are immortal ; But if they reduced , the number of cell replications fell, it means that the way of cultivation, itself , is to be recovered and improved. " We take again the liberty of adding a comment of our own : "Growing cells in culture are immortal "- The multiplication process itself can be continuous. However, the cells probably change ; In this way a human is also immortal- by means of his/her generation or descendants (since Adam till today). Yes, exactly the same process! And don't let Carrel to deceive us. However, as regards the opinion, that "if the number of cell divisions reduced, then the way of cultivation must be improved. " This is right: It's necessary to improve conditions to increase birth-rate in people!).

Carrel's hypothesis (1921) was strengthened by the fact that the scientist had been growing the chicken's fibroblasts in the culture for 34 years. The part of scientists thought this was possible infinitely in vertebrates. However, there was a certain mistake during the experiment (i.e. in accuracy) and most scientists didn't agree with the results. The mistake was in the fact that Carrel daily added chicken's embryonic, axial cells to the culture; This allowed the new cells to multiply and it wasn't multiplication of the initiate, original cells any more; but in this way cells' multiplication was possible unlimitedly. Some researchers are convinced that Carrel knew about this mistake (in the experimental procedure), but he didn't admit it.

Briefly, Alexsis Carrel's theory didn't succeed and his mistake was evident too. However, Alexei Olivnikov's theory is acceptable and corresponds to Hayflick's experiments: Telomerazas' inhibition is a good remedy in malignant cancer treatment.

Ultimately, in reduction of life expectancy the following is important : 1. Reduction of the cell replication i.e. what Hayflick's limit means ; 2. Telomeres' shortening ; 3. Accumulation of cells and reduction of axial cells number; 4. Changes , revealed in the cell with aging: accumulation of free radicals, influence of radiation, generation of oxygen free radical O2 -, modification of albumins, lipids, nuclein acids , reduction of antioxidant mechanisms (vitamin E, glutation peroxidaza) , accumulation of dot mutations; 5. Lowering of the reparation systems, lowering of the DNA helikaza activity i.e. defect (enzyme is involved in DNA replication, reperation and other functions, that are necessary for DNA perfection. Besides Verner syndrome, defect of this enzym is found in Ataxia-Telangiektazia); 6. Strengthened expression of antioxidant enzyme - SOD and katalaza (it has been seen in Drisophila) ; 7.It is thought that proteasome function can be lowered that is called proteolyses mechanisms. Its responsibility is elimination of abnormal and unnecessary intracellular albumen (Lesion of the organels which is one of the reasons for cell aging).

Consequently, with aging, in all the organ systems, there are physiological and structural changes. The rate of aging process is associated with genetic factors, nutrition specialty, social condition , disease development , associated with age. For example, atherosclerosis, diabetes type 2, osteoarthritis.

The most effective way for increasing life expectancy is limitation of calories. It depends on sirtuins. They have hystondeacetilaza activity and probably they promote expression of different genes , products of which increase life expectancy. This products consist of proteins which increase metabolic activity, reduce apoptosis , stimulates albumens' third structure formation (fights with denaturation), inhibits free radicals of oxygen. Sirtuins also rise sensitivity on insulin and strengthen glucose metabolism. They can also be used in diabetes treatment. It's important that red wine activates sirtuins and this prolongs life.

So, probably nothing is impossible, among them defeating cancer disease and increasing life limit... However...

`In spite of the fact that telomeraza is the key to cell immortality i.e. " infinity" of cancer cell is caused by telomeraza, we know and pointed out above that cancer cells (where expression: of this enzym is high and where exactly telomeraza is "accused " in persistent division of the cells), ultimately the condition is achieved when they don't divide any more (more exactly -can't), so their "infinity" is doubtful! Where is the immortality?

We set an example of studies above where there is indicated that aging is possible without telomere shortening or disappearing i.e. nor immortality or "not aging" reverse-process- the death (which follows the aging) entirely depends on telomeres..... Consequently, it is doubtful again that telomeraza is the key to the cell immortality! Then, where is the immortality!

In our opinion the key to immortality should be that "thing" which causes permanent renovation! Though, it's difficult to imagine it in our dimension , where everything has its beginning and the end , still I remember " immortality water" from fairy tales ! - Where is the immortality?

There are such albumens-stress albumens (which appear during different stresses in the cell and protect it from lesion spreading) - Chaperon , Chaperonins, sirtuin molecules are very important and we pointed out above their protecting and " rescuing " occupation ! Red wine turned to be sirtuins action stimulator! There is Resveratrol in the same red wine -plant estrogen, Melatonin's precursor ! Melatonin is a hormone which acts as an obstacle for lesion, "wearing out "; Melatonin has the most expressed regenerative capacity and consequently the ability to restore/maintain living structures!

In the preamble of my first monograph ("melatonini" 2007) Dinara Kasradze wrote : "And in this system too, the most mysterious turned to be the Epiphysis... Epiphysis with its melatonin! However, it is the main thing where the life takes its origin (metaphor) -i.e. it is the "source " of light and darkness, mist and dawn . It causes sleep and waking up, tiredness and relaxing, wearing out and restoration, spring and autumn, summer and winter too .... It gives the world rhythm, biorhythm which gives us a birth, brings us up, breeds, ages or takes us into other..... It causes health and disease... and probably it is not surprising that in a creative way the "third eye" is called Epiphysis, maybe not entirely creatively. It can be so that overwhelming strength of the Lord is incarnated by means of Melatonin in our dimension.... Biological-cosmic key for immortality and constant transformations may probably lay ...... in the very magic molecule of Melatonin.... Who knows...."

6. Centriole, differentiation, senescence

Death is inevitable for any of living organisms, viruses, plants or animals. However, only multicellular animals, including human beings, die from ageing. A multicellulary organism (animal), containing a multitude of irreversibly differentiated cells, develops from only one cell e the totipotential zygote. The potency to differentiate into a certain tissue or tissues (set by the factor which controls the possibility of repression and activation of genes) determines the individual histological state, or morphogenetic "status'" of a cell. The final morphogenetic status means that such a cell is committed to programmed death (apoptosis). A 'zero' morphogenetic status means that the cell has not been committed to any irreversible pathway, i.e. it remains totipotent. Modification of morphogenetic status of a cell changes the whole spectrum of the tissues into which this cell can differentiate. In ontogenesis, this spectrum consequently narrows (totipotential / pluripotential/ multipotential/ unipotential/ non-potential) until the cell reaches the state of final differentiation (Malaitcev et al., 2002).

6.1 Need for a self-replicating controller

It has been established that morphogenetic status of a cell might be changed only through its division. We consider that cell division, differentiation and apoptosis may be controlled by a single intracellular structure. Naturally, this structure has to be self-replicating. Moreover, it has to have some way of counting or recording cell divisions. In a somatic cell potential candidates for this replicable structure are chromosomes, mitochondria (both contain DNA), and centrioles. To date the structures which might count cell divisions e and, therefore, determine the morphogenetical status of a cell e are generally thought to be telomeres (Bodnar et al., 1998; Greider, 1998; Shay and Wright, 2001). However, some data do not confirm the hypothesis that assigns the role of replication 'clock' to these parts of a chromosome.

Thus, the cells of mice bred by Blasco et al. (1997) did not have telomerase activity. Such mice were viable and could produce up to 6 generations, though the chromosomes of each subsequent generation had increasingly shortened telomeres. Only the sixth generation developed abnormalities caused by the extreme shortening of telomeres. The authors emphasised that 'ageing' of cells took place long before the marginal shortening of telomeres. Rudolph et al. (1999) showed that mice with inactivated genes of telomerase had shorter lifetime and increased frequency of oncological diseases, but physiological and biochemical tests did not reveal any signs of early ageing. Animal cloning disproves telomere hypothesis as well as other hypotheses, which suggest that a morphogenetic factor is located in nuclear DNA. In outline, the main point of cloning procedure is injection of the nucleus of a finally differentiated somatic cell into an oocyte with previously removed or destroyed nucleus. It was undoubtedly proved that the pattern of genes expression is changed to comply with the cytoplasm of a 'host' cell (Hardeman et al., 1986; Dominko et al., 1999). Injection of the nucleus of a frog carcinoma cells into an enucleated egg resulted in, not tumor cells, but normal tadpole development.

The key element of gene network controlling the processes of cell differentiation is an external factor for nuclear genome signal, which activates these groups of interactively expressing genes (Kolchanov et al., 2000). We suggest that the processes of cell ageing, differentiation and division are regulated by cytoplasmic factors. The structure, which regulates processes of irreversible differentiation, determination and modification of morphogenetic status, is most likely to be a centriole (centrosome).

Recent data indicate that centriole and nuclear cycles are not nterdependent (Gorgidze and Vorobjev, 1994). It was shown that nucleus controls the synthesis of 'building material' (basically proteins) used by centrioles, thereby having control over the centriole cycle. When a cell has such 'building material' in excess (i.e. oocytes), cycles of centriole duplication may occur even if mitotic cycle has not been launched (Manandkhar et al., 1990). Phillips and Rattner (1976) also demonstrated that inhibition of RNA or RNA/protein synthesis suppresses the duplication of centrioles in cultured cells.

6.2 The rule of cell division

As a rule, somatic cells contain a diploid set of chromosomes and a pair of centrioles (diplosome). This ratio is maintained by the parallel reproduction of nuclear DNA and centrioles, which takes place while cells are being prepared for the next division. In the process of gametogenesis, the number of chromosomes is reduced and the cell becomes haploid. Studies of spermatogenesis performed in insects (Sciara coprphila, Chrysopa carnea, Bombyx mori) and mammals (Heterohyrax syriacus and Memetes berdmorei) discovered that at the first meiotic division spindle poles contain a pair of centrioles, while at the second division e they contain only one centriole; in mammalians spermatocytes get two centrioles after both first and second divisions (Kriouchkova and nishchenco, 1999). On the contrary, oocytes of mammalians (mouse, rat, and rabbit) and Xenopus laevis do not have visible centriolar structures during both the meiotic divisions (Kriouchkova and Onishchenco, 1999). During the process of fertilization, the chromosomal sets of a spermatozoon and an oocyte are mixed. The chromosomal sets/centrioles ratio, typical for somatic cells, may be restored either in a zygote or early blastomeres. Thus, in sea urchins, the spindle pole at first cell division contains a diplosome, while in mice they are centriole-free at both first and second divisions. Only at third division does a centrosome get a pair of centrioles. The literature reveals several hypotheses, which try to explain the formation of centrioles in embryonic cells. These structures may be obtained exclusively from the paternal cell, as in sea urchins. In most mammalians zygotes, the centrosome is of maternal origin, but the centrioles are formed de novo only in the third cell cycle. It should be noted, however, that human centrioles, as well as centrioles of other mammalian species (sheep, cow, and marsupials), belong to the paternal sex cell (Breed et al., 1994; Nijs et al., 1996; Schatten et al., 1996).

Some studies demonstrate that centrioles act as the regulators that control the course of every phase of a cell cycle influencing the processes that take place at least two phases earlier (Neverova et al., 1996; Maniotis and Schliva, 1991).

6.3 Centrioles and cancer

Centrioles seem to play some role in inheritance of tumorigenic properties. Taking into account aforementioned facts, what molecular mechanism underlying the centriolar activity may control determination of morphogenetic status of a somatic cell? Centrioles may contain differently encoded RNA molecules stacked in a definite order. During mitosis these RNA molecules are probably released one by one into cytoplasm. This process presumably changes the status of repressed and potentially active genes and, subsequently, the morphogenetic status of a cell.

Centrioles may have such molecules controlling morphogenetic status contained in their internal chamber (the area of two electron-dense linear structures). It is also possible that they are packed in definite order. Some molecules may differ from the preceding ones and control different morphogenetic status. Other ones can be exact copies, thus determining the same morphogenetic status. In each mitotic division, one of these molecules is released and 'lost' in the cytoplasm, so the centrioles of daughter cells contain one molecule less than the centrioles of the maternal cell. The number of molecules contained in centrioles decreases after each mitotic division. The last molecule triggers the processes of programmed death (i.e. apoptosis). Thus, the number of hypothetic molecules must correspond to the number of possible mitotic divisions, counting down from the cell having the first morphogenetic status to the last offspring cell having the final morphogenetic status (the "Hayflick limit", Hayflick, 1997).

6.4 Importance of small MW RNA (siRNA)

The best candidate for the role of the carrier of information on morphogenetic status seems to be low molecular weight RNA. Indirect evidence for this hypothesis may be the discovery of new classes of small RNA e so-called interfering RNA (siRNA) and micro-RNA (miRNA) e having regulatory activity. The phenomenon of RNA interference occurs to inhibit selectively gene expression in animal cells (Fire et al., 1998; McManus and Sharp, 2002; Montgomery et al., 1998), including mammalian cells (Wianny and Zornicka-Goets, 2000). MicroRNA appeared to act as a regulator of cell differentiation and development in higher organisms. There direct data confirm the role of these molecules in the process of cell division (Lau et al., 2001; Lee and Ambros, 2001; Lagos-Quintana et al., 2001). In 2002, it was found that the influence of siRNA might not be limited to only temporary 'knockout' of genes on RNA level. Small RNA can modify the chromatin structure and make genes active or silent for quite a long period of time (Zilberman et al., 2003). In addition to post-transcriptional and transcriptional homology-dependent gene silencing links between DNA structure and RNA expose themselves in many other phenomena, like dose-dependent compensation in drosophila and mammalian X-chromosome inactivation (Stuckenholz et al., 1999).

The whole body of existing e though sometimes contradictory e data demonstrating that RNA may be located inside of centrosome or linked to this structure (Heath, 1980; Heidemann et al., 1977; Lambert and Nagy, 2000; Nadejdina et al., 1982; Peterson and Berns, 1980) makes it possible to suggest that small RNA (of 20e300 nucleotides) may be an ideal candidate for the role of the molecule if these are inside the centrioles.

6.5 The centriole as the carrier of controlling siRNA

Filling of centrioles with the molecules of RNA in various species apparently takes place in different cells: those, which develop at the first of second meiotic division of gametogenesis (spermatogenesis or oogenesis, depending on species), or in the first blastomeres at the time of centriole formation de novo. Those molecules are transcribed from nuclear DNA and stacked in a definite order within the centrioles. Following this process subsequent release of RNA molecules during mitosis determines the expression of nuclear DNA. Nuclear genome presumably 'chooses' and 'places' into centrioles the information about the sequence of DNA loci activation in the offspring cells. Absence of centrioles in a stage of preleptotenic chromosome condensation in mice may be good illustration of 'zero' morphogenetic status of cells (Hartung and Stahl, 1977). Intracellular 'morphogenetic clocks' seems to be wound up at that moment returning to the initial 'zero' state.

6.6 Conclusions that can be drawn

Should centrioles indeed control the processes of cell differentiation and programmed death, the following may be concluded:

1. When a cell initially does not have centrioles (this situation denotes the absence of morphogenetical status), it will be totipotential;

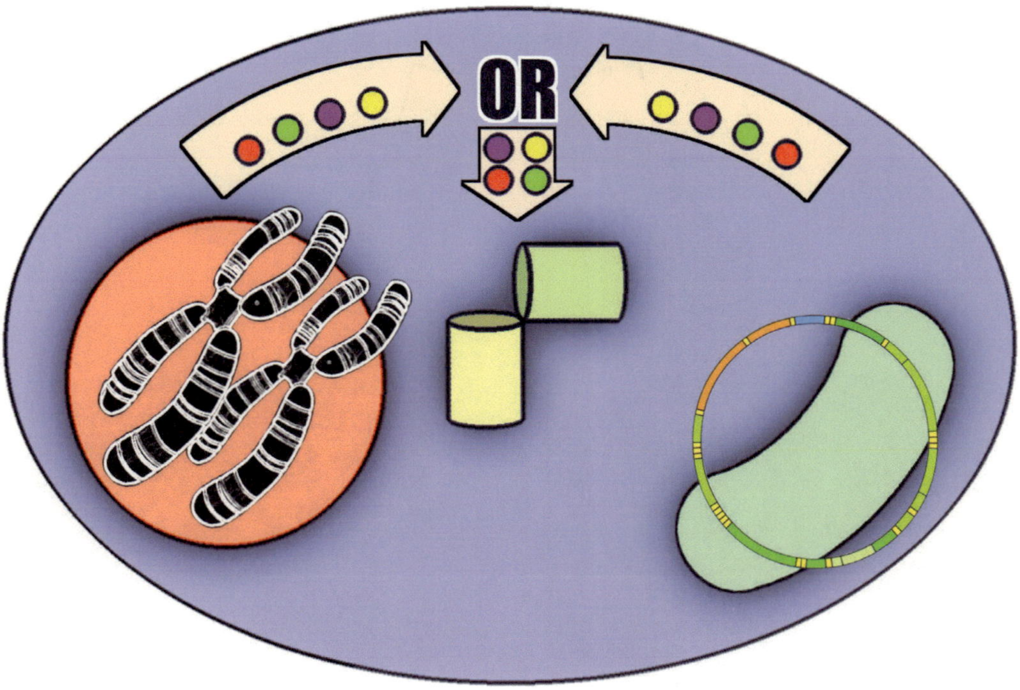

Fig. 1. Causing irrevocable differentiation - Protein or RNA-hypothetical molecular code must be encoded in DNA or mitochondrial or nuclear. It is expected that as many differentiation molecular codes should be encoded in DNA as the quantity of irrevocable differentiation stages, characteristic for each particular species. Molecular structure of the differentiation, complexing at centriol must have the features of matrix - while forming new centriols, it must repeat similar structure.

2. If a cell launches centriole synthesis de novo (the centrioles are considered to be formed de novo as long as the cell is not committed to irreversible differentiation), it will be totipotential and immortal, retaining its initial 'zero' morphogenetic status;

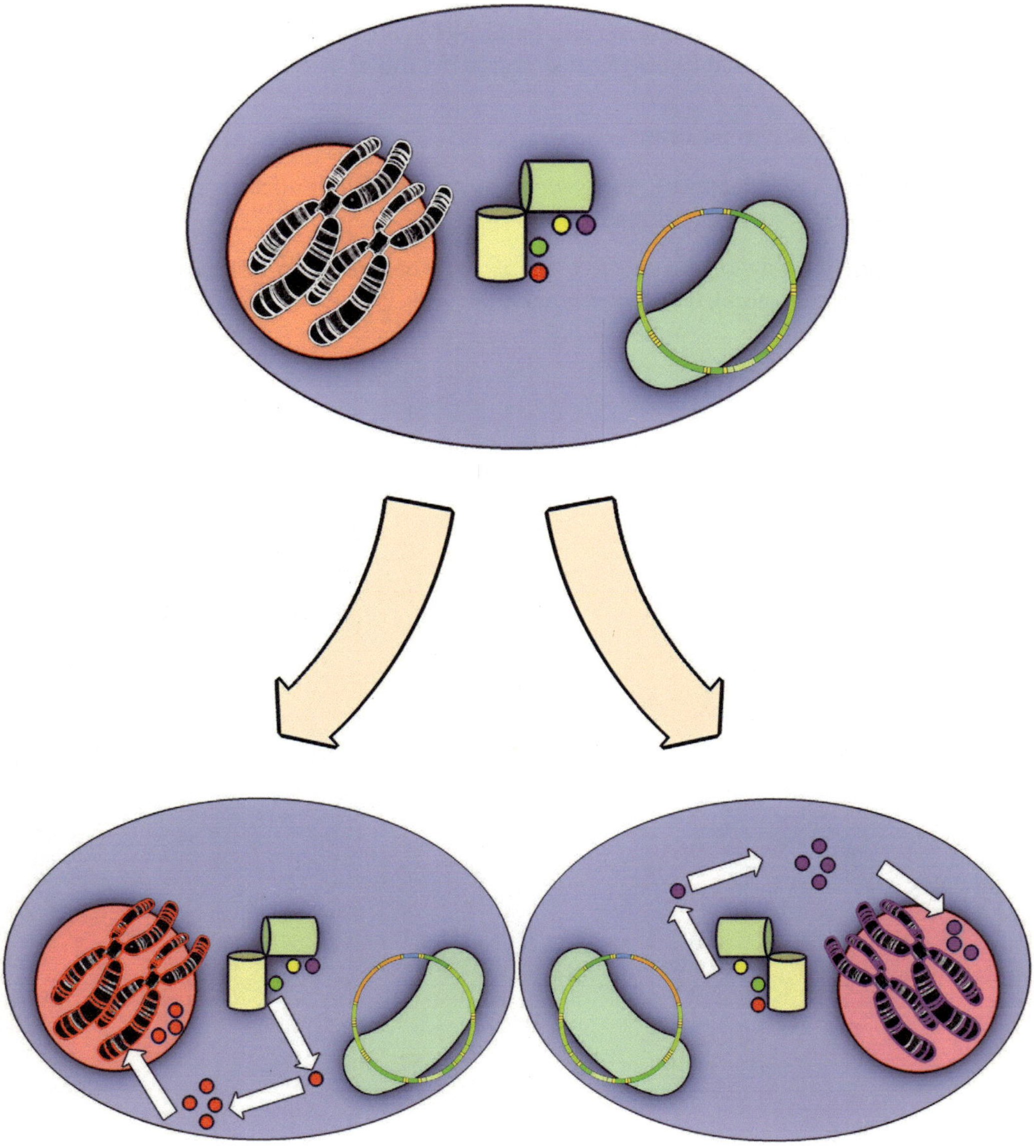

Fig. 2. Cell division, during which release of the molecule, causing differentiation happens, will finish with the irrevocable differentiation of the descendant cells. Probably, the molecule the albumen or RNA differentiation plays the role of the matrix. Ultimately, the small DNA molecule is formed, which enters the nuclear chromosomes, is inserted in them and so changes their structure and function, but not irrevocably.

3. Should a cell not to die due to programmed death when appropriate changes in centrioles do occur, it will be immortal, but not totipotential

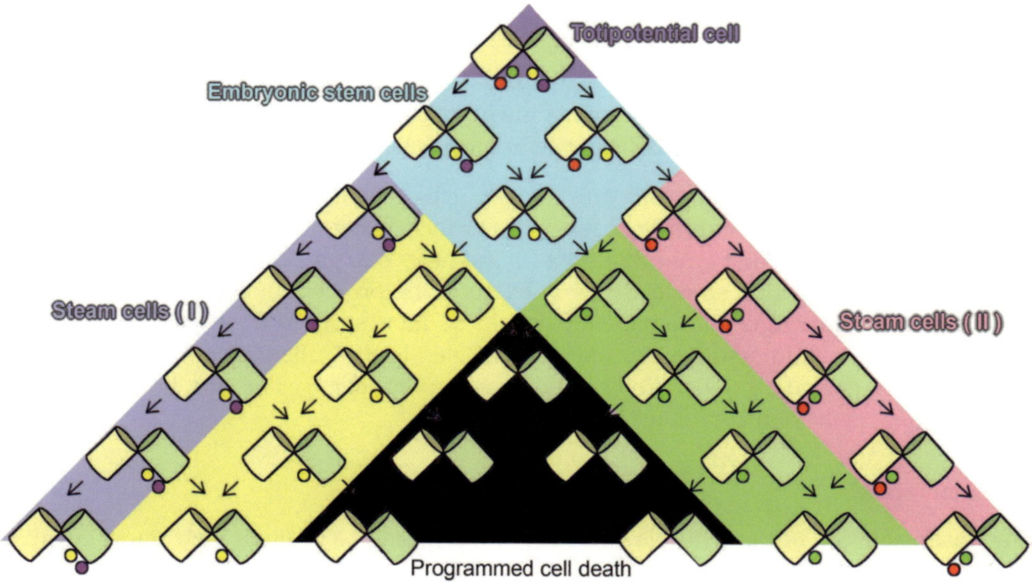

Fig. 3. Maintaining the quantity of the stem cells is explained by the reason, that irrevocable differentiation divisions have asymmetric nature (asymmetric division). Existence of asymmetric division and differentiation structure can also explain the fact that different types of cells give not only different (various), but also similar descendant cells.

Many existing data may be explained on the basis of the proposed hypothesis:

1. Centrioles are initially absent in the cells of higher plants (Sluiman, 1985), zygote and the first blastomeres of some animals (Abumuslimov et al., 1994 Calarco-Gillam et al., 1983). According to our conception they are fully potential and immortal;
2. Centrioles formed de novo in a zygote and the first blastomeres (Maro et al., 1991) belong to the fully potential and immortal cells;
3. Tumor and transformed cells are immortal, but not totipotential. This state may be due to the presence of a certain 'non-zero' morphogenetical status at the moment of transformation.

It is possible that centriolar and nuclear cycles of tumor and transformed cells are irreversibly disengaged. The nucleus looses its ability to perceive some intracellular and extracellular signals, including those which control the morphogenetic status of a cell. The cell becomes immortal, though it has 'non-zero' morphogenetic status.

Based upon the proposed hypothesis, we suggest that centrioles realize their function of 'counting' mitotic divisions. The number of divisions (generations) of a cell is limited; this means that the number of cells of various types is fixed too. Consequently, the possibility of cellular regeneration will be also limited. Sooner or later, regenerating issues experience a lack of cells: then the organism will not be able to further provide its 'homeostatic' support for long-living cells (for instance, neurons). Thus, death from ageing seems to be a phenomenon affecting the whole organism.

Our proposed hypothesis is verifiable, but needs also be tested to destruction. It may be easily checked if the chemical composition of the internal chamber of centrioles is studied more closely. According to the hypothesis, there must be some difference in chemical composition, as well as in ultrastructure (morphology), of the inner chamber of centrioles in different types of somatic cells. Attention should be also paid to monocellular organisms having centrioles.

It should be emphasised that until now the changes of ultrastructure of the centrosome during the processes of maturation of sex cells and their fusion during insemination, as well as in the course of the first embryonic cell cycles, have not yet been studied in any detail. This kind of investigation should throw light upon the problem of centrioles (diplosome) 'inheritance' in embryonic blastomeres. It would be interesting to know how and to what extent the hetero- and homo-gametic states are related to the 'inheritance' of centrioles. It is also important to find out what kind of divisions produce changes in morphogenetic status and how great is the number of such divisions.

6.7 Final remarks

The final resolution of the centriole question, however, can be through their transplantation from differentiated cells of one type into the cells of another type. Today such transplantations are quite possible. To preserve the functional activity of centrioles, they should be extracted immediately after their maturation is finished, i.e. in the middle of metaphase, and injected at the moment the chromosomes are formed. Of course, the centrioles of the recipient cell have to be removed earlier from the spindle poles. Then one could observe whether such 'hybridization' provokes changes in the expression of nuclear genes. In our opinion, the expression of nuclear genes should be changed to resemble that of the donor cell. It would confirm the hypothesis, which states that centrioles (diplosome) are actually the structure controlling the morphogenetical status of a cell.

According to this hypothesis, there must a constant number of stem cells, which is sufficient for regeneration of tissues and organs. However, this doesn't conform with reality. With aging, number of stem cells is reduced. It has to be searched: What is the reason for it? - Influence of the outer factors (e.g.: Gathering mutation in generations, which makes the cell lose the viability) or inner factors, the programmed process (e.g.: Telomeres' shortening in generations, that ends up with transformation in cancer cell or cell death).

7. Centrosomal RNA

In 2006 a group of researchers discovered a specific centrosome-associated RNA, which is called cnRNA. New developments and findings in this direction will clarify the issue whether the differentiation molecules have a protein or RNA nature. It is desirable as well to identify which section of the ovule genome carries the information about these molecules.

8. Conclusion

In spite of the fact, that Telomerase is the key to the cell immortality or that cancer cell "eternity" is caused by Telomerase, we know and have pointed out above that cancer cells (where enzyme expression is high and where every Telomerase is "to be blamed" for constant division of cells), ultimately achieve the condition when they don't divide any more (can't divide is more correct) - i.e. their "eternity" is suspicious! - Where is the immortality?

In our point of view, the "key" to immortality must be "something" which caused constant renovation of the "worn". It's impossible to stop aging, only, it's possible to turn the biological clock back (even for several times). However, it's difficult to imagine in our dimension, where everything has its beginning and end... and still I can remember "water of immortality" from my childhood - Where is the immortality?

The fact that it was possible to induce totipotential qualities in the stem cell, gives us some hope. If we can discover the damaged DNA and replace it with healthy code, it's already possible to return totipotential features to this cell.

If we return this cell to the organism, theoritically, it is expected that the "aged" stem cells "are replaced" by the "rejuvenated" stem cells.

9. References

[1] Abumuslimov SS, Nadezhdina ES, Chentcov YuS. Morphogenesis of centrioles and centrosomes in early mouse development: the Electron microscopic study. Tsitologiia 1994;11:1054e60 [in Russian].

[2] Alliegro M.C., at all. Centrosome-associated RNA in surf clam oocytes. Proc Natl Acad Sci U S A. 2006; 103(24): 9034-9038

[3] Alliegro MC, Satir P., 2009. Origin of the cilium: novel approaches to examine a centriolar evolution hypothesis. Methods Cell Biol. 2009; 94: 53-64

[4] Bartel D., Chen C. Micromanagers of gene expression: the potentially widespread influence of metazoan microRNAs. Nat. Rev. Genet. 2004; 5: 396-400.

[5] Blasco MA, Lee HW, Hande MP, Samper E, Lansdorp PM, DePinho RA, et al. Telomere shortening and tumor formation by mouse cells lacking telomerase RNA. Cell 1997;91:25e34.

[6] Blower MD, Feric E, Weis K, Heald R. Genome-wide analysis demonstrates conserved localization of messenger RNAs to mitotic microtubules. J Cell Biol. 2007; 179(7): 1365-1373.

[7] Blower M.D., Nachury M., Heald R., Weis K. A Rae1-containing ribonucleoprotein complex is required for mitotic spindle assembly. Cell. 2005; 121: 223-234.

[8] Bodnar AG, Ouellette M, Frolkis M, Holt SE, Chiu CP, Morin GB, Harley CB, et al. Extension of life-span by introduction of telomerase into normal human cells. Science 1998 Jan 16;279(5349):334e5.

[9] Breed W, Simerky C, Navara C, Vande Berg J, Schatten G. Distribution of microtubules in eggs and early embtyos of marsupial Monodelphis domestica. Dev Biol 1994;164:230e40.

[10] Calarco-Gillam PD, Siebert MC, Hubble R, Mitchison T, Kirschner M. Centrosome development in early mouse embryos as defined by an autoantibody against pericentriolar material. Cell 1983;35:621e9.

[11] Chang S., Johnston R., Frekjaer-Jensen C. et al. MicroRNAs act sequentially and asymmetrically to control chemosensory laterality in the nematode. Nature. 2004; 430:785-789.

[12] Chapman M.J., Dolan M.F., Margulis L. Centrioles and kinetosomes: form, function, and evolution. Q Rev Biol. 2000; 75(4): 409-429.

[13] Chapman, M.J. and Alliegro, M.A. A symbiotic origin for the centrosome? Symbiosis. 2007; 44: 23-32

[14] Chen C., Li L., Lodish H., Bartel D. MicroRNAs modulate hematopoietic lineange differentiation. Science. 2004; 303: 83-86.

[15] Chu C.Y. and Rana T.M. Small RNAs: regulators and guardians of the genome. J. Cell Physiol. 2007; 213: 412-419.

[16] Dominko T, Mitalipova M, Haley B, Beyhan Z, Memili E, McKusick B, et al. Bovine oocyte cytoplasm supports development of embryos produced by nuclear transfer of somatic cell nuclei from various mammalian species. Biol Reprod 1999;6:1496e502.

[17] Doxsey S., McCollum D., Theurkauf W. Centrosomes in cellular regulation. Ann. Rev. Cell and Dev. Biol. 2005; 21: 411-434.

[18] Etienne-Manneville S. Actin and microtubules in cell motility: which one is in control? Traffic. 2004; 5(7): 470-477.

[19] Filipowicz, W., Bhattacharyya, S.N. and Sonenberg, N. Mechanisms of post-transcriptional regulation by microRNAs: are the answers in sight? Nature Rev. Genet. 2008; 9: 102-114.

[20] Fire A, Xu S, Montgomery MK, Kostas SA, Driver SE, Mello CC. Potent and specific genetic interference by double/stranded RNA in Caenorhabditis elegans. Nature 1998;391:806e11.

[21] Galitskii V.A. Epigenetic nature of ageing. Tsitologiia. 2009; 51(5):388-397. Russian

[22] Gorgidze LA, Vorobjev IA. Centrioles in tissue culture cells are able to replicate in the absence of the nucleus. Tsitologiia 1994;8:837e43 [in Russian].

[23] Gourlay C.W., Ayscough K.R. The actin cytoskeleton: a key regulator of apoptosis and ageing? Nat Rev Mol Cell Biol. 2005; 6(7): 583-589.

[24] Greider CW. Telomerase activity, cell proliferation, and cancer. Proc Natl Acad Sci USA 1998 Jan 6;95(1):90e2.

[25] Hardeman EC, Chiu CP, Minty A, Blau HM. The pattern of actin expression in human fibroblast mouse muscle heterokaryons suggests that human muscle regulatory factors are produces. Cell 1986;47:123e30.

[26] Hiedemann, S.R., Sander, G. and Kirschner, M.W. Evidence for a functional role of RNA in centrioles. Cell. 1977; 10, 337-350.

[27] Hartung M, Stahl A. Preleptotene chromosome condensation in mouse oogenesis. Cytogenet Cell Genet 1977;2:309e19.

[28] Hayflick L. Mortality and Immortality on the cell level. Biochemistry 1997;11:1380e93.

[29] Heath JB. Variant mitosis in lower eucaryotes: indicator of the evolution of mitosis. Int Rev Cytol 1980;64:1e80.

[30] Heidemann SR, Sander G, Kirschner MW. Evidence for a functional role of RNA in centrioles. Cell 1977;10:337e50.

[31] Kim V.N., Han J, Siomi M.C. Biogenesis of small RNAs in animals. Nat Rev Mol Cell Biol. 2009; 10(2): 126-39.

[32] Kingsley E.P., Chan X.Y., Duan Y., Lambert J.D. Widespread RNA segregation in a spiralian embryo. Evol Dev. 2007; 9(6): 527-539.

[33] Kloc M., Zearfoss N.R. and Etkin L.D. Mechanisms of subcellular mRNA localization. Cell. 2002; 108: 533-544.

[34] Kloc M., Etkin L.D. RNA localization mechanisms in oocytes. J Cell Sci. 2005; 118(Pt 2): 269-82.

[35] Klotz, C., Dabauvalle, M.C., Paintrand, M., Weber, T., Bornens, M. and Karsenti, E. Parthenogenesis in Xenopus eggs requires centrosomal integrity. J. Cell Biol. 1990; 110: 405-415.

[36] Kolchanov NA, Anan'ko EA, Kolpakov FA, Podkolodnaia OA, Ignat'eva EV, Goriachkovskaia TN, et al. Gene networks. Mol Biol 2000;4:533e44.

[37] Kriouchkova MM, Onishchenco GE. Structural and functional characteristics of the centrosome in gametogenesis and early embryogenesisi of animals. Intern Rev Cytol 1999;185:107e56.

[38] Lagos-Quintana M, Rauhut R, Lendeckel W, Tuschl T. Identification of novel genes coding for small expressed RNAs. Science 2001; 294:853e8.

[39] Lambert JD, Nagy LM. Asymmetric inheritance of centrosomally localized mRNAs during embryonic cleavages. Nature 2002; 420:682e6.

[40] Lau NC, Lim LP, Weinstein EG, Bartel DP. An abundant class of tiny RNAs with probable regulatory roles in Caenorhabditis elegans. Science 2001;294:858e62.

[41] Lee RC, Ambros V. An extensive class of small RNAs in Caenorhabditis elegans. Science 2001;294:862e4.

[42] Lecuyer E, Yoshida H, Parthasarathy N, Alm C, Babak T, Cerovina T, Hughes TR, Tomancak P, Krause HM. Global analysis of mRNA localization reveals a prominent role in organizing cellular architecture and function. Cell. 2007; 131(1): 174-187.

[43] Lopez de Heredia M, Jansen RP. mRNA localization and the cytoskeleton. Curr Opin Cell Biol. 2004; 16(1): 80-85.

[44] Malaitcev VV, Bogdanov IM, Sukhikh GT. Contemporary introduction of biology of stem cell. Ark Pathol 2002;4:7e11 [in Russian].

[45] Manandkhar G, Khodjakov AL, Onishenko GE. Modified PEGDMSO- Serum method induces high rate of fusion. Cell Biol IntRep 1990;14:82e6.

[46] Maniotis A, Schliva M. Microsurgical removal of centrosomes block cell reproduction and centriole generation in BSC-1 cells. Cell 1991;67:495e504.

[47] Margulis L., Chapman M., Guerrero R., Hall J. The last eukaryotic common ancestor (LECA): acquisition of cytoskeletal motility from aerotolerant spirochetes in the Proterozoic Eon. Proc Natl Acad Sci U S A. 2006; 103(35): 13080-13085

[48] Maro B, Gueth-Hallonet C, Aghion J, Antony C. Cell polarity and microtubule organisation during mouse early embryogenesis. Dev Suppl 1991;1:17e25.

[49] McManus MT, Sharp PA. Gene silencing in mammals by small interfering RNAs. Nat Rev Genet 2002;3:737e47.

[50] Miska E., Alvarez-Saavedra E., Townsend M. et al. Microarray analysis of microRNA expression in the developing mammalian brain. Genome Biol. 2004; 5: R68.

[51] Montgomery MK, Xu S, Fire A. RNA as a target of double/stranded RNA/mediated genetic interference in Caenorhabditis elegans. Proc Natl Acad Sci USA 1998;95:15502e7.

[52] Nadejdina ES, Fais D, Chentsov YuS. Some biomedical aspects of centriole and basal bodies. Macrosomal Funct Cell 2 Sov-Ital. Sympos, Pushchino, 1982, b2, Moscow, p. 163 [in Russian].

[53] Neverova AL, Uzbekov RE, Votchal MS, Vorobjev IA. Effect of microirradiation of the centrosome on cell behaviour. IV. Synthetic activity, spreading and growth of cells with an inactivated centrosome. Tsitologiia 1996;2:145e54 [in Russian].

[54] Nijs M, Vanderswalmen P, Vandamme B, Segal-Bertin G, Lejeune B, Segal L, et al. Fertilizing ability of immotile spermatozoa after intracytoplasmic sperm injection. Hum Reprod 1996;11:2180e5.

[55] Palacios I.M. and St Johnston D. Getting the message across: the intracellular localization of mRNAs in higher eukaryotes. Annu Rev Cell Dev Biol. 2001; 17: 569-614.

[56] Palazzo R.E., Vogel J.M. Isolation of centrosomes from Spisula solidissima oocytes. Methods Cell Biol. 1999; 61: 35-56

[57] Pederson T. The centrosome: built on an mRNA? Nat Cell Biol. 2006; 8(7):652-654

[58] Peterson SP, Berns MW. The centriolar complex. Intern Rev Cytol 1980;64:81e106.

[59] Peterson, S.P., and Berns, M.W. Evidence for centriolar region RNA functioning in spindle formation in dividing PTK2 cells. J. Cell. Sci., 1978; 34; 289-301.

[60] Phillips SG, Rattner JB. Dependence of centriole formation on protein synthesis. J Cell Biol 1976;70:9e19.

[61] Roskelley C.D., Srebrow A., Bissell M.J. A hierarchy of ECM-mediated signalling regulates tissue-specific gene expression. Curr Opin Cell Biol. 1995; 7(5): 736-47.

[62] Rudolph KL, Chang S, Lee H, Blasco M, Gottlieb GJ, Greider C, et al. Longevity, stress response, and cancer in aging telomerasedeficient mice. Cell 1999;96:701e12.

[63] Schatten G. The centrosome and its mode of inheritance: the reduction of the centrosome during gametogenesis and its restoration during fertilization. Dev. Biol. 1994; 165: 299-335.

[64] Schatten H, Schatten G, Mazia D, Balezon R, Simerly C. Behavior of centrosomes during fertilization and cell division in mouse oocytes and sea urchin eggs. Proc Natl Acad Sci U S A 1996;83:105e9.

[65] Shay JW,Wright WE. Ageing and cancdr: the telomere and telomerase connection. Novartis Found Symp 2001;235:116e25.

[66] Sluiman HJ. A cladistic evaluation of the lower and higher green plants (Viridiplantae). Plant Syst Evol 1985;149:217e32.

[67] Stuckenholz C, Kageyama Y, Kuroda MI. Guilt by association: noncoding RNAs, chromosome-specific proteins and dosage compensation in Drosophila. Trends Genet 1999;15:454e8.

[68] Tekotte H., Davis I. Intracellular mRNA localization: motors move messages. Trends Genet. 2002; 18(12): 636-642.

[69] Tkemaladze D., Chichinadze K. Potential role of centrioles in determining the morphogenetic status of animal somatic cells (hypothesis). Cell Biol Int. 2005; 5: 370-374.

[70] Chichinadze K.N., Tkemaladze D.V. Centrosomal hypothesis of cellular ageing and differentiation. Adv Geront. 2008; 21(3): 367-371. Russian.

[71] Tkemaladze J., Chichinadze K. Centriole, Differentiation and Senescence. Rejuven Res. 2010; 13(2-3): 339-342.

[72] Tkemaladze J.V., Chichinadze K.N. Centriolar Mechanisms of Differentiation and Replicative Aging of Higher Animal Cells. Biochemistry (Moscow). 2005; 70(11): 1288-1303.

[73] Wianny F, Zernickab-Goets M. Specific interference with gene function by double-stranded RNA in early mouse development. Nat Cell Biol 2000;2:70e5.

[74] Zilberman D, Cao X, Jacobsen SE. ARGONAUTE4 control of locusspecific siRNA accumulation and DNA and histone methylation. Science 2003;299:716e9.

13

Cellular Degradation Machineries in Age-Related Loss of Muscle Mass (Sarcopenia)

Mikael Altun[1], Max Grönholdt-Klein[1], Lingzhan Wang[1,2] and Brun Ulfhake[1]
[1]*Department of Neuroscience, Karolinska Institutet, Stockholm,*
[2]*Department of Human Anatomy, School of Medicine, Inner Mongolia University for Nationalities, Tongliao City,*
[1]*Sweden*
[2]*P. R. China*

1. Introduction

One of the most characteristic features of the aged is a change in body composition and human cross-sectional and longitudinal studies consistently demonstrate gain in fat mass and decline in lean mass (Attaix et al., 2005). Skeletal muscle mass is gradually reduced through both atrophy and loss of myofibers, and along with this connective tissue and intramyocellular lipids increase (Fig. 1) (St-Onge, 2005). Although sarcopenia is widely recognized it remains poorly understood and has not received appropriate attention until quite recently. Sarcopenia is often assumed to have a multi-factorial background (Adamo and Farrar, 2006; Attaix et al., 2005; Paddon-Jones and Rasmussen, 2009; Roth et al., 2006; Solomon and Bouloux, 2006). A sedentary life-style combined with periods of prolonged bed-rest during illnesses has well-established detrimental effects on muscle mass and function (Janssen et al., 2002). Skeletal muscles do not only generate the power to let us move but collectively they are a highly significant component of the systemic metabolic homeostasis machinery. The progressive loss of muscle mass with advancing age is evident in both the 'healthy' aging population and specialist patient populations. The reduced functional muscle mass is associated with increased morbidity, frailty and reduced quality of life (Baumgartner et al., 1998a). The prevalence of sarcopenia increases with about 5% per year and typically begins in the fourth decade of life (Baumgartner et al., 1998b). After the age of 50 years 1-2 % of the muscle mass is lost annually. Individuals with clinically manifest sarcopenia have 4 times greater risk of disability, three times greater risk of balance impairment, and 3 times greater risk of falling (Baumgartner et al., 1998b). Sarcopenia is the single most common etiology to falls and fall-associated fractures in elderly.

1.1 Regulation of muscle mass and tentative mechanisms in sarcopenia

Myofibers are complex structures build-up by merger of aligned myocytes (myotubes as intermediates). Thus, the myofiber has a common plasma membrane confining multiple sub domains each supported by one myonucleus. According to morphometric analysis the ratio myofiber volume to a myonucleus remains fairly constant suggesting an optimal size of the domain supported by the machinery of one myonucleus. The impressive increase in muscle mass during late fetal and postnatal development but also in conditions of repair in adult muscle across life-span is dependent on recruitment of myogenic progenitors from the resident satellite cells (SC) in the stem cell niche (Kadi et al., 2005). SCs remain quiescent until activation through trophic stimuli e.g. IGF-1 and Notch-related signaling (Carlson et al., 2008). The activity of the SC pool is under the influence of several signaling pathways, enhancing or inhibiting SC proliferation, such as Wnt-β–Catenin, DeltaL/Jagged1-Notch or Smad2/3- TGF-β/Activin/Myostatin (Carlson et al., 2008; Zammit, 2008).

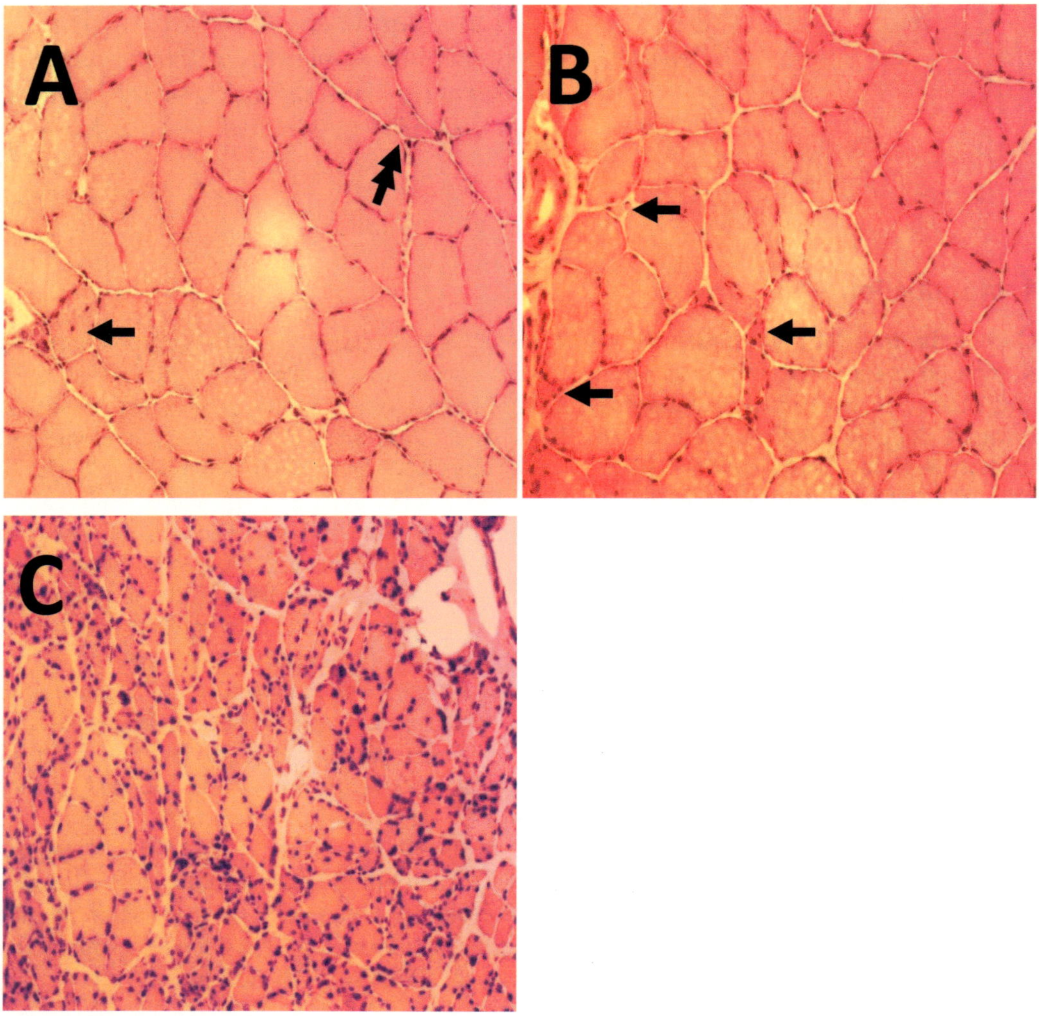

Fig. 1. **Changes in fiber size and occurrence of nuclei with a central location in aged rat soleus muscle.** Eosin-Htx staining of soleus cross sections (8μm) showing (A) young adult muscle where central nuclei (arrow) and very small fibers (double arrow) are infrequent. In early aging (B) fiber size becomes more irregular and the frequency of very small fibers increases (arrows). At advanced age (C) fiber size is highly irregular and centrally located nuclei are frequently occurring. Original micrographs shot with a x20 dry objective.

The signaling events leading to myofiber atrophy converge onto members of the FOXO family of transcription factors, which in an active state induce atrophy by increased proteasome degradation of myofibrillar proteins (Bodine et al., 2001; Sacheck et al., 2007; Sacheck et al., 2004; Sandri et al., 2004; Stitt et al., 2004). Recently, it was discovered that the signaling pathway that activates FOXO also induces an increased degradation through autophagy and lysosomal degradation (Sandri et al., 2006; Solomon and Bouloux, 2006). This "atrophy program" is activated in a range of conditions such as disuse, denervation and systemic diseases (Solomon and Bouloux, 2006). Conversely, myofiber contraction and growth signals (e.g. IGF-1) acting via protein kinase B, mTOR, and pgc-1α induce synthesis of myofibrillar proteins, deactivation of FOXO and, in parallel, adaptation of the energy producing machinery (*idem*). The Activin A/myostatin pathway, acting on Act receptor IIB upstream of Smad, can activate myofibrillar proteolysis (i.e. induce muscle fiber atrophy) and depress SC proliferation (Zhou et al., 2010). This creates a regulatory link between cellular anabolism & catabolism and SC activation & deactivation which should work in concert in conditions with atrophy and hypertrophy, respectively.

A growing body of evidence suggests that loss of muscle mass in elderly occurs through mechanisms more complex than those involved in disuse and disease atrophy in younger individuals (Altun et al., 2010; Edstrom et al., 2007; Edstrom and Ulfhake, 2005). In humans and rodents alike, a number of mechanisms have been suggested to underpin sarcopenia: 1) loss of innervation 2) disuse 3) impaired maintenance and repair including decline in endo-, para- and autocrine signaling (e.g. IGF-1) 4) systemic inflammation 5) imbalance between protein synthesis and degradation and 6) poor nutrition (Adamo and Farrar, 2006; Attaix et al., 2005; Paddon-Jones and Rasmussen, 2009; Roth et al., 2006; Solomon and Bouloux, 2006). However, awaiting more definitive evidence it remains unclear if the mechanism behind loss of muscle mass in elderly is different from that operating in muscle atrophy in young individuals. It should be noted that the progress over the past decade in our understanding changes in muscle mass in health and disease stems mainly from work done in laboratory animals, in particular rodents, and highlights:

1. ***Impaired regeneration of myonuclei from SCs.*** The satellite cell pool has been reported to be reduced in aged individuals and the frequency of myonuclear apoptosis to increase, however, these changes have not been directly associated with the loss of muscle mass in sarcopenia. A reduced SC pool could be consequence of an imbalance of SC recruitment/activation and the replenishment of the SC pool (see above). Furthermore, reports suggest also that age-induced changes in the microenvironment influence utilization of the SC through negative effects on proliferation and differentiation of the SCs and that in the aged the SCs are not activated on demand as in adults (Carlson et al., 2009). Importantly, inhibition of, or failure, to activate SC may augment proliferation of other progenitor cells known to co-exist in the skeletal muscle (Christov et al., 2007). An interplay exists between myogenic cells and fibro/adipogenic cells, and myogenic cells are known to inhibit fibro/adipogenic cells in the SC niche (Rodeheffer, 2010). In animal models this has demonstrated to influence muscle regeneration i.e. the scar tissue formation and fat storage in the skeletal muscle (Fuso et al., 2010), i.e. well-established features of the sarcopenic muscle.
2. ***Loss of innervation.*** Observations in aged human skeletal muscle have shown loss of myofibers, myofiber-atrophy, a selective vulnerability of type IIa fibers and fiber-type grouping suggesting that an underlying mechanism is a progressive age-dependent denervation (Larsson, 1995). Direct observations in animal models have shown both a progressive denervation (Valdez et al., 2010a) and a dramatic increase in fibers re-

expressing the embryonic isoform of myosin (eMyHC; Fig. 2) (Edstrom and Ulfhake, 2005) while the expression levels of adult MyHC isoforms decline (Altun et al., 2007b). In related work using a denervation/re-innervation animal model we have obtained evidence that the re-expression of nicotinic acetylcholine receptor subunit gamma (nAChR-γ) is a reliable marker for muscle denervation (Grönholdt-Klein et al., in preparation) and in animal models on sarcopenia we consistently find a dramatic increase in nAChR-γ expression. Earlier work also showed that spinal motoneurons innervating aged atrophic skeletal muscles show a regenerative phenotype suggesting an impaired contact with the target myofibers (Johnson et al., 1995). Combined, these observations suggest denervation as a significant component of sarcopenia.

3. ***Protein degradation and proteotoxicity.*** Accumulation of damaged proteins is a hallmark of aging that is believed to reflect increased imbalance between generation and scavenging of radicals, and/or decreased ability to degrade damaged proteins (Harriman et al., 1970). A number of studies have reported on an accumulation of oxidatively damaged proteins in aged rodent muscle (Cai et al., 2004; Clavel et al., 2006) as well as increased levels of chaperones that selectively bind unfolded proteins (Clavel et al., 2006; Ferrington et al., 2005). Several groups have published observations suggesting a decreased proteasomal proteolysis as a mechanism for the buildup of worn-out and otherwise damaged proteins in aged rodent skeletal muscle (Ferrington et al., 2005), however, it is hard to reconcile such a reduced rate of proteolysis with the general loss of skeletal muscle mass characteristic of aging (sarcopenia).

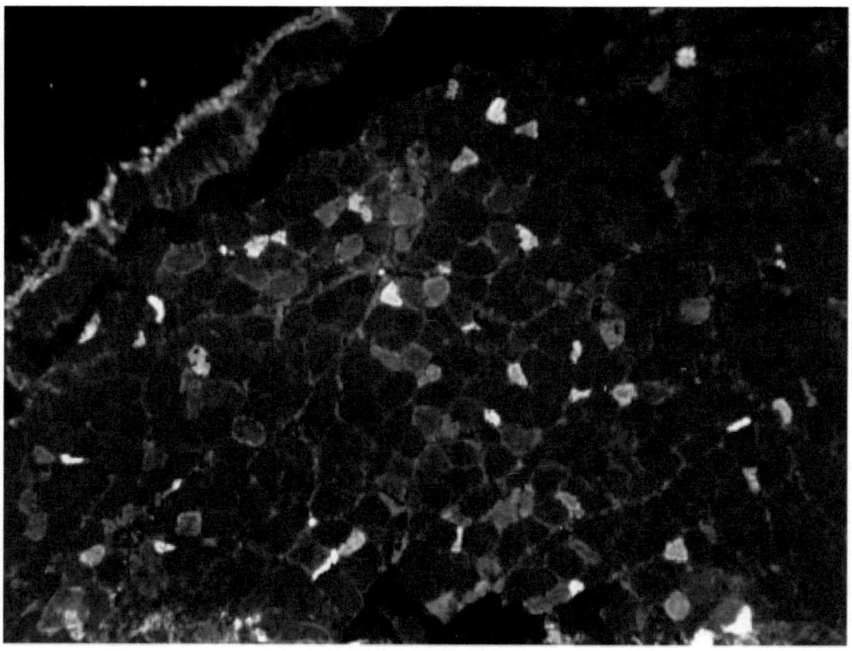

Fig. 2. **Re-expression of the embryonic myosin (eMyHC) in the soleus muscle of an aged mouse.** Immunofluorescence micrograph of an 8 µm thick cross-section through the mid portion of a soleus muscle from a 28 month-old C57BL/6J mouse. Light profiles often with an irregular out-line and small size indicate fibers expressing embryonic MyHC probably caused by an age-related loss of innervation. Original magnification x20.

This chapter will focus on the main cellular degradation machineries and our current understanding of how age-related changes in these systems impact skeletal muscle integrity.

2. Regulated proteolysis

Regulated proteolysis is instrumental for such diverse cellular processes as signaling, cell cycle progression, and apoptosis. Protein and organelle degradation enables recycling of the building blocks and is also an important survival response to starvation, whereby proteins are degraded to supply the organism with fuel for energy production. The accumulation of aggregates of misfolded proteins is a hallmark of cells and tissues of aged organisms, and protein aggregation occurs when damaged or partially unfolded proteins are not efficiently degraded. Disposal of proteins is in most conditions a selective and coordinated process, handled mainly by two cellular proteolytic systems, the ubiquitin-proteasomal system (UPS) and autophagy-lysosomal system (ALS).

2.1 The ubiquitin proteasomal system (UPS)

Work over the last 25 years has established the importance of regulating protein ubiquitination in a wide range of cellular functions including cell cycle control, transcriptional regulation, and diverse aspects of cell signaling. Lysine[48] polyubiquitination targets proteins for degradation by the proteasome, a highly selective mechanism by which multiple cellular processes are being modulated. Collectively, the proteasome and enzymes involved in ubiquitination are referred to as the ubiquitin proteasomal system (UPS) (Fig. 3).

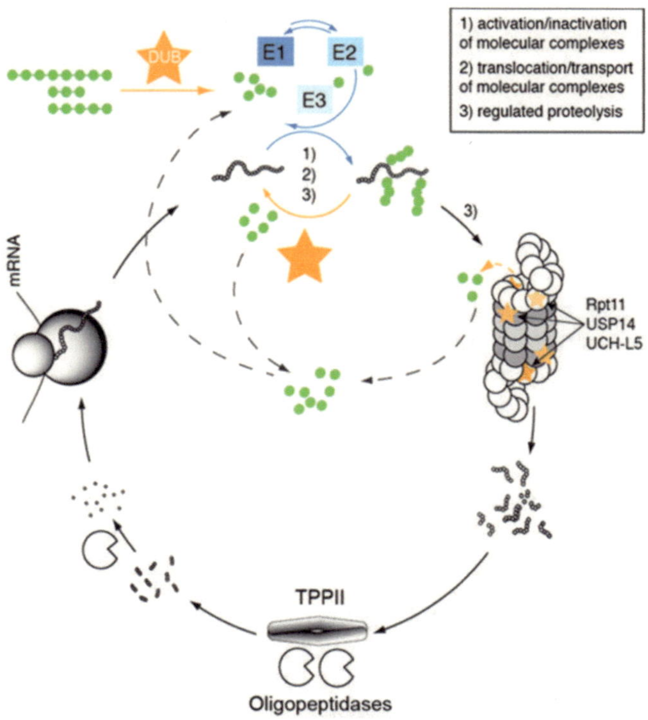

Fig. 3. **The ubiquitin proteasomal system.** Cartoon of the different components of the ubiquitin-proteasomal system described in the text.

However, ubiquitination does not only associate with proteasomal degradation, other forms of ubiquitination play roles in such diverse processes as transcriptional regulation, endocytosis, DNA modifications and stabilization of protein complexes (Harper and Schulman, 2006). Ubiquitin (Ub) is transcribed as precursor proteins from 4 genes and after cleavage to monomeric Ub, Ub-conjugation occurs through an enzymatic cascade where the E3-ligases (>600 E3 ligases have been identified so far) provide for target specificity. Prior to cleavage in the proteasome of a lys^{48} poly-Ub conjugated protein, the Ub-recognition signal is removed (Fig. 3). This serves to enhance passage of the targeted protein into the catalytic chamber and will also free ubiquitin for reuse and hinder the proteasomes to be preoccupied with destroying Ub [itself] (Hanna et al., 2007; Koulich et al., 2008). Hydrolysis of bound Ub and processing of Ub precursor proteins is accomplished by members of the large group of deubiquitinating enzymes (DUBs) (>90 members identified so far); DUBs are cysteine proteases that can be divided into distinct subfamilies based on sequence similarities and likely mechanism of action (reviewed in Nijman et al., 2005). Since DUBs can reshuffle ubiquitin from poly- to mono- or multi-ubiquitin chains, they are not only important for protein half-life but probably all cellular processes that involve ubiquitination of proteins (Clague and Urbe, 2006).

2.2 Activation of the UPS in sarcopenia

Because available data on the integrity of the UPS in the elderly was controversial we examined in 30-month old Sprague-Dawley rats the effects of aging on the content and activity of 26S proteasomes, proteasome-associated regulatory proteins and various other components of the UPS, including multiple DUBs (Altun et al., 2010). Muscles of these aged animals undergo marked atrophy compared to muscles of young adult animals and this age-related atrophy could be impeded if the animals were maintained on a restricted diet (Altun et al., 2007a). Analysis of proteasome protein content and proteasome degradation capacity in these animals revealed a 2-3 fold increase in proteasomes in the aged muscle. The increase in 26S proteasomes was suppressed completely in aged animals maintained on a restricted diet (30% of the consumption recorded for rats having free access to food). Since muscle wasting was reduced in these animals, these findings suggest that the buildup of proteasomes contributes to the loss of muscle mass in aged animals. In support of this notion we found that the levels of proteasome subunits in aged skeletal muscle were inversely correlated with muscle weight (subunits β1: $r=-0.71$, $p<0.05$; β5: $r=-0.69$; $p<0.05$), and no such inverse relationship was found in muscles of adult rats or aged animals maintained on dietary restriction (Altun et al., 2010). However, the underlying mechanism of this accumulation remains unclear. In contrast to muscles atrophying due to disuse, fasting or various systemic diseases, the age-related accumulation of proteasomes occurred without any increase in corresponding mRNAs. Thus, the accumulation of proteasomes in aged muscle must be due to enhanced subunit translation, more efficient assembly of the 26S particles, or slower degradation of the 26S particles (see below under 2.4).

Previous reports suggested that age-related decrease in the proteasome's peptidase activities were due to oxidative modifications (Bulteau et al., 2000; Conconi et al., 1996; Ferrington et al., 2005; Grune et al., 2001; Hayashi and Goto, 1998; Keller et al., 2000). However, we could not observe such defect in degrading capacity towards a range of substrates including ubiquitinated native proteins (Fig. 4). Instead, our data indicates that proteasome content increases during sarcopenia, and that these particles retain their full ability to function in protein breakdown. Together these findings suggest that the enhanced capacity of the UPS may be a response to the increased generation of damaged polypeptides. Strong support for this conclusion is our finding of elevated levels of the ubiquitin ligases, CHIP and E6AP, in muscle of aged animals. CHIP ubiquitinates misfolded or mutated proteins bound to Hsp70 or Hsp90 (Connell et al., 2001), and recently a similar function in cellular quality control has been reported for E6AP (Mishra et al., 2009). Moreover, most of these conclusions about a negative impact of aging on proteasomal degradation in muscle were based exclusively on measurements of the 20S core particle. Although some degradation of unfolded or denatured proteins may occur by the free 20S (Jariel-Encontre et al., 2008), the bulk of proteasome-mediated degradation, even of oxidatively damaged proteins (Medicherla and Goldberg, 2008), seems to require the 26S proteasome and ubiquitylation of the substrate.

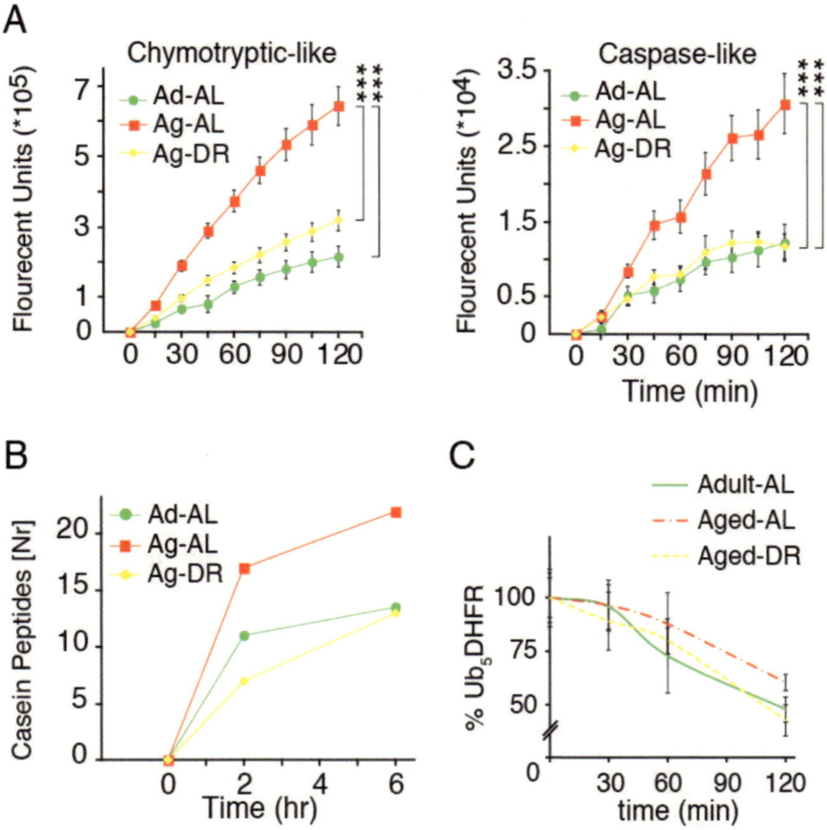

Fig. 4. **Degradation capacity towards different substrates of proteasomes isolated from triceps surae muscle of adult rats (Ad-AL), aged (Ag-AL) and aged rats maintained on dietary restriction (Ag-DR)** (original data reproduced from Altun et al., 2010). The higher content per unit muscle mass of proteasomes in aged (Ag-AL) muscles is paralleled by a corresponding increase in degradation of synthetic peptides designed for the chymotryptic and caspase sites of the proteasome (A) as well as casein (B). In (C) degradation of a native ubiquitinylated protein is shown illustrating that we could not detect any impairment of the degradation capacity of 26S proteasomes isolated from aged rats muscle. Further details on experimental design in Altun at al., 2010.

A decline in the cell's pool of free ubiquitin can limit the rate of proteolysis by the proteasome (Hanna et al., 2003; Kimura et al., 2009) and free ubiquitin is in turn released during degradation of ubiquitylated proteins by the DUBs associated with the 26S proteasome. Thus, in order to achieve high degradation rates, the capacity for deubiquitylation probably needs to be increased too. Using mechanism-based probes to assess the state of DUB activity and expression (Altun et al., 2010), eleven DUB-enzymes were found to be strongly up-regulated in the muscles of aged rats; including USP14 and Uch37 which are known to be associated with the 26S proteasome. USP14 and UCH37 trim off ubiquitin from the polyubiquitin chain and release ubiquitin monomers for re-use. In addition, USP14 controls gate opening into the 20S proteasome and facilitates substrate degradation (Peth et al., 2009). On the other hand, the yeast homolog of USP14, Ubp6, regulates the overall rate of proteolysis and appears critical in replenishing the free ubiquitin pool in yeast (Hanna et al., 2003; Hanna et al., 2007). Similarly, USP5 hydrolyses anchorless ubiquitin chains (Reyes-Turcu et al., 2006; Reyes-Turcu et al., 2008) and appears to work downstream of Rpn11, an intrinsic DUB on the proteasome, to prevent the binding of free ubiquitin chains to the 19S, which would inhibit proteolysis. Together these data illustrate important roles for deubiquitylation in the aged muscle, probably ensuring a supply of ubiquitin for enhanced proteolysis but perhaps also serving additional regulatory functions.

Loss of muscle mass can occur through increased protein degradation but also decreased protein synthesis or through some combination of these responses. With aging, sarcopenia develops over months to years depending on the species, unlike the rapid loss of muscle weight induced by fasting, disuse, and in various catabolic diseases, where marked atrophy (20-50% loss) can occur in rodents in several days. In these latter types of rapid atrophy, as described above, there is a common program of changes in the transcription of a set of atrophy-related genes (Lecker et al., 2006; Lecker et al., 2004; Sacheck et al., 2007). Several of the biochemical changes observed in aged atrophic muscle clearly distinguish them from those undergoing rapid atrophy in adult animals. Upon denervation or fasting, the atrophy-specific ubiquitin ligases, Atrogin-1/MAFbx and MuRF1, are induced by members of the FOXO family of transcription factors, and this induction is essential for the rapid weight loss (Bodine et al., 2001; Lecker et al., 2006; Sandri et al., 2004). Inhibition of FOXOs prevents their induction and the loss of muscle mass upon denervation, fasting, or glucocorticoid treatment (Sandri et al., 2004). In contrast, in the aged muscles, mRNAs for Atrogin-1/MAFbx, MuRF1 and the Ub-conjugating enzyme, E2-14K, were unchanged or lower than adult levels (Edstrom et al., 2006). Also, treatment with the glucocorticoid dexamethasone failed to induce Atrogin-1/MAFbx or MuRF1 or to cause muscle wasting, as it does in adult animals (Bodine et al., 2001; Gomes et al., 2001). However, MuRF1 protein increased in aged muscle, while Atrogin-1/MAFbx protein decreased (in accord with the mRNA data). Another distinction between sarcopenia and rapid atrophy is that the ubiquitin ligases, CHIP and E6AP, increased markedly in the aged muscle, though they do not rise in rapidly atrophying muscles. Their induction may reflect adaptations in the aged muscle to eliminate more efficiently misfolded proteins.

In summary, the finding of increased content of proteasomes and other UPS components (e.g. MuRF1) argues that proteolysis also increases in these muscles and may contribute to muscle wasting in the aged rats. Dietary restriction decreased levels of proteasomes and several other UPS components toward the levels in adult animal and partially inhibited the development of sarcopenia.

2.3 Accumulation of ubiquitinated proteins in sarcopenic muscles

During muscle atrophy in adult animals induced by fasting, disuse or disease, there is a marked increase in protein ubiquitination and proteolysis, especially of myofibrillar components (Lecker et al., 1999; Mitch and Goldberg, 1996). If the rate of ubiquitination exceeds the rate of Ub-dependent proteolysis, Ub-protein will accumulate; this will also occur if proteins are damaged or rearranged (multimeric aggregates) in a way that hinders normal proteasomal degradation. Immunoblotting of muscle extracts with an anti-ubiquitin antibody reveal that the muscles from aged rats contained greater amounts of ubiquitylated proteins than those from adult rats (Fig.5B; see also (Altun et al., 2010)). An increase in free ubiquitin and ubiquitin conjugates with aging was also reported by others in rat muscles (Cai et al., 2004; Clavel et al., 2006). Since the 26S proteasomes isolated from aged muscle are fully active in degrading ubiquitylated proteins, the elevated levels of ubiquitylated proteins strongly suggest higher overall rates of protein ubiquitylation that exceed the rates of conjugate degradation or the formation of nondegradable Ub-protein aggregates. Immunohistochemical analysis (using the same antibody towards ubiquitin) show that some of the fibers in aged skeletal muscles contain Ub+ deposits (Fig. 5A).

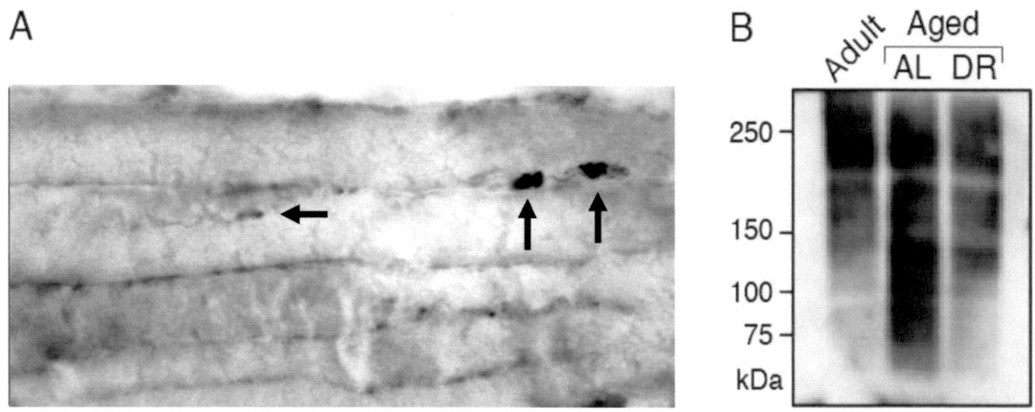

Fig. 5. **Amount of ubiquitylated protein is increased in aged skeletal muscle.** (A) shows micrograph of an aged soleus muscle cut along fiber length and processed with an antibody that recognizes ubiquitylated proteins using the ABC peroxidase technique. Ub+ protein deposits appear in black (arrows) and vary in size but are usually localized to the peripheral domain of the fiber (original micrograph was taken with an x20 dry objective). (B) shows a immunoblot of muscle extract from adult, aged and aged rats maintained on dietary restriction (DR) using the same antibody as in (A). The amount of Ub-proteins is clearly higher in aged fed ad libitum, while aged rats on DR are more similar to adults.

2.4 The autophagy lysosomal system (ALS)

Ubiquitination is also involved in processes leading to abrogation of signal transduction and targeting of the receptors for destruction by the autophagosome lysosomal system (ALS; Fig. 6). One example is the monoubiquitin-dependent endocytosis and degradation of epidermal growth factor receptor (Haglund et al., 2003; Mizuno et al., 2005). Degradation through the LS involves not only proteins but also damaged cell organelles and large complexes (Cuervo et al., 2005; Terman and Brunk, 2006; Terman et al., 2006). Multiple vesicles that constantly fuse and fission constitute the lysosomal system. Lysosomal degradation is initiated through several pathways based on the substrate delivering mechanism (Fig. 6): Endocytosis (clathrin mediated pinching-off of membrane patches with/without inclusion of extracellular material) occurs and the resulting particle is referred to as an endosomes (carrying rab5). Endosomes can then develop into late endosomes, which are equipped with enzymes delivered by secretory vesicles from the trans-Golgi-network and sorted by mannose-6-phosphate receptors, which are markers for late endosomes. Late endosomes may also fuse with lysosomes (then they lose the mannose-6-phosphate receptors).

A second route is chaperone mediated autophagy (CMA), which targets proteins carrying a pentapeptide (KFERQ) motif that is recognized by the chaperon Hsc73 and through binding to the LAMP-2A receptor (lysosome associated membrane protein 2A; a marker of the lysosome), the targeted protein is taken up and degraded in the lysosomal lumen (Fig. 6). The major route for organelles and proteins targeted for lysosomal degradation is via autophagy, a process controlled by the autophagy-conjugase complexes Atg12-Atg5 and Atg8-Atg3 (Atg, autophagy related genes) whereby in-bulk cytoplasm becomes entrapped in a double membrane forming an autophagosome (autophagic vacuole, AV) (Terman and Brunk, 2004).

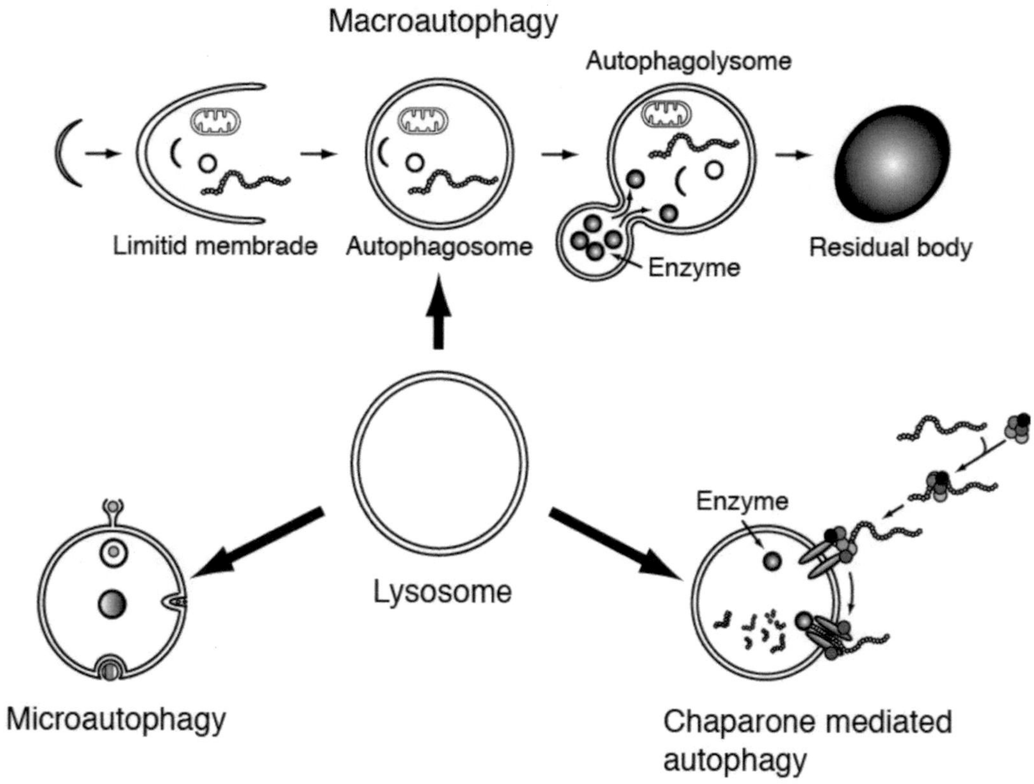

Fig. 6. **Schematic drawing of the autophagy-lysosomal system.** The different cargo routes to lysosomal degradation are illustrated and described in the text.

Subsequently, the autophagosome fuses with a lysosome for degradation under the formation of an autophagolysosome (Fig. 6). With the formation of the AV, the Atg conjugase complexes disassociate, but the Atg 8 (the mammalian homologue is MAP-LC3) remains in the ALS until degradation. While, Atg8 may be a marker for AVs and [by its elimination also] the completion of this degradation route, the autophagy conjugase complexes indicate ongoing ALS formation/autophagy. The role of the autophagy-lysosomal system was not widely recognized until it was demonstrated that cathepsins (D and B+L, respectively; (Felbor et al., 2002)) and autophagy (Hara et al., 2006) were non-redundant for a normal development and that cells rely on a basal level of autophagy to keep them free of worn-out organelles and aberrant proteins.

2.5 Signs of distress of the ALS during aging

There is solid evidence for the engagement of autophagy in major human degenerative diseases and in normal aging. A decreased capacity of the lysosomes to degrade waste will cause a build-up of damaged organelles and proteins disturbing cell homeostasis; and e.g. accumulation of dysfunctional mitochondria in aging cardiomyocytes, myofibers and neurons has been reported. Recently, several studies have shown that the induction of autophagy, by intervention of the above discussed signaling pathways, increase cellular clearance of aberrant proteins also when the normal degradation route operates via the proteasome or through CMA. The load on the ALS in normal aging is evident from the dramatic accumulation of lipofuscin by time (Fig. 7 G-H) and the concomitant upregulation of markers of lysosomal proteolysis. Lipofuscin forms due to iron-catalyzed intralysosomal peroxidation and its accumulation in the lysosomal compartment seems to set down the capacity of autophagy (Brunk and Terman, 2002). Oxidative stress, even mild stress, accelerates the formation/build-up of lipofuscin (Kurz et al., 2008) and stress can cause lysosomes to become leaky due to intralysosomal reactive iron mediated Fenton- reactions with production of hydroxyl radicals and resulting labilization of the lysosomal membrane. Even though the pH is suboptimal, several of the lysosomal enzymes are apparently proteolytically active if released to the cytosol and may then trigger cell degeneration/death (Chu, 2006).

Analysis of atrophic skeletal muscle in aged rats (Altun et al., 2007b) revealed increased levels of molecules involved in iron transport (transferrin), binding (ferritin), as well as iron response element binding protein-1 activity; combined these observations suggest increased load on the iron-handling machinery. Measurements of iron levels revealed a significant accumulation in the aged skeletal muscle, providing further support for iron loading in senescence. Iron-loading increases the risk for common hallmarks of aging such as DNA damage, protein oxidation and misfolding, and lipid peroxidation and may accelerate the accumulation of lipofuscin (see above). Iron-load is not exclusive to aging-related muscle wasting, but is also evident in experimental disuse atrophy (Kondo et al., 1992) and iron-restriction has been shown to be beneficiary in certain inherited myopathies (Bornman et al., 1998).

3. Cross talk between the UPS and the ALS

Until recently the UPS and the ALS were considered as independent pathways for protein degradation. The UPS offers a fast and highly specific mechanism to remove selected proteins. However, the targeted protein must be a monomer and unfolded to be able to enter the proteolytic lumen of the proteasome. The ALS represents a partly overlapping, partly complementary degradation route, taking care of folded and aggregated proteins as well as large complexes and organelles with heterogenic building blocks (carbohydrates, lipids and proteins). However, several lines of evidence indicate intersections between these two pathways. In neurons treated with proteasome inhibitors, aggregate-prone proteins normally degraded by the UPS are degraded by autophagy (Cuervo et al., 2004). Two recent papers also provide evidence that induction of the UPS and LS may occur via a common pathway in skeletal muscle (Mammucari et al., 2007; Zhou et al., 2010).

Several studies report that with increasing age the capacity for lysosomal proteolysis is reduced in postmitotic cells including myofibers, while the capacity to degrade proteins through the UPS is enhanced (see above). Given that transcription of proteasome subunits and the expression of proteins involved in the assembly of the 20S were unaltered in in aged rodents, we hypothesized that proteasome particles accumulate in muscles during aging because they are not degraded at the same rate as in young adults. It is currently unknown which mechanism is responsible for the degradation of proteasomes, although the lysosomal pathway was suggested to accomplish this task in hepatocytes (Cuervo et al., 1995). To test whether this mechanism may be present in skeletal muscle cells, we treated adult rats (Fig.7A-C) and rat muscle derived cell line L6, respectively, with the lysosomal inhibitor chloroquine followed by quantitation of proteasome levels and activity (Fig.7A-F). In these experiments, we observed an accumulation of proteasomes accompanied by increased active site labeling in the muscle extracts from both chloroquine treated animals and L6 cell extracts.

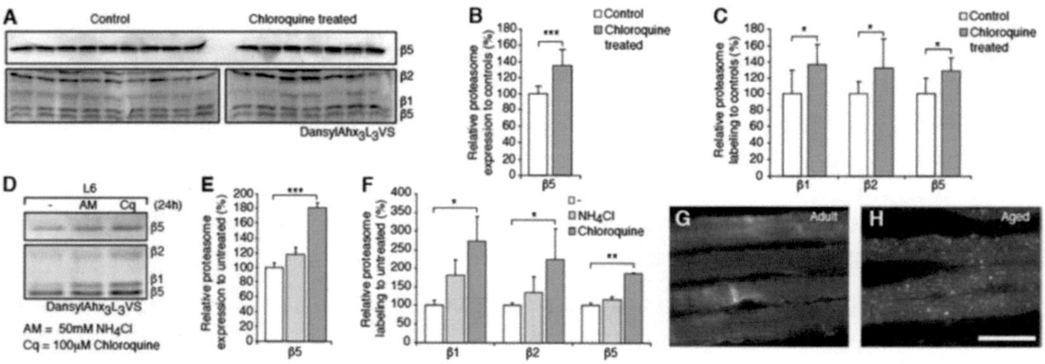

Fig. 7. **Compromised lysosomal proteolysis increases proteasome content and activity.** (**A-C**) Adult animals treated with chloroquine (50mg/kg) for 16 days (1 injection/day). (**A**) Immunoblot against proteasome subunit b5 to assay proteasome content (top) and proteasome labeling (bottom) using the active site directed probe $DansylAhx_3L_3VS$. (**B**) Individual bands were quantified for b5 content and (**C**) active site directed probe $DansylAhx_3L_3VS$ labeling of the b1, b2 and b5 catalytic subunits. (**D-F**) Rat muscle derived cell line L6 was treated when confluence reached about 70% with 50mM NH_4Cl or 100mM chloroquine for 24 hour before lysis. Immunoblot against proteasome subunit b5 to assay proteasome content (**D** top panel, **E**) and active site labeling of the b1, b2 and b5 catalytic subunits (**D** lower panel, **F**). b-actin was used as loading control for immunoblotting (data not shown). All error bars are standard deviations. Statistical significance: * $p<0.05$, ** $p<0.01$ and *** $p<0.001$. (**G, H**) Lipofuscin accumulation in aged skeletal muscle. Unstained longitudinal sections of soleus muscle form adult (A) and aged (B) rats show increased content of lipofuscin autofluorescence in aged sarcopenic muscle. The bar represents 100μm

As in the aged rat muscles, the accumulation of proteasomes following lysosomal inhibition was not induced by a transcriptional up-regulation (data not shown) and therefore results likely from a reduced clearance of proteasomes due to an impairment of lysosomal function. Consistent with this, we observed lipofuscin accumulation in the aged rat muscle tissue (Fig.7 G and H). In addition, Cuervo and colleagues reported that autophagy declines in liver with aging but this effect is reduced by dietary restriction (Hanna et al., 2003; Watts et al., 2004). Activation of autophagy in muscle by dietary restriction could explain our findings that this regime prevented the increase in proteasomes with age without any change in proteasome mRNA levels. Combined these observations suggest the ALS as a candidate pathway for proteasomal degradation awaiting more definitive evidence.

4. Concluding remarks

Human cross-sectional and longitudinal studies have consistently demonstrated a gain in fat mass and decline in lean mass during aging. Although aging-related muscle wasting, or sarcopenia, is widely recognized it still remains poorly understood. The reduced functional muscle mass is associated with increased morbidity and reduced quality of life. To maintain integrity muscle myofibers rely on degradation pathways to keep clean from worn-out organelles and damaged proteins. Our current understanding is that the autophagy-lysosomal system is in distress possibly driven by an age-dependent accumulation of reactive iron, while contrary to the widespread view, the complementary pathway for degradation of proteins, the UPS, is enhanced. The age-dependent increase in the muscle specific ubiquitin-ligase MuRF and ubiquitin-dependent proteasomal proteolysis is expected to occur in the progression of sarcopenia since this route is nonredundant for degradation of myofibrillar proteins. In addition, the UPS in aged skeletal muscle shows adaptations to an increased demand on degradation of aberrant proteins and an accumulation of ubiquitinated proteins. Combined these stigmata suggest that aged myofibers may be at risk to enter a state of proteotoxicity.

Normal skeletal muscles have a good capacity to regenerate following wasting conditions such as disuse. The muscle regenerative response relies on signaling that evokes satellite cell replication and asymmetric division generating offsprings that will differentiate to myocytes via the myoblast stage. Such cells are then incorporated into the myofiber allowing it to grow (for example in response to an exercise stimulus). Poor capacity to regenerate muscle tissue at advanced age may depend on impaired signaling, exhaustion of the SC pool or changes in the extracellular matrix or stem-cell niche impeding the regeneration and incorporation of myoblasts into existing/regenerating myofibers (for references see Introduction). Assessments of the regenerative drive in aged sarcopenic muscle have, however, shown that myogenic differentiation factors are upregulated and that there are overt signs of incorporation of new nuclei into existing fibers (Fig. 1B,C; (Edstrom and Ulfhake, 2005)). Still, regeneration fails and tissue atrophy progresses.

The triggering mechanism for the age-dependent fiber atrophy and fiber loss remains enigmatic. However, several lines of evidence converge towards support of the "neurogenic" theory (Gutman and Hanzlikova, 1972), which stipulates that sarcopenia is driven by a successive drop-out of motoneurons. Early evidence in favor of this theory was the observation of fiber-type grouping and also histological examination revealing regressive changes at the neuro-muscular junctions. The strongest argument against this theory is the absence of unbiased evidence of a significant age-dependent loss of motoneurons. However, as discussed at length elsewhere (Johnson et al., 1995) the denervation may be a peripheral process primarily involving subdomains of the motor axon's terminal arborization within a motor unit (see also (Valdez et al., 2010b)). Failure to maintain the distant axon arbor could cause branches and terminals to degenerate leaving myofibers vacated from innervation. As this process progresses more and more fibers will be denervated and read-outs validating this process are the increase in expression of the nAChR-γ subunit (Gronholdt-Klein et al., in preparation) and embryonic myosin (Edstrom and Ulfhake, 2005); and it should be noted that these proteins are re-expressed by young adult myofibers upon denervation. As denervation becomes significant, it will trigger the atrophy program by which MuRF1 and other enzymes will accelerate proteasomal myofibrillar protein degradation (see above). Recently, further direct histological evidence for this process was obtained by Valdez and coworkers (Valdez et al., 2010b). These authors also showed that exercise and dietary restriction slow-down the progression of age-dependent denervation, at least the latter observation is consistent with our biochemical data on the UPS (see above). It will be important to seek proof of principle for the neurogenic theory in experimental animal models followed by validation in humans since it will impact the development of strategies to impede sarcopenia in humans.

5. Acknowledgements

This work was supported by a grant from the Swedish research council (VR 10820, to B. Ulfhake), Swedish research council post doc grant to M. Altun and a guest researcher stipendship from the PR China government to L. Wang.

6. References

Adamo, M.L., and Farrar, R.P. (2006). Resistance training, and IGF involvement in the maintenance of muscle mass during the aging process. Ageing Res Rev *5*, 310-331.

Altun, M., Bergman, E., Edstrom, E., Johnson, H., and Ulfhake, B. (2007a). Behavioral impairments of the aging rat. Physiol Behav *92*, 911-923.

Altun, M., Besche, H.C., Overkleeft, H.S., Piccirillo, R., Edelmann, M.J., Kessler, B.M., Goldberg, A.L., and Ulfhake, B. (2010). Muscle wasting in aged, sarcopenic rats is associated with enhanced activity of the ubiquitin proteasome pathway. J Biol Chem *285*, 39597-39608.

Altun, M., Edstrom, E., Spooner, E., Flores-Moralez, A., Bergman, E., Tollet-Egnell, P., Norstedt, G., Kessler, B.M., and Ulfhake, B. (2007b). Iron load and redox stress in skeletal muscle of aged rats. Muscle Nerve *36*, 223-233.

Attaix, D., Mosoni, L., Dardevet, D., Combaret, L., Mirand, P.P., and Grizard, J. (2005). Altered responses in skeletal muscle protein turnover during aging in anabolic and catabolic periods. Int J Biochem Cell Biol 37, 1962-1973.

Baumgartner, R.N., Koehler, K.M., Gallagher, D., Romero, L., Heymsfield, S.B., Ross, R.R., Garry, P.J., and Lindeman, R.D. (1998a). Epidemiology of sarcopenia among the elderly in New Mexico. American Journal of Epidemiology *147*, 755-763.

Baumgartner, R.N., Koehler, K.M., Gallagher, D., Romero, L., Heymsfield, S.B., Ross, R.R., Garry, P.J., and Lindeman, R.D. (1998b). Epidemiology of sarcopenia among the elderly in New Mexico. Am J Epidemiol *147*, 755-763.

Bodine, S.C., Latres, E., Baumhueter, S., Lai, V.K., Nunez, L., Clarke, B.A., Poueymirou, W.T., Panaro, F.J., Na, E., Dharmarajan, K., *et al.* (2001). Identification of ubiquitin ligases required for skeletal muscle atrophy. Science *294*, 1704-1708.

Bornman, L., Rossouw, H., Gericke, G.S., and Polla, B.S. (1998). Effects of iron deprivation on the pathology and stress protein expression in murine X-linked muscular dystrophy. Biochem Pharmacol *56*, 751-757.

Brunk, U.T., and Terman, A. (2002). Lipofuscin: mechanisms of age-related accumulation and influence on cell function. Free Radic Biol Med *33*, 611-619.

Bulteau, A.L., Petropoulos, I., and Friguet, B. (2000). Age-related alterations of proteasome structure and function in aging epidermis. Exp Gerontol *35*, 767-777.

Cai, D., Lee, K.K., Li, M., Tang, M.K., and Chan, K.M. (2004). Ubiquitin expression is up-regulated in human and rat skeletal muscles during aging. Arch Biochem Biophys *425*, 42-50.

Carlson, M.E., Silva, H.S., and Conboy, I.M. (2008). Aging of signal transduction pathways, and pathology. Exp Cell Res *314*, 1951-1961.

Carlson, M.E., Suetta, C., Conboy, M.J., Aagaard, P., Mackey, A., Kjaer, M., and Conboy, I. (2009). Molecular aging and rejuvenation of human muscle stem cells. EMBO Mol Med *1*, 381-391.

Christov, C., Chretien, F., Abou-Khalil, R., Bassez, G., Vallet, G., Authier, F.J., Bassaglia, Y., Shinin, V., Tajbakhsh, S., Chazaud, B., *et al.* (2007). Muscle satellite cells and endothelial cells: close neighbors and privileged partners. Mol Biol Cell *18*, 1397-1409.

Chu, C.T. (2006). Autophagic stress in neuronal injury and disease. J Neuropathol Exp Neurol *65*, 423-432.

Clague, M.J., and Urbe, S. (2006). Endocytosis: the DUB version. Trends Cell Biol *16*, 551-559.

Clavel, S., Coldefy, A.S., Kurkdjian, E., Salles, J., Margaritis, I., and Derijard, B. (2006). Atrophy-related ubiquitin ligases, atrogin-1 and MuRF1 are up-regulated in aged rat Tibialis Anterior muscle. Mech Ageing Dev *127*, 794-801.

Conconi, M., Szweda, L.I., Levine, R.L., Stadtman, E.R., and Friguet, B. (1996). Age-related decline of rat liver multicatalytic proteinase activity and protection from oxidative inactivation by heat-shock protein 90. Arch Biochem Biophys *331*, 232-240.

Connell, P., Ballinger, C.A., Jiang, J., Wu, Y., Thompson, L.J., Hohfeld, J., and Patterson, C. (2001). The co-chaperone CHIP regulates protein triage decisions mediated by heat-shock proteins. Nat Cell Biol *3*, 93-96.

Cuervo, A.M., Bergamini, E., Brunk, U.T., Droge, W., Ffrench, M., and Terman, A. (2005). Autophagy and aging: the importance of maintaining "clean" cells. Autophagy *1*, 131-140.

Cuervo, A.M., Palmer, A., Rivett, A.J., and Knecht, E. (1995). Degradation of proteasomes by lysosomes in rat liver. Eur J Biochem *227*, 792-800.

Cuervo, A.M., Stefanis, L., Fredenburg, R., Lansbury, P.T., and Sulzer, D. (2004). Impaired degradation of mutant alpha-synuclein by chaperone-mediated autophagy. Science *305*, 1292-1295.

Edstrom, E., Altun, M., Bergman, E., Johnson, H., Kullberg, S., Ramirez-Leon, V., and Ulfhake, B. (2007). Factors contributing to neuromuscular impairment and sarcopenia during aging. Physiol Behav *92*, 129-135.

Edstrom, E., Altun, M., Hagglund, M., and Ulfhake, B. (2006). Atrogin-1/MAFbx and MuRF1 are downregulated in aging-related loss of skeletal muscle. J Gerontol A Biol Sci Med Sci *61*, 663-674.

Edstrom, E., and Ulfhake, B. (2005). Sarcopenia is not due to lack of regenerative drive in senescent skeletal muscle. Aging Cell *4*, 65-77.

Felbor, U., Kessler, B., Mothes, W., Goebel, H.H., Ploegh, H.L., Bronson, R.T., and Olsen, B.R. (2002). Neuronal loss and brain atrophy in mice lacking cathepsins B and L. Proc Natl Acad Sci U S A *99*, 7883-7888.

Ferrington, D.A., Husom, A.D., and Thompson, L.V. (2005). Altered proteasome structure, function, and oxidation in aged muscle. Faseb J *19*, 644-646.

Fuso, A., Ferraguti, G., Grandoni, F., Ruggeri, R., Scarpa, S., Strom, R., and Lucarelli, M. (2010). Early demethylation of non-CpG, CpC-rich, elements in the myogenin 5'-flanking region: a priming effect on the spreading of active demethylation. Cell Cycle *9*, 3965-3976.

Gomes, M.D., Lecker, S.H., Jagoe, R.T., Navon, A., and Goldberg, A.L. (2001). Atrogin-1, a muscle-specific F-box protein highly expressed during muscle atrophy. Proc Natl Acad Sci U S A *98*, 14440-14445.

Grune, T., Shringarpure, R., Sitte, N., and Davies, K. (2001). Age-related changes in protein oxidation and proteolysis in mammalian cells. J Gerontol A Biol Sci Med Sci *56*, B459-467.

Gutman, B., and Hanzlikova, V. (1972). Age changes in the neuromuscular system. Scientechnica Ltd, Bristol, 1-20.

Haglund, K., Sigismund, S., Polo, S., Szymkiewicz, I., Di Fiore, P.P., and Dikic, I. (2003). Multiple monoubiquitination of RTKs is sufficient for their endocytosis and degradation. Nat Cell Biol *5*, 461-466.

Hanna, J., Leggett, D.S., and Finley, D. (2003). Ubiquitin depletion as a key mediator of toxicity by translational inhibitors. Mol Cell Biol *23*, 9251-9261.

Hanna, J., Meides, A., Zhang, D.P., and Finley, D. (2007). A ubiquitin stress response induces altered proteasome composition. Cell *129*, 747-759.

Hara, T., Nakamura, K., Matsui, M., Yamamoto, A., Nakahara, Y., Suzuki-Migishima, R., Yokoyama, M., Mishima, K., Saito, I., Okano, H., *et al.* (2006). Suppression of basal autophagy in neural cells causes neurodegenerative disease in mice. Nature *441*, 885-889.

Harper, J.W., and Schulman, B.A. (2006). Structural complexity in ubiquitin recognition. Cell *124*, 1133-1136.

Harriman, D.G., Taverner, D., and Woolf, A.L. (1970). Ekbom´s syndrome and burning paraesthesiae. A biopsy study by vital staining and electron microscopy of the intramuscular innervation with a note on age changes in motor nerve endings in distal muscles. Brain *93*, 393-406.

Hayashi, T., and Goto, S. (1998). Age-related changes in the 20S and 26S proteasome activities in the liver of male F344 rats. Mech Ageing Dev *102*, 55-66.

Janssen, I., Heymsfield, S.B., and Ross, R. (2002). Low relative skeletal muscle mass (sarcopenia) in older persons is associated with functional impairment and physical disability. J Am Geriatr Soc *50*, 889-896.

Jariel-Encontre, I., Bossis, G., and Piechaczyk, M. (2008). Ubiquitin-independent degradation of proteins by the proteasome. Biochim Biophys Acta *1786*, 153-177.

Johnson, H., Mossberg, K., Arvidsson, U., Piehl, F., Hökfelt, T., and Ulfhake, B. (1995). Increase in alpha-CGRP and GAP-43 in aged motoneurons: A study of peptides, growth factors, and ChAT mRNA in the lumbar spinal cord of senescent rats with symptoms of hindlimb incapacities. J Comp Neurol *359*, 69-89.

Kadi, F., Charifi, N., Denis, C., Lexell, J., Andersen, J.L., Schjerling, P., Olsen, S., and Kjaer, M. (2005). The behaviour of satellite cells in response to exercise: what have we learned from human studies? Pflugers Arch *451*, 319-327.

Keller, J.N., Huang, F.F., and Markesbery, W.R. (2000). Decreased levels of proteasome activity and proteasome expression in aging spinal cord. Neuroscience *98*, 149-156.

Kimura, Y., Yashiroda, H., Kudo, T., Koitabashi, S., Murata, S., Kakizuka, A., and Tanaka, K. (2009). An inhibitor of a deubiquitinating enzyme regulates ubiquitin homeostasis. Cell *137*, 549-559.

Kondo, H., Miura, M., Kodama, J., Ahmed, S.M., and Itokawa, Y. (1992). Role of iron in oxidative stress in skeletal muscle atrophied by immobilization. Pflugers Arch *421*, 295-297.

Koulich, E., Li, X., and DeMartino, G.N. (2008). Relative structural and functional roles of multiple deubiquitylating proteins associated with mammalian 26S proteasome. Mol Biol Cell *19*, 1072-1082.

Kurz, T., Terman, A., Gustafsson, B., and Brunk, U.T. (2008). Lysosomes in iron metabolism, ageing and apoptosis. Histochem Cell Biol *129*, 389-406.

Larsson, L. (1995). Motor units: remodeling in aged animals. J Gerontol A Biol Sci Med Sci *50 Spec No*, 91-95.

Lecker, S.H., Goldberg, A.L., and Mitch, W.E. (2006). Protein degradation by the ubiquitin-proteasome pathway in normal and disease states. J Am Soc Nephrol *17*, 1807-1819.

Lecker, S.H., Jagoe, R.T., Gilbert, A., Gomes, M., Baracos, V., Bailey, J., Price, S.R., Mitch, W.E., and Goldberg, A.L. (2004). Multiple types of skeletal muscle atrophy involve a common program of changes in gene expression. Faseb J *18*, 39-51.

Lecker, S.H., Solomon, V., Mitch, W.E., and Goldberg, A.L. (1999). Muscle protein breakdown and the critical role of the ubiquitin-proteasome pathway in normal and disease states. J Nutr *129*, 227S-237S.

Mammucari, C., Milan, G., Romanello, V., Masiero, E., Rudolf, R., Del Piccolo, P., Burden, S.J., Di Lisi, R., Sandri, C., Zhao, J., *et al.* (2007). FoxO3 controls autophagy in skeletal muscle in vivo. Cell Metab *6*, 458-471.

Medicherla, B., and Goldberg, A.L. (2008). Heat shock and oxygen radicals stimulate ubiquitin-dependent degradation mainly of newly synthesized proteins. J Cell Biol *182*, 663-673.

Mishra, A., Godavarthi, S.K., Maheshwari, M., Goswami, A., and Jana, N.R. (2009). The ubiquitin ligase E6-AP is induced and recruited to aggresomes in response to proteasome inhibition and may be involved in the ubiquitination of Hsp70-bound misfolded proteins. J Biol Chem *284*, 10537-10545.

Mitch, W.E., and Goldberg, A.L. (1996). Mechanisms of muscle wasting. The role of the ubiquitin-proteasome pathway. N Engl J Med *335*, 1897-1905.

Mizuno, E., Iura, T., Mukai, A., Yoshimori, T., Kitamura, N., and Komada, M. (2005). Regulation of epidermal growth factor receptor down-regulation by UBPY-mediated deubiquitination at endosomes. Mol Biol Cell *16*, 5163-5174.

Nijman, S.M., Luna-Vargas, M.P., Velds, A., Brummelkamp, T.R., Dirac, A.M., Sixma, T.K., and Bernards, R. (2005). A genomic and functional inventory of deubiquitinating enzymes. Cell *123*, 773-786.

Paddon-Jones, D., and Rasmussen, B.B. (2009). Dietary protein recommendations and the prevention of sarcopenia. Curr Opin Clin Nutr Metab Care *12*, 86-90.

Peth, A., Besche, H.C., and Goldberg, A.L. (2009). Ubiquitinated proteins activate the proteasome by binding to Usp14/Ubp6, which causes 20S gate opening. Molecular cell *36*, 794-804.

Reyes-Turcu, F.E., Horton, J.R., Mullally, J.E., Heroux, A., Cheng, X., and Wilkinson, K.D. (2006). The ubiquitin binding domain ZnF UBP recognizes the C-terminal diglycine motif of unanchored ubiquitin. Cell *124*, 1197-1208.

Reyes-Turcu, F.E., Shanks, J.R., Komander, D., and Wilkinson, K.D. (2008). Recognition of polyubiquitin isoforms by the multiple ubiquitin binding modules of isopeptidase T. J Biol Chem *283*, 19581-19592.

Rodeheffer, M.S. (2010). Tipping the scale: muscle versus fat. Nat Cell Biol *12*, 102-104.

Roth, S.M., Metter, E.J., Ling, S., and Ferrucci, L. (2006). Inflammatory factors in age-related muscle wasting. Curr Opin Rheumatol *18*, 625-630.

Sacheck, J.M., Hyatt, J.P., Raffaello, A., Jagoe, R.T., Roy, R.R., Edgerton, V.R., Lecker, S.H., and Goldberg, A.L. (2007). Rapid disuse and denervation atrophy involve transcriptional changes similar to those of muscle wasting during systemic diseases. Faseb J *21*, 140-155.

Sacheck, J.M., Ohtsuka, A., McLary, S.C., and Goldberg, A.L. (2004). IGF-I stimulates muscle growth by suppressing protein breakdown and expression of atrophy-related ubiquitin ligases, atrogin-1 and MuRF1. Am J Physiol Endocrinol Metab *287*, E591-601.

Sandri, M., Lin, J., Handschin, C., Yang, W., Arany, Z.P., Lecker, S.H., Goldberg, A.L., and Spiegelman, B.M. (2006). PGC-1alpha protects skeletal muscle from atrophy by suppressing FoxO3 action and atrophy-specific gene transcription. Proc Natl Acad Sci U S A *103*, 16260-16265.

Sandri, M., Sandri, C., Gilbert, A., Skurk, C., Calabria, E., Picard, A., Walsh, K., Schiaffino, S., Lecker, S.H., and Goldberg, A.L. (2004). Foxo transcription factors induce the atrophy-related ubiquitin ligase atrogin-1 and cause skeletal muscle atrophy. Cell *117*, 399-412.

Solomon, A.M., and Bouloux, P.M. (2006). Modifying muscle mass - the endocrine perspective. J Endocrinol *191*, 349-360.

St-Onge, M.P. (2005). Relationship between body composition changes and changes in physical function and metabolic risk factors in aging. Curr Opin Clin Nutr Metab Care *8*, 523-528.

Stitt, T.N., Drujan, D., Clarke, B.A., Panaro, F., Timofeyva, Y., Kline, W.O., Gonzalez, M., Yancopoulos, G.D., and Glass, D.J. (2004). The IGF-1/PI3K/Akt pathway prevents expression of muscle atrophy-induced ubiquitin ligases by inhibiting FOXO transcription factors. Mol Cell *14*, 395-403.

Terman, A., and Brunk, U.T. (2004). Myocyte aging and mitochondrial turnover. Exp Gerontol *39*, 701-705.

Terman, A., and Brunk, U.T. (2006). Oxidative stress, accumulation of biological 'garbage', and aging. Antioxid Redox Signal *8*, 197-204.

Terman, A., Gustafsson, B., and Brunk, U.T. (2006). The lysosomal-mitochondrial axis theory of postmitotic aging and cell death. Chem Biol Interact *163*, 29-37.

Valdez, G., Tapia, J.C., Kang, H., Clemenson, G.D., Jr., Gage, F.H., Lichtman, J.W., and Sanes, J.R. (2010a). Attenuation of age-related changes in mouse neuromuscular synapses by caloric restriction and exercise. Proc Natl Acad Sci U S A *107*, 14863-14868.

Valdez, G., Tapia, J.C., Kang, H., Clemenson, G.D., Jr., Gage, F.H., Lichtman, J.W., and Sanes, J.R. (2010b). Attenuation of age-related changes in mouse neuromuscular synapses by caloric restriction and exercise. Proc Natl Acad Sci U S A *107*, 14863-14868.

Watts, G.D., Wymer, J., Kovach, M.J., Mehta, S.G., Mumm, S., Darvish, D., Pestronk, A., Whyte, M.P., and Kimonis, V.E. (2004). Inclusion body myopathy associated with Paget disease of bone and frontotemporal dementia is caused by mutant valosin-containing protein. Nat Genet *36*, 377-381.

Zammit, P.S. (2008). All muscle satellite cells are equal, but are some more equal than others? J Cell Sci *121*, 2975-2982.

Zhou, X., Wang, J.L., Lu, J., Song, Y., Kwak, K.S., Jiao, Q., Rosenfeld, R., Chen, Q., Boone, T., Simonet, W.S., *et al.* (2010). Reversal of cancer cachexia and muscle wasting by ActRIIB antagonism leads to prolonged survival. Cell *142*, 531-543.

14

Cell Senescence as Observed by Electron Microscopic Radioautography

Tetsuji Nagata[1,2]
[1]*Department of Anatomy and Cell Biology, Shinshu University School of Medicine, Matsumoto,*
[2]*Shinshu Institute of Alternative Medicine and Welfare, Nagano, Japan*

1. Introduction

The term "cell senescence" initially means how the cells change when they get old due to their aging. It contains 2 meanings, one how a cell changes when it is isolated from in vivo original animals or plants such as in vitro cells in cell culture, while the other means how all the cells of an animal or a plant change in vivo due to the aging of the individual animal or plant. In order to study the cell senescence, we have 2 research techniques to clarify how cells get old, i.e., morphological technique and functional technique. The former employs microscopy either light microscope or electron microscope to observe the structure of cells and tissues, while the latter employs functional techniques such as physiological or biochemical to observe either the electric activities or chemical components. Since I am anatomist and had learned morphological technique, I employed to observe cells by light and electron microscopy. I had first studied the meaning of cell senescence many years ago (more than 50 years) how a cell changed when it was isolated from original experimental animals such as mice and rats by cell culture (Nagata 1956, 1957a,b), and then moved to the study on the latter cell senescence, i.e., how all the cells of an experimental animal change in vivo due to the senescence of the individual animal bodies (Nagata 1959, 1962, Nagata and Momoze 1959, Nagata et al. 1960a,b).

Recently, I have been studying the senescent changes from the viewpoint of the cell nutrients which were incorporated and synthesized into various cells in individual animals during their senescence (Nagata 2010c). Therefore, this article deals with the cell senescence of animal cells in vivo, how the metabolism, i.e., incorporations and syntheses of respective nutrients, the macromolecular precursors, in various kinds of cells change due to the senescence of individual experimental animals such as mice and rats by means of microscopic radioautography. The incorporations and syntheses of various nutrients such as DNA, RNA, proteins, glucides, lipids and others in various kinds of cells of various organ in respective organ systems such as skeletal, muscular, circulatory, digestive, respiratory, urinary, reproductive, endocrine, nervous and sensory systems should be reviewed referring many original papers already published from our laboratory.

When I was first asked early this year (April 2011) from the publisher, named InTech, Open Access Publisher in Croatia, to contribute this article as well as to edit the articles submitted from around 40 authors throughout the world, I initially intended to write only one chapter entitled "Senescence as Analyzed by Microscopic Radioautography." However, when I was almost finishing this article in one chapter which consisted of the text around 140 pages and around 30 figures which might become over 170 pages altogether, the publisher requested me to submit only one chapter within exactly 16, 18, 20, 22, 24 or 26 pages including both text and figures. Since I could not agree with them in submitting such a short chapter dealing with all the research results of myself and my associates, I insisted to submit the large article in one chapter including so much information as the results of my research on senescence for more 50 years since 1955 up to the present time 2011, they requested me to divide the original one chapter into 3 or 4 short chapters.

Thus, I tried to divide the original draft into 4 chapters, including the foundations of radioautography and the results of its application to all the organ systems, i.e., skeletal, muscular, circulatory, digestive, respiratory, urinary, reproductive, endocrine, nervous and sensory organs altogether. As the results of dividing the initial one chapter into 4, the final chapters were consisted of more than 26 pages as the publisher requested. However, I am going to submit the longer chapters to the publisher and insist to publish those chapters as they are, otherwise, I would rather prefer to withdraw them from this book and would like to contribute them to any other suitable publishers in the world.

This first chapter deals with the methodology of microscopic radioautography as well as the first parts of the applications of radioautography to the organ systems, i.e. the organ of movement (skeletal and muscular system) and the circulatory system.

1.1 Method in microscopic radioautography

For the purpose of observing the localizations of the incorporations and syntheses of various nutrients synthesizing macromolecules in the human and animal bodies such as DNA, RNA, proteins, glucides and lipids in various kinds of cells of various organ in respective organ systems such as skeletal, muscular, circulatory, digestive, respiratory, urinary, reproductive, endocrine, nervous and sensory systems, we employed the specific techniques developed in our laboratory during these 50 years (Nagata 2002). The technique is designated as radioautography using RI-labeled compounds. Some scientists use another term autoradiography which is used as the synonym to radioautogarphy. However, the author prefers the term radioautography because of the etymological reason (Nagata 1996b). To demonstrate the localizations of macromolecular synthesis by using such RI-labeled precursors as ^{3}H-thymidine for DNA, ^{3}H-uridine for RNA, ^{3}H-leucine for proteins, ^{3}H-glucosamine or $^{35}SO_4$ for glucides and ^{3}H-glycerol for lipids are divided into macroscopic radioautography and microscopic radioautography. The techniques employ both the physical techniques using RI-labeled compounds and the histochemical techniques treating tissue sections by coating sections containing RI-labeled precursors with photographic emulsions and processing for exposure and development. Such techniques can demonstrate both the soluble compounds diffusible in the cells and tissues and the insoluble compounds bound to the macromolecules (Nagata 1972b). As the results, specimens prepared for EM RAG (electron microscopic radioautography) are very thick than conventional EM specimens and should be observed with high voltage electron microscopes in order to obtain better transmittance and resolution (Nagata 2001a,b). Such radioautographic techniques in details should be referred to other literature (Nagata 2002). On the other hand, the systematic results obtained by radioautography should be designated as radioauographology which means the science of radioautography (Nagata 1998b, 1999e, 2000e). This article deals with the results dealing with the radioautographic changes of individual cell by aging that should be included in radioautographology.

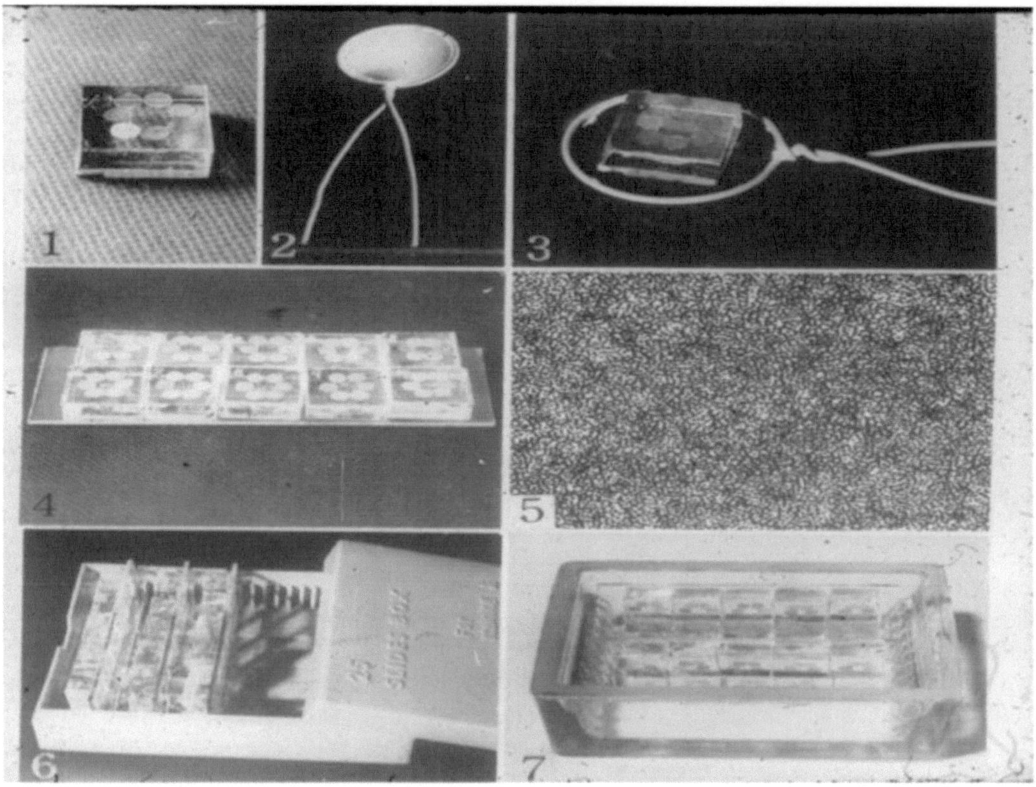

Explanation of Figures. From Nagata, T.: Acta Microsc. Vol. 6: Suppl. B. p. 42, 1997a. Brazil. Soc. Electron Microsc., San Paulo, Brazil

Fig. 1. Photographs showing the standard procedure for preparing EMRAG (electron microscopic radioautograms) by the wire-loop method (Nagata 1982, 1985).
Fig. 1-1. Six grid meshes carrying sections are placed on a square glass block.
Fig. 1-2. A large wire-loop is dipped into the melted radioautographic emulsion and a thin film of the emulsion is obtained.
Fig. 1-3. The emulsion film with the wire-loop (Fig. 1-2) is applied horizontally to the glass block on which 6 grid meshes were placed (Fig. 1-1).
Fig. 1-4. Ten glass blocks carrying 6 grid meshes each (Fig. 1-3) are attached on a glass slide with Scotch tape.
Fig. 1-5. The emulsion film picked up at random is checked by transmission electron microscopy before exposure. Note the monolayer arrangement of the silver bromide crystals in Konica NR-H2 emulsion in this figure. x6,000.
Fig. 1-6. Several glass slides, each carrying 10 glass blocks with grid meshes, are stored in a light tight slide box kept in a refrigerator at 4°C for exposure.
Fig. 1-7. All the grid meshes on glass blocks are developed, fixed and stained simultaneously.

1.2 Macromolecular synthesis

The human body as well as the bodies of any experimental animals such as mice and rats consist of various macromolecules. They are classified into nucleic acids (both DNA and RNA), proteins, glucides and lipids, according to their chemical structures. These macromolecules can be demonstrated by specific histochemical staining for respective molecules such as Feulgen reaction (Feulgen and Rossenbeck 1924) which stains all the DNA contained in the cells. Each compounds of macromolecules such as DNA, RNA, proteins, glucides, lipids can be demonstrated by respective specific histochemical stainings (Pearse 1991) and such reactions can be quantified by microscpectrophotometry using specific wave-lengths demonstrating the total amount of respective compounds (Nagata 1972a). To the contrary, radioautography can only demonstrate the newly synthesized macromolecules such as synthetic DNA or RNA or proteins depending upon the RI-labeled precursors incorporated specifically into these macromolecules such as ^{3}H-thymidine into DNA or ^{3}H-uridine into RNA or ^{3}H-amino acid into proteins (Nagata 2002).

Concerning to the newly synthesized macromolecules, the results of recent studies in our laboratory by the present author and co-workers should be reviewed in this article according to the classification of macromolecules as follows.

1.2.1 The DNA synthesis

The DNA (deoxyribonucleic acid) contained in cells can be demonstrated either by morphological histochemical techniques staining tissue sections such as Feulgen reaction (Feulgen and Rossenbeck 1924) or by biochemical techniques homogenizing tissues and cells. To the contrary, the synthetic DNA or newly synthesized DNA but not all the DNA can be detected as macromolecular synthesis together with other macromolecules such as RNA or proteins in various organs of experimental animals by either morphological or biochemical procedures employing RI-labeled precursors. We have studied the sites of macromolecular synthesis in almost all the organs of mice during their aging from prenatal to postnatal development to senescence by means of microscopic radioautography, one of the morphological methods (Nagata 1992, 1994b,c,d, 1996a,b,c,d, 1997a, 2002, 2010c). The results should be here described according to the order of organ systems in anatomy or histology.

1.2.2 The RNA synthesis

The RNA (ribonucleic acid) contained in cells can be demonstrated either by morphological histochemical techniques staining tissue sections such as methyl green-pyronin staining or by biochemical techniques homogenizing tissues and cells. To the contrary, the synthetic RNA or newly synthesized RNA but not all the RNA in the cells can be detected as macromolecular synthesis together with other macromolecules such as DNA or proteins in various organs of experimental animals by either morphological or biochemical procedures employing RI-labeled precursors. We have studied the sites of macromolecular synthesis in almost all the organs of mice during their aging from prenatal to postnatal development to senescence by means of microscopic radioautography, one of the morphological methods (Nagata 1992, 1994b,c, 1996a,b,c, 1997a, 2002, 2010c). The results obtained from RNA synthesis should be here described according to the order of organ systems in anatomy or histology. In contrast to the results obtained from DNA synthesis of almost all the organs, we have studied only several parts of the organ systems with regards RNA. The skeletal system, the muscular system or the circulatory system were not so much studied.

1.2.3 The protein synthesis

The proteins found in animal cells are composed of various amino-acids which initially form low molecular polypeptides and finally macromolecular compounds designated as proteins. They are chemically classified into two, simple proteins and conjugated proteins. Therefore, the proteins can be demonstrated by showing specific reactions to respective amino-acids composing any proteins. Thus, the proteins contained in cells can be demonstrated either by morphological histochemical techniques staining tissue sections such as Millon reaction (Millon 1849) or tetrazonium reaction or otherwise by biochemical techniques homogenizing tissues and cells. To the contrary, the newly synthesized proteins but not all the proteins in the cells can be detected as macromolecular synthesis together with other macromolecules such as DNA or RNA in various organs of experimental animals by either morphological or biochemical procedures employing RI-labeled precursors. We have studied the sites of macromolecular synthesis in almost all the organs of mice during their aging from prenatal to postnatal development to senescence by means of microscopic radioautography (Nagata 1992, 1994b,c, 1996a,b, 1997a, 2002, 2010c). The results obtained from protein synthesis should be described according to the order of organ systems in anatomy or histology. In contrast to the results obtained from DNA synthesis of almost all the organs, we have studied only several parts of the organ systems.

1.2.4 The glucide synthesis

The glucides found in animal cells and tissues are composed of various low molecular sugars such as glucose or fructose called monosaccharides which form compounds of polysaccharides or complex mucopolysaccharides connecting to sulfated compounds. The former are called simple polysaccharides, while the latter mucopolysubstances. Thus, the glucides are chemically classified into 3 groups, monosaccharides such as glucose or fructose, disaccharides such as sucrose and polysaccharides such as mucosubstances. However, in most animal cells polysaccharides are much more found than monosaccharides or disaccharides. The polysaccharides can be classified into 2, i.e. simple polyscaccharides and mucosubstances. Anyway, they are composed of various low molecular sugars that can be demonstrated by either histochemical reactions or biochemical techniques. To the contrary, the newly synthesized glucides but not all the glucides in the cells and tissues can be detected as macromolecular synthesis together with other macromolecules such as DNA, RNA or proteins in various organs of experimental animals by either morphological or biochemical procedures employing RI-labeled precursors. We have studied the sites of macromolecular synthesis in almost all the organs of mice during their aging from prenatal to postnatal development to senescence by means of microscopic radioautography (Nagata 1992, 1994a,b,c, 1996a, 1997a, 2002, 2010c). The results obtained from glucides synthesis are described according to the order of organ systems in anatomy or histology. In contrast to the results obtained from DNA synthesis of almost all the organs, we have studied only several parts of the organ systems. The skeletal system, the muscular system and the circulatory system were not yet studied.

1.2.5 The lipid synthesis

The lipids found in animal cells are chemically composed of various low molecular fatty acids. They are esters of high fatty acids and glycerol that can biochemically be classified into simple lipids and compound lipids such as phospholipids, glycolipids or proteolipids. The simple lipids are composed of only fatty acids and glycerol, while the latter composed of lipids and other components such as phosphates, glucides or proteins. In order to demonstrate intracellular localization of total lipids, we can employ either histochemical reactions or biochemical techniques. To the contrary, the newly synthesized lipids but not all of the lipids in the cells can be detected as macromolecular synthesis similarly to the other macromolecules such as DNA, RNA, proteins or glucides in various organs of experimental animals by either morphological or biochemical procedures employing RI-labeled precursors. We have studied the sites of macromolecular synthesis in almost all the organs of mice during their aging from prenatal to postnatal development to senescence by means of microscopic radioautography (Nagata 1992, 1994a,b,c,d,e, 1996a, 1997a, 2002, 2010c). However, we have not studied the lipids synthesis so much as compared to other compounds. We have studied only a few organs of the digestive system.

1.3 The intracellular localization of the other substances

The other substances than macromolecules that can also be demonstrated by radioautography are target tracers not the precursors for the macromolecular synthesis. They are hormones such as ^{3}H-methyl prednisolone (Nagata et al. 1978b), neurotransmitters and inhibitors such as ^{14}C-bupranolol, a beta-blocking agent (Tsukahara et al. 1980) or ^{3}H-befunolol (Nagata and Yamabayashi 1983, Yamabayashi et al. 1981), vitamins, drugs such as synthetic anti-allergic agent ^{3}H-tranilast (Nagata et al. 1986b, Nishigaki et al. 1987, 1990a.b, Momose et al. 1989), hypolipidemic agent bezafibrate (Momose et al. 1993a,b, 1995), calmodulin antagonist (Ohno et al. 1982, 1983) or anti-hypertensive agent ^{3}H-benidipine hydrochloride (Suzuki et al. 1994), toxins, inorganic substances such as mercury (Nagata et al. 1977b) and others such as laser beam irradiation (Nagata 1984). The details are referred to the previous publication on the radioatuographology (Nagata 2002). However, their relationships to the cell aging and senescence were not studied.

1.4 Macromolecular synthesis in the normal organ systems

With regards to the macromolecular synthesis such as DNA, RNA, proteins, glucides, lipids etc in various cells and tissues, we have studied various cells and tissues in almost all the organ systems in the experimental animals such as mice and rats. Therefore, the results are classified into the organ systems in anatomy and histology, i.e. the organ of movement including the skeletal system and the muscular system, the circulatory organs, the digestive organs, the respiratory organs, the urinary organs, the reproductive organs, the endocrine organs, the nervous system, and the sensory organs. Thus, the results should be described according to this order in the following chapters divided into 4 chapters.

1.5 Macromolecular synthesis in the tumor cells

As for the tumor cells, on the other hand, which do not belong to any organ systems of the normal organs but grow in any organ systems, the macromolecular synthesis in the tumor cells should be described separately from the normal organ system at the end of this book in chapter 4.

2. Macromolecular synthesis in the organ of movement

The Organ of Movement or locomotive organ of men and experimental animals consists of both the skeletal system and the muscular system. The former consists of many bones, around 200 in case of men while the latter consists of many skeletal muscles around 600 in case of men. We studied the macromolecular synthesis in a part of these locomotive organs in the experimental animals, but not all of them. The results should be described in the following 2 sections, the skeletal system and the muscular system.

2.1 Macromolecular synthesis in the skeletal system

The skeletal system of men and experimental animals consists of bones, joints and ligaments. We studied the DNA synthetic activities of the bones and joints of experimental animals in development and aging (Kobayashi and Nagata 1994, Nagata 1998c).

2.1.1 The DNA synthesis in the skeletal system

We studied the DNA synthetic activities of the bones and joints of experimental animals in development and aging to senescence (Kobayashi and Nagata 1994, Nagata 1998c).

2.1.1.1 The DNA synthesis in the bone

We studied the ossifications of salamander skeletons from hatching to senescence (Nagata 1998c). The fore-limbs (Fig. 2A) and hind-limbs (Fig. 2B) of salamanders were composed of skeletons consisting of bones and cartilages which were covered with skeletal muscles, connective tissues and epidermis consisting of stratified squamous epithelial cells in the outermost layer. The bones of juvenile salamanders at 4 weeks consisted of the hyaline cartilage (Figs. 2A, 2B). The hyaline cartilage consisted of spherical or polygonal cartilage cells or chondrocytes at the center. They were surrounded by rich interstitial ground substance which stained deep blue with toluidine blue staining. The spherical cartilage cells at the center of the bone changed their shapes to flattened shape under the perichondrium or free joint surfaces. Some of the nuclei of the chondrocytes were covered with silver grains when labeled with ^{3}H-thymidine (Figs. 2A, 2B). Mitotic figures were frequently seen in spherical cartilage cells in young animals. Examination of radioautograms at the young stages such as 4 weeks after hatching showed that many spherical cartilage cells and flattened cartilage cells were predominantly labeled. At 6 weeks after hatching, the size of bones enlarged and the number of cartilage cells increased. At this stage, however, the number of labeled cells in the cartilage cells in both fore-limbs (Fig. 2C) and hind-limbs (Fig. 2D) decreased as compared with the previous stage (Figs. 2A, 2B). The size of bones in juvenile animals at 8, 9, 10, and 11 weeks enlarged gradually (Fig. 2E, 2F). Radioautograms at these stages showed that the number of the labeled cells remarkably reduced as compared with those of 4 and 6 weeks. In the adult salamanders at 8 months up to 12 months, the bones showed complete mature structure and examination of radioautograms revealed that the number of labeled cells reached almost zero (Kobayashi and Nagata 1994, Nagata 2006c). No difference was found on the morphology and labeling between the fore-limbs and hind-limbs at any stage.

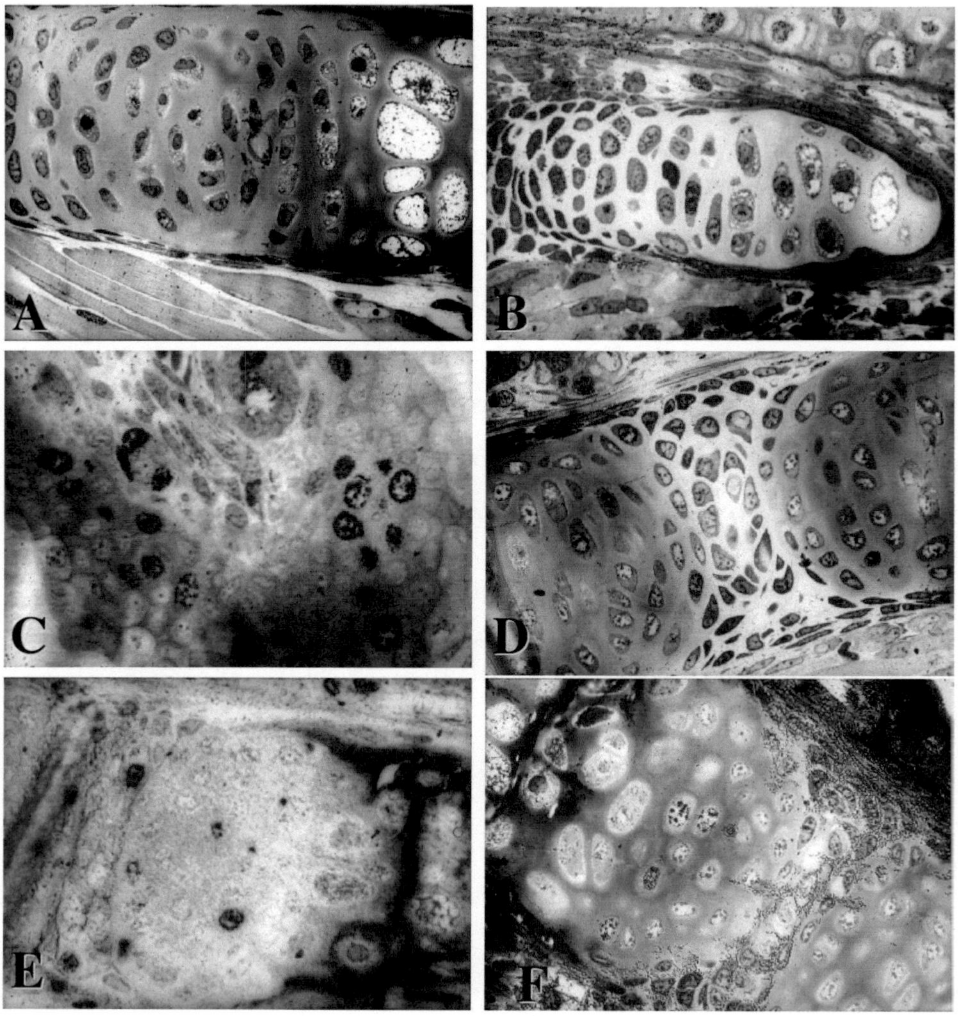

Fig. 2. Light microscopic radioautograms of the bones of either fore-limbs or hind-limbs of salamanders at various ages from 4 weeks to 8 weeks after hatching, injected with ^{3}H-thymidine, fixed and processed for radioautography. Some of the cartilage cells (arrows) are labeled with silver grains due to ^{3}H-thymidine incorporation demonstrating DNA synthesis. From Nagata, T.: Bulletin Shinshu Inst. Alternat. Med. Vol. 2, p. 53, 2006, Nagano, Japan

Fig. 2A. Light microscopic radioautogram of the bone of a fore-limb of a salamander at 4 weeks after hatching. Many cartilage cells (arrows) are labeled with silver grains due to ^{3}H-thymidine. Magnification. x 1200.

Fig. 2B. Light microscopic radioautogram of the bone of a hind-limb of a salamander at 4 weeks after hatching. Many cartilage cells (arrows) are labeled with silver grains due to ^{3}H-thymidine. Magnification. x 1200.

Fig. 2C. Light microscopic radioautogram of the bone of a fore-limb of a salamander at 6 weeks after hatching. Only a few cartilage cells (arrow) are labeled. The numbers of labeled cells are fewer than the bone of a younger salamander at 4 weeks after hatching (Fig. 1A) Magnification x 1200.

Fig. 2D. Light microscopic radioautogram of the bone of a hind-limb of a salamander at 6 weeks after hatching. Only a few cartilage cells (arrow) are labeled. Magnification x 1200.
Fig. 2E. Light microscopic radioautogram of the bone of a fore-limb of a salamander at 8 weeks after hatching. Only a few cartilage cells (arrow) are labeled. Magnification x 1200.
Fig. 2F. Light microscopic radioautogram of the bone of a hind-limb of a salamander at 8 weeks after hatching. Only a few cartilage cells (arrow) are labeled. Magnification x 1200.

The labeling indices of respective cell types changed with aging as expressed by mean in each group. The labeling index of the cartilage cells was lower than the epithelial cells. The peak of the labeling index of the cartilage cells in both fore-limbs and hind-limbs was found about 15-18% at 4 weeks after hatching (Fig. 2). The labeling index of the cartilage cells in both limbs at 6 weeks rapidly decreased to about 4-6%, then increased at 8 weeks to about 7-8% and finally decreased to 2-3% gradually from 8 weeks to 9 weeks with aging and fell down to 0-1% at 10 weeks. The labeling index of cartilage cells from 10 weeks to 12 months kept very low around 0-1% (Fig. 3). Thus, the cartilages and bones of fore-limbs and hind-limbs of salamanders are demonstrated to complete the development by 10 weeks after hatching (Kobayashi and Nagata 1994, Nagata 2006c).

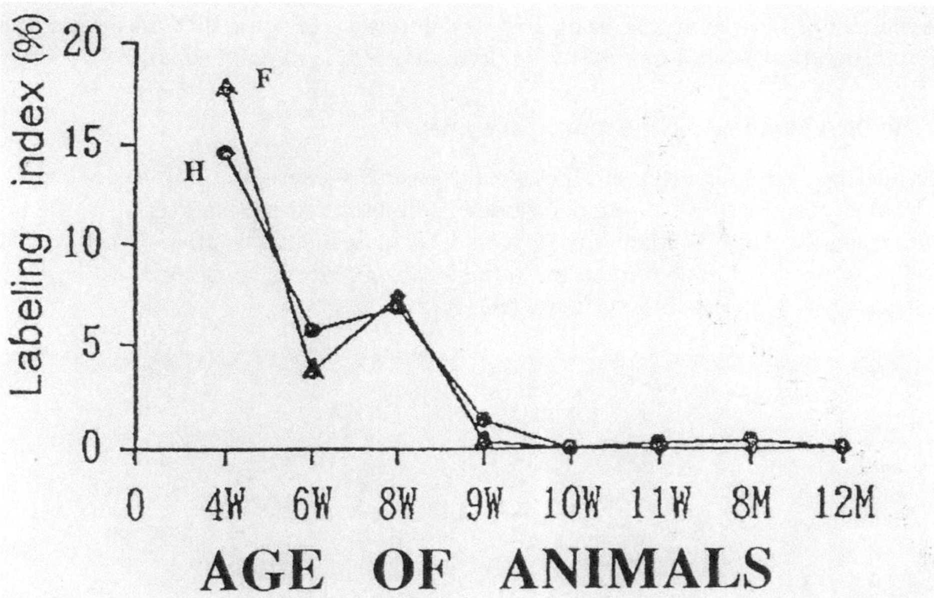

Fig. 3. Transitional curves of the labeling indices of the cartilage cells in the bones of the fore-limbs and the hind-limbs of salamanders labeled with ^{3}H-thymidine at various ages from 4 weeks to 60 months (5 years) after hatching. Mean ± S.D. From Nagata, T.: Bulletin Shinshu Inst. Alternat. Med. Vol. 2, p. 54, 2006, Nagano, Japan,

2.1.1.2 The DNA synthesis in the joint

The joints of an experimental animal such as mouse or human being are consisted of either 2 or 3 bones and the synovial membranes covering the ends of the bones. The synovial membranes are composed of the collagenous fibers interspersed with the synovial cells which are fibroblasts and lining cells. We studied macromolecular synthesis, both DNA and

RNA syntheses of the synovial cells of the joints surgically obtained from 15 elderly human patients of both sexes aged from 50 to 70, suffering from rheumatoid arthritis (Kobayashi and Nagata 1994). Both the normal and rheumatoid cells were cultured and labeled in vitro with media containing precursors such as ^{3}H-thymidine or ^{3}H-uridine, fixed and radioautographed. DNA synthetic cells labeled with silver grains were observed by LM RAG (light microscopic radioautography) in both normal and rheumatoid cells. As the results, some labeled synovial cells with ^{3}H-thymidine were found. However, no significant difference was observed between the labeling indices of normal and rheumatoid cells labeled with ^{3}H-thymidine. From the results, it was concluded that the synovial cells synthesized DNA in both normal and rheumatoid conditions. However, the quantities of these macromolecules synthesized in these synovial cells varied in respective individuals and no significant difference was found between the labeling indices and grain counts in both normal and rheumatoid cells (Kobayashi and Nagata 1994).

2.2 Macromolecular synthesis in the muscular system

The muscular system consists of various skeletal muscles amounting to around 600 in number in men and less in experimental animals such as rats and mice. We studied the aging changes of DNA synthesis in the intercostal muscles of aging ddY mice from prenatal day 13 through postnatal 24 months by ^{3}H-thymidine RAG (Hayashi et al. 1993).

2.2.1 The DNA synthesis in the muscular system

We studied the aging changes of DNA synthesis in the intercostal muscles of aging ddY mice from prenatal day 13 through postnatal 24 months in senescence by ^{3}H-thymidine RAG (Hayashi et al. 1993). Many nuclei were labeled in myotubes at embryonic day 13-17 (Fig. 4C) during development, then the number of labeled nuclei decreased to embryonic day 18-19 (Fig. 4D), and less due to aging after birth.

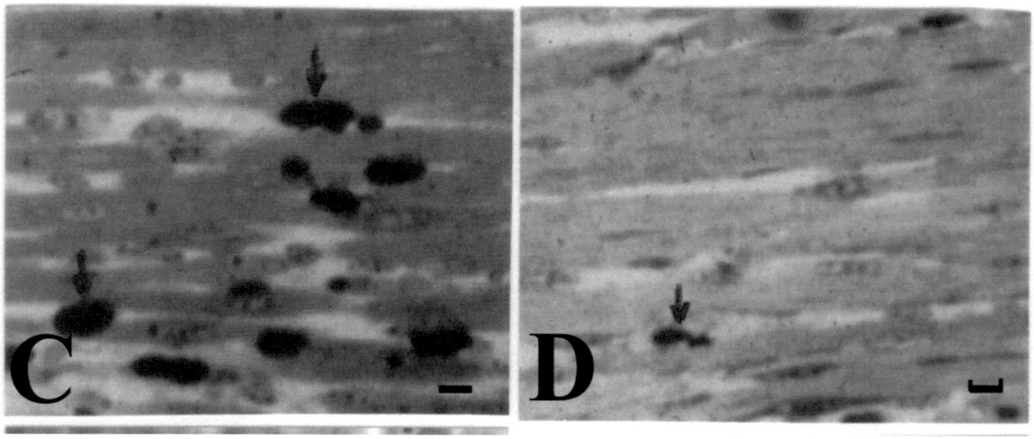

Fig. 4. Light microscopic radioautograms of the skeletal muscle cells in the myotubes labeled with ^{3}H-thymidine at embryonic day 13-17 (Fig. 3C), then the number of labeled nuclei decreased to embryonic day 18-19 (Fig. 3D), and less after birth. x260. From Nagata, T.: Special Cytochemistry in Cell Biology, In, Internat. Rev. Cytol. Vol. 211, No. 1, p. 62, 2001, Academic Press, San Diego, USA, London, UK.

The labeling indices revealed chronological changes, showing a peak at embryonic day 13 and decreasing gradually to 0% at 3 months after birth to month 24 (Fig. 5). We classified the graduation of the embryonic muscle development into 5 stages. Among them, the labeling index (LI) at stage I was the highest, while the LI at stage II was significantly lower than stage I, the LI at stage IV was significantly higher than stage II, and the LI at stage V was significantly lower than stage IV (Fig. 5). These changes accorded well with the primary and secondary myotube formation during the embryonic muscle development. We also studied the DNA synthesis of rat thigh muscles during the muscle regeneration after injury in rats (Sakai et al. 1977). When the skeletal muscles, i.e., the diaphragma, the rectus abdominis muscles and the gastrocnemius femoris muscle of adult Wistar rats were mechanically injured and labeled with ^{3}H-thymidine, satellite cells were labeled during their regeneration. The satellite cells in the muscles of dystrophy chickens and normal control chickens were also labeled with ^{3}H-thymidine, demonstrating DNA synthesis (Oguchi and Nagata 1980, 1981), which was later described in details in the review (Nagata 2002). Briefly, 2 groups of chickens, 4 dystrophy chickens and normal control chickens of both sexes aged 1 day and 21 days after hatching were used. All the animals received every 6 hrs intraperitoneal injections of ^{3}H-thymidine 4 times successively and sacrificed. The superficial pectoral muscles were taken out, fixed, embedded in Epoxy resin and processed for LM and EMRAG. The results demonstrated that many nuclei of the satellite cells in all the experimental groups were labeled but none of the nuclei in the muscle fibers were labeled. The labeling indices of normal chickens at 1 day and 21 days were 4.59 and 3.86%, respectively. These results showed that the LI decreased after hatching due to aging.

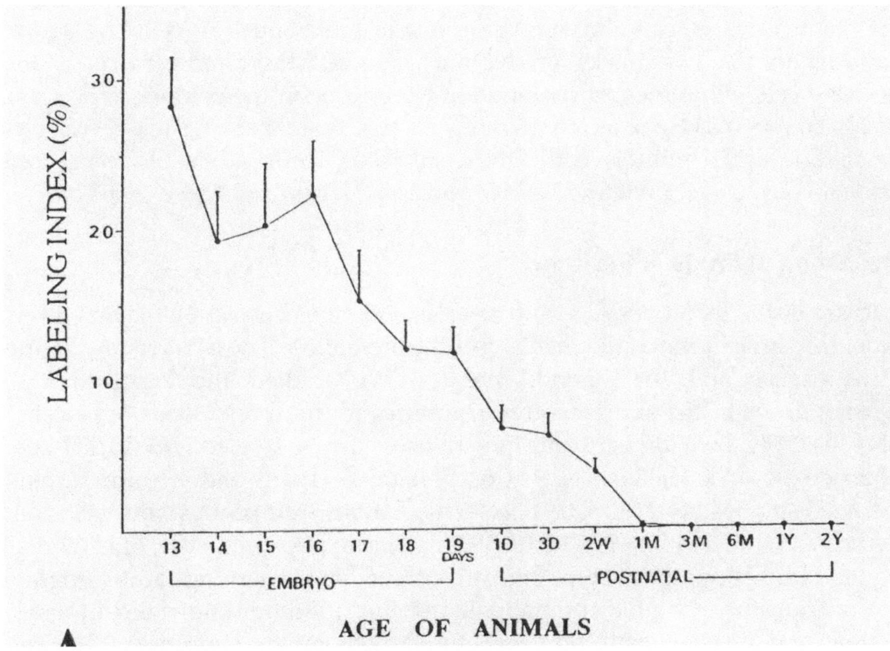

Fig. 5. The labeling indices of the muscular cells labeled with ^{3}H-thymidine revealed chronological changes, showing a peak at embryonic day 13 and decreasing gradually to 0% at 3 months after birth. From Nagata, T.: Radioautographology, General and Special. In, Prog. Histochem. Cytochem. Vol. 37, No. 2, p. 114, 2002, Urban & Fischer, Jena, Germany

2.2.2 The protein synthesis in the muscular system

We studied only ^{3}H-taurin incorporation in the skeletal muscles of both normal and dystrophy adult mice incubated in Eagle's medium containing ^{3}H-taurin in vitro at varying time intervals from 1 min to 5, 10, 30 and 60 min (1 hour). The silver grains were observed over the skeletal muscle cells as well as over the smooth muscle cells and the endothelial cells in the arteries, both the nuclei and cytoplalsm, by LM and EM RAG, showing taurin incorporation into the proteins (Terauch et al. 1988, Terauch and Nagata 1993, 1994). However, the aging changes were not studied yet.

3. Macromolecular synthesis in the circulatory system

The circulatory system or cardiovascular organs consists of the heart, the arteries, the veins, the capillaries, the blood, the lymphatic organs and the spleen. Among these cardiovascular organs, we studied the heart, the artery, some blood cells and the spleen.

3.1 The nucleic acid synthesis in the heart

Among the macromolecular synthesis, the nucleic acid synthesis, both DNA and RNA, in cultured cells from the hearts of chick embryos was studied by LM RAG (Nagata and Nawa 1966a,b). The fibroblasts of chick hearts in culture proliferated extensively and produced many binucleate cells. We compared the nucleic acid synthesis in mononucleate cells and binucleate cells in the heart fibroblasts. The incorporation of ^{3}H-thymidine into each nucleus of a binucleate cell was a little less than that of a mononucleate cell, but the total of the two nuclei of a binucleate cell was almost twice as that of a mononucleate cell. The incorporation of ^{3}H-uridine in the two nuclei of a binucleate cell was almost twice as that of a mononucleate cell, while the incorporation of ^{3}H-uridine in the cytoplasm of a binucleate cell was not so much as twice as a mononucleate cell. From these results, it was concluded that the nucleic acid synthesis both DNA and RNA increased in binucleate cells than mononucleate cells of chick embryo heart fibroblasts (Nagata and Nawa 1966a,b).

3.2 Localization of drugs in the artery

The structure of the blood vessels, both arteries and veins consist of 3 layers, from inside to outside, the tunica intima, the media and the adventitia. Those layers are formed with connective tissues and the smooth muscles. We studied the localization of anti-hypertensive drugs in the supramesenteric arteries of the spontaneous hypertensive rats (Suzuki et al. 1994). Two kinds of anti-hypertensive drugs, labeled with RI, ^{3}H-benidipine hydrochloride (Kyowa Hakko Kogyo Co., Shizuoka, Japan) and ^{3}H-nitrendipine (New England Nuclear, Boston, MA, USA) were used. Both intravenous administrations into rats and in vitro incubation for 10 to 30 min were employed. For light and electron microscopic radioautography, both the conventional wet-mounting radioautograms after chemical fixation for insoluble compounds and the dry-mounting radioautograms after cryo-fixation and freeze-substitution for soluble compounds were prepared. The silver grains due to the anti-hypertensive drugs were localized over the plasma membranes and the cytoplasm of the fibrocytes in the intima and the smooth muscle cells in the media, suggesting the pharmacological active sites. However, the localization of synthetic DNA was not studied.

3.3 The DNA synthesis in the blood cells

The mature blood cells circulating in the blood vessels of mammals are classified into 3 types, the erythrocytes, the leukocytes and the blood platelets. Those mature cells are formed either in the lymphatic tissues in the lymphatic organs or the myeloid tissues in the bone marrow, where various immature cells, lymphoblasts, erythroblasts, myeloblasts, meylocytes, and megakaryocytes can be observed. Among these blood cells, we studied macromolecular synthesis and cytochemical localization in leukocytes, megakaryocytes and blood platelets. As for the granulocytes, normal rabbit granulocytes were shown by EM RAG and X-ray microanalysis to incorporate $^{35}SO_4$ into the Golgi apparatus and to the granules demonstrating glucosaminoglycan synthesis (Murata et al. 1978, 1979).

On the other hand, the DNA, RNA and mucosubstance synthesis of mast cells from Wistar strain rats were studied by ^{3}H-thymidine, ^{3}H-uridine and $^{35}SO_4$ radioautography, demonstrating incorporation changes of those normal mast cells from abnormal mastocytoma cells (Murata et al. 1977a). Mast cells were widely found distributing in the loose connective tissues of most mammals, as well as in the serous exudate in the peritoneal cavity as one of the free cells. We studied the fine structure and nucleic acid and mucosubstance syntheses of normal mast cells and Dunn and Potter's mastocytoma cells in mice and rats by electron microscopic radioautography (Murata et al. 1977b, 1979). As the results, some of the normal mast cells and mastocytoma cells incorporated ^{3}H-thymidine, ^{3}H-uridine and $^{35}SO_4$, demonstrating DNA, RNA and mucosubstance syntheses. The incorporation of ^{3}H-thymidine was observed in the nuclei and mitochondria. The labeling index of ^{3}H-thymidine incorporation in the nuclei and mitochondria of normal mast cells was very low (0.37%) while that of mastocytoma cells was high (2-5%). These results suggested that the macromolecular synthesis such as nucleic acids (DNA, RNA) and mucosubstances were higher in tumor cells than normal blood cells.

3.4 Macromolecular synthesis in the spleen

The spleen is one of the blood cell forming organs and is composed of the lymphatic tissues. Among the macromolecular synthesis, both the DNA, RNA and protein syntheses in the spleen were studied.

3.4.1 The DNA synthesis in the spleen

We studied ^{3}H-thymidine incorporation into the splenic cells of aging mice from newborn to adult and senescence in connection with the lysosomal acid phosphatase activity (Olea 1991, Olea and Nagata 1991, 1992a). The acid phosphatase activity as demonstrated by means of cerium substrate method was observed in the splenic tissues at various ages from postnatal day 1, week 1 and 2, month 1, 2 and 10. Electron dense deposits were localized in the lysosomes of macrophages, reticular cells and littoral cells in all the aging groups. The intensity of the reaction products as visually observed increased from day 1 to week 1, reaching the peak at 1 week, and decreased from week 2 to month 10 due to aging. The incorporation of ^{3}H-thymidine, on the other hand, demonstrating DNA synthesis, was mainly observed in the hematopoietic cells in the spleens from postnatal day 1 to month 10 animals (Olea and Nagata 1991, 1992a). The labeling index was the maximum at day 1 and decreased to week 1, 2, 4, 8 and 40. A correlation between DNA synthesis and AcPase activity was examined by comparing two cell populations in the cell cycle, the S-phase cells which were labeled with ^{3}H-thymidine and the non-S-phase cells or the interphase cells which were not labeled. It was demonstrated that the former showed an increase and decrease of much more AcPase activity with the aging while the latter less activity and no change.

3.4.2 The RNA synthesis in the spleen

On the other hand, the number of labeled cells and the grain counts in the hematopoietic cells in the spleens labeled with ^{3}H-uridine, demonstrating RNA synthesis, from postnatal day 1 increased to 1 and 2 weeks, reaching the maximum, and decreased to 4, 8 and 40 weeks, different from the DNA synthesis (Olea and Nagata 1992b). These results demonstrated that AcPase activity, DNA and RNA synthetic activity changed due to aging.

3.4.3 The protein synthesis in the spleen

Among the circulatory organs, we first studied the protein synthesis in the spleens of aging mice at various ages. Several groups of litter mates, each 3, from fetal day 19 to postnatal day 1, 14, and month 6 to 12 (year 1) were administered with ^{3}H-leucine and sacrificed, the spleens were taken out and processed for LM and EM RAG (Nagata and Olea 1999). The results demonstrated that the sites of incorporations were hematopoietic cells, i.e., lymphoblasts, myeloblasts, erythroblasts and littoral cells in the splenic tissues at every aging stage. In most labeled cells silver grains were observed over the nuclei, nucleoli, endoplasmic reticulum, ribosomes, Golgi apparatus and mitochondria. Quantitative analysis revealed that grain counts in respective cells were higher in young animals than adult aged animals. The grain counts and the labeling index increased from prenatal to postnatal day 14, reaching the maximum, then decreased to month 12. These results showed the increase and decrease due to aging of animals.

4. Conclusion

This chapter deals with the introductory remarks describing the method and procedure of microscopic radioautography as well as the first parts of its application to the organ systems such as the skeletal, muscular and the circulatory organs. The method and the procedure of microscopic radioautography described the detailed technology which was developed by the present author and associates since 1955 in our laboratory. The application of radaioautography to the skeletal, muscular and circulatory systems demonstrated the sites of macromolecular syntheses such as DNA, RNA, proteins, glucides and lipids in various organs as well as the quantitative changes due to aging of the experimental animals. These results should be very important to understand the fundamental changes in the respective bones, the skeletal muscles, and the cardiovascular organs as well as the contributions to the experimental biology and medicine throughout the world.

5. References

Chen, S., Gao, F., Kotani, A., Nagata, T.: Age-related changes of male mouse submandibular gland: A morphometric and radioautographic study. Cell. Mol. Biol. 41, 117-124, 1995.

Clermont Y.: The contractime elements in the limiting membrane of the seminiferous tubules of rats. Exp. Cell Res. 15, 438-342, 1958.

Clermont, Y.: Renewal of spermatogonia in man. Amer. J. Anat. 112, 35-51, 1963.

Cui, H.: Light microscopic radioautographic study on DNA synthesis of nerve cells in the cerebella of aging mice. Cell. Mol. Biol. 41, 1139-1154, 1995.

Cui, H., Gao, F., Nagata, T.: Light microscopic radioautographic study on protein synthesis in perinatal mice corneas. Acta Histochem. Cytochem. 33, 31-37, 2000.

Duan, H., Gao, F., Li, S., Hayashi, K., Nagata, T.: Aging changes and fine structure and DNA synthesis of esophageal epithelium in neonatal, adult and old mice. J. Clin. Electron Microsc. 25, 452-453, 1992.

Duan, H., Gao, F., Li, S., Nagata, T.: Postnatal development of esophageal epithelium in mouse: a light and electron microscopic radioautographic study. Cell. Mol. Biol. 39, 309-316, 1993.

Duan, H., Gao, F., Oguchi, K., Nagata, T.: Light and electron microscopic radioautographic study on the incorporation of ^{3}H-thymidine into the lung by means of a new nebulizer. Drug Res. 44, 880-883, 1994.

Feulgen, R., Rossenbeck, H.: Mikroskopische-chemischer Nachweis einer Nukeinsaeure von Thymus der Thymonukeinsaeure Z. Physik. Chem. 135, 203-248, 1924.

Fujii, Y., Ohno, S., Yamabayashi, S., Usuda, N., Saito, H., Furuta, S., Nagata, T.: Electron microscopic radioautography of DNA synthesis in primary cultured cells from an IgG myeloma patient. J. Clin. Electr. Microsc. 13, 582-583, 1980.

Gao, F.: Study on the macromolecular synthesis in aging mouse seminiferous tubules by light and electron microscopic radioautography. Cell. Mol. Biol. 39, 659-672, 1993.

Gao, F., Toriyama, K., Nagata, T.: Light microscopic radioautographic study on the DNA synthesis of prenatal and postnatal aging mouse retina after labeled thymidine injection. Cell. Mol. Biol. 38, 661-668, 1992a.

Gao, F., Li, S., Duan, H., Ma, H., Nagata, T.: Electron microscopic radioautography on the DNA synthesis of prenatal and postnatal mice retina after labeled thymidine injection. J. Clin. Electron Microsc. 25, 721-722, 1992b.

Gao, F., Toriyama, K., Ma, H., Nagata, T.: Light microscopic radioautographic study on DNA synthesis in aging mice corneas. Cell. Mol. Biol. 39, 435-441, 1993.

Gao, F., Ma, H., Sun, L., Jin, C., Nagata, T.: Electron microscopic radioautographic study on the nucleic acids and protein synthesis in the aging mouse testis. Med. Electron Microsc. 27, 360-362, 1994.

Gao, F., Chen, S., Sun, L., Kang, W., Wang, Z., Nagata, T.: Radioautographic study of the macromolecular synthesis of Leydig cells in aging mice testis. Cell. Mol. Biol. 41, 145-150, 1995a.

Gao, F., Jin, C., Ma, H., Sun, L., Nagata, T.: Ultrastructural and radioautographic studies on DNA synthesis in Leydig cells of aging mouse testis. Cell. Mol. Biol. 41, 151-160, 1995b.

Gunarso, W.: Radioautographic studies on the nucleic acid synthesis of the retina of chick embryo. I. Light microscopic radioautography. Shinshu Med. J. 32, 231-240, 1984a.

Gunarso, W.: Radioautographic studies on the nucleic acid synthesis of the retina of chick embryo. II. Electron microscopic radioautography. Shinshu Med. J. 32, 241-248, 1984b.

Gunarso, W., Gao, F., Cui, H., Ma, H., Nagata, T.: A light and electron microscopic radioautographic study on RNA synthesis in the retina of chick embryo. Acta Histochem. 98, 309-32, 1996.

Gunarso, W., Gao, F., Nagata, T.: Development and DNA synthesis in the retina of chick embryo observed by light and electron microscopic radioautography. Cell. Mol. Biol. 43, 189-201, 1997.

Hanai, T.: Light microscopic radioautographic study of DNA synthesis in the kidneys of aging mice. Cell. Mol. Biol. 39, 81-91, 1993.

Hanai, T., Nagata, T.: Electron microscopic radioautographic study on DNA and RNA synthesis in perinatal mouse kidney. In, Radioautography in Medicine, Nagata, T., Ed., pp. 127-131, Shinshu University Press, Matsumoto, 1994a.

Hanai, T., Nagata, T.: Study on the nucleic acid synthesis in the aging mouse kidney by light and electron microscopic radioautography. In, Radioautography in Medicine, Nagata, T., Ed., pp. 209-214, Shinshu University Press, Matsumoto, 1994b.

Hanai, T., Nagata, T.: Electron microscopic study on nucleic acid synthesis in perinatal mouse kidney tissue. Med. Electron Microsc. 27, 355-357, 1994c.

Hanai, T., Usuda, N., Morita, T., Shimizu, T., Nagata, T.: Proliferative activity in the kidneys of aging mice evaluated by PCNA/cyclin immunohistochemistry. Cell. Mol. Biol. 39, 181-191, 1993.

Hayashi, K., Gao, F., Nagata, T.: Radioautographic study on ^{3}H-thymidine incorporation at different stages of muscle development in aging mice. Cell. Mol. Biol. 39, 553-560, 1993.

Ito, M.: The radioautographic studies on aging change of DNA synthesis and the ultrastructural development of mouse adrenal gland. Cell. Mol. Biol. 42, 279-292, 1996.

Ito, M., Nagata, T.: Electron microscopic radioautographic studies on DNA synthesis and ultrastructure of aging mouse adrenal gland. Med. Electron Microsc. 29, 145-152, 1996.

Izumiyama, K., Kogure, K., Kataoka, S., Nagata, T.: Quantitative analysis of glucose after transient ischemia in the gerbil hippocampus by light and electron microscope radioautography. Brain Res. 416, 175-179, 1987.

Jamieson, J. D., Palade, G. E.: Intracellular transport of secretory proteins in the pancreatic exocrine cells. J. Cell Biol. 34, 577-615, 1967.

Jin, C.: Study on DNA synthesis of aging mouse colon by light and electron microscopic radioautography. Cell. Mol. Biol. 42, 255-268, 1996.

Jin, C., Nagata, T.: Light microscopic radioautographic study on DNA synthesis in cecal epithelial cells of aging mice. J. Histochem. Cytochem. 43, 1223-1228, 1995a.

Jin, C., Nagata, T.: Electron microscopic radioautographic study on DNA synthesis in cecal epithelial cells of aging mice. Med. Electron Microsc. 28, 71-75, 1995b.

Joukura, K.: The aging changes of glycoconjugate synthesis in mouse kidney studied by ^{3}H-glucosamine radioautography. Acta Histochem. Cytochem. 29, 57-63, 1996.

Joukura, K., Nagata, T.: Aging changes of ^{3}H-glucosamine incorporation into mouse kidney observed by radioautography. Acta Histochem. Cytochem. 28, 494-494, 1995.

Joukura, K., Usuda, N., Nagata, T.: Quantitative study on the aging change of glycoconjugates synthesis in aging mouse kidney. Proc. Xth Internat. Cong. Histochem. Cytochem., Acta Histochem. Cytochem. 29, Suppl. 507-508, 1996.

Kobayashi, K., Nagata, T.: Light microscopic radioautographic studies on DNA, RNA and protein syntheses in human synovial membranes of rheumatoid arthritis patients. J. Histochem. Cytochem. 42, 982-982, 1994.

Komiyama, K., Iida, F., Furihara, R., Murata, F., Nagata, T.: Electron microscopic radioautographic study on ^{125}I-albumin in rat gastric mucosal epithelia. J. Clin. Electron Microsc. 11, 428-429, 1978.

Kong, Y.: Electron microscopic radioautographic study on DNA synthesis in perinatal mouse retina. Cell. Mol. Biol. 39, 55-64, 1993.

Kong, Y., Nagata, T.: Electron microscopic radioautographic study on nucleic acid synthesis of perinatal mouse retina. Med. Electron Microsc. 27, 366-368, 1994.

Kong, Y., Usuda, N., Nagata, T.: Radioautographic study on DNA synthesis of the retina and retinal pigment epithelium of developing mouse embryo. Cell. Mol. Biol. 38, 263-272, 1992a.

Kong, Y., Usuda, N., Morita, T., Hanai, T., Nagata, T.: Study on RNA synthesis in the retina and retinal pigment epithelium of mice by light microscopic radioautography. Cell. Mol. Biol. 38, 669-678, 1992b.

Leblond, C. P.: Localization of newly administered iodine in the thyroid gland as indicated by radioiodine. J. Anat. 77, 149-152, 1943.

Leblond, C. P.: The life history of cells in renewing systems. Am. J. Anat. 160, 113-158, 1981.

Leblond, C. P., Messier, B.: Renewal of chief cells and goblet cells in the small intestine as shown by radioautography after injection of thymidine-^{3}H into mice. Anat. Rec. 132: 247-259. 1958.

Li, S.: Relationship between cellular DNA synthesis, PCNA expression and sex steroid hormone receptor status in the developing mouse ovary, uterus and oviduct. Histochemistry 102, 405-413, 1994.

Li, S., Nagata, T.: Nucleic acid synthesis in the developing mouse ovary, uterus and oviduct studied by light and electron microscopic radioautography. Cell. Mol. Biol. 41, 185-195, 1995.

Li, S., Gao, F., Duan, H., Nagata, T.: Radioautographic study on the uptake of $^{35}SO_4$ in mouse ovary during the estrus cycle. J. Clin. Electron Microsc. 25, 709-710, 1992.

Liang, Y.: Light microscopic radioautographic study on RNA synthesis in the adrenal glands of aging mice. Acta Histochem. Cytochem. 31, 203-210, 1998.

Liang, Y., Ito, M., Nagata, T.: Light and electron microscopic radioautographic studies on RNA synthesis in aging mouse adrenal gland. Acta Anat. Nippon. 74, 291-300, 1999.

Ma, H.: Light microscopic radioautographic study on DNA synthesis of the livers in aging mice. Acta Anat. Nippon. 63, 137-147, 1988.

Ma, H., Nagata, T.: Electron microscopic radioautographic study on DNA synthesis of the livers in aging mice. J. Clin. Electron Microsc. 21, 335-343, 1988a.

Ma, H., Nagata, T.: Studies on DNA synthesis of aging mice by means of electron microscopic radioautography. J. Clin. Electron Microsc. 21, 715-716, 1988b.

Ma, H., Nagata, T.: Electron microscopic radioautographic studies on DNA synthesis in the hepatocytes of aging mice as observed by image analysis. Cell. Mol. Biol. 36, 73-84, 1990a.

Ma, H., Nagata, T.: Study on RNA synthesis in the livers of aging mice by means of electron microscopic radioautography. Cell. Mol. Biol. 36, 589-600, 1990b.

Ma, H., Nagata, T.: Collagen and protein synthesis in the livers of aging mice as studied by electron microsopic radioautography. Ann. Microsc. 1, 13-22, 2000.

Ma, H., Gao, F., Olea, M. T., Nagata, T.: Protein synthesis in the livers of aging mice studied by electron microscopic radioautography. Cell. Mol. Biol. 37, 607-615, 1991.

Matsumura, H., Kobayashi, Y., Kobayashi, K., Nagata, T.: Light microscopic radioautographic study of DNA synthesis in the lung of aging salamander, Hynobius nebulosus. J. Histochem. Cytochem. 42, 1004-1004, 1994.

Momose, Y., Nagata, T.: Radioautographic study on the intracellular localization of a hypolipidemic agent, bezafibrate, a peroxisome proliferator, in cultured rat hepatocytes. Cell. Mol. Biol. 39, 773-781, 1993a.

Momose, Y., Naito, J., Nagata, T.: Radioautographic study on the localization of an anti-allergic agent, tranilast, in the rat liver. Cell. Mol. Biol. 35, 347-355, 1989.

Momose, Y., Shibata, N., Kiyosawa, I., Naito, J., Watanabe, T., Horie, S., Yamada, J., Suga, T., Nagata, T.: Morphometric evaluation of species differences in the effects of bezafibrate, a hypolipidemic agent, on hepatic peroxisomes and mitochondria. J. Toxicol. Pathol. 6, 33-45, 1993b.

Momose, Y., Naito, J., Suzawa, H., Kanzawa, M., Nagata, T.: Radioautographic study on the intracellular localization of bezafibrate in cultured rat hepatoctyes. Acta Histochem. Cytochem. 28, 61-66, 1995.

Morita, T.: Radioautographic study on the aging change of ^{3}H-glucosamine uptake in mouse ileum. Cell. Mol. Biol. 39, 875-884, 1993.

Morita, T., Usuda, N. Hanai, T., Nagata, T.: Changes of colon epithelium proliferation due to individual aging with PCNA/cyclin immunostaining comparing with ^{3}H-thymidine radioautography. Histochemistry 101, 13-20, 1994.

Murata, F., Momose,Y. , Yoshida, K., Nagata, T.: Incorporation of ^{3}H-thymidine into the nucleus of mast cells in adult rat peritoneum. Shinshu Med. J. 25, 72-77, 1977a.

Murata, F., Momose, Y., Yoshida, K., Ohno, S., Nagata, T.: Nucleic acid and mucosubstance metabolism of mastocytoma cells by means of electron microscopic radioautography. Acta Pharmacol. Toxicol. 41, 58-59, 1977b.

Murata, F., Yoshida, K., Ohno, S., Nagata, T.: Ultrastructural and electron microscopic radioautographic studies on the mastocytoma cells and mast cells. J. Clin. Electron Microsc. 11, 561-562, 1978.

Murata, F., Yoshida, K., Ohno, S., Nagata, T.: Mucosubstances of rabbit granulocytes studied by means of electron microscopic radioautography and X-ray microanalysis. Histochemistry 61, 139-150, 1979.

Nagata, T.: On the relationship between cell division and cytochrome oxidase in the Yoshida sarcoma cells. Shinshu Med. J. 5: 383-386, 1956.

Nagata, T.: Studies on the amitosis in the Yoshida sarcoma cells. I. Observation on the smear preparation under normal conditions. Med. J. Shinshu Univ. 2: 187-198, 1957a.

Nagata, T.: Studies on the amitosis in the Yoshida sarcoma cells. II. Phase-contrast microscopic observations under normal conditions. Med. J. Shinshu Univ. 2: 199-207, 1957b.

Nagata, T.: Cell divisions in the liver of the fetal and newborn dogs. Med. J. Shinshu Univ. 4: 65-73, 1959.

Nagata, T.: A radioautographic study of the DNA synthesis in rat liver, with special reference to binucleate cells. Med. J. Shinshu Univ. 7, 17-25, 1962.

Nagata, T.: A quantitative study on the ganglion cells in the small intestine of the dog. Med. J. Shinshu Univ. 10, 1-11, 1965.

Nagata, T.: A radioautographic study on the RNA synthesis in the hepatic and the intestinal epithelial cells of mice after feeding with special reference to binuclearity. Med. J. Shinshu Univ. 11, 49-61, 1966.

Nagata, T.: On the increase of binucleate cells in the ganglion cells of dog small intestine due to experimental ischemia. Med. J. Shinshu Univ. 12, 93-113, 1967a.

Nagata, T.: A radioautographic study on the protein synthesis in the hepatic and the intestinal epithelial cells of mice, with special reference to binucleate cells. Med. J. Shinshu Univ. 12, 247-257, 1967b.

Nagata, T.: Chapter 3. Application of microspectrophotometry to various substances. In , Introduction to Microspectrophotometry. Isaka, S., Nagata, T., Inui, N., Eds., Olympus Co., Tokyo, pp. 49-155, 1972a.

Nagata, T.: Electron microscopic dry-mounting autoradiography. Proc. 4th Internat. Cong. Histochem. Cytochem. Kyoto, pp. 43-44, 1972b.

Nagata, T.: Electron microscopic radioautography of intramitochondrial RNA synthesis of HeLa cells in culture. Histochemie 32, 163-170, 1972c.

Nagata, T.: Quantitative electron microscope radioautography of intramitochondrial nucleic acid synthesis. Acta Histochem. Cytochem. 5, 201-203, 1972d.

Nagata, T.: Electron microscopic observation of target cells previously observed by phase-contrast microscopy: Electron microscopic radioautography of laser beam irradiated cultured cells. J. Clin. Electron Microsc. 17, 589-590, 1984.

Nagata, T.: Principles and techniques of radioautography. In, Histo- and Cyto-chemistry 1985, Japan Society of Histochemistry and Cytochemistry, Ed., Gakusai Kikaku Co., Tokyo, pp. 207-226, 1985.

Nagata, T.:. Electron microscopic radioautography and analytical electron microscopy. J. Clin. Electron Microsc. 24, 441-442, 1991.

Nagata, T.: Radiolabeling of soluble and insoluble compounds as demonstrated by light and electron microscopy. Recent Advances in Cellular and Molecular Biology, Wegmann, R. J., Wegmann, M. A., Eds. Peters Press, Leuven, Vol. 6, pp. 9-21, 1992.

Nagata, T.: Quantitative analysis of histochemical reactions: Image analysis of light and electron microscopic radioautograms. Acta Histochem. Cytochem. 26, 281-291, 1993a.

Nagata, T. Quantitative light and electron microscopic radioautographic studies on macromolecular synthesis in several organs of prenatal and postnatal aging mice. Chinese J. Histochem. Cytochem. 2: 106-108, 1993b.

Nagata, T.: Electron microscopic radioautography with cryo-fixation and dry-mounting procedure. Acta Histochem. Cytochem. 27: 471-489, 1994a.

Nagata, T.: Application of electron microscopic radioautography to clinical electron microscopy. Med. Electron Microsc. 27; 191-212, 1994b.

Nagata, T.: Radioautography in Medicine. Shinshu University Press, 268pp, Matsumoto, 1994c.

Nagata, T.: Radioautography, general and special. In, Histo- and Cyto-chemistry 1994, Japan Society of Histochemistry and Cytochemistry, ed, pp. 219-231, Gakusai Kikaku Co., Tokyo, 1994d.

Nagata, T., Application of electron microscopic radioautography to clinical electron microscopy. Med. Electron Microsc. 27, 191-212, 1994e.
Nagata, T.: Light and electron microscopic radioautographic study on macromolecular synthesis in digestive organs of aging mice. Cell. Mol. Biol. 41, 21-38, 1995a.
Nagata, T.: Histochemistry of the organs: Application of histochemistry to anatomy. Acta Anat. Nippon. 70, 448-471, 1995b.
Nagata, T.: Three-dimensional observation of whole mount cultured cells stained with histochemical reactions by ultrahigh voltage electron microscopy. Cell. Mol. Biol. 41, 783-792, 1995c.
Nagata, T.: Morphometry in anatomy: image analysis on fine structure and histochemical reactions with special reference to radioautography. Ital. J. Anat. 100 (Suppl. 1), 591-605, 1995d.
Nagata, T.: Technique and application of electron microscopic radioautography. J. Electron Microsc. 45, 258-274, 1996a.
Nagata, T.: Techniques of light and electron microscopic radioautography. In, Histochemistry and Cytochemistry 1996. Proc. Xth Internat. Congr. Histochem. Cytochem. Acta Histochem. Cytochem. 29 (Suppl.), 343-344, 1996b.
Nagata, T.: Remarks: Radioautographology, general and special. Cell. Mol. Biol. 42 (Suppl.), 11-12, 1996c.
Nagata, T.: On the terminology of radioautography vs. autoradiography. J. Histochem. Cytochem. 44, 1209-1209, 1996d.
Nagata, T.: Techniques and applications of microscopic radioautography. Acta Microsc. Vol. 6: Suppl. B. p. 19-42, 1997a.
Nagata T.: Three-dimensional observation on whole mount cultured cells and thick sections stained with histochemical reactions by high voltage electron microscopy. In, Recent Advances in Microscopy of Cells, Tissues and Organs, Motta, P., Ed., Antonio Delfino Editore, Roma, pp. 37-44, 1997b.
Nagata, T.: Radioautographic study on collagen synthesis in the ocular tissues. J. Kaken Eye Res. 15, 1-9, 1997c.
Nagata, T.: Techniques of radioautography for medical and biological research. Braz. J. Biol. Med. Res. 31, 185-195, 1998a.
Nagata, T.: Radioautographology, the advocacy of a new concept. Braz. J. Biol. Med. Res. 31, 201-241, 1998b.
Nagata, T.: Radioautographic studies on DNA synthesis of the bone and skin of aging salamander. Bull. Nagano Women's Jr. College 6, 1-14, 1998c.
Nagata, T.: 3D observation of cell organelles by high voltage electron microscopy. Microscopy and Analysis, Asia Pacific Edition, 9, 29-32, 1999a.
Nagata, T.: Application of histochemistry to anatomy: Histochemistry of the organs, a novel concept. Proc. XV Congress of the International Federation of Associations of Anatomists, Ital. J. Anat. Embryol. 104 (Suppl. 1), 486-486, 1999b.
Nagata, T.: Aging changes of macromolecular synthesis in various organ systems as observed by microscopic radioautography after incorporation of radiolabeled precursors. Methods Find. Exp. Clin. Pharmacol. 21, 683-706, 1999c.
Nagata, T.: Radioautographic study on protein synthesis in mouse cornea. J. Kaken Eye Res. 8, 8-14, 1999d.

Nagata, T.: Radioautographology, general and special: a novel concept. Ital. J. Anat. Embryol. 104 (Suppl. 1), 487-487, 1999e.
Nagata, T.: Three-dimensional observations on thick biological specimens by high voltage electron microscopy. Image Analysis Stereolog. 19, 51-56, 2000a.
Nagata, T.: Biological microanalysis of radiolabeled and unlabeled compounds by radioautography and X-ray microanalysis. Scanning Microscopy International, 14, on line, 2000b.
Nagata, T.: Electron microscopic radioautographic study on protein synthesis in pancreatic cells of perinatal and aging mice. Bull. Nagano Women's Jr. College 8, 1-22, 2000c.
Nagata, T.: Light microscopic radioautographic study on radiosulfate incorporation into the tracheal cartilage in aging mice. Acta Histochem. Cytochem. 32, 377-383, 2000d.
Nagata, T.: Introductory remarks: Special radioautographology. Cell. Mol. Biol. 46 (Congress Suppl.), 161-161, 2000e.
Nagata, T.: Special radioautographology: the eye. J. Kaken Eye Res. 18, 1-13, 2000f.
Nagata, T.: Three-dimensional high voltage electron microscopy of thick biological specimens. Micron 32, 387-404, 2001a.
Nagata, T.: Three-dimensional and four-dimensional observation of histochemical and cytochemical specimens by high voltage electron microscopy. Acta Histochem. Cytochem. 34, 153-169, 2001b.
Nagata, T. : Special cytochemistry in cell biology. In, Internat. Rev. Cytol. Jeon, K.W., ed., Vol. 211, Chapter 2, Academic Press, New York, pp. 33-154, 2001c.
Nagata, T. : Radioautographology General and Special, In, Prog. Histochem. Cytochem., Graumann, W., Ed., Vol. 37 No. 2, Urban & Fischer, Jena, pp. 57-226, 2002.
Nagata T.: Light and electron microscopic study on macromolecular synthesis in amitotic hepatocyte mitochondria of aging mice. Cell. Mol. Biol. 49, 591-611, 2003.
Nagata, T.: X-ray microanalysis of biological specimens by high voltage electron microscopy. In, Prog. Histochem. Cytochem., Graumann, W., Ed., Vol. 39, No. 4, Urban & Fischer Verlag, Jena, pp. 185-320, 2004.
Nagata T.: Aging changes of macromolecular synthesis in the uro-genital organs as revealed by electron microscopic radioautography. Ann. Rev. Biomed. Sci. 6, 13-78, 2005.
Nagata T.: Electron microscopic radioautographic study on protein synthesis in hepatocyte mitochondria of developing mice. Ann. Microsc. 6, 43-54, 2006a.
Nagata T.: Electron microscopic radioautographic study on nucleic acids synthesis in hepatocyte mitochondria of developing mice. The Sci. World J. 6: 1583-1598, 2006b.
Nagata T.: Macromolecular synthesis in hepatocyte mitochondria of aging mice as revealed by electron microscopic radioautography. I: Nucleic acid synthesis. In, Modern Research and Educational Topics in Microscopy. Mendez-Vilas, A. and Diaz, J. Eds., Formatex Micrscopy Series No. 3, Vol. 1, Formatex, Badajoz, Spain, pp. 245-258, 2007a.
Nagata T.: Macromolecular synthesis in hepatocyte mitochondria of aging mice as revealed by electron microscopic radioautography. II: Protein synthesis. In, Modern Research and Educational Topics in Microscopy. Mendez-Vilas, A. and Diaz, J. eds., Formatex Micrscopy Series No. 3, Vol. 1, Formatex, Badajoz, Spain, pp. 259-271, 2007b.
Nagata, T.: Electron microscopic radioautographic study on macromolecular synthesis in hepatocyte mitochondria of aging mouse. J. Cell Tissue Res. 7, 1019-1029, 2007c.

Nagata, T.; Electron microscopic radioautographic study on nucleic acids synthesis in hepatocyte mitochondria of developing mice. Trends Cell Molec. Biol. 2, 19-33, 2007d.

Nagata, T.; Aging changes of macromolecular synthesis in the mitochondria of mouse hepatocytes as revealed by microscopic radioautography. Ann. Rev. Biomed. Sci. 9, 30-36, 2007e.

Nagata, T.: Radioautographology, Bull. Shinshu Institute Alternat. Med. 2, 3-32, 2007f.

Nagata, T.: Electron microscopic radioautographic study on mitochondrial DNA synthesis in adrenal cortical cells of developing mice. J. Cell. Tis. Res. 8, 1303-1312, 2008a.

Nagata T.: Electron microscopic radioautographic study on mitochondrial DNA synthesis in adrenal cortical cells of developing and aging mice. The Sci. World J. 8, 683-697. 2008b.

Nagata, T.: Sexual difference between the macromolecular synthesis of hepatocyte mitochondria in male and female mice in aging as revealed by electron microscopic radioautography. Chapter 22. In, Women and Aging: New Research, H. T. Bennninghouse, A. D. Rosset, Eds. Nova Biomed. Books, New York, pp. 461-487, 2009a

Nagata, T.: Protein synthesis in hepatocytes of mice as revealed by electron microscopic radioautography. In, Protein Biosynthesis. Esterhouse, T. E. and Petrinos, L. B., Eds., Nova Biomed. Books, New York, pp. 133-161, 2009b.

Nagata, T.: Electron microscopic radioatuographic studies on macromolecular synthesis in mitochondria of various cells. 18EMSM Conference Proc. 9th Asia-Pacific Microscopy Conference (APMC9), Kuala Lumpur, Malaysia, pp. 48-50, 2009c.

Nagata, T.: Recent studies on macromolecular synthesis labeled with ^{3}H-thymidine in various organs as revealed by electron microscopic radioautography. Current Radiopharmaceutics 2, 118-128, 2009d.

Nagata, T.: Electron microscopic radioautographic study on mitochondrial DNA synthesis in adrenal medullary cells of developing and aging mice. J. Cell Tissue Res. 9, 1793-1802, 2009e.

Nagata, T.: Applications of high voltage electron microscopy to thick biological specimens. Ann. Microsc. 9, 4-40, 2009f.

Nagata, T.: Electron microscopic radioautographic study on DNA synthesis of mitochondria in adrenal medullary cells of aging mice. Open Anat. J. 1, 14-24, 2009g.

Nagata, T.: Electron microscopic radioautographic studies on macromolecular synthesis in mitochondria of animal cells in aging. Ann. Rev. Biomed. Sci. 11, 1-17, 2009h.

Nagata, T.: Electron microscopic radioautographic studies on macromoleclular synthesis in mitochondria of some organs in aging animals. Bull. Shinshu Inst. Alternat. Med. Welfare 4, 15-38, 2009i.

Nagata, T.: Electron microscopic radioautographic study on mitochondrial DNA synthesis in adreno-cortical cells of aging ddY mice. Bull. Shinshu Inst. Alternat. Med. Welfare 4, 51-66, 2009j.

Nagata T.: Electron microscopic radioautographic study on mitochondrial RNA synthesis in adrenocortical cells of aging mice. Open Anat J. 2, 91-97, 2010a.

Nagata T. Electron microscopic radioautographic study on mitochondrial RNA synthesis in adrenal medullary cells of aging and senescent mice. J Cell Tissue Res. 10, 2213-2222, 2010b.

Nagata, T.: Macromolecular synthesis in the livers of aging mice as revealed by electron microscopic radioautography. In, Prog. Histochem. Cytochem., Sasse, D., Ed., Elsevier, Amsterdam, Boston, London, New York, Oxford, Paris, Philadelphia, San Diego, St. Louis, Vol. 45, No. 1, pp. 1-80, 2010c.

Nagata, T.: Electron microscopic radioautographic study on protein synthesis of mitochondria in adrenal medullary cells of aging mice. Bulletin Shinshu Inst Alternat Med Welfare 5, 25-37, 2010d.

Nagata, T.: Electron microscopic radioautographic study on mitochondrial RNA synthesis in adrenal cortical and medullary cells of aging mice. J. Biomed. Sci. Enginer. 4, 219-232, 2010e.

Nagata, T.: Electron microscopic radioautographic study on protein synthesis of mitochondria in adrenal cortical cells of aging mice. Bulletin Shinshu Inst. Alternat. Med. Welfare 5, 38-52, 2010f.

Nagata T.: Electron microscopic radioautographic study on mitochondrial DNA, RNA and protein synthesis in adrenal cells of aging mice. Formatex Microscopy Series No. 3, Vol. 3, Formatex, Badajoz, Spain, in press, 2010g.

Nagata, T.: Electron microscopic radioautographic studies on macromolecular synthesis in mitochondria of animal cells in aging. Ann. Rev. Biomed. Sci. 12, 1-29, 2010h.

Nagata, T., Cui, H., Gao, F.: Radioautographic study on glycoprotein synthesis in the ocular tissues. J. Kaken Eye Res. 13, 11-18, 1995.

Nagata, T., Cui, H., Kong, Y.: The localization of TGF-b1 and its mRNA in the spinal cords of prenatal and postnatal aging mice demonstrated with immunohistochemical and in situ hybridization techniques. Bull. Nagano Women's Jr. College, 7, 75-88, 1999a.

Nagata, T., Cui, H., Liang, Y.: Light microscopic radioautographic study on the protein synthesis in the cerebellum of aging mouse. Bull. Nagano Women's Jr. College, 9, 41-60 (2001).

Nagata, T., Fujii, Y., Usuda, N.: Demonstration of extranuclear nucleic acid synthesis in mammalian cells under experimental conditions by electron microscopic radioautography. Proc. 10th Internat. Congr. Electr. Microsc. 2, 305-306, 1982b.

Nagata, T., Hirano, I., Shibata, O., Nagata, T.: A radioautographic study on the DNA synthesis in the hepatic and the pancreatic acinar cells of mice during the postnatal growth, with special reference to binuclearity. Med. J. Shinshu Univ. 11, 35-42, 1966.

Nagata, T., Ito, M., Chen, S.: Aging changes of DNA synthesis in the submandibular glands of mice as observed by light and electron microscopic radioautography. Ann. Microsc. 1, 4-12, 2000a.

Nagata, T. Ito, M., Liang, Y.: Study of the effects of aging on macromolecular synthesis in mouse steroid secreting cells using microscopic radioautography. Methods Find. Exp. Clin. Pharmacol. 22, 5-18, 2000b.

Nagata, T., Iwadare, I., Murata, F.: Electron microscopic radioautography of nucleic acid synthesis in cultured cells treated with several carcinogens. Acta Pharmacol. Toxicol. 41, 64-65, 1977c.

Nagata, T., Kawahara, I.: Radioautographic study of the synthesis of sulfomucin in digestive organs of mice. J. Trace Microprobe Analysis 17, 339-355, 1999.

Nagata, T., Kawahara, I., Usuda, N., Maruyama, M., Ma, H.: Radioautographic studies on the glycoconjugate synthesis in the gastrointestinal mucosa of the mouse. In,

Glycoconjugate in Medicine, Ohyama, M., Muramatsu, T., Eds, pp. 251-256, Professional Postgrad. Service, Tokyo, 1988a.

Nagata, T., Kong, Y.: Distribution and localization of TGFb1 and bFGF, and their mRNAs in aging mice. Bull. Nagano Women's Jr. College 6, 87-105, 1998.

Nagata, T., Ma, H., Electron microscopic radioautographic study on mitochondrial DNA synthesis in hepatocytes of aging mouse. Ann. Microsc. 5, 4-18, 2005a.

Nagata, T., Ma, H., Electron microscopic radioautographic study on RNA synthesis in hepatocyte mitochondria of aging mouse. Microsc. Res. Tech. 67, 55-64, 2005b.

Nagata, T., Momoze, S.: Aging changes of the amitotic and binucleate cells in dog livers. Acta Anat. Nipponica 34, 187-190, 1959.

Nagata, T., Morita, T., I. Kawahara, I.: Radioautographic studies on radiosulfate incorporation in the digestive organs of mice. Histol. Histopathol. 14, 1-8, 1999b.

Nagata, T., Murata, F.: Electron microscopic dry-mounting radioautography for diffusible compounds by means of ultracryotomy. Histochemistry 54, 75-82, 1977.

Nagata, T., Murata, F., Yoshida, K., Ohno, S., Iwadare, N.: Whole mount radioautography of cultured cells as observed by high voltage electron microscopy. Proc. Fifth Internat. Conf. High Voltage Electron Microsc. 347-350, 1977d.

Nagata, T., Nawa, T.: A modification of dry-mounting technique for radioautography of water-soluble compounds. Histochemie 7, 370-371, 1966a.

Nagata, T., Nawa, T.: A radioautographic study on the nucleic acids synthesis of binucleate cells in cultivated fibroblasts of chick embryos. Med. J. Shinshu Univ. 11, 1-5, 1966b.

Nagata, T., Nawa, T., Yokota, S.: A new technique for electron microscopic dry-mounting radioautography of soluble compounds. Histochemie 18, 241-249, 1969.

Nagata, T., Nishigaki, T., Momose, Y.: Localization of anti-allergic agent in rat mast cells demonstrated by light and electron microscopic radioautography. Acta Histochem. Cytochem. 19, 669-683, 1986b.

Nagata, T., Ohno, S., Kawahara, I., Yamabayashi, S., Fujii, Y., Murata, F.: Light and electron microscopic radioautography of nucleic acid synthesis in mitochondria and peroxisomes of rat hepatic cells during and after DEHP administration. Acta Histochem. Cytochem. 16, 610-611, 1979.

Nagata, T., Ohno, S., Murata, F.: Electron microscopic dry-mounting radioautography for soluble compounds. Acta Phamacol. Toxicol. 41, 62-63, 1977a.

Nagata, T., Ohno, S., Yoshida, K., Murata, F.: Nucleic acid synthesis in proliferating peroxisomes of rat liver as revealed by electron microscopical radioautography. Histochem. J. 14, 197-204, 1982a.

Nagata, T., Olea, M. T.: Electron microscopic radioautographic study on the protein synthesis in aging mouse spleen. Bull. Nagano Women's Jr. College 7, 1-9, 1999.

Nagata, T., Shibata, O., Omochi, S.: A new method for radioautographic osbservation on isolated cells. Histochemie 2, 255-259, 1961

Nagata, T., Shibata, O., Nawa, T.: Simplified methods for mass production of radioautograms. -Acta Anat. Nippon.42, 162-166, 1967a.

Nagata, T., Shibata, O., Nawa, T.: Incorporation of tritiated thymidine into mitochondrial DNA of the liver and kidney cells of chickens and mice in tissue culture. Histochemie 10, 305-308, 1967b.

Nagata, T., Shimamura, K., Onozawa, M., Kondo, T., Ohkubo, K., Momoze, S.: Relationship of binuclearity to cell function in some organs. I. Frequencies of binucleate cells in some organs of toads in summer and winter. Med. J. Shinshu Univ. 5, 147-152, 1960a.

Nagata, T., Shimamura, K., Kondo, T., Onozawa, M., Momoze, S., Okubo, M.: Relationship of binuclearity to cell function in some organs. II. Variation of frequencies of binucleate cells in some organs of dogs owing to aging. Med. J. Shinshu Univ. 5, 153-158, 1960b.

Nagata, T., Steggerda, F. R.: Histological study on the deganglionated small intestine of the dog. Physiologist 6, 242-242, 1963.

Nagata, T., Steggerda, F. R.: Observations on the increase of binucleate cells in the ganglion cells of the dog's intestine due to experimental ischemia. Anat. Rec. 148, 315-315, 1964.

Nagata, T., Toriyama, K., Kong, Y., Jin, C., Gao, F.: Radioautographic study on DNA synthesis in the ciliary bodies of aging mice. J. Kaken Eye Res.12, 1-11, 1994.

Nagata, T., Usuda, N.: Image processing of electron microscopic radioautograms in clinical electron microscopy. J. Clin. Electron. Microsc. 18, 451-452, 1985.

Nagata, T., Usuda, N.: Studies on the nucleic acid synthesis in pancreatic acinar cells of aging mice by means of electron microscopic radioautography. J. Clin. Electron Microsc. 19, 486-487, 1986.

Nagata, T., Usuda, N.: Electron microscopic radioautography of protein synthesis in pancreatic acinar cells of aging mice. Acta Histochem. Cytochem. 26, 481-481, 1993a.

Nagata, T., Usuda, N.: In situ hybridization by electron microscopy using radioactive probes. J. Histochem. Cytochem. 41, 1119-1119, 1993b.

Nagata, T., Usuda, N., Ma, H.: Electron microscopic radioautography of nucleic acid synthesis in pancreatic acinar cells of prenatal and postnatal aging mice. Proc. XIth Intern. Cong. Electr. Microsc. 3, 2281-2282, 1984.

Nagata, T., Usuda, N., Ma, H.: Electron microscopic radioautography of lipid synthesis in pancreatic cells of aging mice. J. Clin. Electr. Microsc. 23, 841-842, 1990.

Nagata, T., Usuda, N., Maruyama, M., Ma, H.: Electron microscopic radioautographic study on lipid synthesis in perinatal mouse pancreas. J. Clin. Electr. Microsc. 21, 756-757, 1988b.

Nagata, T., Usuda, N., Suzawa, H., Kanzawa, M.: Incorporation of ^{3}H-glucosamine into the pancreatic cells of aging mice as demonstrated by electron microscopic radioautography. J. Clin. Electron Microsc. 25, 646-647, 1992.

Nagata, T., Yamabayashi, S.: Intracellular localization of ^{3}H-befunolol by means of electron microscopic radioautography of cryo-fixed ultrathin sections. J. Clin. Electron Microsc. 16, 737-738, 1983.

Nagata, T., Yoshida, K., Murata, F.: Demonstration of hot and cold mercury in the human thyroid tissues by means of radioautography and chemography. Acta Pharmacol. Toxicol. 41, 60-61, 1977b.

Nagata, T., Yoshida, K., Ohno, S., Murata, F.: Ultrastructural localization of soluble and insoluble ^{3}H-methyl prednisolone as revealed by electron microscopic dry-mounting radioautography. Proc. 9th Internat. Congr. Electr. Microsc. 2, 40-41, 1978b.

Nishigaki, T., Momose, Y., Nagata, T.: Light microscopic radioautographic study of the localization of anti-allergic agent, tranilast, in rat mast cells. Histochem. J. 19, 533-536, 1987.

Nishigaki, T., Momose, Y., Nagata, T.: Electron microscopic radioautographic study of the localization of an anti-allergic agent, tranilast, in rat mast cells. Cell. Mol. Biol. 36, 65-71, 1990a.

Nishigaki, T., Momose, Y., Nagata, T.: Localization of the anti-allergic agent tranilast in the urinary bladder of rat as demonstrated by light microscopic radioautography. Drug Res. 40, 272-275, 1990b.

Oguchi, K., Nagata, T.: A radioautographic study of activated satellite cells in dystrophic chicken muscle. In, Current Research in Muscular Dystrophy Japan. The Proc. Ann. Meet. Muscular Dystrophy Res. 1980, pp. 16-17, Ministry of Welfare of Japan, Tokyo, 1980.

Oguchi, K., Nagata, T.: Electron microscopic radioautographic observation on activated satellite cells in dystrophy chickens. In, Clinical Studies on the Etiology of Muscular Dystrophy. Annual Report on Neurological Diseases 1981, pp. 30-33, Ministry of Welfare of Japan, Tokyo, 1981.

Ohno, S., Fujii, Y., Usuda, N., Endo, T., Hidaka, H., Nagata, T.: Demonstration of intracellular localization of calmodulin antagonist by wet-mounting radioautography. J. Electron Microsc. 32, 1-12, 1983.

Ohno, S., Fujii, Y., Usuda, N., Nagata, T., Endo, T., Tanaka, T., Hidaka, H.: Intracellular localization of calmodulin antagonists (W-7). In, Calmodulin and intracellular Ca^{2+} receptors. Kakiuchi, S., Hidaka, H, Means, A. R., Eds., pp. 39-48, Plenum Publishing Co., New York, 1982.

Olea, M. T.: An ultrastructural localization of lysosomal acid phosphatase activity in aging mouse spleen: a quantitative X-ray microanalytical study. Acta Histochem. Cytochem. 24, 201-208, 1991.

Olea, M. T., Nagata, T.: X-ray microanalysis of cerium in mouse spleen cells demonstrating acid phosphatase activity using high voltage electron microscopy, Cell. Mol. Biol. 37, 155-163, 1991.

Olea, M. T., Nagata, T. : Simultaneous localization of ^{3}H-thymidine incorporation and acid phosphatase activity in mouse spleen: EM radioautography and cytochemistry. Cell. Mol. Biol. 38, 115-122, 1992a.

Olea, M. T., Nagata, T.: A radioautographic study on RNA synthesis in aging mouse spleen after ^{3}H-uridine labeling in vitro. Cell. Mol. Biol. 38, 399-405, 1992b.

Oliveira, S. F., Nagata, T., Abrahamsohn, P. A., Zorn, T. M. T.: Electron microscopic radioautographic study on the incorporation of ^{3}H-proline by mouse decidual cells. Cell. Mol. Biol. 37, 315-323, 1991.

Oliveira, S. F., Abrahamsohn, P. A., Nagata, T., Zorn, T. M. T.: Incorporation of ^{3}H-amino acids by endometrial stromal cells during decidualization in the mouse. A radioautographical study. Cell. Mol. Biol. 41, 107-116, 1995.

Pearse, A. G. E.: Histochemistry, Theoretical and Applied. 4th Ed. Vol. 1. 439 pp., 1980, Vol. 2. 1055 pp., 1985, Vol. 3. Ed. with P. Stoward, 728 pp. Churchill Livingstone, Edinburgh, London and New York, 1991.

Sakai, Y., Ikado, S., Nagata, T.: Electron microscopic radioautography of satellite cells in regenerating muscles. J. Clin. Electr. Microsc. 10, 508-509, 1977.

Sato, A.: Quantitative electron microscopic studies on the kinetics of secretory granules in G-cells. Cell Tissue Res. 187, 45-59, 1978.

Sato, A., Iida, F., Furihara, R., Nagata, T.: Electron microscopic raioautography of rat stomach G-cells by means of ^{3}H-amino acids. J. Clin. Electron Microsc. 10, 358-359, 1977.

Shimizu, T., Usuda, N., Yamanda, T., Sugenoya, A., Iida, F.: Proliferative activity of human thyroid tumors evaluated by proliferating cell nuclear antigen/cyclin immnohistochemical studies. Cancer 71, 2807-2812, 1993.

Sun, L.: Age related changes of RNA synthesis in the lungs of aging mice by light and electron microscopic radioautography. Cell. Mol. Biol. 41, 1061-1072, 1995.

Sun, L., Gao, F., Duan, H., Nagata, T.: Light microscopic radioautography of DNA synthesis in pulmonary cells in aging mice. In, Radioautography in Medicine, Nagata, T. Ed., pp. 201-205, Shinshu University Press, Matsumoto, 1994.

Sun, L., Gao, F., Nagata, T.: Study on the DNA synthesis of pulmonary cells in aging mice by light microscopic radioautography. Cell. Mol. Biol. 41, 851-859, 1995a.

Sun, L., Gao, F., Jin, C., Duan, H., Nagata, T.: An electron microscopic radioautographic study on the DNA synthesis of pulmonary tissue cells in aging mice. Med. Electron. Microsc. 28, 129-131, 1995b.

Sun, L., Gao, F., Jin, C., Nagata, T.: DNA synthesis in the tracheae of aging mice by means of light and electron microscopic radioautography. Acta Histochem. Cytochem. 30, 211-220, 1997a.

Sun, L., Gao, F., Nagata, T.: A Light Microscopic radioautographic study on protein synthesis in pulmonary cells of aging mice. Acta Histochem. Cytochem. 30, 463-470, 1997b.

Suzuki, K., Imada, T., Gao, F., Ma, H., Nagata, T.: Radioautographic study of benidipine hydrochloride: localization in the mesenteric artery of spontaneously hypertensive rat. Drug Res. 44, 129-133, 1994.

Terauchi, A., Mori, T., Kanda, H., Tsukada, M., Nagata, T.: Radioautographic study of 3H-taurine uptake in mouse skeletal muscle cells. J. Clin. Electron Microsc. 21, 627-628, 1988.

Terauchi, A., Nagata, T.: Observation on incorporation of ^{3}H-taurine in mouse skeletal muscle cells by light and electron microscopic radioautography. Cell. Mol. Biol. 39, 397-404, 1993.

Terauchi, A., Nagata, T.: In corporation of ^{3}H-taurine into the blood capillary cells of mouse skeletal muscle. Radioautography in Medicine, Nagata, T. ed., Shinshu University Press, Matsumoto, 1994.

Toriyama, K.: Study on the aging changes of DNA and protein synthesis of bipolar and photo-receptor cells of mouse retina by light and electron microscopic radioautography. Cell. Mol. Biol. 41, 593-601, 1995.

Tsukahara, S., Yoshida, K., Nagata, T.: A radioautographic study on the incorporation of ^{14}C-bupranolol (beta-blocking agent) into the rabbit eye. Histochemistry 68, 237-244, 1980.

Usuda, N., Nagata, T.: Electron microscopic radioautography of acyl-CoA mRNA by in situ hybridization. J. Clin. Electron Microsc. 25, 332-333, 1992.

Usuda, N., Nagata, T.: The immunohistochemical and in situ hybridization studies on hepatic peroxisomes. Acta Histochem. Cytochem. 28, 169-172, 1995.

Usuda, N., Hanai, T., Morita, T., Nagata, T.: Radioautographic demonstration of peroxisomal acyl-CoA oxidase mRNA by in situ hybridization. In, Recent advances in cellular and molecular biology, Vol. 6. Molecular biology of nucleus, peroxisomes, organelles and cell movement. Wegmann, R. J., Wegmann, M., Eds, pp.181-184, Peeters Press, Leuven, 1992.

Uwa, H., Nagata, T.: Cell population kinetics of the scleroblast during ethisterone-induced anal-fin process formation in adult females of the Medaka. Dev. Growth Different. 9, 693-694, 1976.

Watanabe, I., Makiyama, M. C. K., Nagata, T.: Electron microscopic radioautographic observation of the submandibular salivary gland of aging mouse. Acta Microscopica 6. 130-131, 1997.

Yamabayashi, S., Gunarso, W., Tsukahara, S., Nagata, T.: Incorporation of ^{3}H-befunolol (beta blocking agent) into melanin granules of ocular tissues in the pigmented rabbits. I. Light microscopic radioautography. Histochemistry 73, 371-375, 1981.

Yamada, A. T.: Timely and topologically defined protein synthesis in the periimplanting mouse endometrium revealed by light and electron microscopic radioautography. Cell. Mol. Biol. 39, 1-12, 1993.

Yamada, A., Nagata, T.: Ribonucleic acid and protein synthesis in the uterus of pregnant mouse during activation of implantation window. Med. Electron Microsc. 27, 363-365, 1992a.

Yamada, A., Nagata, T.: Light and electron microscopic raioautography of DNA synthesis in the endometria of pregnant-ovariectomized mice during activation of implantation window. Cell. Mol. Biol. 38, 763-774, 1992b.

Yamada, A., Nagata, T.: Light and electron microscopic raioautography of RNA synthesis of peri-implanting pregnant mouse during activation of receptivity for blastocyst implantation. Cell. Mol. Biol. 38, 211-233, 1993.

Yoshinaga, K.: Uterine receptivity for blastcyst implantation. Ann. N. Y. Acad. Sci. USA, 541, 424-431, 1988.

Yoshizawa, S., Nagata, A., Honma, T., Oda, M., Murata, F., Nagata, T.: Study of ethionine pancreatitis by means of electron microscopic radioautography. J. Clin. Electron Microsc. 7, 349-350, 1974.

Yoshizawa, S., Nagata, A., Honma, T., Oda, M., Murata, F., Nagata, T.: Radioautographic study of protein synthesis in pancreatic exocrine cells of alcoholic rats. J. Clin. Electron. Microsc. 10, 372-373, 1977.

15

Macromolecular Synthesis in the Digestive and Respiratory Systems

Tetsuji Nagata[1,2]
[1]*Department of Anatomy and Cell Biology, Shinshu University School of Medicine, Matsumoto*
[2]*Shinshu Institute of Alternative Medicine and Welfare, Nagano Japan*

1. Introduction

This second chapter deals with the second parts of the application of microscopic radioautography to some of the visceral organ systems. The visceral organs can be divided into 5 organ systems according to anatomy and histology, i.e., the digestive system, the respiratory system, the urinary system, the reproductive system and the endocrine system. Among of them the digestive system consists of 2 parts, i.e., the digestive tract and the digestive glands. The former consists of simple tube structures such as the oral cavity, the esophagus, the stomach and the intestines, while the latter consists of complicated glandular structures such as the large digestive glands , i.e., the liver and the pancreas, while the respiratory system consists of 2 parts, one the respiratory tract such as the nose, the pharynx, the trachea, the bronchus, and final essential part the lungs. This chapter deals with the digestive organs and the respiratory organs, respectively.

1.1 Macromolecular synthesis in the digestive system

The digestive system consists of the digestive tract and the digestive glands. The digestive tract can be divided into several portions, from the upper part to the lower part, i.e., the oral cavity, the pharynx, the esophagus, the stomach, the small and large intestines and the anus, while the digestive glands consist of the large glands such as the salivary glands, the liver and the pancreas and the small glands affiliated to the digestive tracts in the gastrointestinal walls such as the gastric glands including the fundic gland and the pyloric gland, the intestinal glands of Lieberkühn and the duodenal glands of Brunner. We have published many papers from our laboratory dealing with the macromolecular synthesis in respective digestive organs from the oral cavity to the gastrointestinal tracts and the digestive glands (Nagata 1992, 1993a,b, 1994a,b,c,d,e, 1995a,b,c,d, 1996a,b,c, 1999a,b,c, 2002, Nagata et al. 1979, 1982a, 2000a, Chen et al. 1995). The outline of the results concerning to the macromolecular synthesis in the digestive organs should be here described in the order of systematic anatomy and special histology as follows.

1.1.1 Macromolecular synthesis in the oral cavity

The oral cavity consists of the lips, tongue, teeth, and the salivary glands. The DNA synthesis of mucosal epithelia of the 2 upper and lower lips and the tongue as well as the 3 large salivary glands and many small glands of aging mice from fetal day 19 to postnatal 2 years were studied by LM and EM RAG labeled with ^{3}H-thymidine. The glucide and glycoprotein syntheses by ^{3}H-glucosamine and radiosulfate incorporations of the submandibular and sublingual glands of aging mice were also studied.

1.1.2 The DNA synthesis in the oral cavity

We first studied the DNA synthesis of the submandibular glands in 10 groups of aging mice at various ages from embryo to postnatal 2 years (Chen et al. 1995, Nagata et al. 2000a). The submandibular gland of male mouse embryonic day 19 consisted of the glandular acini and duct system (Fig. 5A). The duct system was composed of the juxtaacinar cells (JA), the intercalated duct cells (ICD) and the striated duct cells (SD). Many labeled developing acinar cells (AC), JA and ICD cells were observed. At postnatal day 1 to 3 (Fig. 5B), there was more JA cells and secretory granules than those of former stage. JA cells were cuboidal cells in shape, characterized by small darkly stained granules in the supranuclear cytoplasm and by basophilic mitochondria mostly at the basal half of the cells. JA cells were present at the acinar-intercalated duct junction of the mouse submandibular gland. Many labeled AC, JA, ICD and SD cells were also observed by electron microscopy (Fig. 5C). At postnatal 2 weeks to 3 months, developing immature acinar cells gradually matured to acinar cells, and JA cells increased and granular convoluted duct cells (GCT) appeared.

At postnatal 6 months to 2 years, the GCT cells were very well developed and were composed of the taller cells packed with many granules and became highly convoluted, and only a few labeled cells were found. The aging changes of frequency of 5 main individual cell types in submandibular glands of male mouse from embryonic day 19 to postnatal 2 years of age were counted. On embryonic day 19 of age, the gland consisted of developing acinar cells (49%), intercalated duct cells (37%), juxta-acinar (JA) cells (3%), striated duct (SD) cells (11%). At birth, JA cells increased rapidly to 32%, thereafter decreased gradually. At 1 month of age, JA cells disappeared and granular convoluted tubule (GCT) cells appeared and increased rapidly in number with age. They reached a maximum at 6 months. Then they decreased gradually from 6-21 months. The quantity proportion of acini was relatively stable during these periods. The frequency of ICD cells (Fig. 5C) was the highest (37%) at 1 day after birth. Thereafter it gradually decreased month by month and reached 2.6% at 21 months, while the ratio of SD cells persisted in 7%-12% from embryonic day 19 to postnatal 2 weeks and it disappeared at 3 months after birth. The proliferative activity of the cell population is expressed by the labeling index which is defined as the percentage of labeled nuclei with ^{3}H-thymidine in a given cell population. The labeling index of the entire gland cells increased from 13.6% at embryonic 19 to 18.3% at neonate, when it reached the first peak (Fig. 6A, B). Then it declined to 2.2% at 1 week of age. A second small peak (2.9%) occurred at 2 weeks. Thereafter, the labeling index decreased progressively to less than 1% at 4 weeks of age and then remained low. The analysis of the labeling indices of respective cell types revealed that the first peak at neonate was due to the increased labeling indices of AC, ICD and JA cells, and the second peak at 2 weeks was due to the increase of ICD and SD cells. Thereafter, the labeling index of ICD cells decreased steadily but remained higher than those of any other cell types. Since the labeling index of ICD cells was more than the other cell types and persisted for a long time, it was suggested that ICD cells concerned with the generation of other cell types (Nagata 2002).

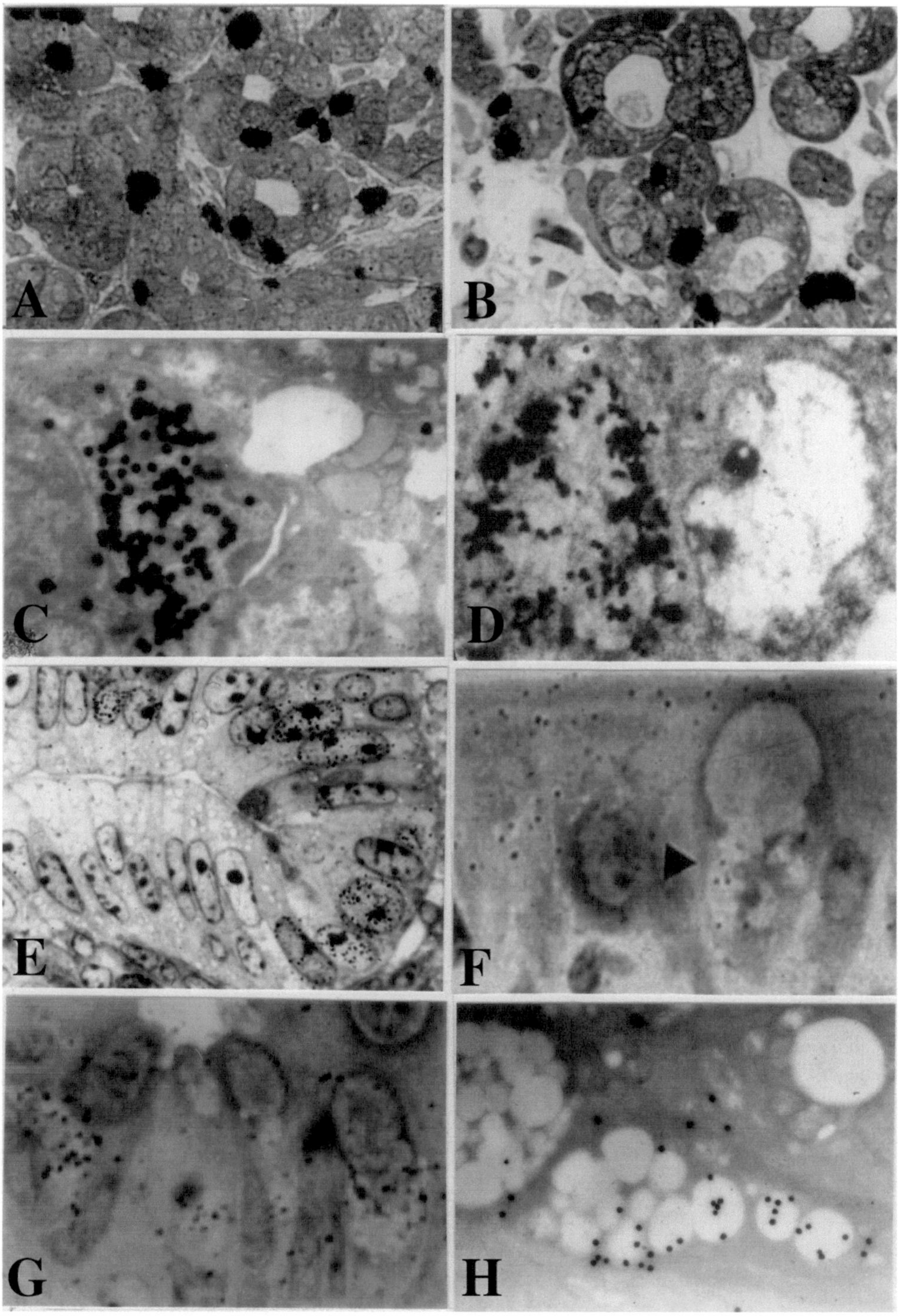

Fig. 6. LM and EM RAG of the digestive organs. From Nagata, T.: Radioautographology, General and Special. In, Prog. Histochem. Cytochem. Vol. 37, No. 2, p. 118, 2002, Urban & Fischer, Jena, Germany

Fig. 6A. LMRAG of the submandibular gland of male mouse embryonic day 19 labeled with ^{3}H-thymidine consisted with the glandular acini and duct system. The duct system was composed of juxtaacinar cells (JA), intercalated duct cells (ICD) and striated duct cells (ICD). Many labeled developing acinar cells (AC), JA and ICD cells were observed. x500.
Fig. 6B. LMRAG of the submandibular gland at postnatal day 3, labeled with ^{3}H-thymidine. There were more JA cells and secretory granules than those of former stage (Fig. 5A). x500.
Fig. 6C. EMRAG of an ICD cell of a mouse at postnatal day 3, labeled with ^{3}H-thymidine observed by electron microscopy. Many silver grains are observed over the nucleus of an ICD. x10,000.
Fig. 6D. EMRAG of the esophageal epithelial cells of a newborn mouse at postnatal day 1, labeled with ^{3}H-thymidine. Many silver grains are observed over one of the nuclei at left. x10,000.
Fig. 6E. LMRAG of the colonic epithelial cells of a mouse embryo at fetal day 19, labeled with ^{3}H-thymidine. Many silver grains are observed over the nuclei of several epithelial cells in the bottom of the crypt. x800.
Fig. 6F. LMRAG of the ileum epithelial cells labeled with ^{3}H-glucosamine of an old mouse at postnatal 6 months. Many silver gains are localized over the Golgi region of the 3 goblet cells as well as over the cytoplasm of several absorptive columnar epithelial cells. x 1,000.
Fig. 6G. LMRAG of the colonic epithelial cells of a mouse at postnatal month 1, labeled with $^{35}SO_4$ in vitro and radioautographed. x1,000.
Fig. 6H. EMRAG of a goblet cell in the deeper crypt of the colonic epithelial cells of an adult mouse after injection of $^{35}SO_4$ and radioautographed. Many silver grains are observed over the Golgi region and mucous droplets of the goblet cell, demonstrating the incorporation of radiosulfate into sulfomucins. x4,800.

1.1.3 The glucide synthesis in the oral cavity

We studied the incorporations of ^{3}H-glucosamine in the submandibular glands of 10 groups of litter mice at various ages. The animals from embryonic day 19, postnatal day 1, 3, 7, 14, and 1, 3, 6 months to 1 and 2 years were sacrificed after administration of ^{3}H-glucosamine and the submandibular glands were processed for LM and EM RAG (Watanabe et al. 1997, Nagata 2002). The results showed that the silver grains appeared over the endoplasmic reticulum, Golgi apparatus and the secretory granules of the acinar cells, demonstrating the glycoprotein synthesis in these cells. Grain counting revealed that the counts increased from the fetal stage at embryonic day 19 to postnatal day 1 to 3, 7, 14, reaching the peak at day 14, then decreased to month 1, 3, 6, to year 1 and 2, showing the aging changes, inverse proportion to DNA synthesis of these cells.

On the other hand, the sulfate uptake and accumulation in sulfomucin in several digestive organs of mice were also studied by light microscopic radioautography (Nagata and Kawahara 1999, Nagata et al. 1999b). Two litters of normal ddY mice 30 days after birth, each consisting of 3 animals, were studied. One litter of animals was sacrificed at 30 min after the intraperitoneal injections with phosphate buffered $Na_2{}^{35}SO_4$, and the other litter animals were sacrificed at 12 hr after the injections. Then the submandibular glands and the sublingual glands were taken out, fixed, embedded in epoxy resin, sectioned, radioautographed and analyzed by light microscopy. As the results, many silver grains were observed on serous cells of the salivary glands at 30 min and 12 hr after the injections

(10-20/cell). The numbers of silver grains at 30 min were less than those at 12 hr. From the results, it was concluded that glycoprotein synthesis was demonstrated in both the submandibular and sublingual glands by radiosulfate incorporation. In the salivary glands the silver grains were more observed in serous cells than mucous cells at 30 min, while in mucous cells more at 12 hr than 30 min after the injection. These results show the time difference of glycoprotein synthesis in the two salivary glands, showing inverse proportion to DNA synthesis of these cells (Watanabe et al. 1997, Nagata 2002).

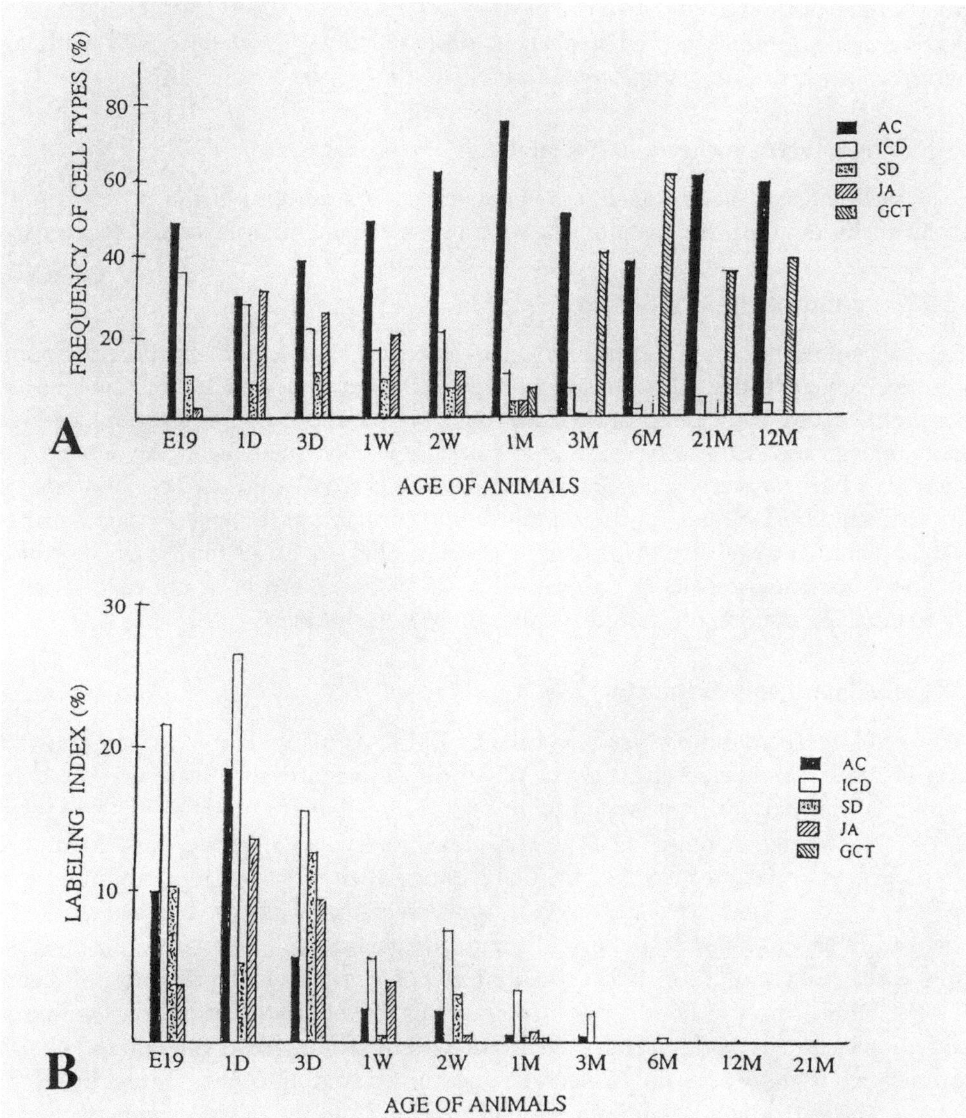

Fig. 7. Histogram showing the frequencies (A) and labeling indices (B) of the five individual cell types in the submandibular glands of male ddY mice at respective ages. From Nagata, T.: Radioautographology, General and Special. In, Prog. Histochem. Cytochem. Vol. 37, No. 2, p.118, 2002, Urban & Fischer, Jena, Germany

1.2 Macromolecular synthesis in the esophagus

The esophagus is the characteristic digestive tract including all the layers, the mucous membrane covered with the stratified squamous epithelia, the submucosa, the muscular layer and the serosa or adventitia. We studied the DNA synthesis of the esophagus of aging mice labeled with ^{3}H-thymidine by LM and EM RAG (Duan et al. 1992, 1993). The labeled cells were mainly found in the basal layer of the esophageal epithelium (Fig. 6D). By electron microscopy the nuclei and nucleoli of labeled cells were larger than those of unlabeled cells, but contained fewer cell organelles (Duan et al. 1993). The labeling indices in respective aging groups showed a peak at postnatal day 1 and decreased with aging keeping a constant level around a few % from 6 months to 2 years after birth.

1.3 Macromolecular synthesis in the stomach

The stomach consists of the mucosa covered with the surface epithelia of the columnar epithelia, including the gastric glands, the submucosa, the muscular layer and the serosa.

1.3.1 DNA synthesis in the stomach

As for the turnover of fundic glandular cells shown by ^{3}H-thymidine radioautography, it was extensively investigated with LM RAG by Leblond and co-workers (Leblond 1981, Leblond et al. 1958). They demonstrated that the DNA synthesis in the stomach increased at perinatal stages and decreased due to aging and senescence. However, the activity never reached zero but low activity continued until senescence. We studied the macromolecular synthesis including DNA, RNA, protein and glycoproteins in the gastric mucosa of both human and animal tissues by LM and EMRAG (Sato et al. 1977). As for the DNA synthesis, we obtained the same results as Leblond et al (1958, 1981). We have not carried out this study so much. Therefore, the minute details will be here omitted.

1.3.2 Protein synthesis in the stomach

We observed the secretion process in G-cells by EM RAG using ^{3}H-amino acid (Sato 1978, Sato et al. 1977, Komiyama et al. 1978). When the stomach tissues were taken out from the adult Wistar rats at postnatal month 1 and were labeled with either ^{3}H-glutamic acid or ^{3}H-glycine in vitro at varying time intervals, silver grains in the EM radioautograms appeared first over the Golgi zones, then migrated to secretory granules and were stored in the cytoplasm, suggesting the secretory kinetics. We also studied the mechanism of serum albumin passing through the gastric epithelial cells into the gastric cells by EM RAG (Sato et al. 1977). When adult Wistar rat stomach tissues were labeled with ^{132}I-albumin in vitro at varying time intervals, silver grains in the radioautograms appeared over rough endoplasmic reticulum within 3 min, then moved to the Golgi apparatus in 10 min, and on to secretory granules and into the lumen in 30 min, suggesting the pathway of serum albumin absorption from the blood vessels through the gastric mucous epithelial cells into the gastric lumen (Komiyama et al. 1978). These results demonstrated that the stomach cells of adult rats synthesized proteins and secreted. However, aging changes of these protein synthesis between the young and senescent animal were not yet completed.

1.3.3 The glucide synthesis in the stomach

When incorporation of radiosulfate into sulfated complex carbohydrate in rat stomach was studied by labeling with $^{35}SO_4$ in vivo, silver grains appeared over the glandular cells of the pyloric gland but not those of the fundic gland, demonstrating the mucous synthesis in the former glands (Nagata et al. 1988a, Nagata and Kawahara 1999). The radiosulfate uptake and accumulation in the stomach of mouse were also studied by light microscopic radioautography (Nagata et al. 1999b). Two litters of normal ddY mice 30 days after birth, each consisting of 3 animals, were studied. One litter animals were sacrificed at 30 min after the intraperitoneal injections with phosphate buffered $Na_2{}^{35}SO_4$, and the other litter animals were sacrificed 12 hr after the injections. Then the antrum and the fundus tissues of the stomachs were taken out. The tissues were fixed, dehydrated, embedded in epoxy resin, sectioned, radioautographed and analyzed. As the results, many silver grains were observed on the mucosa and submucosa of the stomach at 30 min after the injection. Then at 12 hr after the injection silver grains were observed on some of the fundic glands. The numbers of silver grains observed in the stomach especially over the pyloric glands at 30 min (a few per cell) were less than those (several per cell) at 12 hr. The results showed the time difference of glycoprotein synthesis in the stomach, showing inverse proportion to DNA synthesis (Nagata and Kawahara 1999, Nagata 2002).

1.4 Macromolecular synthesis in the intestines

The intestines of mammals are divided into 2 portions, small and large intestines, which can be further divided into several portions, the small intestines into the duodenum, the jejunum and the ileum, while the large intestines into the caecum, the appendix vermiformis, the colon and the rectum. The intestinal tracts in any portions consist of the mucosa covered with columnar epithelial cells including absorptive and secretory cells, the submucosa, the smooth muscular layer and the serosa. We studied the macromolecular synthesis, both the DNA and the proteins in the intestines by LM and EMRAG mainly in the epithelial cells (Nagata 2002).

1.4.1 The DNA synthesis in the intestines

We studied the DNA synthesis in the intestines by LM and EMRAG mainly in the epithelial cells (Nagata 2002). The DNA synthesis of small and large intestines of mice were studied by ^{3}H-thymidine RAG (Fig. 6E). The cells labeled with ^{3}H-thymidine were localized in the crypts of both small and large intestines, a region defined as the proliferative zone. In the colon of aging mice from fetal to postnatal 2 years, the labeled cells in the columnar epithelia were frequently found in the perinatal groups from embryo to postnatal day 1. However, the labeling indices became constant from the suckling period until senescence (Morita 1993, Morita et al. 1994). On the other hand, we examined the labeling indices of respective cell types in each layer of mouse colon such as columnar epithelial cells, lamina propria, lamina muscularis mucosae, tunica submucosa, inner circular muscle layer, outer longitudinal muscle layer, outer connective tissue and serous membrane of the colon and found that most labeling indices decreased after birth to 2 months except the epithelial cells which kept constant value to senescence (Jin and Nagata 1995a,b, Jin 1996) (Fig. 8). Similar results were also obtained from the cecal tissues of mouse by LM and EMRAG. We also studied immunostaining for PCNA/cyclin and compared to the results obtained from RAG (Morita et al. 1994). The colonic tissues of litter mice of six aging groups from the embryonic day 19, to newborn postnatal day 1, 5, 21, adult 2 months and senescent 12 months were fixed in methacarn solution, sectioned and immunostained for cyclin proliferating nuclear antigen (PCNA/cyclin) with the monoclonal antibody and the avidin-biotin peroxidase complex technique. The reaction appeared in the colonic epithelium from G1 to S phase of the cell cycle. The immunostaining positive cells were localized in the crypts of colons similarly to the labeled cells with ^{3}H-thymidine by radioautography, a region defined as the proliferative zone. The positive cells in the columnar epithelia were frequently found in the perinatal groups from embryo to postnatal day 1, and became constant from postnatal day 5 until senescence. Comparing the results by immunostaining with the labeling index by radioautography, it was found that the former was higher in each aging group than the latter. The reason for the difference should be due to that PCNA/cyclin positive cells included not only S-phase cells but also the late G1 cells.

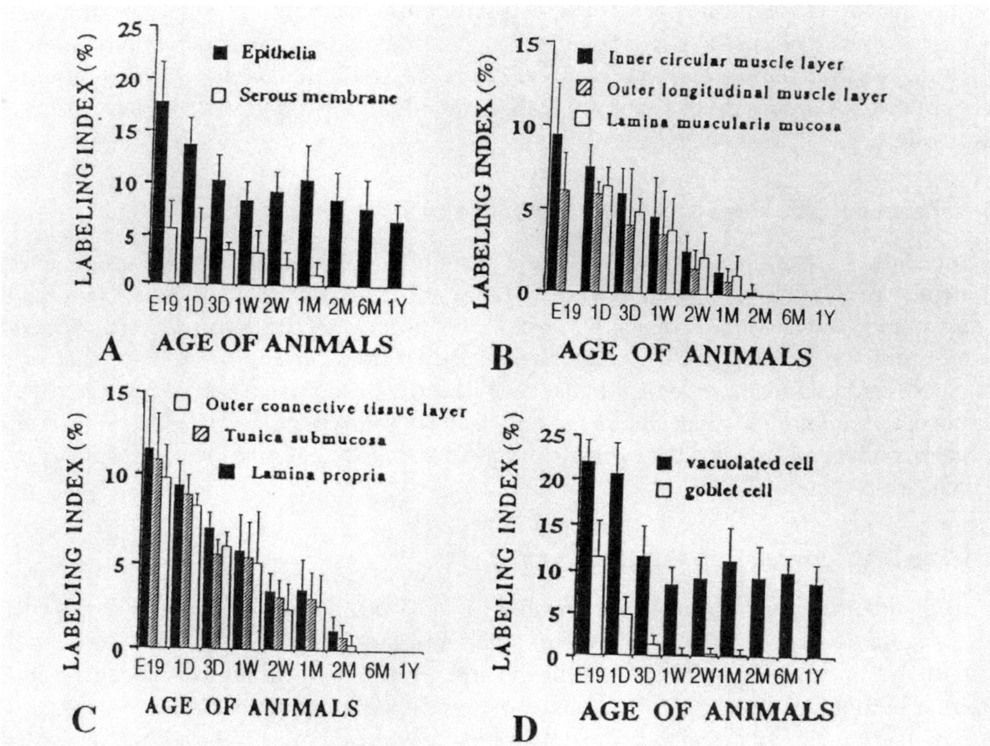

Fig. 8. Histogram showing aging changes of average labeling indices in respective tissue layers and cells of mouse colons at various ages from embryo to postnatal year 1, labeled with ^{3}H-thyidine. From Nagata, T.: Radioautographology, General and Special. In, Prog. Histochem. Cytochem. Vol. 37, No. 2, p. 123, 2002, Urban & Fischer, Jena, Germany

1.4.2 The RNA synthesis in the intestines

We studied the RNA synthesis of the small intestines of mice after feeding or refeeding under the restricted conditions (Nagata 1966). Five groups of ddY mice, each consisting of 5 individuals, total 25, were injected with ^{3}H-uridine, an RNA precursor, and sacrificed at different time intervals after feeding. The animals of the first group were injected with ^{3}H-uridine at 9 a.m. and fed at 10 a.m. for 30 min. and sacrificed at 11 a.m. 1 hour after the feeding and 2 hours after the injection, the 2nd group was sacrificed at 1 p.m. 3 hours after feeding and 4 hours after the injection, the 3rd group at 5 p.m., 7 and 8 hours later, the 4th group at 9 a.m. on the next day 23 and 24 hours later, and finally the 5th group at 1. p.m. on the next day 3 hours after refeeding and 28 hours after the injection. Then, the jejunums obtained from each animal were prepared for isolated cell radioautograms according to Nagata et al. (1961). The results demonstrated that the grain counts in mononucleate villus cells reached the maximum (20-30 grains per cell) 4 hours after injection and decreased (10-20/cell) after 28 hours, while the counts in mononucleate villus cells only increased gradually from 4 hours (10/cell) to 28 hours (20/cell). In contrast to this, the grain counts of binucleate cells which appeared in villus cells increased parallely to the mononucleate villus cells (10-20/cell). It was concluded that the RNA synthesis in the jejunal epithelial cells was high in the following order: mononucleate crypt cells, binucleate cells and mononucleate villus cells. These results revealed that the feeding or refeeding affected the RNA synthesis of the intestinal epithelial cells (Nagata 1966).

1.4.3 The protein synthesis in the intestines

We first studied the incorporations of ^{3}H-leucine and ^{3}H-tryptophane in mouse small intestines in connection to the binuclearity before and after feeding (Nagata 1967b). The results showed that the incorporations of both amino acids were greater in binucleate intestinal epithelial columnar cells than mononucleate villus and crypt cells at both before and after feeding. However, the aging changes of these incorporations were not studied.

1.4.4 The glucide synthesis in the intestines

We also studied the aging changes of glucide synthesis by ^{3}H-glucosamine uptake in the small intestines of mouse (Morita 1993), and found that the silver grains in the ileum columnar epithelial cells were mainly localized over the brush borders and the Golgi regions in these cells (Fig. 6F). The grain counting revealed that the numbers of silver grains over the brush borders and cytoplasm of the columnar epithelial cells increased in the villi (10-15/cell) than in the crypts (1-2/cell) from 6 months up to 2 years due to aging. The grain counting in other cell types also revealed that the number of silver grains in goblet cells, basal granulate cells, Paneth cells increased by aging, but did not in the undifferentiated cells.

The glycoprotein synthesis in goblet cells as well as in absorptive epithelial cells was also studied using $^{35}SO_4$ incorporation in the duodenums, the jejunums and the colons of adult mice at varying time intervals at 30, 60, and 180 min after the administration (Nagata et al. 1988a, Nagata and Kawahara 1999, Nagata et al. 1999b). Silver grains were localized over the columnar absorptive cells and the goblet cells, especially over the Golgi regions and mucous granules of the goblet cells. By EM RAG the intracellular localization of silver grains in goblet cells was clearly shown in the Golgi apparatus. The results from grain counting revealed that the average grain counts were different in the upper and deeper regions of the crypts in the 4 portions and it was shown that silver grains over goblet cells in the lower region of the crypt transferred rapidly from 30 min to 180 min, while they transferred slowly in goblet cells in the upper region of the colonic crypt, leading to the conclusion that the rates of transport and secretion of mucous products of the goblet cells at these two levels in the crypts were different. By EM RAG silver grains first appeared over the Golgi zone at 30 min. and then moved to the secretory granules at 60 and 180 min. The incorporation of $Na_2{}^{35}SO_4$ into sulfated complex carbohydrate was investigated in the mouse small and large intestines by LM and EM RAG as well as in the submandibular glands and the stomachs. Quantitative differences have been observed in the relative uptake of radiosulfate in the various labeled cells of each organ. Incorporation by the colon in goblet cells exceeded that elsewhere in the deep goblet cells of the colonic crypts migration of label progressed during the time tested from the supranuclear Golgi region to the deep position of the goblet and then extended throughout the mucosubstance in the goblet in the superficial goblet cells of the colon. The radioautographic and cytochemical staining differences between secretory cells in the deeper region compared with the upper region of the colonic crypts are considered to reflect differences in the rate of transport of secretory products in the theca and the rate of secretion at the low levels in the crypt (Figs. 6G,H). These results showed the time differences of glycoprotein synthesis in respective organs. The sulfate uptake and accumulation in several mouse digestive organs were also studied by LM RAG. Two litters of normal ddY mice 30 days after birth, each consisting of 3 animals, were studied. One litter of animals was sacrificed 30 min after the intraperitoneal injections with phosphate buffered $Na_2{}^{35}SO_4$, and the other litter animals were sacrificed 12 hr after the injections. Then several digestive organs, the parotid gland, the submandibular gland, the sublingual gland, antrum and fundus of the stomach, the duodenum, the jejunum, the ileum, the caecum, the ascending colon and the descending colon were taken out and radioautographed. As the results, many silver grains were observed on villous cells and crypt cells of the small intestines and whole mucosa of the large intestines at 30 min after the injection. Then at 12 hr after the injection silver grains were observed on mucigen granules of goblet cells in the small intestines and the large intestines. The numbers of silver grains observed in respective organs at 30 min were less than those at 12 hr. From the results, it was concluded that the time difference of the glycoprotein synthesis was demonstrated in several digestive organs by radiosulfate incorporation, in reverse proportion to DNA synthesis. The total S contents in colonic goblet cells in upper and deeper regions of colonic crypts in aging mice were also analyzed by X-ray microanalysis (Nagata et al. 2000b, Nagata 2004). The results accorded well with the results from RAG (Nagata 2002) showing increase and decrease of mucosubstances in these cells due to development and aging to senescence.

1.5 Macromolecular synthesis in the liver

The liver is the largest gland in the human and the mammalian body and consists of several types of cells (Nagata 2010c). The hepatocyte is the main component of the liver, composing the liver parenchyma which form the hepatic lobules, surrounded by other types of cells such as the connective tissue cells, sinusoidal endothelial cells, satellite cells of Kupffer, Ito's fat-storing cells and bile epithelial cells. In the livers of perinatal animals, the liver tissues include hematopoietic cells such as erythroblasts, myeloblasts and magakaryocytes. We studied macromolecular synthesis by LM and EMRAG mainly in hepatocytes of rats and mice (Nagata 1993b, 1994a,b,c,d, 1995a,b,c, 1996a, 1997a, 1999c, 2002, 2003, 2006b, 2007a, 2009a,d,h,i, 2010c,h).

1.5.1 The DNA synthesis in the liver

We first studied the DNA synthesis in the liver tissues at various ages from embryo to postnatal 2 years (Nagata 1993a,b, 1994a,b,c,d, 1995a,b,c,d, 1996a,b,c,d, 1997a,b,c, 1998a,b,c,

1999a,b,c, 2002, Nagata et al. 1977a, Nagata and Nawa 1966b). The results obtained from the tissues of 3 groups of animals injected respectively with 3 kinds of RI-labeled precursors, i.e. ^{3}H-thymidine, ^{3}H-uridine and ^{3}H-leucine, were already reported as several original articles and reviews (Ma 1988, Ma and Nagata 1988a,b, 1990a,b, 2000, Ma et al. 1991, Nagata 1996a,b, 1997a, 1998a, 1999c, 2001c, 2002, 2003, 2006a,b, 2007a,b, 2009a,b,c,d) or as a monograph in the series of Prog. Histochem. Ccytochem (Nagata 2002, 2004, 2010c). Therefore, the results from the livers in aging mice should be briefly summarized in this article.

1.5.1.1 The DNA synthesis in hepatocyte nuclei

As for the nucleic acid synthesis in hepatocytes, we first studied the difference between the mononucleate and binucleate hepatocytes of adult rats, injected with ^{3}H-thymidine and radioautographed (Nagata 1962, 1994d). The results showed that the frequency of labeled cells was greater in the mononucleate cells (Fig. 9A) than in the binucleate cells. The labeled binucleate cells were classified into two types, i.e., a hepatocyte whose one of the two nuclei was labeled and a hepatocyte whose two nuclei were labeled. The former was more frequently observed than the latter. Grain counts revealed that the amount of DNA synthesized in the binucleate cell whose one nucleus was labeled was the same as the mononucleate cell, while the total amount of DNA synthesized in the binucleate cell whose two nuclei were labeled was almost twice as that of the mononucleate cell. These results suggested that the two nuclei of binucleate hepatocytes synthesized DNA independently from each other.

On the other hand, LM and EMRAG of prenatal and postnatal normal mice at various ages labeled with ^{3}H-thymidine revealed that many silver grains were localized over the nuclei of various cell types consisting the liver, i.e., hepatocytes (Fig. 9A), sinusoidal endothelial cells (Fig. 8B), Kupffer's cells, Ito's fat-storing cells, bile ductal epithelia cells, fibroblasts and hematopoietic cells (Ma 1988, Ma and Nagata 1988a,b, 1990, Nagata 1995a). In hematopoietic cells in the livers of perinatal animals, silver grains were observed over the nuclei of erythroblasts, myeloblasts, lymphoblasts and megekaryocytes. However, most hematopoietic cells disappeared on postnatal day 14. At fetal day 19, the liver tissues were chiefly consisted of hepatocytes and haematopoietic cells and no lobular orientation was observed. At postnatal day 1 and 3, lobular formation started and finally the hepatic lobules were formed at day 9 after birth.

During the perinatal period, almost all kinds of cells were labeled with ^{3}H-thymidine. Percentage of labeled hepatocytes was the highest at fetal day 19, and rapidly decreased after birth to day 3. From day 9 to 14, percentage of labeled hepatocytes (labeling index) decreased gradually and finally to the lowest at 24 months (Fig. 10A). When the labeling indices of hepatocytes in 3 hepatic acinar zones were analyzed, the indices decreased in zone 2 (intermediate zone) and zone 3 (peripheral zone) on days 3 and 9 after birth, whereas they increased in zone 1 (central) on day 9, and then they altogether decreased from day 14 to 24 months (Fig. 10B). When the size and number of cell organelles in both labeled and unlabeled hepatocytes were estimated quantitatively by image analysis with an image analyzer, Digigramer G/A (Mutoh Kogyo Co. Ltd., Tokyo, Japan) on EMRAG, the area size of the cytoplasm, nucleus, mitochondria, endoplasmic reticulum, and the number of mitochondria in the unlabeled hepatocytes were more than the labeled cells (Ma and Nagata 1988a,b, Nagata 1995a,d).

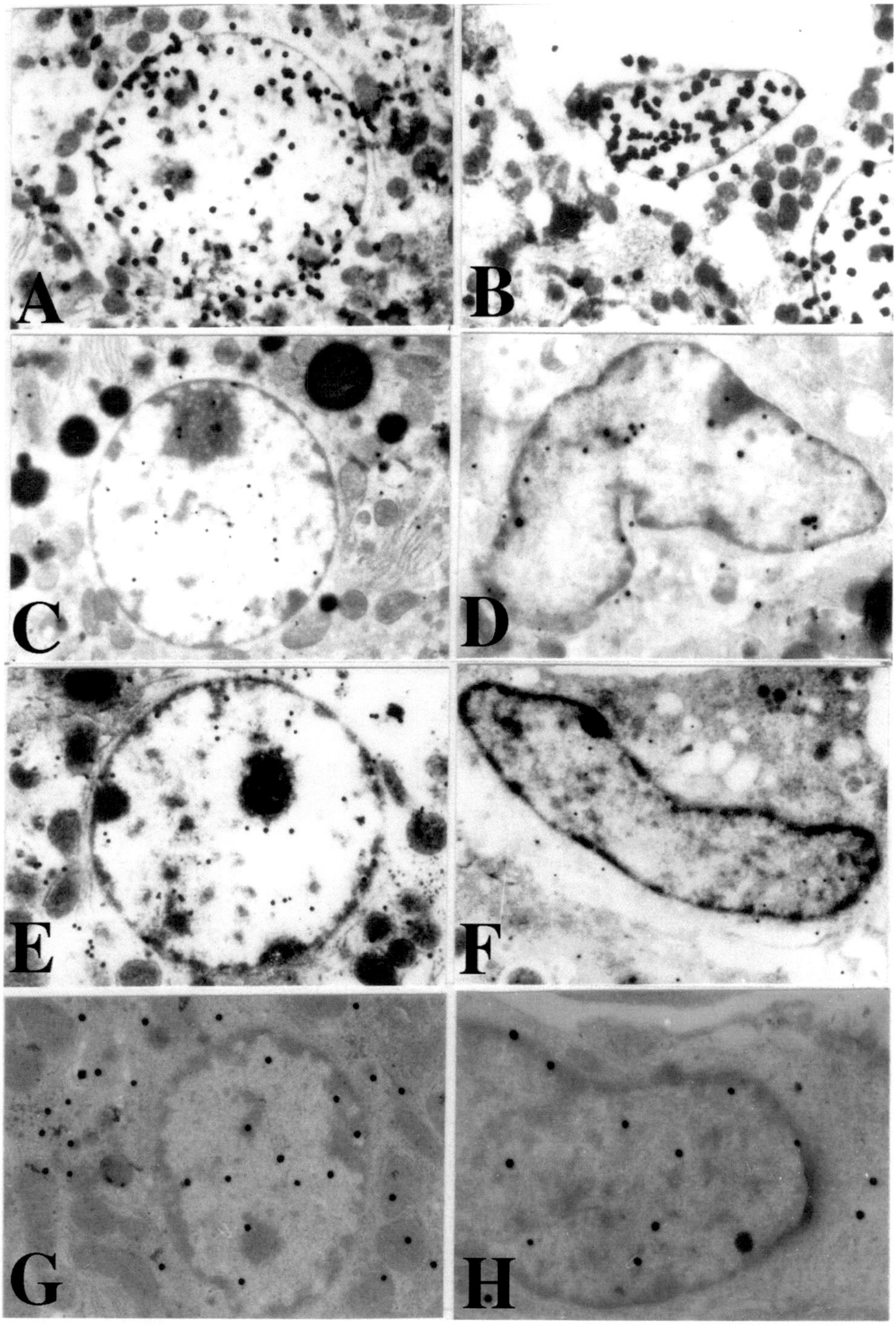

Fig. 9. EM RAG of the liver. From Nagata, T.: Radioautographology, General and Special. In, Prog. Histochem. Cytochem. Vol. 37, No. 2, p. 130, 2002, Urban & Fischer, Jena, Germany
Fig. 9A. EMRAG of a hepatocyte of the liver of a 14 day old mouse labeled with ^{3}H-thymidine. Many silver grains were observed over the nucleus and mitochondria.

Fig. 9B. EM RAG of a sinusoidal endothelial cells of the liver of a 14 day old mouse labeled with ^{3}H-thymidine. Many silver grains were observed over the nucleus and mitochondria.
Fig. 9C. EM RAG of a hepatocyte of the liver of a 14 day old mouse labeled with ^{3}H-uridine. Many silver grains were observed over the nucleus and mitochondria.
Fig. 9D. EM RAG of an Ito's fat-storing cell of the liver of a newborn 14 day old mouse labeled with ^{3}H-uridine. Many silver grains were observed over the nucleus and mitochondria.
Fig. 9E. EM RAG of a hepatocyte of the liver of a 1 month old mouse labeled with ^{3}H-leucine. Many silver grains were observed over the nucleus and mitochondria.
Fig. 9F. EM RAG of a sinusoidal endothelial cells of the liver of a newborn 14 day old mouse labeled with ^{3}H-leucine. Many silver grains were observed over the nucleus and mitochondria.
Fig. 9G. EMRAG of a hepatocyte of the liver of an adult 2 month old mouse labeled with ^{3}H-proline. Many silver grains were observed over the nucleus and mitochondria.
Fig. 9H. EMRAG of a Kupffer cell of the liver of a newborn 1 day old mouse labeled with ^{3}H-proline. Many silver grains were observed over the nucleus and mitochondria.

These data demonstrated that the cell organelles of the hepatocytes which synthesized DNA were not well developed as compared to those not synthesizing DNA during the postnatal development. In some of unlabeled hepatocytes, several silver grains were occasionally observed localizing over mitochondria and peroxisomes as was formerly reported (Nagata et al. 1967a,b, 1982b). The mitochondrial DNA synthesis was first observed in cultured hepatocytes of chickens and mice in vitro (Nagata et al. 1967a,b). The percentages of labeled cells in other cell types in the liver of aging mice such as sinusoidal endothelial cells, Kupffer's cells, Ito's fat-storing cells, bile ductal epithelia cells and fibroblasts showed also decreases from perinatal period to postnatal 24 months.

1.5.1.2 The DNA synthesis in hepatocyte mitochondria

When we observed DNA synthesis in the nuclei of mononucleate and binucleate hepatocytes, we also observed DNA synthesis in hepatocyte mitochondria (Ma 1988, Ma and Nagata 1988a,b, 1990a,b, Nagata and Ma 2005a). The results of visual grain counts on the number of mitochondria labeled with silver grains obtained from 10 mononucleate hepatocytes of each animal labeled with ^{3}H-thymidine demonstrating DNA synthesis in 8 aging groups at perinatal stages, prenatal embryo day 19, postnatal day 3, 9 and 14, month 1, 6, 12 and 24, were obtained. The number of total mitochondria per cell increased from perinatal stage (35-50/cell) to postnatal month 6 (95-105/cell), reaching the maximum, decreased to month 24 (85-90/cell), while the number of labeled mitochondria per cell increased from perinatal stage to postnatal day 14, reaching the maximum, decreased to month 6, then increased again to month 12, reaching the second peak and decreased again to month 24. Thus, the labeling indices in respective aging stages were calculated from the number of labeled mitochondria which showed an increase from perinatal stage to postnatal day 14, reaching the maximum and decreased to month 24. The results showed that the numbers of labeled mitochondria with ^{3}H-thymidine showing DNA synthesis increased from prenatal embryo day 19 (3.8/cell) to postnatal day 14 (6.2/cell), reaching the maximum, and then decreased to month 6 (3.7/cell) and again increased to year 1 (6.0/cell), while the labeling indices increased from prenatal day 19 (11.8%) to postnatal day 14 (16.9%), reaching the maximum, then decreased to month 6 (4.1%), year 1 (6.4%) and year 2 (2.3%). The increase of the total number of mitochondria in mononucleate hepatocytes was stochastically significant ($P<0.01$), while the changes of number of labeled mitochondria and labeling index in mononucleate hepatocytes were not significant ($P<0.01$).

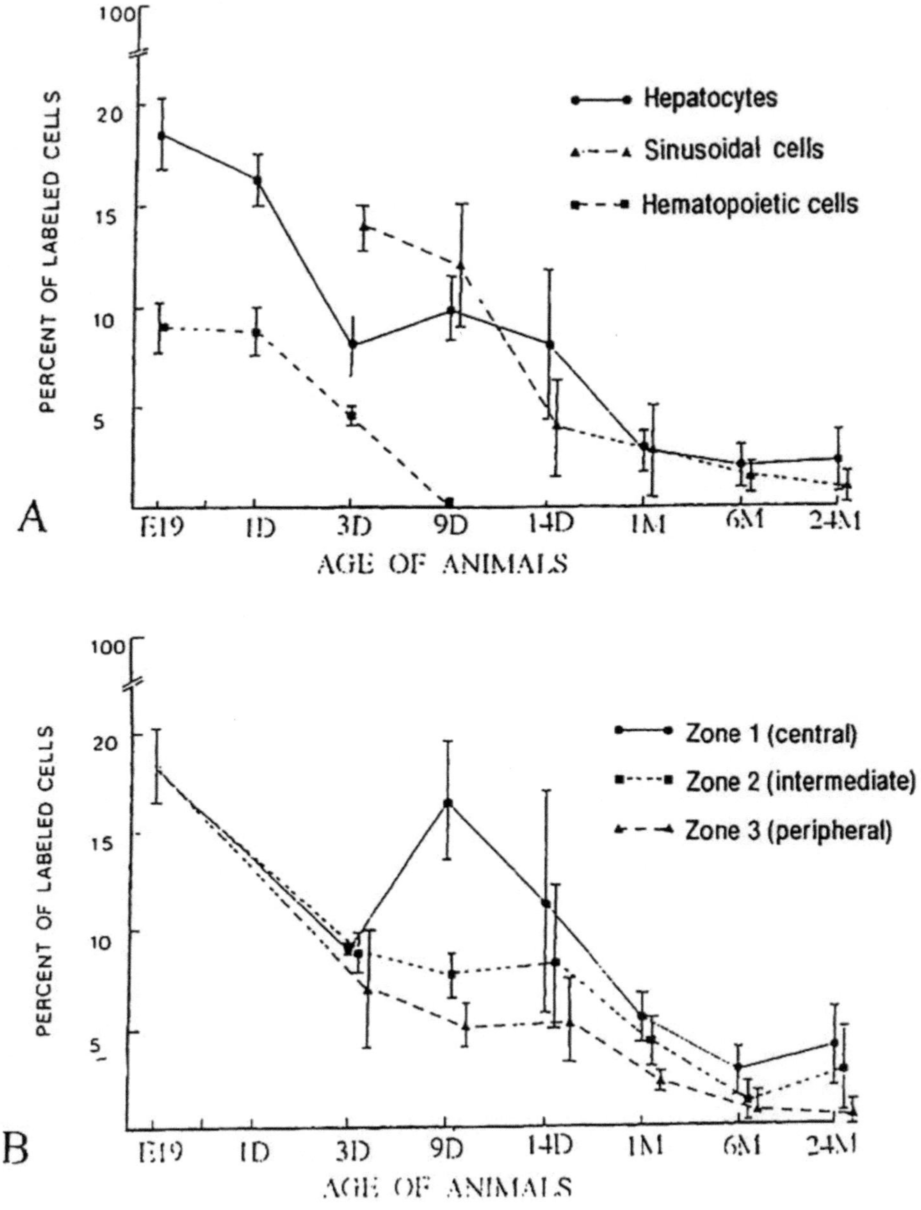

Fig. 10. Transitional curves of the labeling indices in the livers of aging mice after injection of ^{3}H-thymine. Mean ± Standard Deviation. From Nagata, T.: Special Cytochemistry in Cell Biology, In, Internat. Rev. Cytol. Vol. 211, No. 1, p. 92, 2001, Academic Press, San Diego, USA, London, UK.

Fig. 10A. Labeling indices of hepatocytes, sinusoidal endothelial cells and hematopoietic cells, respectively.

Fig. 10B. Labeling indices of hepatocytes, sinusoidal endothelial cells and hematopoietic cells, respectively.

As for the binucleate hepatocytes, on the other hand, because the appearances of binucleate hepatocytes showing silver grains in their nuclei demonstrating DNA synthesis were not so many in the adult and senescent stages from postnatal month 1 to 24, only binucleate cells at perinatal stages when reasonable numbers of labeled hepatocytes were found in respective groups were analyzed. The number of mitochondria in binucleate hepatocytes at postnatal day 1 to 14 kept around 80 (77-84/cell) which did not show such remarkable changes, neither increase nor decrease, as shown in mononucleate cells. Thus, the number of mitochondria per binucleate cell, the number of labeled mitochondria per binucleate cell and the labeling index of binucleate cell in 4 groups from postnatal day 1 to 14 were counted. The number of mitochondria and the number of labeled mitochondria were more in binucleate cells than mononucleate cells (Nagata 2007a,b,c,d,e, Nagata and Ma 2005a,b, Nagata et al. 1977a).

1.5.2 The RNA synthesis in the liver

The RNA synthesis in the liver was studied by ^{3}H-uridine RAG. Silver grains due to RNA synthesis appeared over the nuclei and cytoplasm of hepatocytes.

1.5.2.1 The RNA synthesis in hepatocyte nuclei

When the RI-labeled precursor ^{3}H-uridine was administered to experimental animals, or cultured cells were incubated in a medium containing ^{3}H-uridine in vitro and LM RAG was prepared, silver grains first appeared over the chromatin of the nucleus and nucleolus of all the cells within several minutes, then silver grains spread over the cytoplasm within 30 minutes showing messenger RNA and ribosomal RNA (Nagata 1966, Nagata and Nawa 1966a,b, Nagata et al.1969).

We studied quantitative changes of RNA synthesis in the livers of adult mice before and after feeding by incorporations of ^{3}H-uridine. Five groups of ddY mice, each consisting of 5 individuals, total 25, were injected with ^{3}H-uridine and sacrificed at different time intervals. The animals of the first group were injected with ^{3}H-uridine at 9 a.m. and fed at 10 a.m. for 30 min. and sacrificed at 11 a.m. 1 hour after the feeding and 2 hours after the injection, the 2nd group was sacrificed at 1 p.m. 3 hours after feeding and 4 hours after the injection, the 3rd group at 5 p.m., 7 and 8 hours later, the 4th group at 9 a.m. on the next day 23 and 24 hours later, and finally the 5th group at 1. p.m. on the next day 3 hours after refeeding and 28 hours after the injection. Then, the livers were taken out from each animal, prepared for isolated cell radioautograms according to Nagata et al. (1961). The results demonstrated that the grain counts in both mononucleate and binucleate hepatocytes before feeding (15-25 grains per cell) increased 4 hours after feeding (30-40 grains per cell), reached the maximum in 24 hours (40-50 grains per cell), then decreased on the next day (30-40 grains per cell). It was concluded that the RNA synthesis in the binucleate hepatocytes was a little higher than the mononucleate hepatocytes at the same stages and both increased and decreased after feeding. These results revealed that the feeding or refeeding affected the RNA synthesis of the livers (Nagata 1966).

Then, we studied aging changes of ^{3}H-uridine incorporation in the livers and pancreases of aging mice at various ages from prenatal embryos to postnatal aged mice to senescence at month 12 and 24 by LM and EMRAG (Ma and Nagata 1990b, Nagata 1999c). When aged mice were injected with ^{3}H-uridine, LM and EM RAG showed that silver grains were localized over the nucleoli, nuclear chromatin (both euchromatin and heterochromatin), mitochondria and rough surfaced endoplasmic reticulum of hepatocytes (Fig. 9C) and other types of cells such as sinusoidal endothelial cells, Kupffer's cells, Ito's fat-storing cells (Fig. 9D), ductal epithelial cells, fibroblasts and haematopoietic cells in the livers at various ages. By quantitative analysis, the total number of silver grains in nucleus, nucleolus and cytoplasm of each hepatocyte increased gradually from fetal day 19 to postnatal days, reached the maximum at postnatal day 14 (30%), then decreased to 24 months (5%). The number of silver grains in nucleolus, when classified into two compartments, grains over granular components and those over fibrillar components both increased paralelly after birth, reached the maxima on day 14 (granular 6-7, fibrillar 1-2/per cell), then decreased to 24 months with aging. However, when the ratio (%) of silver grains over euchromatin, heterochromatin of the nuclei and granular components and fibrillar components of the nucleoli are calculated, the ratio remained constant at each aging point.

1.5.2.2 The RNA synthesis in hepatocyte mitochondria

The intramitochondrial RNA synthesis was first found in the cultured HeLa cells and the cultured liver cells in vitro using EM RAG (Nagata 1972c, d). Then, it was also found in any other cells in either in vitro or vivo (Nagata et al. 1977c, Nagata 2002). Observing light microscopic radioautograms labeled with ^{3}H-uridine, the silver grains were found over both the karyoplasm and cytoplasm of almost all the cells not only at the perinatal stages from embryo day 19 to postnatal day 1, 3, 9, 14, but also at the adult and senescent stages from postnatal month 1 to 2, 6, 12 and 24 (Nagata 2007a, c, d, e, f, Nagata and Ma 2005b). By electron microscopic observation, silver grains were detected in most mononucleate hepatocytes in respective aging groups localizing not only over euchromatin and nucleoli in the nuclei but also over many cell organelles such as endoplasmic reticulum, ribosomes, and mitochondria as well as cytoplasmic matrices from perinatal stage at embryonic day 19, postnatal day 1, 3, 9, 14, to adult and senescent stages at postnatal month 1, 2, 12 and 24. The silver grains were also observed in binucleate hepatocytes at postnatal day 1, 3, 9, 14, month 1, 2, 6, 12 and 24. The localizations of silver grains over the mitochondria were mainly on the mitochondrial matrices but a few over the mitochondrial membranes and cristae when observed by high power magnification.

As the results, it was found that almost all the hepatocytes were labeled with silver grains showing RNA synthesis in their nuclei and mitochondria. Preliminary quantitative analysis on the number of mitochondria in 10 mononucleate hepatocytes whose nuclei were intensely labeled with many silver grains (more than 10 per nucleus) and other 10 mononucleate hepatocytes whose nuclei were not so intensely labeled (number of silver grains less than 9) in each aging group revealed that there was no significant difference between the number of mitochondria, number of labeled mitochondria and the labeling indices in both types of hepatocytes ($P<0.01$). Thus, the number of mitochondria and the labeling indices were calculated in 10 hepatocytes selected at random in each animal in respective aging stages regardless whether their nuclei were very intensely labeled or not. The results obtained from the number of mitochondria in mononucleate hepatocytes per cellular profile area showed an increase from the prenatal day (mean ± standard deviation 26.2± /cell) to postnatal day 1 to day 14 (38.4-51.7/cell), then to postnatal month 1-2 (53.7-89.2/cell), reaching the maximum, then decreased to year 1-2 (83.7-80.4/cell) and the increase was stochastically significant ($P<0.01$). The results of visual grain counts on the number of mitochondria labeled with silver grains obtained from 10 mononucleate hepatocytes of each animal labeled with ^{3}H-uridine demonstrating RNA synthesis in 10 aging groups at perinatal stages, prenatal embryo day 19, postnatal day 1, 3, 9 and 14, month 1, 6 and year 1 and 2, were counted. The labeling indices in respective aging stages were calculated from the number of labeled mitochondria and the number of total mitochondria per cellular profile area, respectively. The results showed that the numbers of labeled mitochondria with ^{3}H-uridine showing RNA synthesis increased from prenatal embryo day 19 (3.3/cell) to postnatal month 1 (9.2/cell), reaching the maximum, and then decreased to month 6 (3.5/cell) and again increased to year 1 (4.0/cell) and year 2 (4.3/cell), while the labeling indices increased from prenatal day 19 (12.4%) to postnatal month 1 (16.7%), reaching the maximum, then decreased to year 1 (4.8%) and year 2 (5.3%). Stochastical analysis revealed that the increases and decreases of the number of labeled mitochondria from the perinatal stage to the adult and senescent stage were significant in contrast that the increases and decreases of the labeling indices were not significant ($P<0.01$). As for the binucleate hepatocytes, on the other hand, because the appearances of binucleate hepatocytes were not so many in the embryonic stage, only several binucleate cells (5-8 at least) at respective stages when enough numbers of binucleate cells available from postnatal day 1 to year 2 were analyzed. The results of visual counts on the number of mitochondria labeled with silver grains obtained from several (5 to 8) binucleate hepatocytes labeled with ^{3}H-uridine demonstrating RNA synthesis in 8 aging groups at perinatal stages, postnatal day 1, 9, 14, and month 1, 2, 6, and year 1 and 2, were counted and the labeling indices in respective aging stages were calculated from the number of labeled mitochondria and the number of total mitochondria per cellular profile area calculated, respectively. The results showed that the number of labeled mitochondria increased from postnatal day 1 (2.3/cell) to day 9 (5.2/cell) and remained almost constant around 4-5, but the labeling indices increased from postnatal day 1 (2.1%) to postnatal day 9 (13.6%), remained almost constant around 13% (12.5-13.6%) from postnatal day 9 to month 1, then decreased to month 2 (6.1%) to month 6 (3.9%), and slightly increased to year 1 (6.3%) and 2 (5.3%). The increases and decreases of the number of labeled mitochondria and the labeling indices in binucleate hepatocytes were stochastically not significant ($P<0.01$).

We also studied intracellular localization of mRNA in adult rat hepatocytes localizing over the peroxisomes by means of in situ hybridization technique (Usuda and Nagata 1992, 1995, Usuda et al. 1992). However, its relationship to the aging of animals was not yet studied.

1.5.3 The protein synthesis in the liver

As for the protein synthesis in the liver, we first studied the incorporations of ^{3}H-leucine and ^{3}H-tryptophane in mouse hepatocytes in connection to the binuclearity before and after feeding (Nagata 1967b, Nagata et al. 1967a, Ma et al. 1991). Then, we also studied mitochondrial protein synthesis in the liver later (Nagata 2006a,b, 2007b,c,e, 2009b, 2010c).

1.5.3.1 The protein synthesis in hepatocyte nuclei

We first studied the incorporations of amino-acids, ^{3}H-leucine and ^{3}H-tryptophane, in mouse mononucleate and binucleate hepatocytes before and after feeding (Nagata 1967b, Nagata et al. 1967a, Ma et al. 1991). The results showed that the incorporations of both amino acids were greater in binucleate hepatocytes than mononucleate. When ^{3}H-leucine was injected into several groups of mice at various ages and the liver tissues were processed for LM and EM RAG, silver grains were observed over all cell types of the liver, i.e., hepatocytes (Fig. 9E), sinusoidal endothelial cells (Fig. 9F), ductal epithelial cells, Kupffer's cells, Ito's fat storing cells, fibroblasts and haematopoietic cells. In hepatocytes, number of silver grains in cytoplasm and karyoplasm increased from perinatal animals to postnatal 1 month young adult animals and decreased with aging to senescence at 24 months. Number of silver grains observed over respective cell organelles, the Golgi apparatus, mitochondria and endoplasmic reticulum, changed with aging, reaching the maxima at 1 month but the ratio remained constant at each point. When ^{3}H-proline was injected into mice at various ages from prenatal embryos to postnatal senescence, quantitative changes of collagen and protein synthesis in the livers were studied by electron microscopic radioautography (Ma and Nagata 2000, Nagata 2006a). The silver grains due to ^{3}H-proline showing collagen synthesis were localized over the nuclei, cytoplasmic matrix, endoplasmic reticulum, the Golgi apparatus, mitochondria and peroxisomes of almost all the cells such as hepatocytes (Fig. 9F), sinusoidal endothelial cells, Kupffer's cells (Fig. 9G), Ito's fat-storing cells, ductal epithelial cells, fibroblasts and haematopoietic cells at various ages. The number of silver grains in the cell bodies and nuclei, cytoplasmic matrix, endoplasmic reticulum, mitochondria, the Golgi apparatus and peroxisomes of hepatocytes gradually increased from embryo, reaching the maxima at postnatal month 1 and 6, and decreased with aging until 24 months. The grain counts of the cell bodies reached the maximum at month 6 and the nuclei at month 2, while that of endoplasmic reticulum at month 6 and mitochondria at month 1. The number of silver grains localized over the extracellular collagen fibrils and matrices was not so many in respective aging groups and did not show any remarkable changes with aging. From the results, it was concluded that ^{3}H-proline was incorporated not only into collagen but also into the structural proteins of hepatocytes and increased and decreased due to aging under normal aging conditions.

1.5.3.2 The protein synthesis in hepatocyte mitochondria

When the aging mice at various ages from embryo to senescence were injected with ^{3}H-leucine, it was found that almost all the hepatocytes, from embryonic day 19, postnatal day 1, 3, 9, 14, to adult and senescent stages at postnatal month 1, 2, 6, 12 and 24, incorporated silver grains (Fig. 9E). The silver grains were also observed in binucleate hepatocytes at postnatal day 1, 3, 9, 14, month 1, 2, 6, 12 and 24 (Nagata 2007a,b,c,d, 2006a,b, 2007b,c,e). The localizations of silver grains observed over the mitochondria were mainly on the mitochondrial matrices but a few over their nuclei, cytoplasmic matrix, endoplasmic reticulum, ribosomes, Golgi apparatus and mitochondria (Nagata 2006a, b, 2007b, c, e). In the mitochondria the silver grains were localized over the mitochondrial membranes and cristae when observed by high power magnification. Preliminary quantitative analysis on the number of mitochondria in 20 mononucleate hepatocytes whose nuclei were intensely labeled with many silver grains (more than 10 per nucleus) and other 20 mononucleate hepatocytes whose nuclei were not so intensely labeled (number of silver grains less than 9) in each aging group revealed that there was no significant difference between the number of mitochondria, number of labeled mitochondria and the labeling indices in both types of hepatocytes ($P<0.01$).

On the other hand, the numbers of mitochondria, the numbers of labeled mitochondria and the labeling indices were calculated in 10 binucleate hepatocytes selected at random in each animal in respective aging stages, regardless whether their nuclei were very intensely labeled or not, except the prenatal stage at embryonic day 19, because no binucleate cell was found at this stage, resulted in no significant difference between them. Thus, the numbers of mitochondria, the numbers of labeled mitochondria and the labeling indices were calculated in 20 hepatocytes selected at random in each animal in respective aging stages regardless whether their nuclei were very intensely labeled or not. The results obtained from the total numbers of mitochondria in mononucleate hepatocytes showed an increase from the prenatal day (34.5/cell) to postnatal days 1 (44.6/cell), 3 (45.8/cell), 9 (43.6/cell), 14 (48.5/cell), to postnatal months 1 (51.5/cell), 2 (52.3/cell), reaching the maximum at month 6 (60.7/cell), then decreased to years 1 (54.2/cell) and 2 (51.2/cell). The increase and decrease were stochastically significant ($P<0.01$). The results obtained from visual counting on the numbers of mitochondria labeled with silver grains from 20 mononucleate hepatocytes of each animal labeled with ^{3}H-leucine demonstrating protein synthesis in 10 aging groups at perinatal stages, prenatal embryo day 19, postnatal day 1, 3, 9 and 14, month 1, 2, 6 and year 1 and 2, were counted. The labeling indices in respective aging stages were calculated from the numbers of labeled mitochondria and the numbers of total mitochondria per cell. The results showed that the numbers of labeled mitochondria with ^{3}H-leucine showing protein synthesis increased from prenatal embryo day 19 (8.3/cell) to postnatal days 1 (9.6/cell), 3 (8.1/cell), 9 (8.9/cell), 14 (9.5/cell), and month 1 (11.2/cell), reaching the maximum, and then decreased to months 2 (9.1/cell), 6 (8.8/cell) to years 1 (6.7/cell) and 2 (2.2/cell), while the labeling indices increased from prenatal day 19 (20.1%) to postnatal days 1 (21.2%), 3 (21.6%), 9 (22.2%), 14 (23.1%), reaching the maximum, then decreased to month 1 (21.7%), 2 (17.4%), 6 (14.6%), and years 1 (12.4%) and 2 (4.4%). Stochastical analysis revealed that the increases and decreases of the numbers of labeled mitochondria as well as the labeling indices from the perinatal stage to the adult and senescent stages were significant ($P<0.01$).

The results obtained from the numbers of mitochondria in binucleate hepatocytes showed an increase from the postnatal days 1 (66.2/cell), to 3 (66.4/cell), 14 (81.8/cell), to postnatal months 1 (89.9/cell), 2 (95.1/cell), and 6 (102.1), reaching the maximum at month 12 (128.0/cell), then decreased to years 2 (93.9/cell). The increase and decrease were stochastically significant ($P<0.01$). The results obtained from visual counting on the numbers of mitochondria labeled with silver grains from 10 binucleate hepatocytes of each animal labeled with ^{3}H-leucine demonstrating protein synthesis in 10 aging groups at postnatal day 1, 3, and 14, month 1, 2, 6 and year 1 and 2, were counted. The labeling indices in respective aging stages were calculated from the numbers of labeled mitochondria and the numbers of total mitochondria per cell which showed that the numbers of labeled mitochondria with ^{3}H-leucine showing protein synthesis increased from postnatal day 1 (7.3/cell) to day 3 (6.8/cell), 14 (10.2/cell), and month 1 (15.0/cell), 2 (15.9/cell), reaching the maximum at month 6 (19.6/cell), then decreased to year 1 (8.3/cell) and 2 (5.1/cell), while the labeling indices increased from postnatal day 1 (11.8%) to 3 (10.2%), 14 (12.5%), month 1 (18.3%) and 2 (18.7%), reaching the maximum at month 6 (19.2%), then decreased to year 1 (6.4%) and 2 (5.5%). Stochastical analysis revealed that the increases and decreases of the numbers of labeled mitochondria as well as the labeling indices from the newborn stage to the adult and senescent stages were significant ($P<0.01$). The silver grains due to ^{3}H-leucine were also observed in sinusoidal endothelial cells (Fig. 8F), Kupfer's cells, Ito's fat-storing cells, ductal epithelial cells, fibroblasts and hematopoietic cells at various ages.

When ^{3}H-prolin was injected into aging mice at various ages, silver grains were localized over the nuclei, cytoplasmic matrix, endoplasmic reticulum, the Golgi apparatus, mitochondria and peroxisomes of all the cell such as hepatocytes (Fig. 9G), sinusoidal endothelial cells, Kupfer's cells (Fig. 9H), Ito's fat-storing cells, ductal epithelial cells, fibroblasts and hematopoietic cells at various ages. The number of silver grains in hepatocytes gradually increased from perinatal stage to postnatal month 1 to 6 due to aging, reaching the maximum and decreased to momth 24. The number of silver grains localized the extracellular collage fibrils and matrices was not so great in respective aging groups and did not show any remarkable changes with aging. From the results, it was concluded that ^{3}H-prolin was incorporated not only into collagen but also into the structural proteins of hepatocytes under normal aging conditions (Ma and Nagata 2000).

1.5.4 The glucide synthesis in the liver

We first studied ^{3}H-glucose incorporation into glycogen in the livers of adult mice, in connection to soluble compounds (Nagata and Murata 1977, Nagata et al. 1977a,d). Soluble ^{3}H-glucose, which was demonstrated by cryo-fixation (at -196°C) in combination with dry-mounting radioautography, was localized over the nuclei, nucleoli, all the cell organelles and cytoplasmic ground substance of all the hepatocytes diffusely. On the other hand, by conventional chemical fixation and wet-mounting radioautography, silver grains were localized only over glycogen granules, endoplasmic reticulum and Golgi apparatus showing glycogen synthesis. However, the relationship of glycogen synthesis to aging has not yet been fully clarified.

1.5.5 The lipids synthesis in the liver

We observed lipids synthesis in the liver using ^{3}H-glycerol in connection to soluble compounds (Nagata 1994a,d, Nagata and Murata 1977a, Nagata et al. 1977a,d). When adult mice were injected with ^{3}H-glycerol and the livers were taken out, cryo-fixed in liquid nitrogen at -196°C, then freeze-substituted, embedded in epoxy resin, dry-sectioned, and prepared for dry-mounting radioautography, many silver grains appeared over the nuclei and cytoplasm of hepatocytes diffusely. However, when the same liver tissues were fixed chemically in buffered glutaraldehyde and osmium tetroxide at 4°C, dehydrated, embedded, wet-sectioned and radioautographed by conventional wet-mounting procedures, very few silver grains were observed only over the endoplasmic reticulum and the lipid droplets, which demonstrated insoluble macromolecular lipid synthesis accumulating into the lipid droplets. However, the aging change of the lipid synthesis in the liver has not yet been fully clarified.

1.6 Macromolecular synthesis in the pancreas

The pancreas is a large gland, next to the liver in men and animals, among the digestive glands connected to the intestines. It consists of exocrine and endocrine portions and takes the shape of a compound acinous gland. The exocrine portion is composed of ductal epithelial cells, centro-acinar cells, acinar cells and connective tissue cells, while the endocrine portion, the islet of Langerhans, is composed of 3 types of endocrine cells, A, B, C cells and connective tissue cells. Intracellular transport of secretory proteins in the pancreatic exocrine cells were formerly studied by Jamieson and Palade (1967) by EMRAG. We studied the macromolecular synthesis of the aging mouse pancreas at various ages.

1.6.1 The DNA synthesis in the pancreas

We first studied the DNA synthesis of mouse pancreas by LM and EMRAG using ^{3}H-thymidine (Nagata and Usuda 1984, 1985, 1986, Nagata et al. 1986). Light and electron microscopic radioautograms of the pancreas revealed that the nuclei of pancreatic acinar cells (Fig. 11A), centro-acinar cells (Fig. 11B), ductal epithelial cells, and endocrine cells were labeled with ^{3}H-thymidine. The labeling indices of these cells in 5 groups of litter mate mice, fetal day 15, postnatal day 1, 20, 60 (2 months) and 730 (2 years) were analyzed.

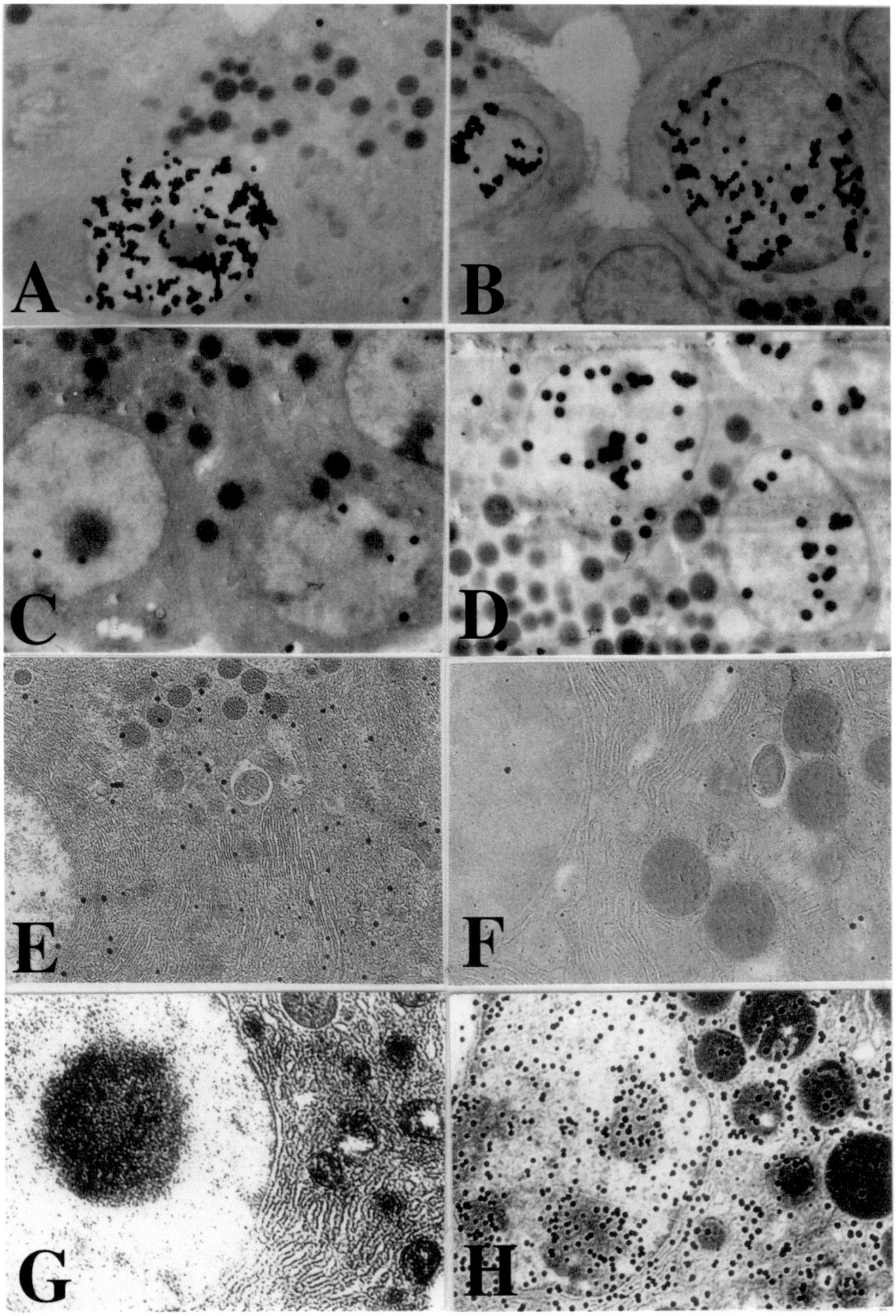

Fig. 11. EM RAG of the pancreas. From Nagata, T.: Radioautographology, General and Special. In, Prog. Histochem. Cytochem. Vol. 37, No. 2, p. 140, 2002, Urban & Fischer, Jena, Germany

Fig. 11A. EM RAG of 2 pancreatic acinar cells of a 14 day old mouse labeled with ^{3}H-thymidine, showing DNA synthesis. x10,000.
Fig. 11B. EM RAG of 2 centro-acinar cells of a 14 day old mouse labeled with ^{3}H-thymidine, showing DNA synthesis. x10,000.
Fig. 11C. EM RAG of 3 pancreatic acinar cells of a 1 day old mouse labeled with ^{3}H-uridine, showing RNA synthesis. x10,000.
Fig. 11D. EM RAG of 3 pancreatic acinar cells of a 14 day old mouse labeled with ^{3}H-uridine, showing RNA synthesis. x10,000.
Fig. 11E. EM RAG of a pancreatic acinar cell of a 30 day old mouse labeled with ^{3}H-leucine, showing protein synthesis. x10,000.
Fig. 11F. EM RAG of a pancreatic acinar cell of a 12 month old mouse labeled with ^{3}H-leucine, showing protein synthesis. x10,000.
Fig. 11G. EM RAG of a pancreatic acinar cell of a 1 day old mouse labeled with ^{3}H-glucosamine, showing glucide synthesis. x10,000.
Fig. 11H. EM RAG of a pancreatic acinar cell of a 14 day old mouse labeled with ^{3}H-glucosamine, showing glucide synthesis. x10,000.

The labeling indices of these cells reached the maxima at day 1 after birth and decreased gradually to 2 years (Fig. 12). The maximum in the acinar cells proceeded to the ductal and centro-acinar cells, suggesting that the acinar cells completed their development earlier than the ductal and centro-acinar cells (Nagata et al. 1986).

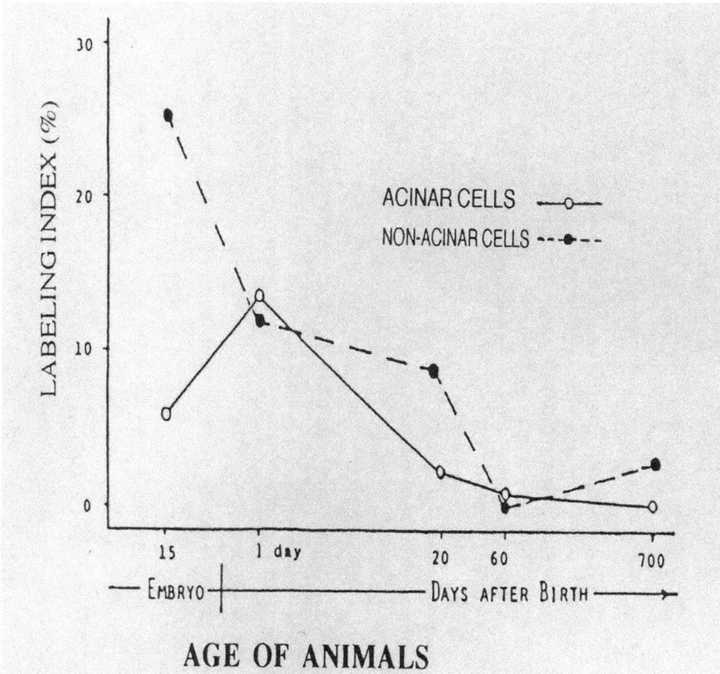

Fig. 12. Transitional curves of the labeling indices of respective cell types of the pancreas of aging mice labeled with ^{3}H-thymidine, showing DNA synthesis. Mean ± Standard Deviation. From Nagata, T.: Radioautographology, General and Special. In, Prog. Histochem. Cytochem. Vol. 37, No. 2, p. 142, 2002, Urban & Fischer, Jena, Germany

1.6.2 The RNA synthesis in the pancreas

On the other hand, LM and EMRAG of pancreas of mouse injected with ^{3}H-uridine demonstrated its incorporation into exocrine and then in endocrine cells, and more in pancreatic acinar cells (Figs. 11C,D) than in ductal or centro-acinar cells (Nagata and Usuda 1986a,b, Nagata et al. 1986). Among the acinar cells, the number of silver grains increased after birth to day 14 and then decreased with aging. Quantification of silver grains in the nucleoli, chromatin, and cell body were carried out by X-ray microanalysis (Nagata 1991, 1993, 2004, Nagata and Usuda 1985), which verified the results obtained by visual grain counting. In EMRAG obtained from the pancreas of fetal day 19 embryos, newborn day 1 and newborn day 14 mice labeled with ^{3}H-uridine, demonstrating RNA synthesis, the number of silver grains in the nucleoli, nuclear chromatin and cytoplasm increased (Nagata 1985, 1991, 1993a,b, 2004, Nagata and Usuda 1985, 1986). In order to quantify the silver contents of grains observed over the nucleoli, nuclei and cytoplasm, X-ray spectra were recorded by energy dispersive X-ray microanalysis (JEM-4000EX TN5400), demonstrating Ag-Ka peaks at higher energies. Thus, P/B ratios expressing relative silver contents were determined and compared between the two age groups. The results obtained by X-ray microanalysis in different cell compartments at postnatal day 1 and day 14 and he results obtained by visual grain counting in different cell compartments in day 1 day and day 14 animals were compared. The number of silver grains was calculated to express the counts per unit area to be compared with the XMA counts. These two results, the silver content analyzed by X-ray microanalysis and the results obtaining from visual grain counting were in good accordance with each other.

1.6.3 The protein synthesis in the pancreas

As for the protein synthesis in the pancreas, ^{3}H-leucine incorporation into endoplasmic reticulum, Golgi apparatus and to secretory granules of pancreatic acinar cells was first demonstrated by Jamieson and Palade (1967). We first studied ^{3}H-glycine incorporation into these cell organelles of mouse pancreatic acinar cells in connection with soluble compounds by EM RAG (Nagata 2000c, 2007a). It was demonstrated that soluble ^{3}H-glycine distributed not only in these cell organelles but also in the karyoplasm and cytoplasm diffusely. Then, the quantitative aspects of protein synthesis with regards the aging from fetal day 19, to postnatal day 1, 3, 7, 14 and 1, 2, 6 and 12 months were also clarified (Nagata and Usuda 1993a, Nagata 2000c). The results showed an increase of silver grain counts labeled with ^{3}H-leucine after birth, reaching a peak from postnatal 2 weeks to 1 month (Fig. 10E), and decreasing from 2 months to 1 year (Fig. 11F).

On the other hand, we also studied ^{3}H-leucine incorporations into the pancreatic acinar cells of both normal adult rats and experimentally pancreatitis induced rats with either ethionine or alcohol (Yoshizawa et al. 1974, 1977). The results showed that the incorporations as indicated silver grain counts in the pancreatitis rats were less than normal control rats. However, its relation to the aging was not yet studied.

1.6.4 The glucide synthesis in the pancreas

Concerning the glucide synthesis of the pancreas, we first studied the incorporation of ^{3}H-glucose into the pancreatic acinar cells of mouse in connection with soluble compounds by

EM RAG (Nagata et al. 1977a). It was demonstrated that soluble ^{3}H-glucose distributed not only in such cell organelles as endoplasmic reticulum, Golgi apparatus, mitochondria but also in the karyoplasm and cytoplasm diffusely. Then, the incorporation of ^{3}H-glucosamine into the pancreases of aging mice at various ages was studied by LM and EM RAG (Nagata et al. 1992). When perinatal baby mice received ^{3}H-glucosamine injections and the pancreatic tissues were radioautographed, silver grains were observed over exocrine and endocrine pancreatic cells. However, the number of silver grains was not so many (Fig. 11G). When juvenile mice at the age of 14 days after birth were examined, many silver grains appeared over the exocrine pancreatic acinar cells (Fig. 11H). Less silver grains were observed over endocrine pancreatic cells and ductal epithelial cells. The grains in the exocrine pancreatic acinar cells were localized over the nucleus, endoplasmic reticulum, Golgi apparatus and secretory granules, demonstrating glycoprotein synthesis. Adult mice at the ages of postnatal 1 month, 6 month or senile mice at the ages of 12 months or 24 months showed very few silver grains on radioautograms. Thus, the glucide synthesis in the pancreatic acinar cells of mice revealed quantitative changes, increase and decrease of ^{3}H-glucosamine incorporation with aging (Nagata 1994a,b,c,d,e, Nagata et al. 1992).

1.6.5 The lipids synthesis in the pancreas

In order to demonstrate the lipids synthesis in the pancreas, several litters of ddY mice aged fetal day 19, postnatal day 1, 3, 7, 14, and 1, 2, 6 up to 12 months, were injected with ^{3}H-glycerol and the pancreas tissues were prepared for LM and EM RAG. The silver grains were observed in both exocrine and endocrine cells of respective ages (Nagata 1995a,b, Nagata et al. 1988b, 1990). In perinatal animals from fetal day 19 to postnatal 1, 3, and 7 days, cell organelles were not well developed in exocrine and endocrine cells and number of silver grains was very few. In 14 day old juvenile animals, cell organelles such as endoplasmic reticulum, Golgi apparatus, mitochondria and secretory granules were well developed and many silver grains were observed over these organelles and nuclei in both exocrine and endocrine cells. The number of silver grains was more in exocrine cells than endocrine cells. In 1, 2, 6 month old adult animals, number of silver grains remained constant. In 12 month old senescent animals, silver grains were fewer than younger animals. It was demonstrated that the number of silver grains expressed the quantity of lipids synthesis, which increased from perinatal atages to adult and senescent stages and finally decreased to senescence.

2. Macromolecular synthesis in the respiratory system

The respiratory system consists of 2 parts, the air-conducting portion and the respiratory portion. The former are the nose, the pharynx, the larynx and the trachea, while the latter the lung. We studied the macromolecular synthesis in the pulmonary tissues as well as the tracheal tissues at various ages from embryo to postnatal 2 years.

2.1 The DNA synthesis in the respiratory system

Among the air-conducting portion and the respiratory portion we studied the macromolecular synthesis in the tracheal tissues as well as the pulmonary tissues at various ages from embryo to postnatal 2 years (Sun et al. 1994, 1995a,b, 1997a,b, Nagata 2000d).

2.1.1 The DNA synthesis in the trachea

The tracheas of mammals are composed of ciliated pseudostratified columnar epithelia, connective tissues, smooth muscles and hyalin cartilages surrounding the epithelia. The changes of DNA synthesis of tracheal cells in aging mice were studied by LM and EMRAG (Sun et al. 1997a, Nagata 2000d). The tracheae of 8 groups of mice from fetal day 18 to 2 years after birth were examined. The results demonstrated that the DNA syntheses and morphology of tracheal cells in the mouse tracheae changed due to aging. The radioautograms revealed that the DNA synthesis in the nuclei of ciliated cells was observed only in the fetal animals (Fig. 13A). However, the DNA synthesis in nonciliated cells and basal cells was observed in both prenatal and postnatal animals (Fig. 13B). The labeling indices of respective cell types were analyzed (Sun et al. 1997a). As the results, the labeling indices of the epithelial cells showed their maxima on fetal day 18, then fell down from postnatal day 3 to 2 years (Fig. 14A). The ciliated cell could not synthesize DNA and proliferate in the postnatal stage. They are supposed to be derived by the division and transformation of the basal cells. On the other hand, the DNA synthesis of chondrocytes was the highest on embryonic day 18, and rapidly declined on postnatal day 3 (Fig. 13C). The chondrocytes lost the ability of synthesizing DNA at 2 months after birth (Fig. 14B). The labeling indices of other cells (including fibroblasts, smooth muscle and glandular cells) were the highest on fetal day 18 and fell down markedly on the third day after birth and decreased progressively due to aging (Fig. 14C).

2.1.2 The DNA synthesis in the lung

We studied the pulmonary tissues at various ages from embryo to postnatal 2 years of mice (Sun et al. 1995a,b). The pulmonary tissues obtained from ddY strain mice at various ages from embryo day 19 to adult postnatal day 30 and to year 2 consisted of several types of cells, i.e., the type I epithelial cells or the small alveolar epithelial cells, type II epithelial cells or large alveolar epithelial cells, interstitial cells and endothelial cells, which incorporated macromolecular precursors respectively (Figs. 13E, F, G, H).

2.1.2.1 The DNA synthesis in the pulmonary cells

The pulmonary tissues obtained from ddY strain mice at embryonic to early postnatal stages consisted of undifferentiated cells (Fig. 13E). However, they differentiated into several types of cells due to aging, the type I epithelial cells or the small alveolar epithelial cells (Fig. 13E), the type II epithelial cells or the large alveolar epithelial cells (Fig. 13F), the interstitial cells (Fig. 13G), the endothelial cells (Fig. 13H) and alveolar phagocytes or dust cells as we had formerly observed (Sun et al. 1995a,b). At embryonic day 16 and 18, the fetal lung tissues appeared as glandular organizations consisting of many alveoli bordering undifferentiated cuboidal cells and no squamous epithelial cells were seen (Figs. 13E, 13G). Mitotic figures were frequently observed in cuboidal epithelial cells. After birth, the structure of the alveoli was characterized by further development of the alveolar-capillary networks from postnatal day 1 to 3 and 7 (Fig. 13H). During the development, the cellular composition of the alveolar epithelium resembled that of the adult lung, with a mixed population of the type I and type II epithelial cells. Up to 1 and 2 weeks after birth, the lung tissues showed complete alveolar structure and single capillary system almost the same as the adult after 1 month (Fig. 13F) to 2 to 6 months, and further to senescent stage over 12 months to 22 months. On electron microscopic radioautograms of the pulmonary tissues labeled with ^{3}H-thymidine, silver grains were observed over the nuclei of some pulmonary cells corresponding to the DNA synthesis in S-phase as observed by light microscopic radioautograpy (Sun et al. 1995a,b, 1997a).

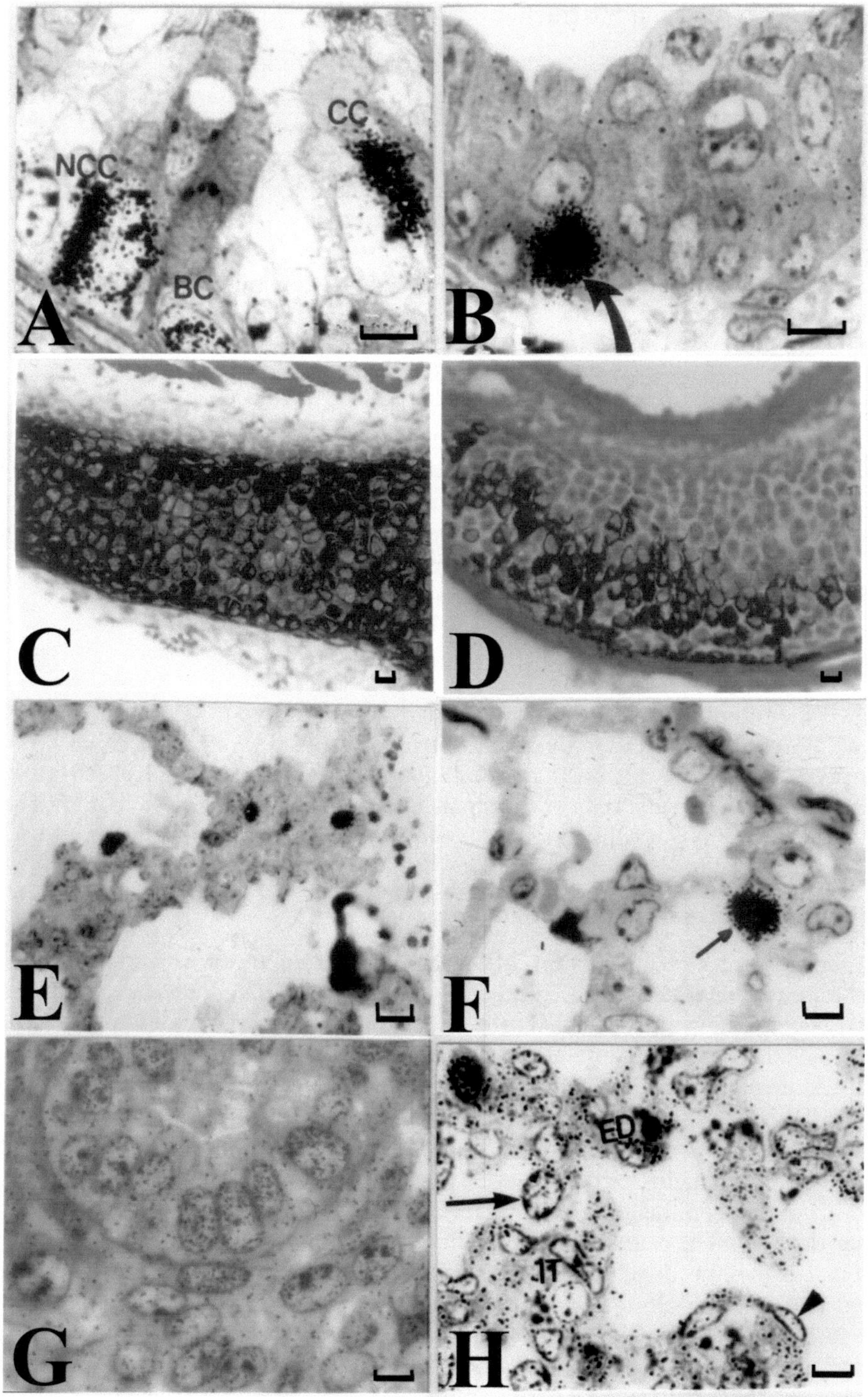

Fig. 13. LM RAG of the respiratory organs. From Nagata, T.: Special Cytochemistry in Cell Biology, In, Internat. Rev. Cytol. Vol. 211, No. 1, p. 102, 2001, Academic Press, San Diego, USA, London, UK.

Fig. 13A. LM RAG of the tracheal epithelial cells of a prenatal day 18 mouse embryo labeled with ^{3}H-thymidine, showing DNA synthesis. x1,125.
Fig. 13B. LM RAG of the tracheal epithelial cells of a postnatal 1 month old mouse labeled with ^{3}H-thymidine, showing DNA synthesis. x1,125.
Fig. 13C. LM RAG of the tracheal cartilage cells of a prenatal day 19 mouse embryo labeled with $^{35}SO_4$ showing mucosubstance synthesis. x400.
Fig. 13D. LM RAG of the tracheal cartilage cells of a postnatal day 3 mouse labeled with $^{35}SO_4$ showing mucosubstance synthesis. x400.
Fig. 13E. LM RAG of the lung of a 1 day old mouse labeled with ^{3}H-thymidine, showing DNA synthesis. x750.
Fig. 13F. LM RAG of the lung of a 1 month old mouse labeled with ^{3}H-thymidine, showing DNA synthesis. x750.
Fig. 13G. LM RAG of the lung of a prenatal day 16 mouse embryo labeled with ^{3}H-uridine, showing RNA synthesis. x750.
Fig. 13H. LM RAG of the lung of a 7 day old mouse labeled with ^{3}H-leucine, showing protein synthesis. x750.

The DNA synthetic activity of respective pulmonary cells as expressed by labeling indices demonstrated increases from perinatal stage to developmental stage and decreased due to aging. We also studied inhalation of ^{3}H-thymidine in air by means of a nebulizer into the lungs of 1 week old young mice as experimental studies and observed by LM and EM RAG (Duan et al. 1994). After 10 min. inhalation, the lung tissues were taken out and processed by either rapid freezing and freeze-substitution for dry-mounting radioautography or conventional chemical fixation for wet-mounting radioautography. By wet-mounting RAG silver grains were observed in the nuclei of a few alveolar type 2 cells and interstitial cells demonstrating DNA synthesis. By dry-mounting RAG, numerous silver grains were located diffusely over all the epithelial cells and interstitial cells demonstrating soluble compounds. The results showed that ^{3}H-thymidine inhaled into the lung distributed over all the pulmonary cells but only some of the alveolar type 2 cells and interstitial cells did synthesize DNA.

On the other hand, we studied the aging changes of DNA synthesis in the lungs of salamanders, *Hynobius nebolosus,* from larvae at 2 month after fertilization, juvenile at 1 month, adults at 10 and 12 months after metamorphosis, and finally to senescence at 5 years by LM RAG after ^{3}H-thymidine injections (Matsumura et at. 1994). The results showed that the labeling indices of in the ciliated cells and mucous cells in the superficial layer of young animals were higher than those of the basal cells and they decreased in adults, demonstrating aging changes in salamanders.

2.1.2.2 The DNA synthesis in mitochondria of mouse pulmonary cells

On electron microscopic radioautograms of the pulmonary tissues labeled with ^{3}H-thymidine, silver grains were observed over not only the nuclei of some pulmonary cells corresponding to the DNA synthesis in S-phase as observed by LM radioautograpy (Sun et al. 1995a,b) but also over the mitochondria by EMRAG (Sun et al. 1995b). Some mitochondria in both S-phase cells and interphase cells which did not show any silver grains over their nuclei were labeled with silver grains showing intramitochondrial DNA synthesis. The intramitochondrial DNA synthesis was observed in all cell types, the type I epithelial cells, the type II epithelial cells (Figs. 13F,G), the interstitial cells (Fig. 13F) and the endothelial cells. Because enough numbers of electron photographs (more than 5) were not obtained from all the cell types in respective aging groups, only some cell types and some aging groups when enough numbers of electron photographs were available were used for quantitative analysis. The numbers of mitochondria per cell profile area, the numbers of labeled mitochondria per cell and the labeling indices of the type I epithelial cells in only a few aging groups were observed and counted. The labeling indices in respective aging stages were calculated from the number of labeled mitochondria and the number of total mitochondria per cellular profile area which were calculated, respectively. These results demonstrated that the labeling indices in these cell types decreased from prenatal stages at embryo day 16 to day 18 (20-25%), and further decreased to postnatal days up to senescent stages due to aging (Fig. 15).

2.2 The RNA synthesis in the respiratory system

We studied the lungs of aging mice among the respiratory organs after administration of ^{3}H-uridine at various ages from prenatal embryonic day 16 to postnatal senescent month 22 as observed by LM and EM RAG (Fig. 13H).

2.2.1 RNA synthesis of mouse pulmonary cells

When the lung tissues of mice were labeled with ^{3}H-uridine, RNA synthesis was observed in all cells of the lungs at various ages by RAG (Sun 1995, Sun et al. 1997b, Nagata 2002). Observing the light microscopic radioautograms labeled with ^{3}H-uridine, the silver grains were found over both the karyoplasm and cytoplasm of almost all the cells not only at the perinatal stages from embryo day 16, 18, to postnatal day 1, 3, 7, 14, but also at the adult and senescent stages from postnatal month 1 to 2, 6, 12 and 22. The number of silver grains, by electron micrography, changed with aging. The grain counts in type I epithelial cells increased from the 1st day after birth and reached a peak at 1 week and decreased gradually to month 22, while the counts in type II epithelial cells (Fig. 13H), interstitial cells and endothelial cells increased from embryo day 16 and reached peaks at 1 week after birth, then decreased to senescence.

2.2.2 The RNA synthesis of mitochondria in pulmonary cells

By electron microscopic radioautography, silver grains were observed in most pulmonary cells in respective aging groups localizing not only over euchromatin and nucleoli in the nuclei but also over many cell organelles such as endoplasmic reticulum, ribosomes, and mitochondria as well as cytoplasmic matrices from perinatal stage at embryonic day 16, 18, to postnatal day 1, 3, 7, 14, to adult and senescent stages at postnatal month 1, 2, 6, 12 and 22 (Sun 1995, Sun et al. 1997b, Nagata 2002). The localizations of silver grains over the mitochondria were mainly on the mitochondrial matrices but a few over the mitochondrial membranes and cristae when observed by high power magnification. However, quantitative analyses on the number of mitochondria, the number of labeled mitochondria and the labeling index were not performed because enough number of EM RAG was not obtained.

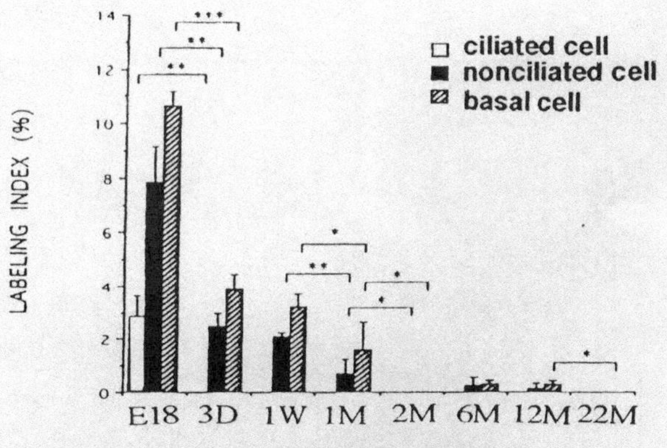

A

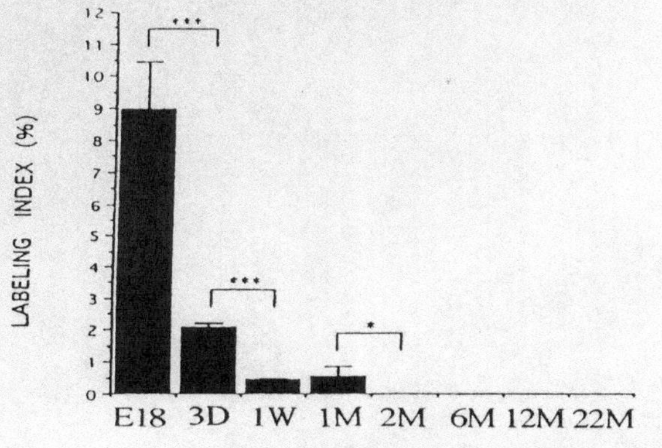

B

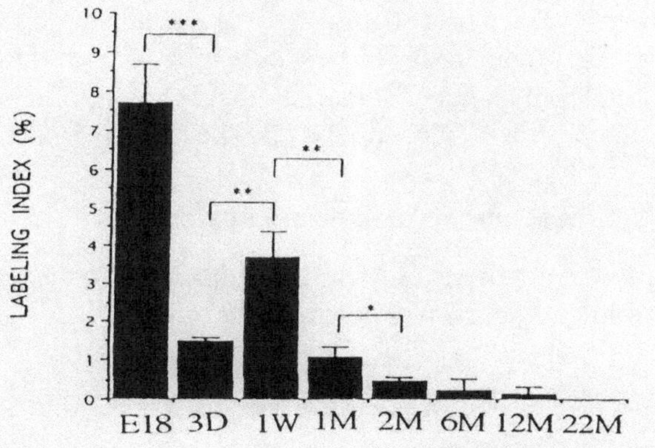

C

Fig. 14. Histogram showing aging changes of average labeling indices in respective cell types of the trachea of aging mice labeled with ^{3}H-thymidine. Mean ± Standard Deviation. From Nagata, T.: Radioautographology, General and Special. In, Prog. Histochem. Cytochem. Vol. 37, No. 2, p. 148, 2002, Urban & Fischer, Jena, Germany

Fig. 14A. Epithelial cells.

Fig. 14B. Chondrocytes in the cartilage.

Fig. 14C. Other cells.

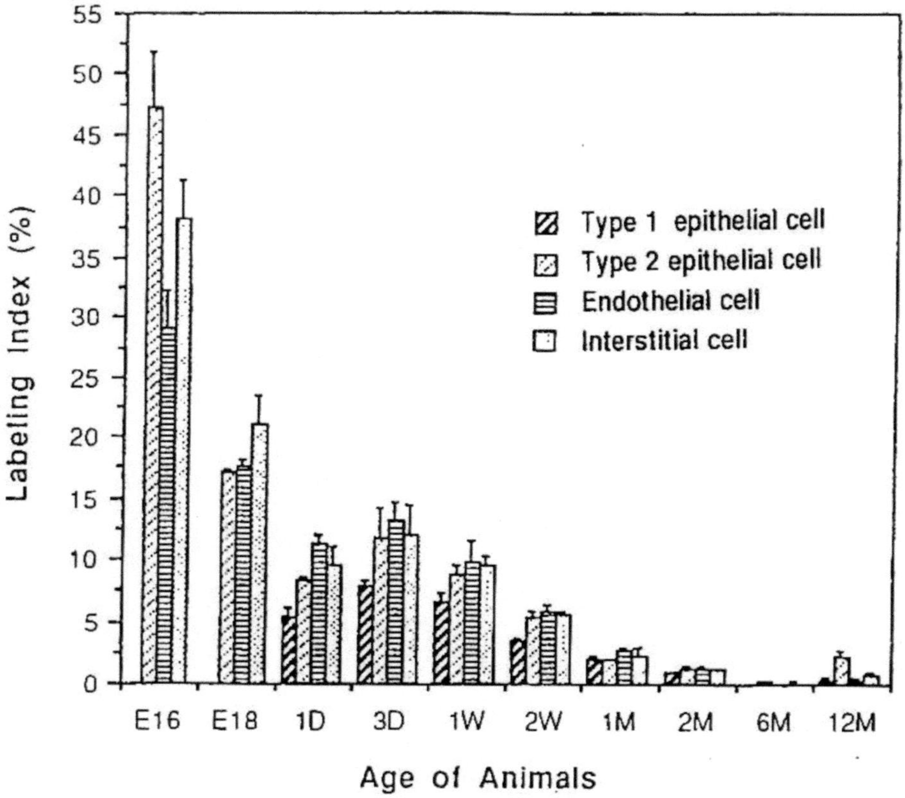

Fig. 15. Histogram showing aging changes of average labeling indices in respective cell types of the tracheal epithelial cells of aging mice labeled with ^{3}H-thymidine. Mean ± Standard Deviation. From Nagata, T.: Radioautographology, General and Special. In, Prog. Histochem. Cytochem. Vol. 37, No. 2, p. 149, 2002, Urban & Fischer, Jena, Germany

2.3 The protein synthesis in the respiratory system

We studied the protein synthesis only in the lungs of aging mice at various ages among the respiratory organs including the respiratory tract.

2.3.1 Protein synthesis of aging mouse pulmonary cells

When the lung tissues of mice at various ages were labeled with ^{3}H-leucine, protein synthesis was observed in all types of cells, type I and type II epithelial cells, interstitial cells and endothelial cells, of the lungs at various ages from embryo to senescence (Sun et al. 1997b). Observing the light microscopic radioautograms, the silver grains were detected over both the karyoplasm and cytoplasm of almost all the cells not only at the perinatal stages from embryo day 16, 18, to postnatal day 1 to 14 (Fig. 13I), but also at the adult and senescent stages from postnatal month 1 to 2, 6, 12 and 22. The number of silver grains, by light microscopic radioautography, changed with aging. The grain counts in type I epithelial cells were the highest on postnatal day 1, decreased on day 3 and increased again at 1 week, then decreased gradually to month 22, while the counts in type II epithelial cells, interstitial cells and endothelial cells reached the highest levels on fetal day 16, declined progressively with aging from fetal day 18 to postnatal day 3, then increased again from postnatal to day 7, reached peaks at 1 week (day 7) after birth, then decreased to senescence. However, grain counting on cell organelles by electron microscopy was not performed because enough numbers of EM RAG were not obtained at that time.

2.4 The glucide synthesis in the respiratory system

The incorporation of $^{35}SO_4$ in the trachea of aging mice was studied among the respiratory organs (Nagata 2000d). As the results, silver grains indicating the incorporations of radiosulfate were found over the cartilage matrices and the cartilage capsules in the hyaline cartilages of the tracheae of fetal (Fig. 13C) and postnatal newborn mice (Fig. 13D). The grain density as analyzed by grain densitometry was the maximum at the fetal day 19 (1200 grains per unit area). The grain density then decreased from the fetal day 19 to the postnatal day 1, 3, 7 (600/area), 14 (200/area) and reached 0 on day 30, and no silver grain was found in the animals aged from 1 to 12 months. The silver grains in the perinatal animals aged at postnatal day 1 and 3, disappearred from the internal layer to the external layer of the cartilage and from the interterritorial matrix to the territorial matrix and the cartilage capsule. In the juvenile animals aged at postnatal day 9 and 14, intense incorporations were observed disseminatedly over several groups of cartilage capsules in the external layer. The results indicated that the glycoproteins constituting the cartilage matrix were synthesized from prenatal to postnatal day 30. To the contrary, no incorporation of silver grains was observed in the aging animals from postnatal 1 to 12 months by both LM and EM RAG. These results demonstrated the aging changes of glycoprotein synthesis in the cartilage matrix of mice at various ages during development and aging.

3. References

Chen, S., Gao, F., Kotani, A., Nagata, T.: Age-related changes of male mouse submandibular gland: A morphometric and radioautographic study. Cell. Mol. Biol. 41, 117-124, 1995.

Clermont Y.: The contractime elements in the limiting membrane of the seminiferous tubules of rats. Exp. Cell Res. 15, 438-342, 1958.

Clermont, Y.: Renewal of spermatogonia in man. Amer. J. Anat. 112, 35-51, 1963.

Cui, H.: Light microscopic radioautographic study on DNA synthesis of nerve cells in the cerebella of aging mice. Cell. Mol. Biol. 41, 1139-1154, 1995.

Cui, H., Gao, F., Nagata, T.: Light microscopic radioautographic study on protein synthesis in perinatal mice corneas. Acta Histochem. Cytochem. 33, 31-37, 2000.

Duan, H., Gao, F., Li, S., Hayashi, K., Nagata, T.: Aging changes and fine structure and DNA synthesis of esophageal epithelium in neonatal, adult and old mice. J. Clin. Electron Microsc. 25, 452-453, 1992.

Duan, H., Gao, F., Li, S., Nagata, T.: Postnatal development of esophageal epithelium in mouse: a light and electron microscopic radioautographic study. Cell. Mol. Biol. 39, 309-316, 1993.

Duan, H., Gao, F., Oguchi, K., Nagata, T.: Light and electron microscopic radioautographic study on the incorporation of ^{3}H-thymidine into the lung by means of a new nebulizer. Drug Res. 44, 880-883, 1994.

Feulgen, R., Rossenbeck, H.: Mikroskopische-chemischer Nachweis einer Nukeinsaeure von Thymus der Thymonukeinsaeure Z. Physik. Chem. 135, 203-248, 1924.

Fujii, Y., Ohno, S., Yamabayashi, S., Usuda, N., Saito, H., Furuta, S., Nagata, T.: Electron microscopic radioautography of DNA synthesis in primary cultured cells from an IgG myeloma patient. J. Clin. Electr. Microsc. 13, 582-583, 1980.

Gao, F.: Study on the macromolecular synthesis in aging mouse seminiferous tubules by light and electron microscopic radioautography. Cell. Mol. Biol. 39, 659-672, 1993.

Gao, F., Toriyama, K., Nagata, T.: Light microscopic radioautographic study on the DNA synthesis of prenatal and postnatal aging mouse retina after labeled thymidine injection. Cell. Mol. Biol. 38, 661-668, 1992a.

Gao, F., Li, S., Duan, H., Ma, H., Nagata, T.: Electron microscopic radioautography on the DNA synthesis of prenatal and postnatal mice retina after labeled thymidine injection. J. Clin. Electron Microsc. 25, 721-722, 1992b.

Gao, F., Toriyama, K., Ma, H., Nagata, T.: Light microscopic radioautographic study on DNA synthesis in aging mice corneas. Cell. Mol. Biol. 39, 435-441, 1993.

Gao, F., Ma, H., Sun, L., Jin, C., Nagata, T.: Electron microscopic radioautographic study on the nucleic acids and protein synthesis in the aging mouse testis. Med. Electron Microsc. 27, 360-362, 1994.

Gao, F., Chen, S., Sun, L., Kang, W., Wang, Z., Nagata, T.: Radioautographic study of the macromolecular synthesis of Leydig cells in aging mice testis. Cell. Mol. Biol. 41, 145-150, 1995a.

Gao, F., Jin, C., Ma, H., Sun, L., Nagata, T.: Ultrastructural and radioautographic studies on DNA synthesis in Leydig cells of aging mouse testis. Cell. Mol. Biol. 41, 151-160, 1995b.

Gunarso, W.: Radioautographic studies on the nucleic acid synthesis of the retina of chick embryo. I. Light microscopic radioautography. Shinshu Med. J. 32, 231-240, 1984a.

Gunarso, W.: Radioautographic studies on the nucleic acid synthesis of the retina of chick embryo. II. Electron microscopic radioautography. Shinshu Med. J. 32, 241-248, 1984b.

Gunarso, W., Gao, F., Cui, H., Ma, H., Nagata, T.: A light and electron microscopic radioautographic study on RNA synthesis in the retina of chick embryo. Acta Histochem. 98, 309-32, 1996.

Gunarso, W., Gao, F., Nagata, T.: Development and DNA synthesis in the retina of chick embryo observed by light and electron microscopic radioautography. Cell. Mol. Biol. 43, 189-201, 1997.

Hanai, T.: Light microscopic radioautographic study of DNA synthesis in the kidneys of aging mice. Cell. Mol. Biol. 39, 81-91, 1993.

Hanai, T., Nagata, T.: Electron microscopic radioautographic study on DNA and RNA synthesis in perinatal mouse kidney. In, Radioautography in Medicine, Nagata, T., Ed., pp. 127-131, Shinshu University Press, Matsumoto, 1994a.

Hanai, T., Nagata, T.: Study on the nucleic acid synthesis in the aging mouse kidney by light and electron microscopic radioautography. In, Radioautography in Medicine, Nagata, T., Ed., pp. 209-214, Shinshu University Press, Matsumoto, 1994b.

Hanai, T., Nagata, T.: Electron microscopic study on nucleic acid synthesis in perinatal mouse kidney tissue. Med. Electron Microsc. 27, 355-357, 1994c.

Hanai, T., Usuda, N., Morita, T., Shimizu, T., Nagata, T.: Proliferative activity in the kidneys of aging mice evaluated by PCNA/cyclin immunohistochemistry. Cell. Mol. Biol. 39, 181-191, 1993.

Hayashi, K., Gao, F., Nagata, T.: Radioautographic study on ^{3}H-thymidine incorporation at different stages of muscle development in aging mice. Cell. Mol. Biol. 39, 553-560, 1993.

Ito, M.: The radioautographic studies on aging change of DNA synthesis and the ultrastructural development of mouse adrenal gland. Cell. Mol. Biol. 42, 279-292, 1996.

Ito, M., Nagata, T.: Electron microscopic radioautographic studies on DNA synthesis and ultrastructure of aging mouse adrenal gland. Med. Electron Microsc. 29, 145-152, 1996.

Izumiyama, K., Kogure, K., Kataoka, S., Nagata, T.: Quantitative analysis of glucose after transient ischemia in the gerbil hippocampus by light and electron microscope radioautography. Brain Res. 416, 175-179, 1987.

Jamieson, J. D., Palade, G. E.: Intracellular transport of secretory proteins in the pancreatic exocrine cells. J. Cell Biol. 34, 577-615, 1967.

Jin, C.: Study on DNA synthesis of aging mouse colon by light and electron microscopic radioautography. Cell. Mol. Biol. 42, 255-268, 1996.

Jin, C., Nagata, T.: Light microscopic radioautographic study on DNA synthesis in cecal epithelial cells of aging mice. J. Histochem. Cytochem. 43, 1223-1228, 1995a.

Jin, C., Nagata, T.: Electron microscopic radioautographic study on DNA synthesis in cecal epithelial cells of aging mice. Med. Electron Microsc. 28, 71-75, 1995b.

Joukura, K.: The aging changes of glycoconjugate synthesis in mouse kidney studied by ^{3}H-glucosamine radioautography. Acta Histochem. Cytochem. 29, 57-63, 1996.

Joukura, K., Nagata, T.: Aging changes of ^{3}H-glucosamine incorporation into mouse kidney observed by radioautography. Acta Histochem. Cytochem. 28, 494-494, 1995.

Joukura, K., Usuda, N., Nagata, T.: Quantitative study on the aging change of glycoconjugates synthesis in aging mouse kidney. Proc. Xth Internat. Cong. Histochem. Cytochem., Acta Histochem. Cytochem. 29, Suppl. 507-508, 1996.

Kobayashi, K., Nagata, T.: Light microscopic radioautographic studies on DNA, RNA and protein syntheses in human synovial membranes of rheumatoid arthritis patients. J. Histochem. Cytochem. 42, 982-982, 1994.

Komiyama, K., Iida, F., Furihara, R., Murata, F., Nagata, T.: Electron microscopic radioautographic study on ^{125}I-albumin in rat gastric mucosal epithelia. J. Clin. Electron Microsc. 11, 428-429, 1978.

Kong, Y.: Electron microscopic radioautographic study on DNA synthesis in perinatal mouse retina. Cell. Mol. Biol. 39, 55-64, 1993.

Kong, Y., Nagata, T.: Electron microscopic radioautographic study on nucleic acid synthesis of perinatal mouse retina. Med. Electron Microsc. 27, 366-368, 1994.

Kong, Y., Usuda, N., Nagata, T.: Radioautographic study on DNA synthesis of the retina and retinal pigment epithelium of developing mouse embryo. Cell. Mol. Biol. 38, 263-272, 1992a.

Kong, Y., Usuda, N., Morita, T., Hanai, T., Nagata, T.: Study on RNA synthesis in the retina and retinal pigment epithelium of mice by light microscopic radioautography. Cell. Mol. Biol. 38, 669-678, 1992b.

Leblond, C. P.: Localization of newly administered iodine in the thyroid gland as indicated by radioiodine. J. Anat. 77, 149-152, 1943.

Leblond, C. P.: The life history of cells in renewing systems. Am. J. Anat. 160, 113-158, 1981.

Leblond, C. P., Messier, B.: Renewal of chief cells and goblet cells in the small intestine as shown by radioautography after injection of thymidine-^{3}H into mice. Anat. Rec. 132: 247-259. 1958.

Li, S.: Relationship between cellular DNA synthesis, PCNA expression and sex steroid hormone receptor status in the developing mouse ovary, uterus and oviduct. Histochemistry 102, 405-413, 1994.

Li, S., Nagata, T.: Nucleic acid synthesis in the developing mouse ovary, uterus and oviduct studied by light and electron microscopic radioautography. Cell. Mol. Biol. 41, 185-195, 1995.

Li, S., Gao, F., Duan, H., Nagata, T.: Radioautographic study on the uptake of $^{35}SO_4$ in mouse ovary during the estrus cycle. J. Clin. Electron Microsc. 25, 709-710, 1992.

Liang, Y.: Light microscopic radioautographic study on RNA synthesis in the adrenal glands of aging mice. Acta Histochem. Cytochem. 31, 203-210, 1998.

Liang, Y., Ito, M., Nagata, T.: Light and electron microscopic radioautographic studies on RNA synthesis in aging mouse adrenal gland. Acta Anat. Nippon. 74, 291-300, 1999.

Ma, H.: Light microscopic radioautographic study on DNA synthesis of the livers in aging mice. Acta Anat. Nippon. 63, 137-147, 1988.

Ma, H., Nagata, T.: Electron microscopic radioautographic study on DNA synthesis of the livers in aging mice. J. Clin. Electron Microsc. 21, 335-343, 1988a.

Ma, H., Nagata, T.: Studies on DNA synthesis of aging mice by means of electron microscopic radioautography. J. Clin. Electron Microsc. 21, 715-716, 1988b.

Ma, H., Nagata, T.: Electron microscopic radioautographic studies on DNA synthesis in the hepatocytes of aging mice as observed by image analysis. Cell. Mol. Biol. 36, 73-84, 1990a.

Ma, H., Nagata, T.: Study on RNA synthesis in the livers of aging mice by means of electron microscopic radioautography. Cell. Mol. Biol. 36, 589-600, 1990b.

Ma, H., Nagata, T.: Collagen and protein synthesis in the livers of aging mice as studied by electron microsopic radioautography. Ann. Microsc. 1, 13-22, 2000.

Ma, H., Gao, F., Olea, M. T., Nagata, T.: Protein synthesis in the livers of aging mice studied by electron microscopic radioautography. Cell. Mol. Biol. 37, 607-615, 1991.

Matsumura, H., Kobayashi, Y., Kobayashi, K., Nagata, T.: Light microscopic radioautographic study of DNA synthesis in the lung of aging salamander, Hynobius nebulosus. J. Histochem. Cytochem. 42, 1004-1004, 1994.

Momose, Y., Nagata, T.: Radioautographic study on the intracellular localization of a hypolipidemic agent, bezafibrate, a peroxisome proliferator, in cultured rat hepatocytes. Cell. Mol. Biol. 39, 773-781, 1993a.

Momose, Y., Naito, J., Nagata, T.: Radioautographic study on the localization of an anti-allergic agent, tranilast, in the rat liver. Cell. Mol. Biol. 35, 347-355, 1989.

Momose, Y., Shibata, N., Kiyosawa, I., Naito, J., Watanabe, T., Horie, S., Yamada, J., Suga, T., Nagata, T.: Morphometric evaluation of species differences in the effects of bezafibrate, a hypolipidemic agent, on hepatic peroxisomes and mitochondria. J. Toxicol. Pathol. 6, 33-45, 1993b.

Momose, Y., Naito, J., Suzawa, H., Kanzawa, M., Nagata, T.: Radioautographic study on the intracellular localization of bezafibrate in cultured rat hepatoctyes. Acta Histochem. Cytochem. 28, 61-66, 1995.

Morita, T.: Radioautographic study on the aging change of ^{3}H-glucosamine uptake in mouse ileum. Cell. Mol. Biol. 39, 875-884, 1993.

Morita, T., Usuda, N. Hanai, T., Nagata, T.: Changes of colon epithelium proliferation due to individual aging with PCNA/cyclin immunostaining comparing with ^{3}H-thymidine radioautography. Histochemistry 101, 13-20, 1994.

Murata, F., Momose,Y. , Yoshida, K., Nagata, T.: Incorporation of ^{3}H-thymidine into the nucleus of mast cells in adult rat peritoneum. Shinshu Med. J. 25, 72-77, 1977a.

Murata, F., Momose, Y., Yoshida, K., Ohno, S., Nagata, T.: Nucleic acid and mucosubstance metabolism of mastocytoma cells by means of electron microscopic radioautography. Acta Pharmacol. Toxicol. 41, 58-59, 1977b.

Murata, F., Yoshida, K., Ohno, S., Nagata, T.: Ultrastructural and electron microscopic radioautographic studies on the mastocytoma cells and mast cells. J. Clin. Electron Microsc. 11, 561-562, 1978.

Murata, F., Yoshida, K., Ohno, S., Nagata, T.: Mucosubstances of rabbit granulocytes studied by means of electron microscopic radioautography and X-ray microanalysis. Histochemistry 61, 139-150, 1979.

Nagata, T.: On the relationship between cell division and cytochrome oxidase in the Yoshida sarcoma cells. Shinshu Med. J. 5: 383-386, 1956.

Nagata, T.: Studies on the amitosis in the Yoshida sarcoma cells. I. Observation on the smear preparation under normal conditions. Med. J. Shinshu Univ. 2: 187-198, 1957a.

Nagata, T.: Studies on the amitosis in the Yoshida sarcoma cells. II. Phase-contrast microscopic observations under normal conditions. Med. J. Shinshu Univ. 2: 199-207, 1957b.

Nagata, T.: Cell divisions in the liver of the fetal and newborn dogs. Med. J. Shinshu Univ. 4: 65-73, 1959.

Nagata, T.: A radioautographic study of the DNA synthesis in rat liver, with special reference to binucleate cells. Med. J. Shinshu Univ. 7, 17-25, 1962.

Nagata, T.: A quantitative study on the ganglion cells in the small intestine of the dog. Med. J. Shinshu Univ. 10, 1-11, 1965.

Nagata, T.: A radioautographic study on the RNA synthesis in the hepatic and the intestinal epithelial cells of mice after feeding with special reference to binuclearity. Med. J. Shinshu Univ. 11, 49-61, 1966.

Nagata, T.: On the increase of binucleate cells in the ganglion cells of dog small intestine due to experimental ischemia. Med. J. Shinshu Univ. 12, 93-113, 1967a.

Nagata, T.: A radioautographic study on the protein synthesis in the hepatic and the intestinal epithelial cells of mice, with special reference to binucleate cells. Med. J. Shinshu Univ. 12, 247-257, 1967b.

Nagata, T.: Chapter 3. Application of microspectrophotometry to various substances. In , Introduction to Microspectrophotometry. Isaka, S., Nagata, T., Inui, N., Eds., Olympus Co., Tokyo, pp. 49-155, 1972a.

Nagata, T.: Electron microscopic dry-mounting autoradiography. Proc. 4th Internat. Cong. Histochem. Cytochem. Kyoto, pp. 43-44, 1972b.

Nagata, T.: Electron microscopic radioautography of intramitochondrial RNA synthesis of HeLa cells in culture. Histochemie 32, 163-170, 1972c.

Nagata, T.: Quantitative electron microscope radioautography of intramitochondrial nucleic acid synthesis. Acta Histochem. Cytochem. 5, 201-203, 1972d.

Nagata, T.: Electron microscopic observation of target cells previously observed by phase-contrast microscopy: Electron microscopic radioautography of laser beam irradiated cultured cells. J. Clin. Electron Microsc. 17, 589-590, 1984.

Nagata, T.: Principles and techniques of radioautography. In, Histo- and Cyto-chemistry 1985, Japan Society of Histochemistry and Cytochemistry, Ed., Gakusai Kikaku Co., Tokyo, pp. 207-226, 1985.

Nagata, T.:. Electron microscopic radioautography and analytical electron microscopy. J. Clin. Electron Microsc. 24, 441-442, 1991.

Nagata, T.: Radiolabeling of soluble and insoluble compounds as demonstrated by light and electron microscopy. Recent Advances in Cellular and Molecular Biology, Wegmann, R. J., Wegmann, M. A., Eds. Peters Press, Leuven, Vol. 6, pp. 9-21, 1992.

Nagata, T.: Quantitative analysis of histochemical reactions: Image analysis of light and electron microscopic radioautograms. Acta Histochem. Cytochem. 26, 281-291, 1993a.

Nagata, T. Quantitative light and electron microscopic radioautographic studies on macromolecular synthesis in several organs of prenatal and postnatal aging mice. Chinese J. Histochem. Cytochem. 2: 106-108, 1993b.

Nagata, T.: Electron microscopic radioautography with cryo-fixation and dry-mounting procedure. Acta Histochem. Cytochem. 27: 471-489, 1994a.

Nagata, T.: Application of electron microscopic radioautography to clinical electron microscopy. Med. Electron Microsc. 27; 191-212, 1994b.

Nagata, T.: Radioautography in Medicine. Shinshu University Press, 268pp, Matsumoto, 1994c.

Nagata, T.: Radioautography, general and special. In, Histo- and Cyto-chemistry 1994, Japan Society of Histochemistry and Cytochemistry, ed, pp. 219-231, Gakusai Kikaku Co., Tokyo, 1994d.

Nagata, T., Application of electron microscopic radioautography to clinical electron microscopy. Med. Electron Microsc. 27, 191-212, 1994e.

Nagata, T.: Light and electron microscopic radioautographic study on macromolecular synthesis in digestive organs of aging mice. Cell. Mol. Biol. 41, 21-38, 1995a.

Nagata, T.: Histochemistry of the organs: Application of histochemistry to anatomy. Acta Anat. Nippon. 70, 448-471, 1995b.

Nagata, T.: Three-dimensional observation of whole mount cultured cells stained with histochemical reactions by ultrahigh voltage electron microscopy. Cell. Mol. Biol. 41, 783-792, 1995c.

Nagata, T.: Morphometry in anatomy: image analysis on fine structure and histochemical reactions with special reference to radioautography. Ital. J. Anat. 100 (Suppl. 1), 591-605, 1995d.

Nagata, T.: Technique and application of electron microscopic radioautography. J. Electron Microsc. 45, 258-274, 1996a.

Nagata, T.: Techniques of light and electron microscopic radioautography. In, Histochemistry and Cytochemistry 1996. Proc. Xth Internat. Congr. Histochem. Cytochem. Acta Histochem. Cytochem. 29 (Suppl.), 343-344, 1996b.

Nagata, T.: Remarks: Radioautographology, general and special. Cell. Mol. Biol. 42 (Suppl.), 11-12, 1996c.

Nagata, T.: On the terminology of radioautography vs. autoradiography. J. Histochem. Cytochem. 44, 1209-1209, 1996d.

Nagata, T.: Techniques and applications of microscopic radioautography. Histol. Histopathol. 12, 1091-1124, 1997a.

Nagata T.: Three-dimensional observation on whole mount cultured cells and thick sections stained with histochemical reactions by high voltage electron microscopy. In,

Recent Advances in Microscopy of Cells, Tissues and Organs, Motta, P., Ed., Antonio Delfino Editore, Roma, pp. 37-44, 1997b.
Nagata, T.: Radioautographic study on collagen synthesis in the ocular tissues. J. Kaken Eye Res. 15, 1-9, 1997c.
Nagata, T.: Techniques of radioautography for medical and biological research. Braz. J. Biol. Med. Res. 31, 185-195, 1998a.
Nagata, T.: Radioautographology, the advocacy of a new concept. Braz. J. Biol. Med. Res. 31, 201-241, 1998b.
Nagata, T.: Radioautographic studies on DNA synthesis of the bone and skin of aging salamander. Bull. Nagano Women's Jr. College 6, 1-14, 1998c.
Nagata, T.: 3D observation of cell organelles by high voltage electron microscopy. Microscopy and Analysis, Asia Pacific Edition, 9, 29-32, 1999a.
Nagata, T.: Application of histochemistry to anatomy: Histochemistry of the organs, a novel concept. Proc. XV Congress of the International Federation of Associations of Anatomists, Ital. J. Anat. Embryol. 104 (Suppl. 1), 486-486, 1999b.
Nagata, T.: Aging changes of macromolecular synthesis in various organ systems as observed by microscopic radioautography after incorporation of radiolabeled precursors. Methods Find. Exp. Clin. Pharmacol. 21, 683-706, 1999c.
Nagata, T.: Radioautographic study on protein synthesis in mouse cornea. J. Kaken Eye Res. 8, 8-14, 1999d.
Nagata, T.: Radioautographology, general and special: a novel concept. Ital. J. Anat. Embryol. 104 (Suppl. 1), 487-487, 1999e.
Nagata, T.: Three-dimensional observations on thick biological specimens by high voltage electron microscopy. Image Analysis Stereolog. 19, 51-56, 2000a.
Nagata, T.: Biological microanalysis of radiolabeled and unlabeled compounds by radioautography and X-ray microanalysis. Scanning Microscopy International, 14, on line, 2000b.
Nagata, T.: Electron microscopic radioautographic study on protein synthesis in pancreatic cells of perinatal and aging mice. Bull. Nagano Women's Jr. College 8, 1-22, 2000c.
Nagata, T.: Light microscopic radioautographic study on radiosulfate incorporation into the tracheal cartilage in aging mice. Acta Histochem. Cytochem. 32, 377-383, 2000d.
Nagata, T.: Introductory remarks: Special radioautographology. Cell. Mol. Biol. 46 (Congress Suppl.), 161-161, 2000e.
Nagata, T.: Special radioautographology: the eye. J. Kaken Eye Res. 18, 1-13, 2000f.
Nagata, T.: Three-dimensional high voltage electron microscopy of thick biological specimens. Micron 32, 387-404, 2001a.
Nagata, T.: Three-dimensional and four-dimensional observation of histochemical and cytochemical specimens by high voltage electron microscopy. Acta Histochem. Cytochem. 34, 153-169, 2001b.
Nagata, T. : Special cytochemistry in cell biology. In, Internat. Rev. Cytol. Jeon, K.W., ed., Vol. 211, Chapter 2, Academic Press, New York, pp. 33-154, 2001c.
Nagata, T. : Radioautographology General and Special, In, Prog. Histochem. Cytochem., Graumann, W., Ed., Vol. 37 No. 2, Urban & Fischer, Jena, pp. 57-226, 2002.
Nagata T.: Light and electron microscopic study on macromolecular synthesis in amitotic hepatocyte mitochondria of aging mice. Cell. Mol. Biol. 49, 591-611, 2003.
Nagata, T.: X-ray microanalysis of biological specimens by high voltage electron microscopy. In, Prog. Histochem. Cytochem., Graumann, W., Ed., Vol. 39, No. 4, Urban & Fischer Verlag, Jena, pp. 185-320, 2004.

Nagata T.: Aging changes of macromolecular synthesis in the uro-genital organs as revealed by electron microscopic radioautography. Ann. Rev. Biomed. Sci. 6, 13-78, 2005.

Nagata T.: Electron microscopic radioautographic study on protein synthesis in hepatocyte mitochondria of developing mice. Ann. Microsc. 6, 43-54, 2006a.

Nagata T.: Electron microscopic radioautographic study on nucleic acids synthesis in hepatocyte mitochondria of developing mice. The Sci. World J. 6: 1583-1598, 2006b.

Nagata T.: Macromolecular synthesis in hepatocyte mitochondria of aging mice as revealed by electron microscopic radioautography. I: Nucleic acid synthesis. In, Modern Research and Educational Topics in Microscopy. Mendez-Vilas, A. and Diaz, J. Eds., Formatex Micrscopy Series No. 3, Vol. 1, Formatex, Badajoz, Spain, pp. 245-258, 2007a.

Nagata T.: Macromolecular synthesis in hepatocyte mitochondria of aging mice as revealed by electron microscopic radioautography. II: Protein synthesis. In, Modern Research and Educational Topics in Microscopy. Mendez-Vilas, A. and Diaz, J. eds., Formatex Micrscopy Series No. 3, Vol. 1, Formatex, Badajoz, Spain, pp. 259-271, 2007b.

Nagata, T.: Electron microscopic radioautographic study on macromolecular synthesis in hepatocyte mitochondria of aging mouse. J. Cell Tissue Res. 7, 1019-1029, 2007c.

Nagata, T.; Electron microscopic radioautographic study on nucleic acids synthesis in hepatocyte mitochondria of developing mice. Trends Cell Molec. Biol. 2, 19-33, 2007d.

Nagata, T.; Aging changes of macromolecular synthesis in the mitochondria of mouse hepatocytes as revealed by microscopic radioautography. Ann. Rev. Biomed. Sci. 9, 30-36, 2007e.

Nagata, T.: Radioautographology, Bull. Shinshu Institute Alternat. Med. 2, 3-32, 2007f.

Nagata, T.: Electron microscopic radioautographic study on mitochondrial DNA synthesis in adrenal cortical cells of developing mice. J. Cell. Tis. Res. 8, 1303-1312, 2008a.

Nagata T.: Electron microscopic radioautographic study on mitochondrial DNA synthesis in adrenal cortical cells of developing and aging mice. The Sci. World J. 8, 683-697. 2008b.

Nagata, T.: Sexual difference between the macromolecular synthesis of hepatocyte mitochondria in male and female mice in aging as revealed by electron microscopic radioautography. Chapter 22. In, Women and Aging: New Research, H. T. Bennninghouse, A. D. Rosset, Eds. Nova Biomed. Books, New York, pp. 461-487, 2009a

Nagata, T.: Protein synthesis in hepatocytes of mice as revealed by electron microscopic radioautography. In, Protein Biosynthesis. Esterhouse, T. E. and Petrinos, L. B., Eds., Nova Biomed. Books, New York, pp. 133-161, 2009b.

Nagata, T.: Electron microscopic radioatuographic studies on macromolecular synthesis in mitochondria of various cells. 18EMSM Conference Proc. 9th Asia-Pacific Microscopy Conference (APMC9), Kuala Lumpur, Malaysia, pp. 48-50, 2009c.

Nagata, T.: Recent studies on macromolecular synthesis labeled with ^{3}H-thymidine in various organs as revealed by electron microscopic radioautography. Current Radiopharmaceutics 2, 118-128, 2009d.

Nagata, T.: Electron microscopic radioautographic study on mitochondrial DNA synthesis in adrenal medullary cells of developing and aging mice. J. Cell Tissue Res. 9, 1793-1802, 2009e.

Nagata, T.: Applications of high voltage electron microscopy to thick biological specimens. Ann. Microsc. 9, 4-40, 2009f.

Nagata, T.: Electron microscopic radioautographic study on DNA synthesis of mitochondria in adrenal medullary cells of aging mice. Open Anat. J. 1, 14-24, 2009g.

Nagata, T.: Electron microscopic radioautographic studies on macromolecular synthesis in mitochondria of animal cells in aging. Ann. Rev. Biomed. Sci. 11, 1-17, 2009h.

Nagata, T.: Electron microscopic radioautographic studies on macromoleclular synthesis in mitochondria of some organs in aging animals. Bull. Shinshu Inst. Alternat. Med. Welfare 4, 15-38, 2009i.

Nagata, T.: Electron microscopic radioautographic study on mitochondrial DNA synthesis in adreno-cortical cells of aging ddY mice. Bull. Shinshu Inst. Alternat. Med. Welfare 4, 51-66, 2009j.

Nagata T.: Electron microscopic radioautographic study on mitochondrial RNA synthesis in adrenocortical cells of aging mice. Open Anat J. 2, 91-97, 2010a.

Nagata T. Electron microscopic radioautographic study on mitochondrial RNA synthesis in adrenal medullary cells of aging and senescent mice. J Cell Tissue Res. 10, 2213-2222, 2010b.

Nagata, T.: Macromolecular synthesis in the livers of aging mice as revealed by electron microscopic radioautography. In, Prog. Histochem. Cytochem., Sasse, D., Ed., Elsevier, Amsterdam, Boston, London, New York, Oxford, Paris, Philadelphia, San Diego, St. Louis, Vol. 45, No. 1, pp. 1-80, 2010c.

Nagata, T.: Electron microscopic radioautographic study on protein synthesis of mitochondria in adrenal medullary cells of aging mice. Bulletin Shinshu Inst Alternat Med Welfare 5, 25-37, 2010d.

Nagata, T.: Electron microscopic radioautographic study on mitochondrial RNA synthesis in adrenal cortical and medullary cells of aging mice. J. Biomed. Sci. Enginer. 4, 219-232, 2010e.

Nagata, T.: Electron microscopic radioautographic study on protein synthesis of mitochondria in adrenal cortical cells of aging mice. Bulletin Shinshu Inst. Alternat. Med. Welfare 5, 38-52, 2010f.

Nagata T.: Electron microscopic radioautographic study on mitochondrial DNA, RNA and protein synthesis in adrenal cells of aging mice. Formatex Microscopy Series No. 3, Vol. 3, Formatex, Badajoz, Spain, in press, 2010g.

Nagata, T.: Electron microscopic radioautographic studies on macromolecular synthesis in mitochondria of animal cells in aging. Ann. Rev. Biomed. Sci. 12, 1-29, 2010h.

Nagata, T., Cui, H., Gao, F.: Radioautographic study on glycoprotein synthesis in the ocular tissues. J. Kaken Eye Res. 13, 11-18, 1995.

Nagata, T., Cui, H., Kong, Y.: The localization of TGF-b1 and its mRNA in the spinal cords of prenatal and postnatal aging mice demonstrated with immunohistochemical and in situ hybridization techniques. Bull. Nagano Women's Jr. College, 7, 75-88, 1999a.

Nagata, T., Cui, H., Liang, Y.: Light microscopic radioautographic study on the protein synthesis in the cerebellum of aging mouse. Bull. Nagano Women's Jr. College, 9, 41-60 (2001).

Nagata, T., Fujii, Y., Usuda, N.: Demonstration of extranuclear nucleic acid synthesis in mammalian cells under experimental conditions by electron microscopic radioautography. Proc. 10th Internat. Congr. Electr. Microsc. 2, 305-306, 1982b.

Nagata, T., Hirano, I., Shibata, O., Nagata, T.: A radioautographic study on the DNA synthesis in the hepatic and the pancreatic acinar cells of mice during the postnatal growth, with special reference to binuclearity. Med. J. Shinshu Univ. 11, 35-42, 1966.

Nagata, T., Ito, M., Chen, S.: Aging changes of DNA synthesis in the submandibular glands of mice as observed by light and electron microscopic radioautography. Ann. Microsc. 1, 4-12, 2000a.

Nagata, T. Ito, M., Liang, Y.: Study of the effects of aging on macromolecular synthesis in mouse steroid secreting cells using microscopic radioautography. Methods Find. Exp. Clin. Pharmacol. 22, 5-18, 2000b.

Nagata, T., Iwadare, I., Murata, F.: Electron microscopic radioautography of nucleic acid synthesis in cultured cells treated with several carcinogens. Acta Pharmacol. Toxicol. 41, 64-65, 1977c.

Nagata, T., Kawahara, I.: Radioautographic study of the synthesis of sulfomucin in digestive organs of mice. J. Trace Microprobe Analysis 17, 339-355, 1999.

Nagata, T., Kawahara, I., Usuda, N., Maruyama, M., Ma, H.: Radioautographic studies on the glycoconjugate synthesis in the gastrointestinal mucosa of the mouse. In, Glycoconjugate in Medicine, Ohyama, M., Muramatsu, T., Eds, pp. 251-256, Professional Postgrad. Service, Tokyo, 1988a.

Nagata, T., Kong, Y.: Distribution and localization of TGFb1 and bFGF, and their mRNAs in aging mice. Bull. Nagano Women's Jr. College 6, 87-105, 1998.

Nagata, T., Ma, H., Electron microscopic radioautographic study on mitochondrial DNA synthesis in hepatocytes of aging mouse. Ann. Microsc. 5, 4-18, 2005a.

Nagata, T., Ma, H., Electron microscopic radioautographic study on RNA synthesis in hepatocyte mitochondria of aging mouse. Microsc. Res. Tech. 67, 55-64, 2005b.

Nagata, T., Momoze, S.: Aging changes of the amitotic and binucleate cells in dog livers. Acta Anat. Nipponica 34, 187-190, 1959.

Nagata, T., Morita, T., I. Kawahara, I.: Radioautographic studies on radiosulfate incorporation in the digestive organs of mice. Histol. Histopathol. 14, 1-8, 1999b.

Nagata, T., Murata, F.: Electron microscopic dry-mounting radioautography for diffusible compounds by means of ultracryotomy. Histochemistry 54, 75-82, 1977.

Nagata, T., Murata, F., Yoshida, K., Ohno, S., Iwadare, N.: Whole mount radioautography of cultured cells as observed by high voltage electron microscopy. Proc. Fifth Internat. Conf. High Voltage Electron Microsc. 347-350, 1977d.

Nagata, T., Nawa, T.: A modification of dry-mounting technique for radioautography of water-soluble compounds. Histochemie 7, 370-371, 1966a.

Nagata, T., Nawa, T.: A radioautographic study on the nucleic acids synthesis of binucleate cells in cultivated fibroblasts of chick embryos. Med. J. Shinshu Univ. 11, 1-5, 1966b.

Nagata, T., Nawa, T., Yokota, S.: A new technique for electron microscopic dry-mounting radioautography of soluble compounds. Histochemie 18, 241-249, 1969.

Nagata, T., Nishigaki, T., Momose, Y.: Localization of anti-allergic agent in rat mast cells demonstrated by light and electron microscopic radioautography. Acta Histochem. Cytochem. 19, 669-683, 1986b.

Nagata, T., Ohno, S., Kawahara, I., Yamabayashi, S., Fujii, Y., Murata, F.: Light and electron microscopic radioautography of nucleic acid synthesis in mitochondria and peroxisomes of rat hepatic cells during and after DEHP administration. Acta Histochem. Cytochem. 16, 610-611, 1979.

Nagata, T., Ohno, S., Murata, F.: Electron microscopic dry-mounting radioautography for soluble compounds. Acta Phamacol. Toxicol. 41, 62-63, 1977a.

Nagata, T., Ohno, S., Yoshida, K., Murata, F.: Nucleic acid synthesis in proliferating peroxisomes of rat liver as revealed by electron microscopical radioautography. Histochem. J. 14, 197-204, 1982a.

Nagata, T., Olea, M. T.: Electron microscopic radioautographic study on the protein synthesis in aging mouse spleen. Bull. Nagano Women's Jr. College 7, 1-9, 1999.

Nagata, T., Shibata, O., Omochi, S.: A new method for radioautographic osbservation on isolated cells. Histochemie 2, 255-259, 1961

Nagata, T., Shibata, O., Nawa, T.: Simplified methods for mass production of radioautograms. -Acta Anat. Nippon.42, 162-166, 1967a.

Nagata, T., Shibata, O., Nawa, T.: Incorporation of tritiated thymidine into mitochondrial DNA of the liver and kidney cells of chickens and mice in tissue culture. Histochemie 10, 305-308, 1967b.

Nagata, T., Shimamura, K., Onozawa, M., Kondo, T., Ohkubo, K., Momoze, S.: Relationship of binuclearity to cell function in some organs. I. Frequencies of binucleate cells in some organs of toads in summer and winter. Med. J. Shinshu Univ. 5, 147-152, 1960a.

Nagata, T., Shimamura, K., Kondo, T., Onozawa, M., Momoze, S., Okubo, M.: Relationship of binuclearity to cell function in some organs. II. Variation of frequencies of binucleate cells in some organs of dogs owing to aging. Med. J. Shinshu Univ. 5, 153-158, 1960b.

Nagata, T., Steggerda, F. R.: Histological study on the deganglionated small intestine of the dog. Physiologist 6, 242-242, 1963.

Nagata, T., Steggerda, F. R.: Observations on the increase of binucleate cells in the ganglion cells of the dog's intestine due to experimental ischemia. Anat. Rec. 148, 315-315, 1964.

Nagata, T., Toriyama, K., Kong, Y., Jin, C., Gao, F.: Radioautographic study on DNA synthesis in the ciliary bodies of aging mice. J. Kaken Eye Res.12, 1-11, 1994.

Nagata, T., Usuda, N.: Image processing of electron microscopic radioautograms in clinical electron microscopy. J. Clin. Electron. Microsc. 18, 451-452, 1985.

Nagata, T., Usuda, N.: Studies on the nucleic acid synthesis in pancreatic acinar cells of aging mice by means of electron microscopic radioautography. J. Clin. Electron Microsc. 19, 486-487, 1986.

Nagata, T., Usuda, N.: Electron microscopic radioautography of protein synthesis in pancreatic acinar cells of aging mice. Acta Histochem. Cytochem. 26, 481-481, 1993a.

Nagata, T., Usuda, N.: In situ hybridization by electron microscopy using radioactive probes. J. Histochem. Cytochem. 41, 1119-1119, 1993b.

Nagata, T., Usuda, N., Ma, H.: Electron microscopic radioautography of nucleic acid synthesis in pancreatic acinar cells of prenatal and postnatal aging mice. Proc. XIth Intern. Cong. Electr. Microsc. 3, 2281-2282, 1984.

Nagata, T., Usuda, N., Ma, H.: Electron microscopic radioautography of lipid synthesis in pancreatic cells of aging mice. J. Clin. Electr. Microsc. 23, 841-842, 1990.

Nagata, T., Usuda, N., Maruyama, M., Ma, H.: Electron microscopic radioautographic study on lipid synthesis in perinatal mouse pancreas. J. Clin. Electr. Microsc. 21, 756-757, 1988b.

Nagata, T., Usuda, N., Suzawa, H., Kanzawa, M.: Incorporation of ^{3}H-glucosamine into the pancreatic cells of aging mice as demonstrated by electron microscopic radioautography. J. Clin. Electron Microsc. 25, 646-647, 1992.

Nagata, T., Yamabayashi, S.: Intracellular localization of ^{3}H-befunolol by means of electron microscopic radioautography of cryo-fixed ultrathin sections. J. Clin. Electron Microsc. 16, 737-738, 1983.

Nagata, T., Yoshida, K., Murata, F.: Demonstration of hot and cold mercury in the human thyroid tissues by means of radioautography and chemography. Acta Pharmacol. Toxicol. 41, 60-61, 1977b.

Nagata, T., Yoshida, K., Ohno, S., Murata, F.: Ultrastructural localization of soluble and insoluble ^{3}H-methyl prednisolone as revealed by electron microscopic dry-mounting radioautography. Proc. 9th Internat. Congr. Electr. Microsc. 2, 40-41, 1978b.

Nishigaki, T., Momose, Y., Nagata, T.: Light microscopic radioautographic study of the localization of anti-allergic agent, tranilast, in rat mast cells. Histochem. J. 19, 533-536, 1987.

Nishigaki, T., Momose, Y., Nagata, T.: Electron microscopic radioautographic study of the localization of an anti-allergic agent, tranilast, in rat mast cells. Cell. Mol. Biol. 36, 65-71, 1990a.

Nishigaki, T., Momose, Y., Nagata, T.: Localization of the anti-allergic agent tranilast in the urinary bladder of rat as demonstrated by light microscopic radioautography. Drug Res. 40, 272-275, 1990b.

Oguchi, K., Nagata, T.: A radioautographic study of activated satellite cells in dystrophic chicken muscle. In, Current Research in Muscular Dystrophy Japan. The Proc. Ann. Meet. Muscular Dystrophy Res. 1980, pp. 16-17, Ministry of Welfare of Japan, Tokyo, 1980.

Oguchi, K., Nagata, T.: Electron microscopic radioautographic observation on activated satellite cells in dystrophy chickens. In, Clinical Studies on the Etiology of Muscular Dystrophy. Annual Report on Neurological Diseases 1981, pp. 30-33, Ministry of Welfare of Japan, Tokyo, 1981.

Ohno, S., Fujii, Y., Usuda, N., Endo, T., Hidaka, H., Nagata, T.: Demonstration of intracellular localization of calmodulin antagonist by wet-mounting radioautography. J. Electron Microsc. 32, 1-12, 1983.

Ohno, S., Fujii, Y., Usuda, N., Nagata, T., Endo, T., Tanaka, T., Hidaka, H.: Intracellular localization of calmodulin antagonists (W-7). In, Calmodulin and intracellular Ca^{2+} receptors. Kakiuchi, S., Hidaka, H, Means, A. R., Eds., pp. 39-48, Plenum Publishing Co., New York, 1982.

Olea, M. T.: An ultrastructural localization of lysosomal acid phosphatase activity in aging mouse spleen: a quantitative X-ray microanalytical study. Acta Histochem. Cytochem. 24, 201-208, 1991.

Olea, M. T., Nagata, T.: X-ray microanalysis of cerium in mouse spleen cells demonstrating acid phosphatase activity using high voltage electron microscopy, Cell. Mol. Biol. 37, 155-163, 1991.

Olea, M. T., Nagata, T. : Simultaneous localization of ^{3}H-thymidine incorporation and acid phosphatase activity in mouse spleen: EM radioautography and cytochemistry. Cell. Mol. Biol. 38, 115-122, 1992a.

Olea, M. T., Nagata, T.: A radioautographic study on RNA synthesis in aging mouse spleen after ^{3}H-uridine labeling in vitro. Cell. Mol. Biol. 38, 399-405, 1992b.

Oliveira, S. F., Nagata, T., Abrahamsohn, P. A., Zorn, T. M. T.: Electron microscopic radioautographic study on the incorporation of ^{3}H-proline by mouse decidual cells. Cell. Mol. Biol. 37, 315-323, 1991.

Oliveira, S. F., Abrahamsohn, P. A., Nagata, T., Zorn, T. M. T.: Incorporation of ^{3}H-amino acids by endometrial stromal cells during decidualization in the mouse. A radioautographical study. Cell. Mol. Biol. 41, 107-116, 1995.

Pearse, A. G. E.: Histochemistry, Theoretical and Applied. 4th Ed. Vol. 1. 439 pp., 1980, Vol. 2. 1055 pp., 1985, Vol. 3. Ed. with P. Stoward, 728 pp. Churchill Livingstone, Edinburgh, London and New York, 1991.

Sakai, Y., Ikado, S., Nagata, T.: Electron microscopic radioautography of satellite cells in regenerating muscles. J. Clin. Electr. Microsc. 10, 508-509, 1977.

Sato, A.: Quantitative electron microscopic studies on the kinetics of secretory granules in G-cells. Cell Tissue Res. 187, 45-59, 1978.

Sato, A., Iida, F., Furihara, R., Nagata, T.: Electron microscopic raioautography of rat stomach G-cells by means of ^{3}H-amino acids. J. Clin. Electron Microsc. 10, 358-359, 1977.

Shimizu, T., Usuda, N., Yamanda, T., Sugenoya, A., Iida, F.: Proliferative activity of human thyroid tumors evaluated by proliferating cell nuclear antigen/cyclin immnohistochemical studies. Cancer 71, 2807-2812, 1993.

Sun, L.: Age related changes of RNA synthesis in the lungs of aging mice by light and electron microscopic radioautography. Cell. Mol. Biol. 41, 1061-1072, 1995.

Sun, L., Gao, F., Duan, H., Nagata, T.: Light microscopic radioautography of DNA synthesis in pulmonary cells in aging mice. In, Radioautography in Medicine, Nagata, T. Ed., pp. 201-205, Shinshu University Press, Matsumoto, 1994.

Sun, L., Gao, F., Nagata, T.: Study on the DNA synthesis of pulmonary cells in aging mice by light microscopic radioautography. Cell. Mol. Biol. 41, 851-859, 1995a.

Sun, L., Gao, F., Jin, C., Duan, H., Nagata, T.: An electron microscopic radioautographic study on the DNA synthesis of pulmonary tissue cells in aging mice. Med. Electron. Microsc. 28, 129-131, 1995b.

Sun, L., Gao, F., Jin, C., Nagata, T.: DNA synthesis in the tracheae of aging mice by means of light and electron microscopic radioautography. Acta Histochem. Cytochem. 30, 211-220, 1997a.

Sun, L., Gao, F., Nagata, T.: A Light Microscopic radioautographic study on protein synthesis in pulmonary cells of aging mice. Acta Histochem. Cytochem. 30, 463-470, 1997b.

Suzuki, K., Imada, T., Gao, F., Ma, H., Nagata, T.: Radioautographic study of benidipine hydrochloride: localization in the mesenteric artery of spontaneously hypertensive rat. Drug Res. 44, 129-133, 1994.

Terauchi, A., Mori, T., Kanda, H., Tsukada, M., Nagata, T.: Radioautographic study of 3H-taurine uptake in mouse skeletal muscle cells. J. Clin. Electron Microsc. 21, 627-628, 1988.

Terauchi, A., Nagata, T.: Observation on incorporation of ^{3}H-taurine in mouse skeletal muscle cells by light and electron microscopic radioautography. Cell. Mol. Biol. 39, 397-404, 1993.

Terauchi, A., Nagata, T.: In corporation of ^{3}H-taurine into the blood capillary cells of mouse skeletal muscle. Radioautography in Medicine, Nagata, T. ed., Shinshu University Press, Matsumoto, 1994.

Toriyama, K.: Study on the aging changes of DNA and protein synthesis of bipolar and photo-receptor cells of mouse retina by light and electron microscopic radioautography. Cell. Mol. Biol. 41, 593-601, 1995.

Tsukahara, S., Yoshida, K., Nagata, T.: A radioautographic study on the incorporation of ^{14}C-bupranolol (beta-blocking agent) into the rabbit eye. Histochemistry 68, 237-244, 1980.

Usuda, N., Nagata, T.: Electron microscopic radioautography of acyl-CoA mRNA by in situ hybridization. J. Clin. Electron Microsc. 25, 332-333, 1992.

Usuda, N., Nagata, T.: The immunohistochemical and in situ hybridization studies on hepatic peroxisomes. Acta Histochem. Cytochem. 28, 169-172, 1995.

Usuda, N., Hanai, T., Morita, T., Nagata, T.: Radioautographic demonstration of peroxisomal acyl-CoA oxidase mRNA by in situ hybridization. In, Recent advances in cellular and molecular biology, Vol. 6. Molecular biology of nucleus, peroxisomes, organelles and cell movement. Wegmann, R. J., Wegmann, M., Eds, pp.181-184, Peeters Press, Leuven, 1992.

Uwa, H., Nagata, T.: Cell population kinetics of the scleroblast during ethisterone-induced anal-fin process formation in adult females of the Medaka. Dev. Growth Different. 9, 693-694, 1976.

Watanabe, I., Makiyama, M. C. K., Nagata, T.: Electron microscopic radioautographic observation of the submandibular salivary gland of aging mouse. Acta Microscopica 6. 130-131, 1997.

Yamabayashi, S., Gunarso, W., Tsukahara, S., Nagata, T.: Incorporation of ^{3}H-befunolol (beta blocking agent) into melanin granules of ocular tissues in the pigmented rabbits. I. Light microscopic radioautography. Histochemistry 73, 371-375, 1981.

Yamada, A. T.: Timely and topologically defined protein synthesis in the periimplanting mouse endometrium revealed by light and electron microscopic radioautography. Cell. Mol. Biol. 39, 1-12, 1993.

Yamada, A., Nagata, T.: Ribonucleic acid and protein synthesis in the uterus of pregnant mouse during activation of implantation window. Med. Electron Microsc. 27, 363-365, 1992a.

Yamada, A., Nagata, T.: Light and electron microscopic raioautography of DNA synthesis in the endometria of pregnant-ovariectomized mice during activation of implantation window. Cell. Mol. Biol. 38, 763-774, 1992b.

Yamada, A., Nagata, T.: Light and electron microscopic raioautography of RNA synthesis of peri-implanting pregnant mouse during activation of receptivity for blastocyst implantation. Cell. Mol. Biol. 38, 211-233, 1993.

Yoshinaga, K.: Uterine receptivity for blastcyst implantation. Ann. N. Y. Acad. Sci. USA, 541, 424-431, 1988.

Yoshizawa, S., Nagata, A., Honma, T., Oda, M., Murata, F., Nagata, T.: Study of ethionine pancreatitis by means of electron microscopic radioautography. J. Clin. Electron Microsc. 7, 349-350, 1974.

Yoshizawa, S., Nagata, A., Honma, T., Oda, M., Murata, F., Nagata, T.: Radioautographic study of protein synthesis in pancreatic exocrine cells of alcoholic rats. J. Clin. Electron. Microsc. 10, 372-373, 1977.

16

Macromolecular Synthesis in the Urinary and Reproductive Systems

Tetsuji Nagata[1,2]
[1]*Department of Anatomy and Cell Biology, Shinshu University School of Medicine, Matsumoto*
[2]*Shinshu Institute of Alternative Medicine and Welfare, Nagano*
Japan

1. Introduction

This chapter deals with the third parts of the application of microscopic radioautography to the organ systems, including the urinary organs, the reproductive organs and the endocrine organs.

2. Macromolecular synthesis in the urinary system

The urinary system consists of the kidney and the urinary tract. We studied only the macromolecular synthesis in the kidneys of several groups of aging mice by LM and EM RAG, while the localization of an anti-allergic agent was observed in the urinary bladders of adult rats (Nagata 2005).

2.1 Macromolecular synthesis in the kidney

We studied only the DNA, RNA and glucides syntheses in the kidneys of several groups of aging mice by LM and EM RAG.

2.1.1 The DNA synthesis in the kidney

The kidneys of mammals microscopically consist of the nephrons, which can be divided into two portions, the renal corpuscles and the uriniferous tubules. The renal corpuscles are composed of the glomeruli which are covered with the Bowman's capsules. They are localized in the outer zone of the kidney, the renal cortex, while the uriniferous tubules are composed of two portions, the proximal portions and the distal portions which can further be divided into several portions which run from the outer zone of the kidney, the renal cortex, to the inner zone, the medulla. We studied the DNA synthesis by ^{3}H-thymidine radioautography in 3 groups of ddY mouse embryos from prenatal day 13 (Fig. 16A), day 15 (Fig. 16B) to day 19 in vitro, as well as perinatal mice from embryonic day 19 to postnatal day 1, 8, 30, 60 and 365 (1 year) in vivo (Hanai 1993, Hani et al. 1993, Hanai and Nagata 1994a,b).

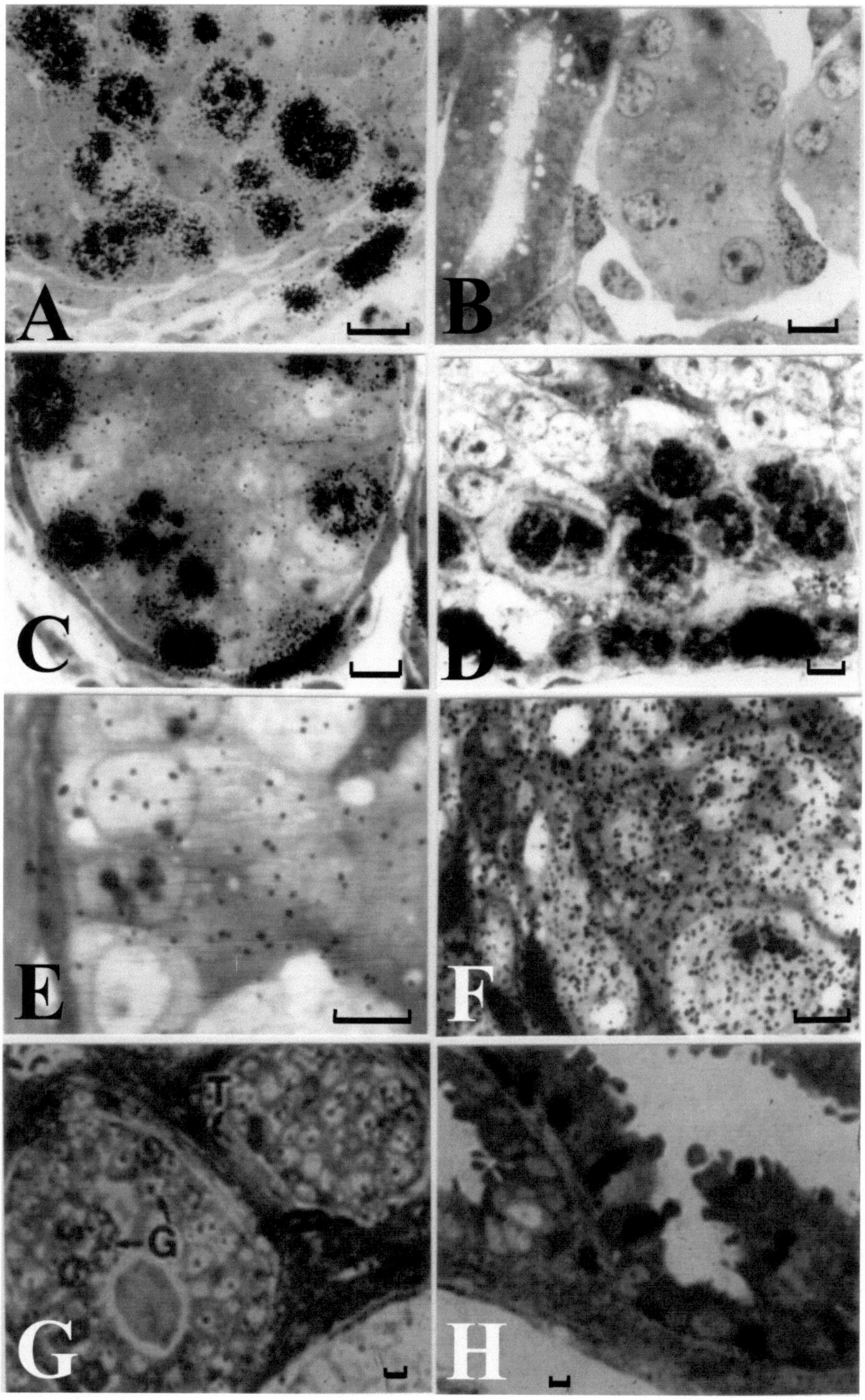

Fig. 16. LM RAG of the uro-genital organs. From Nagata, T.: Special Cytochemistry in Cell Biology, In, Internat. Rev. Cytol. Vol. 211, No. 1, p. 108, 2001, Academic Press, San Diego, USA, London, UK.

Fig. 16A. LM RAG of the metanephros of a prenatal day 13.5 mouse embryo labeled with ^{3}H-thymidine, showing DNA synthesis. x1,200.
Fig. 16B. LM RAG of the metanephros cortex of a prenatal day 15.5 mouse embryo labeled with ^{3}H-thymidine, showing DNA synthesis. x1,200.
Fig. 16C. LM RAG of the testis of a postnatal day 7 male mouse labeled with ^{3}H-thymidine, showing DNA synthesis. x800.
Fig. 16D. LM RAG of the testis of a postnatal year 1 male mouse labeled with ^{3}H-thymidine, showing DNA synthesis. x800.
Fig. 16E. LM RAG of the testis of a postnatal day 3 male mouse labeled with ^{3}H-uridine in vitro, showing RNA synthesis. x1,500.
Fig. 16F. LM RAG of the testis of a male mouse at postnatal day 1 labeled with ^{3}H-leucine in vitro, showing protein synthesis. x1,125.
Fig. 16G. LM RAG of the ovary of a postnatal day 3 female mouse labeled with ^{3}H-thymidine in vitro, showing DNA synthesis in granulosa cells (G) and theca cells (T). x400.
Fig. 16H. LM RAG of the oviduct of a postnatal day 30 female mouse labeled with ^{3}H-thymidine in vitro, showing DNA synthesis in epithelial cells. x400.

The labeling indices by LM RAG in glomeruli (28 to 32%) and uriniferous tubules (31 to 33%) in the superficial layer were higher than those of labeling indices (10 to 12%) and (8 to 16%) in the deeper layer from the late fetal to the suckling period, then decreased with aging from weaning to senescence (Fig. 17). EM RAG revealed the same results (Hanai and Nagata 1994a,b,c). At the same time, immunocytochemical staining of PCNA/cyclin was carried out in the same animals in several aging groups as ^{3}H-thymidine RAG (Hanai 1993, Hanai et al. 1993). The results from the PCNA/cyclin positive indices in respective aging groups were almost the same as the labeling indices with ^{3}H-thymidine RAG. The incorporation of ^{3}H-thymidine was formerly observed by EM RAG in mitochondrial matrix of cultured kidney cells from chickens and mice in vitro demonstrating mitochondrial DNA synthesis (Nagata et al. 1967b).

2.1.2 The RNA synthesis in the kidney

The RNA synthesis by incorporation of ^{3}H-uridine into the kidneys of aging mice was studied by LM and EM RAG (Hanai and Nagata 1994a,b, Nagata 2002). When the kidneys of several groups of aging mice from embryo to postnatal 1 year were radioautographed with ^{3}H-uridine either in vitro (embryonic day 15, 19 and postnatal day 1) and in vivo (embryonic day 19, postnatal day 1, 7, month 1, 2, 12), RNA synthesis was observed in all the cells of the kidney at various ages. The numbers of silver grains demonstrating the incorporation of ^{3}H-uridine in glomeruli (34.6 per cell) and uriniferous tubules (56.4 per cell) were higher in the superficial layer than those (15.6 and 18.6 per cell) in the deeper layer at embryonic day 15 and decreased gradually with aging. These results demonstrated the aging changes of RNA synthesis in the kidney.

2.1.3 Glucide synthesis in the kidney

The incorporations of ^{3}H-glucosamine in the kidneys of aging mice were studies by LM RAG (Joukura 1996, Joukura and Nagata 1995) and EM RAG (Joukura et al. 1996). Silver grains were observed over all the cell type nephrons at embryonic day 19, i.e., glomerular epithelial cells, endothelial cells, mesangial cells, Bowman's capsular cells and tubule cells.

In newborn and suckling stages, from postnatal day 1, 3, 7 to 14, both the renal corpuscles and urinary tubules were well differentiated and the number of silver grains increased (Figs. 36 C, D, E F, G, H in Nagata 2002). The results from grain counting revealed that the numbers of silver grains in both the renal corpuscles and the uriniferous tubules were less in the embryonic stage, but increased postnatally and reached peaks at day 1 and 3, then decreased to senescence at 1 year. These results showed that glucide synthesis in the kidney cells also changed with aging of animals.

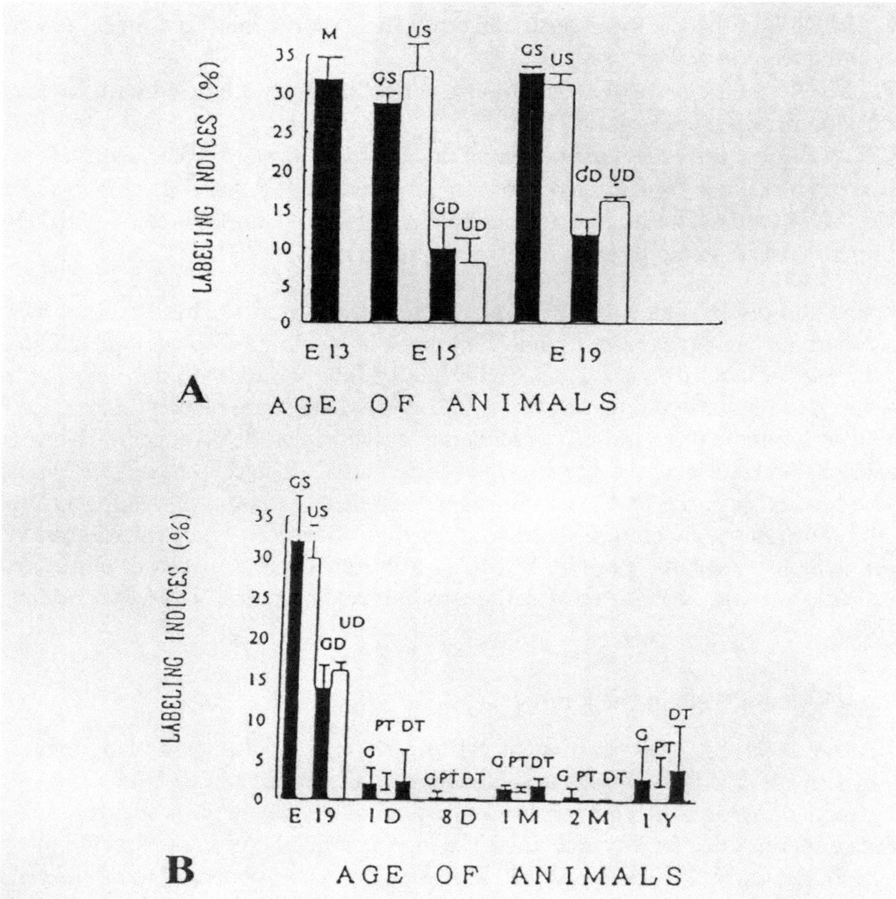

Fig. 17. Histogram showing aging changes of average labeling indices in respective cell types of the kidneys of aging mice labeled with ^{3}H-thyidine. Mean ± Standard Deviation. From Nagata, T.: Radioautographology, General and Special. In, Prog. Histochem. Cytochem. Vol. 37, No. 2, p. 156, 2002, Urban & Fischer, Jena, Germany
Fig. 17A. Labeling indices of the glomeruli and the uriniferous tubules of of mouse embryo from prenatal day 13 and 19.
Fig. 17B. Labeling indices of the glomeruli and the proximal and distal tubules of mouse embryo from prenatal day 19 to postnatal year 1. Abbreviations: GS=glomeruli of the superficial layer. US=uriniferous tubules of the superficial layer. GD=glomeruli of the deeper layer. UD=uriniferous tubules of the deeper layer. G=glomeruli. PT=proximal tubules. DT=distal tubules.

2.2 Localization of drugs in the urinary tract

The urinary tract is composed of the ureter, the urinary bladder and the urethra. We studied the urinary bladder of adult rats by LM RAG after oral administration of ^{3}H-tranilast, an anti-allergic agent produced by Kissei Pharmaceutical Co. (Momose et al. 1989, Nishigaki et al. 1987, 1990a,b). It was found that this agent specifically localized over the transitional epithelium and the endothelium of the veins in the mucosa of normal adult rats. However, any study on the DNA synthesis in the ureter, the urinary bladder and the urethra was not carried out.

3. Macromolecular synthesis in the reproductive system

The reproductive system or genital organs can be divided into two parts, the male genital organs and female genital organs. We studied the DNA and RNA syntheses and protein synthesis in several groups of aging mice, both male and female, by LM and EM RAG (Nagata 2002).

3.1 Macromolecular synthesis in the male genital organs

The male genital organs consist of the testis and its excretory ducts such as ductuli efferentes, ductus epididymidis, ductus deferens, ejaculatory ducts, auxiliary glands and penis. We studied both DNA and RNA syntheses in these organs of several groups of ddY aging mice by LM and EMRAG using macromolecular precursors.

3.1.1 The DNA synthesis in the male genital organs

Among the male genital organs, the testis was the main target of the scientific interests. Formerly, Clermont (1958, 1963) demonstrated using ^{3}H-thymidine radioautography that several stages of development of the spermatogonia were found at different levels in the germinal epithelium of mature men and rodents, with the most primitive germ cells found at the base and the more differentiated cells located at higher levels. We studied the DNA synthesis in the testis of several groups of aging mice.

3.1.1.1 The DNA synthesis in the testis

The structure of the testis of mammals is a compound tubular gland enclosed in tunica albuginea, a thick fibrous capsule. The parenchyma of the testis is composed of around 250 pyramidal compartments in men and animals, named lobules. Each lobule is made of convoluted seminiferous tubules, consisting of many spermatogenic cells differentiatiang to sperms among the supporting cells of Sertoli in the seminiferous epithelium, surrounded by the interstitial cells of Leydig. We first studied the macromolecular synthesis in the testis of aging male ddY mice at various ages (Gao 1993, Gao et al. 1994,1995a,b). When testicular tissues were labeled with ^{3}H-thymidine and observed by LM and EM RAG, many spermatogonia and myoid cells as well as Leydig cells were labeled with ^{3}H-thymidine at various ages from embryonic day 19 to postnatal day 1, 3, 7 (Fig. 16C), 14, month 1, 2, 6, 12 (Fig. 16D) and 24 (2 years). Silver grains were localized over the nuclei and several mitochondria of the spermatogonia showing DNA synthesis. Among of the aging groups, we counted the numbers of mitochondria per cell profile area, the numbers of labeled mitochondria per cell of the spermatogonia from 4 aging groups, prenatal embryonic day 19, postnatal day 3, and adults at month 1 and 6, and the labeling indices were calculated.

The results showed that the LI of the spermatogonia increased from embryonic day 19 (17%) to postnatal day 7 (25%) and month 1 (30%), reaching the maximum, then decreased to month 6 (20%) to year 2.

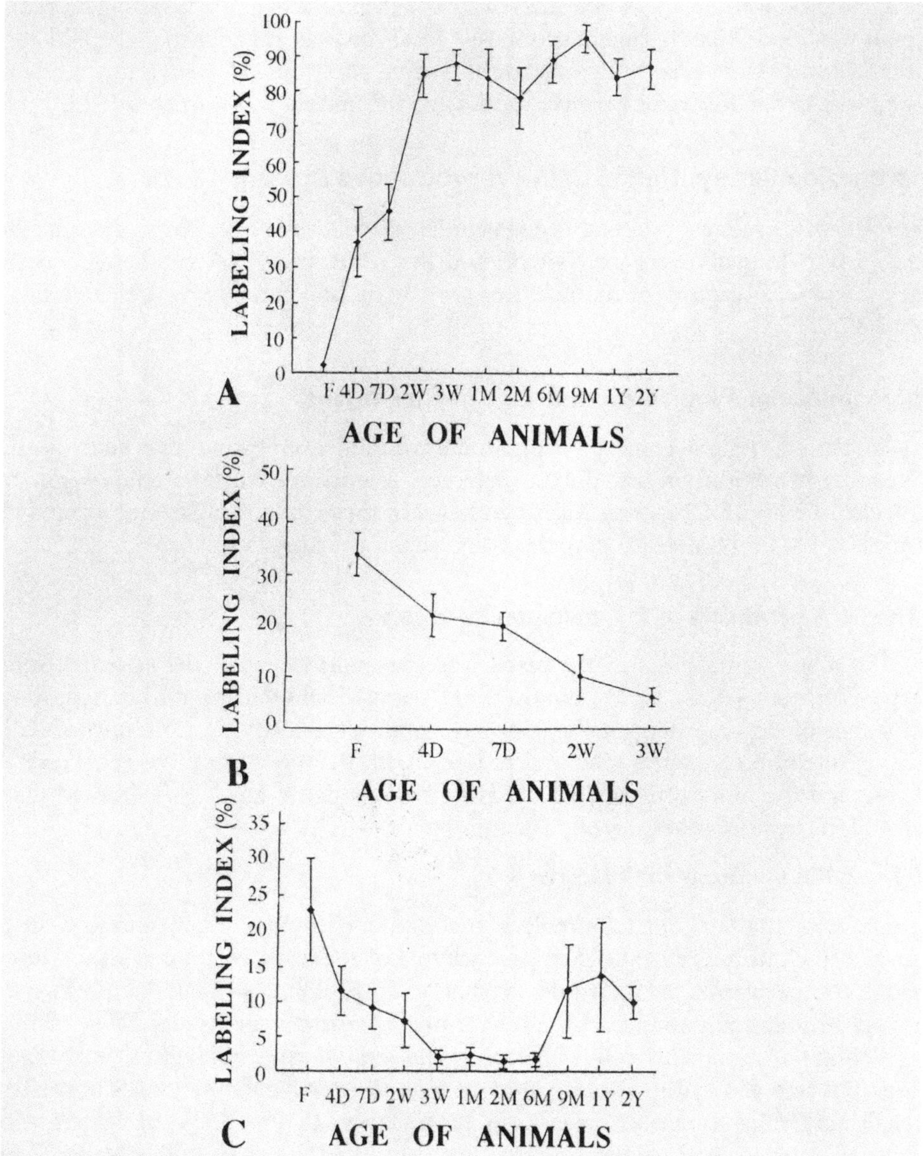

Fig. 18. Transitional curves of the labeling indices of respective cell types in the testis of aging mice labeled with ^{3}H-thymidine, showing DNA synthesis. Mean ± Standard Deviation. From Nagata, T.: Radioautographology, General and Special. In, Prog. Histochem. Cytochem. Vol. 37, No. 2, p. 160, 2002, Urban & Fischer, Jena, Germany

Fig. 18A. The spermatogonia.

Fig. 18B. The Sertoli cells.

Fig. 18C. The myoid cells.

At embryonic and neonatal stages, DNA synthesis of spermatocytes was weak and only a few labeled spermatogonia could be observed during the perinatal stages. The labeled spermatocytes were recognized at postnatal day 4 and 7 (Fig. 16C) and the number of labeled spermatogonia and spermatocytes increased from 2 and 3 weeks, keeping high level from month 1 to year 1 and 2 until senescence (Fig. 18A). However, the Sertoli's cells (Fig. 18B) and myoid cells (Fig. 18C) labeled with ^{3}H-thymidine were frequently observed at perinatal stages from embryo to postnatal day 7, while the labeling indices of both cells decreased from young adulthood (postnatal 2 weeks) to senescence (Gao 1993, Gao et al. 1994,1995a). The interstitial cells of Leydig in the testis surrounding the seminiferous tubules shall be described in the following section of the endocrine system in detail.

3.1.2 The RNA synthesis in the male genital organs

Among of the male genital organs, we studied the RNA synthesis in the testis of several groups of aging mice.

3.1.2.1 The RNA synthesis in the testis

We studied the RNA syntheses in aging mouse testis by LM and EM RAG, demonstrating the incorporations of ^{3}H-uridine into various cells of the seminiferous tubules (Gao 1993, Gao et al. 1994, Nagata 2002). The RNA synthesis of various cells in the seminiferous tubules was studied using ^{3}H-uridine. Silver grains due to ^{3}H-uridine demonstrating RNA synthesis were observed over the nuclei and cytoplasm of all spermatogonia, spermatocytes, Sertoli's cells, myoid cells of immature mice at perinatal stages at day 1 and 3 (Fig. 16E), as well as in mature and senescent mice from month 1, 6 to year 1 and 2. The synthetic activities of spermatogonia, Sertoli's cells and myoid cells as shown by grain counting with ^{3}H-uridine, as expressed by grain counting, were low (2-8 grain counts per 10 mm^2) at the embryonic and neonatal stages but increased at adult stages and maintained high levels (10-20 grain counts per 10 mm^2) until senescence. These results showed that DNA synthesis in myoid cells and Sertoli's cells increased at the perinatal stages and decreased from postnatal 2 weeks as described previously (Fig. 16A), while the RNA synthesis (Fig. 16E) in spermatogonia increased from postnatal 2 weeks together with DNA and protein syntheses (Fig. 16F) to senescence.

3.1.3 The protein synthesis in the male genital organs

We studied the protein synthesis of the reproductive system in both the male and female reproductive organs.

3.1.3.1 The protein synthesis in the testis

We studied the protein syntheses in aging mouse testis by LM and EM RAG, demonstrating the incorporations of ^{3}H-leucine into various cells of the seminiferous tubules (Gao 1993, Gao et al. 1994, Nagata 2002). The protein synthesis of various cells in the seminiferous tubules was first studied after administration of ^{3}H-leucine into aging male mice at various ages from perinatal to senescence at postnatal 2 years. Silver grains due to ^{3}H-leucine incorporation demonstrating protein synthesis were observed over the nuclei and cytoplasm of all the cells, spermatogonia, spermatocytes, Sertoli's cells, myoid cells of all male mice at respective stages from perinatal to senescence. The synthetic activities of spermatogonia, Sertoli's cells and myoid cells as shown by the number of silver grains due to ^{3}H-leucine, as expressed by grain counting, were low at the embryonic and neonatal stages but increased at adult stages and maintained high levels until senescence. These results showed that DNA synthesis in Sertoli's cells (Fig. 18B) and myoid cells (Fig. 18C) that increased at the perinatal stages and decreased from postnatal 2 weeks, while the DNA synthesis in spermatogonia increased from postnatal 2 weeks (Fig. 18A) together with RNA and protein syntheses to senescence.

3.2 Macromolecular synthesis in the female genital organs

The female genital organs consist of the ovary, the oviduct, the uterus, the vagina and the external genitals. We studied the macromolecular synthesis in the ovary, oviduct and uterus of several litters of ddY mice in aging.

3.2.1 The DNA synthesis in the female genital organ

Among the female genital organs, we studied the DNA synthesis in the ovary, oviduct and uterus of several litters of ddY mice in aging.

3.2.1.1 The DNA synthesis in the ovary

The ovary consists of the germinal epithelium covering the surface and the stroma containing many developing ovarian follicles depending upon the age of animals.

The nucleic acids, DNA and RNA, syntheses in the developing virgin mice ovaries of 6 litters, each 3 individuals, consisting of 36 female mice at various ages in respective precursors were studied by ^{3}H-thymidine and ^{3}H-uridine radioautography (Li 1994, Li and Nagata 1995, Li et al. 1992). The ^{3}H-thymidine incorporations were active in all surface epithelial cells, stromal and follicular cells of the ovaries between postnatal days 1 to 7 and decreased from day 14 (Fig. 16G) and maintained a lower level to day 60, while ^{3}H-uridine incorporations were active in all surface epithelial cells, stromal and follicular cells of the ovaries between postnatal days 1 to 7 and maintained medium levels from day 14 on.

The labeling indices with ^{3}H-thymidine showing DNA synthetic activity were high in all the surface epithelial cells, follicular cells and stromal cells of mice at neonatal stage from postnatal day 1 to 7, but decreased from day 40 to day 60 at mature stage (Fig. 19A). The grain counts showing RNA synthetic activity were high at neonatal stage from day 1 to day 7, and maintained medium levels from day 14 to day 60 at mature stage.

3.2.1.2 The DNA synthesis in the oviduct

The nucleic acids, DNA and RNA, syntheses in the oviducts of developing virgin mice at various ages were studied by ^{3}H-thymidine and ^{3}H-uridine radioautography (Li 1994, Li and Nagata 1995). The silver grains with ^{3}H-thymidine showing the DNA synthesis were observed over many nuclei in all surface epithelial cells, stromal and smooth muscle cells at neonatal stage between postnatal day 1 to 3 and decreased from day 7 to 30 (Fig. 16H) and 60, while the silver grains showing the RNA synthesis with ^{3}H-uridine were observed over the nuclei and cytoplasm of all the epithelial and stromal cells from postnatal day 1 to day 60. The labeling indices with ^{3}H-thymidine were high at neonatal stage from postnatal day 1 to 3 but decreased from day 7 to day 60 (Fig. 19C). The grain counts with ^{3}H-uridine were high at neonatal stage from postnatal day 1 to 3 and increased from day 7 to day 14 and decreased from day 30 to day 60. These results demonstrated an unparalleled alternation of DNA and RNA syntheses in the oviduct (Li and Nagata 1995).

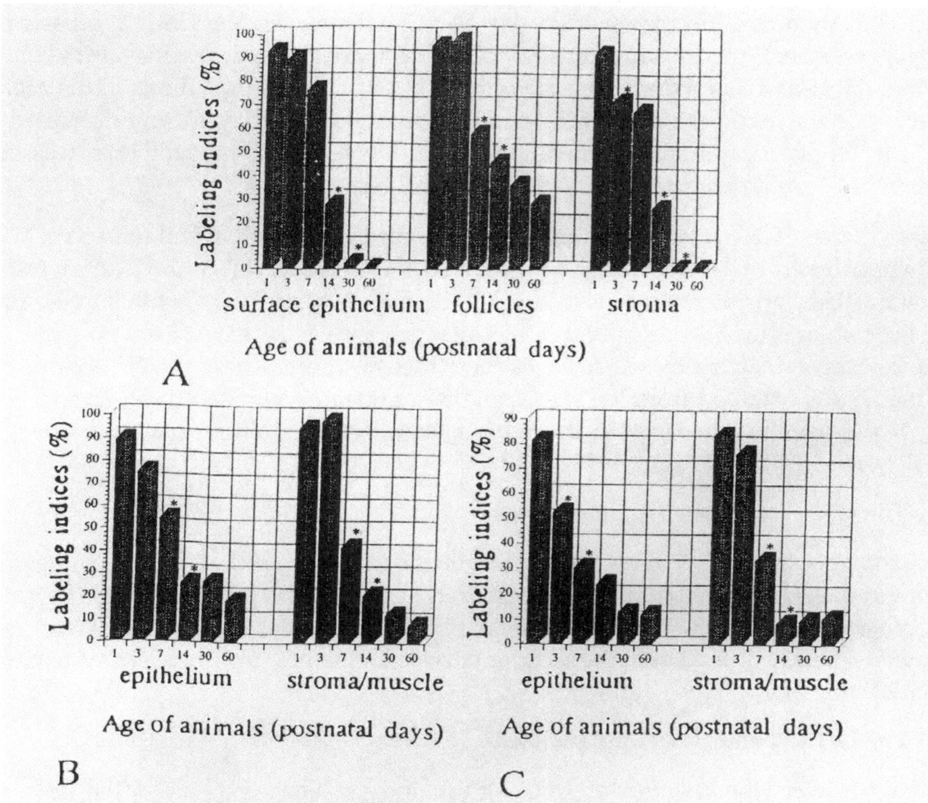

Fig. 19. Histogram showing aging changes of average labeling indices in respective cell types of female genital organs of aging mice labeled with ^{3}H-thymidine. Mean ± Standard Deviation. From Nagata, T.: Radioautographology, General and Special. In, Prog. Histochem. Cytochem. Vol. 37, No. 2, p. 166, 2002, Urban & Fischer, Jena, Germany
Fig. 19A. The ovary.
Fig. 19B. The uterus.
Fig. 19C. The oviduct.

3.2.1.3 The DNA synthesis in the uterus

The silver grains with ^{3}H-thymidine showing DNA synthesis of the uterus was observed over some of the nuclei of all the cells in the epithelia, stroma and smooth muscles from postnatal day 1 to 60 (Li 1994, Li and Nagata 1995). The labeling indices with ^{3}H-thymidine (Fig. 19B) were high (80-95%) at postnatal day 1 and decreased from day 3 to 60 (>10%). The silver grains showing RNA synthesis of the uterus were observed over all the nuclei and cytoplasm of all the cells in the uterine epithelia, stroma and smooth muscles from day 1 to 60. The number of silver grains in the uterine epithelium increased from postnatal day 1 to 7 and decreased from day 14 to 60, while they increased in the stroma from day 1 to 3 and decreased from day 7 to 60.

These results from the female genital organs showed that both DNA and RNA syntheses, as expressed by labeling indices and grain counting, were active in all kinds of cells, such as surface epithelial cells, stromal cells and follicular cells of the ovaries between postnatal days 1 to 7, then they decreased from day 14 to 60. However, the DNA synthesis in the epithelial cells and the stromal cells of both the uteri and the oviducts was active at postnatal day 1 and 3 and decreased from day 7 to 60. The RNA synthesis in the uteri and oviducts was active at postnatal day 1, increased from day 1 to day 14, and decreased from day 30 to 60. The unparalleled alteration of the DNA and RNA syntheses was shown between the ovary and the uterus or oviduct (Li and Nagata 1995).

We also studied PCNA/cyclin immunostaining in the ovary, oviduct and uterus (Li 1994). It was demonstrated that PCNA/cyclin positive cells were observed in the ovarian follicular epithelium, ovarian interstitial cells, tubal epithelial cells, tubal interstitial cells, uterine epithelial cells and uterine interstitial cells. The positive cells increased from postnatal 1 day to 3 and 7 days, then decreased from 14 days to senescence. These results accorded well with the results obtained from the ^{3}H-thymidine radioautography (Li 1994, Li and Nagata 1995). Moreover, the mucosubstance synthesis incorporating sulfuric acid was also carried out (Oliveira et al. 1991, Li et al. 1995).

3.2.1.4 The DNA synthesis in gametogenesis

The gametogenesis consists of both spermatogenesis in male germ cells and the oogenesis in female germ cells, leading to the implantation and further development of blastcysts. The macromolecular synthesis, DNA, RNA and protein synthesis, in both the testis and the ovary were already described in the sections of male and female reproductive systems (3.7.1. and 3.7.2.) previously.

3.2.1.5 The DNA synthesis in implantaion

In order to detect the changes of DNA, RNA and protein synthesis of the developing blastcysts in mouse endometrium during activation of the implantation, ovulations of female BALB/C strain mice were controlled by pregnant mare serum gonadotropin and human chorionic gonadotropin, then pregnant female mice were ovariectomized on the 4th day of pregnancy (Yamada 1993, Yamada and Nagata 1992a,b, 1993). The delay implantation state was maintained for 48 hrs and after 0 to 18 hrs of estrogen supply ^{3}H-thymidine was injected. The three regions of the endometrium, i. e. the interinplantation site, the antimesometrial and mesometrial sides of implantation site, were taken out and processed for LM and EM RAG. It was well known that the uterus of the rodent becomes receptive to blastcyst implantation only for a restricted period. This is called the implantation window which is intercalated between refractory states of the endometrium whose cycling is regulated by ovarian hormones (Yoshinaga 1988). We studied the changes of DNA synthesis by ^{3}H-thymidine (Yamada and Nagata 1992a,b) incorporations in the endometrial cells of pregnant-ovariectomized mice after time-lapse effect of nidatory estradiol. As the results, the endometrial cells showed topographical and chronological differences in the nucleic acid synthesis. The cells labeled with ^{3}H-thymidine increased after nidatory estradiol effects in the stromal cells around the blastocyst, but not in the epithelial cells. The results suggested that the presence of the blastocysts in the uterine lumen induced selective changes in the behavior of endometrial cells after nidatory estradiol effect showing the changes of DNA synthesis.

As for a lower vertebrate, cell proliferation and migration of scleroblasts and their precursor cells during ethisterone-induced anal-fin process formation of the medaka, orizias latipes, was studied by LM RAG labeled with ^{3}H-thymidine (Uwa and Nagata 1976). The results showed that the labeling index in the posterior margin of the joint plate rapidly increased and the scleroblast population in the central portion increased simultaneously from the 3rd to 5th day of ethisterone treatment. These results indicated that the scleroblasts and their precursor cells migrated from the peripheral portion to the central portion along the proxi-distal axis of the joint plate.

3.2.2 The RNA synthesis in the female genital organs

We studied the RNA synthesis of female reproductive organs of aging mice after the administration of ^{3}H-uridine at various ages.

3.2.2.1 The RNA synthesis in the ovary

The ovary consists of the germinal epithelium covering the surface and the stroma containing many developing ovarian follicles depending upon the age of animals.

The nucleic acids, DNA and RNA, syntheses in the developing virgin mice ovaries of 6 litters, each 3 individuals, consisting of 36 female mice at various ages in 2 groups were studied by ^{3}H-thymidine and ^{3}H-uridine radioautography (Li 1994, Li and Nagata 1995, Li et al. 1992). The ^{3}H-thymidine incorporations were active in all surface epithelial cells, stromal and follicular cells of the ovary between postnatal days 1 to 7 and decreased from day 14 (Fig. 16G) and maintained a lower level to day 60, while ^{3}H-uridine incorporations were active in all surface epithelial cells, stromal and follicular cells of the ovary between postnatal days 1 to 7 and maintained medium levels from day 14 on.

The labeling indices with ^{3}H-thymidine showing DNA synthetic activity were high in all the surface epithelial cells, follicular cells and stromal cells of mice at neonatal stage from postnatal day 1 to 7, but decreased from day 40 to day 60 at mature stage. The grain counts showing RNA synthetic activity were high at neonatal stage from day 1 to day 7, and maintained medium levels from day 14 to day 60 at mature stage.

3.2.2.2 The RNA synthesis in the oviduct

The nucleic acids, DNA and RNA, syntheses in the oviducts of developing virgin mice at various ages were studied by ^{3}H-thymidine and ^{3}H-uridine radioautography (Li 1994, Li and Nagata 1995). The silver grains with ^{3}H-thymidine showing the DNA synthesis were observed over many nuclei in all surface epithelial cells, stromal and smooth muscle cells at neonatal stage between postnatal day 1 to 3 and decreased from day 7 to 30 (Fig. 16H) and 60, while the silver grains showing the RNA synthesis with ^{3}H-uridine were observed over the nuclei and cytoplasm of all the epithelial and stromal cells from postnatal day 1 to day 60. The labeling indices with ^{3}H-thymidine were high at neonatal stage from postnatal day 1 to 3 but decreased from day 7 to day 60. The grain counts with ^{3}H-uridine were high at neonatal stage from postnatal day 1 to 3 and increased from day 7 to day 14 and decreased from day 30 to day 60. These results demonstrated an unparalleled alternation of DNA and RNA syntheses in the oviduct (Li and Nagata 1995).

3.2.2.3 The RNA synthesis in the uterus

The silver grains with ^{3}H-uridine showing RNA synthesis of the uterus was observed over almost all the nuclei and cytoplasm of all the cells in the epithelia, stroma and smooth muscles from postnatal day 1 to 60 (Li 1994, Li and Nagata 1995). The labeling indices with

^{3}H-thymidine were high (80-95%) at postnatal day 1 and decreased from day 3 to 60 (>10%). The silver grains showing RNA synthesis of the uterus were observed over all the nuclei and cytoplasm of all the cells in the uterine epithelia, stroma and smooth muscles from day 1 to 60. The number of silver grains in the uterine epithelium increased from postnatal day 1 to 7 and decreased from day 14 to 60, while they increased in the stroma from day 1 to 3 and decreased from day 7 to 60.

These results from the female genital organs showed that both DNA and RNA syntheses, as expressed by labeling indices and grain counting, were active in all kinds of cells, such as surface epithelial cells, stromal cells and follicular cells of the ovaries between postnatal days 1 to 7, then they decreased from day 14 to 60. However, the DNA synthesis in the epithelial cells and the stromal cells of both the uteri and the oviducts was active at postnatal day 1 and 3 and decreased from day 7 to 60. The RNA synthesis in the uteri and oviducts was active at postnatal day 1, increased from day 1 to day 14, and decreased from day 30 to 60. The unparalleled alteration of the DNA and RNA syntheses was shown between the ovary and the uterus or oviduct (Li and Nagata 1995).

We also studied PCNA/cyclin immunostaining in the ovary, oviduct and uterus (Li 1994). It was demonstrated that PCNA/cyclin positive cells were observed in the ovarian follicular epithelium, ovarian interstitial cells, tubal epithelial cells, tubal interstitial cells, uterine epithelial cells and uterine interstitial cells. The positive cells increased from postnatal 1 day to 3 and 7 days, then decreased from 14 days to senescence. These results accorded well with the results obtained from the ^{3}H-thymidine radioautography (Li 1994, Li and Nagata 1995). Moreover, the mucosubstance synthesis incorporating sulfuric acid was also carried out (Oliveira et al. 1991, 1995, Li et al. 1992).

3.2.2.4 The RNA synthesis in gametogenesis

The gametogenesis consists of both spermatogenesis in male germ cells and the oogenesis in female germ cells, leading to the implantation and further development of blastcysts. The macromolecular synthesis, DNA, RNA and protein synthesis, in both the testis and the ovary were already described in the sections of male and female reproductive systems (8.1.1. and 8.1.2.) previously.

3.2.2.5 The RNA synthesis in implantation

In order to detect the changes of DNA, RNA and protein synthesis of the developing blastcysts in mouse endometrium during activation of the implantation, ovulations of female BALB/C strain mice were controlled by pregnant mare serum gonadotropin and human chorionic gonadotropin, then pregnant female mice were ovariectomized on the 4th day of pregnancy (Yamada 1993, Yamada and Nagata 1992a,b, 1993). The delay implantation state was maintained for 48 hrs and after 0 to 18 hrs of estrogen supply ^{3}H-thymidine was injected. The three regions of the endometrium, i. e. the interinplantation site, the antimesometrial and mesometrial sides of implantation site, were taken out and processed for LM and EM RAG. It was well known that the uterus of the rodent becomes receptive to blastcyst implantation only for a restricted period. This is called the implantation window which is intercalated between refractory states of the endometrium whose cycling is regulated by ovarian hormones (Yoshinaga 1988). We studied the changes of DNA synthesis by ^{3}H-thymidine (Yamada and Nagata 1992a,b) incorporations in the endometrial cells of pregnant-ovariectomized mice after time-lapse effect of nidatory estradiol. As the results, the endometrial cells showed topographical and chronological differences in the nucleic acid synthesis. The cells labeled with ^{3}H-thymidine increased after nidatory estradiol effects in the stromal cells around the blastocyst, but not in the epithelial cells. The results suggested that the presence of the blastocysts in the uterine lumen induced selective changes in the behavior of endometrial cells after nidatory estradiol effect showing the changes of DNA synthesis.

As for a lower vertebrate, cell proliferation and migration of scleroblasts and their precursor cells during ethisterone-induced anal-fin process formation of the medaka, orizias latipes, was studied by LM RAG labeled with ^{3}H-thymidine (Uwa and Nagata 1976). The results showed that the labeling index in the posterior margin of the joint plate rapidly increased and the scleroblast population in the central portion increased simultaneously from the 3rd to 5th day of ethisterone treatment. These results indicated that the scleroblasts and their precursor cells migrated from the peripheral portion to the central portion along the proxi-distal axis of the joint plate.

3.2.3 The protein synthesis of the female genital organs

We studied the protein synthesis of female reproductive organs of aging mice after the administration of ^{3}H-leucine at various ages.

3.2.3.1 The protein synthesis in the uterus

We studied the protein synthesis of the developing blastocysts in female mouse endometrium during activation of the implantation. The ovulations of female BALB/C strain adult mice were controlled by pregnant mare serum gonadotropin and human chorionic gonadotropin, then pregnant female mice were ovariectomized on the 4th day of pregnancy (Yamada 1993, Yamada and Nagata 1992a,b, 1993). The delay implantation state was maintained for 48 hrs and after 0 to 18 hrs of estrogen supply. After the mice were injected with ^{3}H-leucine, they were sacrificed and the uteri were processed for LM and EMRAG. We studied the changes of protein synthesis by ^{3}H-leucine incorporations (Yamada 1993, Yamada and Nagata 1992a). As the results, the endometrial cells showed topographical and chronological differences in the protein synthesis. The cells labeled with ^{3}H-leucine were observed in both epithelial cells and stromal cells. Quantitative analysis revealed that the number of silver grains increased from 0 hr to 3 and 6 hr, reaching the peak at 6 hr and decreased from 12 to 18 hr. The protein synthesis in the decidual cells of pregnant mice uteri was compared to the endometrial cells of virgin mice uteri using ^{3}H-proline and ^{3}H-tryptophane incorporations. The results demonstrated that silver grains were localized over the endoplasmic reticulum and the Golgi apparatus of fibroblasts and accumulated over collagen fibrils in the extracellular matrix suggesting that the decidual cells produced collagen in the matrix. The collagen synthesis in the mouse decidual cells by ^{3}H-proline showed that silver grains were localized over the endoplasmic reticulum and Golgi apparatus of fibroblasts and accumulated over collagen fibrils in the extracellular matrix (Oliveira et al. 1991, 1995). However, analytical studies on protein synthesis in aging mice at various ages were not yet carried out.

3.2.3.2 The protein synthesis in the implantation

In order to detect the changes of DNA, RNA and protein synthesis of the developing blastocysts in female mouse endometrium during activation of the implantation, ovulations of female BALB/C strain mice were controlled by pregnant mare serum gonadotropin and human chorionic gonadotropin, then pregnant female mice were ovariectomized on the 4th day of pregnancy (Yamada 1993, Yamada and Nagata 1992a,b, 1993). The delay implantation state was maintained for 48 hrs and after 0 to 18 hrs of estrogen supply and ^{3}H-leucine was injected. The three regions of the endometrium, i. e. the interinplantation site, the antimesometrial and mesometrial sides of implantation site, were taken out and processed for LM and EM RAG. It was well known that the uterus of the rodent becomes receptive to blastocyst implantation only for a restricted period. This is called the implantation window which is intercalated between refractory states of the endometrium whose cycling is regulated by ovarian hormones (Yoshinaga 1988). We studied the changes of protein synthesis by ^{3}H-leucine (Yamada 1993, Yamada and Nagata 1992a) incorporations in the endometrial cells of pregnant-ovariectomized mice after time-lapse effect of nidatory estradiol. As the results, the endometrial cells showed topographical and chronological differences in the nucleic acid and protein synthesis. The cells labeled with ^{3}H-leucine were observed in both epithelial cells and stromal cells. Quantitative analysis revealed that the number of silver grains as expressed by grain counting per mm^2 in both the stromal and epithelial cells on the antimesometrial side with ^{3}H-leucine increased from 0 hr to 3 and 6 hr, reaching the peak at 6 hr and decreased from 12 to 18 hr. These results suggested that the presence of the blastocysts in the uterine lumen induced selective changes in the behavior of endometrial cells after nidatory estradiol effect showing the changes of DNA, RNA and protein synthesis. The time coincident peak of RNA and protein synthesis detected in the endometrial cells at the anti-mesometrial side of the implantation site, probably reflected the activation moment of the implantation window. The protein synthesis in the decidual cells of pregnant mice uteri was compared to the endometrial cells of virgin mice uteri using ^{3}H-proline and ^{3}H-tryptophane incorporations. The results demonstrated that silver grains were localized over the endoplasmic reticulum and the Golgi apparatus of fibroblasts and accumulated over collagen fibrils in the extracellular matrix suggesting that the decidual cells produced collagen in the matrix. On the other hand, collagen synthesis in the mouse decidual cells was studied by LM and EM RAG using ^{3}H-proline (Oliveira et al. 1991, 1995). Silver grains were localized over the endoplasmic reticulum and Golgi apparatus of fibroblasts and accumulated over collagen fibrils in the extracellular matrix. The results suggested that the decidual cells produced collagen into the matrix. The quantitative analysis showed that both incorporations in the decidual cells and the matrix increased in the pregnant mice than the endometrial cells in virgin mice.

3.2.4 The glucide synthesis in the reproductive system

Among the reproductive organs, only the mucosubstance synthesis with radiosulfate, $^{35}SO_4$, was studied in the ovaries of mice during the estrus cycle.

3.2.4.1 The glucide synthesis in the ovary

Litter mate groups of female ddY mice, aged 8-10 weeks, were divided into 4 groups, diestrus, proestrus, estrus and metestrus according to the vaginal smears. The ovaries were taken out, labeled with $^{35}SO_4$ in vitro and radioautographed. In all the animals, silver grains were localized over the granulosa and theca cells. Almost all compartments of the ovaries were labeled. The grain counts per cell changed according to cell cycle. From the results, it was concluded that all the cells of the ovary incorporated mucosubstances throughout the estrus cycle (Li et al. 1992).

4. References

Chen, S., Gao, F., Kotani, A., Nagata, T.: Age-related changes of male mouse submandibular gland: A morphometric and radioautographic study. Cell. Mol. Biol. 41, 117-124, 1995.

Clermont Y.: The contractime elements in the limiting membrane of the seminiferous tubules of rats. Exp. Cell Res. 15, 438-342, 1958.

Clermont, Y.: Renewal of spermatogonia in man. Amer. J. Anat. 112, 35-51, 1963.

Cui, H.: Light microscopic radioautographic study on DNA synthesis of nerve cells in the cerebella of aging mice. Cell. Mol. Biol. 41, 1139-1154, 1995.

Cui, H., Gao, F., Nagata, T.: Light microscopic radioautographic study on protein synthesis in perinatal mice corneas. Acta Histochem. Cytochem. 33, 31-37, 2000.

Duan, H., Gao, F., Li, S., Hayashi, K., Nagata, T.: Aging changes and fine structure and DNA synthesis of esophageal epithelium in neonatal, adult and old mice. J. Clin. Electron Microsc. 25, 452-453, 1992.

Duan, H., Gao, F., Li, S., Nagata, T.: Postnatal development of esophageal epithelium in mouse: a light and electron microscopic radioautographic study. Cell. Mol. Biol. 39, 309-316, 1993.

Duan, H., Gao, F., Oguchi, K., Nagata, T.: Light and electron microscopic radioautographic study on the incorporation of ^{3}H-thymidine into the lung by means of a new nebulizer. Drug Res. 44, 880-883, 1994.

Feulgen, R., Rossenbeck, H.: Mikroskopische-chemischer Nachweis einer Nukeinsaeure von Thymus der Thymonukeinsaeure Z. Physik. Chem. 135, 203-248, 1924.

Fujii, Y., Ohno, S., Yamabayashi, S., Usuda, N., Saito, H., Furuta, S., Nagata, T.: Electron microscopic radioautography of DNA synthesis in primary cultured cells from an IgG myeloma patient. J. Clin. Electr. Microsc. 13, 582-583, 1980.

Gao, F.: Study on the macromolecular synthesis in aging mouse seminiferous tubules by light and electron microscopic radioautography. Cell. Mol. Biol. 39, 659-672, 1993.

Gao, F., Toriyama, K., Nagata, T.: Light microscopic radioautographic study on the DNA synthesis of prenatal and postnatal aging mouse retina after labeled thymidine injection. Cell. Mol. Biol. 38, 661-668, 1992a.

Gao, F., Li, S., Duan, H., Ma, H., Nagata, T.: Electron microscopic radioautography on the DNA synthesis of prenatal and postnatal mice retina after labeled thymidine injection. J. Clin. Electron Microsc. 25, 721-722, 1992b.

Gao, F., Toriyama, K., Ma, H., Nagata, T.: Light microscopic radioautographic study on DNA synthesis in aging mice corneas. Cell. Mol. Biol. 39, 435-441, 1993.

Gao, F., Ma, H., Sun, L., Jin, C., Nagata, T.: Electron microscopic radioautographic study on the nucleic acids and protein synthesis in the aging mouse testis. Med. Electron Microsc. 27, 360-362, 1994.

Gao, F., Chen, S., Sun, L., Kang, W., Wang, Z., Nagata, T.: Radioautographic study of the macromolecular synthesis of Leydig cells in aging mice testis. Cell. Mol. Biol. 41, 145-150, 1995a.

Gao, F., Jin, C., Ma, H., Sun, L., Nagata, T.: Ultrastructural and radioautographic studies on DNA synthesis in Leydig cells of aging mouse testis. Cell. Mol. Biol. 41, 151-160, 1995b.

Gunarso, W.: Radioautographic studies on the nucleic acid synthesis of the retina of chick embryo. I. Light microscopic radioautography. Shinshu Med. J. 32, 231-240, 1984a.

Gunarso, W.: Radioautographic studies on the nucleic acid synthesis of the retina of chick embryo. II. Electron microscopic radioautography. Shinshu Med. J. 32, 241-248, 1984b.

Gunarso, W., Gao, F., Cui, H., Ma, H., Nagata, T.: A light and electron microscopic radioautographic study on RNA synthesis in the retina of chick embryo. Acta Histochem. 98, 309-32, 1996.

Gunarso, W., Gao, F., Nagata, T.: Development and DNA synthesis in the retina of chick embryo observed by light and electron microscopic radioautography. Cell. Mol. Biol. 43, 189-201, 1997.

Hanai, T.: Light microscopic radioautographic study of DNA synthesis in the kidneys of aging mice. Cell. Mol. Biol. 39, 81-91, 1993.

Hanai, T., Nagata, T.: Electron microscopic radioautographic study on DNA and RNA synthesis in perinatal mouse kidney. In, Radioautography in Medicine, Nagata, T., Ed., pp. 127-131, Shinshu University Press, Matsumoto, 1994a.

Hanai, T., Nagata, T.: Study on the nucleic acid synthesis in the aging mouse kidney by light and electron microscopic radioautography. In, Radioautography in Medicine, Nagata, T., Ed., pp. 209-214, Shinshu University Press, Matsumoto, 1994b.

Hanai, T., Nagata, T.: Electron microscopic study on nucleic acid synthesis in perinatal mouse kidney tissue. Med. Electron Microsc. 27, 355-357, 1994c.

Hanai, T., Usuda, N., Morita, T., Shimizu, T., Nagata, T.: Proliferative activity in the kidneys of aging mice evaluated by PCNA/cyclin immunohistochemistry. Cell. Mol. Biol. 39, 181-191, 1993.

Hayashi, K., Gao, F., Nagata, T.: Radioautographic study on ^{3}H-thymidine incorporation at different stages of muscle development in aging mice. Cell. Mol. Biol. 39, 553-560, 1993.

Ito, M.: The radioautographic studies on aging change of DNA synthesis and the ultrastructural development of mouse adrenal gland. Cell. Mol. Biol. 42, 279-292, 1996.

Ito, M., Nagata, T.: Electron microscopic radioautographic studies on DNA synthesis and ultrastructure of aging mouse adrenal gland. Med. Electron Microsc. 29, 145-152, 1996.

Izumiyama, K., Kogure, K., Kataoka, S., Nagata, T.: Quantitative analysis of glucose after transient ischemia in the gerbil hippocampus by light and electron microscope radioautography. Brain Res. 416, 175-179, 1987.

Jamieson, J. D., Palade, G. E.: Intracellular transport of secretory proteins in the pancreatic exocrine cells. J. Cell Biol. 34, 577-615, 1967.

Jin, C.: Study on DNA synthesis of aging mouse colon by light and electron microscopic radioautography. Cell. Mol. Biol. 42, 255-268, 1996.

Jin, C., Nagata, T.: Light microscopic radioautographic study on DNA synthesis in cecal epithelial cells of aging mice. J. Histochem. Cytochem. 43, 1223-1228, 1995a.

Jin, C., Nagata, T.: Electron microscopic radioautographic study on DNA synthesis in cecal epithelial cells of aging mice. Med. Electron Microsc. 28, 71-75, 1995b.

Joukura, K.: The aging changes of glycoconjugate synthesis in mouse kidney studied by ^{3}H-glucosamine radioautography. Acta Histochem. Cytochem. 29, 57-63, 1996.

Joukura, K., Nagata, T.: Aging changes of ^{3}H-glucosamine incorporation into mouse kidney observed by radioautography. Acta Histochem. Cytochem. 28, 494-494, 1995.

Joukura, K., Usuda, N., Nagata, T.: Quantitative study on the aging change of glycoconjugates synthesis in aging mouse kidney. Proc. Xth Internat. Cong. Histochem. Cytochem., Acta Histochem. Cytochem. 29, Suppl. 507-508, 1996.

Kobayashi, K., Nagata, T.: Light microscopic radioautographic studies on DNA, RNA and protein syntheses in human synovial membranes of rheumatoid arthritis patients. J. Histochem. Cytochem. 42, 982-982, 1994.

Komiyama, K., Iida, F., Furihara, R., Murata, F., Nagata, T.: Electron microscopic radioautographic study on ^{125}I-albumin in rat gastric mucosal epithelia. J. Clin. Electron Microsc. 11, 428-429, 1978.

Kong, Y.: Electron microscopic radioautographic study on DNA synthesis in perinatal mouse retina. Cell. Mol. Biol. 39, 55-64, 1993.

Kong, Y., Nagata, T.: Electron microscopic radioautographic study on nucleic acid synthesis of perinatal mouse retina. Med. Electron Microsc. 27, 366-368, 1994.

Kong, Y., Usuda, N., Nagata, T.: Radioautographic study on DNA synthesis of the retina and retinal pigment epithelium of developing mouse embryo. Cell. Mol. Biol. 38, 263-272, 1992a.

Kong, Y., Usuda, N., Morita, T., Hanai, T., Nagata, T.: Study on RNA synthesis in the retina and retinal pigment epithelium of mice by light microscopic radioautography. Cell. Mol. Biol. 38, 669-678, 1992b.

Leblond, C. P.: Localization of newly administered iodine in the thyroid gland as indicated by radioiodine. J. Anat. 77, 149-152, 1943.

Leblond, C. P.: The life history of cells in renewing systems. Am. J. Anat. 160, 113-158, 1981.

Leblond, C. P., Messier, B.: Renewal of chief cells and goblet cells in the small intestine as shown by radioautography after injection of thymidine-^{3}H into mice. Anat. Rec. 132: 247-259. 1958.

Li, S.: Relationship between cellular DNA synthesis, PCNA expression and sex steroid hormone receptor status in the developing mouse ovary, uterus and oviduct. Histochemistry 102, 405-413, 1994.

Li, S., Nagata, T.: Nucleic acid synthesis in the developing mouse ovary, uterus and oviduct studied by light and electron microscopic radioautography. Cell. Mol. Biol. 41, 185-195, 1995.

Li, S., Gao, F., Duan, H., Nagata, T.: Radioautographic study on the uptake of $^{35}SO_4$ in mouse ovary during the estrus cycle. J. Clin. Electron Microsc. 25, 709-710, 1992.

Liang, Y.: Light microscopic radioautographic study on RNA synthesis in the adrenal glands of aging mice. Acta Histochem. Cytochem. 31, 203-210, 1998.

Liang, Y., Ito, M., Nagata, T.: Light and electron microscopic radioautographic studies on RNA synthesis in aging mouse adrenal gland. Acta Anat. Nippon. 74, 291-300, 1999.

Ma, H.: Light microscopic radioautographic study on DNA synthesis of the livers in aging mice. Acta Anat. Nippon. 63, 137-147, 1988.

Ma, H., Nagata, T.: Electron microscopic radioautographic study on DNA synthesis of the livers in aging mice. J. Clin. Electron Microsc. 21, 335-343, 1988a.

Ma, H., Nagata, T.: Studies on DNA synthesis of aging mice by means of electron microscopic radioautography. J. Clin. Electron Microsc. 21, 715-716, 1988b.

Ma, H., Nagata, T.: Electron microscopic radioautographic studies on DNA synthesis in the hepatocytes of aging mice as observed by image analysis. Cell. Mol. Biol. 36, 73-84, 1990a.

Ma, H., Nagata, T.: Study on RNA synthesis in the livers of aging mice by means of electron microscopic radioautography. Cell. Mol. Biol. 36, 589-600, 1990b.

Ma, H., Nagata, T.: Collagen and protein synthesis in the livers of aging mice as studied by electron microsopic radioautography. Ann. Microsc. 1, 13-22, 2000.

Ma, H., Gao, F., Olea, M. T., Nagata, T.: Protein synthesis in the livers of aging mice studied by electron microscopic radioautography. Cell. Mol. Biol. 37, 607-615, 1991.

Matsumura, H., Kobayashi, Y., Kobayashi, K., Nagata, T.: Light microscopic radioautographic study of DNA synthesis in the lung of aging salamander, Hynobius nebulosus. J. Histochem. Cytochem. 42, 1004-1004, 1994.

Momose, Y., Nagata, T.: Radioautographic study on the intracellular localization of a hypolipidemic agent, bezafibrate, a peroxisome proliferator, in cultured rat hepatocytes. Cell. Mol. Biol. 39, 773-781, 1993a.

Momose, Y., Naito, J., Nagata, T.: Radioautographic study on the localization of an anti-allergic agent, tranilast, in the rat liver. Cell. Mol. Biol. 35, 347-355, 1989.

Momose, Y., Shibata, N., Kiyosawa, I., Naito, J., Watanabe, T., Horie, S., Yamada, J., Suga, T., Nagata, T.: Morphometric evaluation of species differences in the effects of bezafibrate, a hypolipidemic agent, on hepatic peroxisomes and mitochondria. J. Toxicol. Pathol. 6, 33-45, 1993b.

Momose, Y., Naito, J., Suzawa, H., Kanzawa, M., Nagata, T.: Radioautographic study on the intracellular localization of bezafibrate in cultured rat hepatoctyes. Acta Histochem. Cytochem. 28, 61-66, 1995.

Morita, T.: Radioautographic study on the aging change of ^{3}H-glucosamine uptake in mouse ileum. Cell. Mol. Biol. 39, 875-884, 1993.

Morita, T., Usuda, N. Hanai, T., Nagata, T.: Changes of colon epithelium proliferation due to individual aging with PCNA/cyclin immunostaining comparing with ^{3}H-thymidine radioautography. Histochemistry 101, 13-20, 1994.

Murata, F., Momose,Y. , Yoshida, K., Nagata, T.: Incorporation of ^{3}H-thymidine into the nucleus of mast cells in adult rat peritoneum. Shinshu Med. J. 25, 72-77, 1977a.

Murata, F., Momose, Y., Yoshida, K., Ohno, S., Nagata, T.: Nucleic acid and mucosubstance metabolism of mastocytoma cells by means of electron microscopic radioautography. Acta Pharmacol. Toxicol. 41, 58-59, 1977b.

Murata, F., Yoshida, K., Ohno, S., Nagata, T.: Ultrastructural and electron microscopic radioautographic studies on the mastocytoma cells and mast cells. J. Clin. Electron Microsc. 11, 561-562, 1978.

Murata, F., Yoshida, K., Ohno, S., Nagata, T.: Mucosubstances of rabbit granulocytes studied by means of electron microscopic radioautography and X-ray microanalysis. Histochemistry 61, 139-150, 1979.

Nagata, T.: On the relationship between cell division and cytochrome oxidase in the Yoshida sarcoma cells. Shinshu Med. J. 5: 383-386, 1956.

Nagata, T.: Studies on the amitosis in the Yoshida sarcoma cells. I. Observation on the smear preparation under normal conditions. Med. J. Shinshu Univ. 2: 187-198, 1957a.

Nagata, T.: Studies on the amitosis in the Yoshida sarcoma cells. II. Phase-contrast microscopic observations under normal conditions. Med. J. Shinshu Univ. 2: 199-207, 1957b.

Nagata, T.: Cell divisions in the liver of the fetal and newborn dogs. Med. J. Shinshu Univ. 4: 65-73, 1959.

Nagata, T.: A radioautographic study of the DNA synthesis in rat liver, with special reference to binucleate cells. Med. J. Shinshu Univ. 7, 17-25, 1962.

Nagata, T.: A quantitative study on the ganglion cells in the small intestine of the dog. Med. J. Shinshu Univ. 10, 1-11, 1965.

Nagata, T.: A radioautographic study on the RNA synthesis in the hepatic and the intestinal epithelial cells of mice after feeding with special reference to binuclearity. Med. J. Shinshu Univ. 11, 49-61, 1966.

Nagata, T.: On the increase of binucleate cells in the ganglion cells of dog small intestine due to experimental ischemia. Med. J. Shinshu Univ. 12, 93-113, 1967a.

Nagata, T.: A radioautographic study on the protein synthesis in the hepatic and the intestinal epithelial cells of mice, with special reference to binucleate cells. Med. J. Shinshu Univ. 12, 247-257, 1967b.

Nagata, T.: Chapter 3. Application of microspectrophotometry to various substances. In , Introduction to Microspectrophotometry. Isaka, S., Nagata, T., Inui, N., Eds., Olympus Co., Tokyo, pp. 49-155, 1972a.

Nagata, T.: Electron microscopic dry-mounting autoradiography. Proc. 4th Internat. Cong. Histochem. Cytochem. Kyoto, pp. 43-44, 1972b.

Nagata, T.: Electron microscopic radioautography of intramitochondrial RNA synthesis of HeLa cells in culture. Histochemie 32, 163-170, 1972c.

Nagata, T.: Quantitative electron microscope radioautography of intramitochondrial nucleic acid synthesis. Acta Histochem. Cytochem. 5, 201-203, 1972d.

Nagata, T.: Electron microscopic observation of target cells previously observed by phase-contrast microscopy: Electron microscopic radioautography of laser beam irradiated cultured cells. J. Clin. Electron Microsc. 17, 589-590, 1984.

Nagata, T.: Principles and techniques of radioautography. In, Histo- and Cyto-chemistry 1985, Japan Society of Histochemistry and Cytochemistry, Ed., Gakusai Kikaku Co., Tokyo, pp. 207-226, 1985.

Nagata, T.:. Electron microscopic radioautography and analytical electron microscopy. J. Clin. Electron Microsc. 24, 441-442, 1991.

Nagata, T.: Radiolabeling of soluble and insoluble compounds as demonstrated by light and electron microscopy. Recent Advances in Cellular and Molecular Biology, Wegmann, R. J., Wegmann, M. A., Eds. Peters Press, Leuven, Vol. 6, pp. 9-21, 1992.

Nagata, T.: Quantitative analysis of histochemical reactions: Image analysis of light and electron microscopic radioautograms. Acta Histochem. Cytochem. 26, 281-291, 1993a.

Nagata, T. Quantitative light and electron microscopic radioautographic studies on macromolecular synthesis in several organs of prenatal and postnatal aging mice. Chinese J. Histochem. Cytochem. 2: 106-108, 1993b.

Nagata, T.: Electron microscopic radioautography with cryo-fixation and dry-mounting procedure. Acta Histochem. Cytochem. 27: 471-489, 1994a.

Nagata, T.: Application of electron microscopic radioautography to clinical electron microscopy. Med. Electron Microsc. 27; 191-212, 1994b.

Nagata, T.: Radioautography in Medicine. Shinshu University Press, 268pp, Matsumoto, 1994c.

Nagata, T.: Radioautography, general and special. In, Histo- and Cyto-chemistry 1994, Japan Society of Histochemistry and Cytochemistry, ed, pp. 219-231, Gakusai Kikaku Co., Tokyo, 1994d.

Nagata, T., Application of electron microscopic radioautography to clinical electron microscopy. Med. Electron Microsc. 27, 191-212, 1994e.
Nagata, T.: Light and electron microscopic radioautographic study on macromolecular synthesis in digestive organs of aging mice. Cell. Mol. Biol. 41, 21-38, 1995a.
Nagata, T.: Histochemistry of the organs: Application of histochemistry to anatomy. Acta Anat. Nippon. 70, 448-471, 1995b.
Nagata, T.: Three-dimensional observation of whole mount cultured cells stained with histochemical reactions by ultrahigh voltage electron microscopy. Cell. Mol. Biol. 41, 783-792, 1995c.
Nagata, T.: Morphometry in anatomy: image analysis on fine structure and histochemical reactions with special reference to radioautography. Ital. J. Anat. 100 (Suppl. 1), 591-605, 1995d.
Nagata, T.: Technique and application of electron microscopic radioautography. J. Electron Microsc. 45, 258-274, 1996a.
Nagata, T.: Techniques of light and electron microscopic radioautography. In, Histochemistry and Cytochemistry 1996. Proc. Xth Internat. Congr. Histochem. Cytochem. Acta Histochem. Cytochem. 29 (Suppl.), 343-344, 1996b.
Nagata, T.: Remarks: Radioautographology, general and special. Cell. Mol. Biol. 42 (Suppl.), 11-12, 1996c.
Nagata, T.: On the terminology of radioautography vs. autoradiography. J. Histochem. Cytochem. 44, 1209-1209, 1996d.
Nagata, T.: Techniques and applications of microscopic radioautography. Histol. Histopathol. 12, 1091-1124, 1997a.
Nagata T.: Three-dimensional observation on whole mount cultured cells and thick sections stained with histochemical reactions by high voltage electron microscopy. In, Recent Advances in Microscopy of Cells, Tissues and Organs, Motta, P., Ed., Antonio Delfino Editore, Roma, pp. 37-44, 1997b.
Nagata, T.: Radioautographic study on collagen synthesis in the ocular tissues. J. Kaken Eye Res. 15, 1-9, 1997c.
Nagata, T.: Techniques of radioautography for medical and biological research. Braz. J. Biol. Med. Res. 31, 185-195, 1998a.
Nagata, T.: Radioautographology, the advocacy of a new concept. Braz. J. Biol. Med. Res. 31, 201-241, 1998b.
Nagata, T.: Radioautographic studies on DNA synthesis of the bone and skin of aging salamander. Bull. Nagano Women's Jr. College 6, 1-14, 1998c.
Nagata, T.: 3D observation of cell organelles by high voltage electron microscopy. Microscopy and Analysis, Asia Pacific Edition, 9, 29-32, 1999a.
Nagata, T.: Application of histochemistry to anatomy: Histochemistry of the organs, a novel concept. Proc. XV Congress of the International Federation of Associations of Anatomists, Ital. J. Anat. Embryol. 104 (Suppl. 1), 486-486, 1999b.
Nagata, T.: Aging changes of macromolecular synthesis in various organ systems as observed by microscopic radioautography after incorporation of radiolabeled precursors. Methods Find. Exp. Clin. Pharmacol. 21, 683-706, 1999c.
Nagata, T.: Radioautographic study on protein synthesis in mouse cornea. J. Kaken Eye Res. 8, 8-14, 1999d.
Nagata, T.: Radioautographology, general and special: a novel concept. Ital. J. Anat. Embryol. 104 (Suppl. 1), 487-487, 1999e.

Nagata, T.: Three-dimensional observations on thick biological specimens by high voltage electron microscopy. Image Analysis Stereolog. 19, 51-56, 2000a.

Nagata, T.: Biological microanalysis of radiolabeled and unlabeled compounds by radioautography and X-ray microanalysis. Scanning Microscopy International, 14, on line, 2000b.

Nagata, T.: Electron microscopic radioautographic study on protein synthesis in pancreatic cells of perinatal and aging mice. Bull. Nagano Women's Jr. College 8, 1-22, 2000c.

Nagata, T.: Light microscopic radioautographic study on radiosulfate incorporation into the tracheal cartilage in aging mice. Acta Histochem. Cytochem. 32, 377-383, 2000d.

Nagata, T.: Introductory remarks: Special radioautographology. Cell. Mol. Biol. 46 (Congress Suppl.), 161-161, 2000e.

Nagata, T.: Special radioautographology: the eye. J. Kaken Eye Res. 18, 1-13, 2000f.

Nagata, T.: Three-dimensional high voltage electron microscopy of thick biological specimens. Micron 32, 387-404, 2001a.

Nagata, T.: Three-dimensional and four-dimensional observation of histochemical and cytochemical specimens by high voltage electron microscopy. Acta Histochem. Cytochem. 34, 153-169, 2001b.

Nagata, T. : Special cytochemistry in cell biology. In, Internat. Rev. Cytol. Jeon, K.W., ed., Vol. 211, Chapter 2, Academic Press, New York, pp. 33-154, 2001c.

Nagata, T. : Radioautographology General and Special, In, Prog. Histochem. Cytochem., Graumann, W., Ed., Vol. 37 No. 2, Urban & Fischer, Jena, pp. 57-226, 2002.

Nagata T.: Light and electron microscopic study on macromolecular synthesis in amitotic hepatocyte mitochondria of aging mice. Cell. Mol. Biol. 49, 591-611, 2003.

Nagata, T.: X-ray microanalysis of biological specimens by high voltage electron microscopy. In, Prog. Histochem. Cytochem., Graumann, W., Ed., Vol. 39, No. 4, Urban & Fischer Verlag, Jena, pp. 185-320, 2004.

Nagata T.: Aging changes of macromolecular synthesis in the uro-genital organs as revealed by electron microscopic radioautography. Ann. Rev. Biomed. Sci. 6, 13-78, 2005.

Nagata T.: Electron microscopic radioautographic study on protein synthesis in hepatocyte mitochondria of developing mice. Ann. Microsc. 6, 43-54, 2006a.

Nagata T.: Electron microscopic radioautographic study on nucleic acids synthesis in hepatocyte mitochondria of developing mice. The Sci. World J. 6: 1583-1598, 2006b.

Nagata T.: Macromolecular synthesis in hepatocyte mitochondria of aging mice as revealed by electron microscopic radioautography. I: Nucleic acid synthesis. In, Modern Research and Educational Topics in Microscopy. Mendez-Vilas, A. and Diaz, J. Eds., Formatex Micrscopy Series No. 3, Vol. 1, Formatex, Badajoz, Spain, pp. 245-258, 2007a.

Nagata T.: Macromolecular synthesis in hepatocyte mitochondria of aging mice as revealed by electron microscopic radioautography. II: Protein synthesis. In, Modern Research and Educational Topics in Microscopy. Mendez-Vilas, A. and Diaz, J. eds., Formatex Micrscopy Series No. 3, Vol. 1, Formatex, Badajoz, Spain, pp. 259-271, 2007b.

Nagata, T.: Electron microscopic radioautographic study on macromolecular synthesis in hepatocyte mitochondria of aging mouse. J. Cell Tissue Res. 7, 1019-1029, 2007c.

Nagata, T.; Electron microscopic radioautographic study on nucleic acids synthesis in hepatocyte mitochondria of developing mice. Trends Cell Molec. Biol. 2, 19-33, 2007d.

Nagata, T.; Aging changes of macromolecular synthesis in the mitochondria of mouse hepatocytes as revealed by microscopic radioautography. Ann. Rev. Biomed. Sci. 9, 30-36, 2007e.

Nagata, T.: Radioautographology, Bull. Shinshu Institute Alternat. Med. 2, 3-32, 2007f.

Nagata, T.: Electron microscopic radioautographic study on mitochondrial DNA synthesis in adrenal cortical cells of developing mice. J. Cell. Tis. Res. 8, 1303-1312, 2008a.

Nagata T.: Electron microscopic radioautographic study on mitochondrial DNA synthesis in adrenal cortical cells of developing and aging mice. The Sci. World J. 8, 683-697. 2008b.

Nagata, T.: Sexual difference between the macromolecular synthesis of hepatocyte mitochondria in male and female mice in aging as revealed by electron microscopic radioautography. Chapter 22. In, Women and Aging: New Research, H. T. Bennninghouse, A. D. Rosset, Eds. Nova Biomed. Books, New York, pp. 461-487, 2009a

Nagata, T.: Protein synthesis in hepatocytes of mice as revealed by electron microscopic radioautography. In, Protein Biosynthesis. Esterhouse, T. E. and Petrinos, L. B., Eds., Nova Biomed. Books, New York, pp. 133-161, 2009b.

Nagata, T.: Electron microscopic radioatuographic studies on macromolecular synthesis in mitochondria of various cells. 18EMSM Conference Proc. 9th Asia-Pacific Microscopy Conference (APMC9), Kuala Lumpur, Malaysia, pp. 48-50, 2009c.

Nagata, T.: Recent studies on macromolecular synthesis labeled with ^{3}H-thymidine in various organs as revealed by electron microscopic radioautography. Current Radiopharmaceutics 2, 118-128, 2009d.

Nagata, T.: Electron microscopic radioautographic study on mitochondrial DNA synthesis in adrenal medullary cells of developing and aging mice. J. Cell Tissue Res. 9, 1793-1802, 2009e.

Nagata, T.: Applications of high voltage electron microscopy to thick biological specimens. Ann. Microsc. 9, 4-40, 2009f.

Nagata, T.: Electron microscopic radioautographic study on DNA synthesis of mitochondria in adrenal medullary cells of aging mice. Open Anat. J. 1, 14-24, 2009g.

Nagata, T.: Electron microscopic radioautographic studies on macromolecular synthesis in mitochondria of animal cells in aging. Ann. Rev. Biomed. Sci. 11, 1-17, 2009h.

Nagata, T.: Electron microscopic radioautographic studies on macromoleclular synthesis in mitochondria of some organs in aging animals. Bull. Shinshu Inst. Alternat. Med. Welfare 4, 15-38, 2009i.

Nagata, T.: Electron microscopic radioautographic study on mitochondrial DNA synthesis in adreno-cortical cells of aging ddY mice. Bull. Shinshu Inst. Alternat. Med. Welfare 4, 51-66, 2009j.

Nagata T.: Electron microscopic radioautographic study on mitochondrial RNA synthesis in adrenocortical cells of aging mice. Open Anat J. 2, 91-97, 2010a.

Nagata T. Electron microscopic radioautographic study on mitochondrial RNA synthesis in adrenal medullary cells of aging and senescent mice. J Cell Tissue Res. 10, 2213-2222, 2010b.

Nagata, T.: Macromolecular synthesis in the livers of aging mice as revealed by electron microscopic radioautography. In, Prog. Histochem. Cytochem., Sasse, D., Ed., Elsevier, Amsterdam, Boston, London, New York, Oxford, Paris, Philadelphia, San Diego, St. Louis, Vol. 45, No. 1, pp. 1-80, 2010c.

Nagata, T.: Electron microscopic radioautographic study on protein synthesis of mitochondria in adrenal medullary cells of aging mice. Bulletin Shinshu Inst Alternat Med Welfare 5, 25-37, 2010d.

Nagata, T.: Electron microscopic radioautographic study on mitochondrial RNA synthesis in adrenal cortical and medullary cells of aging mice. J. Biomed. Sci. Enginer. 4, 219-232, 2010e.

Nagata, T.: Electron microscopic radioautographic study on protein synthesis of mitochondria in adrenal cortical cells of aging mice. Bulletin Shinshu Inst. Alternat. Med. Welfare 5, 38-52, 2010f.

Nagata T.: Electron microscopic radioautographic study on mitochondrial DNA, RNA and protein synthesis in adrenal cells of aging mice. Formatex Microscopy Series No. 3, Vol. 3, Formatex, Badajoz, Spain, in press, 2010g.

Nagata, T.: Electron microscopic radioautographic studies on macromolecular synthesis in mitochondria of animal cells in aging. Ann. Rev. Biomed. Sci. 12, 1-29, 2010h.

Nagata, T., Cui, H., Gao, F.: Radioautographic study on glycoprotein synthesis in the ocular tissues. J. Kaken Eye Res. 13, 11-18, 1995.

Nagata, T., Cui, H., Kong, Y.: The localization of TGF-b1 and its mRNA in the spinal cords of prenatal and postnatal aging mice demonstrated with immunohistochemical and in situ hybridization techniques. Bull. Nagano Women's Jr. College, 7, 75-88, 1999a.

Nagata, T., Cui, H., Liang, Y.: Light microscopic radioautographic study on the protein synthesis in the cerebellum of aging mouse. Bull. Nagano Women's Jr. College, 9, 41-60 (2001).

Nagata, T., Fujii, Y., Usuda, N.: Demonstration of extranuclear nucleic acid synthesis in mammalian cells under experimental conditions by electron microscopic radioautography. Proc. 10th Internat. Congr. Electr. Microsc. 2, 305-306, 1982b.

Nagata, T., Hirano, I., Shibata, O., Nagata, T.: A radioautographic study on the DNA synthesis in the hepatic and the pancreatic acinar cells of mice during the postnatal growth, with special reference to binuclearity. Med. J. Shinshu Univ. 11, 35-42, 1966.

Nagata, T., Ito, M., Chen, S.: Aging changes of DNA synthesis in the submandibular glands of mice as observed by light and electron microscopic radioautography. Ann. Microsc. 1, 4-12, 2000a.

Nagata, T. Ito, M., Liang, Y.: Study of the effects of aging on macromolecular synthesis in mouse steroid secreting cells using microscopic radioautography. Methods Find. Exp. Clin. Pharmacol. 22, 5-18, 2000b.

Nagata, T., Iwadare, I., Murata, F.: Electron microscopic radioautography of nucleic acid synthesis in cultured cells treated with several carcinogens. Acta Pharmacol. Toxicol. 41, 64-65, 1977c.

Nagata, T., Kawahara, I.: Radioautographic study of the synthesis of sulfomucin in digestive organs of mice. J. Trace Microprobe Analysis 17, 339-355, 1999.

Nagata, T., Kawahara, I., Usuda, N., Maruyama, M., Ma, H.: Radioautographic studies on the glycoconjugate synthesis in the gastrointestinal mucosa of the mouse. In, Glycoconjugate in Medicine, Ohyama, M., Muramatsu, T., Eds, pp. 251-256, Professional Postgrad. Service, Tokyo, 1988a.

Nagata, T., Kong, Y.: Distribution and localization of TGFb1 and bFGF, and their mRNAs in aging mice. Bull. Nagano Women's Jr. College 6, 87-105, 1998.

Nagata, T., Ma, H., Electron microscopic radioautographic study on mitochondrial DNA synthesis in hepatocytes of aging mouse. Ann. Microsc. 5, 4-18, 2005a.
Nagata, T., Ma, H., Electron microscopic radioautographic study on RNA synthesis in hepatocyte mitochondria of aging mouse. Microsc. Res. Tech. 67, 55-64, 2005b.
Nagata, T., Momoze, S.: Aging changes of the amitotic and binucleate cells in dog livers. Acta Anat. Nipponica 34, 187-190, 1959.
Nagata, T., Morita, T., I. Kawahara, I.: Radioautographic studies on radiosulfate incorporation in the digestive organs of mice. Histol. Histopathol. 14, 1-8, 1999b.
Nagata, T., Murata, F.: Electron microscopic dry-mounting radioautography for diffusible compounds by means of ultracryotomy. Histochemistry 54, 75-82, 1977.
Nagata, T., Murata, F., Yoshida, K., Ohno, S., Iwadare, N.: Whole mount radioautography of cultured cells as observed by high voltage electron microscopy. Proc. Fifth Internat. Conf. High Voltage Electron Microsc. 347-350, 1977d.
Nagata, T., Nawa, T.: A modification of dry-mounting technique for radioautography of water-soluble compounds. Histochemie 7, 370-371, 1966a.
Nagata, T., Nawa, T.: A radioautographic study on the nucleic acids synthesis of binucleate cells in cultivated fibroblasts of chick embryos. Med. J. Shinshu Univ. 11, 1-5, 1966b.
Nagata, T., Nawa, T., Yokota, S.: A new technique for electron microscopic dry-mounting radioautography of soluble compounds. Histochemie 18, 241-249, 1969.
Nagata, T., Nishigaki, T., Momose, Y.: Localization of anti-allergic agent in rat mast cells demonstrated by light and electron microscopic radioautography. Acta Histochem. Cytochem. 19, 669-683, 1986b.
Nagata, T., Ohno, S., Kawahara, I., Yamabayashi, S., Fujii, Y., Murata, F.: Light and electron microscopic radioautography of nucleic acid synthesis in mitochondria and peroxisomes of rat hepatic cells during and after DEHP administration. Acta Histochem. Cytochem. 16, 610-611, 1979.
Nagata, T., Ohno, S., Murata, F.: Electron microscopic dry-mounting radioautography for soluble compounds. Acta Phamacol. Toxicol. 41, 62-63, 1977a.
Nagata, T., Ohno, S., Yoshida, K., Murata, F.: Nucleic acid synthesis in proliferating peroxisomes of rat liver as revealed by electron microscopical radioautography. Histochem. J. 14, 197-204, 1982a.
Nagata, T., Olea, M. T.: Electron microscopic radioautographic study on the protein synthesis in aging mouse spleen. Bull. Nagano Women's Jr. College 7, 1-9, 1999.
Nagata, T., Shibata, O., Omochi, S.: A new method for radioautographic osbservation on isolated cells. Histochemie 2, 255-259, 1961
Nagata, T., Shibata, O., Nawa, T.: Simplified methods for mass production of radioautograms. -Acta Anat. Nippon.42, 162-166, 1967a.
Nagata, T., Shibata, O., Nawa, T.: Incorporation of tritiated thymidine into mitochondrial DNA of the liver and kidney cells of chickens and mice in tissue culture. Histochemie 10, 305-308, 1967b.
Nagata, T., Shimamura, K., Onozawa, M., Kondo, T., Ohkubo, K., Momoze, S.: Relationship of binuclearity to cell function in some organs. I. Frequencies of binucleate cells in some organs of toads in summer and winter. Med. J. Shinshu Univ. 5, 147-152, 1960a.
Nagata, T., Shimamura, K., Kondo, T., Onozawa, M., Momoze, S., Okubo, M.: Relationship of binuclearity to cell function in some organs. II. Variation of frequencies of

binucleate cells in some organs of dogs owing to aging. Med. J. Shinshu Univ. 5, 153-158, 1960b.

Nagata, T., Steggerda, F. R.: Histological study on the deganglionated small intestine of the dog. Physiologist 6, 242-242, 1963.

Nagata, T., Steggerda, F. R.: Observations on the increase of binucleate cells in the ganglion cells of the dog's intestine due to experimental ischemia. Anat. Rec. 148, 315-315, 1964.

Nagata, T., Toriyama, K., Kong, Y., Jin, C., Gao, F.: Radioautographic study on DNA synthesis in the ciliary bodies of aging mice. J. Kaken Eye Res.12, 1-11, 1994.

Nagata, T., Usuda, N.: Image processing of electron microscopic radioautograms in clinical electron microscopy. J. Clin. Electron. Microsc. 18, 451-452, 1985.

Nagata, T., Usuda, N.: Studies on the nucleic acid synthesis in pancreatic acinar cells of aging mice by means of electron microscopic radioautography. J. Clin. Electron Microsc. 19, 486-487, 1986.

Nagata, T., Usuda, N.: Electron microscopic radioautography of protein synthesis in pancreatic acinar cells of aging mice. Acta Histochem. Cytochem. 26, 481-481, 1993a.

Nagata, T., Usuda, N.: In situ hybridization by electron microscopy using radioactive probes. J. Histochem. Cytochem. 41, 1119-1119, 1993b.

Nagata, T., Usuda, N., Ma, H.: Electron microscopic radioautography of nucleic acid synthesis in pancreatic acinar cells of prenatal and postnatal aging mice. Proc. XIth Intern. Cong. Electr. Microsc. 3, 2281-2282, 1984.

Nagata, T., Usuda, N., Ma, H.: Electron microscopic radioautography of lipid synthesis in pancreatic cells of aging mice. J. Clin. Electr. Microsc. 23, 841-842, 1990.

Nagata, T., Usuda, N., Maruyama, M., Ma, H.: Electron microscopic radioautographic study on lipid synthesis in perinatal mouse pancreas. J. Clin. Electr. Microsc. 21, 756-757, 1988b.

Nagata, T., Usuda, N., Suzawa, H., Kanzawa, M.: Incorporation of ^{3}H-glucosamine into the pancreatic cells of aging mice as demonstrated by electron microscopic radioautography. J. Clin. Electron Microsc. 25, 646-647, 1992.

Nagata, T., Yamabayashi, S.: Intracellular localization of ^{3}H-befunolol by means of electron microscopic radioautography of cryo-fixed ultrathin sections. J. Clin. Electron Microsc. 16, 737-738, 1983.

Nagata, T., Yoshida, K., Murata, F.: Demonstration of hot and cold mercury in the human thyroid tissues by means of radioautography and chemography. Acta Pharmacol. Toxicol. 41, 60-61, 1977b.

Nagata, T., Yoshida, K., Ohno, S., Murata, F.: Ultrastructural localization of soluble and insoluble ^{3}H-methyl prednisolone as revealed by electron microscopic dry-mounting radioautography. Proc. 9th Internat. Congr. Electr. Microsc. 2, 40-41, 1978b.

Nishigaki, T., Momose, Y., Nagata, T.: Light microscopic radioautographic study of the localization of anti-allergic agent, tranilast, in rat mast cells. Histochem. J. 19, 533-536, 1987.

Nishigaki, T., Momose, Y., Nagata, T.: Electron microscopic radioautographic study of the localization of an anti-allergic agent, tranilast, in rat mast cells. Cell. Mol. Biol. 36, 65-71, 1990a.

Nishigaki, T., Momose, Y., Nagata, T.: Localization of the anti-allergic agent tranilast in the urinary bladder of rat as demonstrated by light microscopic radioautography. Drug Res. 40, 272-275, 1990b.

Oguchi, K., Nagata, T.: A radioautographic study of activated satellite cells in dystrophic chicken muscle. In, Current Research in Muscular Dystrophy Japan. The Proc. Ann. Meet. Muscular Dystrophy Res. 1980, pp. 16-17, Ministry of Welfare of Japan, Tokyo, 1980.

Oguchi, K., Nagata, T.: Electron microscopic radioautographic observation on activated satellite cells in dystrophy chickens. In, Clinical Studies on the Etiology of Muscular Dystrophy. Annual Report on Neurological Diseases 1981, pp. 30-33, Ministry of Welfare of Japan, Tokyo, 1981.

Ohno, S., Fujii, Y., Usuda, N., Endo, T., Hidaka, H., Nagata, T.: Demonstration of intracellular localization of calmodulin antagonist by wet-mounting radioautography. J. Electron Microsc. 32, 1-12, 1983.

Ohno, S., Fujii, Y., Usuda, N., Nagata, T., Endo, T., Tanaka, T., Hidaka, H.: Intracellular localization of calmodulin antagonists (W-7). In, Calmodulin and intracellular Ca^{2+} receptors. Kakiuchi, S., Hidaka, H, Means, A. R., Eds., pp. 39-48, Plenum Publishing Co., New York, 1982.

Olea, M. T.: An ultrastructural localization of lysosomal acid phosphatase activity in aging mouse spleen: a quantitative X-ray microanalytical study. Acta Histochem. Cytochem. 24, 201-208, 1991.

Olea, M. T., Nagata, T.: X-ray microanalysis of cerium in mouse spleen cells demonstrating acid phosphatase activity using high voltage electron microscopy, Cell. Mol. Biol. 37, 155-163, 1991.

Olea, M. T., Nagata, T. : Simultaneous localization of ^{3}H-thymidine incorporation and acid phosphatase activity in mouse spleen: EM radioautography and cytochemistry. Cell. Mol. Biol. 38, 115-122, 1992a.

Olea, M. T., Nagata, T.: A radioautographic study on RNA synthesis in aging mouse spleen after ^{3}H-uridine labeling in vitro. Cell. Mol. Biol. 38, 399-405, 1992b.

Oliveira, S. F., Nagata, T., Abrahamsohn, P. A., Zorn, T. M. T.: Electron microscopic radioautographic study on the incorporation of ^{3}H-proline by mouse decidual cells. Cell. Mol. Biol. 37, 315-323, 1991.

Oliveira, S. F., Abrahamsohn, P. A., Nagata, T., Zorn, T. M. T.: Incorporation of ^{3}H-amino acids by endometrial stromal cells during decidualization in the mouse. A radioautographical study. Cell. Mol. Biol. 41, 107-116, 1995.

Pearse, A. G. E.: Histochemistry, Theoretical and Applied. 4th Ed. Vol. 1. 439 pp., 1980, Vol. 2. 1055 pp., 1985, Vol. 3. Ed. with P. Stoward, 728 pp. Churchill Livingstone, Edinburgh, London and New York, 1991.

Sakai, Y., Ikado, S., Nagata, T.: Electron microscopic radioautography of satellite cells in regenerating muscles. J. Clin. Electr. Microsc. 10, 508-509, 1977.

Sato, A.: Quantitative electron microscopic studies on the kinetics of secretory granules in G-cells. Cell Tissue Res. 187, 45-59, 1978.

Sato, A., Iida, F., Furihara, R., Nagata, T.: Electron microscopic raioautography of rat stomach G-cells by means of ^{3}H-amino acids. J. Clin. Electron Microsc. 10, 358-359, 1977.

Shimizu, T., Usuda, N., Yamanda, T., Sugenoya, A., Iida, F.: Proliferative activity of human thyroid tumors evaluated by proliferating cell nuclear antigen/cyclin immnohistochemical studies. Cancer 71, 2807-2812, 1993.

Sun, L.: Age related changes of RNA synthesis in the lungs of aging mice by light and electron microscopic radioautography. Cell. Mol. Biol. 41, 1061-1072, 1995.

Sun, L., Gao, F., Duan, H., Nagata, T.: Light microscopic radioautography of DNA synthesis in pulmonary cells in aging mice. In, Radioautography in Medicine, Nagata, T. Ed., pp. 201-205, Shinshu University Press, Matsumoto, 1994.

Sun, L., Gao, F., Nagata, T.: Study on the DNA synthesis of pulmonary cells in aging mice by light microscopic radioautography. Cell. Mol. Biol. 41, 851-859, 1995a.

Sun, L., Gao, F., Jin, C., Duan, H., Nagata, T.: An electron microscopic radioautographic study on the DNA synthesis of pulmonary tissue cells in aging mice. Med. Electron. Microsc. 28, 129-131, 1995b.

Sun, L., Gao, F., Jin, C., Nagata, T.: DNA synthesis in the tracheae of aging mice by means of light and electron microscopic radioautography. Acta Histochem. Cytochem. 30, 211-220, 1997a.

Sun, L., Gao, F., Nagata, T.: A Light Microscopic radioautographic study on protein synthesis in pulmonary cells of aging mice. Acta Histochem. Cytochem. 30, 463-470, 1997b.

Suzuki, K., Imada, T., Gao, F., Ma, H., Nagata, T.: Radioautographic study of benidipine hydrochloride: localization in the mesenteric artery of spontaneously hypertensive rat. Drug Res. 44, 129-133, 1994.

Terauchi, A., Mori, T., Kanda, H., Tsukada, M., Nagata, T.: Radioautographic study of 3H-taurine uptake in mouse skeletal muscle cells. J. Clin. Electron Microsc. 21, 627-628, 1988.

Terauchi, A., Nagata, T.: Observation on incorporation of ^{3}H-taurine in mouse skeletal muscle cells by light and electron microscopic radioautography. Cell. Mol. Biol. 39, 397-404, 1993.

Terauchi, A., Nagata, T.: In corporation of ^{3}H-taurine into the blood capillary cells of mouse skeletal muscle. Radioautography in Medicine, Nagata, T. ed., Shinshu University Press, Matsumoto, 1994.

Toriyama, K.: Study on the aging changes of DNA and protein synthesis of bipolar and photo-receptor cells of mouse retina by light and electron microscopic radioautography. Cell. Mol. Biol. 41, 593-601, 1995.

Tsukahara, S., Yoshida, K., Nagata, T.: A radioautographic study on the incorporation of ^{14}C-bupranolol (beta-blocking agent) into the rabbit eye. Histochemistry 68, 237-244, 1980.

Usuda, N., Nagata, T.: Electron microscopic radioautography of acyl-CoA mRNA by in situ hybridization. J. Clin. Electron Microsc. 25, 332-333, 1992.

Usuda, N., Nagata, T.: The immunohistochemical and in situ hybridization studies on hepatic peroxisomes. Acta Histochem. Cytochem. 28, 169-172, 1995.

Usuda, N., Hanai, T., Morita, T., Nagata, T.: Radioautographic demonstration of peroxisomal acyl-CoA oxidase mRNA by in situ hybridization. In, Recent advances in cellular and molecular biology, Vol. 6. Molecular biology of nucleus, peroxisomes, organelles and cell movement. Wegmann, R. J., Wegmann, M., Eds, pp.181-184, Peeters Press, Leuven, 1992.

Uwa, H., Nagata, T.: Cell population kinetics of the scleroblast during ethisterone-induced anal-fin process formation in adult females of the Medaka. Dev. Growth Different. 9, 693-694, 1976.

Watanabe, I., Makiyama, M. C. K., Nagata, T.: Electron microscopic radioautographic observation of the submandibular salivary gland of aging mouse. Acta Microscopica 6. 130-131, 1997.

Yamabayashi, S., Gunarso, W., Tsukahara, S., Nagata, T.: Incorporation of ^{3}H-befunolol (beta blocking agent) into melanin granules of ocular tissues in the pigmented rabbits. I. Light microscopic radioautography. Histochemistry 73, 371-375, 1981.

Yamada, A. T.: Timely and topologically defined protein synthesis in the periimplanting mouse endometrium revealed by light and electron microscopic radioautography. Cell. Mol. Biol. 39, 1-12, 1993.

Yamada, A., Nagata, T.: Ribonucleic acid and protein synthesis in the uterus of pregnant mouse during activation of implantation window. Med. Electron Microsc. 27, 363-365, 1992a.

Yamada, A., Nagata, T.: Light and electron microscopic raioautography of DNA synthesis in the endometria of pregnant-ovariectomized mice during activation of implantation window. Cell. Mol. Biol. 38, 763-774, 1992b.

Yamada, A., Nagata, T.: Light and electron microscopic raioautography of RNA synthesis of peri-implanting pregnant mouse during activation of receptivity for blastocyst implantation. Cell. Mol. Biol. 38, 211-233, 1993.

Yoshinaga, K.: Uterine receptivity for blastcyst implantation. Ann. N. Y. Acad. Sci. USA, 541, 424-431, 1988.

Yoshizawa, S., Nagata, A., Honma, T., Oda, M., Murata, F., Nagata, T.: Study of ethionine pancreatitis by means of electron microscopic radioautography. J. Clin. Electron Microsc. 7, 349-350, 1974.

Yoshizawa, S., Nagata, A., Honma, T., Oda, M., Murata, F., Nagata, T.: Radioautographic study of protein synthesis in pancreatic exocrine cells of alcoholic rats. J. Clin. Electron. Microsc. 10, 372-373, 1977.

17

Macromolecular Synthesis in the Endocrine, Nervous and Sensory Systems

Tetsuji Nagata[1,2]
[1]*Department of Anatomy and Cell Biology, Shinshu University School of Medicine, Matsumoto*
[2]*Shinshu Institute of Alternative Medicine and Welfare, Nagano*
Japan

1. Introduction

This chapter deals with the last forth part of the application of microscopic radioautography to the organ systems, including the endocrine system, the nervous system and the sensory organs. The endocrine system includes the hypophysis, the pineal body, the thyroid gland, the parathyroid gland, the thymus, the adrenal gland, the islet of Langerhans and the reproductive glands, i. e. the testis and the ovary. The nervous system includes the central nervous system, i.e. the brains and spinal cord and the peripheral nerves, i.e. the ganglion and nerves, while the sensory system includes, the skin, the visual, the stato-acoustic, the olfactory and the gustatory organs. We have studied some of these organs, not all of them yet.

2. Macromolecular synthesis in the endocrine system

Among the endocrine organs, we studied macromolecular synthesis in the adrenal gland and the steroid secreting cells of both sexes, the Leydig cells of the testis and the ovarian follicular cells in mice. On the other hand, incorporation of mercury chloride into the human thyroid tissues was also studied (Nagata 2002).

2.1 The DNA synthesis in the endocrine system

Among the endocrine organs, we studied DNA synthesis in the adrenal glands and steroid secreting cells of both sexes, the Leydig cells of the testis and the ovarian follicular cells in mice.

2.1.1 The DNA synthesis in the adrenal gland

We studied the adrenal tissues of aging mice, both the adrenal cortex and the medulla, from embryo to postnatal 2 years in senescence. Some of the results were already published in several original articles (Ito 1996, Ito and Nagata 1996, Liang 1998, Liang et al. 1999, Nagata 1994, 1999c, 2000a,b, 2008a,b, 2009c,d,e,f,g,h,i,j, 2010a, Nagata et al. 2000b). The results shall be summarized in this review.

2.1.1.1 The DNA synthesis in the adrenal cortex

We studied the adrenal tissues of mice at various ages from embryo to postnatal 2 years (Ito 1996, Ito and Nagata 1996, Nagata 2008a,b, 2009c,d,e,f,g,h,i,j). The adrenal tissues obtained from ddY strain mice at various ages from embryo day 19 to postnatal day 30 of both sexes, consisted of the adrenal cortex and the adrenal medulla. The former consisted of 3 layers, zona glomerulosa (Fig. 20A), zona fasciculata (Fig. 20B) and zona reticularis (Fig. 20C), developing gradually with aging from perinatal stage at embryonic day 19 to postnatal stages as day 1, 3, 9, 14, month 1, 2, 6, 12, 24 as observed by light microscopy.

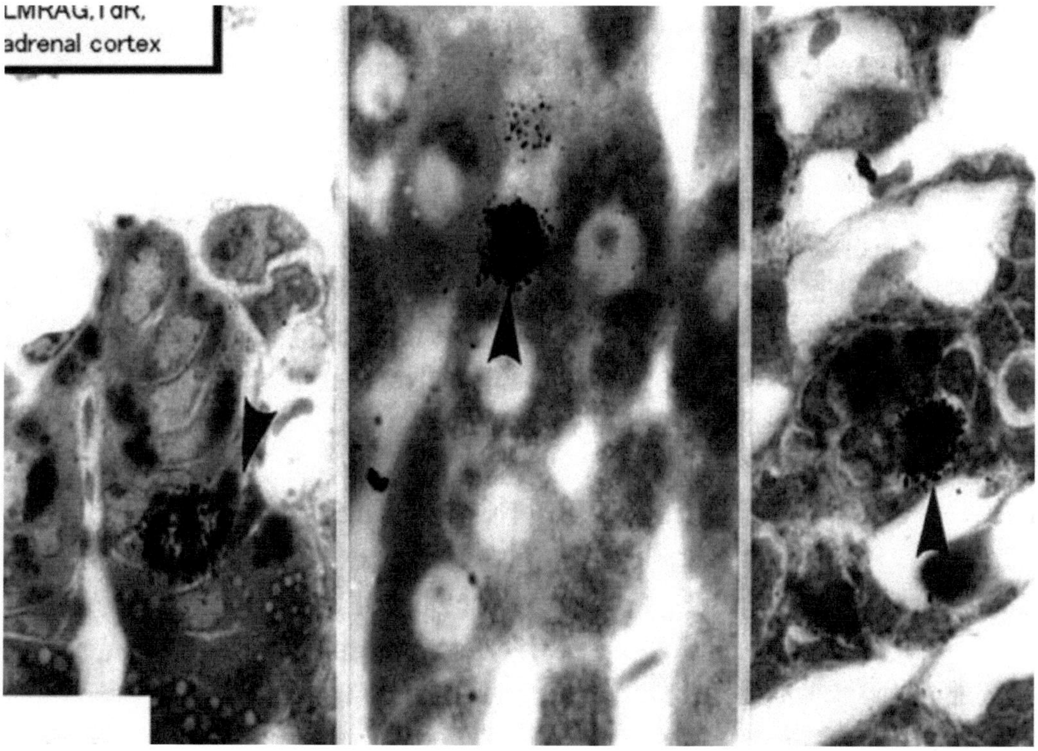

Fig. 20. LM RAG of a young mouse adrenal cortex, labeled with ^{3}H-thymine, showing DNA synthesis (arrow) in 3 layers, zona glomerulosa (left), zona fasciculate (middle), zona reticularis (right). From Nagata, T.: Annals Microsc. Vol. 10, p. 61, 2010, Microsc. Soc. Singapore.

At embryonic day 19 and postnatal day 1, the 3 layers of the adreno-cortical cells, zona glomerulosa (Fig. 21D), zona fasciculate (Fig. 21E) and zona reticularis were composed mainly of polygonal cells, while the specific orientation of the 3 layers was not yet well established as observed by EMRAG. At postnatal day 3, orientation of 3 layers, especially the zona glomerulosa became evident. At postnatal day 9 and 14, the specific structure of the 3 layers was completely formed and the arrangements of the cells in respective layers became typical especially at day 14 (Fig. 21D) and month 1 (Fig. 21E) to 24. Observing the ultrastructure of the adreno-cortical cells by electron microscopy, cell organelles including mitochondria were not so well developed at perinatal and early postnatal stages from embryonic day 19 to postnatal day 9. However, these cell organelles, mitochondria, endoplasmic reticulum, Golgi apparatus, appeared well developed similarly to the adult stages at postnatal day 14. The zona glomerulosa is the thinnest layer found at the outer zone, covered by the capsule, consisted of closely packed groups of columnar or pyramidal cells forming arcades of cell columns. The cells contained many spherical mitochondria and well developed smooth surfaced endoplasmic reticulum but a compact Golgi apparatus in day 14 animals. The zona fasciculate was the thickest layer, consisted of polygonal cells that were larger than the glomerulosa cells, arranged in long cords disposed radially to the medulla containing many lipid droplets. The mitochondria were less numerous and were more variable in size and shape than those of the glomerulosa cells, while the smooth surfaced endoplasmic reticulum were more developed and the Golgi apparatus was larger than the glomerulosa. In the zona reticularis, the parallel arrangement of cell cords were anastomosed showing networks continued to the medullar cells. The mitochondria were less numerous and were more variable in size and shape than those of the glomerulosa cells like the fasciculata cells, as well as the smooth surfaced endoplasmic reticulum were developed and the Golgi apparatus was large like the fasciculata cells. However, the structure of the adrenal cortex tissues showed changes due to development and aging at respective developmental stages.

Observing both LM and EM RAG of the adrenal cortex labeled with ^{3}H-thymidine, demonstrating DNA synthesis, the silver grains were found over the nuclei of some adreno-cortical cells in S-phase of cell cycle mainly in perinatal stages at embryonic day 19, postnatal day 1 and day 3, while less at day 9 and day 14 to month 1-24 (Ito 1996, Ito and Nagata 1996, Nagata 2008a,b,c,d, 2009c,d,e). Those labeled cells were found in all the 3 layers (Fig. 20), the zona glomerulosa (Fig. 20 left), the zona fasciculata (Fig. 20 middle) and the zona reticularis (Fig. 20 right), at respective aging stages. In labeled adreno-cortical cells in the 3 layers the silver grains were mainly localized over the euchromatin of the nuclei and only a few or several silver grains were found over the mitochondria of these cells as observed by EM RAG (Fig. 21D,E).

To the contrary, most adreno-cortical cells were not labeled with any silver grains in their nuclei nor cytoplasm, showing no DNA synthesis after labeling with ^{3}H-thymidine. The labeling indices in respective 3 zones in the cortex as well as the medulla showed the maxima at perinatal stages and decreased due to aging (Fig. 22A,B). Among many unlabeled adreno-cortical cells, however, most cells in the 3 layers were observed to be labeled with several silver grains over their mitochondria due to the incorporations of ^{3}H-thymidine especially at the perinatal stages from embryonic day 19 to postnatal day 1, day 3, day 9 and 14 (Fig. 21D). The ultrastructural localizations of silver grains over the mitochondria were mainly on the mitochondrial matrices and some over the cristae or membranes.

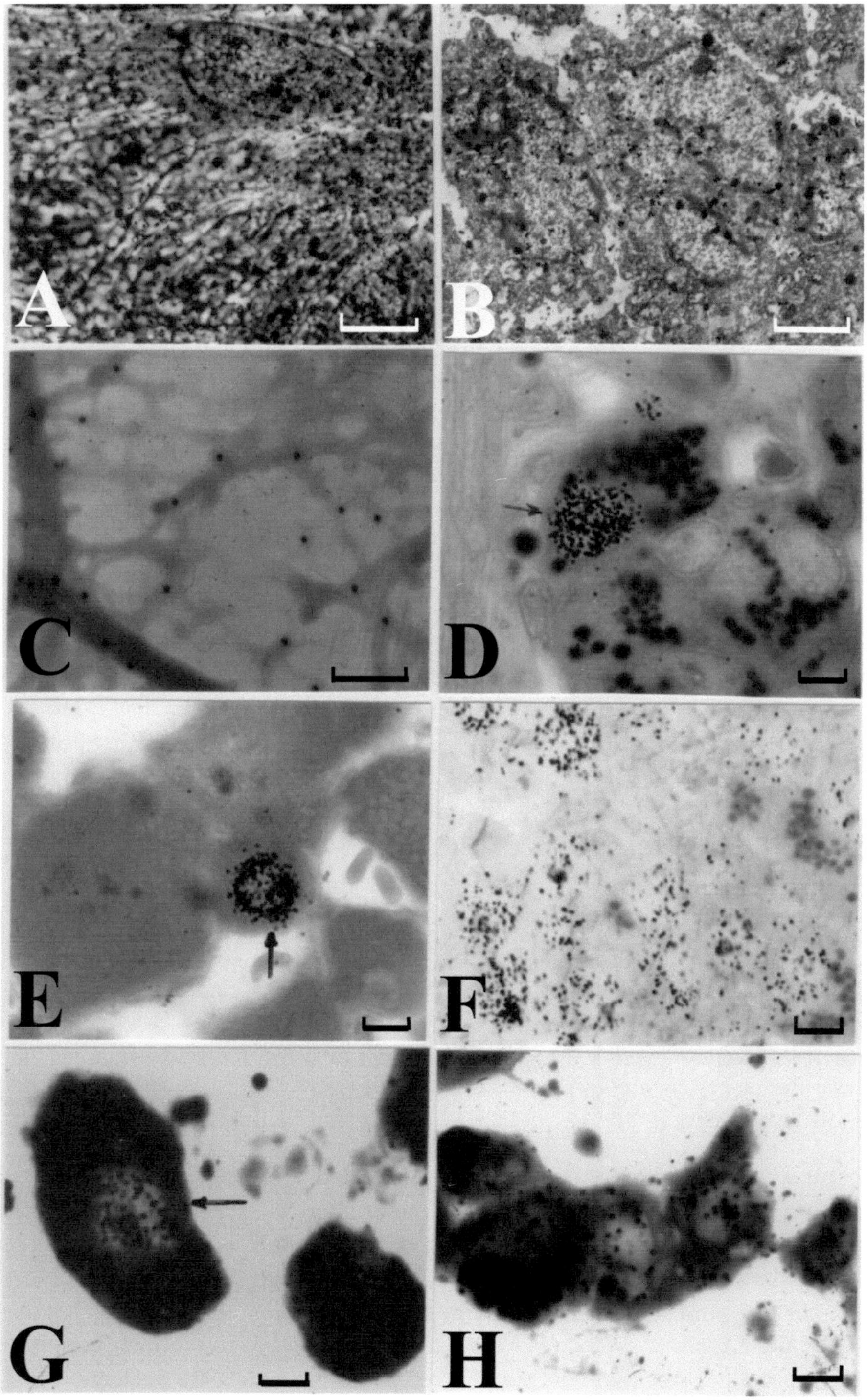

Fig. 21. LM and EM RAG of the endocrine organs. From Nagata, T.: Special Cytochemistry in Cell Biology, In, Internat. Rev. Cytol. Vol. 211, No. 1, p. 115, 2001, Academic Press, San Diego, USA, London, UK.

Fig. 21A. EM RAG of human thyroid cancer cells, labeled with $^{205}HgCl_2$ in vitro, quick frozen, freeze-dried, embedded in Epoxy resin, dry-sectioned, and radioautographed by dry-mounting procedure for demonstrating soluble compounds, many silver grains showing soluble $^{205}HgCl_2$ incorporations. x15,000.
Fig. 21B. EM RAG of human thyroid cancer cells, labeled with $^{205}HgCl_2$ in vitro, chemically fixed doubly in buffered glutaraldehyde and osmium tetroxide, dehydrated, embedded in Epoxy resin, wet-sectioned, and radioautographed by wet-mounting procedure for demonstrating insoluble compounds, less silver grains showing insoluble $^{205}HgCl_2$ incorporations. x15,000.
Fig. 21C. EM photo of a human thyroid cancer cell, fixed in paraformaldehyde and glutaraldehyde mixture, embedded in Lowicryl K4M, sectioned and immuno-stained with anti-keratin antibody by the protein-A gold technique, demonstrating keratin filaments. x15,000.
Fig. 21D. LM RAG of the zona glomelurosa of the adrenal cortex of a postnatal day 14 mouse labeled with ^{3}H-thymidine, showing DNA synthesis. x900.
Fig. 21E. LM RAG of the zona fasciculata of the adrenal cortex of a postnatal month 6 mouse labeled with ^{3}H-thymidine, showing DNA synthesis. x900.
Fig. 21F. LM RAG of the zona gromeulosa of the adrenal cortex of a prenatal day 19 mouse labeled with ^{3}H-uridine, showing RNA synthesis. x1,000.
Fig. 21G. LM RAG of the interstitial tissues of a postnatal month 12 male mouse labeled with ^{3}H-thymidine, showing DNA synthesis in Leydig cells. x1,000.
Fig. 21H. LM RAG of the interstitial tissues of a postnatal day 3 male mouse labeled with ^{3}H-uridine, showing RNA synthesis in Leydig cells. x1,000.

2.1.1.1.1 The number of mitochondria of mouse adreno-corticl cells

Preliminary quantitative analysis on the number of mitochondria in 10 adreno-cortical cells whose nuclei were labeled with silver grains and other 10 cells whose nuclei were not labeled in each aging group revealed that there was no significant difference between the number of mitochondria and the labeling indices ($P<0.01$). Thus, the number of mitochondria and the labeling indices were later calculated regardless whether their nuclei were labeled or not (Ito 1996, Ito and Nagata 1996, Nagata 2008a,b,c,d, 2009c,d,e). The results obtained from the number of mitochondria in adreno-cortical cells in the 3 layers of respective animals in 10 aging groups at perinatal stages, prenatal embryo day 19, postnatal day 1, 3, 9 and 14, showed an gradual increase from the prenatal day 19 (glomerulosa 12.5, fasciculata 14.9, reticularis 15/2/cell) to postnatal day 14 and month 1, 2 (glomerulosa 62.2, fasciculata 64.0, reticularis 68.2/cell) to month 6 and 12. The increase from embryo day 19 to postnatal month 2 was stochastically significant ($P <0.01$). Then, they did not change significanctly from month 12 to 24 (Fig. 22A).

2.1.1.1.2 The DNA synthesis in the mitochondria of mouse adreno-cortical cells

The results of visual grain counts on the number of mitochondria labeled with silver grains obtained from 10 adreno-cortical cells in the 3 layers of each animal labeled with ^{3}H-thymidine demonstrating DNA synthesis in 10 aging groups at perinatal stages, prenatal embryo day 19, postnatal day 1, 3, 9 and 14, and month 1, 2, 6, 12 and 24 were reported previously (Ito 1996, Ito and Nagata 1996, Nagata 2008a,b, 2009c,d,e). The results demonstrated that the numbers of labeled mitochondria with ^{3}H-thymidine showing DNA synthesis gradually increased from prenatal embryo day 19 (glomerulosa 0.3, fasciculata 0.5, reticularis 0.4/cell) to postnatal day 14, month 1 and 2 (glomerulosa 5.3, fasciculata 5.0, reticularis 6.2/cell), reaching the maximum, then decreased to month 6, 12 and 24 (Fig. 22A). The increase and decrease were stochastically significant (P <0.01).

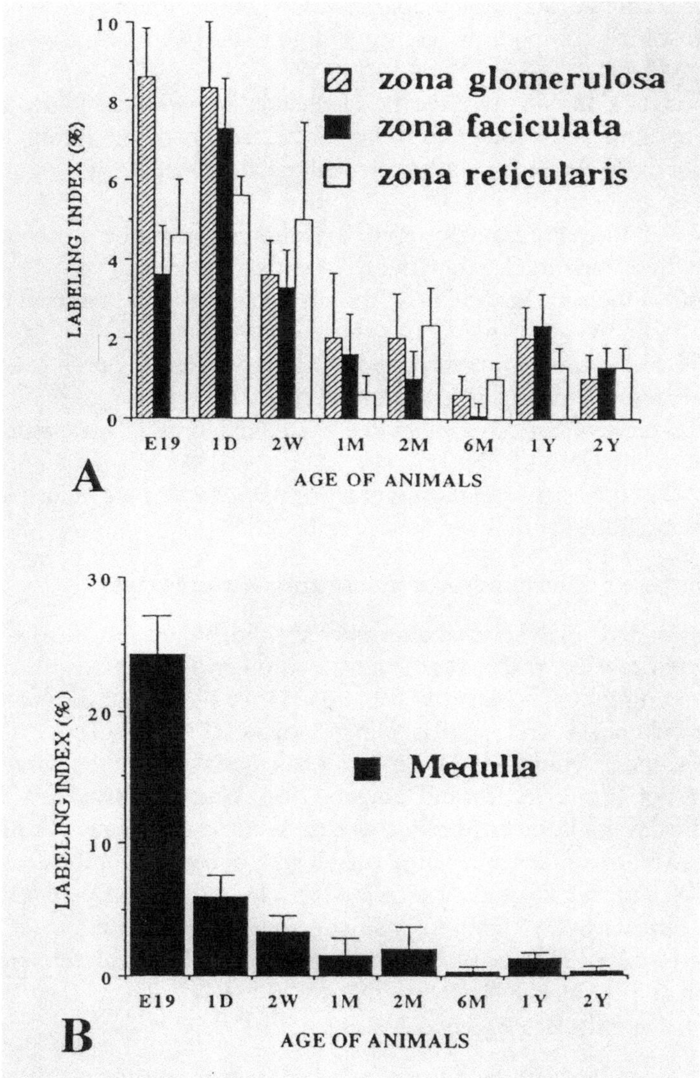

Fig. 22. Histogram showing aging changes of average labeling indices in respective cell types of the adrenal glands of aging mice labeled with ^{3}H-thymidine showing DNA synthesis. Mean ± Standard Deviation. From Nagata, T.: Radioautographology, General and Special. In, Prog. Histochem. Cytochem. Vol. 37, No. 2, p. 171, 2002, Urban & Fischer, Jena, Germany

Fig. 22A. The adrenal cortex.

Fig. 22B. The adrenal medulla.

2.1.1.1.3 The labeling index of DNA synthesis in mouse adreno-cortical mitochondria

On the other hand, the labeling indices in respective aging stages were calculated from the number of labeled mitochondria, dividing by the number of total mitochondria per cell which were mentioned previously (Ito 1996, Ito and Nagata 1996, Nagata 2008a,b, 2009c,d,e,j, 2010e). The results showed that the labeling indices gradually increased from prenatal day 19 (glomerulosa 2.4, fasciculata 2.7, reticularis 2.6%) to postnatal day 14, month 1 and 2 (glomerulosa 8.5, fasciculata 7.8, reticularis 8.8%), reaching the maximum and decreased to month 6 (glomerulosa 4.1, fasciculata 4.2, reticularis 3.8%), 12 and 24 (Fig. 23C). The increase and decrease were stochastically significant (P <0.01).

2.1.1.2 The DNA synthesis in mouse adreno-medullary cells

We studied the adrenal tissues of mice at various ages from embryo to postnatal 2 years. The adrenal tissues obtained from ddY strain mice at various ages from embryo day 19 to postnatal day 30 of both sexes, consisted of the adrenal cortex and the adrenal medulla (Ito 1996, Ito and Nagata 1996, Nagata 2008a,b, 2009c,d,e,g, 2010d,e,f,g). The former consited of 3 layers, zona glomerulosa, zona fasciculata and zona reticularis, developing gradually with aging as observed by light microscopy (Fig. 20), while the latter consisted of 2 cell types in one layer when observed by electron microscopy (Nagata 2009c,d,e, 2010d,e,f,g). At embryonic day 19 and postnatal day 1, the 3 layers of the adreno-cortical cells, zona glomerulosa, zona fasciculate and zona reticularis were composed mainly of polygonal cells, while the specific orientation of the 3 layers was not yet well established. However, the orientation of 3 layers became evident at day 3 and completely formed at day 14 (Fig. 20) and to month 1-24 (Fig. 21D,E,F). On the other hand, the medulla consisted of only one layer containing 2 types of cells, adrenalin cell and noradrenalin cell. The former contains adrenalin granlules with low electron density, while the latter contains noradrenalin granules with high electron density.

The adrenal medulla is the deepest layer in the adrenal glands, surrounded by the 3 layers of the adrenal cortex as observed by light and electron microscopy (Ito 1996, Ito and Nagata 1996, Nagata 2008a,b,c,d, 2009c,d,e, 2010d,e,f,g), containing either adrenalin granules or noradrenalin granules. Quantitative analysis revealed that the numbers of mitochondria in both adrenalin and noradrenalin cells at various ages increased from fetal day 19 to postnatal month 1 due to aging of animals, respectively, but did not decrease to month 24, while the number of labeled mitochondria and the labeling indices of intramitochondrial DNA synthesis changed due to aging. When they were labeled with ^{3}H-thymidine silver grains appeared over some nuclei of both cell types at perinatal stages, but they appeared almost all the cell bodies containing mitochondria. Quantitative analysis revealed that the numbers of mitochondria in both adrenalin and noradrenalin cells at various ages increased from fetal day 19 to postnatal month 1 due to aging of animals, respectively, while the number of labeled mitochondria and the labeling indices of intramitochondrial DNA synthesis incorporating ^{3}H-thymidine increased from fetal day 19 to postnatal day 14 (2 weeks), reaching the maxima, and decreased to month 24. It was shown that the activity of intramitochnodrial DNA synthesis in the adrenal medullary cells in aging mice increased and decreased due to aging of animals.

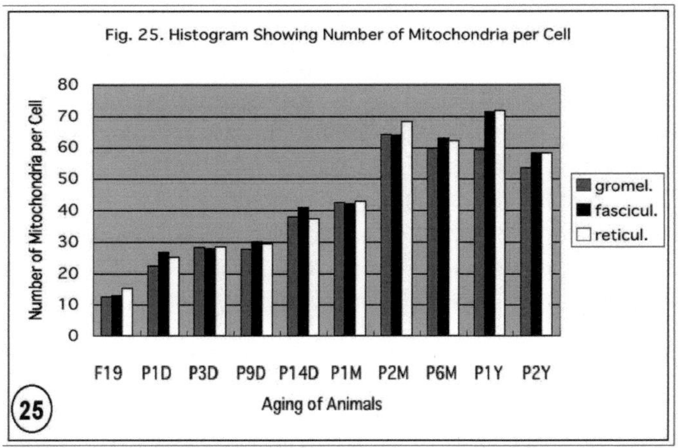

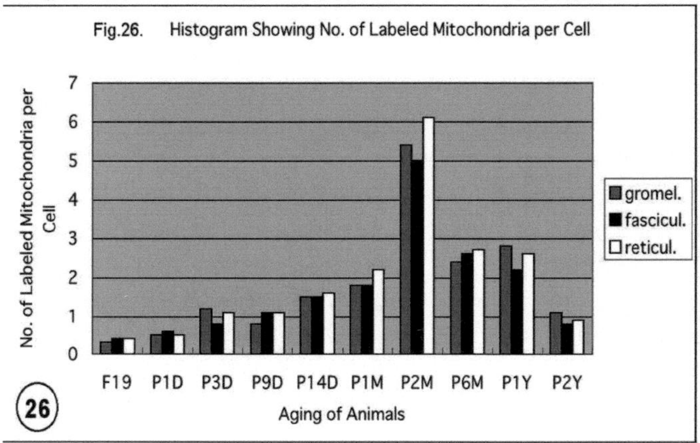

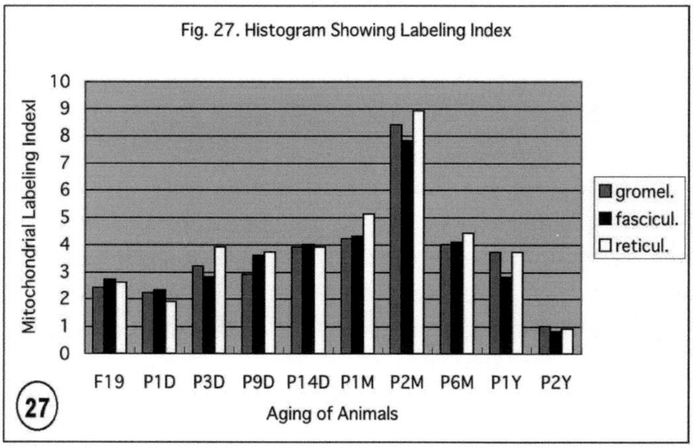

Fig. 23. Histogram showing aging changes of the respective cell types of the adrenal glands of aging mice labeled with ^{3}H-thymidine showing DNA synthesis. Mean ± Standard Deviation. From Nagata, T.: Current Radiopharmaceutics, Vol. 2, p. 173, 2002.
Fig. 23A(25). The number of mitochondria per cell.
Fig. 23B(26). The number of labeled mitochondria per cell.
Fig. 23C(27). The mitochondrial labeling index.

2.1.2 The DNA synthesis in the islets of Langerhans

When we studied macromolecular synthesis in the exocrine pancreatic cells of aging mice by LM and EMRAG we also studied the islet cells of Langerhans together with the exocrine cells, using RI labeled precursors such as ^{3}H-thymidine for DNA (Nagata and Usuda 1985, 1986, Nagata et al. 1986a,b), ^{3}H-uridine for RNA (Nagata and Usuda 1985, 1993b, Nagata et al. 1986a,b), ^{3}H-leucine for proteins (Nagata 2000, Nagata and Usuda 1993a, 1995), ^{3}H-glucosamine for glucides (Nagata et al. 1992), ^{3}H-glycerol for lipids (Nagata et al. 1988b, 1990). The results showed that the islets cells, A, B and C cells, incorporated those precursors to synthesize DNA, RNA, proteins and glucides. The labeling index of DNA synthesis and the densities of silver grains showing RNA, proteins and glucides syntheses were high at prenatal and earlier postnatal stages from day 1 to day 14, then decreased from 1 month to 1 years due to aging. However, the labeling indices by ^{3}H-thymidine and the grain counts by ^{3}H-uridine and ^{3}H-leucine in the endocrine cells were less than those in the exocrine cells at the same ages.

2.1.3 The DNA synthesis in the Leydig cells of the testis

The cells of Leydig can be found in the interstitial tissues between the seminiferous tubules of the testis of mammals (Gao 1993, Gao et al. 1994, 1995a,b, Nagata et al. 2000b). They are identified as spherical, oval, or irregular in shape and their cytoplasms contain lipid droplets. We studied the macromolecular synthesis of the cells in the testis of several groups of litter ddY mice at various ages from fetal day 19 to postnatal aging stages up to 2 years senescence by LM and EMRAG using ^{3}H-thymidine, ^{3}H-uridine and ^{3}H-leucine incorporations.

The Leydig cells from embryonic stage to senescent stages were labeled with ^{3}H-thymidine as observed by LMRAG (Fig. 21G). The changes of the numbers of labeled Leydig cells with the ^{3}H-thymidine incorporation into the nuclei showing the DNA synthesis were found in these cells at different aging stages. Only a few cells were labeled after ^{3}H-thymidine at embryonic day 19. At early postnatal stages, there was a slight increase of the number of labeled cells. The number of labeled cells from perinatal stage to postnatal 14 days and 1, 2, 6 months were similar to the values found at prenatal and early postnatal stages. The notable increases in the number of labeled cells of Leydig were found from 9 months to 2 years in senescence. The labeling indices with ^{3}H-thymidine in perinatal stages to postnatal 6 months were low (5-10%) but increased at 9 months and maintained high level (50-60%) to 2 years (Gao 1993, Gao et al. 1994, 1995a, Nagata et al. 2000b). The labeling indices at senescent stages still maintained a relatively high level and they were obviously higher than those of young animals. By electron microscopy, typical Leydig cells contained abundant cell organelles such as smooth surfaced endoplasmic reticulum, Golgi apparatus and mitochondria with tubular cristae. The silver grains were mainly localized over the euchromatin of labeled nucleus. Some of the grains were also localized over some of the mitochondria in both the nuclei labeled and unlabeled cells.

2.1.4 The DNA synthesis in the ovarian follicles

The ovarian follicles in the ovaries of mature mice are one of the steroid secreting organs in female animals. We studied the DNA and RNA synthesis of the follicular cells in the developing ddY mice ovaries in several aging groups at postnatal day 1, 3, 7, 14, 30 and 60 by LM and EMRAG using ^{3}H-thymidine and ^{3}H-uridine (Li 1994, Li and Nagata 1995). From the results it was shown that both DNA and RNA synthesis in the ovarian follicular cells were observed (Fig. 16G). Quantitative analysis, as expressed with labeling indices and grain counts, revealed that both increased significantly from postnatal day 1 to 3, then decreased from day 7 to 60 (Fig. 19A). Comparing the results to other female genital cells, a paralleled alteration of both DNA and RNA synthesis was revealed between the ovarian follicular cells and other uterine or oviductal cells (Fig. 19B,C). On the other hand, the glycoconjugate synthesis as shown by the uptake of $^{35}SO_4$ in mouse ovary during the estrus cycle was also demonstrated (Li et al. 1992).

2.2 The RNA synthesis in the endocrine system

We studied the RNA synthesis of the adrenal glands and the cells of Leydig in the testis of aging mice among the endocrine organs after the administration of ^{3}H-uridine at various ages.

2.2.1 The RNA synthesis in the adrenal glands

The RNA synthesis in the adrenal glands in aging mice was studied in both the adrenal cortex and the adrenal medulla after administration of ^{3}H-uridine in many groups of mice at various ages from perinatal stages to senescence at year 2.

2.2.1.1 The RNA synthesis in aging mouse adreno-cortical cells

Observing both LM and EM RAG labeled with ^{3}H-uridine, demonstrating RNA synthesis, the silver grains were found over the nuclei and cytoplasm of almost all the adreno-cortical cells from perinatal stages to postnatal month 1-24 (Liang 1998, Liang et al. 1999, Nagata et al. 2000b, Nagata 2010a). Those labeled cells were found in all the 3 layers, the zona glomerulosa (Fig. 21F), the zona fasciculata and the zona reticularis, at respective aging stages. In labeled adreno-cortical cells in the 3 layers the silver grains were mainly localized over the euchromatin of the nuclei and several silver grains were found over the endoplasmic reticulum, ribosomes and mitochondria of these cells. The ultrastructural localizations of silver grains over the mitochondria were mainly on the mitochondrial matrices and some over the cristae or membranes.

2.2.1.2 The RNA synthesis in the mitochondria of mouse adreno-cortical cells

The results of visual grain counts on the number of mitochondria labeled with silver grains obtained from 10 adreno-cortical cells in the 3 layers of each animal labeled with ^{3}H-uridine demonstrating RNA synthesis in 10 aging groups at perinatal stages, prenatal embryo day 19, postnatal day 1, 3, 9 and 14, and month 1, 2, 6, 12 and 24 were reported previously (Liang 1998, Liang et al. 1999, Nagata et al. 2000b, Nagata 2010a). The results demonstrated that the numbers of labeled mitochondria with ^{3}H-uridine showing RNA synthesis gradually increased from prenatal embryo day 19 (glomerulosa 0.3, fasciculata 0.5, reticularis 0.4/cell) to postnatal day 14, month 1 and 2 (glomerulosa 5.3, fasciculata 5.0, reticularis 6.2/cell), reaching the maximum, then decreased to month 6, 12 and 24 (Fig. 23B). The increase and decrease were stochastically significant ($P < 0.01$).

2.2.1.3 The labeling index of RNA synthesis in mouse adreno-cortical mitochondria

On the other hand, the labeling indices in respective aging stages were calculated from the number of labeled mitochondria (Fig. 14B), dividing by the number of total mitochondria per cell (Fig. 24A) which were mentioned previously (Liang 1998, Liang et al. 1999, Nagata et al. 2000b, Nagata 2010a). The results showed that the labeling indices gradually increased from prenatal day 19 (glomerulosa 10.4, fasciculata 12.1, reticularis 13.1%) to postnatal day 1 (glomerulosa 12.6, fasciculata 11.4, reticularis 11.1%), 3, 9 (glomerulosa 16.6, fasciculata 18.0, reticularis 18.0%), reaching the maximum and decreased to day 14, month 1 (glomerulosa 11.4, fasciculata 11.0, reticularis 10.7%) 2 (glomerulosa 8.5, fasciculata 7.8, reticularis 8.8%), month 6 (glomerulosa 4.1, fasciculata 4.2, reticularis 3.8%), 12 and 24 (Fig. 24C). The increase and decrease were stochastically significant (P <0.01).

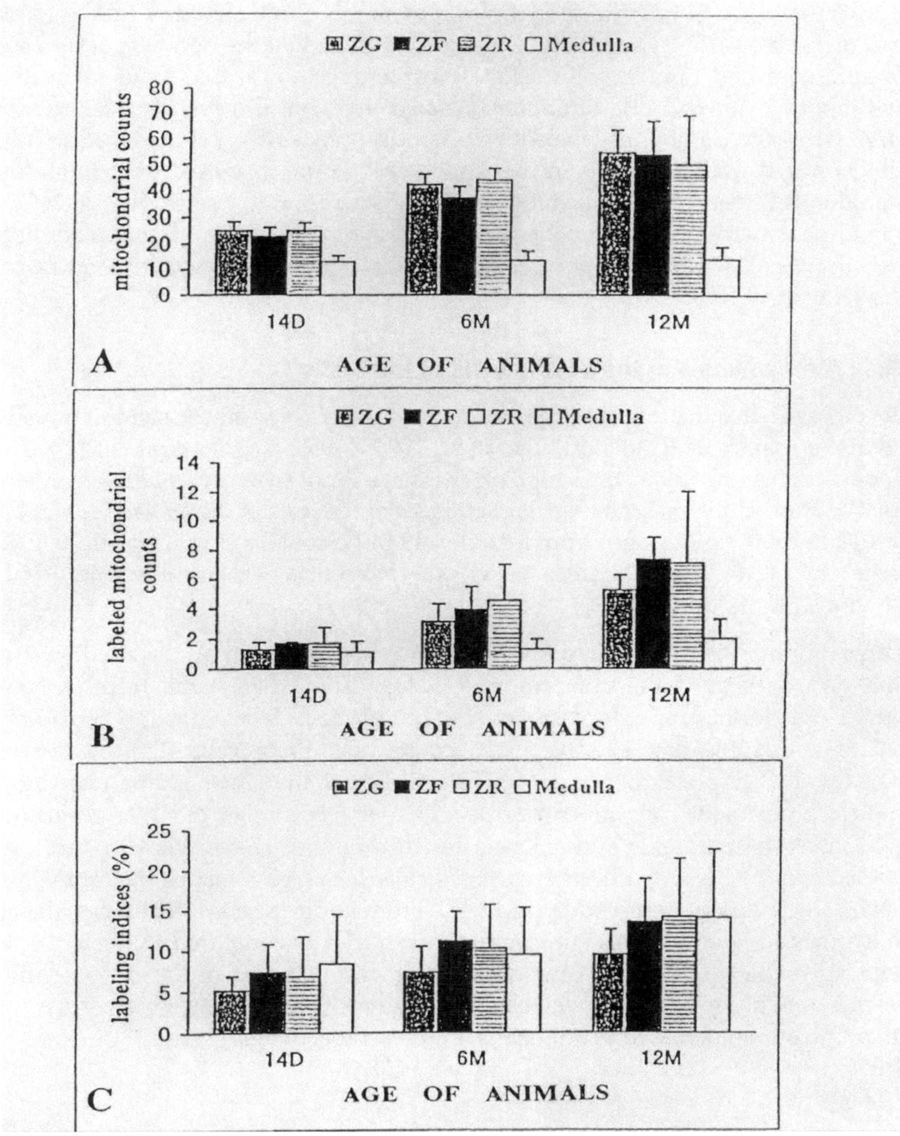

Fig. 24. Histogram showing aging changes of the respective cell types of the adrenal glands of aging mice labeled with ^{3}H-uridine showing RNA synthesis. Mean ± Standard Deviation. From Nagata, T.: Radioautographology, General and Special. In, Prog. Histochem. Cytochem. Vol. 37, No. 2, p. 173, 2002, Urban & Fischer, Jena, Germany

Fig. 24A. The number of mitochondria per cell.
Fig. 24B. The number of labeled mitochondria per cell.
Fig. 24C. The mitochondrial labeling index.

2.2.2 The RNA synthesis in aging mouse adreno-medullary cells

The adrenal medulla consists of 2 cell types, the adrenalin cells and noradrenalin cells. When they were labeled with ^{3}H-uridine, an RNA precursor, silver grains appeared over almost all the cells, both nuclei and cytoplasm containing mitochondria (Liang et al. 1999, Nagata et al. 2000b, 2010b). Quantitative analysis revealed that the numbers of mitochondria in both adrenalin and noradrenalin cells at various ages increased from fetal day 19 to postnatal month 1 due to aging of animals, respectively, but did not decrease to month 24 (Fig. 24A), while the number of labeled mitochondria (Fig. 24B) and the labeling indices of intramitochondrial RNA synthesis incorporating ^{3}H-uridine increased from fetal day 19 to postnatal month 1, reaching the maxima, but did not decrease to month 24 (Fig. 24C). It was shown that the activity of intramitochnodrial RNA synthesis in the adrenal medullary cells in aging mice increased but did not decrease due to aging of animals in contrast to DNA synthesis (Nagata 2010b).

2.2.3 The RNA synthesis in the Leydig cells of the testis

The cells of Leydig can be found in the interstitial tissues between the seminiferous tubules of the testis of mammals (Gao 1993, Gao et al. 1994, 1995a, Nagata et al. 2000b). They are identified as spherical, oval, or irregular in shape and their cytoplasms contain lipid droplets. We studied the macromolecular synthesis of the cells in the testis of several groups of litter ddY mice at various ages from fetal day 19 to postnatal aging stages up to 2 years in senescence by LM and EMRAG using ^{3}H-thymidine, ^{3}H-uridine and ^{3}H-leucine incorporations.

The incorporation of ^{3}H-uridine into RNA was observed in almost all the Leydig cells in the interstitial tissues of the testis from embryonic day 19 to 2 years after birth. A few silver grains over the nuclei and cytoplasm of the Leydig cells labeled with ^{3}H-uridine were observed at embryonic day 19. The silver grains over those cells slightly decreased at postnatal day 1, 3 (Fig. 21H), 7 and 14. The number of the silver grains over the nuclei increased from postnatal 1 months onwards. The average number of silver grains over the cytoplasm increased gradually and reached the maximum at 12 months after birth. At each stage, the activity of RNA synthesis was specifically localized over the euchromatin in the nucleus and nucleolus as observed by EMRAG. From adult to senescent stages, the activity of RNA synthesis maintained a high level in their nuclei as compared to the cytoplasm. In the cytoplasm of Leydig cells in respective aging groups some of the mitochondria and endoplasmic reticulum were also labeled with silver grains. It is noteworthy that the average grain counts increased prominently in the senescent aging groups at 1 and 2 years after birth.

2.3 The protein synthesis in the endocrine system

We studied the protein synthesis of the adrenal glands and the cells of Leydig in the testis of aging mice among the endocrine organs after the administration of ^{3}H-leucine at various ages.

2.3.1 The protein synthesis in the adrenal gland

Observing both LM and EM RAG labeled with ^{3}H-leucine, demonstrating protein synthesis, the silver grains were found over the nuclei and cytoplasm of almost all the adreno-cortical and adreno-medullary cells from perinatal stages to postnatal month 1-24 (Nagata 2010c,d,e,f,g). Those labeled cells were found in all the 3 layers, the zona glomerulosa, the zona fasciculata and the zona reticularis, as well as in all the cells in the adreno-medullae at respective aging stages.

2.3.1.1 Protein synthesis in mitochondria of mouse adrenal cells

In order to study the aging changes of intramitochondrial protein synthesis of mouse adrenal cells, 10 groups of developing and aging mice, each consisting of 3 individuals, total 30, from fetal day 19 to postnatal newborn at day 1, 3, 9, 14, adult at month 1, 2, 6 and senescent animals at month 12 (year 1) and 24 (year 2) were injected with ^{3}H-leucine, an protein precursor, sacrificed 1 hr later and the adrenal tissues were fixed and processed for electron microscopic radioautography. On electron microscopic radioautograms obtained from each animal, the number of mitochondria per cell, the number of labeled mitochondria with ^{3}H-leucine showing protein synthesis per cell and the mitochondrial labeling index in each adreno-cortical cells, in 3 zones, as well as in each adreno-medullary cells, 2 types of cells in the medulla, the adrenalin cells and the noradrenalin cells, were calculated and the results in respective aging groups were compared with each others (Nagata 2010c,d,e,f,g). Preliminary quantitative analysis on the number of mitochondria in either 10 adreno-cortical cells or adreno-medullary cells whose nuclei and cytoplasm were labeled with silver grains and other 10 cells whose nuclei and cytoplasm were not labeled in each aging group revealed that there was no significant difference between the number of mitochondria and the labeling indices ($P<0.01$). Thus, the number of mitochondria and the labeling indices were calculated regardless whether their nuclei were labeled or not (Nagata 2010d,e,f,g). The results demonstrated that the number of mitochondria in adreno-cortical cells in 3 zones, the zona glomerulosa, fasciculata and reticularis of respective mice at various ages increased from fetal day 19 to postnatal month 1 reaching the plateau from month 1 to 24 due to development and aging of animals, respectively, while the number of labeled mitochondria per cell and the labeling index of intramitochondrial protein synthesis incorporating ^{3}H-leucine increased from fetal day 19 to postnatal day 3 to month 2 and decreased to month 24. We carried out the quantitative analysis of these incorporations into nuclei and cell organelles of adrenal cells, both adrenal cortical cells and medullary cells, in aging mice from prenatal to postnatal newborn, juvenile, adult and senescent individuals (Nagata 2010a,b).

Observing EM radioautograms, the silver grains were found over the nuclei of some adreno-cortical cells labeled with ^{3}H-leucine demonstrating protein synthesis in all aging stages from perinatal stages at embryonic day 19, postnatal day 1 and day 3, day 9 and day 14 and adults at month 1, month 2, month 6, month 12 and month 24. Those labeled cells were found in all the 3 layers, the zona glomerulosa (Fig. 25A), the zona fasciculata and the zona reticularis (Fig. 25B, C), at respective aging stages. In the labeled adreno-cortical cells in 3 layers the silver grains were mainly localized over the euchromatin of the nuclei or a few or several silver grains were found over cytoplasmic organelles, especially over some of the mitochondria showing protein synthesis incorporating ^{3}H-leucine. The localizations of silver grains over the mitochondria were mainly on the mitochondrial matrices and some over the mitochondrial membranes as observed by high power magnification (Fig. 25C).

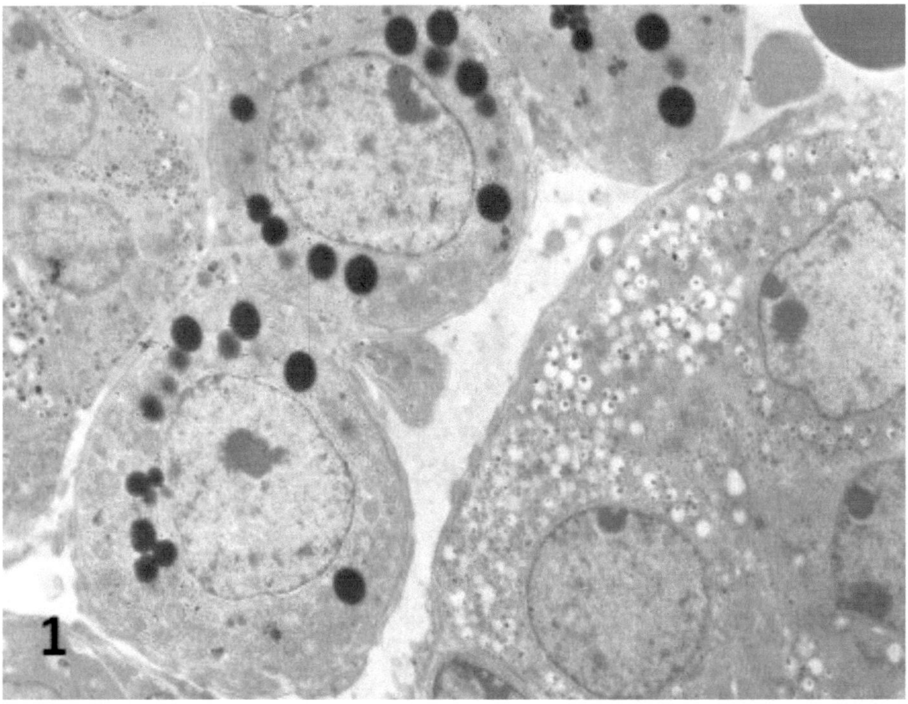

25A

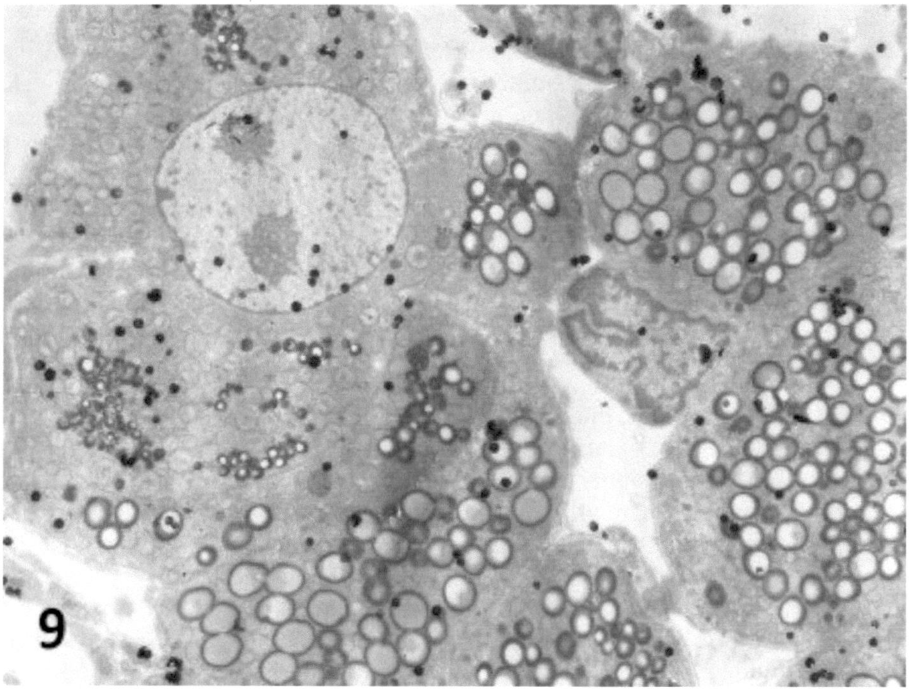

25B

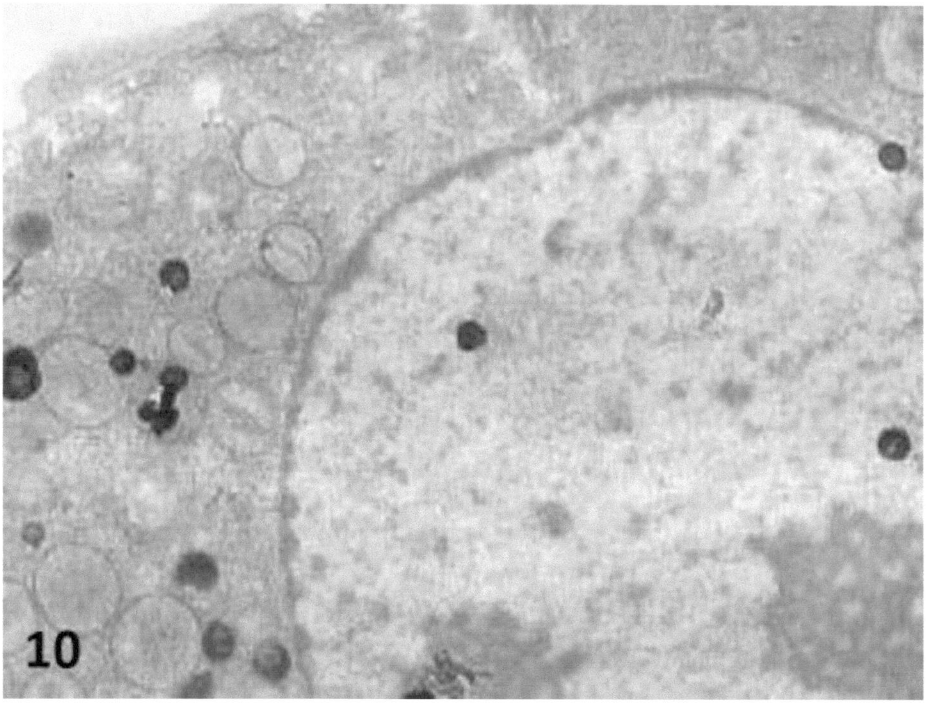

25C

Fig. 25. EMRAG of the adrenal cortical cells aging mice labeled with ^{3}H-leucine showing protein synthesis in the nucleus as well as in a few mitochondria. From Nagata, T.: Annals of Microscopy Vol. 4, p. 54-71, 2011.

Fig. 25A. EMRAG of the zona glomerulosa of a juvenile mouse at postnatal day 14, labeled with ^{3}H-leucine showing protein synthesis (several silver grains) in the nucleus as well as in a few mitochondria. x 3,000.

Fig. 25B. EMRAG of the zona reticularis of an old adult mouse aged at postnatal month 12, labeled with ^{3}H-leucine showing protein synthesis in the nucleus and a few mitochondria. x 3,000

Fig. 25C. High power magnification EMRAG of Fig. 24B, the zona reticularis of an old adult mouse aged at postnatal month 12, showing protein synthesis in a few mitochondria at upper left corner. x15,000.

2.3.1.1.1 Number of mitochondria of adreno-cortical cells in aging mice labeled with ^{3}H-leucine

Preliminary quantitative analysis on the number of mitochondria in either 10 adreno-cortical cells whose nuclei and cytoplasm were labeled with ^{3}H-leucine showing silver grains and other 10 cells whose nuclei were not labeled in each aging group revealed that there was no significant difference between the number of mitochondria and the labeling indices ($P<0.01$). Thus, the number of mitochondria and the labeling indices were calculated regardless whether their nuclei were labeled or not (Fig. 26A). The results obtained from the number of mitochondria in adreno-cortical cells in the 3 layers of respective animals in 10 aging groups at perinatal stages, prenatal embryo day 19, postnatal day 1, 3, 9 and 14, showed an gradual increase from the prenatal day 19 (glomerulosa 13.5, fasciculata 14.9, reticularis 15.2/cell) to postnatal day 14 (glomerulosa 37.7, fasciculata 37.8, reticularis 39.8/cell), and to adult stages at postnatal month 1 (glomerulosa 41.5, fasciculata 42.3, reticularis 42.9/cell), then increased at month 2 (glomerulosa 64.2, fasciculata 65.1, reticularis 67.2/cell), but kept plateau from month 6 (glomerulosa 61.7, fasciculata 62.9, reticularis 62.1/cell), to month 12 (glomerulosa 59.4, fasciculata 70.5, reticularis 71.4/cell) and month 24 (glomerulosa 59.5, fasciculata 62.2, reticularis 63.3/cell). The increase from embryo day 19 to postnatal month 1 was stochastically significant ($P < 0.01$).

2.3.1.1.2 Number of labeled mitochondria of adreno-cortical cells in aging mice labeled with ^{3}H-leucine

The results of visual grain counting on the number of mitochondria labeled with silver grains obtained from 10 adreno-cortical cells in the 3 layers of each animal labeled with ^{3}H-leucine demonstrating protein synthesis in 10 aging groups at perinatal stages, prenatal embryo day 19, postnatal day 1, 3, 9 and 14, month 1, 3, 6, 12 and 24, showed that the numbers of labeled mitochondria with ^{3}H-leucine showing protein synthesis per cell gradually increased from prenatal embryo day 19 (glomerulosa 0.3, fasciculata 0.4, reticularis 0.4/cell) to postnatal day 1 (glomerulosa 0.5, fasciculata 0.6, reticularis 0.5/cell), day 3 (glomerulosa 1.2, fasciculata 0.8, reticularis 1.1/cell), day 9 (glomerulosa 0.8, fasciculata 1.1, reticularis 1.1/cell), day 14 (glomerulosa 1.5, fasciculata 1.5, reticularis 1.6/cell), and month 1 (glomerulosa 1.8, fasciculata 1.8, reticularis 2.2/cell) and month 2 (glomerulosa 5.4, fasciculata 5.3, reticularis 5.8/cell), reaching the maximum, then decreased to month 6 (glomerulosa 4.5, fasciculata 4.8, reticularis 5.1/cell), month 12 (glomerulosa 5.2, fasciculata 5.8, reticularis 6.0/cell) and 24 (glomerulosa 3.8, fasciculata 4.1, reticularis 4.3/cell), as demonstrated in Fig. 26B.

2.3.1.1.3 Labeling index of mitochondria of adrenal cortical cells in aging mice labeled with ^{3}H-leucine

Finally, the labeling indices of adreno-cortical cells showing protein synthesis in respective aging stages were calculated from the number of labeled mitochondria (Fig. 26B) dividing by the number of total mitochondria per cell (Fig.26A), which were plotted in Fig. 26C, respectively.

The results showed that the labeling indices gradually increased from prenatal day 19 (glomerulosa 2.2, fasciculata 2.7, reticularis 2.6%) to postnatal newborn stage at postnatal day 1 (glomerulosa 2.2, fasciculate 2.4, reticularis 2.0%) and day 3 (glomerulosa 4.5 fasciculata 2.9, reticularis 3.9%), and to juvenile stage at postnatal day 9 (glomerulosa 2.8, fasciculate 3.7, reticularis 3.7%), day 14 (glomerulosa 3.9, fasciculate 3.9, reticularis 4.0%) and to the adult stage at month 1 (glomerulosa 4.3, fasciculate 4.2 reticularis 5.1%) and month 2 (glomerulosa 8.5, fasciculate 8.1, reticularis 8.6%), reaching the maximum, and decreased to month 6 (glomerulosa 7.3, fasciculate 7.6, reticularis 8.1%) to month 12 (glomerulosa 8.4, fasciculate 8.2, reticularis 8.4%) and finally to senescence at month 24 (glomerulosa 6.1, fasciculate 6.6 reticularis 6.8%), as is shown in the histogram (Fig. 26C).

From the results obtained it was shown that the labeling indices of the adreno-cortical cells in 3 layers of each animal labeled with ^{3}H-leucine demonstrating protein synthesis in 10 groups gradually increased from prenatal embryo day 19 to postnatal day 1, 3, 9, and 14, month 1, 2, reaching the maximum, and decreased to 6, 12 and 24, due to aging and senescence.

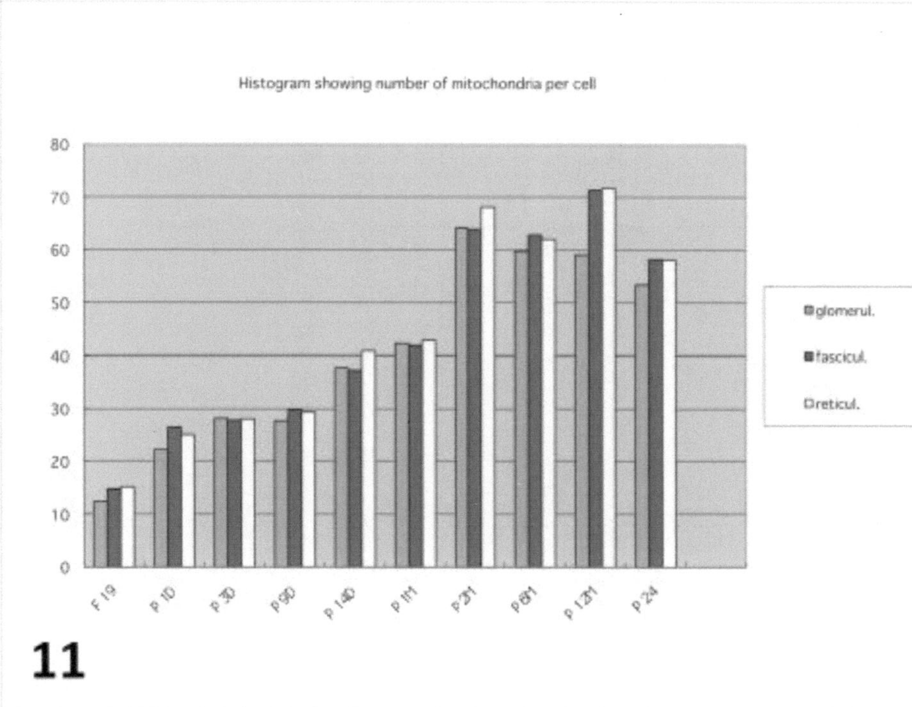

Fig. 26A.

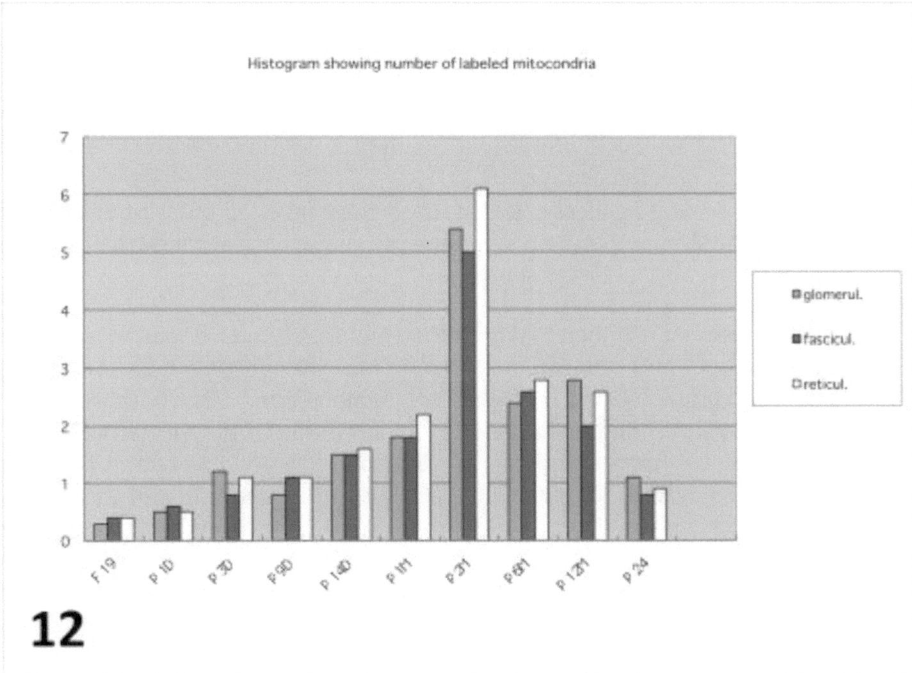

Fig. 26B.

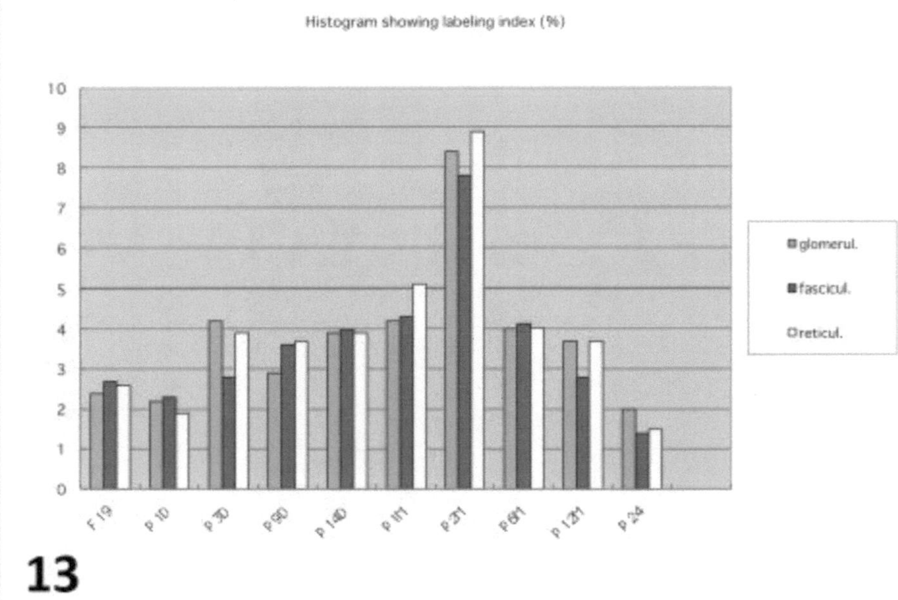

Fig. 26C.

Fig. 26. Histogram showing aging changes of the mitochondria in each adreno-cortical cell in the 3 layers of respective animals in 10 aging groups. From Nagata, T.: Annals of Microscopy Vol. 4, p. 54-71, 2011.
Fig. 26A. Histogram showing aging changes of the average numbers of mitochondria per cell in each adreno-cortical cell in the 3 layers of respective animals in 10 aging groups
Fig. 26B. Histogram showing aging changes of the average numbers of labeled mitochondria with ^{3}H-leucine showing protein synthesis per cell in each adrenocortical cell in the 3 layers of respective animals in 10 aging groups.
Fig. 26C. Histogram showing aging changes of the average labeling index of mitochondria labeled with ^{3}H-leucine showing protein synthesis per cell in each adreno-cortical cell in the 3 layers of respective animals in 10 aging groups.

As for the macromolecular synthesis in various cells in various organs of experimental animals observed by light and electron microscopic radioautography, it is well known that the silver grains due to radiolabeled ^{3}H-thymidine demonstrated DNA synthesis, while the grains due to ^{3}H-uridine demonstrated RNA synthesis. On the other hand, the radioautograms showing incorporations of ^{3}H-leucine into mitochondria indicating mitochondrial protein synthesis (Nagata 2002, 2009c,d,e, 2010a,b,c). It was shown from the results that the silver grains localized over the mitochondria independently from the nuclei whether the nuclei were labeled with silver grains or not in almost all the cells in the 3 layers of the adreno-cortical cells from prenatal embryo day 19 to postnatal month 24, administered with ^{3}H-leucine during the development and aging. The numbers of labeled mitochondria showing protein synthesis increased from perinatal day to postnatal adult stage at month 2, then kept plateau, while the labeled mitochondria with ^{3}H-leucine showing protein synthesis increased from perinatal stage to postnatal adult stage at month

2, then decreased at month 24, while the labeling indices increased from perinatal embryonic day to postnatal newborn and juvenile stages at day 9, then decreased from day 14 to senescence at month 24, then decreased to the adult stages at month 1 and 2, to month 6, 12 and 24. These changes demonstrate the chronological aging changes. The results obtained previously (Nagata 2008a,b,c,d, 2009a, Nagata & Ito 1996) indicated that mitochondria in the adreno-cortical cells proliferated from newborn to adult stages around month 1 and 2, showing mitochondrial DNA synthesis, while the mitochondrial RNA synthesis increased from newborn stage to postnatal day 9, then decreased from day 14, reaching the maximum, then decreased to month 24, but the RNA synthetic activity was kept plateau from day 14 to month 12, then decreased to senescent at month 24 due to aging (Nagata 2010e).

2.3.1.2 Protein synthesis in mitochondria of mouse adreno-medullary cells

The adreno-medullary tissues obtained from ddY strain mice at various ages from embryo day 19 to postnatal day 30, consisted mainly of 2 cell types, as observed by electron microscopy, adrenalin cells and noradrenalin cells, developing gradually (Nagata 2010a,b). At embryonic day 19 and postnatal day 1, the adreno-medullary cells were composed mainly of polygonal epitheloid cells, surrounded by blood capillaries and fibroblasts. The medullary cells can be divided into 2 types by the ultrastructure of granules. Some of the medullary cells possessed many granules of medium electron density which were believed to correspond to the adrenalin granules, while some other cells possessed many granules of very high electron density which were believed to correspond to the noradrenalin granules. However, the numbers of mitochondria found in their cytoplasm were not so many. At postnatal day 1, day 3 and day 9, the 2 types of cells differentiated and the numbers of granules, both adrenalin and noradrenalin granules, increased respectively. Likewise, the numbers of mitochondria also increased from prenatal day to postnatal days. At postnatal day 14 to month 1, month 2, month 6, month 12 and month 24 the numbers of adrenalin and noradrenalin granules as well as mitochondria increased. At postnatal month 1 and 2, the ultrastructures of 2 cell types were completely developed and the arrangements of the cells in the medulla became typical as adult tissues. Thus, the ultrastructure of the adrenal medullary cells showed changes due to development and aging at respective developmental stages. The number of mitochondria per cell increased from perinatal stage to postnatal stages due to aging. The data were stochastically analyzed using variance and Student's t-test. The increases of mitochondrial numbers in both adrenalin and noradrenalin cells from embryonic day 19 to postnatal month 6 were considered to be significant at P value <0.01.

Observing electron microscopic radioautograms, the silver grains were found over the nuclei of some adreno-medullary cells labeled with ^{3}H-leucine, demonstrating protein synthesis less in perinatal stages at embryonic day 19, postnatal day 1, day 3, day 9, while more day 14 and adults at month 1, month 2, month 6, month 12 and month 24.

However, those labeled cells were found in all the 2 cell types, adrenalin cells and noradrenalin cells, at respective aging stages. In the labeled adreno-medullary cells the silver grains were mainly localized over the euchromatin of the nuclei and only a few or several silver grains were found over the mitochondria of adrenalin cells. Likewise, most noradrenalin cells were also labeled with several silver grains in their nuclei as well as in their cytoplasm not only over the mitochondria but also over ribosomes, showing protein synthesis due to the incorporations of ^{3}H-leucine especially at the senescent stages from postnatal month 12 when observed at high power magnifications by high voltage electron microscopy. The localizations of silver grains over the mitochondria were not only on the mitochondrial matrices but also over mitochondrial membranes (Nagata 2010a,b).

2.3.1.2.1 Number of mitochondria of adreno-medullary cells in aging mice labeled with ^{3}H-leucine

Preliminary quantitative analysis on the number of mitochondria in 10 adreno-medullary cells whose nuclei were labeled with silver grains and other 10 cells whose nuclei were not labeled in each aging group revealed that there was no significant difference between the number of mitochondria and the labeling indices (P<0.01). Thus, the number of mitochondria and the labeling indices were calculated in 10 adreno-medullary cells regardless whether their nuclei were labeled or not. The results obtained from the number of mitochondria in adreno-medullary cells of respective animals in 10 aging groups at perinatal stages, from prenatal embryo day 19 to postnatal day 1, 3, 9, 14, and month 1, 2, 6, 12, showed an gradual increase from the prenatal day 19 (adrenalin 17.8, noradrenalin 18.2/cell) to postnatal day 1 (adrenalin 21.5, noradrenalin 22.4/cell), day 3 (adrenalin 22.5, noradrenalin 22.9/cell), day 9 (adrenalin 23.5, noradrenalin 23.9/cell), day 14 (adrenalin 24.1, noradrenalin 24.4/cell), and to adult stages at postnatal month 1 (adrenalin 24.7, noradrenalin 23.9/cell), month 2 (adrenalin 25.1, noradrenalin 24.5/cell) and month 6 (adrenalin 24.8, noradrenalin 24.3/cell), month 12 (adrenalin 24.5, noradrenalin 24.1/cell), and month 24 (adrenalin 23.5, noradrenalin 23.3/cell). The increases of mitochondrial numbers in both adrenalin and noradrenalin cells from embryonic day 19 to postnatal month 2 were considered to be significant at P value <0.01. However, the slight decrease from month 6 to 24 was not significant (Nagata 2010a or b).

2.3.1.2.2 Number of labeled mitochondria of adrenal medullary cells in aging mice labeled with ^{3}H-leucine

We counted the number of mitochondria labeled with silver grains obtained from 10 adreno-medullary cells in the 3 layers of each animal labeled with ^{3}H-leucine demonstrating protein synthesis in 10 aging groups at perinatal stages, prenatal embryo day 19, postnatal day 1, 3, 9 and 14, month 1, 3, 6, 12 and 24, as well as the number of all the mitochondria and calculated the labeling index.

The results demonstrated that the numbers of labeled mitochondria with ^{3}H-leucine showing protein synthesis per cell gradually increased from prenatal embryo day 19 (adrenalin 0.5, noradrenalin 0.5/cell), to postnatal day 1 (adrenalin 0.65, noradrenalin 0.6/cell), day 3 (adrenalin 0.7, noradrenalin 0.75/cell), day 9 (adrenalin 0.8, noradrenalin 0.8/cell), day 14 (adrenalin 0.8, noradrenalin 0.9/cell), reaching the maxima at month 1 (adrenalin 0.9, noradrenalin 0.85/cell), and decreased to month 2 (adrenalin 0.8, noradrenalin 0.82/cell), month 6 (adrenalin 0.81, noradrenalin 0.8/cell) month 12 (adrenalin 0.7, noradrenalin 0.75/cell) and month 24 (adrenalin 0.7, noradrenalin 0.65/cell). The data were stochastically analyzed using variance and Student's t-test. The increases of the numbers of labeled mitochondria in both adrenalin and noradrenalin cells from embryo day 19 to postnatal day 14 and month 1, as well as the decreases from month 1 to month 24 were stochastically significant (P <0.01).

2.3.1.2.3 Labeling index of mitochondria of adreno-medullary cells in aging mice labeled with ^{3}H-leucine

From the results, the labeling indices of mitochondrial protein synthesis in 2 cell types in respective aging stages were calculated from the number of labeled mitochondria dividing by the number of total mitochondria per cell.

The results showed that the labeling indices gradually increased from prenatal day 19 (adrenalin 2.8, noradrenalin 2.6%) to postnatal newborn day 1 (adrenalin 2.8, noradrenalin 2.4%), day 3 (adrenalin 3.3, noradrenalin 2.9%), day 9 (adrenalin 3.4, noradrenalin 3.3%) to juvenile stage at day 14 (adrenalin 3.6, noradrenalin 3.8%), reaching the maximum, and decreased to adult stages at month 1 (adrenalin 3.6, noradrenalin 3.5%), month 2 (adrenalin 3.1, noradrenalin 3.3%), month 6 (adrenalin 3.2, noradrenalin 3.3%), month 12 (adrenalin 2.8, noradrenalin 3.1%) and month 24 (adrenalin 2.9, noradrenalin 2.8%). From the results, the increases of the mitochondrial labeling indices in both the adrenalin and noradrenalin cells from embryo day 19 to postnatal day 14, as well as the decreases from day 14 to month 24 were stochastically significant ($P < 0.01$).

From the results obtained it was shown that intramitochondrial protein synthesis was observed in adreno-medullary cells, both the adrenalin cells and noradrenalin cells of developing and aging mice at various ages from prenatal embryos to postnatal newborn, young juvenile, adult and senescent stages and the number of mitochondria per cell showed increases due to aging, while the number of labeled mitochondria per cell and the labeling indices showed increases and slight decreases due to aging.

As for the macromolecular synthesis in various cells in various organs of experimental animals observed by light and electron microscopic radioautography, it is well known that the silver grains due to radiolabeled ^{3}H-thymidine demonstrate DNA synthesis, while the grains due to ^{3}H-uridine demonstrate RNA synthesis and ^{3}H-leucine protein synthesis (Nagata 1996, 1997, 2002, 2010). We formerly observed the intramitochondrial DNA synthesis as well as RNA synthesis in various cells in mice and rats (Nagata 1972a,b,c,d, 1974, 1984, 2001, 2001, Nagata et al. 1975, 1976, 1977). Lately we observed in the intramitochondrial DNA synthesis as well as RNA synthesis in the adrenal cortical and medullary cells, both the adrenalin cells and the noradrenalin cells at various ages from fetal day 19 to postnatal newborn day 1, 3, 9, juvenile day 14 and to adult month 1, 2, 6, 12 and 24 (Nagata 2008a,b, 2009a, 2010b,e), as well as the intramitochondrial protein synthesis during the aging and senescence (Nagata 2010d,f,g,h).

These results demonstrated that the numbers of silver grains showing nuclear protein synthesis did not give any significant difference between the 2 cells types in the same aging groups from perinatal to senescent stages. The radioautograms showing incorporations of ^{3}H-leucine into mitochondria indicating mitochondrial protein synthesis resulted in silver grain localization over the mitochondria independently from the nuclei whether the nuclei were labeled with silver grains or not in both cell types, adrenalin and noradrenalin cells, in the medullae from prenatal embryo day 19 to postnatal day 1, 3, 9 and 14, to postnatal month 1, 2, 6, 12 and 24, during the development and aging. The numbers of labeled mitochondria showing protein synthesis as well as the labeling indices increased from perinatal embryonic day to postnatal newborn and juvenile stages at day 14 to month 12, reaching the maxima, and then did not decrease to the senescent stages at month 24 (year 2).

From the results obtained, it was shown that intramitochondrial protein synthesis was observed in adreno-medullary cells, both the adrenalin cells and noradrenalin cells of developing and aging mice at various ages from prenatal embryos to postnatal newborn, young juvenile, adult and senescent stages and the number of mitochondria per cell showed increases due to aging, while the number of labeled mitochondria per cell and the labeling indices showed increases and slight decreases due to aging (Nagata 2010a,b,c,d,e,f,g,h).

As for the macromolecular synthesis in various cells in various organs of experimental animals observed by light and electron microscopic radioautography, it is well known that the silver grains due to radiolabeled ^{3}H-thymidine demonstrate DNA synthesis, while the grains due to ^{3}H-uridine demonstrate RNA synthesis and ^{3}H-leucine protein synthesis (Nagata et al. 1967a, b, Nagata 1972a, b, c, 2001, 2002). The previous results obtained from the studies on the adreno-cortical cells of aging mice by light microscopic radioautography revealed that silver grains indicating DNA synthesis incorporating ^{3}H-thymidine were observed over the nuclei of some adreno-cortical cells at perinatal stages from postnatal day 1 to day 14 (Ito 1996, Ito & Nagata 1996). However, they did not observe the intramitochondrial RNA synthesis. We formerly observed the intramitochondrial DNA synthesis (Nagata et al. 1967a, b, Nagata 1972a, b, c, 2001, 2002) as well as RNA synthesis (Nagata 1972a,b,c,d, 1974, 1984, 2001, 2002, Nagata et al. 1975, 1976, 1977, Nagata & Murata 1977) in the adrenal medullary cells, both the adrenalin cells and the noradrenalin cells at various ages from fetal day 19 to postnatal newborn day 1, 3, 9, juvenile day 14 and to adult month 1, 2, 6, 12 and 24. In the present study, we also observed the intramitochondrial protein synthesis during the aging and senescence. The numbers of silver grains showing nuclear protein synthesis did not give any significant difference between the 2 cells types in the same aging groups from perinatal to senescent stages. The radioautograms showing incorporations of ^{3}H-leucine into mitochondria indicating mitochondrial protein synthesis resulted in silver grain localization over the mitochondria independently from the nuclei whether the nuclei were labeled with silver grains or not in both cell types, adrenalin and noradrenalin cells, in the medullae from prenatal embryo day 19 to postnatal day 1, 3, 9 and 14, to postnatal month 1, 2, 6, 12 and 24, during the development and aging. The numbers of labeled mitochondria showing protein synthesis as well as the labeling indices increased from perinatal embryonic day to postnatal newborn and juvenile stages at day 14 to month 12, reaching the maxima, and then did not decrease to the senescent stages at month 24 (year 2).

With regards to DNA in mitochondria in animal cells or plastids in plant cells, many studies have been reported in various cells of various plants and animals since 1960s (Nass 1966, Nass and Nass 1963, Gibor and Granick 1964, Gahan and Chayen 1965). Most of these authors observed DNA fibrils in mitochondria which were histochemically extracted by DN'ase. Electron microscopic observation of the DNA molecules isolated from the mitochondria revealed that they were circular in shape, with a circumference of 5-6 μm. It was calculated that such a single molecule had a molecular weight of about 10^7 daltons (van Bruggen et al. 1966). Mitochondria of various cells also contained a DNA polymerase, which was supposed to function in the replication of the mitochondrial DNA. On the other hand, the incorporations of ^{3}H-thymidine into mitochondria demonstrating DNA synthesis were observed by means of electron microscopic radioautography in lower organism such as slime mold (Guttes and Guttes 1964, Schuster 1965), tetrahymena (Stone and Miller Jr.

1965) or chicken fibroblasts in tissue culture under abnormal conditions (Chévremont 1963). However, these authors used old-fashioned developers consisting of methol and hydroquinone (MQ-developer) which produced coarse spiral silver grains resulting in inaccurate localization over cell organelles when observed by electron microscopy. All of these authors showed photographs of electron radioautographs with large spiral-formed silver grains (2-3 µm in diameter) localizing not only over the mitochondria but also outside the mitochondria. In order to obtain smaller silver grains, we first used elon-ascorbic acid developer after gold latensification, which produced comma-shaped smaller silver grains (0.4-0.8 µm in diameter), then later we used phenidon developer after gold latensification, producing dot-like smaller silver grains (0.2-0.4 µm in diameter) localizing only inside the mitochondria showing ultrahigh resolution of radioautograms. These papers were the first which demonstrated intramitochondrial DNA synthesis incorporating ^{3}H-thymidine with accurate intramitochondrial localization in avian and mammalian cells. With regards the resolution of electron microscopic radioautography, on the other hand, many authors discussed the sizes of silver grains under various conditions and calculated various values of resolutions (Salpeter et al. 1969, Nadler 1971, Uchida & Mizuhira 1971, Nagata 1972b,c). Those authors who used the M-Q developers maintained the resolution to be 100-160 nm (Salpeter et al. 1969, Nadler 1971), while those authors who used the elon-ascorbic acid developer (Nagata 1972b, , Uchida & Mizuhira 1971) calculated it to be 25-50 nm. When we used phenidon developer at 16°C for 1 min after gold latensification, we could produce very fine dot-shaped silver grains and obtained the resolution around 25 nm (Nagata 1992, 1996, 1997, 2001, 2002, Murata et al. 1979). For the analysis of electron radioautographs, Salpeter et al. (1969) proposed to use the half-distance and very complicated calculations through which respective coarse spiral-shaped silver grains were judged to be attributable to the radioactive source in a certain territory within a resolution boundary circle. However, since we used phenidon developer after gold latensification to produce very fine dot-shaped silver grains, we judged only the silver grains which were located in the mitochondria which were dot-shaped very fine ones to be attributable to the mitochondria without any problem as was formerly discussed (Nagata 1972a,b, c, 1996, 1997, 2001, 2002).

Then we also demonstrated intramitochondrial DNA synthesis incorporating ^{3}H-thymidine in some other established cell lines originated from human being such as HeLa cells (Nagata 1972a,b,c,d) or mitochondrial fractions prepared from in vivo mammalian cells such as rat and mouse (Nagata 1974, Nagata et al. 1975, 1976). It was later commonly found in various cells and tissues not only in vitro obtained from various organs in vivo such as the cultured human HeLa cells (Nagata et al. 1966, 1986, Nagata 1984), cultured rat sarcoma cells (Nagata et al. 1977), mouse liver and pancreas cells in vitro (Nagata & Murata 1977, Nagata et al. 1977, 1986), but also in vivo cells obtained from various organs such as the salivary glands (Nagata et al. 2000), the liver (Nagata 2003, 2006a,b, 2007a,b,c,d,e, Nagata & Ma 2005, Nagata et al. 1979, 1982a,b, Ma & Nagata 1988a,b, Ma et al. 1994), the pancreas (Nagata 1992, Nagata et al. 1986), the trachea (Sun et al. 1997), the lung (Sun et al. 1994, 1995a,b, Nagata 2007), the kidneys (Hanai & Nagata 1994, Nagata 2005), the testis (Gao et al. 1994, 1995), the uterus (Yamada et al. 1993, 1994), the adrenal glands (Ito 1996, Ito et al. 1996, Nagata 2008a,b, 2009g,j, 2010a,b), the brains (Cui et al. 1996), and the retina (Gunarso 1984, Gunarso et al. 1996, 1997, Kong & Nagata 1994, Nagata 1996) of mice, rats and chickens. Thus, it is clear that all the cells in various organs of various animals synthesize DNA not only in their nuclei but also in their mitochondria.

The relationship between the intramitochondrial DNA synthesis and cell cycle was formerly studied in synchronized cells and it was clarified that the intramitochondrial DNA synthesis was performed without nuclear involvement (Nagata 1972b). However, the relationship between the DNA synthesis and the aging of individual animals and men has not yet been clarified except a few papers recently published by Korr and associates on mouse brain (Korr et al. 1997, 1998, Schmitz et al. 1999a,b,). They reported both nuclear DNA repair, measured as nuclear unscheduled DNA synthesis, and cytoplasmic DNA synthesis labeled with ^{3}H-thymidine in several types of cells in brains such as pyramidal cells, Purkinje cells, granular cells, glial cells, endothelial cells, ependymal cells, epithelial cells as observed by light microscopic radioautography using paraffin sections observed by LMRAG. They observed silver grains over cytoplasm of these cells by light microscopy and maintained that it was reasonable to interpret these labeling as ^{3}H-DNA outside the nuclei, which theoretically belonged to mitochondrial DNA without observing the mitochondria by electron microscopy. From the results, they concluded that distinct types of neuronal cells showed a decline of both unscheduled DNA and mitochondrial DNA syntheses with age in contrast that other cell types, glial and endothelial cells, did not show such age-related changes neither counting the number of mitochondria in respective cells nor counting the labeling indices at respective aging stages. Thus, their results from the statistics obtained from the cytoplasmic grain counting seems to be not accurate without observing mitochondria directly. To the contrary, we had studied DNA synthesis in the livers of aging mice (Nagata et al. 1979, Nagata 1982a,b, 2003, 2005, 2006a,b,c,d,e, 2010c, Ma et al. 1988, 1994, Ma & Nagata 1988) and clearly demonstrated that the number of mitochondria in each hepatocytes, especially mononucleate hepatocytes, increased with the ages of animals from the perinatal stages to adult and senescent stages, while the number of labeled mitochondria and the labeling indices increased from the perinatal stages, reaching a maximum at postnatal day 14, then decreased. We also demonstrated that the number of mitochondria and labeled mitochondria with ^{3}H-thymidine, ^{3}H-uridine and ^{3}H-leucine in the adrenal glands in aging mice increased due to aging (Nagata 2009j, 2010a,b,d,e,f,g,h).

2.3.2 The protein synthesis in the Leydig cells of the testis

We studied the macromolecular synthesis of the cells in the testis of several groups of litter ddY mice at various ages from fetal day 19 to postnatal aging stages up to 2 years senescence by LM and EM RAG using ^{3}H-thymidine, ^{3}H-uridine and ^{3}H-leucine incorporations (Gao 1993, Gao et al. 1994, 1995a, Nagata 2000b). The incorporation of ^{3}H-leucine into proteins was observed in almost all the Leydig cells in the interstitial tissues of the testis. The silver grains were located over the nuclei and cytoplasm of respective Leydig cells. The aging change of protein synthesis of Leydig cells among different aging groups was also found (Nagata 2001c, 2002). At embryonic day 19, the silver grains of Leydig cells labeled with ^{3}H-leucine was observed in both nucleus and cytoplasm and there was no obvious difference between the number of silver grains on the cytoplasm and the nucleus. The number of silver grains decreased at postnatal day 1 and then increased at day 3 and 7. However, the number of silver grains on both the nucleus and cytoplasm decreased from 1 month to 3 months and increased again from 6 months onwards maintaining a high level from adult to senescent stages. Some of the silver grains were also localized over some of the mitochondria in respective aging groups as observed by EM RAG. These results indicate that the DNA, RNA and protein syntheses in Leydig cells are maintained at rather high level even at senescent stages at postnatal 1 and 2 years when the animals survived for longer lives.

2.4 The localization of mercury in the thyroid gland

We studied incorporations of mercury chloride into human thyroid tissues of both normal and cancer cells obtained from human patients (Nagata et al. 1977b, Nagata 1994a,b,c,d,e). The tissues were obtained surgically from human patients of both sexes in various ages suffering from the cancer of thyroids and the both normal and cancer cells were cut into small pieces (3x3 mm) aseptically which were incubated in a medium (Eagle's MEM) containing RI-mercury chloride ($^{203}HgCl_2$) and fixed either cryo-fixation at -196°C and freeze-dried or chemically fixed with buffered glutaraldehyde and osmium tetroxide. The former tissue blocks were processed for dry-mounting radioautography, while the latter were processed for conventional wet-mounting radioautography. The results revealed that the silver grains appeared much more in the cancer cells processed for freeze-fixation and dry-mounting radioatuography (Fig. 21A) than the cancer cells processed for chemical fixation and wet-mounting radioatuography (Fig. 21B), as well as much more in the cancer cells than the normal cells under the same conditions. On the other hand, PCNA/cycline and both keratin kinase C and vimentin were immunostained in connection to DNA synthetic activity. It was found that PCNA/cycline, keratin kinase C and vimentin antibodeis were localized around the filaments in the thyroid cancer cells (Fig. 21C), demonstrating the relation between those antigens and DNA synthetic activity in cell cycle (Shimizu et al. 1993, Nagata 1994b,c, Gao et al. 1994).

3. Macromolecular synthesis in the nervous system

The nervous system consists of the central nervous system and the peripheral nervous system. The former is divided into the brains and the spinal cord, while the latter into the cerebrospinal system and the autonomous system. We studied macromolecular synthesis of the brains, the spinal cord in the cerebrospinal system and the autonomic peripheral nerves in the autonomous system by LM and EM RAG.

3.1 The DNA synthesis in the nervous system

We studied the DNA synthesis of the brains, the spinal cord in the cerebrospinal system and the autonomic peripheral nerves in the autonomous system by LM and EM RAG (Cui 1995, Cui et al. 1996, Izumiyama et al. 1987, Nagata 1965, 1967a, Nagata and Stegerda 1963, 1964, Nagata et al. 1999a).

3.1.1 The DNA synthesis in the brains

The brains of mammals consist of the cerebrum, the cerebellum and the brain stem. We studied on DNA synthesis and protein synthesis in the cerebellum of aging mouse (Cui 1995, Cui et al. 1996) as well as the glucose incorporation in the cerebrum of adult gerbils (Izumiyama et al. 1987). The DNA synthesis was examined in the cerebella of 9 groups of aging ddY strain mice from fetal day 19, to postnatal day 1, 3, 8, 14 and month 1, 2, 6, 12, each consisting of 3 litter animals, using ^{3}H-thymidine, a DNA precursor, by LM and EM RAG (Cui 1995, Cui et al. 1996). The labeled nuclei, by the precursor, in both the neurons and glias, i.e., neuroblasts and glioblasts, were observed in the external granular layers of the cerebella of perinatal mice from embryonic day 19 (Fig. 27A) to postnatal day 1, 3, 7 and day 14 by LMRAG and EMRAG. The labeled nuclei disappeared at postnatal 1 month. The peak of labeling index was at postnatal day 3 in both neuroblasts and glioblasts (Fig. 28A, B). The glioblasts of the external granular layer migrated inward, some of them formed the Bergmann glia cells located between Purkinje cells. Labeled nuclei of neuroblasts and glioblasts in the internal granular layers were observed at perinatal stages. The maximum of the labeling index in the internal granular layer was at postnatal day 3, similarly to the external granular layer. The endothelial cells of the cerebellar vessels were progressively labeled from embryos to neonates, reaching the peak at 1 week after birth and decreasing thereafter.

3.1.2 The DNA synthesis in the peripheral nerves

We first studied the degeneration and regeneration of autonomous nerve cells in the plexuses of Auerbach and Meissner of the jejunums of 15 dogs which were operated upon to produce experimental ischemia of the jejunal loops by perfusing with Tyrode's solution via the mesenteric arteries for 1, 2, 3 and 4 hours (Nagata 1965, 1967, Nagata and Steggerda 1963, 1964). Tissue blocks were obtained from the deganglionated portions and the adjoining normal portions, which were fixed in Carnoy's fluid, embedded in paraffin, sectioned and stained with buffered thionine, methyl-green and pyronine and PAS. Some animals were injected with either ^{3}H-thymidine or ^{3}H-cytidine and the intestinal tissues obtained from ischemic portions and normal portions were processed for LM RAG. The results revealed that the ganglion cells in Auerbach's plexus showed various degenerative changes in accordance with the duration of ischemia. After 4 hours ischemia, most of the ganglion cells in Auerbach's plexus were completely destroyed. The degenerative changes in Auerbach's plexus after 4 hours ischemia were irreversible after 1 week recovery. The ganglion cells in the Meissner's plexus, on the other hand, were less sensitive to the ischemia. They recovered completely even after 4 hours ischemia. The PAS positive substances in degenerative ganglion cells in both plexuses decreased immediately after 4 hours ischemia. The DNA contents of ganglion cells in both Auerbach's and Meissner's plexus did not show any change before and after ischemia. The RNA contents decreased immediately after the ischemia (Nagata and Steggerda 1963, 1964). The number of binucleate cells in ganglion cells in both Auerbach's and Meissner's plexuses after 4 hours ischemia increased to 4.6% and 5.7% respectively. In contrast, in the non-ischemic normal control preparations, the binucleate cells occurred only 0.5% and 1.8% in Auerbach's and Meissner's plexus respectively. The high frequency of binucleate cells in the ganglion cells persisted for more than 100 days after the ischemia, indicating a possible regeneration of ganglion cells. The radioautographic study revealed that there was no evidence for DNA synthesis in both Auerbach's and Meissner's plexus from either ischemic or normal loops. The RNA synthesis was observed to be higher in gaglion cells in normal loop than ischemic loop and higher in Auerbach's than in Meissner's as expressed by grain counting. It was higher in binucleate ganglion cells than in mononucleate cells.

3.2 The RNA synthesis in the nervous system

We studied only messenger RNA in the spinal cords of aging mice from perinatal to postnatal adult stages by means of in situ hybridizaion.

3.2.1 The RNA synthesis in the spinal cord

The localization of TGF-β1 mRNA in the segments of the spinal cords of mice was investigated by means of in situ hybridization techniques together with immunohistochemical staining (Nagata et al. 1999). The tissues of lower cervical segments of the spinal cords of BALB/c mice, from embryonic day 12, 14, 16, 19 and postnatal day 1, 3, 7, 14, 21, 28, 42 and 70, were used. For in situ hybridization, ^{35}S-labeled oligonucleotide probes for TGF-β1 were used to detect their messenger RNA. Cryosections were incubated under silicon cover slides with 100 μl of pre-incubation solution plus final concentration of 2.4 x 10^6 cpm/ml probes and 100 mM DTT for 16 hours. After washing with SSC and DTT, the slides were dried and processed for radioautography by dipping in Konica NR-M2 emulsion, which were exposed and developed. The results showed that TGF-β1 mRNA was detectable in the meninges surrounding the spinal cord, but scarcely detected in spinal cord parenchyma (Fig. 27B). The localization of TGF-β1 mRNA in the spinal cord suggested that TGF- β1 acted through paracrine mechanism in the morphogenesis of the spinal cord in mice. The localization of TGF-β1 and its mRNA in the segments of the spinal cords of mice was also investigated with immunocytochemical techniques (Nagata et al. 1999). The tissues of lower cervical segments of the spinal cords of BALB/c mice, from embryonic day 12, 14, 16, 19 and postnatal day 1, 3, 7, 14, 21, 28, 42 and 70, the same as in situ hybridization were used. For immunocytochemistry, transverse cryosections of the spinal cords were cut and stained with rabbit anti-TGF-β1 polyclonal antibody followed with ABC method. The results showed that positive immunoreactivities arose in the ventral horn motoneurons from the embryonic stage to postnatal neonates (Fig. 27B) up to the adults. The extracellular matrix of the white matter, however, showed positive immunocytochemical staining from postnatal day 14, and thereafter, and the immunoreactivity remained with aging. The whole white matter showed only background level of staining before postnatal day 14. The results indicated that TGF-β1 regulates motoneuron growth and differentiation as well as they were probably correlated with formation, differentiation and regeneration of myelin of nerve tracts. The immunostaining with βFGF antibody presented the same basal pattern as shown in TGFβ1 immunohistochemistry (Nagata and Kong 1988). The positive immunoreactivities were detected in ganglion cell layer, inner and outer plexiform layers, retinal pigment epithelial layer, choroidal and scleral layers. Since TGF-β1 mRNA was detectable in the meninges surrounding the spinal cord by in situ hybridization but scarcely detected in spinal cord parenchyma, the disparate localization of TGF-β1 polypeptide and TGF-β1 mRNA in the spinal cord suggest that TGF-β1 acts through paracrine mechanism in the morphogenesis of the spinal cord in mice. The negative control abolished virtually all reactivity when using the normal rabbit serum instead of primary antibody or using avidin-biotin-peroxidase complex solution only.

3.3 The protein synthesis in the cerebellum

When 10 groups of aging ddY mice from fetal day 19, to postnatal day 1, 3, 7, 14 and month 1, 2, 6, 12 and 24, each consisting of 3 litter mates, using ^3H-leucine, protein syntheses of both neuroblasts and glioblasts were observed by LM and EM RAG in the extragranular layers of perinatal animals (Cui 1995, Cui et al. 1996, 2000, Nagata et al. 2001). The silver grains due to ^3H-leucine demonstrating protein synthesis were localized over the nuclei and cytoplasm of neuroblasts and glioblasts of embryos at fetal day 19 and the number of silver grains increased after birth from postnatal day 1, 3 to day 7 and onward. On day 3, some Purkinje cells were recognized incorporating silver grains. The number of silver grains in these cells increased from neonatal stages to mature adult stage at postnatal day 14 and 30, then decreased from month 1, 2, 6, 12 to 24. The increase and decrease of the silver grains were due to the aging changes of protein synthesis in the cerebella due to development and senescence of individual animals.

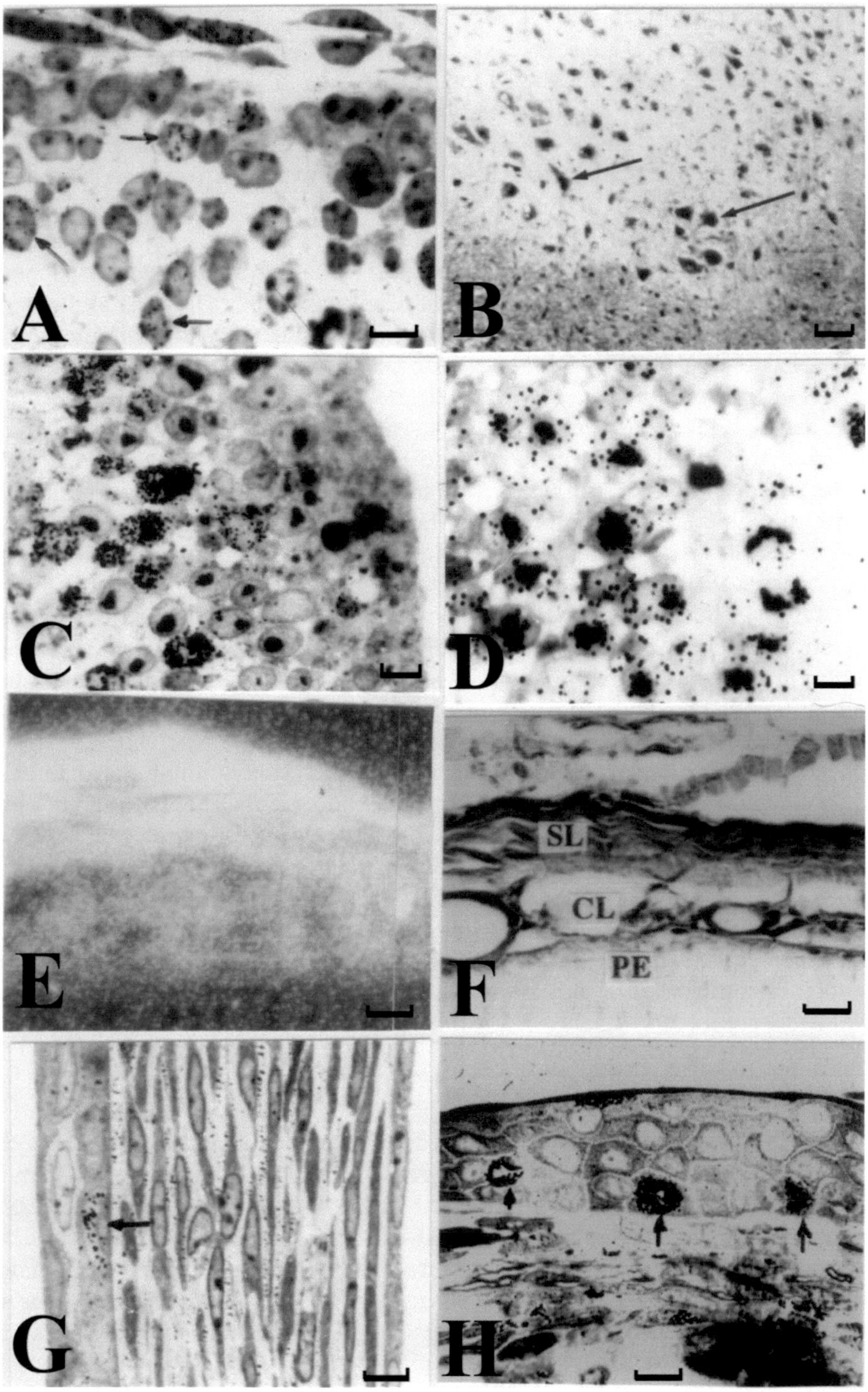

Fig. 27. LM RAG of the neuro-sensory cells. From Nagata, T., Special Cytochemistry in Cell Biology, In, Internat. Rev. Cytol. Jeon, K. W. Ed., Academic Press, San Diego, USA, London, UK, Vol. 211, No. 1, p. 122, 2001.

Fig. 27A. LM RAG of a prenatal day 19 mouse cerebellum labeled with ^{3}H-thymidine, showing DNA synthesis. x900.
Fig. 27B. LM RAG of the spinal cord of a postnatal day 14 mouse immunostained with rabbit anti-TGF-β1 polyclonal IgG followed by ABC method, showing that the ventral horn motoneurons are strongly positive. x70.
Fig. 27C. LM RAG of the optic vesicle of a day 2 chick embryo labeled with ^{3}H-thymidine, showing DNA synthesis. x750.
Fig. 27D. LM RAG of the optic vesicle of a day 2 chick embryo labeled with ^{3}H-uridine, showing RNA synthesis. x750.
Fig. 27E. Dark-field LM photo of the scleral layer (top), choroid layer (middle) and pigment epithelium (bottom) of an adult 1 month old mouse demonstrating intense silver grains by in situ hybridization for TGF-β1 mRNA. x450.
Fig. 27F. Bright-field LM photo of the scleral layer (top), choroid layer (middle) and pigment epithelium (bottom) of an adult 1 month old mouse demonstrating intense silver grains by in situ hybridization for TGF-β1 mRNA. x450.
Fig. 27G. LM RAG of the cornea of a postnatal day 14 mouse labeled with ^{3}H-thymidine, showing DNA synthesis in the epithelial nucleus (arrow) as well as in the stroma. x900.
Fig. 27H. LM RAG of the skin of the fore-limb of a salamander at 6weeks after hatching labeled with ^{3}H-thymidine, showing DNA synthesis. x900.

3.4 The glucide synthesis in the brains

The incorporation of ^{3}H-deoxyglucose was studied in the adult gerbil brains among the nervous system of experimental animals (Izumiyama et al. 1987). The changes of soluble deoxyglucose uptake in the hippocampus were studied after ^{3}H-deoxyglucose injections by means of cryo-fixation, freeze-substitution and dry-mounting radioautography to demonstrate soluble compounds under normal and post-ischemic conditions. The results demonstrated that the neurons in the hippocampus subjected to ischemia revealed higher uptake of soluble glucose than normal control. The concentration of soluble ^{3}H-deoxyglucose was higher than the chemically fixed and wet-mounted radioautograms that demonstrated only insoluble compounds. However, the relation of glycogen synthesis to aging has not yet been fully clarified.

4. Macromolecular synthesis in the sensory system

The sensory system consists of five organs, i.e., the visual organ or the eye, the stato-acoustic organ or the ear, the gustatory organ or the tongue, the olfactory organ or the nose, and the dermis or the skin. Among these sensory organs, we mainly studied the visual organ and the skin (Gunarso 1983a,b, Gunarso et al. 1996, 1997, Gao et al. 1992a,b, 1993, Kong 1993, Kong and Nagata 1994, Kong et al. 1992a,b, Nagata 1998, 1999, 2000, Nagata et al. 1994, Toriyama 1995).

4.1 The DNA synthesis in the sensory organs

Among the sensory organs, we mainly studied the DNA synthesis of the visual organ and the skin. They should be described separately.

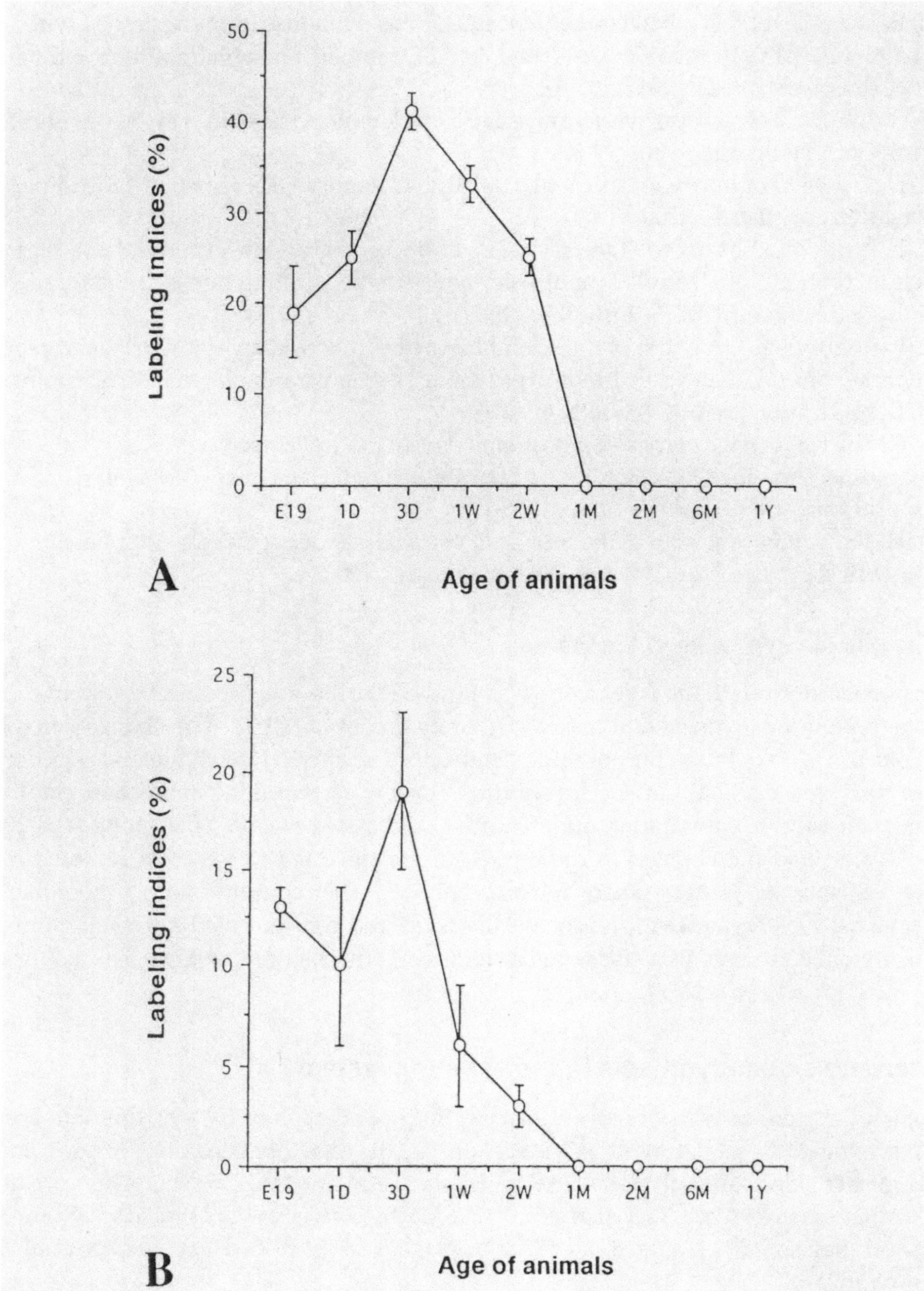

Fig. 28. Transitional curves of the labeling indices of respective cell types in the cerebella of aging mice labeled with ^{3}H-thymidine, showing DNA synthesis. Mean ± Standard Deviation. From Nagata, T.: Radioautographology, General and Special. In, Prog. Histochem. Cytochem. Vol. 37, No. 2, p. 186, 2002, Urban & Fischer, Jena, Germany

Fig. 28A. The neuroblasts in the extragranular layer of the cerebella.
Fig. 28B. The glioblasts in the extragranular layer of the cerebella.

4.1.1 The DNA synthesis in the visual organ

The visual organ consists of the eye and its accessory organs. The eye of mammals consists of the cornea, iris, cilliary body, lens, retina, choroid and sclera. We studied mainly the macromolecular synthesis in the retina of chickens and mice (Nagata 2000f). The nucleic acid syntheses, both DNA and RNA, were first studied in the ocular tissues of white Leghorn chick embryos from day 1 to day 14 incubations by LM and EMRAG (Gunarso 1984a,b, Gunarso et al. 1997, Gao et al. 1992a,b, 1993, Kong 1993, Kong and Nagata 1994, Kong et al. 1992a,b, Nagata et al. 1994). It was shown that the labeled cells with silver grains due to ^{3}H-thymidine were most frequently observed in the nuclei of the retinal cells in the posterior region of the day 2 chick embryo optic vesicle (Fig. 27C) and the labeled cells moved from anterior to posterior regions due to aging by incubation in vitro. The number of labeled cells as expressed by labeling index (%), was more in the posterior regions than the anterior and the equatorial regions and more in the outer portions than in the inner portions at day 2, but the labeling index became more in the anterior regions than the equatorial and posterior regions at day 3, 4 and 7 and it became more in the inner portions than in the outer portions at day 7, decreasing from day 2 to 3, 4 and 7 in each regions (Fig. 28). On the other hand, the silver grains due to ^{3}H-uridine were observed over the nuclei and cytoplasm of all retinal cells from day 2 to 7 (Fig. 27D) and the number of silver grains incorporating ^{3}H-uridine increased from day 1 to day 7 and it was more in the anterior regions than in the posterior regions at the same stage (Gunarso et al. 1996). On the other hand, DNA and RNA syntheses in the ocular tissues of aging ddY mice were also studied (Gao et al. 1993, Kong and Nagata 1994, Kong et al. 1992a,b). The ocular tissues taken out from several groups of litter ddY mice at ages varying from fetal day 9, 12, 14, 16, 19 to postnatal day 1, 3, 7, 14 were labeled with ^{3}H-thymidine in vitro and radioautographed (Gao et al. 1992a,b, 1993, Kong 1993, Kong et al. 1992a,b, Toriyama 1995). Silver grains showing DNA synthesis were localized over the nuclei of retinal cells and pigment epithelial cells in the anterior, equatorial and posterior regions of perinatal animals (Fig. 27A). The labeling indices of the retina and pigment epithelium were higher in earlier stages than in later stages, during which they steadily declined (Fig. 28A,B). However, the retina and the pigment epithelium followed different courses in their changes of labeling indices during embryonic development. In the retina, the labeling indices in the vitreal portions were more than those in the scleral portions during the earlier stages. However, the indices of scleral portions were more than those in the vitreal portions in the later stages. Comparing the three regions of the retinae of mice, the anterior, equatorial and posterior regions, the labeling indices of the anterior region were generally higher than those of the equatorial and posterior regions (Fig. 28A). In the pigment epithelium (Fig. 28B), the labeling indices gradually increased in the anterior region, but decreased in the equatorial and the posterior regions through all developmental stages. These results suggest that the proliferation of both the retina and pigment epithelium in the central region occurred earlier than those of the peripheral regions (Nagata 1999a, Gao et al. 1992a,b, Kong 1993, Kong and Nagata 1994, Kong et al. 1992a, b). In the juvenile and adult stages, however, the labeled cells were localized at the middle of the bipolar-photoreceptor layer of the retina, where was supposed to be the undifferentiated zone.

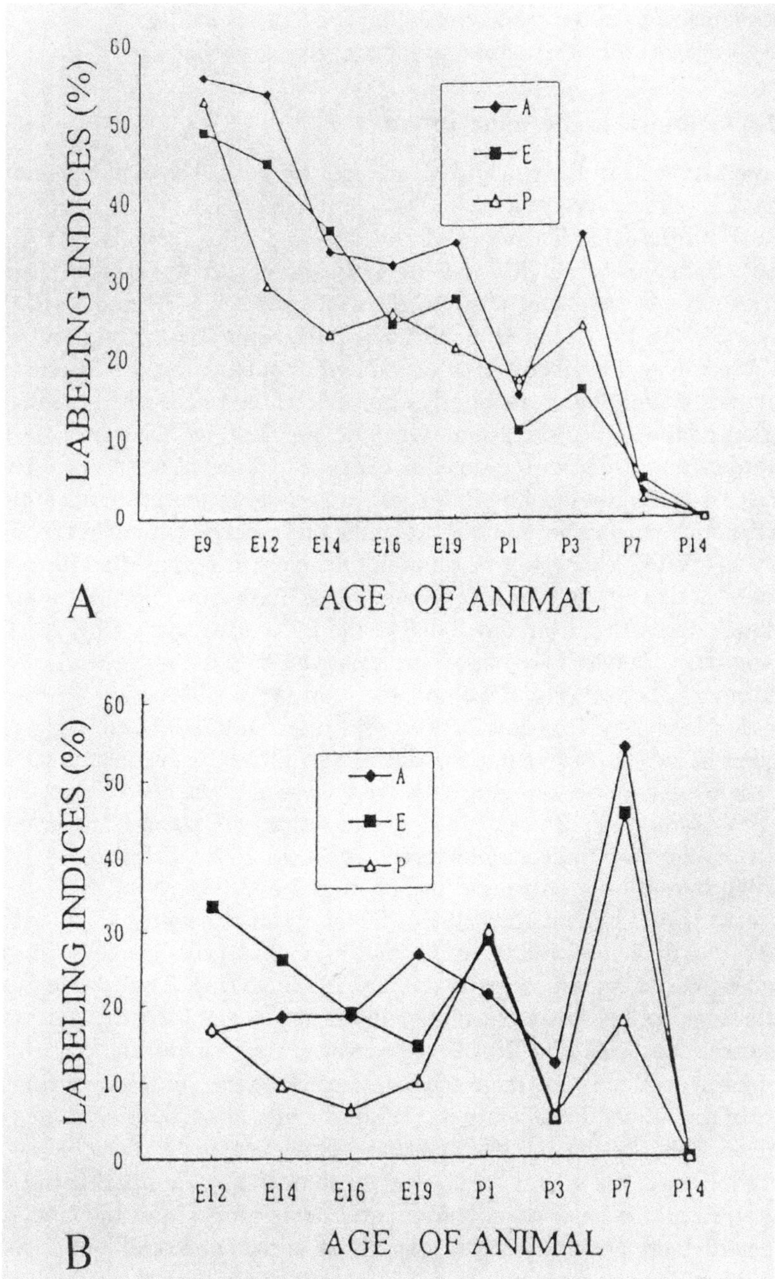

Fig. 29. Transitional curves of the labeling indices in the three regions (A: anterior, E: eqauator, P: posterior) of the retina and the pigment epithelium of aging mice labeled with ^{3}H-thymidine, showing DNA synthesis. Mean ± Standard Deviation. From Nagata, T.: Radioautographology, General and Special. In, Prog. Histochem. Cytochem. Vol. 37, No. 2, p. 191, 2002, Urban & Fischer, Jena, Germany

Fig. 29A. The labeling index in the retina.

Fig. 29B. The labeling index in the pigment epithelium.

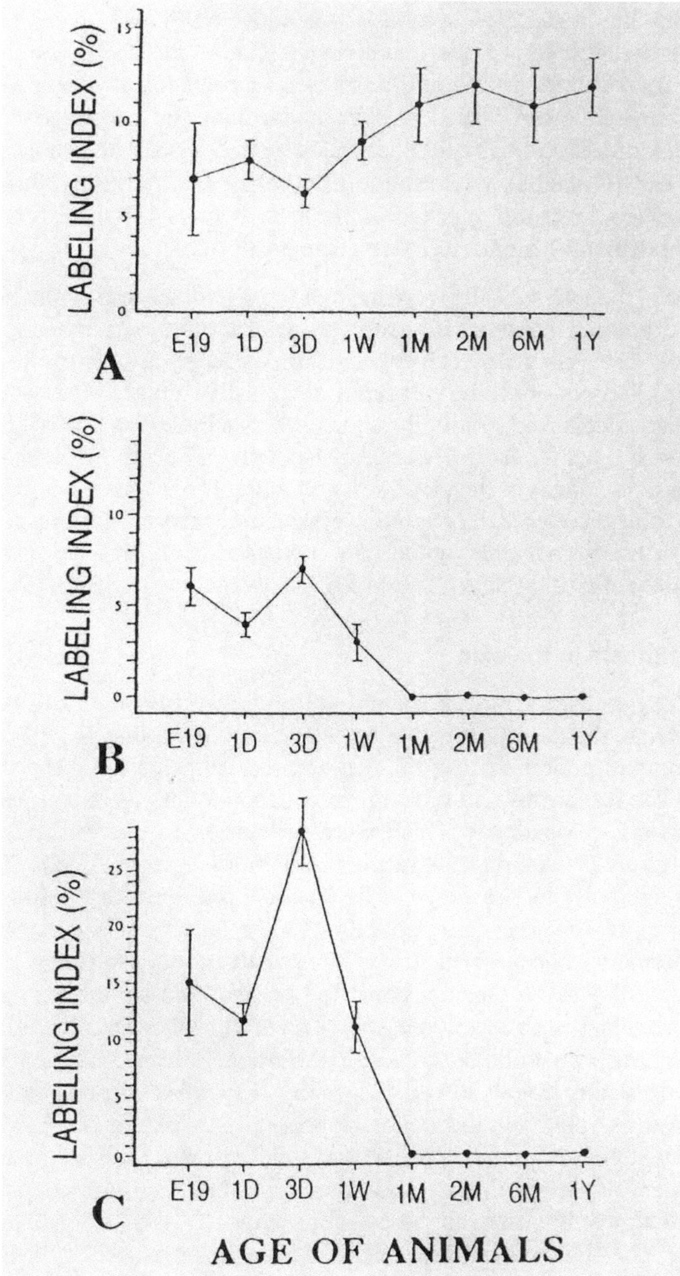

Fig. 30. Transitional curves of the labeling indices in the three layers of the central area of the cornea of aging mice labeled with ^{3}H-thymidine, showing DNA synthesis. Mean ± Standard Deviation. From Nagata, T.: Radioautographology, General and Special. In, Prog. Histochem. Cytochem. Vol. 37, No. 2, p. 192, 2002, Urban & Fischer, Jena, Germany

Fig. 30A. The labeling index in the epithelium.

Fig. 30B. The labeling index in the stroma.

Fig. 30C. The labeling index in the endothelium.

In the corneas of aging mice, DNA synthesis was observed in all 3 layers, i.e., the epithelial, stromal and endothelial layers, at perinatal stages (Gao et al. 1993). The labeled cells with ^{3}H-thymidine were localized in the epithelial cells at prenatal day 19, postnatal day 1, 14 (Fig. 27G) to 1 year, while the labeled cells in the stromal and endothelial layers were less. The labeling index of the corneal epithelial cells reached a peak at 1 month after birth and decreased to 1 year, (Fig. 30A), while the indices of the stromal (Fig. 30B) and endothelial (Fig. 30C) cells were low and reached a peak at 3 days after birth and disappeared completely from postnatal 1 month to 1 year (Nagata 1999c).

In the cilliary body, the labeled cells were located in the cilliary and pigment epithelial cells, stromal cells and smooth muscle cells from prenatal day 19 to postnatal 1 week, but no labeled cells were observed in any cell types from postnatal day 14 to 1 year (Nagata et al. 1994). The labeling indices of all the cell types in the cilliary body were at the maximum at prenatal day 19 and decreased gradually after birth reaching 0 at postnatal day 14. On the other hand, when the ocular tissues were labeled with ^{3}H-uridine, silver grains appeared over all cell types at all stages of development and aging (Toriyama 1995, Nagata 2000f). The grain counts in the retina and the pigment epithelium increased from prenatal day 9 to postnatal day 1 in the retinal cells, while they increased from prenatal day 12 to postnatal day 7 in the pigment epithelial cells (Nagata 1999a,b, Nagata et al. 1994)

4.2 The DNA synthesis in the skin

The skin which covers the surface of the animal body can histologically be divided into 3 layers, the epidermis, the dermis and the hypodermis. We studied only the epidermal cells of young salamanders after hatching to 24 months during the aging by radioautography (Nagata 1998c). The fore-limbs and hind-limbs of salamanders were composed of skeletons consisting of bones and cartilages which were covered with skeletal muscles, connective tissues and epidermis consisting of stratified squamous epithelial cells in the outermost layer. We observed both the cartilage cells in the bone and the epithelial cells in the epidermis to compare the two cell populations. The skin of a salamander consisted of epidermis and dermis or corium which was lined with connective tissue layers designated as the subcutaneous layer. The former consisted of stratified squamous epithelium, while the latter consisted of dense connective tissues. The epithelial cells in the juvenile animals at 4 weeks after hatching were cuboidal in shape and not keratinized. Radioautograms labeled with ^{3}H-thymidine at this stage showed that many cells were labeled demonstrating DNA synthesis at both the superficial and deeper layers (Fig. 27H), resulting very high labeling index. At 6 weeks after hatching, the superficial cells changed their shape from cuboidal to flattened squamous, while the deeper and basal cells remained cuboidal. The numbers of labeled cells were almost the same as the previous stage at 4 weeks, but they were localized at the basal layer. The shape of epithelial cells in juvenile animals at 8, 9, 10, and 11 weeks differentiated gradually forming the superficial corneum layer which appeared keratinized and the deeper basal layer. Radioautograms at these stages showed that the labeled cells remarkably reduced as compared with that of 4 and 6 weeks. In the adult salamanders at 8 months up to 12 months, the dermal and epidermal cells showed complete mature structure and examination of radioautograms revealed that the labeled cells were localized at only the basal cell layer and their number reached very low but at constant level. No difference was found on the morphology and labeling between the fore-limbs and hind-limbs at any stages. Comparing the labeling indices of both epidermal cells and the cartilage cells in the limbs, the labeling index of the epidermal cells was higher than the cartilage cells. The index of the dermal cells in the hind-limbs was at its maximum about 25% at 4 weeks, and fell down markedly with time from 6 weeks to 9 weeks. The labeling index of epidermal cells of the hind-limbs, on the other hand, had its maximum about 23% at 6 weeks, increasing from 20% at 4 weeks, and decreasing to about 18% at 8 weeks, then fell progressively with time, dropped to 5% at 9 weeks (Fig. 31). The labeling indices of the epidermal cells of both fore-limbs and hind-limbs were almost the same from 9 weeks to 12 months, keeping low constant level about 4-5%, but never reaching 0. These results indicated that the cutaneous cells belonged to the renewing cell population (Nagata 1998c).

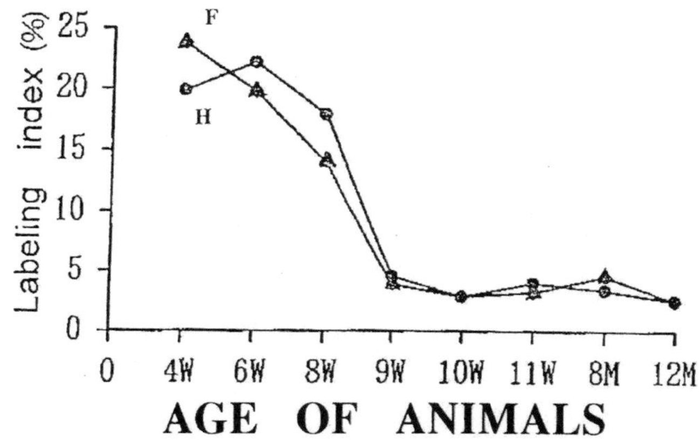

Fig. 31. Transitional curves of the labeling indices of the epithelial cells in the epidermis of the fore-limbs (F) and the hind-limbs (H) of the salamanders at various ages from 4 weeks to 12 months after hatching labeled with ^{3}H-thymidine. From Nagata, T.: Radioautographology, General and Special. In, Prog. Histochem. Cytochem. Vol. 37, No. 2, p.197, 2002, Urban & Fischer, Jena, Germany

4.3 The RNA synthesis in the sensory organs

We studied only the RNA synthesis in the chicken and mouse eyes among of the sensory organs.

4.3.1 The RNA synthesis in the eye

The RNA synthesis in the chicken eyes was studied with the ocular tissues of chicken embryos in incubation (Fig. 27D). Silver grains due to the incorporations of ^{3}H-uridine were observed over all the nuclei, cell organelles, cytoplasm of all the cells in the optic cups in development showing the RNA synthesis (Gunarso 1984a,b, Gunarso et al. 1969). Grain counting revealed that the counts gradually increased from day 2 to 7 and the numbers of silver grains were the most in the nuclei, while the numbers between the 3 portions of the optic cups, the anterior, equator and the posterior portions decreased from the anterior to the posterior at the same developmental stages (Gunarso 1984a).

On the other hand, the ocular tissues of aging mice were also labeled with ^{3}H-uridine. The silver grains demonstrating RNA synthesis appeared over all the cell types at all the stages of development and aging. The grain counts in the retina and the pigment epithelium increased from prenatal day 9 to postnatal day 1 in the retinal cells, while they increased from prenatal day 12 to postnatal day 7 in the pigment epithelial cells (Kong et al. 1992b).

On the other hand, the distribution and localization of TGF-β1 and βFGF and their mRNA in the ocular tissues of aging mice were also studied (Nagata and Kong 1998). The posterior segment of BALB/c mouse eyes from embryonic day 14, 16, 19 and postnatal 1, 3, 5, 7, 14, 28, 42 and 70 were used. For in situ hybridization, ^{35}S-labeled oligonucleotide probes for TGF-β1 and βFGF were used to detect their mRNA. Cryo-sections were picked up on glass slides which were processed for in situ hybridization and for radioautography. As the results, silver grains mainly located in the scleral layers and some in the choroidal and pigment epithelial layers, but only background level of grains were found in the whole retina. In the radioautograms from embryonic day 14 to adult mice at week 10 (day 70), the significant distribution of silver grains representing TGF-β1 mRNA was not detected in the whole retina. However, the significant silver grains were detected in scleral and chorioidal layers and mesenchymal cells at embryonic day 14, then the number of grains increased in these layers particularly in sclera from prenatal to postnatal neonate until adult (Fig. 27E). These results suggest that mRNA for TGF-β1 and βFGF were synthesized in scleral, choroidal and pigment epithelial layers, but their proteins were transferred to the target cells of the retina and elsewhere. Furthermore, it is suggested that TGF-β1 and βFGF may play important roles on retinal differentiation, development and aging, particularly during the late embryonic and newborn stages (Nagata and Kong 1998).

These results showed that RNA synthetic activities in the ocular cells changed due to the aging of individual animals.

4.4 The protein synthesis in the sensory organs

We studied only the protein synthesis in the mouse eyes among of the sensory organs.

4.4.1 The protein synthesis of the eye

The protein synthesis in the ocular tissues of aging mouse were studied in all the 3 layers of the eye, the tunica fibrosa, the tunica vasculosa and the tunica intima, or the cornea, cilliary bodies and the retina of the aging mouse at various stages after the administration of several precursors (Toriyama 1995, Nagata 1997c, 1999b,c,d, 2000e,f, 2001c, Nagata and Kong 1998, Cui et al. 2000).

The protein synthesis of the retina in aging mouse as revealed by ^{3}H-leucine incorporation demonstrated that number of silver grains in bipolar cells and photoreceptor cells was the most intense at embryonic stage and early postnatal days. The peak was 1 day after birth and decreased from 14 days to 1 year after birth. (Toriyama 1995). The protein synthesis of the cornea as revealed by ^{3}H-leucine incorporation (Nagata 1997c, 1999d, 2000f, 2001c, Nagata and Kong 1998, Cui et al. 2000) and the glycoprotein synthesis demonstrated by ^{3}H-glucosamine (Nagata et al. 1995) were also studied in several groups of aging ddY mice. Silver grains of both ^{3}H-leucine and ^{3}H-glucosamine incorporations were located in the epithelial cells, the stromal fibroblasts and the endothelial cells from prenatal day 19 to postnatal 6 months. No silver grains were observed in the lamina limitans anterior (Bowman's membrane) and the lamina limitans posterior (Descemet's membrane). The grain densities by ^{3}H-leucine incorporation in 3 layers, i. e., epithelial, stromal and endothelial layers, increased from embryonic stage to postnatal day 3 and 7, then decreased to 2 weeks and 1 year. The grain densities due to the glycoprotein synthesis with ^{3}H-glucosamine were more observed in the endothelial cells of prenatal day 19 animals, but more in the epithelial cells of postnatal day 1, 3 and 7 animals. From the results, it was shown that the glycoprotein synthetic activity in respective cell types in the cornea of mouse changed with aging of the animals.

The collagen synthesis in the ocular tissues was also demonstrated by the incorporation of ^{3}H-proline in 4 groups of mice at various ages, from prenatal day 20, postnatal day 3, 7 and 30. The results showed that the sites of ^{3}H-proline incorporation were located in the stromal fibroblasts in both cornea and the trabecular meshworks in the iridocorneal angle in prenatal and postnatal newborn mice. No silver grains were observed in the epithelial and endothelial cells. On EM RAG, silver grains were localized over the endoplasmic reticulum and Golgi apparatus of fibroblasts and over intercellular matrices consisting of collagen fibrils. From the quantitative analysis, the grain densities were more observed in the fibroblasts in postnatal day 7 animals than younger animals at fetal day 20 and postnatal day 3, 7 and 30. In the same aging groups, the grain densities were more in the cornea than the iridocorneal angle. It was concluded that the collagen synthetic activity was localized in the fibroblasts in the cornea and the trabecular meshworks in the iridocorneal angle and the activity changed with aging, reaching the maximum at postnatal day 7.

On the other hand, the distributions of some of the ophthalmological drugs used for the treatment of human glaucoma patients were examined in the ocular tissues by LM and EM RAG (Nagata 2000f). However, its relationship to the aging was not studied.

4.5 The glucide synthesis in the sensory organs

We studied the aging changes of glucide synthesis by ^{3}H-glucosamine uptake in the ocular tissues of aging mice.

4.5.1 The glucide synthesis in the eye

The glycoprotein synthesis of the cornea in aging mouse as revealed by ^{3}H-glucosamine incorporation was studied in several groups of aging mice at various ages from prenatal stages to senescence (Nagata et al. 1995). Silver grains were located in the epithelial cells, the stromal fibroblasts and the endothelial cells from prenatal day 19 to postnatal 6 months. No silver grains were observed in the lamina limitans anterior (Bowman's membrane) and the lamina limitans posterior (Descemet's membrane). On the other hand, the grain densities by ^{3}H-leucine incorporation in 3 layers, i.e., epithelial, stromal and endothelial layers, increased from embryonic stage to postnatal day 3 and 7, then decreased to week 2 and year 1. The grain densities due to the glycoprotein synthesis with ^{3}H-glucosamine were more observed in the endothelial cells of prenatal day 19 animals, but more in the epithelial cells of postnatal day 1, 3 and 7 animals. From the results, it was shown that the glycoprotein synthetic activity in respective cell types in the cornea of mouse changed with aging of the animals.

5. Macromolecular synthesis in the tumor cells

We carried out several experiments dealing with the nucleic acid synthesis in some malignant tumor cells by means of LM and EM RAG.

5.1 The DNA synthesis in the tumor cells

The DNA synthesis in nuclei and mitochondria of cultured HeLa cells, an established cell line obtained from the carcinoma of the human uterus, or IgG myeloma cells from a human patient, labeled with ^{3}H-thymidine were demonstrated (Nagata 1972b,c,d, Fujii et al. 1980). The incorporations of these precursors increased or decreased depending upon the aging of isolated cells in vitro, i.e., the days of incubation in vitro. The incorporations of ^{3}H-thymidine demonstrating DNA synthesis increased immediately after the incubation and then gradually decreased due to incubation days, reaching zero within several days.

5.2 The RNA synthesis in the tumor cells

The RNA synthesis in nuclei and mitochondria of cultured HeLa cells, or IgG myeloma cells from a human patient, labeled with ^{3}H-uridine were demonstrated (Nagata 1972b,c,d, Fujii et al. 1980). The incorporations of these precursors increased or decreased depending upon the aging of isolated cells in vitro. The incorporations of ^{3}H-uridine demonstrating RNA synthesis increased immediately after the incubation and then gradually decreased due to incubation days.

6. Conclusions

From the results obtained, it was concluded that almost all the cells in various organs of all the organ systems of experimental animals at various ages from prenatal to postnatal development and senescence during the aging of cells and individual animals demonstrated to incorporate various macromolecular precursors such as ^{3}H-thymidine, ^{3}H-uridine, ^{3}H-leucine, ^{3}H-glucose or glucosamine, ^{3}H-glycerol and others localizing in the nuclei, cytoplasmic cell organelles showing silver grains due to DNA, RNA, proteins, glucides, lipids and others those which the cells synthesized during the cell aging. Quantitative analysis carried out on the numbers of silver grains in respective cell organelles demonstrated quantitative changes, increases and decreases, of these macromolecular synthesis in connection to cell aging of respective organs. In general, DNA synthesis with ^{3}H-thymidine incorporations in most organs showed maxima at perinatal stages and gradually decreased due to aging. To the contrary, the other syntheses such as RNA, proteins, glucides and lipids increased due to aging and did not remarkably decrease until senescence. Anyway, these results indicated that macromolecular synthetic activities of respective compounds in various cells were affected from the aging of the individual animals.

Thus, the results obtained from the various cells of various organs should form a part of special radioautographology that I had formerly proposed (Nagata 1999e, 2002), i.e., application of radioautography to the aging of cells, as well as a part of special cytochemistry (Nagata 2001), as was formerly reviewed. We expect that such special radioautographology and special cytochemistry should be further developed in all the organs in the future.

7. Acknowledgments

This study was supported in part by Grant-in-Aids for Scientific Research from the Ministry of Education, Science and Culture of Japan (No. 02454564) while the author worked at Shinshu University School of Medicine by 1996 as well as Grants for Promotion of Characteristic Research and Education from the Japan Foundation for Promotion of Private Schools (No. 1997, 1998 1999, 2000) while the author worked at Nagano Women's Jr. College from 1996 to 2002. The author is also grateful to Grant-in-Aids for Scientific Research from the Japan Society for Promotion of Sciences (No. 18924034, 19924204, 20929003) while the author has been working at Shinshu Institute of Alternative Medicine and Welfare since 2005 up to the present time. The author thanks Dr. Kiyokazu Kametani, Technical Official, Department of Instrumental Analysis, Research Center for Human and Environmental Sciences, Shinshu University, for his technical assistance in electron microscopy during the course of this study.

8. References

Chen, S., Gao, F., Kotani, A., Nagata, T.: Age-related changes of male mouse submandibular gland: A morphometric and radioautographic study. Cell. Mol. Biol. 41, 117-124, 1995.

Clermont Y.: The contractime elements in the limiting membrane of the seminiferous tubules of rats. Exp. Cell Res. 15, 438-342, 1958.

Clermont, Y.: Renewal of spermatogonia in man. Amer. J. Anat. 112, 35-51, 1963.

Cui, H.: Light microscopic radioautographic study on DNA synthesis of nerve cells in the cerebella of aging mice. Cell. Mol. Biol. 41, 1139-1154, 1995.

Cui, H., Gao, F., Nagata, T.: Light microscopic radioautographic study on protein synthesis in perinatal mice corneas. Acta Histochem. Cytochem. 33, 31-37, 2000.

Duan, H., Gao, F., Li, S., Hayashi, K., Nagata, T.: Aging changes and fine structure and DNA synthesis of esophageal epithelium in neonatal, adult and old mice. J. Clin. Electron Microsc. 25, 452-453, 1992.

Duan, H., Gao, F., Li, S., Nagata, T.: Postnatal development of esophageal epithelium in mouse: a light and electron microscopic radioautographic study. Cell. Mol. Biol. 39, 309-316, 1993.

Duan, H., Gao, F., Oguchi, K., Nagata, T.: Light and electron microscopic radioautographic study on the incorporation of ^{3}H-thymidine into the lung by means of a new nebulizer. Drug Res. 44, 880-883, 1994.

Feulgen, R., Rossenbeck, H.: Mikroskopische-chemischer Nachweis einer Nukeinsaeure von Thymus der Thymonukeinsaeure Z. Physik. Chem. 135, 203-248, 1924.

Fujii, Y., Ohno, S., Yamabayashi, S., Usuda, N., Saito, H., Furuta, S., Nagata, T.: Electron microscopic radioautography of DNA synthesis in primary cultured cells from an IgG myeloma patient. J. Clin. Electr. Microsc. 13, 582-583, 1980.

Gao, F.: Study on the macromolecular synthesis in aging mouse seminiferous tubules by light and electron microscopic radioautography. Cell. Mol. Biol. 39, 659-672, 1993.

Gao, F., Toriyama, K., Nagata, T.: Light microscopic radioautographic study on the DNA synthesis of prenatal and postnatal aging mouse retina after labeled thymidine injection. Cell. Mol. Biol. 38, 661-668, 1992a.

Gao, F., Li, S., Duan, H., Ma, H., Nagata, T.: Electron microscopic radioautography on the DNA synthesis of prenatal and postnatal mice retina after labeled thymidine injection. J. Clin. Electron Microsc. 25, 721-722, 1992b.

Gao, F., Toriyama, K., Ma, H., Nagata, T.: Light microscopic radioautographic study on DNA synthesis in aging mice corneas. Cell. Mol. Biol. 39, 435-441, 1993.

Gao, F., Ma, H., Sun, L., Jin, C., Nagata, T.: Electron microscopic radioautographic study on the nucleic acids and protein synthesis in the aging mouse testis. Med. Electron Microsc. 27, 360-362, 1994.

Gao, F., Chen, S., Sun, L., Kang, W., Wang, Z., Nagata, T.: Radioautographic study of the macromolecular synthesis of Leydig cells in aging mice testis. Cell. Mol. Biol. 41, 145-150, 1995a.

Gao, F., Jin, C., Ma, H., Sun, L., Nagata, T.: Ultrastructural and radioautographic studies on DNA synthesis in Leydig cells of aging mouse testis. Cell. Mol. Biol. 41, 151-160, 1995b.

Gunarso, W.: Radioautographic studies on the nucleic acid synthesis of the retina of chick embryo. I. Light microscopic radioautography. Shinshu Med. J. 32, 231-240, 1984a.

Gunarso, W.: Radioautographic studies on the nucleic acid synthesis of the retina of chick embryo. II. Electron microscopic radioautography. Shinshu Med. J. 32, 241-248, 1984b.

Gunarso, W., Gao, F., Cui, H., Ma, H., Nagata, T.: A light and electron microscopic radioautographic study on RNA synthesis in the retina of chick embryo. Acta Histochem. 98, 309-32, 1996.

Gunarso, W., Gao, F., Nagata, T.: Development and DNA synthesis in the retina of chick embryo observed by light and electron microscopic radioautography. Cell. Mol. Biol. 43, 189-201, 1997.

Hanai, T.: Light microscopic radioautographic study of DNA synthesis in the kidneys of aging mice. Cell. Mol. Biol. 39, 81-91, 1993.

Hanai, T., Nagata, T.: Electron microscopic radioautographic study on DNA and RNA synthesis in perinatal mouse kidney. In, Radioautography in Medicine, Nagata, T., Ed., pp. 127-131, Shinshu University Press, Matsumoto, 1994a.

Hanai, T., Nagata, T.: Study on the nucleic acid synthesis in the aging mouse kidney by light and electron microscopic radioautography. In, Radioautography in Medicine, Nagata, T., Ed., pp. 209-214, Shinshu University Press, Matsumoto, 1994b.

Hanai, T., Nagata, T.: Electron microscopic study on nucleic acid synthesis in perinatal mouse kidney tissue. Med. Electron Microsc. 27, 355-357, 1994c.

Hanai, T., Usuda, N., Morita, T., Shimizu, T., Nagata, T.: Proliferative activity in the kidneys of aging mice evaluated by PCNA/cyclin immunohistochemistry. Cell. Mol. Biol. 39, 181-191, 1993.

Hayashi, K., Gao, F., Nagata, T.: Radioautographic study on ^{3}H-thymidine incorporation at different stages of muscle development in aging mice. Cell. Mol. Biol. 39, 553-560, 1993.

Ito, M.: The radioautographic studies on aging change of DNA synthesis and the ultrastructural development of mouse adrenal gland. Cell. Mol. Biol. 42, 279-292, 1996.

Ito, M., Nagata, T.: Electron microscopic radioautographic studies on DNA synthesis and ultrastructure of aging mouse adrenal gland. Med. Electron Microsc. 29, 145-152, 1996.

Izumiyama, K., Kogure, K., Kataoka, S., Nagata, T.: Quantitative analysis of glucose after transient ischemia in the gerbil hippocampus by light and electron microscope radioautography. Brain Res. 416, 175-179, 1987.

Jamieson, J. D., Palade, G. E.: Intracellular transport of secretory proteins in the pancreatic exocrine cells. J. Cell Biol. 34, 577-615, 1967.

Jin, C.: Study on DNA synthesis of aging mouse colon by light and electron microscopic radioautography. Cell. Mol. Biol. 42, 255-268, 1996.

Jin, C., Nagata, T.: Light microscopic radioautographic study on DNA synthesis in cecal epithelial cells of aging mice. J. Histochem. Cytochem. 43, 1223-1228, 1995a.

Jin, C., Nagata, T.: Electron microscopic radioautographic study on DNA synthesis in cecal epithelial cells of aging mice. Med. Electron Microsc. 28, 71-75, 1995b.

Joukura, K.: The aging changes of glycoconjugate synthesis in mouse kidney studied by ^{3}H-glucosamine radioautography. Acta Histochem. Cytochem. 29, 57-63, 1996.

Joukura, K., Nagata, T.: Aging changes of ^{3}H-glucosamine incorporation into mouse kidney observed by radioautography. Acta Histochem. Cytochem. 28, 494-494, 1995.

Joukura, K., Usuda, N., Nagata, T.: Quantitative study on the aging change of glycoconjugates synthesis in aging mouse kidney. Proc. Xth Internat. Cong. Histochem. Cytochem., Acta Histochem. Cytochem. 29, Suppl. 507-508, 1996.

Kobayashi, K., Nagata, T.: Light microscopic radioautographic studies on DNA, RNA and protein syntheses in human synovial membranes of rheumatoid arthritis patients. J. Histochem. Cytochem. 42, 982-982, 1994.

Komiyama, K., Iida, F., Furihara, R., Murata, F., Nagata, T.: Electron microscopic radioautographic study on ^{125}I-albumin in rat gastric mucosal epithelia. J. Clin. Electron Microsc. 11, 428-429, 1978.

Kong, Y.: Electron microscopic radioautographic study on DNA synthesis in perinatal mouse retina. Cell. Mol. Biol. 39, 55-64, 1993.

Kong, Y., Nagata, T.: Electron microscopic radioautographic study on nucleic acid synthesis of perinatal mouse retina. Med. Electron Microsc. 27, 366-368, 1994.

Kong, Y., Usuda, N., Nagata, T.: Radioautographic study on DNA synthesis of the retina and retinal pigment epithelium of developing mouse embryo. Cell. Mol. Biol. 38, 263-272, 1992a.

Kong, Y., Usuda, N., Morita, T., Hanai, T., Nagata, T.: Study on RNA synthesis in the retina and retinal pigment epithelium of mice by light microscopic radioautography. Cell. Mol. Biol. 38, 669-678, 1992b.

Leblond, C. P.: Localization of newly administered iodine in the thyroid gland as indicated by radioiodine. J. Anat. 77, 149-152, 1943.

Leblond, C. P.: The life history of cells in renewing systems. Am. J. Anat. 160, 113-158, 1981.

Leblond, C. P., Messier, B.: Renewal of chief cells and goblet cells in the small intestine as shown by radioautography after injection of thymidine-^{3}H into mice. Anat. Rec. 132: 247-259. 1958.

Li, S.: Relationship between cellular DNA synthesis, PCNA expression and sex steroid hormone receptor status in the developing mouse ovary, uterus and oviduct. Histochemistry 102, 405-413, 1994.

Li, S., Nagata, T.: Nucleic acid synthesis in the developing mouse ovary, uterus and oviduct studied by light and electron microscopic radioautography. Cell. Mol. Biol. 41, 185-195, 1995.

Li, S., Gao, F., Duan, H., Nagata, T.: Radioautographic study on the uptake of $^{35}SO_4$ in mouse ovary during the estrus cycle. J. Clin. Electron Microsc. 25, 709-710, 1992.
Liang, Y.: Light microscopic radioautographic study on RNA synthesis in the adrenal glands of aging mice. Acta Histochem. Cytochem. 31, 203-210, 1998.
Liang, Y., Ito, M., Nagata, T.: Light and electron microscopic radioautographic studies on RNA synthesis in aging mouse adrenal gland. Acta Anat. Nippon. 74, 291-300, 1999.
Ma, H.: Light microscopic radioautographic study on DNA synthesis of the livers in aging mice. Acta Anat. Nippon. 63, 137-147, 1988.
Ma, H., Nagata, T.: Electron microscopic radioautographic study on DNA synthesis of the livers in aging mice. J. Clin. Electron Microsc. 21, 335-343, 1988a.
Ma, H., Nagata, T.: Studies on DNA synthesis of aging mice by means of electron microscopic radioautography. J. Clin. Electron Microsc. 21, 715-716, 1988b.
Ma, H., Nagata, T.: Electron microscopic radioautographic studies on DNA synthesis in the hepatocytes of aging mice as observed by image analysis. Cell. Mol. Biol. 36, 73-84, 1990a.
Ma, H., Nagata, T.: Study on RNA synthesis in the livers of aging mice by means of electron microscopic radioautography. Cell. Mol. Biol. 36, 589-600, 1990b.
Ma, H., Nagata, T.: Collagen and protein synthesis in the livers of aging mice as studied by electron microsopic radioautography. Ann. Microsc. 1, 13-22, 2000.
Ma, H., Gao, F., Olea, M. T., Nagata, T.: Protein synthesis in the livers of aging mice studied by electron microscopic radioautography. Cell. Mol. Biol. 37, 607-615, 1991.
Matsumura, H., Kobayashi, Y., Kobayashi, K., Nagata, T.: Light microscopic radioautographic study of DNA synthesis in the lung of aging salamander, Hynobius nebulosus. J. Histochem. Cytochem. 42, 1004-1004, 1994.
Momose, Y., Nagata, T.: Radioautographic study on the intracellular localization of a hypolipidemic agent, bezafibrate, a peroxisome proliferator, in cultured rat hepatocytes. Cell. Mol. Biol. 39, 773-781, 1993a.
Momose, Y., Naito, J., Nagata, T.: Radioautographic study on the localization of an anti-allergic agent, tranilast, in the rat liver. Cell. Mol. Biol. 35, 347-355, 1989.
Momose, Y., Shibata, N., Kiyosawa, I., Naito, J., Watanabe, T., Horie, S., Yamada, J., Suga, T., Nagata, T.: Morphometric evaluation of species differences in the effects of bezafibrate, a hypolipidemic agent, on hepatic peroxisomes and mitochondria. J. Toxicol. Pathol. 6, 33-45, 1993b.
Momose, Y., Naito, J., Suzawa, H., Kanzawa, M., Nagata, T.: Radioautographic study on the intracellular localization of bezafibrate in cultured rat hepatoctyes. Acta Histochem. Cytochem. 28, 61-66, 1995.
Morita, T.: Radioautographic study on the aging change of ^{3}H-glucosamine uptake in mouse ileum. Cell. Mol. Biol. 39, 875-884, 1993.
Morita, T., Usuda, N. Hanai, T., Nagata, T.: Changes of colon epithelium proliferation due to individual aging with PCNA/cyclin immunostaining comparing with ^{3}H-thymidine radioautography. Histochemistry 101, 13-20, 1994.
Murata, F., Momose,Y. , Yoshida, K., Nagata, T.: Incorporation of ^{3}H-thymidine into the nucleus of mast cells in adult rat peritoneum. Shinshu Med. J. 25, 72-77, 1977a.
Murata, F., Momose, Y., Yoshida, K., Ohno, S., Nagata, T.: Nucleic acid and mucosubstance metabolism of mastocytoma cells by means of electron microscopic radioautography. Acta Pharmacol. Toxicol. 41, 58-59, 1977b.

Murata, F., Yoshida, K., Ohno, S., Nagata, T.: Ultrastructural and electron microscopic radioautographic studies on the mastocytoma cells and mast cells. J. Clin. Electron Microsc. 11, 561-562, 1978.

Murata, F., Yoshida, K., Ohno, S., Nagata, T.: Mucosubstances of rabbit granulocytes studied by means of electron microscopic radioautography and X-ray microanalysis. Histochemistry 61, 139-150, 1979.

Nagata, T.: On the relationship between cell division and cytochrome oxidase in the Yoshida sarcoma cells. Shinshu Med. J. 5: 383-386, 1956.

Nagata, T.: Studies on the amitosis in the Yoshida sarcoma cells. I. Observation on the smear preparation under normal conditions. Med. J. Shinshu Univ. 2: 187-198, 1957a.

Nagata, T.: Studies on the amitosis in the Yoshida sarcoma cells. II. Phase-contrast microscopic observations under normal conditions. Med. J. Shinshu Univ. 2: 199-207, 1957b.

Nagata, T.: Cell divisions in the liver of the fetal and newborn dogs. Med. J. Shinshu Univ. 4: 65-73, 1959.

Nagata, T.: A radioautographic study of the DNA synthesis in rat liver, with special reference to binucleate cells. Med. J. Shinshu Univ. 7, 17-25, 1962.

Nagata, T.: A quantitative study on the ganglion cells in the small intestine of the dog. Med. J. Shinshu Univ. 10, 1-11, 1965.

Nagata, T.: A radioautographic study on the RNA synthesis in the hepatic and the intestinal epithelial cells of mice after feeding with special reference to binuclearity. Med. J. Shinshu Univ. 11, 49-61, 1966.

Nagata, T.: On the increase of binucleate cells in the ganglion cells of dog small intestine due to experimental ischemia. Med. J. Shinshu Univ. 12, 93-113, 1967a.

Nagata, T.: A radioautographic study on the protein synthesis in the hepatic and the intestinal epithelial cells of mice, with special reference to binucleate cells. Med. J. Shinshu Univ. 12, 247-257, 1967b.

Nagata, T.: Chapter 3. Application of microspectrophotometry to various substances. In , Introduction to Microspectrophotometry. Isaka, S., Nagata, T., Inui, N., Eds., Olympus Co., Tokyo, pp. 49-155, 1972a.

Nagata, T.: Electron microscopic dry-mounting autoradiography. Proc. 4th Internat. Cong. Histochem. Cytochem. Kyoto, pp. 43-44, 1972b.

Nagata, T.: Electron microscopic radioautography of intramitochondrial RNA synthesis of HeLa cells in culture. Histochemie 32, 163-170, 1972c.

Nagata, T.: Quantitative electron microscope radioautography of intramitochondrial nucleic acid synthesis. Acta Histochem. Cytochem. 5, 201-203, 1972d.

Nagata, T.: Electron microscopic observation of target cells previously observed by phase-contrast microscopy: Electron microscopic radioautography of laser beam irradiated cultured cells. J. Clin. Electron Microsc. 17, 589-590, 1984.

Nagata, T.: Principles and techniques of radioautography. In, Histo- and Cyto-chemistry 1985, Japan Society of Histochemistry and Cytochemistry, Ed., Gakusai Kikaku Co., Tokyo, pp. 207-226, 1985.

Nagata, T.:. Electron microscopic radioautography and analytical electron microscopy. J. Clin. Electron Microsc. 24, 441-442, 1991.

Nagata, T.: Radiolabeling of soluble and insoluble compounds as demonstrated by light and electron microscopy. Recent Advances in Cellular and Molecular Biology, Wegmann, R. J., Wegmann, M. A., Eds. Peters Press, Leuven, Vol. 6, pp. 9-21, 1992.

Nagata, T.: Quantitative analysis of histochemical reactions: Image analysis of light and electron microscopic radioautograms. Acta Histochem. Cytochem. 26, 281-291, 1993a.

Nagata, T. Quantitative light and electron microscopic radioautographic studies on macromolecular synthesis in several organs of prenatal and postnatal aging mice. Chinese J. Histochem. Cytochem. 2: 106-108, 1993b.

Nagata, T.: Electron microscopic radioautography with cryo-fixation and dry-mounting procedure. Acta Histochem. Cytochem. 27: 471-489, 1994a.

Nagata, T.: Application of electron microscopic radioautography to clinical electron microscopy. Med. Electron Microsc. 27; 191-212, 1994b.

Nagata, T.: Radioautography in Medicine. Shinshu University Press, 268pp, Matsumoto, 1994c.

Nagata, T.: Radioautography, general and special. In, Histo- and Cyto-chemistry 1994, Japan Society of Histochemistry and Cytochemistry, ed, pp. 219-231, Gakusai Kikaku Co., Tokyo, 1994d.

Nagata, T., Application of electron microscopic radioautography to clinical electron microscopy. Med. Electron Microsc. 27, 191-212, 1994e.

Nagata, T.: Light and electron microscopic radioautographic study on macromolecular synthesis in digestive organs of aging mice. Cell. Mol. Biol. 41, 21-38, 1995a.

Nagata, T.: Histochemistry of the organs: Application of histochemistry to anatomy. Acta Anat. Nippon. 70, 448-471, 1995b.

Nagata, T.: Three-dimensional observation of whole mount cultured cells stained with histochemical reactions by ultrahigh voltage electron microscopy. Cell. Mol. Biol. 41, 783-792, 1995c.

Nagata, T.: Morphometry in anatomy: image analysis on fine structure and histochemical reactions with special reference to radioautography. Ital. J. Anat. 100 (Suppl. 1), 591-605, 1995d.

Nagata, T.: Technique and application of electron microscopic radioautography. J. Electron Microsc. 45, 258-274, 1996a.

Nagata, T.: Techniques of light and electron microscopic radioautography. In, Histochemistry and Cytochemistry 1996. Proc. Xth Internat. Congr. Histochem. Cytochem. Acta Histochem. Cytochem. 29 (Suppl.), 343-344, 1996b.

Nagata, T.: Remarks: Radioautographology, general and special. Cell. Mol. Biol. 42 (Suppl.), 11-12, 1996c.

Nagata, T.: On the terminology of radioautography vs. autoradiography. J. Histochem. Cytochem. 44, 1209-1209, 1996d.

Nagata, T.: Techniques and applications of microscopic radioautography. Histol. Histopathol. 12, 1091-1124, 1997a.

Nagata T.: Three-dimensional observation on whole mount cultured cells and thick sections stained with histochemical reactions by high voltage electron microscopy. In, Recent Advances in Microscopy of Cells, Tissues and Organs, Motta, P., Ed., Antonio Delfino Editore, Roma, pp. 37-44, 1997b.

Nagata, T.: Radioautographic study on collagen synthesis in the ocular tissues. J. Kaken Eye Res. 15, 1-9, 1997c.

Nagata, T.: Techniques of radioautography for medical and biological research. Braz. J. Biol. Med. Res. 31, 185-195, 1998a.

Nagata, T.: Radioautographology, the advocacy of a new concept. Braz. J. Biol. Med. Res. 31, 201-241, 1998b.

Nagata, T.: Radioautographic studies on DNA synthesis of the bone and skin of aging salamander. Bull. Nagano Women's Jr. College 6, 1-14, 1998c.

Nagata, T.: 3D observation of cell organelles by high voltage electron microscopy. Microscopy and Analysis, Asia Pacific Edition, 9, 29-32, 1999a.

Nagata, T.: Application of histochemistry to anatomy: Histochemistry of the organs, a novel concept. Proc. XV Congress of the International Federation of Associations of Anatomists, Ital. J. Anat. Embryol. 104 (Suppl. 1), 486-486, 1999b.

Nagata, T.: Aging changes of macromolecular synthesis in various organ systems as observed by microscopic radioautography after incorporation of radiolabeled precursors. Methods Find. Exp. Clin. Pharmacol. 21, 683-706, 1999c.

Nagata, T.: Radioautographic study on protein synthesis in mouse cornea. J. Kaken Eye Res. 8, 8-14, 1999d.

Nagata, T.: Radioautographology, general and special: a novel concept. Ital. J. Anat. Embryol. 104 (Suppl. 1), 487-487, 1999e.

Nagata, T.: Three-dimensional observations on thick biological specimens by high voltage electron microscopy. Image Analysis Stereolog. 19, 51-56, 2000a.

Nagata, T.: Biological microanalysis of radiolabeled and unlabeled compounds by radioautography and X-ray microanalysis. Scanning Microscopy International, 14, on line, 2000b.

Nagata, T.: Electron microscopic radioautographic study on protein synthesis in pancreatic cells of perinatal and aging mice. Bull. Nagano Women's Jr. College 8, 1-22, 2000c.

Nagata, T.: Light microscopic radioautographic study on radiosulfate incorporation into the tracheal cartilage in aging mice. Acta Histochem. Cytochem. 32, 377-383, 2000d.

Nagata, T.: Introductory remarks: Special radioautographology. Cell. Mol. Biol. 46 (Congress Suppl.), 161-161, 2000e.

Nagata, T.: Special radioautographology: the eye. J. Kaken Eye Res. 18, 1-13, 2000f.

Nagata, T.: Three-dimensional high voltage electron microscopy of thick biological specimens. Micron 32, 387-404, 2001a.

Nagata, T.: Three-dimensional and four-dimensional observation of histochemical and cytochemical specimens by high voltage electron microscopy. Acta Histochem. Cytochem. 34, 153-169, 2001b.

Nagata, T. : Special cytochemistry in cell biology. In, Internat. Rev. Cytol. Jeon, K.W., ed., Vol. 211, Chapter 2, Academic Press, New York, pp. 33-154, 2001c.

Nagata, T. : Radioautographology General and Special, In, Prog. Histochem. Cytochem., Graumann, W., Ed., Vol. 37 No. 2, Urban & Fischer, Jena, pp. 57-226, 2002.

Nagata T.: Light and electron microscopic study on macromolecular synthesis in amitotic hepatocyte mitochondria of aging mice. Cell. Mol. Biol. 49, 591-611, 2003.

Nagata, T.: X-ray microanalysis of biological specimens by high voltage electron microscopy. In, Prog. Histochem. Cytochem., Graumann, W., Ed., Vol. 39, No. 4, Urban & Fischer Verlag, Jena, pp. 185-320, 2004.

Nagata T.: Aging changes of macromolecular synthesis in the uro-genital organs as revealed by electron microscopic radioautography. Ann. Rev. Biomed. Sci. 6, 13-78, 2005.

Nagata T.: Electron microscopic radioautographic study on protein synthesis in hepatocyte mitochondria of developing mice. Ann. Microsc. 6, 43-54, 2006a.

Nagata T.: Electron microscopic radioautographic study on nucleic acids synthesis in hepatocyte mitochondria of developing mice. The Sci. World J. 6: 1583-1598, 2006b.

Nagata T.: Macromolecular synthesis in hepatocyte mitochondria of aging mice as revealed by electron microscopic radioautography. I: Nucleic acid synthesis. In, Modern Research and Educational Topics in Microscopy. Mendez-Vilas, A. and Diaz, J. Eds., Formatex Micrscopy Series No. 3, Vol. 1, Formatex, Badajoz, Spain, pp. 245-258, 2007a.

Nagata T.: Macromolecular synthesis in hepatocyte mitochondria of aging mice as revealed by electron microscopic radioautography. II: Protein synthesis. In, Modern Research and Educational Topics in Microscopy. Mendez-Vilas, A. and Diaz, J. eds., Formatex Micrscopy Series No. 3, Vol. 1, Formatex, Badajoz, Spain, pp. 259-271, 2007b.

Nagata, T.: Electron microscopic radioautographic study on macromolecular synthesis in hepatocyte mitochondria of aging mouse. J. Cell Tissue Res. 7, 1019-1029, 2007c.

Nagata, T.; Electron microscopic radioautographic study on nucleic acids synthesis in hepatocyte mitochondria of developing mice. Trends Cell Molec. Biol. 2, 19-33, 2007d.

Nagata, T.; Aging changes of macromolecular synthesis in the mitochondria of mouse hepatocytes as revealed by microscopic radioautography. Ann. Rev. Biomed. Sci. 9, 30-36, 2007e.

Nagata, T.: Radioautographology, Bull. Shinshu Institute Alternat. Med. 2, 3-32, 2007f.

Nagata, T.: Electron microscopic radioautographic study on mitochondrial DNA synthesis in adrenal cortical cells of developing mice. J. Cell. Tis. Res. 8, 1303-1312, 2008a.

Nagata T.: Electron microscopic radioautographic study on mitochondrial DNA synthesis in adrenal cortical cells of developing and aging mice. The Sci. World J. 8, 683-697. 2008b.

Nagata, T.: Sexual difference between the macromolecular synthesis of hepatocyte mitochondria in male and female mice in aging as revealed by electron microscopic radioautography. Chapter 22. In, Women and Aging: New Research, H. T. Bennninghouse, A. D. Rosset, Eds. Nova Biomed. Books, New York, pp. 461-487, 2009a

Nagata, T.: Protein synthesis in hepatocytes of mice as revealed by electron microscopic radioautography. In, Protein Biosynthesis. Esterhouse, T. E. and Petrinos, L. B., Eds., Nova Biomed. Books, New York, pp. 133-161, 2009b.

Nagata, T.: Electron microscopic radioatuographic studies on macromolecular synthesis in mitochondria of various cells. 18EMSM Conference Proc. 9th Asia-Pacific Microscopy Conference (APMC9), Kuala Lumpur, Malaysia, pp. 48-50, 2009c.

Nagata, T.: Recent studies on macromolecular synthesis labeled with ^{3}H-thymidine in various organs as revealed by electron microscopic radioautography. Current Radiopharmaceutics 2, 118-128, 2009d.

Nagata, T.: Electron microscopic radioautographic study on mitochondrial DNA synthesis in adrenal medullary cells of developing and aging mice. J. Cell Tissue Res. 9, 1793-1802, 2009e.

Nagata, T.: Applications of high voltage electron microscopy to thick biological specimens. Ann. Microsc. 9, 4-40, 2009f.

Nagata, T.: Electron microscopic radioautographic study on DNA synthesis of mitochondria in adrenal medullary cells of aging mice. Open Anat. J. 1, 14-24, 2009g.

Nagata, T.: Electron microscopic radioautographic studies on macromolecular synthesis in mitochondria of animal cells in aging. Ann. Rev. Biomed. Sci. 11, 1-17, 2009h.

Nagata, T.: Electron microscopic radioautographic studies on macromoleclular synthesis in mitochondria of some organs in aging animals. Bull. Shinshu Inst. Alternat. Med. Welfare 4, 15-38, 2009i.

Nagata, T.: Electron microscopic radioautographic study on mitochondrial DNA synthesis in adreno-cortical cells of aging ddY mice. Bull. Shinshu Inst. Alternat. Med. Welfare 4, 51-66, 2009j.

Nagata T.: Electron microscopic radioautographic study on mitochondrial RNA synthesis in adrenocortical cells of aging mice. Open Anat J. 2, 91-97, 2010a.

Nagata T. Electron microscopic radioautographic study on mitochondrial RNA synthesis in adrenal medullary cells of aging and senescent mice. J Cell Tissue Res. 10, 2213-2222, 2010b.

Nagata, T.: Macromolecular synthesis in the livers of aging mice as revealed by electron microscopic radioautography. In, Prog. Histochem. Cytochem., Sasse, D., Ed., Elsevier, Amsterdam, Boston, London, New York, Oxford, Paris, Philadelphia, San Diego, St. Louis, Vol. 45, No. 1, pp. 1-80, 2010c.

Nagata, T.: Electron microscopic radioautographic study on protein synthesis of mitochondria in adrenal medullary cells of aging mice. Bulletin Shinshu Inst Alternat Med Welfare 5, 25-37, 2010d.

Nagata, T.: Electron microscopic radioautographic study on mitochondrial RNA synthesis in adrenal cortical and medullary cells of aging mice. J. Biomed. Sci. Enginer. 4, 219-232, 2010e.

Nagata, T.: Electron microscopic radioautographic study on protein synthesis of mitochondria in adrenal cortical cells of aging mice. Bulletin Shinshu Inst. Alternat. Med. Welfare 5, 38-52, 2010f.

Nagata T.: Electron microscopic radioautographic study on mitochondrial DNA, RNA and protein synthesis in adrenal cells of aging mice. Formatex Microscopy Series No. 3, Vol. 3, Formatex, Badajoz, Spain, in press, 2010g.

Nagata, T.: Electron microscopic radioautographic studies on macromolecular synthesis in mitochondria of animal cells in aging. Ann. Rev. Biomed. Sci. 12, 1-29, 2010h.

Nagata, T., Cui, H., Gao, F.: Radioautographic study on glycoprotein synthesis in the ocular tissues. J. Kaken Eye Res. 13, 11-18, 1995.

Nagata, T., Cui, H., Kong, Y.: The localization of TGF-b1 and its mRNA in the spinal cords of prenatal and postnatal aging mice demonstrated with immunohistochemical and in situ hybridization techniques. Bull. Nagano Women's Jr. College, 7, 75-88, 1999a.

Nagata, T., Cui, H., Liang, Y.: Light microscopic radioautographic study on the protein synthesis in the cerebellum of aging mouse. Bull. Nagano Women's Jr. College, 9, 41-60 (2001).

Nagata, T., Fujii, Y., Usuda, N.: Demonstration of extranuclear nucleic acid synthesis in mammalian cells under experimental conditions by electron microscopic radioautography. Proc. 10th Internat. Congr. Electr. Microsc. 2, 305-306, 1982b.

Nagata, T., Hirano, I., Shibata, O., Nagata, T.: A radioautographic study on the DNA synthesis in the hepatic and the pancreatic acinar cells of mice during the postnatal growth, with special reference to binuclearity. Med. J. Shinshu Univ. 11, 35-42, 1966.

Nagata, T., Ito, M., Chen, S.: Aging changes of DNA synthesis in the submandibular glands of mice as observed by light and electron microscopic radioautography. Ann. Microsc. 1, 4-12, 2000a.

Nagata, T. Ito, M., Liang, Y.: Study of the effects of aging on macromolecular synthesis in mouse steroid secreting cells using microscopic radioautography. Methods Find. Exp. Clin. Pharmacol. 22, 5-18, 2000b.

Nagata, T., Iwadare, I., Murata, F.: Electron microscopic radioautography of nucleic acid synthesis in cultured cells treated with several carcinogens. Acta Pharmacol. Toxicol. 41, 64-65, 1977c.

Nagata, T., Kawahara, I.: Radioautographic study of the synthesis of sulfomucin in digestive organs of mice. J. Trace Microprobe Analysis 17, 339-355, 1999.

Nagata, T., Kawahara, I., Usuda, N., Maruyama, M., Ma, H.: Radioautographic studies on the glycoconjugate synthesis in the gastrointestinal mucosa of the mouse. In, Glycoconjugate in Medicine, Ohyama, M., Muramatsu, T., Eds, pp. 251-256, Professional Postgrad. Service, Tokyo, 1988a.

Nagata, T., Kong, Y.: Distribution and localization of TGFb1 and bFGF, and their mRNAs in aging mice. Bull. Nagano Women's Jr. College 6, 87-105, 1998.

Nagata, T., Ma, H., Electron microscopic radioautographic study on mitochondrial DNA synthesis in hepatocytes of aging mouse. Ann. Microsc. 5, 4-18, 2005a.

Nagata, T., Ma, H., Electron microscopic radioautographic study on RNA synthesis in hepatocyte mitochondria of aging mouse. Microsc. Res. Tech. 67, 55-64, 2005b.

Nagata, T., Momoze, S.: Aging changes of the amitotic and binucleate cells in dog livers. Acta Anat. Nipponica 34, 187-190, 1959.

Nagata, T., Morita, T., I. Kawahara, I.: Radioautographic studies on radiosulfate incorporation in the digestive organs of mice. Histol. Histopathol. 14, 1-8, 1999b.

Nagata, T., Murata, F.: Electron microscopic dry-mounting radioautography for diffusible compounds by means of ultracryotomy. Histochemistry 54, 75-82, 1977.

Nagata, T., Murata, F., Yoshida, K., Ohno, S., Iwadare, N.: Whole mount radioautography of cultured cells as observed by high voltage electron microscopy. Proc. Fifth Internat. Conf. High Voltage Electron Microsc. 347-350, 1977d.

Nagata, T., Nawa, T.: A modification of dry-mounting technique for radioautography of water-soluble compounds. Histochemie 7, 370-371, 1966a.

Nagata, T., Nawa, T.: A radioautographic study on the nucleic acids synthesis of binucleate cells in cultivated fibroblasts of chick embryos. Med. J. Shinshu Univ. 11, 1-5, 1966b.

Nagata, T., Nawa, T., Yokota, S.: A new technique for electron microscopic dry-mounting radioautography of soluble compounds. Histochemie 18, 241-249, 1969.

Nagata, T., Nishigaki, T., Momose, Y.: Localization of anti-allergic agent in rat mast cells demonstrated by light and electron microscopic radioautography. Acta Histochem. Cytochem. 19, 669-683, 1986b.

Nagata, T., Ohno, S., Kawahara, I., Yamabayashi, S., Fujii, Y., Murata, F.: Light and electron microscopic radioautography of nucleic acid synthesis in mitochondria and peroxisomes of rat hepatic cells during and after DEHP administration. Acta Histochem. Cytochem. 16, 610-611, 1979.

Nagata, T., Ohno, S., Murata, F.: Electron microscopic dry-mounting radioautography for soluble compounds. Acta Phamacol. Toxicol. 41, 62-63, 1977a.

Nagata, T., Ohno, S., Yoshida, K., Murata, F.: Nucleic acid synthesis in proliferating peroxisomes of rat liver as revealed by electron microscopical radioautography. Histochem. J. 14, 197-204, 1982a.

Nagata, T., Olea, M. T.: Electron microscopic radioautographic study on the protein synthesis in aging mouse spleen. Bull. Nagano Women's Jr. College 7, 1-9, 1999.

Nagata, T., Shibata, O., Omochi, S.: A new method for radioautographic osbservation on isolated cells. Histochemie 2, 255-259, 1961

Nagata, T., Shibata, O., Nawa, T.: Simplified methods for mass production of radioautograms. -Acta Anat. Nippon.42, 162-166, 1967a.

Nagata, T., Shibata, O., Nawa, T.: Incorporation of tritiated thymidine into mitochondrial DNA of the liver and kidney cells of chickens and mice in tissue culture. Histochemie 10, 305-308, 1967b.

Nagata, T., Shimamura, K., Onozawa, M., Kondo, T., Ohkubo, K., Momoze, S.: Relationship of binuclearity to cell function in some organs. I. Frequencies of binucleate cells in some organs of toads in summer and winter. Med. J. Shinshu Univ. 5, 147-152, 1960a.

Nagata, T., Shimamura, K., Kondo, T., Onozawa, M., Momoze, S., Okubo, M.: Relationship of binuclearity to cell function in some organs. II. Variation of frequencies of binucleate cells in some organs of dogs owing to aging. Med. J. Shinshu Univ. 5, 153-158, 1960b.

Nagata, T., Steggerda, F. R.: Histological study on the deganglionated small intestine of the dog. Physiologist 6, 242-242, 1963.

Nagata, T., Steggerda, F. R.: Observations on the increase of binucleate cells in the ganglion cells of the dog's intestine due to experimental ischemia. Anat. Rec. 148, 315-315, 1964.

Nagata, T., Toriyama, K., Kong, Y., Jin, C., Gao, F.: Radioautographic study on DNA synthesis in the ciliary bodies of aging mice. J. Kaken Eye Res.12, 1-11, 1994.

Nagata, T., Usuda, N.: Image processing of electron microscopic radioautograms in clinical electron microscopy. J. Clin. Electron. Microsc. 18, 451-452, 1985.

Nagata, T., Usuda, N.: Studies on the nucleic acid synthesis in pancreatic acinar cells of aging mice by means of electron microscopic radioautography. J. Clin. Electron Microsc. 19, 486-487, 1986.

Nagata, T., Usuda, N.: Electron microscopic radioautography of protein synthesis in pancreatic acinar cells of aging mice. Acta Histochem. Cytochem. 26, 481-481, 1993a.

Nagata, T., Usuda, N.: In situ hybridization by electron microscopy using radioactive probes. J. Histochem. Cytochem. 41, 1119-1119, 1993b.

Nagata, T., Usuda, N., Ma, H.: Electron microscopic radioautography of nucleic acid synthesis in pancreatic acinar cells of prenatal and postnatal aging mice. Proc. XIth Intern. Cong. Electr. Microsc. 3, 2281-2282, 1984.

Nagata, T., Usuda, N., Ma, H.: Electron microscopic radioautography of lipid synthesis in pancreatic cells of aging mice. J. Clin. Electr. Microsc. 23, 841-842, 1990.

Nagata, T., Usuda, N., Maruyama, M., Ma, H.: Electron microscopic radioautographic study on lipid synthesis in perinatal mouse pancreas. J. Clin. Electr. Microsc. 21, 756-757, 1988b.

Nagata, T., Usuda, N., Suzawa, H., Kanzawa, M.: Incorporation of ^{3}H-glucosamine into the pancreatic cells of aging mice as demonstrated by electron microscopic radioautography. J. Clin. Electron Microsc. 25, 646-647, 1992.
Nagata, T., Yamabayashi, S.: Intracellular localization of ^{3}H-befunolol by means of electron microscopic radioautography of cryo-fixed ultrathin sections. J. Clin. Electron Microsc. 16, 737-738, 1983.
Nagata, T., Yoshida, K., Murata, F.: Demonstration of hot and cold mercury in the human thyroid tissues by means of radioautography and chemography. Acta Pharmacol. Toxicol. 41, 60-61, 1977b.
Nagata, T., Yoshida, K., Ohno, S., Murata, F.: Ultrastructural localization of soluble and insoluble ^{3}H-methyl prednisolone as revealed by electron microscopic dry-mounting radioautography. Proc. 9th Internat. Congr. Electr. Microsc. 2, 40-41, 1978b.
Nishigaki, T., Momose, Y., Nagata, T.: Light microscopic radioautographic study of the localization of anti-allergic agent, tranilast, in rat mast cells. Histochem. J. 19, 533-536, 1987.
Nishigaki, T., Momose, Y., Nagata, T.: Electron microscopic radioautographic study of the localization of an anti-allergic agent, tranilast, in rat mast cells. Cell. Mol. Biol. 36, 65-71, 1990a.
Nishigaki, T., Momose, Y., Nagata, T.: Localization of the anti-allergic agent tranilast in the urinary bladder of rat as demonstrated by light microscopic radioautography. Drug Res. 40, 272-275, 1990b.
Oguchi, K., Nagata, T.: A radioautographic study of activated satellite cells in dystrophic chicken muscle. In, Current Research in Muscular Dystrophy Japan. The Proc. Ann. Meet. Muscular Dystrophy Res. 1980, pp. 16-17, Ministry of Welfare of Japan, Tokyo, 1980.
Oguchi, K., Nagata, T.: Electron microscopic radioautographic observation on activated satellite cells in dystrophy chickens. In, Clinical Studies on the Etiology of Muscular Dystrophy. Annual Report on Neurological Diseases 1981, pp. 30-33, Ministry of Welfare of Japan, Tokyo, 1981.
Ohno, S., Fujii, Y., Usuda, N., Endo, T., Hidaka, H., Nagata, T.: Demonstration of intracellular localization of calmodulin antagonist by wet-mounting radioautography. J. Electron Microsc. 32, 1-12, 1983.
Ohno, S., Fujii, Y., Usuda, N., Nagata, T., Endo, T., Tanaka, T., Hidaka, H.: Intracellular localization of calmodulin antagonists (W-7). In, Calmodulin and intracellular Ca^{2+} receptors. Kakiuchi, S., Hidaka, H, Means, A. R., Eds., pp. 39-48, Plenum Publishing Co., New York, 1982.
Olea, M. T.: An ultrastructural localization of lysosomal acid phosphatase activity in aging mouse spleen: a quantitative X-ray microanalytical study. Acta Histochem. Cytochem. 24, 201-208, 1991.
Olea, M. T., Nagata, T.: X-ray microanalysis of cerium in mouse spleen cells demonstrating acid phosphatase activity using high voltage electron microscopy, Cell. Mol. Biol. 37, 155-163, 1991.
Olea, M. T., Nagata, T. : Simultaneous localization of ^{3}H-thymidine incorporation and acid phosphatase activity in mouse spleen: EM radioautography and cytochemistry. Cell. Mol. Biol. 38, 115-122, 1992a.

Olea, M. T., Nagata, T.: A radioautographic study on RNA synthesis in aging mouse spleen after ^{3}H-uridine labeling in vitro. Cell. Mol. Biol. 38, 399-405, 1992b.

Oliveira, S. F., Nagata, T., Abrahamsohn, P. A., Zorn, T. M. T.: Electron microscopic radioautographic study on the incorporation of ^{3}H-proline by mouse decidual cells. Cell. Mol. Biol. 37, 315-323, 1991.

Oliveira, S. F., Abrahamsohn, P. A., Nagata, T., Zorn, T. M. T.: Incorporation of ^{3}H-amino acids by endometrial stromal cells during decidualization in the mouse. A radioautographical study. Cell. Mol. Biol. 41, 107-116, 1995.

Pearse, A. G. E.: Histochemistry, Theoretical and Applied. 4th Ed. Vol. 1. 439 pp., 1980, Vol. 2. 1055 pp., 1985, Vol. 3. Ed. with P. Stoward, 728 pp. Churchill Livingstone, Edinburgh, London and New York, 1991.

Sakai, Y., Ikado, S., Nagata, T.: Electron microscopic radioautography of satellite cells in regenerating muscles. J. Clin. Electr. Microsc. 10, 508-509, 1977.

Sato, A.: Quantitative electron microscopic studies on the kinetics of secretory granules in G-cells. Cell Tissue Res. 187, 45-59, 1978.

Sato, A., Iida, F., Furihara, R., Nagata, T.: Electron microscopic raioautography of rat stomach G-cells by means of ^{3}H-amino acids. J. Clin. Electron Microsc. 10, 358-359, 1977.

Shimizu, T., Usuda, N., Yamanda, T., Sugenoya, A., Iida, F.: Proliferative activity of human thyroid tumors evaluated by proliferating cell nuclear antigen/cyclin immnohistochemical studies. Cancer 71, 2807-2812, 1993.

Sun, L.: Age related changes of RNA synthesis in the lungs of aging mice by light and electron microscopic radioautography. Cell. Mol. Biol. 41, 1061-1072, 1995.

Sun, L., Gao, F., Duan, H., Nagata, T.: Light microscopic radioautography of DNA synthesis in pulmonary cells in aging mice. In, Radioautography in Medicine, Nagata, T. Ed., pp. 201-205, Shinshu University Press, Matsumoto, 1994.

Sun, L., Gao, F., Nagata, T.: Study on the DNA synthesis of pulmonary cells in aging mice by light microscopic radioautography. Cell. Mol. Biol. 41, 851-859, 1995a.

Sun, L., Gao, F., Jin, C., Duan, H., Nagata, T.: An electron microscopic radioautographic study on the DNA synthesis of pulmonary tissue cells in aging mice. Med. Electron. Microsc. 28, 129-131, 1995b.

Sun, L., Gao, F., Jin, C., Nagata, T.: DNA synthesis in the tracheae of aging mice by means of light and electron microscopic radioautography. Acta Histochem. Cytochem. 30, 211-220, 1997a.

Sun, L., Gao, F., Nagata, T.: A Light Microscopic radioautographic study on protein synthesis in pulmonary cells of aging mice. Acta Histochem. Cytochem. 30, 463-470, 1997b.

Suzuki, K., Imada, T., Gao, F., Ma, H., Nagata, T.: Radioautographic study of benidipine hydrochloride: localization in the mesenteric artery of spontaneously hypertensive rat. Drug Res. 44, 129-133, 1994.

Terauchi, A., Mori, T., Kanda, H., Tsukada, M., Nagata, T.: Radioautographic study of 3H-taurine uptake in mouse skeletal muscle cells. J. Clin. Electron Microsc. 21, 627-628, 1988.

Terauchi, A., Nagata, T.: Observation on incorporation of ^{3}H-taurine in mouse skeletal muscle cells by light and electron microscopic radioautography. Cell. Mol. Biol. 39, 397-404, 1993.

Terauchi, A., Nagata, T.: In corporation of ^{3}H-taurine into the blood capillary cells of mouse skeletal muscle. Radioautography in Medicine, Nagata, T. ed., Shinshu University Press, Matsumoto, 1994.

Toriyama, K.: Study on the aging changes of DNA and protein synthesis of bipolar and photo-receptor cells of mouse retina by light and electron microscopic radioautography. Cell. Mol. Biol. 41, 593-601, 1995.

Tsukahara, S., Yoshida, K., Nagata, T.: A radioautographic study on the incorporation of ^{14}C-bupranolol (beta-blocking agent) into the rabbit eye. Histochemistry 68, 237-244, 1980.

Usuda, N., Nagata, T.: Electron microscopic radioautography of acyl-CoA mRNA by in situ hybridization. J. Clin. Electron Microsc. 25, 332-333, 1992.

Usuda, N., Nagata, T.: The immunohistochemical and in situ hybridization studies on hepatic peroxisomes. Acta Histochem. Cytochem. 28, 169-172, 1995.

Usuda, N., Hanai, T., Morita, T., Nagata, T.: Radioautographic demonstration of peroxisomal acyl-CoA oxidase mRNA by in situ hybridization. In, Recent advances in cellular and molecular biology, Vol. 6. Molecular biology of nucleus, peroxisomes, organelles and cell movement. Wegmann, R. J., Wegmann, M., Eds, pp.181-184, Peeters Press, Leuven, 1992.

Uwa, H., Nagata, T.: Cell population kinetics of the scleroblast during ethisterone-induced anal-fin process formation in adult females of the Medaka. Dev. Growth Different. 9, 693-694, 1976.

Watanabe, I., Makiyama, M. C. K., Nagata, T.: Electron microscopic radioautographic observation of the submandibular salivary gland of aging mouse. Acta Microscopica 6. 130-131, 1997.

Yamabayashi, S., Gunarso, W., Tsukahara, S., Nagata, T.: Incorporation of ^{3}H-befunolol (beta blocking agent) into melanin granules of ocular tissues in the pigmented rabbits. I. Light microscopic radioautography. Histochemistry 73, 371-375, 1981.

Yamada, A. T.: Timely and topologically defined protein synthesis in the periimplanting mouse endometrium revealed by light and electron microscopic radioautography. Cell. Mol. Biol. 39, 1-12, 1993.

Yamada, A., Nagata, T.: Ribonucleic acid and protein synthesis in the uterus of pregnant mouse during activation of implantation window. Med. Electron Microsc. 27, 363-365, 1992a.

Yamada, A., Nagata, T.: Light and electron microscopic raioautography of DNA synthesis in the endometria of pregnant-ovariectomized mice during activation of implantation window. Cell. Mol. Biol. 38, 763-774, 1992b.

Yamada, A., Nagata, T.: Light and electron microscopic raioautography of RNA synthesis of peri-implanting pregnant mouse during activation of receptivity for blastocyst implantation. Cell. Mol. Biol. 38, 211-233, 1993.

Yoshinaga, K.: Uterine receptivity for blastcyst implantation. Ann. N. Y. Acad. Sci. USA, 541, 424-431, 1988.

Yoshizawa, S., Nagata, A., Honma, T., Oda, M., Murata, F., Nagata, T.: Study of ethionine pancreatitis by means of electron microscopic radioautography. J. Clin. Electron Microsc. 7, 349-350, 1974.

Yoshizawa, S., Nagata, A., Honma, T., Oda, M., Murata, F., Nagata, T.: Radioautographic study of protein synthesis in pancreatic exocrine cells of alcoholic rats. J. Clin. Electron. Microsc. 10, 372-373, 1977.

18

Cellular Senescence and Its Relation with Telomere

Diego Julio Arenas-Aranda[1],
Elena Hernández-Caballero[2] and Fabio Salamanca-Gómez[1]
[1]*Unit of Medical Research in Human Genetics, Medical National Center 21st Century, Mexican Institute of Social Insurance,*
[2]*Section of Posgrado's Studies and Investigation, High School of Medicine, Technical National Institute. Mexico City, Mexico*

1. Introduction

For years it was thought that cells under culture conditions were immortal; however, from the publication of the works of Leonard Hayflick, this concept changed. Hayflick demonstrated that somatic cells under culture conditions had a limited capacity to proliferate; they stop dividing and enter into permanent arrest in the cell cycle, known as senescence. A particular characteristic of this state is that the cell maintains its viability and metabolic activity, and despite the presence of nutrients and mitogens, it does not divide (Ouellette et al., 2000). There are reports of cells that have been maintained in this state during several decades (Michaloglou et al., 2005). Regarding the origin of this process in mammalian cells, two different and apparently contradictory hypotheses have been proposed: senescence as a mechanism that suppresses tumor development, and senescence as the loss of the cells' regenerative capacity *in vivo*. In terms of the first hypothesis, senescence possesses a beneficial effect for the organism because it would avoid the development of cancer; otherwise, the second hypothesis would exert a harmful effect on organisms in that it would favor aging. Commentary will appear later on that both hypotheses joined together in the antagonist pleiotropic hypothesis (Williams, 1957; Campisi & Adda di Fagagna, 2007; Campisi, 2011).

2. Hayflick experiments

It was 50 years ago that Hayflick first reported on the condition of mortality that cells maintain (Hayflick & Moorhead, 1961), which the researcher himself cited in 1998 (Hayflick, 1998). To the present day, few have dared to enter into the study of Biogerontology. The generalized belief was that cells kept under culture conditions could replicate themselves indefinitely; if this were not possible, it would be due to lack of knowledge on the appropriate conditions for maintaining cells under culture (Hayflick, 2003). Carrel in 1921 stated that it was possible to keep chicken-heart fibroblasts indefinitely, maintaining these with embryonic tissue extract. However, as Hayflick noted, this experiment involved a great technical error because the extract with which the culture was nourished throughout 34 years was supplied with fresh cells throughout the entire time that the experiment lasted (Hayflick, 1998).

Hayflick identified three phases in his cellular proliferation experiments: phase I or that of primary culture, in which cells initiate their proliferation; phase II, that of rapid and continuous proliferation, and phase III, in which proliferation velocity diminishes and is finally detained (Hayflick & Moorhead, 1961). Hayflick concludes that cells possess some type of counting mechanism because they stop dividing after a certain number of duplications, between 40 and 60. This counting mechanism is conserved even after the cells are frozen and cultured anew (Hayflick & Moorhead, 1961; Hayflick, 1965).

Some years later, thanks to the work of McClintock on chromosomal ends (McClintock, 1941), Olovnikov formulated his theory concerning the problem of replication and the solution to this. Suggesting that the inability of polymerase to replicate chromosomal ends totally was what could lead to cellular senescence, he proposed that the ends could function as a buffer, avoiding the loss of important sequences, but that in turn, this buffer function could also could be lost with successive replications (Olovnikov, 1996). Later, with the discovery of the telomeric repeats sequence of and telomerase by Blackburn, the study of telomeres and their participation in the senescence process began.

Currently, the existence is accepted of a limit of normal somatic cell replication, denominated the Hayflick limit. However, once the importance is established of telomerase as the enzyme that synthesizes telomeres (Greider & Blackburn, 1985), it was discovered that this enzyme is found to be active in immortalized cell lines (Morin, 1989), tumor cells (Kim et al., 1994), stem cells (Chiu et al., 1996), and embryonic and germinal cell lines (Mantell & Greider, 1994; Wright et al., 1996).

3. The antagonistic pleiotropy hypothesis

Antagonistic pleiotropy is a concept pertaining to Evolutionary Biology that proposes that some genes can have an impact on the physical state of the organism differentially throughout its lifetime (Williams, 1957; Tuminello & Han, 2011). It is suggested that senescence evolved as an example of antagonistic pleiotropy; thus, its characteristics are beneficial in a reproductively active organism; later in this organism's lifespan, these characteristics become deteriorating. That is, senescence is the result of the random accumulation, whether passive or active, of harmful mutations (Kirkwood, 1977), reducing vigor and longevity, after the individual has passed reproductive age (Walker, 2011), although there is no definitive evidence that supports the negative effect of senescence in old persons.

Diverse processes have been found that are considered examples of antagonistic pleiotropy. Inflammation is a vital process to fight against infections and for cicatrization at all ages, but is also a process that can have negative effects if it becomes chronic in old age (Hornsby, 2010). On analyzing the influence of TP53 polymorphisms on cancer with respect to age, Cherdyntseva et al. (2010) found a relationship between the presence of polymorphisms in both genes and the increase of the risk of lung cancer in young, but not in older, smokers, while the combination of wild-type alleles increased the risk of lung cancer in individuals aged >60 years. The researchers concluded that p53 protects the organism against cancer at the beginning of life, but that it promotes the aging phenotype in older persons, including the appearance of cancer at the end of life. Another recent study suggests that allele ε4 carriers enjoy a beneficial cognitive effect in youth, and that later at an advanced age present cognitive diminution, which could increase the risk of presenting Alzheimer disease, although it could be that this allele is not pleiotropically antagonistic, but rather that it interacts with other risk factors for Alzheimer disease (Tuminello & Han, 2011). Feltes et al. (2011) suggest that aging and age-associated diseases could be the result of a program of development that is activated from the embryo stage, that persists throughout life, and that is regulated by the interaction of protein networks that connect environmental with molecular signals. The protein networks of the immune system, the epigenetic network, and aerobic metabolism are subject to great selection pressure during embryogenesis. However, this pressure becomes more relaxed in the adult, which allows the initiation of aging-associated diseases.

4. Somatic cells and senescence

After gametes are fused during the fertilization process, that primordial cell denominated the zygote begins a long journey in the formation of the individual. However, this journey begins with an accelerated expansion in the number of cells, which later decelerates. Once the organism has been formed, it will utilize cellular replication during its entire lifetime to grow, regenerate its tissues, cure wounds, or during the immune response.

Somatic cells possess a limited number of possible cell divisions, after which these become refractory to mitogeneic stimuli and enter into replicative senescence. In 2001, Sin et al. cite that aging at the cellular level is the result of cell function alterations, such as the response to DNA structural changes that is reflected in the expression of genes. A senescent cell remains arrested at cell cycle stage G1, and although it does not divide again, it remains metabolically active for a long time. The accumulation of mutations and damage to the DNA, together with inefficient repair mechanisms, become critical with each cell division and cause genetic heterogeneity in aging cells (De, 2011). There are somatic cells that possess the capacity to renew themselves, such as epithelial and blood cells, while there are cells that once differentiated, do not divide again, such as neurons. The equilibrium in death maintains homeostasis in the individual; thus, excessive death can lead to tissue degeneration and the inability to die can lead to hyperplasia and finally, cancer. The accumulated errors in a senescent cell's DNA can alter this balance and cause diverse diseases (Hotchkiss et al., 2009).

5. Senescent phenotype

To date, there is no senescence marker that is totally specific for this stage because not all senescent cells express the same markers. These cells can exhibit diverse changes that in their entirety can aid us in defining the senescent phenotype (Rodier & Campisi, 2011).

Change in cell volume is one of the most evident characteristics of a senescent cell, because cells may be observed that range from 1,000 μm^2 in an early passage of human fetal fibroblasts up to 9,000 μm² in terminal passages of the culture. Size increase has been correlated with changes in cytoskeletal organization (Wang & Gundersen, 1984), which leads to modification in cell shape. For example, fibroblasts lose their typical tapered form to acquire a flat appearance (Greenberg et al., 1977), apparently due to changes in the expression of diverse cytoskeletal proteins. Nishio et al. (2001) found that senescent fibroblasts contain three times the amount of the cytoskeletal protein vimentin as embryonic fibroblasts. Vimentin presents as dense filament bundles that are parallel to the longest cell-body axis in senescent cells, while in young cells vimentin formation is observed as a network of short and thin filaments. The authors also demonstrated that young fibroblasts acquire a senescent phenotype once they are transfected with a vector that over expresses the vimentin gene, while actin levels diminish in senescent fibroblasts (Nishio & Inoue, 2005). This diminution causes rigidity in old donor cells and increases in the kinesis of cell reorganization (Zahn et al., 2011). On the other hand, cellular adhesion of aging fibroblasts increases. It was found recently that the senescence of vascular epithelial cells induces an increase in cell adhesion proteins, which in turn increases the adhesion of monocytes to endothelial cells through their binding with Intracellular adhesion molecule 1 (ICAM1), contributing to the appearance of atherosclerosis (Yanaka et al., 2011).

Another characteristic of cellular senescence is change in diverse organelles; a very common occurrence comprises the increase in lysosome number and size. In lysosomes, granules of lipofuscin, the so-called aging pigment, accumulate (Brunk & Terman, 2002; Gutteridge, 1984). This material cannot be degraded by the cell's proteolytic machinery, is highly toxic, and inhibits the degradation of oxidized proteins (Bader et al., 2007; Höhn et al., 2011). Another lysosome-linked senescence biomarker is β-galactosidase, which is derived from the β-D-galactosidase and whose activity increases in senescent cells. In non-senescent cells, lysosomes possess a pH4-optimal function, while when the cell ages, the lysosomal compartment expands and β-galactosidase increases; thus, it is possible to detect a suboptimal pH of 6, a change known as senescence-associated β-galactosidase activity (Dimri et al., 1995; Lee et al., 2006). Senescence is also implicated in the deterioration of mitochondrial function and in the appearance of mutations in mitochondrial DNA, due to the lack of a repair system (Percy et al., 2008), and it is considered that aberrant production of Reactive oxygen species (ROS) can increase the mitochondrial mass (Hwang et al., 2009) and on the other hand accelerate telomere shortening and contribute to cellular aging (Liu et al., 2002) due to damage to the DNA. With respect to the nucleus, the increase in chromatin condensation is the most evident nuclear change. Regions are formed that are known as Senescence-associated heterochromatin foci (SAHF); these DNA regions are associated with heterochromatin proteins such as HP1 and H3K9m (Narita et al., 2003). SAHF are also evident in cells that become senescent because of oncogenic stress with H-Ras (Kosar et al., 2011).

Changes in senescent cells are also reflected in their functions; for example, fibroblasts under culture conditions adopt a matrix-degrading phenotype, while adrenal cortex epithelial cells produce an altered steroid-hormone profile (Campisi, 2000). Due to the increase in the secretion of pro-inflammatory proteins such as interleukins and chemokines, it is said that senescent cells are found in a pro-inflammatory state (Freund et al., 2010), which in an aging organism can favor tissue deterioration.

5.1 Changes in gene expression, growth arrest, and apoptosis resistance

Cell cycle arrest-associated replicative senescence is related with telomere shortening and, as previously noted, is a response for suppressing tumor formation and that can have aging of the organism as a side effect (Harley et al., 1990; Campisi, 2011). The cell population gradually stops dividing. (Thomas et al., 1997). Cell growth inhibition can be the result of cellular quiescence, whether due to lack of growth or nutrient factors or to other in- and extrinsic factors. This leads to the cell's exhibiting a low metabolic rate, low protein synthesis and cell functions, and the absence of growth (Blagosklonny, 2011). The senescent cell is defined by the permanent lack of replicative potential despite receiving a mitogenic stimulus (Rodier & Campisi, 2011). The cells remain arrested in G1, although on some occasions can be stopped in G2 (Harley et al., 1990). The central signaling pathways for senescence are represented by the p16-pRb Retinoblastoma (Rb) protein and the p53 tumor suppressor (Lowe & Sherr, 2003). The p14-p53-p21 pathway is partially telomere-dependent, while the p16-pRb pathway is independent of the presence of dysfunctional telomeres (Campisi & d'Adda di Fagagna, 2007). The product of *p53* gene accumulates in response to cellular stress, which activates a specific gene target program to restrict the growth of abnormal or damaged cells; the result can be apoptosis, transitory cell cycle arrest, or permanent arrest (Beausejour et al., 2003). Thus, the product of *p53 gene* possesses anti-cancerous as well as pro-aging effects depending upon the context of the individual's age (Campisi, 2005). Among p53 target genes are found the Cyclin-dependent kinase (CDK) inhibitor p21, the pro-apoptotic genes *BAX* and *APAF1*, and the E3 ubiquitin ligase, MDM2 (Vousden & Lu, 2002). *p53* expression is controlled by p19 (Arf). On the other hand, Rb expression is controlled by p16Ink4a, whose protein levels increase in senescent cells. p16Ink4a maintains pRb in a hypophosphorylated state, which inhibits cell proliferation and induces growth arrest through the pRB effect on E2F; this is necessary to activate the genes implicated in cell cycle progression (Campisi & d'Adda di Fagagna, 2007). Both signaling pathways interact and are reciprocally regulated. However, each can interrupt the cell cycle independently.

As Blagosklonny (2011) cites, cell arrest is only one part of the senescence equation, because senescent cells also become resistant to apoptosis. There are mechanisms of defense that augment apoptosis resistance, increasing anti-apoptotic signaling and avoiding the death of damaged cells. The increase of apoptosis resistance is a cell safety mechanism, because if cells have an acute stress due to some damage, they possess the capacity of recovering their homeostasis. However, in aging, when stress becomes persistent apoptosis resistance can cause the survival of undesired cells (Hampel et al., 2004; Salminen et al., 2011). It has been observed that the equilibrium between apoptotic and pro-apoptotic proteins changes with age. Bcl-2 and Bcl-xL protein levels are higher in aging than in young fibroblasts, while pro-apoptotic Bax levels are higher in young cells (Rochette & Brash, 2008). Apoptosis markers such as FasL and cytochrome C decrease in serum and, on the other hand, levels of soluble Fas (an apoptosis inhibitor) increase (Kavathia et al., 2009). Salminen et al. (2011) suggest that apoptosis resistance can affect the host's defenses in age-related fashion, a situation that meets promoted by the chronic inflammation that senescent cells develop.

6. Senescence markers

There are some molecular senescence markers that are characteristic of damage to DNA, including the nuclear foci of phosphorylated histones H2AX and DNA damage response factors such as 53BP1, MDC1, and NBS1 (d'Adda di Fagagna, 2008), which explains why culture shock can trigger senescence without the participation of telomeres. p16 is used for identification of senescent cells due to that it is overexpressed in the majority of these cells (Krishnamurthy et al., 2004). Although it has been demonstrated that in *Caenorhabditis elegans* alterations in microRNA´s (miRNAs) expression are associated with aging, the role that these could play in mammals remains unknown. In *C. elegans,* lin-4 over expression leads to an extension in its life span, while loss of lin-4 reduces the life span (Boehm & Slack, 2005). Lin-4 acts on the lin-14 messenger, affecting not only the life span, but also the insulin signaling pathway (Hung et al., 2010).

7. Causes of cellular senescence

In stem cells, it has been observed that premature differentiation and senescence are alternatives to DNA damage repair that can exert a beneficial effect on restricting the accumulation of defective stem cells. However, sensitivity to DNA damage and p53-related apoptosis induction differ widely among stem cells (Blanpain et al., 2011). The stem cells of melanocytes, for example, undergo premature differentiation, which reduces the stem cell pool and causes graying of the hair (Inomata et al., 2009). On the other hand, loss of TP63 (a member of the p53 family) in dermal precursors leads to skin ulceration and cicatrization defects due to genomic instability and the induction of senescence (Su et al., 2009).

Recently, a chromatin remodeling factor was found to be implicated in replicative senescence, the Jun 2 dimerization protein (JDP2), which binds to histones and inhibits the binding of Polycomb repressor complexes (PRC1 and PRC2) to p16 gene promotor (Huang et al., 2011).

7.1 Telomere-induced senescense

The loss of proliferative potential can be a genetically programmed process. The telomere-associated aging theory suggests that progressive telomere sequence loss triggers chronic p53 activation, which consequently leads the cell to halt its proliferation (Lee et al., 1998). Telomere shortening is a stochastic event; thus, telomere length varies greatly among individuals (Halaschek-Wiener et al., 2008).

Dysfunctional telomeres trigger the response to DNA damage, which includes activation of ATM, 53BP1, Mdc1, Chk2, and H2AX, in addition to over expression of cell cycle inhibitors p21Cip1/Waf1 and p16INK4a and under expression of different cell cycle proteins (Herbig et al., 2004).

7.2 Senescence induced by non-telomeric chromatin alterations

Non-genotoxic stress can cause perturbations in chromatin, that is, epigenetic changes that can alter the genetic schema of the cell. It has been demonstrated that global genome methylation diminishes with age. However, it has also been observed that the promoters of certain genes can be hypermethylated, thus silenced. Histones themselves undergo modifications during aging, whether because of methylation or hypoacetylation; all of these chromatin regions in senescent cells are observed as transcriptionally inactive domains

(SAHF) (Funayama, 2007). One characteristic of the senescence program is observed in cultured fibroblasts in chromatin reorganization through H3 methylation in the Lys9 residue and by protein recruitment in the heterochromatin. Some agents that interact with DNA, such as doxorubicin, cisplatin, taxol, vincristine, cytarabine, and etoposide, can produce the senescent phenotype in tumor cells (Chang et al., 1999).

It has been suggested that the condensation of genes implicated in proliferation through SAHF formation can contribute directly to senescence-associated silencing. However, it was recently suggested that SAHF are the result of persistent damage to the DNA and that it is condensation of the genes that promote proliferation, to a greater extent than large-scale SAHF, which detains senescence-associated proliferation (Rai & Adams, 2011).

7.3 Senescence induced by stress and other factors

Cellular senescence can additionally be induced prior to telomere shortening, which is also known as premature senescence or stress-induced premature senescence. One example are fibroblasts under culture, which are exposed to stress by abnormal concentrations of nutrients and growth factors, in addition to the absence of neighbor cells and extracellular matrix, which can lead to the senescent phenotype (Sherr & DePinho, 2000). It also results from exposure to mutagens, such as ionizing radiation, ROS, chemotherapeutic agents, or bacterial toxins (Campisi & d'Adda di Fagagna, 2007); thus, the molecular mechanisms of induction are nearly identical to replicative senescence, that is, it is mediated by ATM-p53-p21. Another type is oncogene-induced senescence (Vavrova & Rezacova, 2011). However, it has been observed that moderate stress leads to telomere shortening and that the main cause of shortening is due to the presence of damaged bases, which interferes with the replication fork in telomeres, increasing the extension of the non-replicated ends (von Zglinicki, 2002; Duan et al., 2005). Non-genotoxic stress induces senescence by means of a telomere-independent mechanism, which involves p16-pRB pathway activation by $p16_{INK4a}$ over regulation (Ben-Porath & Weinberg, 2005).

Matos et al. (2011) recently analyzed the role of copper in inducing senescence in WI-38 fibroblasts and found that on exposing these to subcytotoxic copper sulfate concentrations, the fibroblasts exhibited the appearance of the senescent phenotype and an increase in senescence-associated genes such as *p21, apoJ*, fibronectin, *TGF β1, IGFBP3*, and Hemo oxigenase-1 (*HO-1*). These results are interesting because of the participation that copper can have in the establishment and progression of diseases such as Alzheimer and that of Wilson. On the other hand, it is possible that oxidative stress produces telomere shortening, therefore senescence, as confirmed by Brandl et al. (2011), because on exposing articular chondrocytes to oxidative stress with a sublethal dose of H_2O_2, the authors observed accelerated telomere exhaustion with over regulation of p21 expression and sub expression of SIRT1 and XRCC5, once the cells had acquired the senescent phenotype. Cellular senescence also can be induced by stress in the cultured cells, such as continuous mitogenic stimulation (Serrano & Blasco, 2001). Sustained exposure of melanocytes to an aberrant mitotic stimulus causes senescence after an initial proliferative burst, such as that observed by Michaloglou et al. (2005) suggesting that oncogene-induced senescence represents a factor of protection against cancer.

8. The mammalian telomere

Telomeres are restricted to chromosomal ends and present in eukaryotes as diverse protozoans, fungi, flagellates, plants, and animals. The greater part of telomere DNA is double-stranded; however, the terminal 3′ end is single-stranded. Each telomere is composed of a great region of short repeats rich in G. The sequence comprising a telomere varies in length and complexity depending on the organism (Greider, 1996). In the case of humans and other mammals, the sequence is TTAGGG, while organisms such as yeasts possess irregular repeat sequences in which a T is followed by one, two, or three Gs (TG_{1-3}), while other organisms lack A in their repeats, as occurs in the ciliate Tetrahymena, which presents the TTGGGG sequence, and the Paramecium, which is distinguished by the TTGGGG and TTTGGG alteration.

Telomere DNA consists of two regions: one is double-stranded, and the other is single-stranded at its terminal end. The G-rich chain is that which projects further than the C-rich chain in the 3′ direction. This salient is essential for telomere formation, due to that linear chromosomes need to protect their ends from degradation. The 3′-OH salient invades double-stranded telomere repeats, forming a loop-like structure called the T-loop (Telomere loop), in such a way that the salient remains hidden in the double chain (Griffith et al., 1999). The T-loop avoids that the ends are considered as DNA breaks and preserves genome integrity. The exact structure of the T-loop's base is unknown, but there is a short, double-stranded DNA segment that forms a D-loop (Displaced loop) of TTAGGG repeats, which is displaced by the invasion of the 3′ salient (De Lange, 2002). The D-loop region can include Holliday-type binding (the intermediate state in homolog recombination) or a quadruple G fold (Neidle & Parkinson, 2003). The 3′ salient, which in humans is between 35 and 600 nucleotides long, is the result of the impossibility of replicating the last fragment of Okasaki and of post-replicative processing events (Stewart et al., 2003).

9. The shelterin

Maintenance of telomeric structure and regulation of its functions are supplied by diverse proteins that stabilize it and that permit the cell to distinguish between a natural chromosomal end and a DNA break. Shelterin or Telosome is a six-protein complex whose function is to form and maintain the T-loop. TRF1 and TRF2 are the main shelterin proteins. TRF1 modules telomere length, while TRF2 stabilizes T-loop structure (Xin et al., 2008). Other proteins have been described that, in addition to associating with the telomere, possess other cellular functions, such as XRCC5, which participates in double-stranded DNA damage repair (Thacker & Zdzienicka, 2004). SIRT1 is a negative regulator of p53 and that which avoids growth arrest, senescence, and apoptosis (Guarente, 1999). Double-stranded telomere DNA is wrapped in protein complexes that specifically bind to double-stranded proteins and that participate in the regulation of their length, while the 3′ salient is wrapped in one or more single-stranded binding proteins that protect it (McEachern et al., 2000). The TRF protein family has a similar architecture, defined by two characteristic sequences: both have a DNA-binding motif in their helix-turn-helix carboxyl-terminus (highly related with the Myb domain of cMyb), and both possess a centrally localized sequence motif known as the TRF homolog domain (TRFH), unique for this protein family, which allows it to form homodimers (Fairall et al., 2001). However, the TRFH domain does not form heterodimers, which leads to the presence of two protein complexes on the telomeres: one formed through TRF1, and the other by means of a paralog, TRF2 (Karlseder, 2003). TRF1 forms homodimers in order to bind stably to the DNA thanks to its Myb domain and, by means of T-loop formation, its binding with Rap1 at telomere repeats induces superficial double-strand folding, which indicates that it participates in loop formation (Bianchi et al., 1999). In cis, TRF1 acts in as a negative telomere length regulator. Its over expression produces telomere shortening and a dominant negative allele produces inappropriate lengthening in such a way that the amount of protein affects telomere size (Smogorzewska & de Lange, 2002). TRF1 can control telomerase access through its interaction with proteins TIN2, PTOP/PIP1, and POT1 and regulates their activity on interacting with PINX1 (Zhou et al., 2001). It also binds to TANK1 and 2 (Smith et al., 1998). Elimination of TRF1 produces telomere lengthening, but the extension stabilizes eventually due to that now the TIN2/TINT1 complex associates with TRF2, blocking access to telomerase (Houghtaling et al., 2004).

On the other hand, the complex formed by TRF2 is particularly important for protecting single-strand of the degradation and DNA repair processes (van Steensel et al., 1998; Smogorzewska & De Lange, 2004). TRF2 couples in the binding between double- and single-stranded repeats to facilitate T-loop formation, thus protecting its ends. In this manner, it is responsible for linear telomeric folding for T-loop formation (Griffith et al., 1999) and is found in >100 copies per chromosome (de Lange, 2002); additionally, given that it is the stabilizer of this structure, a lesser amount of TRF2 leads to T-loop opening, an event that can lead to senescence (Karlseder, 2003). Additionally, loss of TRF2 activates the Ataxia-Telangiectasia protein (ATM) kinase pathway, because while this is present it impedes autophosphorylation. ATM activation leads to p53 over regulation and G1/S arrest by means of p21 (Karlseder et al., 1999). When this is displaced from the telomere employing a dominant negative allele, the cell loses its ability to recognize the difference between a natural DNA end and a broken end. On the other hand, its over expression accelerates telomere shortening, which can be the result of the increase in the activity of a nuclease, whose activity is mediated by TRF2 (van Steelsen et al., 1998); Karlseder et al. (2002) suggest that an increase in TRF2 can protect critically short telomeres, delaying induction of cellular senescence even when the telomeres have been reduced. It can protect the single chain indirectly on recruiting Pot1.

It can bind to proteins such as Rap1 and to others involved in DNA damage repair responses, such as the MRE11/RAD50/NBS1 complex, Ku86, and ERCC1/XPF. Among its activities in blocking DNA repair is found that of avoiding that the T-loop insertion site is treated as a Holliday structure. On the other hand, inhibiting the binding of Non-homologous end-joining (NHEJ) and homologous recombination in telomeres and probably in non-telomeric breaks allows determination of which repair pathway the cell should use (Wright & Shay, 2005). On the other hand, TRF2 facilitates the degradation of telomeric DNA on interacting with the WRN exonuclease, whose loss-of-function is implicated in premature cellular senescence, increasing the frequency of cancer and genomic instability (Machwe et al., 2004).

There are diverse proteins that bind indirectly with telomeres; TIN2 has emerged as an important component of the telomere complex. It interacts with the telomere through the

TRFH domain of TRF1, negatively regulating telomere length. A truncated form of TIN2 produces abnormal telomerase-independent telomere lengthening; therefore, it is a TRF1-function mediator on potentiating the pairing of telomere repeats in a TRF1-dependent manner; in addition, it can lead to the telomerase-inhibiting telomere (Kanoh & Ishikawa, 2003). In addition to this telomere-size regulator function, another mutant form generates DNA damage response and senescence (Kim et al., 2004). Through this protein, TRF1 and TRF2 can interact, while TIN2 can stabilize TRF2-complex binding to the telomere on acting as a liaison between this and TRF1. On the other hand, thanks to its third domain, it binds to PIP1/PTOP/TINT1, which in turn serves to recruit POT1 (Liu et al., 2004; Ye & de Lang, 2004). On controlling the Poly (ADP-ribose) polymerase (PARP) activity of tankirase 1, TIN2 protects TRF1 on its removal from the telomere (Ye & de Lang, 2004).

Tankirase 1 interacts with the TRF1. It is a PARP telomere that adds poly ADP-ribose to TRF1, diminishing its affinity for telomeric DNA (Smith & de Lange, 2000). More than diminishing TRF1 affinity for telomere repeats, what TANK1 does on separating TRF1 from the DNA is to expose its myb domain, which is recognized and marked by ubiquitin, leading to degradation of the protein by the proteosome. If this were performed otherwise, TRF1 would bind again to the telomere and its separation would permit the telomerase to gain access to and extend it (Chang et al., 2003). TIN2 is what stabilizes TANK1 binding to the TRF1 complex, and although TANK1 is the lesser abundant of these two proteins, it is necessary for controlled dismantling of the telomere complex during S phase (Ye & de Lange, 2004).

TANK 2, recently identified as a Golgi-associated protein, shares 80% identity in the amino-acid sequence with TANK1, in addition to similar distribution; however, when this is over expressed, it induces rapid cell death with necrotic characteristics (Kaminker et al., 2001). In addition and similar to TANK1, it is a PARP modifier of TRF1 and possibly possesses little effect on telomerase activity (d'Adda di Fagagna et al., 2004).

There are a variety of other proteins that bind to telomeres, such as Ku, Rap1, PIP1/PTOP/TINT1, WRN, PINX1 (Stellwagen et al., 2003; Espejel et al., 2002; Kanoh & Ishikawa, 2003; Köning & Rhodes, 1997; Lei et al., 2000; Ye & de Lange, 2004; Crabbe et al., 2004), and ATM. On the other hand, repair-machinery proteins such as the Mre11/Rad50/ /Nsb1 complex (the MRN complex), which participates in double-stranded DNA repair, can play a role in telomere maintenance, although it does not directly bind with it but rather interacts through TRF2 and possibly participates in T-loop formation (Saldanha et al., 2003). Among these single-stranded binding proteins is found POT1; this binds to a telomeric salient with exceptionally high specificity. It adopts an oligosaccharide-oligonucleotide (OB) joining fold with two forks that overhang to form a clamp for binding to DNA (Lei et al., 2003). When the PTO1 binding domain is mutated, there is no telomeric end fusion, but rather an increase in telomere extension by the telomerase; thus, one of its functions is to block the access of this enzyme to the DNA. TRF1 interacts with POT1; thus, it is the length control terminal transductor for TRF1. The more TRF1, more POT1, which leads to an increase in telomerase inhibition (Mattern et al., 2004). POT1 is necessary to maintain structure in telomere salients, protecting the cell against apoptosis, avoiding chromosomal instability and senescence, and interacting with TRF2 at the T-loop formation point, with which it cooperates for maintaining telomere integrity (Yan et al., 2005).

Recently, it was discovered that Rap1 is an important factor for avoiding telomere recombination and fragility (Martínez & Blasco, 2011).

10. The telomerase

Telomerase is a Ribonucleoprotein (RNP) composed of two units: the catalytic subunit, TERT, and a RNA template, TERC. TERT is a member of the family of reverse transcriptases related with non-LTR retrotransposons and group II introns. Its reverse transcriptase domain is found at the middle of the carboxyl-terminus and it supplies the active site for catalysis (Cech, 2004). TERC, also called TR, is highly expressed in all tissues, it not being important whether they possess telomerase activity or not, and it contains a short sequence that acts as a template from which DNA repeats are copied (Cong et al., 2002). Telomerase carries its own template and is restricted to copying solely a small segment of its RNA. Thus, implicit in telomerase polymerization activity is its ability to specify the template region and its limits, and also a mechanism for maintaining itself as a stable RNP while carrying out synthesis, because it allows the template to move through the active site during the synthesis process of a repeat, to later translocate itself and initiate the synthesis of another repeat. (O'Reilly et al., 1999; Cech, 2004).

When the telomere catalytic subunit in mouse mutates, the first generation that lacks telomerase activity is phenotypically normal, with long telomeres. After four to six generations, its telomeres become very short, and the mice suffer from infertility, proliferation defects, and the risk of apoptosis in organs that undergo constant turnover, which diminishes their life span, while a *TERC* gene mutation causes Dyskeratosis congenita (DKC), a disease in which, among other characteristics, the telomeres are abnormally short (Blasco, 2005).

There are accessory factors that aid the telomerase in acting on the telomere, such as dyskerin and TP1. Dyskerin is important for ribosomal processing because it binds to many small nucleolar RNA, and it is implicit in TERC and even TERT processing or stability because its small nucleolar RNP domain reached maturation in the nucleolus and later binds to the dyskerin (Cech, 2004). TP1 can form one or more structures that mediate interactions with other telomerase- or telomere-binding proteins such as TRF. The TP1 pattern of expression is not restricted to tissues and cell lines that express telomerase activity; therefore, it is not an essential subunit (Harrington et al., 1997).

Chai et al. (2006) found that it is possible that telomerase preferentially extends the leader chain of 20-30 nucleotides per replication round in order to produce a salient similar to that of the delayed chain, because the leader-chain salient is smaller, which otherwise would affect the conformation of telomere structure.

Telomerase-to-telomere access regulation is carried out by telomere-associated proteins, for example, TRF1 and TRF2; on forming the T-loop, these inhibit telomerase binding, while POT1 binding to the salient does not permit coupling of the enzyme so that this would extend it.

Mutations in telomerase components produce premature dysfunctions in adult stem cells and reduce longevity (Mitchell et al., 1999).

11. Telomere position effect (TPE)

At present, it is accepted that telomere clipping can affect gene expression in subtelomeric regions, which can lead to modification of the Biology of the cell prior to initiation of replicative senescence (Baur et al., 2001).

The Position variegation effect (PVE) refers to inactivation of a gene, which occurs when it is removed from its normal context by means of a rearrangement or by transgene insertion. The best known example of this is the result of the expression of the euchromatic white gene in Drosophila, which is responsible for the red color of the eye. Provoked by a rearrangement in chromosome X that causes its relocation near the heterochromatin region, it eliminates function in some cells, which produces mottled pigmentation. The explanation for silencing of the white gene in some cells and not in others is that condensed and inactive conformation of pericentric heterochromatin is dispersed on the rearrangement break and randomly inactivates nearby genes (Henikoff, 1990). This chromosomal position effect affects up to a distance of approximately 1Mb and reflects a genetic inactivation gradient that is inversely correlated with distance (Wakimoto, 1998). The PVE phenomenon suggests that heterochromatin forms a transcriptionally repressor environment within which the presence of heterochromatically active resident genes is somewhat paradoxical, because these genes exhibit reciprocal heterochromatic PVE, that is, a heterochromatic gene will undergo variation if it is translocated to an euchromatic ambit. From this arises the suggestion that these genes have developed transcriptional dependence in factors that normally silence the expression of other genes (Schulze et al., 2005). Among proteins known to possess an important function in gene silencing in Drosophila is found HP1, which is a protein associated with pericentric heterochromatin. It has unequal distribution through the genome and is principally associated with the fourth chromosome. Specifically, it exerts an impact on structural organization and does not only cover the DNA or serves to direct all repetitive DNA sequences toward the repressive structure (Cryderman et al., 1999).

In the case of *Saccharomyces cerevisiae,* the heterochromatin is not cytologically visible; however, it presents position effects in three places: the telomeres; the rDNA locus, and the silent "mating-type" loci (HML and HMR). When a gene is found in one of these sites, its transcription is repressed. As in PVE, silencing depends on gene localization and not on its sequence (Chen & Widom, 2004). Several proteins are involved in the repressive chromatin, including H3 and H4 histones, their acetylases and associated deacetylases, the molecular regulators Sir1-Sir4, and the Origin recognition complex (ORC) (Pryde & Louis, 1999). The four Sir proteins are necessary for transcriptional silencing in HML and HMR, while only Sir2p, Sir3p, and Sir4p are required for telomere silencing and only Sir2p is required for rDNA silencing (Chen & Widom, 2004). TPE was described for the first time in 1990 through generation of a terminal deletion that caused the *URA3* gene (the gene necessary for uracil synthesis) to be localized 6 kb from a telomere. This new gene position provoked its transcriptional repression, which was lost when this was localized 20 kb from the telomere (Gottschling et al., 1990).

It was in 1992 that Wright and Shay set forth the possibility that TPE exists in humans. However, the first experimental proposal to identify TPE in humans, carried out by Bayne et al. (1994), did not yield positive results because changes were not found in the hygromycin-resistant gene on generating deletions in the long arm of chromosome X. Again, this time in

1996, Sprung et al. (1996) sought to study the telomere-length effect on HSV-tk promotor expression, utilizing the KB319 cell line (SV40-transformed fibroblasts); the authors integrated a plasmid with the neo-gene at the end of chromosome 13 and found no effect on neo-gene expression when telomere length ranged from 25-0.5 kb; this leads them to suggest that chromatin structural differences conferred by telomere length do not affect the expression of nearby genes. A 130-kb microdeletion in the end of chromosome 22q in cells from a child with mental retardation; the broken end had been repaired by telomere addition, and consequently a unique DNA region that was normally localized at a distance of >100 kb from the telomere was now adjacent to it. This was the model employed by Ofir et al. in 1999 to demonstrate that telomeric sequences influence the activation of nearby replication origins, delaying the synchronization of replication at mid-S phase. The latter suggests that if human telomere repeats silence genes adjacent to repaired ends, then it is also conceivable that nearby genes may be epigenetically inactivated. On the other hand, Kilburn et al. (2001) found that the presence of a telomere sequence in an *APRT* gene intron in hamster ovary cells only had a modest effect on its expression. Finally, it was Baur et al. in 2001 who, employing a luciferase reporter, supplied convincing evidence of transcriptional silencing near telomeres in humans. The authors found that on placing the reporter adjacent to telomere repeats, there was 10-times lower expression than when they placed it at non-telomeric sites. However, the authors also found that TPE in humans required a histone deacetylase, because on treating the telomeric clones with trichostatin A (a histone deacetylase inhibitor), luciferase expression was restored. Koering et al. (2002) obtained similar results utilizing the *EGFP* reporter gene in C33-A cells (undifferentiated cervical carcinoma), reverting the repressor effect on employing trichostatin A, and they suggested that the position effect depends on the organization of telomeric chromatin, due to that they encountered the release of heterochromatin proteins HP1α and HP1β. Pedram et al. (2006) developed embryonic stem cell clones of mouse with unique-copy gene markers and found that telomeric transgenes were not silenced in cells obtained from 3-day-old embryos as a result of their demethylation during early development, which led the authors to suggest that TPE also plays a role in embryo development. On the other hand, Wright and Shay (1992) also propose that progressive changes in presenescent cells can be the result of the reorganization of telomere chromatin and of the corresponding silencing or desilencing of subtelomere genes. This hypothesis has been extended to include the possibility that silenced proteins can be released from telomeres when the latter are shortened, in order to affect the expression of genes at internal non-telomere sites (Wood and Sinclair, 2002). This idea was based on studies with *S. cerevisiae,* in which it was demonstrated that gene markers inserted <4 kb from telomere repeats are frequently repressed and replicated at the end of the S phase (Dubrana et al., 2001). Although the loss of TPE is not the senescence trigger, it can be responsible for progressive changes in gene expression as a function of replicative age (Wood and Sinclair, 2002).

12. Role of telomere length in subtelomeric gene expression and its possible relation to cellular senescence

To date, there is only one report to our knowledge that studies *in vivo* TPE in human subtelomere genes. The results obtained suggest that the expression of these genes can be influenced by alterations in local heterochromatin structure so that this obstructs access to transcriptional factors (Ning et al., 2003). Due to the fact that few evidence exist about of how age-related telomere length affects the expression of specific human subtelomeric genes, we analyzed the relationship between telomere length and gene expression levels in fibroblasts derived from human donors at ages ranging from 0-70 years. We studied three groups of genes localized 100-150 kb, 200-250 kb, and >300kb away from telomeres. We found that chromatin modifier-encoding genes *Eu-HMTase1*, *ZMYND11*, and *RASA3* were over expressed in adults and implicated in chromatin restructuring (Hernández-Caballero et al., 2009). These genes are interesting because can participate in cellular senescence through the p53-p21Cip1 pathway and can also participate in chromatin restructuring, interacting with remodeling factors including ATP-dependent helicases, histone deacetylases, and histone methyltransferases (Velasco et al., 2006; Zhang et al., 2007). On the other hand, *Eu-HMTase1* can regulate H3-K9 mono- and dimethylation in euchromatin (Tachibana et al., 2005).

13. Conclusions

Undoubtedly the Antagonistic pleiotropy helped to understand the seemingly contradictory functions of the cellular senescence, nevertheless still it is not clear how does the senescence response balance tumour suppression, tissue regeneration and ageing phenotypes, for which it will be needed of a major number of studies.

Our results suggest that the expression of the subtelomeric genes modifies with the age, probably as result of decrease of the telomere length. How the changes on telomere length affected the expression of subtelomeric genes? Recently Martínez et al (2010) demonstrated that the RAP1 protein associated with the telomere, also it associates to the subtelomeric genes. Probably this protein might be involved in TPE.

The Senescence is a complex phenomenon where different factors are involved, the changes in expression of subtelomeric genes, as result of the age, is another variable that will help to the understanding cellular senescence.

14. Acknowledgment

The authors are grateful to Dra. Martha Ruíz and Maggie Brunner for the support in the preparation of the manuscript. This work was supported by grant Salud-2009-C01-115296, from Consejo Nacional de Ciencia y Tecnología (CONACyT, Mexico).

15. References

Bader, N., Jung, T. & Grune, T. (2007). The proteasome and its role in nuclear protein maintenance. *Exp Gerontol*, Vol.42, No.9, pp. 864-870, ISSN 1873-6815

Baur, JA., Zou, Y., Shay, JW. & Wright, WE. (2001). Telomere position effect in human cells. *Science*, Vol.292, No.5524, pp. 2075-2077, ISSN 1095-9203

Bayne, RA., Broccoli, D., Taggart, MH., Thomson, EJ., Farr, CJ. & Cooke, HJ. (1994). Sandwiching of a gene within 12 kb of a functional telomere and alpha satellite does not result in silencing. *Hum Mol Genet*, Vol.3, No.4, pp. 539-546, ISSN 0964-6906

Beausejour, CM., Krtolica, A., Galimi, F., Narita, M., Lowe, SW., Yaswen, P. & Campisi, J. (2003). Reversal of human cellular senescence: roles of the p53 and p16 pathways. *EMBO J*, Vol. 22, No.16, pp. 4212–4222, ISSN 1460-2075

Ben-Porath, I & Weinberg, RA. (2005). The signals and pathways activating cellular senescence. *Int J Biochem Cell Biol*, Vol.37, No.5, (Epub2004 Dec 30), pp. 961-976, ISSN 1878-5875

Bianchi, A., Stansel, RM., Fairall, L., Griffith, JD., Rhodes, D. & de Lange, T. (1999). TRF1 binds a bipartite telomeric site with extreme spatial flexibility. *EMBO J*, Vol.18, No.20, pp. 5735-5744, ISSN 1460-2075

Blagosklonny, M. (2011). Cell cycle arrest is not senescence. *Aging*, Vol.3, No.2, pp. 94-101, ISSN 1945-4589

Blanpain, C., Mohrin, M., Sotiropoulou, PA. & Passegue, E. (2011). DNA-damage response in tissue-specific and cancer stem cells. *Cell Stem Cell*, Vol.8, No.1, pp. 16–29, ISSN 1875-9777

Blasco, MA. (2005). Telomeres and human disease: ageing, cancer and beyond. *Nat Rev Genet*, Vol. 6, No.8, pp. 611–622, ISSN 1471-0064

Boehm, M. & Salck, F. (2005). A developmental timing microRNA and its target regulate life span in C. elegants. *Science*, Vol.310, No.5756, pp. 1954-1957, ISSN 0036-8075

Brandl, A., Hartmann, A., Bechmann, V., Graf, B., Nerlich, M. & Angele, P. (2011). Oxidative Stress Induces Senescence in Chondrocytes. *J Orthop Res*, Vol.29, No.7, (Epub 2011 Jan 31), pp. 1114–1120, ISSN 1554-527X

Brunk, UT. & Terman, A. (2002). Lipofuscin: mechanisms of age-related accumulation and influence on cell function. *Free Radic Biol Med*, Vol.33, No.5, (Sep 1), pp. 611–619, ISSN 1873-4596

Campisi, J. (2000). Cancer, aging and celular senescence. *In vivo*, Vol.14, No.1, (Jan-Feb), pp. 183-188, ISSN 1791-7549

Campisi, J. (2005). Aging, tumor suppression and cancer: high wire-act! *Mech Ageing Dev*, Vol.126, No.1, (Jan), pp. 51–58, ISSN 1872-6216

Campisi, J. & d'Adda di Fagagna, F. (2007). Cellular senescence: when bad things happen to good cells. *Nat Rev Mol Cell Biol*, Vol. 8, No.9, (Sep), pp. 729-740, ISSN 1471-0080

Campisi, J. (2011). Cellular senescence: Putting the paradoxes in perspective. *Curr opin Genet Dev*, Vol.21, No.1, (Feb), pp. 107- 112, ISSN 1879-0380

Cech, TR. (2004). Beginning to understand the end of the chromosome. *Cell*, Vol.116, No.2, (Jan 23), pp. 273-279, ISSN 1097- 4172

Chai, W., Du, Q,, Shay, JW. & Wright, WE. (2006). Human telomeres have different overhang sizes al leading versus lagging strands. *Mol Cell*, Vol.21, No.3, (Feb 3), pp. 427-435, ISSN 1097-4164

Chang, BD., Xuan, Y., Broude, EV., Zhu, H., Schott, B., Fang, J. & Roninson, IB. (1999). Role of p53 and p21waf1/cip1 in senescence-like terminal proliferation arrest induced in human tumor cells by chemotherapeutic drugs. *Oncogene*, Vol.18, No.34, (Aug 28), pp.4808-4818, ISSN 1476-5594

Chang, W., Dynek, JN. & Smith, S. (2003). TRF1 is degraded by ubiquitina-mediated proteolysis after release from telomeres. *Genes Dev*, Vol.17, No.11, (Jun 1), pp. 1328-1333, ISSN 1549-5477

Chen, L. & Widom, J. (2004). Molecular basis of transcriptional silencing in budding yeast. Biochem *Cell Biol*, Vol.82, No.4, (Aug), pp. 413-418, ISSN 1208-6002

Cherdyntseva, NV., Gervas, PA., Litvyakov, NV., Stakcheeva, MN., Ponomaryeva, AA., Dobrodeev, AY., Denisov, EV., Belyavskaya, VA. & Choinzonov, EL. (2010). Age-related function of tumor suppressor gene tp53: contribution to cancer risk and progression. *Exp Oncol*, Vol.32, No.3, (Sep), pp. 205-208, ISSN 1812-9269

Chiu, CP., Dragowska, W., Kim, NW., Vaziri, H., Yui, J., Thomas, TE., Harley, CB. & Lansdorp, PM. (1996). Differential expression of telomerase activity in hematopoietic progenitors from adult human bone marrow. *Stem Cells*, Vol.14, No.2, pp. 239-248, ISSN 0250-6793

Cong, Y., Wright, WE. & Shay, JW. (2002). Human telomerase and its regulation. *Microb Mol Biol Rev*, Vol.66, No.3, pp. 407- 425, ISSN 1098-5557

Crabbe, L., Verdun, RE., Haggblom, CI. & Karlseder, J. (2004). Defective telomere lagging strand synthesis in cells lacking WRN helicase activity. *Science*, Vol.306, No.5703, (Dec 10), pp. 1951-1953, ISSN 1095-9203

Cryderman, DE., Morris, EJ., Biessmann, H., Elgin, S. & Wallrath, LL. (1999). Silencing at Drosophila telomeres: Nuclear organization and chromatin structure play critical roles. *EMBO J*, Vol.18, No.13, (Jul 1), pp. 3724-3735, ISSN 1460- 2075

d'Adda di Fagagna, F., Teo, S. & Jackson, SP. (2004). Functional links between telomeres and proteins of the DNA-damage response. *Genes Dev*, Vol.18, No.15, (Aug 1), pp. 1781-1799, ISSN 1549-5477

d'Adda di Fagagna, F. (2008). Living on a break: cellular senescence as a DNA-damage response. *Nat Rev Cancer*, Vol.8, No.7, pp. 512-522, ISSN 1474-1768

de Lange, T. (2002). Protection of mammalian telomeres. *Oncogene*, Vol.21, No.4, (Jan 21), pp. 532-540, ISSN 1476-5594

De, S. (2011). Somatic mosaicism in healthy human tissues. *Trends Genet* Vol.27, No. 6, pp. 217-223, ISSN 1476-5594

Dimri, GP., Lee, X., Basile, G., Acosta, M., Scott, G., Roskelley, C., Medrano, EE., Linskens, M., Rubelj, I., Pereira-Smith, O., Peacocke, M. & Campisi, J. (1995). A biomarker that identifies senescent human cells in culture and in aging skin in vivo. *Proc Natl Acad Sci USA*, Vol.92, No.20, (Sep 26), pp. 9363–9367, ISSN 1091-6490

Duan, J., Zhang, Z. & Tong, T. (2005). Irreversible cellular senescence induced by prolonged exposure to H2O2 involves DNA-damage and- repair genes and telomere shortening. *Int J Biochem Cell Biol*, Vol.37, No. 7, pp. 1407–1420, ISSN 1878-5875

Dubrana, K., Perrod, S. & Gasser, SM. (2001). Turning telomeres on and off. *Curr Opin Cell Biol*, Vol.13, No.3, pp. 281-289, ISSN 1879-0410

Espejel, S., Franco, S., Rodríguez-Perales, S., Bouffler, SD., Cigudosa, JC. & Blasco, MA. (2002). Mammalian Ku86 mediates chromosomal fusions and apoptosis caused by critically short telomeres. *EMBO J*, Vol.21, pp. 2207-2219, ISSN 1460-2075

Fairall, L., Chapman, L., Moss, H., de Lange, T. & Rhodes, D. (2001). Structure of the TRFH dimerization domain of the human telomeric proteins TRF1 and TRF2. *Mol Cell*, Vol.8, No.2, pp. 351-361, ISSN 1097-4164

Feltes, BC., de Faria Poloni, J. & Bonatto, D. (2011). The developmental aging and origins of health and disease hypotheses explained by different protein networks. *Biogerontology*, Vol.12, No.4, (Epub 2011 Mar 5), pp. 293-308, ISSN 1389- 5729

Freund, A., Orjalo, AV., Desprez, PY. & Campisi, J. (2010). Inflammatory networks during cellular senescence: causes and consequences. *Trends Mol Med*, Vol.16, No.5, (Epub 2010 May 3), pp. 238–246, ISSN 1471-499X

Funayama, R. & Ishikawa, F. (2007). Cellular senescence and chromatin structure. *Chromosoma*, Vol.116, No.5, (Epub 2007 Jun 20), pp. 431–440, ISSN 1432-0886

Gottschling, DE., Aparicio, OM., Billington, BL. & Zakian, VA. (1990). Position effect at S. cerevisiae telomeres: Reversible repression of Pol II transcription. *Cell*, Vol.63, No.4, pp. 751-762, ISSN 1097-4172

Greenberg, SB., Grove, GL. & Cristofalo, VJ. (1977). Cell size in aging monolayer cultures. *In Vitro*, Vol.13, No. 5, pp. 297–300, ISSN 0073-5655

Greider, CW. & Blackburn, EH. (1985). Identification of a specific telomere terminal transferase enzyme with two kinds of primer specificity. *Cell*, Vol.51, No.6, pp. 405–413, ISSN 1097-4172

Greider, CW. (1996). Telomere length regulation. *Annu Rev Biochem*, Vol.65, pp. 337-365, ISSN 1545-4509

Griffith, JD., Comeau, L., Rosenfield, S., Stansel, RM., Bianchi, A., Moss, H. & de Lange, T. (1999). Mammalian telomeres end in a large duplex loop. *Cell*, Vol. 97, No.4, pp. 503-514, ISSN 1097-4172

Guarente, L. (1999). Mutant mice live longer. *Nature*, Vol.402, No.6759, pp. 243-245, ISNN 1476-4687

Guarente, L. (1999). Diverse and dynamic functions of the Sir silencing complex. *Nat Genet*, Vol.23, No.3, pp. 281–285, ISSN 1546-1718

Gutteridge, JM. (1984). Age pigments: role of iron and copper salts in the formation of fluorescent lipid complexes. *Mech Ageing Dev*, Vol.25, No.1-2, pp. 205–214, ISSN 1872-6216

Halaschek-Wiener, J., Vulto, I., Fornika, D., Collins, J., Connors, JM., Le, ND., Lansdorp, PM. & Brooks-Wilson, A. (2008). Reduced telomere length variation in healthy oldest old. *Mech Ageing Dev*, Vol.29, No.11, (Epub 2008 Aug 14), pp. 638–641, ISSN 1872-6216

Hampel, B., Malisan, F., Niederegger, H., Testi, R. & Jansen-Durr, P. (2004). Differential regulation of apoptotic cell death in senescent human cells. *Exp Gerontol*, Vol.39, No.11-12, pp. 1713–1721, ISSN 1873-6815

Harley, CB., Futcher, AB. & Greider, CW. (1990). Telomeres shorten during ageing of human fibroblasts. *Nature*, Vol.345, No.6274, pp. 458–460, ISSN 1476-4687

Harrington, L., McPhhail, T., Mar, V., Zhou, W., Oulton, R., Bass, MB., Arruda, I. & Robinson, M. (1997). A mammalian telomerase-associated protein. *Science*, Vol.275, No.5302, pp. 973-977, ISSN 1095-9203

Hayflick, L. & Moorhead, PS. (1961). The serial cultivation of human diploid cell strains. *Exp Cell Res* 1961; Vol.25, pp. 585- 621, ISSN 1090-2422

Hayflick, L. (1998). A brief history of the mortality and immortality of cultured cells. *Keio J Med*, Vol.47, No.3, pp. 174-182, ISSN 1880-1293

Hayflick, L. (2003). Living for ever and dying in the attempt. *Exp Gerontol*, Vol.38, No.11-12, pp. 1231-1241, ISSN 1873-6815

Henikoff, S. (1990). Position-effect variegation after 60 years. *Trends Genet*, Vol.6, No.12, pp. 422–426, ISSN 0168-9525

Herbig, U., Jobling, WA., Chen, BP., Chen, DJ. & Sedivy, JM. (2004). Telomere shortening triggers senescence of human cells through a pathway involving ATM, p53, and p21(CIP1), but not p16(INK4a). *Mol Cell*, Vol.14, No.4, pp. 501-513, ISSN 1097-4164

Hernández-Caballero, E., Herrera-González, NE., Salamanca-Gómez, F. & Arenas-Aranda, DJ. (2009). Role of telomere length in subtelomeric gene expression and its possible relation to cellular senescence. *BMB Rep*, Vol.42, No.11, pp. 747- 751, ISSN 1976-670X

Höhn, A., Jung, T., Grimm, S., Catalgol, B., Weber, D. & Grune, T. (2011). Lipofuscin inhibits the proteasome by binding to surface motifs. *Free Radic Biol Med*, Vol.50, No.5, (Epub 2010 Dec 16), pp. 585-591, ISSN 1873-4596

Hornsby, PJ. (2011). Cellular aging and cancer. *Crit Rev Oncol Hematol*, Vol.79, No.2, pp. 189-195, ISSN 1040-8428

Hotchkiss, RS., Strasser, A., McDunn, JE. & Swanson, PE. (2009). Cell death. *N Engl J Med*, Vol.361, No.16, pp. 1570-1583, ISSN 1533-4406

Houghtaling, BR., Cuttonaro, L., Chang, W. & Smith, S. (2004). A dynamic molecular link between the telomere length regulator TRF1 and the chromosome end protector TRF2. *Current Biology*, Vol.14, No.18, pp. 1621–1631, ISSN 1879- 0445

Huang, YC., Hasegawa, H., Wang, SW., Ku, CC., Lin, YC., Chiou, SS., Hou, MF., Wu, DC., Tsai, EM., Saito, S., Yamaguchi, N. & Yokoyama, KK. (2011). Jun dimerization protein 2 controls senescence and differentiation via regulating histone modification. *J Biomed Biotechnol*, Epub 2010 Dec 12, ISSN 1110-7251

Hung, YC., Lee, JH., Chen, HM. & Huang, GS. (2010). Effects of static magnetic fields on the development and aging of Caenorhabditis elegans. *J Exp Biol*, Vol.213, No.12, pp. 2079-2085, ISSN 1477-9145

Hwang, ES., Yoon, G. & Kang, HT. (2009). A comparative analysis of the cell biology of senescence and aging. *Cell Mol Life Sci*, Vol.66, No.15,(Epub 2009 May 7), pp. 2503-2524, ISSN 1420-9071

Inomata, K., Aoto, T., Binh, NT., Okamoto, N., Tanimura, S., Wakayama, T., Iseki, S., Hara, E., Masunaga, T., Shimizu, H. & Nishimura, EK. (2009). Genotoxic stress abrogates renewal of melanocyte stem cells by triggering their differentiation. *Cell*, Vol.137, No.6, pp. 1088–1099, ISSN 1097-4172

Kaminker, PG., Kim, S., Taylor, RD., Zebarjadian, Y., Funk, WD., Morin, GB., Yaswen. P. & Campisi, J. (2001). TANK2, a new TRF1-associated Poly(ADP-ribose) polymerase, causes rapid induction of cell death upon overexpression. *J Biol Chem*, Vol.276, No.38, (Epub 2001 Jul 13), pp. 35891–35899, ISSN 1083-351X

Kanoh, J. & Ishikawa, F. (2003). Composition and conservation of the telomeric complex. *Cell Mol Life Sci*, Vol.60, No.11, pp. 2295-2302, ISSN 1420-9071

Karlseder, J., Broccoli, D., Day, D., Hardy, S. & de Lange, T. (1999). p53- and ATM-dependent apoptosis induced by telomeres lacking TRF2. *Science*, Vol.283, No.5406, pp. 1321-1325, ISSN 1095-9203

Karlseder, J., Smogorzweska, A. & de Lange, T. (2002). Senescence induced by altered telomere state, not telomere loss. *Science*, Vol.295, No.5564, pp. 2446-2449, ISSN 1095-9203

Karlseder, J. (2003). Telomere repeat binding factors: Keeping the ends in check. *Cancer Letters*, vol.194, No.2, pp. 189-197, ISSN 1872-7980

Kavathia, N., Jain, A., Walston, J., Beamer, BA., Fedarko, NS. (2009). Serum markers of apoptosis decrease with age and cancer stage. *Aging* Vol.1, No.7, pp. 652–663, ISSN 1945-4589

Kilburn, AE., Shea, MJ., Sargent, G. & Wilson. JH. (2001). Insertion of a telomere repeat sequence into a mammalian gene causes chromosome instability. *Mol Cell Biol*, Vol.21, No.1, pp. 126-135, ISSN 1097-4164

Kim, NW., Piatyszek, MA., Prowse, KR., Harley, CB., West, MD., Ho, PL., Coviello. GM., Wright, WE., Weinrich, SL. & Shay, JW. (1994). Specific association of human telomerase activity with immortal cells and cancer. *Science*, Vol.266, No.5193, pp. 2011–2015, ISSN 1095-9203

Kim, S., Beausejour, C., Davalos, AR., Kaminker, P., Heo, S. & Campisi, J. (2004). TIN2 mediates functions of TRF2 at Human Telomeres. *J Biol Chem*, Vol. 279, No.42, (Epub 2004 Aug 3) pp. 43799–43804, ISSN 1083-351X

Kirkwood, TB. (1977). Evolution of ageing. *Nature*, Vol.170, No.5635, pp. 201–204, ISSN 1476-4687

Koering, CS., Pollice A., Zibella, MP., Bauwens, S. Puisieux, A., Brunori, M., Brun, C., Martins, L., Sabatier, L., Pulitzer, JF. & Gilson, E. (2002). Human telomeric position effect is determined by chromosomal context and telomeric chromatin integrity. *EMBO Rep*, Vol.3, No. 11, pp. 1055-1061, ISSN 1469-221X

König, P. & Rhodes, D. (1997). Recognition of telomeric DNA. *TIBS*, Vol.22, No.2, pp. 43-47, ISSN 0968-0004

Kosar, M., Bartkova, J., Hubackova, S., Hodny, Z., Lukas, J. & Bartek, J. (2011). Senescence-associated heterochromatin foci are dispensable for cellular senescence, occur in a cell type- and insult-dependent manner and follow expression of p16 (ink4a). *Cell Cycle*, Vol.10, No.3, pp. 457-468, ISSN 1551-4005

Krishnamurthy, J., Torrice, C., Ramsey, MR., Kovalev, GI., Al-Regaiey, K., Su, L. & Sharpless, NE. (2004). Ink4a/Arf expression is a biomarker of aging. *J Clin Invest*, Vol.114, No.9, pp. 1299-1307, ISSN 1558-8238

Lee, BY., Han, JA., Im, JS., Morrone, A., Johung, K., Goodwin, EC., Kleijer, WJ., DiMaio, D. & Hwang, ES. (2006). Senescence-associated b-galactosidase is lysosomal b-galactosidase. *Aging Cell*, Vol.5, No.2, pp. 187–195, ISSN 1474-9726

Lee, HW., Blasco, MA., Gottlieb, GJ., Horner, JW., Greider, CW. & DePinho, RA. (1998). Essential role of mouse telomerase in highly proliferative organs. *Nature*, Vol.392, No. 6676, pp. 569–574, ISSN 1476-4687

Lei, M., Podell, ER., Baumann, P. & Cech, TR. (2003). DNA self-recognition in the structure of Pot1 bound to telomeric single-stranded DNA. *Nature*, Vol.426, No.6963, pp. 198-203, ISSN 1476-4687

Liu, D., O'Connor, M., Qin, J. & Songyang, Z. (2004). Telosome. A mammalian telomere associated complex formed by multiple telomeric proteins. *J Biol Chem*, Vol.279, No.49, (Epub 2004 Sep 20), pp. 51338-51342, ISSN 1083-351X

Liu, L., Trimarchi, JR., Smith, PJ. & Keefe, DL. (2002). Mitochondrial dysfunction leads to telomere attrition and genomic instability. *Aging Cell*, Vol.1, No.1, pp. 40–46, ISSN 1097-4172

Lowe, SW. & Sherr, CJ. (2003). Tumor suppression by Ink4a-Arf: progress and puzzles. *Curr Opin Genet Dev*, Vol.13, No.1, pp. 77–83, ISSN 1879-0380

Machwe, A., Xiao, L. & Orren, DK. (2004). TRF2 recruits the Werner syndrome (WRN) exonuclease for processing of telomeric DNA. *Oncogene*, Vol.23, No.1, pp. 149-156, ISSN 1476-5594

Mantell, LL. & Greider, CW. (1994). Telomerase activity in germline and embryonic cells of Xenopus. *EMBO J*, Vol.13, No.13, pp. 3211-3217, ISSN 1460-2075

Martínez, P., Thanasoula, M., Caslos, AR., Gómez-López, G., Tejera, AM., Schoefther, S., Dominguez, O., Pisano, DG., Tarsounas, M. & Blasco, MA. (2010). Mammalian Rap1 controls telomere function and gene expression through binding to telomeric and extratelomeric sites. *Nat Cell Biol*, Vol.12, No.8, pp. 768-780, ISSN 1097-6256

Martínez, P. & Blasco MA. (2011). Telomeric and extra-telomeric roles for telomerase and the telomere-binding proteins. *Nat Rev Cancer*, Vol.11, pp. 161-176, ISSN 1474-175X

Matos, L., Gouveia, A. & Almeida, H. (2011). Copper ability to induce premature senescence in human fibroblasts. *Age (Dordr)*, Jun 22, ISSN 1574-1587

Mattern, KA., Swiggers, JJ., Nigg, AL., Löwenberg, B., Houtsmuller, AB. & Zijlmans, JM. (2004). Dynamics of protein binding to telomeres in living cells: Implications for telomere structure and function. *Mol Cell Biol*, Vol.24, No.12, pp. 5587-5594, ISNN 1098-5549

McClintock, B. (1941). The stability of broken ends of chromosomes in Zea mays. *Genetics*, Vol.26, No.2, pp. 234-282, ISSN 1943-2631

McEachern, MJ., Krauskopf, A. & Blackburn, EH. (2000). Telomeres and their control. *Annu Rev Genet*, Vol. 34, pp. 331-358, ISSN 1545-2948

Michaloglou, C., Vredeveld, LC., Soengas, MS., Denoyelle, C., Kuilman, T., van der Horst, CM., Majoor, DM., Shay, JW., Mooi, WJ. & Peeper, DS. (2005). BRAFE600-associated senescence-like cell cycle arrest of human naevi. *Nature*, Vol.436, No.7051, pp. 720-724, ISSN 1476-4687

Mitchell, JR., Wood, E. & Collins, K. (1999). A telomerase component is defective in the human disease dyskeratosis congenita. *Nature*, Vol.402, No.6761, pp. 551-555, ISSN 1476-4687

Morin, GB. (1989). The human telomere terminal transferase enzyme is a ribonucleoprotein that synthesizes TTAGGG repeats. *Cell*, Vol.59, No.3, pp. 521-529, ISSN 1097-4172

Narita, M., Nuñez, S., Heard, E., Narita, M., Lin, AW., Hearn, SA., Spector, DL., Hannon, GL. & Lowe, SW. (2003). Rb- mediated heterochromatin formation and silencing of E2F target genes during cellular senescence. *Cell*, Vol.113, No.6, pp. 703-716, ISSN 1097-4172

Neidle, S. & Parkinson, GN. (2003). The structure of telomeric DNA. *Curr Opin Struct Biol*, Vol.13, No.3, pp. 275-283, ISSN 1879-033X

Ning, Y., Xu, JF., Li, Y., Chavez, L., Riethman, HC., Lansdorp, PM. & Weng, NP. (2003). Telomere length and the expression of natural telomeric genes in human fibroblasts. *Hum Mol Genet*, Vol.12, No.11, pp. 1329-1336, ISSN 1460-2083

Nishio, K., Inoue, A., Qiao, S., Kondo, H. & Mimura, A. (2001). Senescence and cytoskeleton: overproduction of vimentin induces senescent-like morphology in human fibroblasts. *Histochem Cell Biol*, Vol.116, No.4, pp. 321–327, ISSN 1432-119X

Nishio, K. & Inoue, A. (2005) Senescence-associated alterations of cytoskeleton: extraordinary production of vimentin that anchors cytoplasmic p53 in senescent human fibroblasts. *Histochem Cell Biol*, Vol.123, No.3, pp. 263–273, ISSN 1432-119X

O'Reilly, M., Teichmann, SA. & Rhodes, D. (1999). Telomerases. *Curr Opin Struc Biol*, Vol.9, No.1, pp. 56-65, ISSN 1879-033X

Ofir, R., Wong, AC., McDermind, HE., Skorecki, KL. & Selig, S. (1999). Position effect of human telomeric repeats on replication timing. *Proc Natl Acad Sci USA*, Vol.96, No.20, pp. 11434-11439, ISSN 1091-6490

Olovnikov, AM. (1996). Telomeres, telomerase and aging: Origin of the Theory. *Exp Gerontol*, Vol.31, No.4, pp. 443-448, ISSN 1873-6815

Ouellette, MM., Liao, M., Herbert, BS., Johnson, M., Holt, SE., Liss, HS., Shay, JW. & Wright WE. (2000). Subsenescent telomere lengths in fibroblasts immortalized by limiting amounts of telomerase. *J Biol Chem*, Vol.275, No.14, pp. 10072-10076, ISSN 0021-9258

Pedram, M., Sprung, CN., Gao, Q., Lo, AW., Reynolds, GE. & Murnane JP. (2006). Telomere position effect and silencing of transgenes near telomeres in the mouse. *Mol Cell Biol*, Vol.26, No.5, pp. 1865-1878, ISSN 1098-5549

Percy, CJ., Power, D. & Gobe, GC. (2008). Renal ageing: changes in the cellular mechanism of energy metabolism and oxidant handling. *Nephrology*, Vol.13, No.2, pp. 147–152, ISNN 1440-1797

Pryde, FE. & Louis, EJ. (1999). Limitations of silencing at native yeast telomeres. *EMBO J*, Vol.18, No.9, pp. 2538-2550, ISSN 1460-2075

Rai, TS. & Adams, PD. (2011). Lessons from senescence: Chromatin maintenance in non-proliferating cells. *Biochim Biophys Acta.* Aug 3, ISSN 0006-3002

Riley, T., Sontag, E., Chen, P. & Levine, A. (2008). Transcriptional control of human p53-regulated genes. *Nat Rev Mol Cell Biol*, Vol. 9, No.5, pp. 402–412, ISSN 1097-4164

Rochette, PJ. & Brash, DE. (2008). Progressive apoptosis resistance prior to senescence and control by the anti-apoptotic protein BCL-xL. *Mech Ageing Dev*, Vol.129, No.4, pp. 207–214, ISSN 1872-6216

Rodier, F. & Campisi, J. (2011). Four faces of cellular senescence. *J Cell Biol*, Vol.192, No.4, (Epub 2011 Feb 14), pp. 547-556, ISSN 1540-8140

Saldanha, SN., Andrews, LG. & Tollefsbol, TO. (2003). Assessment of telomere length and factors that contribute to its stability. *Eur J Biochem*, Vol.270, No.3, pp. 389-403, ISSN 1432-1033

Salminen, A., Ojala, J. & Kaarniranta, K. (2011). Apoptosis and aging: increased resistance to apoptosis enhances the aging process. *Cell Mol Life Sci*, Vol.68, No.6, (Epub 2010 Nov 30), pp. 1021-1031, ISSN 1420-9071

Schulze, SR., Sinclair, D., Fitzpatrick, KA. & Honda, BM. (2005). A Genetic and molecular characterization of two Proximal heterochromatic genes on chromosome 3 of Drosophila melanogaster. *Genetics*, Vol.169, No.4, pp. 2165–2177, ISSN 1943-2631

Serrano, M. & Blasco, MA. (2001). Putting the stress on senescence. *Curr Opin Cell Biol*, Vol.13, No.6, pp. 748–753, ISSN 1879-0410

Sherr, CJ. & DePinho, RA. (2000). Cellular senescence: Mitotic clock or culture shock? *Cell*, Vol.102, No.4, pp. 407–410, ISSN 1097-4172

Sin, D., Kucia, M. & Ratajcsak, MZ. (2011). Nuclear and chromatin reorganization during cell senescence and aging- A mini-review. *Gerontology*, Vol.57, No.1, (Epub 2010 Feb 4), pp. 76-84, ISSN 1423-0003

Smith, S., Giriat, I., Schmitt, A. & de Lange, T. (1998). Tankyrase, a poly (ADP-ribose) polymerase at human telomeres. *Science*, Vol.282, No.5393, pp. 1484-1487, ISSN 1095-9203

Smith, S. & de Lange, T. (2000). Tankyrase promotes telomere elongation in human cells. *Curr Biol*, Vol.10, No.20, pp. 1299-1302, ISSN 1879-0445

Smogorzewska, A. & de Lange, T. (2002). Different telomere damage signaling pathways in human and mouse cells. *EMBO J*, Vol.21, No.16, pp. 4338-4348, ISSN 1460-2075

Smogorzewska, A. & de Lange, T. (2004). Regulation of telomerase by telomeric proteins. *Annu Rev Biochem*, Vol.73, pp. 177-208, ISSN 0066-4154

Sprung, CN., Sabatier, L. & Murnane, JP. (1996). Effect of telomere length on telomeric gene expression. Nucleic Acids Res, Vol.24, No.21, pp. 4336-4340, ISSN 1362-4962

Stellwagen, AE., Haimberger, ZW., Veatch, JR. & Gottschling, DE. (2003). Ku interacts with telomerase RNA to promote telomere addition at native and broken chromosome ends. *Genes Dev*, Vol.17, No.19, (Epub 2003 Sep 15), pp. 2384-2395, ISSN 1549-5477

Stewart, SA., Ben-Porath, I., Carey, VJ., O'Connor, BF., Hahn, WC. & Weinberg, RA. (2003). Erosion of the telomeric single-strand overhang at replicative senescence. *Nat Genet*, Vol.33, No.4, (Epub 2003 Mar 24), pp. 492-496, ISSN 1546-1718

Su, X., Paris, M., Gi, YJ., Tsai, KY., Cho, MS., Lin, YL., Biernaskie, JA., Sinha, S., Prives, C., Pevny, LH., Miller. FD. & Flores ER. (2009). TAp63 prevents premature aging by promoting adult stem cell maintenance. *Cell Stem Cell*, Vol.5, No.1, pp. 64–75, ISSN 1875-9777

Tachibana, M., Ueda, J., Fukuda, M., Takeda, N., Ohta, T., Iwanari, H., Sakihama, T., Kodama, T., Hamakubo, T. & Shinkai, Y. (2005). Histone methyltransferases G9a and GLP form heteromeric complexes and are both crucial for methylation of euchromatin at H3-K9. *Genes & Dev*. Vol.19, No.7, pp. 815-826, ISSN 1549-5477

Thacker, J. & Zdzienicka, MZ. (2004). The XRCC genes: expanding roles in DNA double-strand break repair. *DNA Repair*, Vol.3, No. 8-9, pp. 1081-1090, ISNN 1568-7856

Thomas, E., al-Baker, E., Dropcova, S., Denyer, S., Ostad, N., Lloyd, A., Kill, IR. & Faragher, RG. (1997). Different kinetics of senescence in human fibroblasts and peritoneal mesothelial cells. *Exp Cell Res*, Vol.236, No.1, pp. 355-358, ISSN 1090-2422

Tuminello ER & Han SD. (2011). The apolipoprotein e antagonistic pleiotropy hypothesis: review and recommendations. *Int J Alzheimers Dis*, Vol.24, pp. 1-12, ISSN 2090-0252

Van Steensel, B., Smogorzewska, A. & de Lange, T. (1998). TRF2 protects human telomeres from end-to-end fusions. *Cell*, Vol.92, No.3, pp. 401-413, ISSN 1097-4172

Vavrova, J. & Rezacova, M. (2011). The importance of senescence in ionizing radiation-induced tumour suppression. *Folia Biologica,* Vol.57, No.2, pp. 41-46, ISSN 0015-5500

Velasco, G., Grkovic, S. & Ansieau, S. (2006). New insights into BS69 functions. *J Biol Chem,* Vol.281, No.24, (Epub 2006 Mar 24), pp. 16546-16550, ISSN 1083-351X

von Zglinicki, T. (2002). Oxidative stress shortens telomeres. *Trends Biochem Sci,* Vol.27, No.7, pp.339-344, ISSN 0968-0004

Vousden, KH. & Lu, L. (2002). Live or let die: the cell's response to p53. *Nat Rev Cancer,* Vol.2, No.8, pp. 594-604, ISSN 1474-1768

Wakimoto, BT. (1998). Beyond the nucleosome: Epigenetic aspects of position-effect variegation in Drosophila. *Cell,* Vol.93, No.3, pp. 321-324, ISSN 1097-4172

Walker, RF. (2011). Developmental theory of aging revisited: focus on causal and mechanistic links between development and senescence. *Rejuvenation Res,* Vol.14, No.4, (Epub 2011 Jul 18), pp. 429-36, ISSN 1557-8577

Wang, E. & Gundersen, D. (1984). Increased organization of cytoskeleton accompanying the aging of human fibroblasts in vitro. *Exp Cell Res,* Vol.154, No.1, pp. 191–202, ISSN 1090-2422

Williams, G. (1957). Pleiotropy, natural selection, and the evolution of senescence. *Evolution,* Vol.11, pp. 398-411, ISSN 1558-5646

Wood, JG. & Sinclair, DA. (2002). TPE or not TPE? It's no longer a question. *TRENDS Pharmacol Sci,* Vol.23, No.1, pp. 1-4, ISSN 1873-3735

Wright, WE. & Shay, JW. (1992). Telomere positional effects and the regulation of cellular senescence. *Trends Genet,* Vol.8, No.6, pp. 193-197, ISSN 0168-9525

Wright, WE., Piatyszek, MA., Rainey, WE., Byrd, W. & Shay, JW. (1996). Telomerase activity in human germline and embryonic tissues and cells. *Dev Genet,* Vol.18, No.2, pp. 173-179, ISSN 0192-253X

Wright, WE. & Shay, JW. (2005). Telomere-binding factors and general DNA repair. *Nat Genet,* Vol.37, No.2, pp. 116-118, ISSN 1546-1718

Xin, H., Liu, D. & Songyang, Z. (2008). The telosome/shelterin complex and its functions. *Genome Biol,* Vol.9, No.9, (Epub 2008 Sep 18), pp. 232-236, ISSN 1465-6914

Yan, Q., Zheng, Y. & Harris. CC. (2005). POT1 and TRF2 cooperate to maintain telomeric integrity. *Mol Cell Biol,* Vol.25, No.3, pp. 1070-1080, ISSN 1098-5549

Yanaka, M., Honma, T., Sato, K., Shinohara, N., Ito, J., Tanaka, Y., Tsuduki, T. & Ikeda, I. (2011). Increased monocytic adhesion by senescence in human umbilical vein endothelial cells. *Biosci Biotechnol Biochem,* Vol.75, No.6, (Epub 2011 Jun 13), pp. 1098-1103, ISSN 1347-6947

Ye, JZ. & de Lange, T. (2004). TIN2 is a tankyrase 1 PARP modulator in the TRF1 telomere length control complex. *Nat Genet,* Vol.36, No.6, pp. 618-623, ISSN 1546-1718

Zahn, JT., Louban, I., Jungbauer, S., Bissinger, M., Kaufmann, D., Kemkemer, R. & Spatz, JP. (2011). Age-dependent changes in microscale stiffness and mechanoresponses of cells. *Small,* Vol.7, No.10, (Epub 2011 May 2), pp. 1480-1487, ISSN 1613-6829

Zhang, W., Chan, HM., Gao, Y., Poon, R. & Wu, Z. (2007). BS69 is involved in cellular senescence through the p53-p21Cip1 pathway. *EMBO Rep,* Vol.8, No.10, (Epub 2007 Aug 24), pp.952-958, ISSN 1469-3178

Zhou, XZ. & Lu, KP. (2001). The PIN2/TRF1 interacting protein PinX1 is a potent telomerase inhibitor. *Cell*, Vol.107, No.3, pp. 347-359, ISSN 1097-4172

19

Caveolar Vesicles in Cellular Senescence

Keith Wheaton
Department of Biology, York University, Toronto
Canada

1. Introduction

The replicative limit of human fibroblasts has long provided a model to assess the molecular mechanisms which underlie cellular aging. In culture, fibroblasts which reach the end of their proliferative lifespan acquire profound molecular changes that limit their response to growth factors, and cause permanent exit from the cell cycle. Part of the senescence programme is due to a well established link between telomere attrition which occurs with each population doubling and the subsequent activation of the p53 tumour suppressor. Critical shortening of telomeres is thought to cause a form of DNA damage, that leads to the activation of caretaker proteins ATM, ATR or DNA-PK which activate p53, leading to the initiation of senescence through p53 effector genes. In addition, p53 mediates senescence by many other stimuli including oxidative stress, DNA damaging agents and oncogenic activation.

Caveolins are the main scaffolding proteins driving the formation of caveolae (50-100 nm wide cave like invaginations at the plasma membrane) from lipid rafts and allows the organization of many signalling cascades. This compartmentalization concentrates receptors, proteins with lipid anchors, and the lipids from which second messengers are derived. In this capacity caveolin has also been shown to bind and inactivate many key components of mitogenic pathways through the caveolin scaffolding domain (CSD) and thus is often considered a tumour suppressor. About a decade ago, the original investigations into the relationship between caveolae and senescence showed elevated levels of the caveolin proteins during replicative senescence. Both the ectopic expression or endogenous upregulation of caveolin was shown to lead to p53 mediated senescent arrest. However, this upregulation has not been proven to lead to an increase of caveolae at the cell surface, but does lead to increased number of internalized structures. The mislocalized caveolar vesicles likely influence the regulation of mitogenic signals that normally are integrated through caveolae. In addition the caveolin protein has been shown to regulate many signalling cascades that have an impact on senescence, and on the activation of p53.

1.1 Fibroblast model of senescence

Primary human diploid fibroblasts (HDFs) have traditionally served as an experimental model to investigate cellular and molecular aspects of aging. Normal fibroblasts derived from human donors are neither immortal or transformed and are limited in the number of times they are capable of dividing *in vitro* and *in vivo*. This finite replicative lifespan terminates with the acquisition of a phenotype having distinct morphological and biochemical characteristics termed replicative senescence (Hayflick, 1965a; Hayflick and

Moorhead, 1961). This is a cell fate distinct from apoptosis or differentiation since the cells remain viable but are refractory to mitogenic signals. Senescing fibroblasts progressively acquire a flattened morphology with an increased cellular volume, an irregular shape, and increased accumulation of debris (Hayflick, 1965a; Hayflick and Moorhead, 1961).

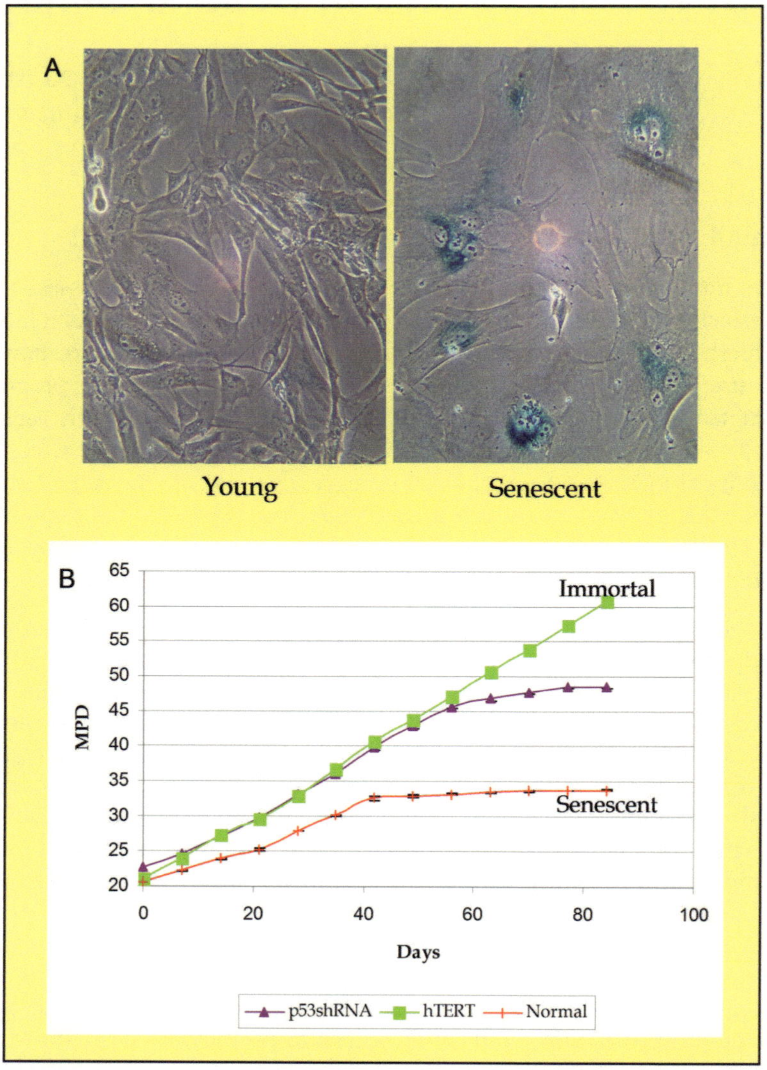

Fig. 1. Cellular Senescence
A) Young and senescent primary fibroblasts prepared with an acidic β-galactosidase assay, staining senescent cells blue. Note the enlarged and flattened morphology of senescent cells compared to young fibroblasts. **B)** A growth curve of AG08470 primary fibroblasts virally transfected with empty vector (Normal), human telomerase (hTERT) or p53 short hairpin RNA (p53 shRNA). This strain of fibroblasts undergo replicative senescence at a mean population doubling (MPD) of 34 (Normal). The knockdown of p53 protein levels using p53 shRNA extends the proliferative lifespan by 13 MPDs. The ectopic expression of hTERT immortalizes the fibroblast strain.

Additional phenotypic changes include increased actin stress fibers and an increase in cells containing irregular and multiple nuclei (Wheaton et al., 1996). These morphological changes were further shown to be dependent on the innate property of the number of mean population doublings of a particular cell strain, and were not influenced by proximity to lower passage cells, splitting ratio, viral contamination, media composition, or periods of storage in liquid nitrogen (Hayflick, 1965b; Hayflick and Moorhead, 1961). Senescent cells can be distinguished from low passage fibroblasts by the innate property to stain blue (Fig. 1A) when processed with an acidic β-galactosidase (β-gal) assay (Dimri, 1995).

Although HDFs in culture are separated from their normal cellular environment, several observations support the use of HDFs grown *in vitro* as a valid model of biological aging. These include: 1) Fibroblasts isolated from young individuals are reproducibly able to undergo more mean population doublings (MPDs) then cells from old donors of the same species (Martin et al., 1970). 2) Fibroblasts from longer lived species undergo more population doublings than short lived species, indicating a relationship between the maximum lifespan of a species and the proliferative capacity of their fibroblasts grown in culture (Goldstein and Singal, 1974; Rohme, 1981). 3) Fibroblasts from individuals with premature aging syndromes such as progeria and Werner's syndrome undergo fewer population doublings in culture than normal cells (Brown, 1990). 4) Normal human fibroblasts in tissues stain with β-gal, indicating senescence *in vivo* (Dimri et al., 1995). These and other observations regarding biochemical differences that accompany senescent HDFs suggest that the HDF model of cellular aging reflects the normal biological processes that occur during *in vivo* aging. In addition to this evidence it has become increasingly apparent that senescence is a natural barrier to oncogenic transformation in many different tumour types (Collado and Serrano, 2010).

2. The post-receptor block

As a result of the refractory nature of senescent fibroblasts to mitogenic stimuli, many of the original studies exploring the molecular details of replicative senescence focused on various growth factor signalling pathways. The growth factors which have been reported to give optimal proliferative response in human fibroblasts are the epidermal growth factor (EGF), insulin like growth factor 1 (IGF-1) and dexamethasone (Phillips and Cristofalo, 1988). Although these tyrosine kinase receptors (RTKs) have many potential down stream mediators, the classical example is a cascade through the small GTPase Ras that leads to the mitogen-activated protein kinase (MAPK) cascade. Early studies investigating the loss of mitogenic response of senescent human diploid fibroblasts focused upon the growth factor receptor:ligand interactions (Gerhard et al., 1991; Phillips et al., 1983; Sell et al., 1993). In the cases of EGF, dexamethasone and IGF-1, it was found that the number of receptors remained the same per unit surface area in senescent cells and that the ligand affinity remained unchanged (Sell et al., 1993). Similarly, the binding kinetics of the glucocorticoid receptor and the insulin receptor have been shown to remain unaltered in senescent cells (Chua et al., 1986). The degradation process of EGF receptor has been shown to be largely unchanged with fibroblast age (Phillips et al., 1984). Studies have also looked at tyrosine autophosphorylation of EGF and PDGF and found no significant differences (Chua et al., 1986; Gerhard et al., 1991). Thus, the general consensus is that decrease in mitogen response is not due to alterations of receptor function or processing (Rattan and Derventzi, 1991).

However, it has been established that the downstream responses of growth factors, such as the induction of the immediate early genes *c-fos* and *egr-1*, are blunted in senescent cells (Meyyappan et al., 1999; Riabowol et al., 1992; Seshadri and Campisi, 1990). Thus, the senescence-specific growth block is thought not to be due to alterations in growth factor-receptor engagement or processing, but to a postreceptor block which leads to reduced immediate early gene responsiveness. Many studies have attempted to identify the points where signalling cascades are modified in senescent cells to account for this block.

2.1 EGFR-Ras-MAPK cascade in senescence

The signal transduction pathway through the epidermal growth factor receptor (EGFR) (and other RTKs) begins with ligand engagement, which initiates dimerization and autophosphorylation within the cytoplasmic domains of the receptors (Fantl et al., 1993). This, in turn, is followed by Src homology 2 domain (SH2) containing molecules interacting with the receptor and recruiting other factors including adaptors. The classic adaptor molecule is Grb2, which binds to the growth factor receptor directly or indirectly through Shc and is associated constitutively with the son of sevenless (SOS) protein. The SOS guanine nucleotide exchange factor catalyses the transformation of inactive GDP-ras to active GTP-ras (Boguski and McCormick, 1993). Activated Ras recruits Raf1 to the membrane allowing its activation (Moodie and Wolfman, 1994). Appropriately localized and activated Raf1 then initiates a kinase cascade through the MAPK cascade. Raf 1 phosphorylates MEK (MAP kinase kinase) which activates Erk1 and Erk2 (MAPK) and leads to MAPK nuclear localization. In the nucleus MAPK phosphorylates transcription factors such as Elk-1 & serum response factor (SRF), stimulating cell proliferation (reviewed in (Wheaton et al., 1996)).

Many studies have attempted to elucidate the role of signalling cascades in senescence, and investigations into the signalling pathways downstream of the EGFR are the most common. It is unclear whether these pathways are compromised in senescence, or whether they need to be intact to promote senescence. Considering that EGFR has been localized to caveolae it is of interest to evaluate studies that have seen a differential regulation in senescent cells. First, it has been found that the EGFR is cleaved to a 100 kD fragment in non-ionic detergent isolates from senescent but not from young primary fibroblasts. This activity appears to be confined to a specialized region of the plasma membrane in senescent cells and was independent of receptor turnover (Carlin et al., 1994). However, it is unclear whether this proteolytic processing is an artefact of the isolation procedure or is physiologically relevant. Second, several studies have reported an age dependent decline in mitogenic stimulation of rat hepatocytes which may be caused by a reduced association between Shc and the EGFR (Hutter et al., 2000; Palmer et al., 1999). Although total tyrosine phosphorylation levels on EGFR appear equivalent after serum stimulation in young and senescent cells, there is a specific reduction of phosphorylation on tyrosine 1173 (a known phosphotyrosine binding (PTB) domain that interacts with Shc (Okabayashi et al., 1994)) in senescent cells. The 1173 residue is known as an autophosphorylation site (Downward et al., 1985), but can also be targeted by Src kinase *in vitro* (Wright et al., 1996) and also is recognized by the SHP-1 phosphatase (Keilhack et al., 1998). This site was subsequently shown to be dephosphorylated by an upregulation of SHP-1 and other phosphatases in senescent human fibroblasts (Tran et al., 2003). Thus, the EGFR in senescence is regulated by differential interaction of adapter molecule Shc at the plasma membrane, which likely compromises its downstream signalling. Interestingly, different splice forms of Shc may have a role in cellular senescence and longevity (Migliaccio et al., 1999).

Studies have also focused on the downstream effectors of EGFR in senescence, particularly on the MAPK (erk 1/2). MAPK is pivotal in transactivation of various transcription factors that drive the cell through proliferation. Although a general reduction in MAPK (Erk1/2) activation has not been seen in senescence (Kim et al., 2000; Tresini et al., 2001), there is a dramatic reduction in localization of activated Erk to the nucleus of senescent fibroblasts (Bose et al., 2004; Kim et al., 2000; Lim et al., 2000; Tresini et al., 2001). However, it has also been found that a phosphatase MKP-2 is stabilized and acts on Erk in senescent cells (Torres et al., 2003), explaining the reduction in active MAPK. This reduced MAPK activity leads to a lack of Elk-1 activation, which loses its ability to bind to the adjacent ets region of the serum response element in *c-fos* promoter. These studies also concede that the reduction in binding of elk-1 alone cannot explain the entire loss of binding at the *c-fos* promoter, or the repression of its transcription. Interestingly, there is an equal amount of non-phosphorylated MAPK (activated) in the nucleus of young and senescent cells, and although reduced, there is still some localization of phospho-MAPK to the senescent cell nucleus. Therefore, these studies raise the question of whether the reduction in MAPK and Elk-1 represents a significant threshold to suppress *c-fos* transcription and explain the post receptor block. This was confirmed when SRF, the primary transcription factor of c-fos and Egr-1, was shown to be hyper-phosphorylated in senescent cells by PKCδ, and suppress immediate early gene transcription (Atadja et al., 1994; Wheaton and Riabowol, 2004). It was shown that immediate early genes could be restored in senescent cells by blocking PKCδ activity independent of MAPK. However, even though immediate early genes could be restored, this was insufficient to allow senescent cells to re-enter the cell cycle (Wheaton and Riabowol, 2004). Not surprisingly, other factors are clearly involved in senescent arrest besides the refractory mitogenic response.

Premature senescence can be induced by the introduction of oncogenic Ras (Serrano et al., 1997) or Raf (Zhu et al., 1998) or constitutively active MAPK (Lin et al., 1998) in primary fibroblasts. In every case, there is an upregulation of p21 and p16 and an induction of senescence which depends on p53 activity. Also the inducible levels of the *c-fos* transcript were found to be repressed in oncogenic Ras induced senescence (Serrano et al., 1997). This oncogenic Ras/Raf/MAPK pathway has been shown to impinge on the $p38^{MAPK}$ stress activated kinase, which is required for the induction of premature senescence (Debacq-Chainiaux et al., 2010). The p38 activity likely impinges directly on p53, or the Rb/p16 pathway to lead to this arrest. The induction of premature senescence likely represents a natural mechanism to block oncogenesis when there is an inappropriately sustained mitogenic signal. Thus, the perturbations of the cellular system as a whole induced by hyperactive Ras/Raf/MAPK are important to inducing premature senescence and only indirectly produce the post receptor block.

2.2 Protein kinase C activity during senescence

Conventional PKCs (α, β, & γ isoforms) and novel PKCs (δ, ε, η, & θ isoforms) are activated by the lipid second messenger 1,2 diacylglycerol (DAG) which is generated downstream of many G-protein-coupled receptors and tyrosine-kinase receptors (Dempsey et al., 2000; Newton, 2001). PKC family members are activated in response to a large number of extracellular signals, and regulate a large number of effectors including receptors, kinases, cytoskeletal components and transcription factors. The outcomes of these signals include changes in proliferation, gene expression, differentiation, permeability, migration, hypertrophy, apoptosis and exocytosis. Each outcome depends on the cellular context, the originating signal and the particular isoform activated (Dempsey et al., 2000). Altered PKC activity has been observed in senescent fibroblasts where a change in serum-induced translocation of PKC from the cytosol to the plasma membrane was reported (De Tata et al., 1993). In contrast, exogenously added phorbol 12-myristate 13-acetate (PMA, a DAG analog) stimulated this translocation identically in young and old cells, implying that the difference in response to serum was due to changes in the production of DAG (De Tata et al., 1993). A similar differential response to serum vs. PMA was also reported for the induction of the *c-fos* gene (Riabowol et al., 1992). Although old fibroblasts have a higher basal level of DAG (Vannini et al., 1994; Venable et al., 1994), the response due to serum induction was reported to be much lower in senescent cells (Chang and Huang, 1994). It should be noted that the specific isoforms were not noted in these studies, but are likely PKC α or β. Attenuated PKC response could contribute to the senescent phenotype in several ways. For example, decreased phosphorylation of substrates that are downstream of PKC could affect the expression of many growth-regulatory genes such as *c-fos* or other MAPK substrates. Alternatively, the higher basal amount of DAG in the resting state of senescent cells compared to young cells may also allow constitutive activation of some kinases. One such kinase, PKCα was found to be required in oxidative stress induced senescence in human fibroblasts. PKCα was shown to induce the senescent phenotype by acting on erk1/2 and Sp1, which converge on and up regulate transcription from the p21 promoter (Kim and Lim, 2009). Interestingly the knockdown of PKCα restored proliferative capacity of senescent cells, implying that the increased basal levels in DAG in senescence constitutively activate PKCα.

The PKCδ isoform has a multifunctional role in various processes including growth inhibition, differentiation, apoptosis and tumour suppression (Basu and Pal, 2010). Many groups have reported that PKC δ activation leads to growth inhibition, including CHO cells, smooth muscle, NIH 3T3 fibroblasts, human glioma cells, and capillary endothelial cells (reviewed in (Gschwendt, 1999)). Studies using ectopic PKCδ implicate p27 as part of the cellular arrest phenotype (Ashton et al., 1999). PKCδ also assists in the sustained up-regulation of p21 message and protein levels in a p53-independent manner (Zezula et al., 1997). However, PKCδ is also capable of phosphorylating and activating p53 in response to genotoxic stress (Johnson et al., 2002; Yoshida et al., 2006). The activity of PKCδ is substantially higher in senescent cells, and has been shown to hyper-phosphorylate SRF, which prevents it from binding to DNA and transactivating the immediate early genes *egr-1* and *c-fos* (Wheaton and Riabowol, 2004). Similarly, increased PKCδ activity during senescence was shown to indirectly inactivate WARTS, a kinase required to exit cytokinesis, and arrest cells after nuclear fission but not before division (Takahashi et al., 2006). A subsequent report also established that constitutively active PKCδ can induce senescent phenotype when introduced to young fibroblasts (Katakura et al., 2009). Interestingly, the activation of PKCδ by PMA is known to be localized to caveolae in cardiomyocytes (Rybin et al., 2008). PKCδ has also been found in the caveolar membrane microdomains of human fibroblasts (Wheaton, 2002). The high activity of PKCδ in senescence may be due to the loss of Src activity in caveolae, which normally inactivates PKCδ through degradation (Blake et al., 1999).

2.3 Phospholipase D activity during senescence

Phospholipase D (PLD) activity is required for an integrated mitogenic response from a variety of receptors including RTKs (reviewed in (Exton, 1998)). PLD catalyses the hydrolysis of phosphatidylcholine (PC) to yield phosphatidic acid (PA) and choline. PA is an important second messenger in many biological processes (Exton, 1997) such as in a membrane localization of Raf-1 (Ghosh et al., 1996). PA can be modified further to the mitogenic lyso-PA by phospholipase A2 or to DAG by PA phosphohydrolase (McDermott et al., 2004). Activation of PLD is complex, involving phosphatidylinositol 4,5-bisphosphate (PIP_2), PKCα/β, Rho family GTPases and ARF GTPase (Exton, 1999). PLD activity has been correlated with mitogenic activity (reviewed in (Foster and Xu, 2003)) and has been shown to be reduced in senescent cells (Venable et al., 1994), possibly due to the reduction of PKC activity or inhibition by ceramide (Venable and Obeid, 1999).

Ceramide acts as a second messenger in a variety of biological processes after being generated from membrane associated sphingomyelin by neutral sphingomyelinase (reviewed in (Foster and Xu, 2003)). The ceramide levels remain stable with fibroblast age, but rise 2-4 fold relative to young cells upon the onset of senescence and are accompanied by an increase in the neutral Mg^{2+} dependent sphingomyelinase activity. The addition of a synthetic, cell permeable analog of ceramide to young cells led to growth arrest and cellular senescence (Venable et al., 1995). These cells showed cellular arrest, lack of Rb phosphorylation, no AP-1 production (Venable et al., 1995) and stained positive with the β-gal test for senescence (Mouton and Venable, 2000). Ceramide acts to inhibit the activation of PLD, by possibly three mechanisms, inhibiting activation by PKC, translocation to the membrane and gene expression, but none of these has been clearly defined (Exton, 1999). Exogenous ceramide inhibits PLD activity in primary fibroblasts (Venable et al., 1994) and this inhibition was shown to depend on PKC interaction but not on phosphorylation or translocation in cell free systems (Venable et al., 1996). However, ceramide has been shown to disrupt the liquid order of lipid rafts, which leads to PLD inhibition (Gidwani et al., 2003). To this end, recent work has identified that the deficiency in PLD activity is specific to the senescent membrane fractions, and not to changes in the cytosol (Webb et al., 2010). The increase in ceramide in senescent membranes likely changes the properties of lipid rafts, which no longer supports an integrated PLD response. Thus, the elevated ceramide levels and PKC regulation are important factors in reduced PLD activity in senescent cell membranes.

2.4 The phosphoinositide 3-kinase pathway during senescence

Due to the role of IGF-1 in the optimal proliferative response of primary fibroblasts (Phillips and Cristofalo, 1988), a common downstream effector of this pathway, phosphoinositide 3-kinase (PI3K) was assessed for its role during senescence. PI3K consists of a p85 regulatory subunit and a p110 catalytic subunit which selectively phosphorylates the 3-OH position of phophoinositides. The enzyme is implicated in both mitogenic and survival signals which are propagated through down stream effectors such as PKB/Akt, IRS-1 and p70 S6K (reviewed in (Vanhaesebroeck et al., 1997). Application of a specific PI3K inhibitor (LY294002) to young primary fibroblasts resulted in cell arrest and the senescent phenotype. Conversely, in the same study, inactivation of the Ras/Raf/MAPK pathway by PD98059 also arrested cell growth, but no induction of senescence was noted (Tresini et al., 1998). Another group using the same approach showed that p27 was highly up-regulated, but that the presumed mediators of senescence, p21, p16, and p53 were all down-regulated. They additionally showed that p27 was the only mediator of the response, since p27-/- mouse embryonic fibroblasts did not become senescent with application of the drug (Collado et al., 2000). Overall, the role of PI3K seems to be in maintaining continued growth, and its inhibition leads to senescence through a non-traditional mechanism of p27 up-regulation.

One of the main effectors of the PI3K pathway is the mammalian target of rapamycin (mTOR), a kinase that integrates signals from multiple mitogenic pathways. The mTOR protein is activated by PI3K through the pathway of PKB/Akt leading to TSC1/TSC2 inactivation, which normally acts as a guainine exchange protein for the small GTPase Rheb. Rheb-GDP holds mTOR in an inactive state, until it is activated through PI3K-Akt-TSC1/2, allowing GTP exchange (Li et al. 2004). The increased mTOR activity has a global effect on translation and cell growth, which is required for rapid cell proliferation (Guertin and Sabatini, 2007). However, it has been shown that serum mitogens are required for the full development of the senescent phenotype (Satyanarayana et al., 2004). The mitogen based induction of senescence has been shown to involve the activation of mTOR, because its inactivation by rapamycin prevents senescence, even in the presence of DNA damage (Leontieva and Blagosklonny, 2010). Recently, treatment with rapamycin has even been shown to extend the proliferative lifespan of human fibroblasts (Cao et al., 2011). These effects were shown to depend on increased autophagic degradation of proteins that enforce senescence, but may also involve a disconnection between mitogen induced translational control and promotion of the cell cycle. Thus, the roles of PI3K and mTOR in senescence would seem to oppose each other, even though they are in the same pathway. These divergent results are difficult to reconcile, but possibly can be explained by other downstream PI3K targets that promote proliferation over senescence. This is supported by the finding that transcriptional targets of the PI3K/PKB are not properly regulated in replicative senescence (Lorenzini et al., 2002). Conversely, in stress or oncogenic induced senescence the PI3K pathway has been shown to have a positive role in the onset of senescence (Binet et al., 2009; Matuoka et al., 2003), consistent with a role for mTOR.

3. P53 and telomere attrition

Replicative senescence is widely accepted to be triggered by critically short telomeres. Stress-induced senescence (also called premature senescence) occurs when cells are exposed to sub-lethal cellular stress such as DNA damage (Di Leonardo et al., 1994; Resnick-Silverman et al., 1998), oxidative stress (Chen and Ames, 1994), or oncogenic stress (Serrano et al., 1997). Both replicative and stress-induced senescence result in the accumulation of cells that are incapable of further divisions and arrest primarily in the G1 phase of the cell cycle. Thus, senescence is thought to represent an intrinsic barrier to oncogenesis by limiting proliferation.

The p53 tumour suppressor protein is a transcription factor that under normal cellular conditions is unstable and inactive. In response to many forms of cellular stress, p53 becomes activated by post-translational modification and is able to transactivate target genes that regulate diverse cellular processes including, cell cycle progression, senescence, DNA repair, metabolism and cell survival (Appella and Anderson, 2001; Vousden and Lane, 2007). Active p53 protein promotes cell cycle arrest through transcriptional activation of many genes including: *p21WAF1* (el-Deiry et al., 1993), *GADD45α* (Kastan et al., 1992), *BTG2* (Rouault et al., 1996), *REPRIMO* (Ohki et al., 2000), *14-3-3σ* (Hermeking et al., 1997), and Prl-3 (Basak et al., 2008). Different subsets of p53-responsive genes regulate DNA repair, metabolism, survival and apoptosis. The p53 protein has been implicated as one of the key mediators of both the onset (Hara et al., 1991; Shay et al., 1991) and maintenance (Beausejour et al., 2003; Gire and Wynford-Thomas, 1998) of cellular senescence. The transcriptional targets of p53 shown to initiate replicative senescence include *p21WAF1* (Brown et al., 1997; el-Deiry et al., 1993; Noda et al., 1994), BTG2 (Wheaton et al., 2010), GADD45α (Jackson and Pereira-Smith, 2006) and PAI (Kortlever et al., 2006). When p53 is knocked down by shRNA (or other method) in fibroblasts it extends the proliferative lifespan by 10-20 population doublings, by avoiding p53 induced senescent program (Fig. 1B).

Various chemical agents and gamma irradiation can cause DNA double stranded breaks, which also lead to premature senescence. The biological process that occurs at a doubled stranded break involves hundreds of H2AX histones becoming phosphorylated (γH2AX) as the signal propagates from the break site. This DNA damage can visualized in the nucleus of a cell as foci by immunofluorescence using a γH2AX phospho-specific antibody (Rogakou et al., 1999; Rogakou et al., 1998). The kinase Ataxia telangiectasia mutated (ATM) acts as a sensor of DNA damage, becomes activated at the γH2AX foci and phosphorylates p53 (Bakkenist and Kastan, 2003). This phosphorylation stabilizes and activates p53, and allows it to transactivate its effector genes.

Telomeres consist of a tandem repeat of 6 nucleotides (TTAGGG) that cap the ends of linear double stranded DNA in mammals. Human telomeres consist of 5-10 kilobase pairs at the end of every chromosome arm and have an overhang of single-stranded telomeric repeat of several hundred bases. If ends of chromosomes were not protected by telomeres the cell would detect the end of the DNA as a double stranded break and initiate a DNA damage response. Telomeres normally protect the double stranded chromosome ends by the formation of telomere-loops (t-loops) in which the telomeric single-stranded overhang hybridizes within the double-stranded telomeric region of a chromosome. T-loops are maintained and stabilized by a complex of proteins referred to as shelterin (de Lange, 1994). Telomeres are know to shorten with each round of DNA replication because of the "end-replication problem"; the inability of DNA polymerases to completely replicate the 3′ end of linear DNA molecules (Harley et al., 1990). Telomeres will shorten to a critical length after a finite number of DNA replication cycles, and lose the ability to form the sheltern/t-loop cap at the ends of chromosomes. The DNA damage signal arising from eroded telomeres will activate ATM, leading in turn to p53 activation (Herbig et al., 2004). Thus, t-loop disruption as a consequence of telomere shortening exposes telomeric DNA that leads to p53 activation and the initiation of replicative senescence (Herbig et al., 2004; Karlseder et al., 2002; Li et al., 2003; Li et al., 2004; Stewart et al., 2003). This model is supported by studies that ectopically expressed telomerase (hTERT) allowing fibroblasts to bypass senescence (Figure 1B) and become immortalized by preventing telomere shortening (Bodnar et al., 1998; Vaziri and

Benchimol, 1998). Hence, critically short telomeres provide a physiological signal for activation of the p53-dependent replicative senescence program in human cells.

4. Caveolae

Caveolae are flask shaped invaginations which form at the plasma membrane from lateral assemblies of cholesterol and sphingolipids known as lipid rafts (reviewed in (Harder and Simons, 1997)). Lipid rafts are composed of sphingomyelin, glycosphingolipids and cholesterol which form microdomain rafts surrounded by the phosphatidylcholine rich plasma membrane. These rafts sequester a specific subset of transmembrane associated proteins (Simons and Ikonen, 1997). Thus, lipid rafts are organelle like environments which have been postulated to have specific functions in various cell types (Simons and Toomre, 2000). Lipid rafts are also found to form higher order structures, caveolae (little caves), when associated with the scaffolding transmembrane proteins (Figure 2A & B). Caveolae are distinct from other vesicle-like invaginations, such as clathrin coated pits, due to their small size and lipid raft composition (Kurzchalia and Parton, 1999). The catalyst of caveolar formation is the oligomerization of a class of sphingolipid and cholesterol binding proteins known as caveolins (Monier et al., 1996), which stabilize and induce the lipid rafts to coalesce (reviewed in (Harder and Simons, 1997)). Three caveolin genes have been identified encoding caveolin proteins 1, 2, and 3 (Glenney, 1992; Kurzchalia et al., 1992; Scherer et al., 1996; Tang et al., 1996 ; Way and Parton, 1996). Both the N- and C-termini of caveolins are exposed to the cytoplasm forming a hairpin structure in the membrane, and are palmitoylated (Dietzen et al., 1995). Caveolin monomers oligomerize into hetero- and homo-dimers and trimers as they are translated in the cytoplasm (Lisanti et al., 1993), traffic through the trans-Golgi network and associate at the plasma membrane (reviewed in (Rietveld and Simons, 1998)). Due to their unique lipid raft composition caveolae can be biochemically purified based on their insolubility in the detergent Triton X-100 as well as on their low buoyant density on sucrose gradients (reviewed in (Anderson, 1998)). The insolubility of caveolae is likely due to the enrichment in sphingolipids and cholesterol in contrast to the glycerophospholipid rich plasma membrane (Hanada et al., 1995).

Recent advances in the characterization of lipid rafts have identified a new class of proteins which are essential to the biogenesis and regulation of caveolae; cavins 1 to 4. Cavin 1 (or polymerase I and transcript release factor: PTRF) has been shown to be essential for the stability and organization of caveolar structures (Hill et al., 2008; Liu and Pilch, 2008). Cavins 1-4 are part of a heterologous complex which bind to mature caveolin proteins (Figure 2B) that have emerged as caveolae after being processed through the trans-golgi system (Hayer et al., 2010). This interaction is cavin 1 and caveolin dependent and is thought to be due to a cavin phosphatidyl-serine interaction domain in all cavin proteins; a lipid which is enriched in caveolae (Bastiani et al., 2009). Cavin-2 is thought to play a role in the curvature of caveolar structures (Hansen et al., 2009). Cavin-3 is known to be involved in caveolae endocytosis and coordinates internalization on microtubules (McMahon et al., 2009). Cavin-4 is specifically expressed in striated muscle and has been shown to have specific roles related to myogenesis (Tagawa et al., 2008) and contraction (Ogata et al., 2008). Caveolin and cavin expression are interdependent on one another, since the depletion of one leads to the suppression of the other. Thus, cavins have emerged as an essential component of caveolae regulation, stability, and biogenesis.

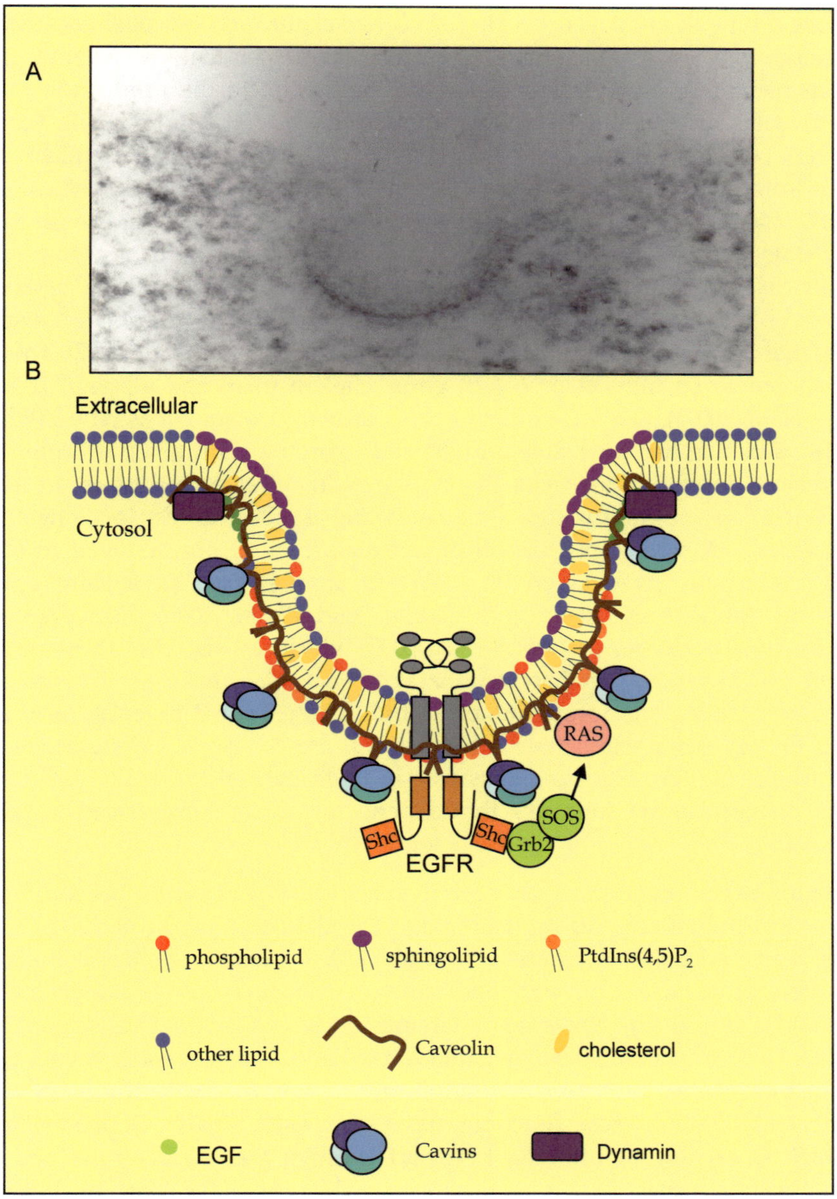

Fig. 2. Caveolae Structure

A) Electron micrograph of a caveolae at the membrane surface of 3T3 L1 fibroblasts.

B) Schematic diagram of the lipid and protein composition of caveolae. Phospholipids and PtdIns(4,5)P2 are concentrated on the inner leaflet, while sphingolipid is found in the outer leaflet of caveolae. Cholesterol is required for the caveolin proteins to bind and create a multimeric scaffold that forms the caveolar structure. Dynamin proteins surround the neck of the caveolae, and play a role in the fission of caveolar vesicles during endocytosis. Many receptor and signalling cascades are compartmentalized in caveolae, including the epidermal growth factor receptor (EGFR), the adaptors Shc, Grb & SOS, and Ras small GTPase. Cavins 1 to 4 bind to caveolin and regulate caveolae biogenesis, shape and trafficking.

Caveolae are a type of endocytic vesicle (much like clathrin coated pits) and can undergo internalization with particular stimuli. The process is dependent on dynamin (a GTPase involved in membrane fission) and cholesterol and leads to the production of enclosed vesicular caveolar structures with in the cytoplasm of the cell (Fig. 3A & B). For example, caveolae can be generated in transformed NIH 3T3 cells when a dominant negative dynamin is introduced, and is blocked in the presence of cholesterol sequestering agent (Li et al., 2001). This implies that even in cells that normally have no detectable caveolae, there is a steady state of caveolar invagination that is stabilized with dominant negative dynamin. Pinched off caveolae can be visualized as self contained vesicles (called cavicles) using electron microscopy (Mundy et al., 2002), and have been shown to fuse with a specialized endosome (that is caveolin positive) called caveosomes (Pelkmans et al., 2002). This pathway has been shown to be utilized by SV-40 virus, cholera toxin and albumin (reviewed in (Lajoie and Nabi, 2007)). Caveolae utilizing this pathway are known as type I (Fig. 3B) and this cavicle trafficking has been shown to depend upon transport along microtubles. These caveolar vesicles form into alternate morphologies in different cell types; in adipocytes, caveolar vesicles cluster into rosettes, and in endothelial cells, the vesicles elongate and fuse to form channels. A second population of caveolae (type 2) are involved in continuous rounds of fusion and invagination (Fig. 3B) but are restricted to remain near the cell membrane by the actin cytoskeleton (Pelkmans and Zerial, 2005). This cycle is highly regulated by various kinases (del Pozo et al., 2005) which can also shift these caveolae into long range type I transport. It is theorized that type 2 caveolae are largely responsible for the potocytosis of vitamins and ions (Anderson et al., 1992). Type 3 caveolae form elongated tubes from the cell surface in certain cell types and are not as well characterized. Several types of caveolae can be seen simultaneously in the same cell lineage (Fig. 3A & B), and often carry out specialized functions that depend on cell type (reviewed in (White and Anderson, 2005)).

In addition to the endocytic transport described above, it has recently been found that the EGFR has a functional role during trafficking through caveolar system. Under normal conditions, activated EGFR is recycled through clathrin coated pit mediated endocytosis and degraded or recycled through endosomes or lysomes respectively (reviewed in (Madshus and Stang, 2009)). However, in circumstances of sustained EGF signalling levels or the presence of oxidative stress or gamma irradiation, the caveolar system transports the EGFR through an endosomal endoplasmic route to the nucleus (reviewed in (Dittmann et al., 2009)). These functions have been shown to be dependent on active EGFR, which is capable of utilizing transport through the nuclear pore and becomes soluble in the nucleoplasm. This localization is thought to be very important in the resolution of DNA damage. To this end, nuclear EGFR has been shown to phosphorylate and activate DNA dependent protein kinase (DNA-PK), an important mediator of non-homologous end joining (Dittmann et al., 2005). In addition, nuclear EGFR has been shown to regulate transcription of cyclin D1, iNOS and B-myb, and regulate PCNA by phosphorylation, all of which correlate with entry into the cell cycle (Dittmann et al., 2009). Many tumours have been reported to have a nuclear population of EGFR, and its presence is linked to continued proliferation. Thus, this cellular transport system is the target of chemotherapy agents that either inactivate EGF signalling by inhibition of src kinase or antibody therapies that promote the uptake of EGFR through caveolae and thus block its activation (Dittmann et al., 2009).

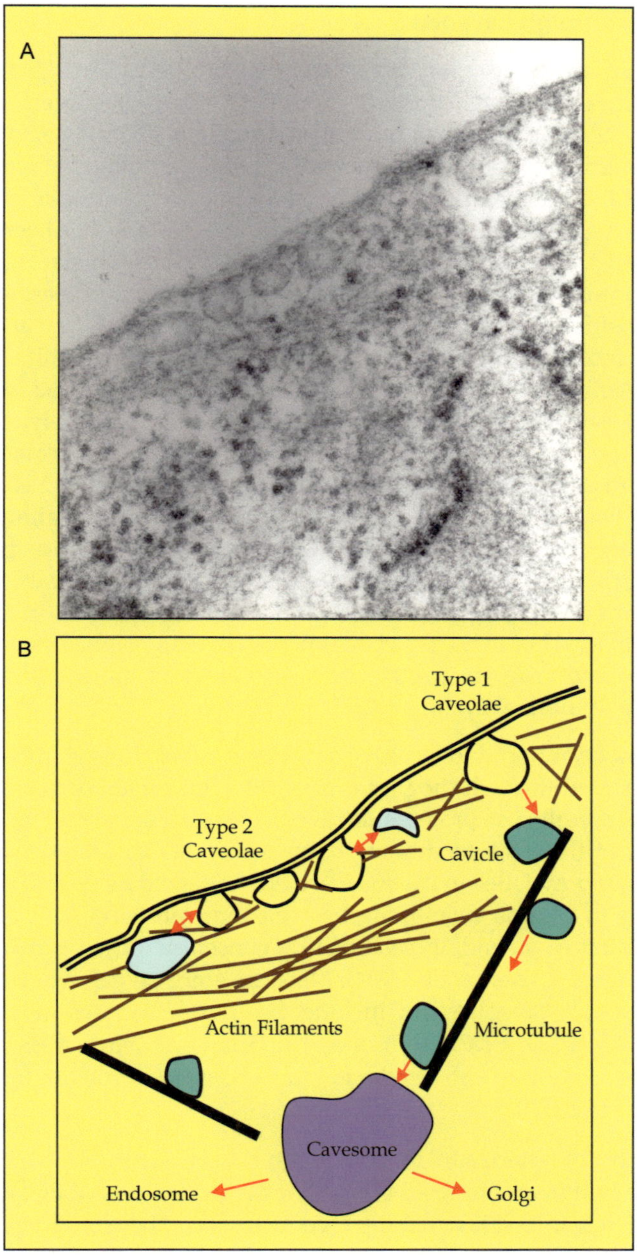

Fig. 3. Caveolar Endocytosis
A) Electron micrograph of caveolar structures at the membrane surface of differentiated 3T3 L1 fibroblasts. **B)** A schematic diagram showing caveolar endocytosis. Type I caveolae invaginate in response to various stimulae and form caveolar vesicles (cavicles) that are transported on microtubules. Cavicles can fuse together in cavesomes, where various contents may be recycled, or are transported to endosomes or the Golgi. Type II caveolae invaginate, fuse, and transport back to the cell surface. They are confined by the actin cytoskeleton and are important for potocytosis.

4.1 Cell signalling through caveolae

There is significant evidence that many well-studied receptor signalling systems are localized and operate through caveolae. Caveolin protein has been shown to directly interact with many of these signalling molecules through a 20 amino acid domain known as the caveolin scaffolding domain (CSD: (Couet et al., 1997)). Interaction with this domain has been shown to hold the signalling molecules in an inactive conformation (Okamoto et al., 1998). The pepitide sequence is rich in aromatic amino acids and has been shown to bind to adenylyl cyclase (AC), heterotrimeric Gα and Gβγ, PI3K, endothelial nitric oxide synthase (eNOS), protein kinase A (PKA), PKC, ERK1/2 and Src family kinases. In each case, the CSD is associated with the inactivation of the particular pathway (reviewed in (Patel et al., 2008)). However, since the CSD also binds lipids, there is the possibility that there are two populations of caveolin, one integral with rafts and another associated with the membrane that is not part of caveolae (Parton and Simons, 2007). Alternatively, the CSD has been conjectured to release the signalling proteins it binds to upon conformational change with activation (Okamoto et al., 1998). Although the exact role of the CSD is controversial, it is clear that it is involved in regulating and possibly sequestering signalling molecules to the caveolae. The inhibitory signalling associated with caveolin proteins has been challenged by many studies which show a requirement for Caveolin 1 in activating signal cascades (Kurzchalia and Parton, 1999, White, 2005 #707). This theory is based on the caveolin driven generation of caveolae, which acts to compartmentalize many signalling cascades. Thus, the caveolar structures and caveolin protein act as a center of cross talk and integration of mitogenic responses in normal cycling cells.

Many proteins have been found to localize to caveolae either through direct interaction with caveolins or sequestered through the properties of the lipid microdomains (Zajchowski and Robbins, 2002). Localization of proteins to caveolae is also enhanced by palmitoylation. A significant number of these are membrane bound receptors and kinase cascades with their adaptor proteins. Lipid moieties in caveolae are often utilized as second messengers (figure 2B) or for docking to plasma membrane by signalling proteins. This allows caveolae to regulate the activation of signalling cascades by concentration or proximity of substrates and second messengers (Cohen et al., 2004). Many receptor signalling systems are localized to and operate through caveolae and include; Src family kinases, nitric oxide synthase, EGFR, PDGFR, PLCγ, PLD, PKCα & β, Ras, trimeric G-proteins, MEK and Erk2, among others. Some of these proteins can also be found to be concentrated in lipid rafts (reviewed in (de Laurentiis et al., 2007)).

The most thoroughly characterized RTK residing in caveolae is EGFR, which is also crucial to mitogenic reposnse in human fibroblasts. Whether the localization of EGFR in caveolae has a negative or positive role in EGFR signalling is controversial. There is strong evidence for both, and it may be difficult to reconcile the observations definitively. The first evidence of the MAPK pathway in caveolae found H-Ras, Grb2 and SOS in Rat-1 cells (Mineo et al., 1996). The EGFR was present in the caveolin fraction in unstimulated Rat-1 cells, but declined rapidly after stimulation by EGF. The same migration was found in human fibroblasts and depended on EGF engagement, active EGFR tyrosine kinase, and phosphorylation of the EGFR receptor (Mineo et al., 1999). These observations implied that the activation of EGFR occurred within the caveolae, and is required to migrate in order to attenuate the EGF response. This was supported by the finding that some common mutations in EGFR that are oncogenic are also incapable of migrating from caveolae when stimulated.

In addition to the MAPK pathway, EGFR has been shown to activate other downstream effectors such as phospholipase Cγ (PLCγ) through PI3K (Jang et al., 2001) and PLD1 (Han et al., 2002)) in caveolae. PLCγ hydrolyses phosphatidylinositol- 4,5-bisphosphate (PIP_2) to produce diacylglycerol and inositol 1,3,5,-trisphosphate (IP_3), which activates PKC and mobilizes intracellular calcium respectively. PLD catalyses the hydrolysis of phosphatidylcholine to yield phosphatidic acid. These second messengers lead to the activation of Akt and mTOR which promote cellular proliferation (reviewed in (de Laurentiis et al., 2007)).

5. Caveolae and cavicles in senescence

The first report examining caveolin protein in replicative senescence (Park et al., 2000) found that the protein was highly elevated as human fibroblasts reached high population doublings. This upregulation was correlated to an increased number of caveolar structures seen in the EM of senescent cells, which were thought to be caveolae. Additionally, the group found EGFR signalling was attenuated in senescence through the binding to caveolin. However, these studies did not address whether caveolin generated bona-fide functional caveolar structures or whether it represented a differential regulation of caveolar pathway. Unfortunately, the EM chosen to examine the senescent cells did not have a clear cross section of the outer membrane, and it was unclear whether the structures being scored were caveolae or cavicles. The paradigm then (as now) was that increased caveolin drives the formation of caveolae and the regulation of cavicle generation had not yet been fully elucidated. This lead to the interpretation that the number of caveolae increase in senescent cells. Additionally, the low numbers of caveolae counted in low passage fibroblasts was in direct contrast to what had been previously seen in human fibroblasts by EM (Rothberg et al., 1992) or by freeze fracture EM (Fujimoto et al., 2000). Since this initial report, other groups have visualized a similar elevation of caveolar structures, which appear to be vesicles, and not classical caveolae in senescent cells (Bai et al., 2011; Volonte and Galbiati, 2011). Figure 3A shows structures consistent with caveolae in differentiated 3T3 L1 fibroblasts. Note the flask like invaginations within the outer membrane and the opening to the extracellular space through a smaller pore like neck. Thus, classically defined caveolae do not increase during senescence, and potentially are lost, while cavicles consistent with increased endocytosis have been seen in all senescent cells examined so far (Figure 3A & B). Although our own work examining caveolae (Wheaton and Riabowol, 2004) originally appeared to radically differ from other published reports, it does support the idea of increased caveolar vesicles in senescent fibroblasts. A comparison of young and senescent cells indicated that senescent cells contained a higher total amount of caveolins 1 and 2, but had significantly less of both proteins in the caveolar fraction obtained by sucrose density centrifugation. Additionally, caveolar fractions from senescent cells completely lacked the tyrosine kinase activity associated with functional caveolae and the EGF response. Furthermore, old cells had little caveolar protein exposed to the outer plasma membrane as estimated by an *in vivo* biotinoylation assay and there was no caveolin 1 detected on the cell surface using immunofluorescence (Fig. 4A & B) and confocal microscopy. Together, these data suggest that a fundamental loss of signal integration at the plasma membrane of senescent cells is due to the loss of signalling competent caveolae. However, they do not rule out the possibility that increased caveolar vesicles are present within the cytoplasm, as has been conjectured above. In fact, the poor response of EGFR and tyrosine phosphorylation of its targets in caveolae could be due the separation of these structures from the extracellular space. Therefore, the increase in caveolar structures in senescence may represent a misregulation of the normal functional caveolae during the aging process. This implies that some part of the endocytic process is blocked, leading to accumulation and stabilization of cavicles during senescence. This is supported by the finding that endocytosis is reduced in senescent cells and is correlated with an upregulation of caveolin 1 (Park et al., 2002).

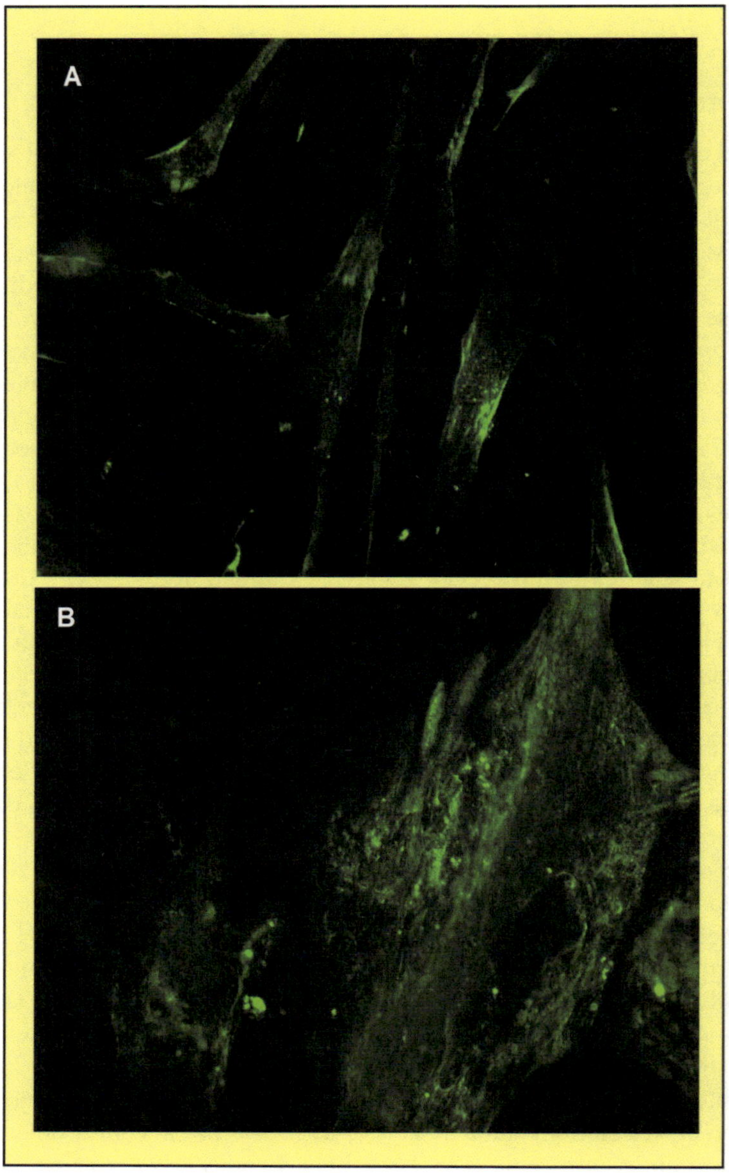

Fig. 4. Caveolin-1 Localization in Young and Senescent Fibroblasts
Young (A) and senescent (B) Hs68 fibroblasts were immuno-stained with anti-caveolin-1 and Alexa 488 flourescent secondary antibodies. Caveolin-1 is concentrated at the cell periphery in young cells (A) and is largely internalized in senescent cells (B).

These data suggest a model in which senescent cells are unable to organize and localize the components of functional caveolae to the plasma membrane. The pinched off caveolar vesicles observed in senescent cells may represent a unique misregulation of caveolae that could explain both the functional differences and the increase in caveolar structures seen previously (Wheaton, 2011). Thus, although increased expression of cavin-1 and caveolin proteins drive the biogenesis of caveolar structures, they unbalance the normal equilibrium between cavicles and cavaolae. This unbalance could promote invagination, but stall cavicle migration at some point in their migration along microtubles before they fuse with caveosomes or endosomes. Consistent with this idea, caveolin 1 staining is found at the cell periphery in young cells, but not at the membrane of senescent cells. However, there is very intense staining of caveolin within the interior of senescent cells (Fig. 4A & B). Using confocal microscopy with a deconvolution algorithm found intense caveolin-1 staining in senescent cells that was associated with fibre like structures (Fig. 5B). Confocal analysis of young cell caveolin -1 found it concentrated in regions of the cell periphery (Fig. 5A). This pattern of fibres is consistent with the caveolae associating with microtubules, and becoming stalled after internalization. The increased number of cavicles could represent a natural response to stress, in which cell arrest is maintained by sequestering key signalling receptors away from their ligands in the extracellular space. This would have a similar effect to EGFR antibody based chemotherapies which drive internalization of the EGFR through caveolae, but prevent its localization to the nucleus and activation (Dittmann et al., 2009). Considering internalization of EGFR through caveolae is a response to gentoxic agents, it is possible that DNA damage downstream of telomere attrition may do the same. Thus, the cell may respond to stress by down regulating mitogen activated cascades through internalization of caveolae. Recent studies in which caveolae are found to be redistributed by internalization during mitosis support this idea (Boucrot et al., 2011) . The caveolae in this case internalize through microtubules and could be a mechanism to block mitogenic signals after the commitment to divide.

5.1 Physical changes in senescent membranes and lipids

It is possible that some of the changes seen in caveolar structures can be explained by the unique properties and composition of the plasma membrane of old cells (Rutter et al., 1996; Schroeder et al., 1984). Rafts are comprised of a high concentration of sphingolipids and cholesterol, which have strong cohesive forces that counteract the entropic force inherent in a fluid mosaic membrane (reviewed in (Harder and Simons, 1997)). Examining senescent cells using proton magnetic resonance has shown that the ratio of cholesterol/ phosphatidylcholine increases as human fibroblasts age in culture, indicating an increased amount of mobile cholesterol (Rutter et al., 1996). Another early report sought to probe the lipid composition of these fibroblasts by using fluorescent probes. These labelled lipids can be used to determine the limiting anisotropy (fluidity) of membranes and showed that the microsomal fraction increased in fluidity with donor age (Schroeder et al., 1984). Lipid composition changes during fibroblast aging lead to higher lipid fluidity and may reflect the inability of significant raft domains to form with age, since rafts by nature are islands of less fluid lipid. This is in part is due to the levels of a species of phosphatidylcholine comprised of stearic acid and arachidonic acid becoming elevated in senescent fibroblasts (Naru et al., 2008). This dilutes the components of lipid rafts in the membrane of senescent cells.

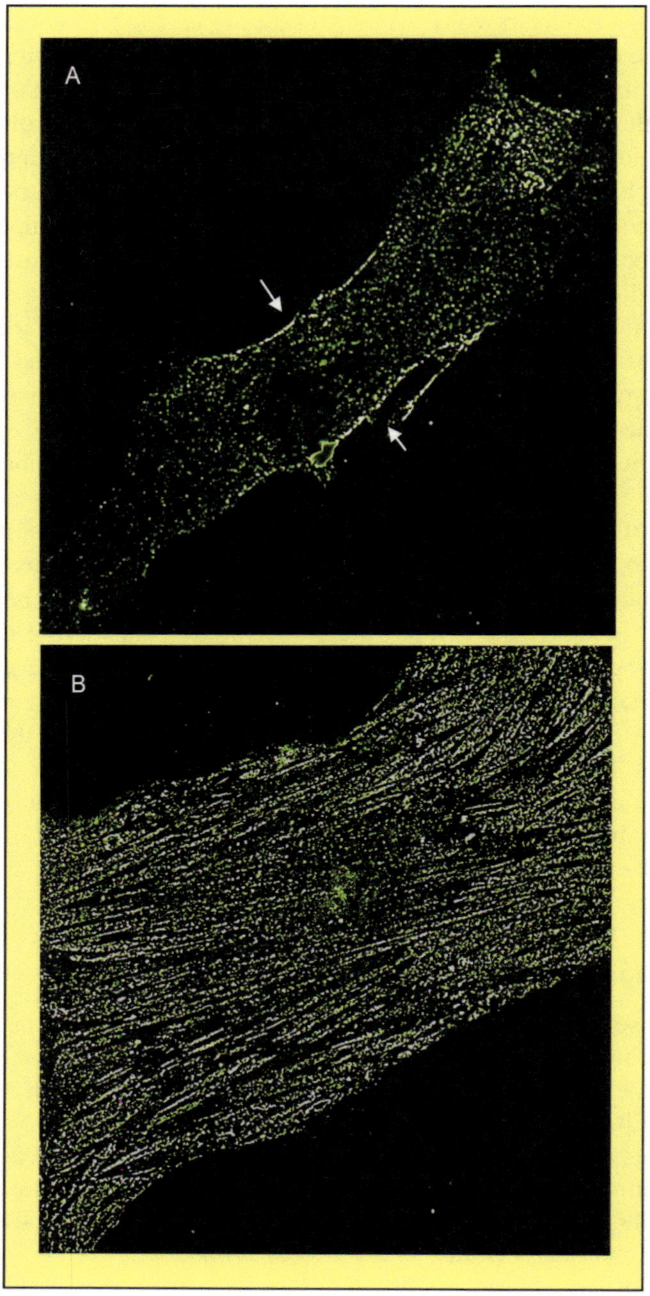

Fig. 5. Confocal Microscopy of Caveolin-1 Staining in Young and Senescent Fibroblasts. Young (A) and senescent (B) Hs68 fibroblasts were immuno-stained with anit-caveolin-1 and Alexa 488 fluorescent secondary antibodies. The images show a single confocal layer that was filtered through a de-convolution protocol to show the localization in sharper detail. The young cells have a high concentration of caveolin at the cell periphery, indicated by arrows. In senescent cells, caveolin is concentrated through out the cell on filaments consistent with microtubules.

In addition, senescent cell membranes are characterized by the specific loss of cholesterol from the microsomal fraction (Nakamura et al., 2003), even if the overall cholesterol may rise with age (Park et al., 2000). As previously mentioned, cholerterol is essential for lipid raft and caveolae formation (Fig. 2B). The altered cholesterol in the membrane also likely affects various signal transduction pathways (Fielding and Fielding, 2004). Alteration of the raft composition or dynamics may interfere with raft coalescence or its ability to sequester caveolin proteins. The loss of caveolae at the surface of the plasma membrane in old cells supports this model, since it would indicate that the proteins are unable to associate with rafts due to altered dynamics or composition, and subsequently they are not transported to the cell surface.

5.2 Upregulation of caveolin proteins and its effect on caveolar signalling

Key signalling pathways that operate through caveolar structures which are inactivated or misregulated could lead to aspects of the senescent phenotype. Since many growth receptors have been found to be localized within, and to signal through caveolar structures, it is possible that one or more of these may modulate the mitogenic response in primary fibroblasts. Many signalling pathways shown to be altered in senescence, including MAPK, PI3K, PLD and PKCδ (reviewed in (Caino et al., 2009)) are localized to caveolae. Since a significant post receptor block of mitogenic signalling is associated with the development of senescence, the existence of microdomains where receptors and signalling cascades are believed to be linked offers a promising functional connection to these observations. Indeed, the absence of a membrane population of caveolae may prevent mitogenic signal propagation. Thus, the post receptor block could be the result of receptors being either uncoupled from internalized caveolae or sequestered from access to ligands in the extracellular space. These kinase cascades would subsequently be unable to maintain integrated downstream responses to ligand and contribute to senescent arrest. Alternatively, the increases in caveolin protein itself may lead directly to the attenuation of many kinase cascades by virtue of the tumour suppressive function of CSD binding to key components of the cascade. Thus, a mechanism linking the post receptor block to caveolae is either through misregulated caveolar internalization or the inhibitory CSD of caveolin, both of which are characterized by increased caveolin-1 protein expression.

The initial observation linking caveolae to repressed signal propagation in senescence noted that EGF signalling was attenuated (Park et al., 2000). These first studies observed an increase in caveolin-1 & 2 proteins, and therefore the CSD domain (Park et al., 2000; Wheaton et al., 2001). Consistent with this observation, ectopic caveolin 1 expression in fibroblasts was shown to induce premature senescence and thus lead directly to cellular arrest (Volonte et al., 2002). This was further supported by the suppression of caveolin-1 using small inferring RNA or antisense oligos in senescent fibroblasts. Knockdown of caveolin in fibroblasts restores the response to EGF and the cells are capable of entering the cell cycle (Cho et al., 2003). It is thought that this response works primarily through the interaction of the caveolin CSD with erk1/2, leading to attenuation of kinase activity (Engelman et al., 1998). Supporting this, the erk1/2 kinase has been previously reported to be misregulated during senescence (see section 2.1).

Oxidative stress has been shown to cause irreversible growth arrest in NIH 3T3 cells and is dependent on the upregulation of caveolin-1 (Volonte et al., 2002). Such stress also leads to tyrosine phosphorylation of caveolin-1 which depends on p38 and Src (Volonte et al., 2001) and drives the internalization of caveolae. The same stress (H_2O_2) was shown to cause premature senescence in human fibroblasts, with a relocalization of caveolin to the cytoplasm and nucleus that required p38 activity (Chretien et al., 2008). Thus stress induced senescence appears to upregulate caveolin and redistribute the protein (and likely caveolar structures). This is similar to what is seen in replicative senescence where caveolin protein is found in the cytoplasm (Wheaton et al., 2001) or when cavicles accumulate (Bai et al., 2011; Park et al., 2000; Volonte and Galbiati, 2011). Thus, p38 activated by stress may drive internalization of caveolae and causes receptor tyrosine receptor signalling to be attenuated.

Senescent cells have a flattened and enlarged morphology that is characterized by an increase in focal adhesions (Cho et al., 2004) and which lead to increased amount of actin stress fibres (Wheaton et al., 1996). Caveolin has also been reported to localize to focal adhesions through integrin and likely plays a role in mitogen signalling during cell adhesion. This interaction appears to be upregulated during senescence since caveolin-1 and paxillin (a focal adhesion marker) co-localize strongly in senescent cells (Cho et al., 2004). Furthermore, when caveolin-1 is knocked down in senescent cells, there is an inhibition of focal adhesion kinase, depolarization of anchored actin and reversion of the cells to a younger morphology (Cho et al., 2004). The origin of these morphological alterations is difficult to verify since caveolin repression affects other aspects of mitogenic signalling. However, it has been shown that breaking cell adhesion contacts influences the internalization of lipid rafts within transformed cells (del Pozo et al., 2004; del Pozo et al., 2005). In addition, the clustering of integrins is known to activate Fyn in a caveolin-1 dependent manner to allow anchorage dependent growth (Wary et al., 1998). Consistent with these studies it has been shown that localization of caveolin-1 to cholesterol enriched microdomains decreases in senescent fibroblasts when they are liberated from the substratum by scraping or trypsin (Inomata et al., 2006). This implies that internalization of lipid rafts occurs in senescent cells when there detached and reflects caveolae misregulation in senescent cells. The absence of caveolae when senescent cells are establishing new focal contacts could represent another way in which mitogenic signals are blocked.

In summary, inappropriate caveolin regulation in senescent cells may contribute to the senescence associated post receptor block in three ways. First, the CSD may bind and neutralize various signalling molecules, and prevent signal propagation. Second, caveolin drives internalization of caveolae which prevents receptors access to ligands. Third, caveolin may no longer be sequestered to lipid rafts preventing the development of caveolae to allow signal integration.

5.3 P53, DNA damage and caveolae

Although the most common interpretation in the literature is that telomere attrition is the origin of DNA damage in replicative senescence, a considerable amount of damage foci (γH2AX) are not localized to telomeres in senescent cells (Sedelnikova et al., 2004). The γH2AX-telomere foci are also dependent on whether these cells are cultured in normoxic (2% O_2) conditions (Herbig et al., 2004). Thus, the possibility exists that other forms of stress cause DNA damage in parallel with telomere erosion, such as elevated reactive oxygen species (ROS) or replication fork collapse. These forms of stress may result from the misregulation of caveolae or the upregulation of caveolin. The upregulation of caveolin leading to a increase in caveolar vesicles causes both the attenuation of the EGFR signalling (de Laurentiis et al., 2007) and an increase in the activity of the p53 tumour suppressor through elevated ROS (Volonte and Galbiati, 2009a). Both of these mechanisms may lead to DNA damage that is not localized to telomeres. This is also consistent with studies in senescent cells which demonstrate higher p53 activity and p21 expression (see section 3).

Overexpression of caveolin 1 protein has been shown to cause G1 arrest, which is dependent on p21 expression induced by increased p53 activity. Mouse embryonic fibroblasts expressing caveolin-1 have a reduced proliferative lifespan and a senescent morphology (Volonte et al., 2002). The aberrant caveolin-1 levels lead to G0/G1 cell cycle arrest, activation of p53 and upregulation of p21 (Galbiati et al., 2001). This shows that caveolin-1 expression mediates premature senescence through a p53/p21 dependent pathway. This pathway is further enhanced by caveolin 1 mediated inactivation of MDM2 and PP2A-C which act as negative regulators of p53 and ATM, respectively (Bartholomew et al., 2009; Volonte et al., 2009). The MDM2 protein is an ubiquitin ligase which targets p53 for degradation and keeps p53 at basal levels in unstressed conditions. Upon activation by stress p53 is phosphorylated at residues which prevent MDM2 association and in turn stabilizes p53. It has been shown during oxidative stress induced senescence that MDM2 is neutralized by caveolin and stabilizes p53 (Volonte et al., 2009). It is thought that the activation of p53 is usually achieved by the kinase ATM, which is sensor of DNA damage (see section 3). Auto-phosphorylation of ATM occurs when it binds to regions of DNA damage and dissociates as active monomers (Bakkenist and Kastan, 2003). ATM is turned off after repair is completed by the phosphatase PP2A-C. When modeling pulmonary emphysema in murine fibroblasts, it was found that oxidative stress caused the sequestration and neutralization of PP2A-C into caveolar enriched microdomains (Bartholomew et al., 2009). Thus, there appears to be a role for CSD in caveolin for the activation of p53 at many levels. To further demonstrate a role for the CSD in caveolin, it was shown that introduction of the peptide of this domain was able to cause premature senescence by itself (Volonte et al., 2009).

The family of cavin proteins have recently been investigated for their potential role during senescence. Cavin-1 (PTRF) and Cavin-3 (SRBC) both appear to be elevated through protein stabilization during replicative senescence, but not quiescence (Bai et al., 2011; Cong et al., 2006) Additionally, it has been shown that cavin-1 is upregulated during oxidative stress induced premature senescence (Volonte and Galbiati, 2011). The ectopic expression of cavin-1 leads to activation of p53, a decrease in MAPK activity, and induced premature senescence. Interestingly, the cavin-1 expression also induced DNA foci that were visualized by γH2AX and did not colocalize with telomeres. The knockdown of cavin-1 extended proliferative lifespan, and reversed the γH2AX in high passage cells (Bai et al., 2011). Similarly, the knockdown of PTRF prevented oxidative stress from inducing senescence and was shown to prevent the MDM2:caveolin 1 interaction leading to p53 activation (Volonte and Galbiati, 2011). Cavin-1 expression is known to have a direct affect on the levels of caveolin (Hansen and Nichols, 2010) and therefore the upregulation of cavin-1 in these systems likely explains the upregulation of caveolin observed during senescence. Although these two studies focused on PTRF, much of the data can be explained by the elevation of caveolin and caveolar vesicles. What is most significant is the generation of DNA damage seen downstream of caveolar vesicles (Wheaton, 2011).

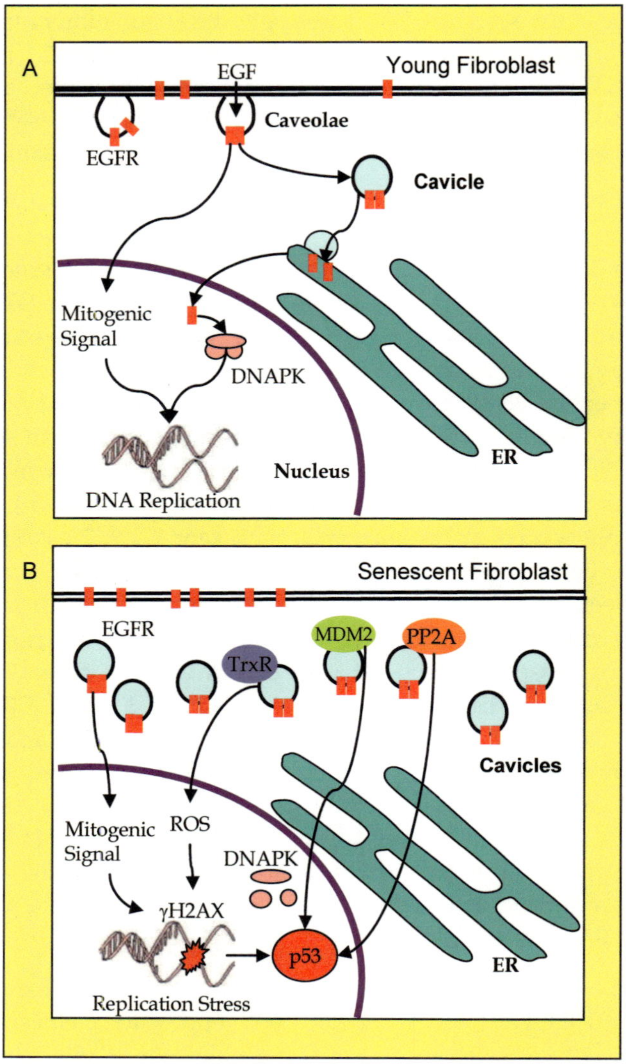

Fig. 6 Model for Cavicle Induced Senescence.
A) In young fibroblasts mitogenic signalling is achieved through a caveolae localized EGFR cascade that activates transcription of growth promoting genes. Signalling competent caveolae are capable of internalizing and traffic to the endoplasmic reticulum (ER) in response to cellular stress. EGFR is transported via cavicles to the ER followed by localization to the nucleus where it can activate DNA protein kinase (DNA-PK). DNA-PK is required to repair DNA damage that is generated by stress or during replication.
B) In senescence fibroblasts mitogenic signalling occurs through EGFR, but is unable to initiate DNA replication. The majority of caveolae are internalized as cavicles, and the increased caveolin protein levels inactivate many signalling molecules or negative regulators of the p53 tumour suppressor (MDM2 and PP2A-C). In theory the EGFR is no longer able to localize to the nucleus and therefore DNA damage generated by reactive oxygen species (ROS), replication stress, and cellular aging cannot be repaired. The activation of p53 through DNA damage causes cellular senescence.

The upregulation of caveolin was shown to block thioredoxin reductase I activity, and thus raise the ROS levels within fibroblasts (Volonte and Galbiati, 2009b). Elevated ROS production is well known to damage DNA, activate p53 and lead to senescence (Chen et al., 1995). Thus, DNA damage could be caused by the presence of ROS being produced in cells that over express caveolin 1 or reach replicative senescence. Furthermore, the negative regulation by caveolin 1 of many key regulatory proteins involved in the p53 mediated DNA damage response could be ensuring that damage signals that lead to a senescent outcome are reinforced.

The transfer of EGFR to the nucleus is well known to influence the resolution of γH2AX damage foci. As previously described (section 4), EGFR is internalized in response to gamma radiation or oxidative stress through a caveolar mediated endocytotic pathway. This pathway leads to EGFR localization to the nucleus and phosphorylates targets such as DNA-PK which facilitate the completion of DNA repair (Dittmann et al., 2005). This function depends on EGFR kinase activity and is blocked by a class of radio-sensitizing agents that work by antagonizing EGFR such as Cetuximab or Gefitinib. Such drugs enhance DNA damage and lead to apoptosis of malignant cells because of unrepaired DNA damage. The EGF signalling pathway is also upstream of the survival kinases MAPK and Akt which assist in the resolution of DNA damage (Golding et al., 2009). Additionally, EGFR activity was found to modulate non-homologous end joining after gamma radiation (Kriegs et al., 2010). Taken together, EGFR signalling plays a major role in controlling cell cycle arrest in response to cellular stress and DNA damage. In support of the role of caveolae in this model, EGFR was found to transport to the nucleus in a caveolin and Src dependent mechanism after oxidative stress (Khan et al., 2006). Similarly, gamma radiation causes Src induced association between caveolin-1 and EGFR leading to internalization. This leads to nuclear localization and to control of DNA-PK activity (Dittmann et al., 2008). Caveolin-1 expression has been demonstrated to be up regulated by ionizing radiation and is required for both homologous recombination and non-homologous end joining (Zhu et al., 2010). In this case, caveolin-1 is pivotal in forming the caveolar vesicles that allow transport of the EGFR, and nuclear DNA-PK activation. Lastly, Gefitinib (an EGFR kinase inhibitor) can generate premature senescence in non-small lung cancer cells (Hotta et al., 2007). Thus, the current evidence strongly suggests mitogenic signals and EGFR internalization to the nucleus are required to resolve DNA damage. Furthermore, blocked EGFR activity leads to apoptosis or senescence.

Although primary fibroblasts are genetically stable, they do undergo transient DNA damage foci as a result of mitogenic stimulation (Ichijima et al., 2005; McManus and Hendzel, 2005). These γH2AX foci occur as a natural part of the synthesis of DNA or division, and are resolved by the time the cell returns to G0 of the cell cycle. Thus, it is possible that a signal from the EGFR could assist cycling cells to resolve this DNA damage. Therefore, EGFR would promote both the initiation of the cell cycle and its continued signalling would be required to resolve DNA damage arising from progress through the cell cycle. However, in senescent cells, the up regulation of caveolin antagonizes EGFR signalling (see section 5.2). Thus, the attenuation of the EGFR pathway during senescence could perpetuate the normally transient DNA damage foci in fibroblasts. The blocking of EGF signalling in this case would prevent the resolution of damage induced by replication stress during normal growth. This could explain the DNA damage seen downstream of increased caveolar vesicles during aging as a form of replication stress (Fig. 6A & B).

6. Conclusion

The inhibition or reduction of components of mitogenic signaling cascades in senescent cell caveolar fractions is consistent with the loss of caveolae playing a causal role in the blunted growth response seen during cellular senescence. Collectively, these observations suggest that localization and integration of signalling cascades in caveolae are disrupted in senescent cells. The mitogenic pathways leading to MAPK, PLD, PKC isoforms and PI3K are all localized to caveolae and have been shown to have deficiencies in senescent cells. In the case of EGFR, the proper coordination with shc is disrupted, the CSD of caveolin blocks kinase activity, and inappropriate retention or internalization in caveolae occurs. It is unclear whether this difference influences the downstream localization of activated erk1/2 to the senescent nucleus, however several groups have noted a decreased erk stimulation by EGF with age. Evidence suggests that the composition of lipid rafts likely change in senescent cells and that this may influence how PI3K, PLD and PKC are regulated. Cholesterol levels are decreased in lipid raft fractions, PC levels increase in the plasma membrane, and ceramide levels increase with fibroblast age. These observations suggest an increase in fluidity of the membrane, which changes the properties of lipid rafts. The increases in ceramide disrupt PLD, and the increase in DAG constitutively activates PKCα in caveolae. The decrease in src kinase activity in caveolae may prevent the inactivation of the PKCδ and induce senescence. The loss of PI3K signal integration through caveolae may be a part of the induction of senescence, explaining why inhibitors of the pathway induce premature senescence. These examples indicate that signal transduction pathways rely upon caveolae for signal integration and propagation that they become disorganized in senescent cells. Collectively, these signalling changes may explain their reduced or absent response to mitogens in senescent cells.

There has been a shift in the understanding of how the DNA damage occurring in senescence is generated. Remarkably, the increase of caveolar vesicles observed in the senescent state can itself lead to the generation of DNA damage foci in parallel with the well known DNA damage localized to eroded telomeres. The exact mechanism by which this is achieved is still unknown, but likely involves the strong inhibitory activities of the scaffolding protein caveolin 1. The proteins theoridoxin, MDM2 and PP2A-C are all inhibited or sequestered by increases in caveolin protein during senescence. Inhibition of theoridoxin leads to an increase in ROS, which leads to DNA damage and p53 activation. The activation of p53 in turn is augmented by inhibition of the negative regulators of p53, MDM2 and PP2A-C by caveolin. The DNA damage that leads to p53 mediated senescence may also be generated through failure to resolve γH2AX foci that occur during normal replication. The increase of caveolin and cavin-1 proteins shift the balance of caveolar structures to internalized cavicles. These cavicles are no longer capable of integrating the EGFR cascade, which is required to transfer EGFR to the nucleus and resolve replication dependent DNA damage through proteins such as DNA-PK. The failure to repair DNA leads to replication stress, the activation of p53 and thus cellular senescence (Fig. 6A & B). Thus, the misregulation of caveolar vesicles interferes with the essential role of these structures in repairing DNA damage.

7. Acknowledgements

I would like to thank Dr. S. Robbins and Dr. Kari Sampsel (University of Calgary) for use of the electron microscopy images. I would also like to thank Densie Campuzano for editing this manuscript.

8. References

Anderson, R.G. (1998). The caveolae membrane system. Annu Rev Biochem *67*, 199-225.

Anderson, R.G., Kamen, B.A., Rothberg, K.G., and Lacey, S.W. (1992). Potocytosis: sequestration and transport of small molecules by caveolae. Science *255*, 410-411.

Appella, E., and Anderson, C.W. (2001). Post-translational modifications and activation of p53 by genotoxic stresses. Eur J Biochem *268*, 2764-2772.

Ashton, A.W., Watanabe, G., Albanese, C., Harrington, E.O., Ware, J.A., and Pestell, R.G. (1999). Protein kinase Cdelta inhibition of S-phase transition in capillary endothelial cells involves the cyclin-dependent kinase inhibitor p27(Kip1). J Biol Chem *274*, 20805-20811.

Atadja, P.W., Stringer, K.F., and Riabowol, K.T. (1994). Loss of serum response element-binding activity and hyperphosphorylation of serum response factor during cellular aging. Mol Cell Biol *14*, 4991-4999.

Bai, L., Deng, X., Li, J., Wang, M., Li, Q., An, W., A, D., and Cong, Y.S. (2011). Regulation of cellular senescence by the essential caveolar component PTRF/Cavin-1. Cell Res *21*, 1088-1101.

Bakkenist, C.J., and Kastan, M.B. (2003). DNA damage activates ATM through intermolecular autophosphorylation and dimer dissociation. Nature *421*, 499-506.

Bartholomew, J.N., Volonte, D., and Galbiati, F. (2009). Caveolin-1 regulates the antagonistic pleiotropic properties of cellular senescence through a novel Mdm2/p53-mediated pathway. Cancer Res *69*, 2878-2886.

Basak, S., Jacobs, S.B., Krieg, A.J., Pathak, N., Zeng, Q., Kaldis, P., Giaccia, A.J., and Attardi, L.D. (2008). The metastasis-associated gene Prl-3 is a p53 target involved in cell-cycle regulation. Mol Cell *30*, 303-314.

Bastiani, M., Liu, L., Hill, M.M., Jedrychowski, M.P., Nixon, S.J., Lo, H.P., Abankwa, D., Luetterforst, R., Fernandez-Rojo, M., Breen, M.R., *et al.* (2009). MURC/Cavin-4 and cavin family members form tissue-specific caveolar complexes. J Cell Biol *185*, 1259-1273.

Basu, A., and Pal, D. (2010). Two faces of protein kinase Cdelta: the contrasting roles of PKCdelta in cell survival and cell death. ScientificWorldJournal *10*, 2272-2284.

Beausejour, C.M., Krtolica, A., Galimi, F., Narita, M., Lowe, S.W., Yaswen, P., and Campisi, J. (2003). Reversal of human cellular senescence: roles of the p53 and p16 pathways. Embo J *22*, 4212-4222.

Binet, R., Ythier, D., Robles, A.I., Collado, M., Larrieu, D., Fonti, C., Brambilla, E., Brambilla, C., Serrano, M., Harris, C.C., *et al.* (2009). WNT16B is a new marker of cellular senescence that regulates p53 activity and the phosphoinositide 3-kinase/AKT pathway. Cancer Res *69*, 9183-9191.

Blake, R.A., Garcia-Paramio, P., Parker, P.J., and Courtneidge, S.A. (1999). Src promotes PKCdelta degradation. Cell Growth Differ *10*, 231-241.

Bodnar, A.G., Ouellette, M., Frolkis, M., Holt, S.E., Chiu, C.P., Morin, G.B., Harley, C.B., Shay, J.W., Lichtsteiner, S., and Wright, W.E. (1998). Extension of life-span by introduction of telomerase into normal human cells [see comments]. Science *279*, 349-352.

Boguski, M.S., and McCormick, F. (1993). Proteins regulating Ras and its relatives. Nature *366*, 643-654.

Bose, C., Bhuvaneswaran, C., and Udupa, K.B. (2004). Altered mitogen-activated protein kinase signal transduction in human skin fibroblasts during in vitro aging:

differential expression of low- density lipoprotein receptor. J Gerontol A Biol Sci Med Sci *59*, 126-135.

Boucrot, E., Howes, M.T., Kirchhausen, T., and Parton, R.G. (2011). Redistribution of caveolae during mitosis. J Cell Sci *124*, 1965-1972.

Brown, J.P., Wei, W., and Sedivy, J.M. (1997). Bypass of senescence after disruption of p21CIP1/WAF1 gene in normal diploid human fibroblasts. Science *277*, 831-834.

Brown, W.T. (1990). Genetic diseases of premature aging as models of senescence. Annu Rev Gerontol Geriatr *10*, 23-42.

Caino, M.C., Meshki, J., and Kazanietz, M.G. (2009). Hallmarks for senescence in carcinogenesis: novel signaling players. Apoptosis *14*, 392-408.

Cao, K., Graziotto, J.J., Blair, C.D., Mazzulli, J.R., Erdos, M.R., Krainc, D., and Collins, F.S. (2011). Rapamycin reverses cellular phenotypes and enhances mutant protein clearance in Hutchinson-Gilford progeria syndrome cells. Sci Transl Med *3*, 89ra58.

Carlin, C., Phillips, P.D., Brooks-Frederich, K., Knowles, B.B., and Cristofalo, V.J. (1994). Cleavage of the epidermal growth factor receptor by a membrane-bound leupeptin-sensitive protease active in nonionic detergent lysates of senescent but not young human diploid fibroblasts. J Cell Physiol *160*, 427-434.

Chang, Z.F., and Huang, D.Y. (1994). Decline of protein kinase C activation in response to growth stimulation during senescence of IMR-90 human diploid fibroblasts. Biochem Biophys Res Commun *200*, 16-27.

Chen, Q., and Ames, B.N. (1994). Senescence-like growth arrest induced by hydrogen peroxide in human diploid fibroblast F65 cells. Proc Natl Acad Sci U S A *91*, 4130-4134.

Chen, Q., Fischer, A., Reagan, J.D., Yan, L.J., and Ames, B.N. (1995). Oxidative DNA damage and senescence of human diploid fibroblast cells. Proc Natl Acad Sci U S A *92*, 4337-4341.

Cho, K.A., Ryu, S.J., Oh, Y.S., Park, J.H., Lee, J.W., Kim, H.P., Kim, K.T., Jang, I.S., and Park, S.C. (2004). Morphological adjustment of senescent cells by modulating caveolin-1 status. J Biol Chem *279*, 42270-42278.

Cho, K.A., Ryu, S.J., Park, J.S., Jang, I.S., Ahn, J.S., Kim, K.T., and Park, S.C. (2003). Senescent phenotype can be reversed by reduction of caveolin status. J Biol Chem *278*, 27789-27795.

Chretien, A., Piront, N., Delaive, E., Demazy, C., Ninane, N., and Toussaint, O. (2008). Increased abundance of cytoplasmic and nuclear caveolin 1 in human diploid fibroblasts in H(2)O(2)- induced premature senescence and interplay with p38alpha(MAPK). FEBS Lett *582*, 1685- 1692.

Chua, C.C., Geiman, D.E., and Ladda, R.L. (1986). Receptor for epidermal growth factor retains normal structure and function in aging cells. Mech Ageing Dev *34*, 35-55.

Cohen, A.W., Hnasko, R., Schubert, W., and Lisanti, M.P. (2004). Role of caveolae and caveolins in health and disease. Physiol Rev *84*, 1341-1379.

Collado, M., Medema, R.H., Garcia-Cao, I., Dubuisson, M.L., Barradas, M., Glassford, J., Rivas, C., Burgering, B.M., Serrano, M., and Lam, E.W. (2000). Inhibition of the phosphoinositide 3- kinase pathway induces a senescence-like arrest mediated by p27Kip1. J Biol Chem *275*, 21960-21968.

Collado, M., and Serrano, M. (2010). Senescence in tumours: evidence from mice and humans. Nat Rev Cancer *10*, 51-57.

Cong, Y.S., Fan, E., and Wang, E. (2006). Simultaneous proteomic profiling of four different growth states of human fibroblasts, using amine-reactive isobaric tagging reagents and tandem mass spectrometry. Mech Ageing Dev *127*, 332-343.

Couet, J., Li, S., Okamoto, T., Ikezu, T., and Lisanti, M.P. (1997). Identification of peptide and protein ligands for the caveolin-scaffolding domain. Implications for the interaction of caveolin with caveolae-associated proteins. J Biol Chem *272*, 6525-6533.

de Lange, T. (1994). Activation of telomerase in a human tumor. Proc Natl Acad Sci U S A *91*, 2882-2885.

de Laurentiis, A., Donovan, L., and Arcaro, A. (2007). Lipid rafts and caveolae in signaling by growth factor receptors. Open Biochem J *1*, 12-32.

De Tata, V., Ptasznik, A., and Cristofalo, V.J. (1993). Effect of the tumor promoter phorbol 12-myristate 13-acetate (PMA) on proliferation of young and senescent WI-38 human diploid fibroblasts. Exp Cell Res *205*, 261-269.

Debacq-Chainiaux, F., Boilan, E., Dedessus Le Moutier, J., Weemaels, G., and Toussaint, O. (2010). p38(MAPK) in the senescence of human and murine fibroblasts. Adv Exp Med Biol *694*, 126-137.

del Pozo, M.A., Alderson, N.B., Kiosses, W.B., Chiang, H.H., Anderson, R.G., and Schwartz, M.A. (2004). Integrins regulate Rac targeting by internalization of membrane domains. Science *303*, 839-842.

del Pozo, M.A., Balasubramanian, N., Alderson, N.B., Kiosses, W.B., Grande-Garcia, A., Anderson, R.G., and Schwartz, M.A. (2005). Phospho-caveolin-1 mediates integrin-regulated membrane domain internalization. Nat Cell Biol *7*, 901-908.

Dempsey, E.C., Newton, A.C., Mochly-Rosen, D., Fields, A.P., Reyland, M.E., Insel, P.A., and Messing, R.O. (2000). Protein kinase C isozymes and the regulation of diverse cell responses. Am J Physiol Lung Cell Mol Physiol *279*, L429-438.

Di Leonardo, A., Linke, S.P., Clarkin, K., and Wahl, G.M. (1994). DNA damage triggers a prolonged p53-dependent G1 arrest and long-term induction of Cip1 in normal human fibroblasts. Genes Dev *8*, 2540-2551.

Dietzen, D.J., Hastings, W.R., and Lublin, D.M. (1995). Caveolin is palmitoylated on multiple cysteine residues. Palmitoylation is not necessary for localization of caveolin to caveolae. J Biol Chem *270*, 6838-6842.

Dimri, G.P., Lee, X., Basile, G., Acosta, M., Scott, G., Roskelley, C., Medrano, E.E., Linskens, M., Rubelj, I., Pereira-Smith, O., *et al.* (1995). A biomarker that identifies senescent human cells in culture and in aging skin in vivo. Proc Natl Acad Sci U S A *92*, 9363-9367.

Dittmann, K., Mayer, C., Fehrenbacher, B., Schaller, M., Raju, U., Milas, L., Chen, D.J., Kehlbach, R., and Rodemann, H.P. (2005). Radiation-induced epidermal growth factor receptor nuclear import is linked to activation of DNA-dependent protein kinase. J Biol Chem *280*, 31182-31189.

Dittmann, K., Mayer, C., Kehlbach, R., and Rodemann, H.P. (2008). Radiation-induced caveolin-1 associated EGFR internalization is linked with nuclear EGFR transport and activation of DNA-PK. Mol Cancer *7*, 69.

Dittmann, K., Mayer, C., and Rodemann, H.P. (2009). Nuclear EGFR as novel therapeutic target: insights into nuclear translocation and function. Strahlenther Onkol *186*, 1-6.

Downward, J., Waterfield, M.D., and Parker, P.J. (1985). Autophosphorylation and protein kinase C phosphorylation of the epidermal growth factor receptor. Effect on tyrosine kinase activity and ligand binding affinity. J Biol Chem *260*, 14538-14546.

el-Deiry, W.S., Tokino, T., Velculescu, V.E., Levy, D.B., Parsons, R., Trent, J.M., Lin, D., Mercer, W.E., Kinzler, K.W., and Vogelstein, B. (1993). WAF1, a potential mediator of p53 tumor suppression. Cell *75*, 817-825.

Engelman, J.A., Chu, C., Lin, A., Jo, H., Ikezu, T., Okamoto, T., Kohtz, D.S., and Lisanti, M.P. (1998). Caveolin-mediated regulation of signaling along the p42/44 MAP kinase cascade in vivo. A role for the caveolin-scaffolding domain. FEBS Lett *428*, 205-211.

Exton, J.H. (1997). New developments in phospholipase D. J Biol Chem *272*, 15579-15582.

Exton, J.H. (1998). Phospholipase D. Biochim Biophys Acta *1436*, 105-115.

Exton, J.H. (1999). Regulation of phospholipase D. Biochim Biophys Acta *1439*, 121-133.

Fantl, W.J., Johnson, D.E., and Williams, L.T. (1993). Signalling by receptor tyrosine kinases. Annu Rev Biochem *62*, 453-481.

Fielding, C.J., and Fielding, P.E. (2004). Membrane cholesterol and the regulation of signal transduction. Biochem Soc Trans *32*, 65-69.

Foster, D.A., and Xu, L. (2003). Phospholipase D in cell proliferation and cancer. Mol Cancer Res *1*, 789- 800.

Fujimoto, T., Kogo, H., Nomura, R., and Une, T. (2000). Isoforms of caveolin-1 and caveolar structure. J Cell Sci *113 Pt 19*, 3509-3517.

Galbiati, F., Volonte, D., Liu, J., Capozza, F., Frank, P.G., Zhu, L., Pestell, R.G., and Lisanti, M.P. (2001). Caveolin-1 expression negatively regulates cell cycle progression by inducing G(0)/G(1) arrest via a p53/p21(WAF1/Cip1)-dependent mechanism. Mol Biol Cell *12*, 2229-2244.

Gerhard, G.S., Phillips, P.D., and Cristofalo, V.J. (1991). EGF- and PDGF-stimulated phosphorylation in young and senescent WI-38 cells. Exp Cell Res *193*, 87-92.

Ghosh, S., Strum, J.C., Sciorra, V.A., Daniel, L., and Bell, R.M. (1996). Raf-1 kinase possesses distinct binding domains for phosphatidylserine and phosphatidic acid. Phosphatidic acid regulates the translocation of Raf-1 in 12-O-tetradecanoylphorbol-13-acetate-stimulated Madin-Darby canine kidney cells. J Biol Chem *271*, 8472-8480.

Gidwani, A., Brown, H.A., Holowka, D., and Baird, B. (2003). Disruption of lipid order by short-chain ceramides correlates with inhibition of phospholipase D and downstream signaling by FcepsilonRI. J Cell Sci *116*, 3177-3187.

Gire, V., and Wynford-Thomas, D. (1998). Reinitiation of DNA synthesis and cell division in senescent human fibroblasts by microinjection of anti-p53 antibodies. Mol Cell Biol *18*, 1611-1621.

Glenney, J.R., Jr. (1992). The sequence of human caveolin reveals identity with VIP21, a component of transport vesicles. FEBS Lett *314*, 45-48.

Golding, S.E., Morgan, R.N., Adams, B.R., Hawkins, A.J., Povirk, L.F., and Valerie, K. (2009). Pro- survival AKT and ERK signaling from EGFR and mutant EGFRvIII enhances DNA double- strand break repair in human glioma cells. Cancer Biol Ther *8*, 730-738.

Goldstein, S., and Singal, D.P. (1974). Senescence of cultured human fibroblasts: mitotic versus metabolic time. Exp Cell Res *88*, 359-364.

Gschwendt, M. (1999). Protein kinase C delta. Eur J Biochem *259*, 555-564.

Guertin, D.A., and Sabatini, D.M. (2007). Defining the role of mTOR in cancer. Cancer Cell *12*, 9-22.

Han, J.M., Kim, Y., Lee, J.S., Lee, C.S., Lee, B.D., Ohba, M., Kuroki, T., Suh, P.G., and Ryu, S.H. (2002). Localization of phospholipase D1 to caveolin-enriched membrane via palmitoylation: implications for epidermal growth factor signaling. Mol Biol Cell *13*, 3976-3988.

Hanada, K., Nishijima, M., Akamatsu, Y., and Pagano, R.E. (1995). Both sphingolipids and cholesterol participate in the detergent insolubility of alkaline phosphatase, a glycosylphosphatidylinositol-anchored protein, in mammalian membranes. J Biol Chem *270*, 6254-6260.

Hansen, C.G., Bright, N.A., Howard, G., and Nichols, B.J. (2009). SDPR induces membrane curvature and functions in the formation of caveolae. Nat Cell Biol *11*, 807-814.

Hansen, C.G., and Nichols, B.J. (2010). Exploring the caves: cavins, caveolins and caveolae. Trends Cell Biol *20*, 177-186.

Hara, E., Tsurui, H., Shinozaki, A., Nakada, S., and Oda, K. (1991). Cooperative effect of antisense-Rb and antisense-p53 oligomers on the extension of life span in human diploid fibroblasts, TIG-1. Biochem Biophys Res Commun *179*, 528-534.

Harder, T., and Simons, K. (1997). Caveolae, DIGs, and the dynamics of sphingolipid-cholesterol microdomains. Curr Opin Cell Biol *9*, 534-542.

Harley, C.B., Futcher, A.B., and Greider, C.W. (1990). Telomeres shorten during ageing of human fibroblasts. Nature *345*, 458-460.

Hayer, A., Stoeber, M., Bissig, C., and Helenius, A. (2010). Biogenesis of caveolae: stepwise assembly of large caveolin and cavin complexes. Traffic *11*, 361-382.

Hayflick, L. (1965a). The Limited in Vitro Lifetime of Human Diploid Cell Strains. Exp Cell Res *37*, 614- 636.

Hayflick, L. (1965b). The limited in vitro lifetime of human diploid cell strians. Exp Cell Res *37*, 614-636.

Hayflick, L., and Moorhead, P.S. (1961). The serial cultivation of human diploid cel strains. Exp Cell Res *25*, 585-621.

Herbig, U., Jobling, W.A., Chen, B.P., Chen, D.J., and Sedivy, J.M. (2004). Telomere shortening triggers senescence of human cells through a pathway involving ATM, p53, and p21(CIP1), but not p16(INK4a). Mol Cell *14*, 501-513.

Hermeking, H., Lengauer, C., Polyak, K., He, T.C., Zhang, L., Thiagalingam, S., Kinzler, K.W., and Vogelstein, B. (1997). 14-3-3 sigma is a p53-regulated inhibitor of G2/M progression. Mol Cell *1*, 3-11.

Hill, M.M., Bastiani, M., Luetterforst, R., Kirkham, M., Kirkham, A., Nixon, S.J., Walser, P., Abankwa, D., Oorschot, V.M., Martin, S., *et al.* (2008). PTRF-Cavin, a conserved cytoplasmic protein required for caveola formation and function. Cell *132*, 113-124.

Hotta, K., Tabata, M., Kiura, K., Kozuki, T., Hisamoto, A., Katayama, H., Takigawa, N., Fujimoto, N., Fujiwara, K., Ueoka, H., *et al.* (2007). Gefitinib induces premature senescence in non-small cell lung cancer cells with or without EGFR gene mutation. Oncol Rep *17*, 313-317.

Hutter, D., Yo, Y., Chen, W., Liu, P., Holbrook, N.J., Roth, G.S., and Liu, Y. (2000). Age-related decline in Ras/ERK mitogen-activated protein kinase cascade is linked to a reduced association between Shc and EGF receptor. J Gerontol A Biol Sci Med Sci *55*, B125-134.

Ichijima, Y., Sakasai, R., Okita, N., Asahina, K., Mizutani, S., and Teraoka, H. (2005). Phosphorylation of histone H2AX at M phase in human cells without DNA damage response. Biochem Biophys Res Commun *336*, 807-812.

Inomata, M., Shimada, Y., Hayashi, M., Kondo, H., and Ohno-Iwashita, Y. (2006). Detachment- associated changes in lipid rafts of senescent human fibroblasts. Biochem Biophys Res Commun *343*, 489-495.

Jackson, J.G., and Pereira-Smith, O.M. (2006). p53 is preferentially recruited to the promoters of growth arrest genes p21 and GADD45 during replicative senescence of normal human fibroblasts. Cancer Res *66*, 8356-8360.

Jang, I.H., Kim, J.H., Lee, B.D., Bae, S.S., Park, M.H., Suh, P.G., and Ryu, S.H. (2001). Localization of phospholipase C-gamma1 signaling in caveolae: importance in EGF-induced phosphoinositide hydrolysis but not in tyrosine phosphorylation. FEBS Lett *491*, 4-8.

Johnson, C.L., Lu, D., Huang, J., and Basu, A. (2002). Regulation of p53 stabilization by DNA damage and protein kinase C. Mol Cancer Ther *1*, 861-867.

Karlseder, J., Smogorzewska, A., and de Lange, T. (2002). Senescence induced by altered telomere state, not telomere loss. Science *295*, 2446-2449.

Kastan, M.B., Zhan, Q., el-Deiry, W.S., Carrier, F., Jacks, T., Walsh, W.V., Plunkett, B.S., Vogelstein, B., and Fornace, A.J., Jr. (1992). A mammalian cell cycle checkpoint pathway utilizing p53 and GADD45 is defective in ataxia-telangiectasia. Cell *71*, 587-597.

Katakura, Y., Udono, M., Katsuki, K., Nishide, H., Tabira, Y., Ikei, T., Yamashita, M., Fujiki, T., and Shirahata, S. (2009). Protein kinase C delta plays a key role in cellular senescence programs of human normal diploid cells. J Biochem *146*, 87-93.

Keilhack, H., Tenev, T., Nyakatura, E., Godovac-Zimmermann, J., Nielsen, L., Seedorf, K., and Bohmer, F.D. (1998). Phosphotyrosine 1173 mediates binding of the protein-tyrosine phosphatase SHP- 1 to the epidermal growth factor receptor and attenuation of receptor signaling. J Biol Chem *273*, 24839-24846.

Khan, E.M., Heidinger, J.M., Levy, M., Lisanti, M.P., Ravid, T., and Goldkorn, T. (2006). Epidermal growth factor receptor exposed to oxidative stress undergoes Src- and caveolin-1-dependent perinuclear trafficking. J Biol Chem *281*, 14486-14493.

Kim, H.S., and Lim, I.K. (2009). Phosphorylated extracellular signal-regulated protein kinases 1 and 2 phosphorylate Sp1 on serine 59 and regulate cellular senescence via transcription of p21Sdi1/Cip1/Waf1. J Biol Chem *284*, 15475-15486.

Kim, K., Nose, K., and Shibanuma, M. (2000). Significance of nuclear relocalization of ERK1/2 in reactivation of c-fos transcription and DNA synthesis in senescent fibroblasts. J Biol Chem *275*, 20685-20692.

Kortlever, R.M., Higgins, P.J., and Bernards, R. (2006). Plasminogen activator inhibitor-1 is a critical downstream target of p53 in the induction of replicative senescence. Nat Cell Biol *8*, 877-884.

Kriegs, M., Kasten-Pisula, U., Rieckmann, T., Holst, K., Saker, J., Dahm-Daphi, J., and Dikomey, E. (2010). The epidermal growth factor receptor modulates DNA double-strand break repair by regulating non-homologous end-joining. DNA Repair (Amst) *9*, 889-897.

Kurzchalia, T.V., Dupree, P., Parton, R.G., Kellner, R., Virta, H., Lehnert, M., and Simons, K. (1992). VIP21, a 21-kD membrane protein is an integral component of trans-Golgi-network-derived transport vesicles. J Cell Biol *118*, 1003-1014.

Kurzchalia, T.V., and Parton, R.G. (1999). Membrane microdomains and caveolae. Curr Opin Cell Biol *11*, 424-431.

Lajoie, P., and Nabi, I.R. (2007). Regulation of raft-dependent endocytosis. J Cell Mol Med *11*, 644-653.

Leontieva, O.V., and Blagosklonny, M.V. (2010). DNA damaging agents and p53 do not cause senescence in quiescent cells, while consecutive re-activation of mTOR is associated with conversion to senescence. Aging (Albany NY) *2*, 924-935.

Li, G.Z., Eller, M.S., Firoozabadi, R., and Gilchrest, B.A. (2003). Evidence that exposure of the telomere 3' overhang sequence induces senescence. Proc Natl Acad Sci U S A *100*, 527-531.

Li, G.Z., Eller, M.S., Hanna, K., and Gilchrest, B.A. (2004). Signaling pathway requirements for induction of senescence by telomere homolog oligonucleotides. Exp Cell Res *301*, 189-200.

Li, W.P., Liu, P., Pilcher, B.K., and Anderson, R.G. (2001). Cell-specific targeting of caveolin-1 to caveolae, secretory vesicles, cytoplasm or mitochondria. J Cell Sci *114*, 1397-1408.

Lim, I.K., Won Hong, K., Kwak, I.H., Yoon, G., and Park, S.C. (2000). Cytoplasmic retention of p-Erk1/2 and nuclear accumulation of actin proteins during cellular senescence in human diploid fibroblasts. Mech Ageing Dev *119*, 113-130.

Lin, A.W., Barradas, M., Stone, J.C., van Aelst, L., Serrano, M., and Lowe, S.W. (1998). Premature senescence involving p53 and p16 is activated in response to constitutive MEK/MAPK mitogenic signaling. Genes Dev *12*, 3008-3019.

Lisanti, M.P., Tang, Z.L., and Sargiacomo, M. (1993). Caveolin forms a hetero-oligomeric protein complex that interacts with an apical GPI-linked protein: implications for the biogenesis of caveolae. J Cell Biol *123*, 595-604.

Liu, L., and Pilch, P.F. (2008). A critical role of cavin (polymerase I and transcript release factor) in caveolae formation and organization. J Biol Chem *283*, 4314-4322.

Lorenzini, A., Tresini, M., Mawal-Dewan, M., Frisoni, L., Zhang, H., Allen, R.G., Sell, C., and Cristofalo, V.J. (2002). Role of the Raf/MEK/ERK and the PI3K/Akt(PKB) pathways in fibroblast senescence. Exp Gerontol *37*, 1149-1156.

Madshus, I.H., and Stang, E. (2009). Internalization and intracellular sorting of the EGF receptor: a model for understanding the mechanisms of receptor trafficking. J Cell Sci *122*, 3433-3439.

Martin, G.M., Sprague, C.A., and Epstein, C.J. (1970). Replicative life-span of cultivated human cells. Effects of donor's age, tissue, and genotype. Lab Invest *23*, 86-92.

Matuoka, K., Chen, K.Y., and Takenawa, T. (2003). A positive role of phosphatidylinositol 3-kinase in aging phenotype expression in cultured human diploid fibroblasts. Arch Gerontol Geriatr *36*, 203-219.

McDermott, M., Wakelam, M.J., and Morris, A.J. (2004). Phospholipase D. Biochem Cell Biol *82*, 225-253.

McMahon, K.A., Zajicek, H., Li, W.P., Peyton, M.J., Minna, J.D., Hernandez, V.J., Luby-Phelps, K., and Anderson, R.G. (2009). SRBC/cavin-3 is a caveolin adapter protein that regulates caveolae function. Embo J *28*, 1001-1015.

McManus, K.J., and Hendzel, M.J. (2005). ATM-dependent DNA damage-independent mitotic phosphorylation of H2AX in normally growing mammalian cells. Mol Biol Cell *16*, 5013-5025.

Meyyappan, M., Wheaton, K., and Riabowol, K.T. (1999). Decreased expression and activity of the immediate-early growth response (Egr-1) gene product during cellular senescence. J Cell Physiol *179*, 29-39.

Migliaccio, E., Giorgio, M., Mele, S., Pelicci, G., Reboldi, P., Pandolfi, P.P., Lanfrancone, L., and Pelicci, P.G. (1999). The p66shc adaptor protein controls oxidative stress response and life span in mammals. Nature *402*, 309-313.

Mineo, C., Gill, G.N., and Anderson, R.G. (1999). Regulated migration of epidermal growth factor receptor from caveolae. J Biol Chem *274*, 30636-30643.

Mineo, C., James, G.L., Smart, E.J., and Anderson, R.G. (1996). Localization of epidermal growth factor- stimulated Ras/Raf-1 interaction to caveolae membrane. J Biol Chem *271*, 11930-11935.

Monier, S., Dietzen, D.J., Hastings, W.R., Lublin, D.M., and Kurzchalia, T.V. (1996). Oligomerization of VIP21-caveolin in vitro is stabilized by long chain fatty acylation or cholesterol. FEBS Lett *388*, 143-149.

Moodie, S.A., and Wolfman, A. (1994). The 3Rs of life: Ras, Raf and growth regulation. Trends Genet *10*, 44-48.

Mouton, R.E., and Venable, M.E. (2000). Ceramide induces expression of the senescence histochemical marker, beta-galactosidase, in human fibroblasts. Mech Ageing Dev *113*, 169-181.

Mundy, D.I., Machleidt, T., Ying, Y.S., Anderson, R.G., and Bloom, G.S. (2002). Dual control of caveolar membrane traffic by microtubules and the actin cytoskeleton. J Cell Sci *115*, 4327-4339.

Nakamura, M., Kondo, H., Shimada, Y., Waheed, A.A., and Ohno-Iwashita, Y. (2003). Cellular aging- dependent decrease in cholesterol in membrane microdomains of human diploid fibroblasts. Exp Cell Res *290*, 381-390.

Naru, E., Takanezawa, Y., Kobayashi, M., Misaki, Y., Kaji, K., and Arakane, K. (2008). Increased levels of a particular phosphatidylcholine species in senescent human dermal fibroblasts in vitro. Hum Cell *21*, 70-78.

Newton, A.C. (2001). Protein kinase C: structural and spatial regulation by phosphorylation, cofactors, and macromolecular interactions. Chem Rev *101*, 2353-2364.

Noda, A., Ning, Y., Venable, S.F., Pereira-Smith, O.M., and Smith, J.R. (1994). Cloning of senescent cell- derived inhibitors of DNA synthesis using an expression screen. Exp Cell Res *211*, 90-98.

Ogata, T., Ueyama, T., Isodono, K., Tagawa, M., Takehara, N., Kawashima, T., Harada, K., Takahashi, T., Shioi, T., Matsubara, H., *et al.* (2008). MURC, a muscle-restricted coiled-coil protein that modulates the Rho/ROCK pathway, induces cardiac dysfunction and conduction disturbance. Mol Cell Biol *28*, 3424-3436.

Ohki, R., Nemoto, J., Murasawa, H., Oda, E., Inazawa, J., Tanaka, N., and Taniguchi, T. (2000). Reprimo, a new candidate mediator of the p53-mediated cell cycle arrest at the G2 phase. J Biol Chem *275*, 22627-22630.

Okabayashi, Y., Kido, Y., Okutani, T., Sugimoto, Y., Sakaguchi, K., and Kasuga, M. (1994). Tyrosines 1148 and 1173 of activated human epidermal growth factor receptors are binding sites of Shc in intact cells. J Biol Chem *269*, 18674-18678.

Okamoto, T., Schlegel, A., Scherer, P.E., and Lisanti, M.P. (1998). Caveolins, a family of scaffolding proteins for organizing "preassembled signaling complexes" at the plasma membrane. J Biol Chem *273*, 5419-5422.

Palmer, H.J., Tuzon, C.T., and Paulson, K.E. (1999). Age-dependent decline in mitogenic stimulation of hepatocytes. Reduced association between Shc and the epidermal growth factor receptor is coupled to decreased activation of Raf and extracellular signal-regulated kinases. J Biol Chem *274*, 11424-11430.

Park, S.C., Park, J.S., Park, W.Y., Cho, K.A., Ahn, J.S., and Jang, I.S. (2002). Down-regulation of receptor- mediated endocytosis is responsible for senescence-associated hyporesponsiveness. Ann N Y Acad Sci *959*, 45-49.

Park, W.Y., Park, J.S., Cho, K.A., Kim, D.I., Ko, Y.G., Seo, J.S., and Park, S.C. (2000). Up-regulation of Caveolin Attenuates Epidermal Growth Factor Signaling in Senescent Cells. J Biol Chem *275*, 20847-20852.

Parton, R.G., and Simons, K. (2007). The multiple faces of caveolae. Nat Rev Mol Cell Biol *8*, 185-194.

Patel, H.H., Murray, F., and Insel, P.A. (2008). Caveolae as organizers of pharmacologically relevant signal transduction molecules. Annu Rev Pharmacol Toxicol *48*, 359-391.

Pelkmans, L., Puntener, D., and Helenius, A. (2002). Local actin polymerization and dynamin recruitment in SV40-induced internalization of caveolae. Science *296*, 535-539.

Pelkmans, L., and Zerial, M. (2005). Kinase-regulated quantal assemblies and kiss-and-run recycling of caveolae. Nature *436*, 128-133.

Phillips, P.D., and Cristofalo, V.J. (1988). Classification system based on the functional equivalency of mitogens that regulate WI-38 cell proliferation. Exp Cell Res *175*, 396-403.

Phillips, P.D., Kaji, K., and Cristofalo, V.J. (1984). Progressive loss of the proliferative response of senescing WI-38 cells to platelet-derived growth factor, epidermal growth factor, insulin, transferrin, and dexamethasone. J Gerontol *39*, 11-17.

Phillips, P.D., Kuhnle, E., and Cristofalo, V.J. (1983). [125I]EGF binding ability is stable throughout the replicative life-span of WI-38 cells. J Cell Physiol *114*, 311-316.

Rattan, S.I., and Derventzi, A. (1991). Altered cellular responsiveness during ageing. Bioessays *13*, 601- 606.

Resnick-Silverman, L., St Clair, S., Maurer, M., Zhao, K., and Manfredi, J.J. (1998). Identification of a novel class of genomic DNA-binding sites suggests mechanism for selectivity in target gene activation by the tumor suppressor protein p53. Genes Dev *12*, 2102-2107.

Riabowol, K., Schiff, J., and Gilman, M.Z. (1992). Transcription factor AP-1 activity is required for initiation of DNA synthesis and is lost during cellular aging. Proc Natl Acad Sci U S A *89*, 157-161.

Rietveld, A., and Simons, K. (1998). The differential miscibility of lipids as the basis for the formation of functional membrane rafts. Biochim Biophys Acta *1376*, 467-479.

Rogakou, E.P., Boon, C., Redon, C., and Bonner, W.M. (1999). Megabase chromatin domains involved in DNA double-strand breaks in vivo. J Cell Biol *146*, 905-916.

Rogakou, E.P., Pilch, D.R., Orr, A.H., Ivanova, V.S., and Bonner, W.M. (1998). DNA double-stranded breaks induce histone H2AX phosphorylation on serine 139. J Biol Chem *273*, 5858-5868.

Rohme, D. (1981). Ageing and the fusion sensitivity potential of human cells in culture: relation to tissue origin, donor age, and in vitro culture level and condition. Mech Ageing Dev *16*, 241-253.

Rothberg, K.G., Heuser, J.E., Donzell, W.C., Ying, Y.S., Glenney, J.R., and Anderson, R.G. (1992). Caveolin, a protein component of caveolae membrane coats. Cell *68*, 673-682.

Rouault, J.P., Falette, N., Guehenneux, F., Guillot, C., Rimokh, R., Wang, Q., Berthet, C., Moyret-Lalle, C., Savatier, P., Pain, B., *et al.* (1996). Identification of BTG2, an antiproliferative p53- dependent component the DNA damage cellular response pathway. Nat Genet *14*, 482-486.

Rutter, A., Mackinnon, W.B., Huschtscha, L.I., and Mountford, C.E. (1996). A proton magnetic resonance spectroscopy study of aging and transformed human fibroblasts. Exp Gerontol *31*, 669-686.

Rybin, V.O., Guo, J., Gertsberg, Z., Feinmark, S.J., and Steinberg, S.F. (2008). Phorbol 12-myristate 13- acetate-dependent protein kinase C delta-Tyr311 phosphorylation in cardiomyocyte caveolae. J Biol Chem *283*, 17777-17788.

Satyanarayana, A., Greenberg, R.A., Schaetzlein, S., Buer, J., Masutomi, K., Hahn, W.C., Zimmermann, S., Martens, U., Manns, M.P., and Rudolph, K.L. (2004). Mitogen stimulation cooperates with telomere shortening to activate DNA damage responses and senescence signaling. Mol Cell Biol *24*, 5459-5474.

Scherer, P.E., Okamoto, T., Chun, M., Nishimoto, I., Lodish, H.F., and Lisanti, M.P. (1996). Identification, sequence, and expression of caveolin-2 defines a caveolin gene family. Proc Natl Acad Sci U S A *93*, 131-135.

Schroeder, F., Goetz, I., and Roberts, E. (1984). Age-related alterations in cultured human fibroblast membrane structure and function. Mech Ageing Dev *25*, 365-389.

Sedelnikova, O.A., Horikawa, I., Zimonjic, D.B., Popescu, N.C., Bonner, W.M., and Barrett, J.C. (2004). Senescing human cells and ageing mice accumulate DNA lesions with unrepairable double- strand breaks. Nat Cell Biol *6*, 168-170.

Sell, C., Ptasznik, A., Chang, C.D., Swantek, J., Cristofalo, V.J., and Baserga, R. (1993). IGF-1 receptor levels and the proliferation of young and senescent human fibroblasts. Biochem Biophys Res Commun *194*, 259-265.

Serrano, M., Lin, A.W., McCurrach, M.E., Beach, D., and Lowe, S.W. (1997). Oncogenic ras provokes premature cell senescence associated with accumulation of p53 and p16INK4a. Cell *88*, 593- 602.

Seshadri, T., and Campisi, J. (1990). Repression of c-fos transcription and an altered genetic program in senescent human fibroblasts. Science *247*, 205-209.

Shay, J.W., Pereira-Smith, O.M., and Wright, W.E. (1991). A role for both RB and p53 in the regulation of human cellular senescence. Exp Cell Res *196*, 33-39.

Simons, K., and Ikonen, E. (1997). Functional rafts in cell membranes. Nature *387*, 569-572.

Simons, K., and Toomre, D. (2000). Lipid rafts and signal transduction. Nat Rev Mol Cell Biol *1*, 31-39.

Stewart, S.A., Ben-Porath, I., Carey, V.J., O'Connor, B.F., Hahn, W.C., and Weinberg, R.A. (2003). Erosion of the telomeric single-strand overhang at replicative senescence. Nat Genet *33*, 492- 496.

Tagawa, M., Ueyama, T., Ogata, T., Takehara, N., Nakajima, N., Isodono, K., Asada, S., Takahashi, T., Matsubara, H., and Oh, H. (2008). MURC, a muscle-restricted coiled-coil protein, is involved in the regulation of skeletal myogenesis. Am J Physiol Cell Physiol *295*, C490-498.

Takahashi, A., Ohtani, N., Yamakoshi, K., Iida, S., Tahara, H., Nakayama, K., Nakayama, K.I., Ide, T., Saya, H., and Hara, E. (2006). Mitogenic signalling and the p16INK4a-Rb pathway cooperate to enforce irreversible cellular senescence. Nat Cell Biol *8*, 1291-1297.

Tang, Z., Scherer, P.E., Okamoto, T., Song, K., Chu, C., Kohtz, D.S., Nishimoto, I., Lodish, H.F., and Lisanti, M.P. (1996). Molecular cloning of caveolin-3, a novel member of the caveolin gene family expressed predominantly in muscle. J Biol Chem *271*, 2255-2261.

Torres, C., Francis, M.K., Lorenzini, A., Tresini, M., and Cristofalo, V.J. (2003). Metabolic stabilization of MAP kinase phosphatase-2 in senescence of human fibroblasts. Exp Cell Res *290*, 195-206.

Tran, K.T., Rusu, S.D., Satish, L., and Wells, A. (2003). Aging-related attenuation of EGF receptor signaling is mediated in part by increased protein tyrosine phosphatase activity. Exp Cell Res *289*, 359-367.

Tresini, M., Lorenzini, A., Frisoni, L., Allen, R.G., and Cristofalo, V.J. (2001). Lack of Elk-1 phosphorylation and dysregulation of the extracellular regulated kinase signaling pathway in senescent human fibroblast. Exp Cell Res *269*, 287-300.

Tresini, M., Mawal-Dewan, M., Cristofalo, V.J., and Sell, C. (1998). A phosphatidylinositol 3-kinase inhibitor induces a senescent-like growth arrest in human diploid fibroblasts [see comments]. Cancer Res *58*, 1-4.

Vanhaesebroeck, B., Leevers, S.J., Panayotou, G., and Waterfield, M.D. (1997). Phosphoinositide 3- kinases: a conserved family of signal transducers. Trends Biochem Sci *22*, 267-272.

Vannini, F., Meacci, E., Vasta, V., Farnararo, M., and Bruni, P. (1994). Involvement of protein kinase C and arachidonate signaling pathways in the alteration of proliferative response of senescent IMR-90 human fibroblasts. Mech Ageing Dev *76*, 101-111.

Vaziri, H., and Benchimol, S. (1998). Reconstitution of telomerase activity in normal human cells leads to elongation of telomeres and extended replicative life span. Curr Biol *8*, 279-282.

Venable, M.E., Bielawska, A., and Obeid, L.M. (1996). Ceramide inhibits phospholipase D in a cell-free system. J Biol Chem *271*, 24800-24805.

Venable, M.E., Blobe, G.C., and Obeid, L.M. (1994). Identification of a defect in the phospholipase D/diacylglycerol pathway in cellular senescence. J Biol Chem *269*, 26040-26044.

Venable, M.E., Lee, J.Y., Smyth, M.J., Bielawska, A., and Obeid, L.M. (1995). Role of ceramide in cellular senescence. J Biol Chem *270*, 30701-30708.

Venable, M.E., and Obeid, L.M. (1999). Phospholipase D in cellular senescence. Biochim Biophys Acta *1439*, 291-298.

Volonte, D., and Galbiati, F. (2009a). Caveolin-1, cellular senescence and pulmonary emphysema. Aging (Albany NY) *1*, 831-835.

Volonte, D., and Galbiati, F. (2009b). Inhibition of thioredoxin reductase 1 by caveolin 1 promotes stress- induced premature senescence. EMBO Rep *10*, 1334-1340.

Volonte, D., and Galbiati, F. (2011). Polymerase I and Transcript Release Factor (PTRF)/Cavin-1 Is a Novel Regulator of Stress-induced Premature Senescence. J Biol Chem *286*, 28657-28661.

Volonte, D., Galbiati, F., Pestell, R.G., and Lisanti, M.P. (2001). Cellular stress induces the tyrosine phosphorylation of caveolin-1 (Tyr(14)) via activation of p38 mitogen-activated protein kinase and c-Src kinase. Evidence for caveolae, the actin cytoskeleton, and focal adhesions as mechanical sensors of osmotic stress. J Biol Chem *276*, 8094-8103.

Volonte, D., Kahkonen, B., Shapiro, S., Di, Y., and Galbiati, F. (2009). Caveolin-1 expression is required for the development of pulmonary emphysema through activation of the ATM-p53-p21 pathway. J Biol Chem *284*, 5462-5466.

Volonte, D., Zhang, K., Lisanti, M.P., and Galbiati, F. (2002). Expression of caveolin-1 induces premature cellular senescence in primary cultures of murine fibroblasts. Mol Biol Cell *13*, 2502-2517.

Vousden, K.H., and Lane, D.P. (2007). p53 in health and disease. Nat Rev Mol Cell Biol *8*, 275-283.

Wary, K.K., Mariotti, A., Zurzolo, C., and Giancotti, F.G. (1998). A requirement for caveolin-1 and associated kinase Fyn in integrin signaling and anchorage-dependent cell growth. Cell *94*, 625-634.

Way, M., and Parton, R.G. (1996). M-caveolin, a muscle-specific caveolin-related protein [corrected and republished with original paging, article originally printed in FEBS Lett 1995 Nov 27;376(1- 2):108-12]. FEBS Lett *378*, 108-112.

Webb, L.M., Arnholt, A.T., and Venable, M.E. (2010). Phospholipase D modulation by ceramide in senescence. Mol Cell Biochem *337*, 153-158.

Wheaton, K. (2002). Regulation of Serum Response Factor during Cellular Senescence. In Biochemistry & Molecular Biology (Calgary, University of Calgary), pp. 208.

Wheaton, K. (2011). Caveolar vesicles generate DNA damage and perpetuate cellular aging. Cell Res *21*, 993-994.

Wheaton, K., Atadja, P., and Riabowol, K. (1996). Regulation of transcription factor activity during cellular aging. Biochem Cell Biol *74*, 523-534.

Wheaton, K., Muir, J., Ma, W., and Benchimol, S. (2010). BTG2 antagonizes Pin1 in response to mitogens and telomere disruption during replicative senescence. Aging Cell *9*, 747-760.

Wheaton, K., and Riabowol, K. (2004). Protein kinase C delta blocks immediate-early gene expression in senescent cells by inactivating serum response factor. Mol Cell Biol *24*, 7298-7311.

Wheaton, K., Sampsel, K., Boisvert, F.M., Davy, A., Robbins, S., and Riabowol, K. (2001). Loss of functional caveolae during senescence of human fibroblasts. J Cell Physiol *187*, 226-235.

White, M.A., and Anderson, R.G. (2005). Signaling networks in living cells. Annu Rev Pharmacol Toxicol *45*, 587-603.

Wright, J.D., Reuter, C.W., and Weber, M.J. (1996). Identification of sites on epidermal growth factor receptors which are phosphorylated by pp60src in vitro. Biochim Biophys Acta *1312*, 85-93.

Yoshida, K., Liu, H., and Miki, Y. (2006). Protein kinase C delta regulates Ser46 phosphorylation of p53 tumor suppressor in the apoptotic response to DNA damage. J Biol Chem *281*, 5734-5740.

Zajchowski, L.D., and Robbins, S.M. (2002). Lipid rafts and little caves. Compartmentalized signalling in membrane microdomains. Eur J Biochem *269*, 737-752.

Zezula, J., Sexl, V., Hutter, C., Karel, A., Schutz, W., and Freissmuth, M. (1997). The cyclin-dependent kinase inhibitor p21cip1 mediates the growth inhibitory effect of phorbol esters in human venous endothelial cells. J Biol Chem *272*, 29967-29974.

Zhu, H., Yue, J., Pan, Z., Wu, H., Cheng, Y., Lu, H., Ren, X., Yao, M., Shen, Z., and Yang, J.M. (2010). Involvement of Caveolin-1 in repair of DNA damage through both homologous recombination and non-homologous end joining. PLoS One *5*, e12055.

Zhu, J., Woods, D., McMahon, M., and Bishop, J.M. (1998). Senescence of human fibroblasts induced by oncogenic Raf. Genes Dev *12*, 2997-3007.

20

Alternative Splicing in Endothelial Senescence: Role of the TGF-β Co-Receptor Endoglin

Francisco J. Blanco and Carmelo Bernabéu
Centro de Investigaciones Biológicas, CSIC,
Centro de Investigación Biomédica en Red de Enfermedades Raras,
Spain

1. Introduction

The vascular endothelium is the thin monolayer of specialized cells that line the blood vessels of the cardiovascular system. This endothelium is more than a simple protective barrier since it possesses anticoagulatory properties, mediates the metabolites exchange and regulates the vascular tone and homeostasis maintenance. These functions are finely tuned by endothelial cells that, in the absence of any stimuli, remain in a quiescent stage (Conway & Carmeliet, 2004). In fact, endothelial cells occasionally divide in a normal vessel, displaying a very low turnover rate except for localized areas (Foteinos et al., 2008). Thus, the endothelium is quite sensitive to a variety of signals including shear stress and circulating factors that lead to endothelial activation. As a result of their own physiology along the lifespan, endothelial cells progressively accumulate reactive oxygen species and pro-oxidant metabolites due to an increased oxidative stress, damages in DNA and advanced cellular replication involving shortening of telomeres. Altogether, these alterations lead endothelial cells to reach senescence (Brandes et al., 2005; Foreman & Tang, 2003), which has been proposed to be at the cellular basis of most of the vascular pathologies associated with ageing, such as atherosclerosis or hypertension (Minamino & Komuro, 2008; Rodríguez-Mañas et al., 2009).

The major aspect of endothelial physiology implies the growth or formation of new blood vessels from pre-existing ones, process named angiogenesis which is mainly induced by metabolic requests (Fraisl et al., 2009). Angiogenesis plays a key role from the first steps during the embryonic development to the adult stage, and is involved in numerous physiological processes such as wound repair or the growth of the tissues (Carmeliet & Jain, 2011). However, angiogenesis and vascular remodelling decline with age and several lines of evidence indicate that ageing and endothelial dysfunction progress in parallel (Brandes et al., 2005; Ferrari et al., 2003; Minamino et al., 2004). In this sense, numerous efforts are addressed to elucidate the molecular mechanisms that underlie vascular ageing.

2. TGF-β in angiogenesis - Role of endoglin

The angiogenesis process consists of two separate but balanced phases, activation and resolution, that are finely arranged by a suite of cytokines, among which the transforming growth factor (TGF)-β plays a dual role (Pardali et al., 2010). TGF-β is the prototypic member of a large family of multifunctional and evolutionarily conserved cytokines, including also activins and bone morphogenetic proteins (BMPs). Upon proteolytic activation, TGF-β circulates as a 25 kDa homodimer that elicits its cellular functions by binding to a membrane complex of type II (TβRII) and type I (TβRI or ALKs) receptors with cytoplasmic serine-threonine kinase activity (Kang et al., 2009). Endothelial cells express two different TβRIs, named ALK5 and ALK1, with distinct affinity for the ligand and different signalling pathways mediated mainly by Smad proteins (Smad2/3 and Smad1/5/8, respectively) (Massague et al., 2005). Moreover, endothelial cells also express endoglin, or CD105, an auxiliary TGF-β receptor that modulates the balance between ALK1 and ALK5 signalling. Endoglin is mainly expressed as a homodimeric protein of 180 kDa and is associated to the activation phase of angiogenesis, acting as a modulator between both phases. In this context, endoglin interacts with ALK1 and promotes the TGF-β/ALK1 signalling pathway (Blanco et al., 2005; Lebrin et al., 2004).

The TGF-β/endoglin pairing has been studied in different contexts such as differentiation (Tang et al., 2011), cancer (Bernabeu et al., 2009; Perez-Gomez et al., 2010) and other pathologies including liver fibrosis (Meurer et al., 2011) or preeclampsia (Venkatesha et al., 2006). However, endoglin plays a major role in angiogenesis as well as in vascular remodelling and homeostasis (Lopez-Novoa & Bernabeu, 2010; ten Dijke et al., 2008). Heterozygous mutations in the endoglin gene (*ENG*) are responsible for the vascular dysplasia named hereditary haemorrhagic telangiectasia (HHT) type 1 (McAllister et al., 1994; Shovlin, 2010), a rare genetic disease with autosomal dominant inheritance. These mutations lead to the development of abnormal vascular structures that are the basis of the characteristic HHT symptoms, including frequent and recurrent nosebleeds, telangiectases in the nasal and gastrointestinal tracts and large arteriovenous malformations in different organs such as lung, liver or brain (Mahmoud et al., 2010; Shovlin, 2010). Nonetheless, the HHT symptoms are not present at birth and normally appear during adolescence, getting worse with age. This is in line with the functional role of endoglin in angiogenesis and with previous observation that angiogenesis becomes impaired with ageing (Rivard et al., 1999).

2.1 Two alternatively spliced endoglin isoforms

Most of published studies about endoglin are referred to L-endoglin (long endoglin) that is the predominantly expressed isoform. However, the expression of a short variant (S-endoglin) was described first in humans (Bellon et al., 1993) and later in mouse (Perez-Gomez et al., 2005). In humans, both isoforms share the identical large extracellular region and the transmembrane domain, so that the only difference resides in their cytoplasmic tails (Figure 1A). In the case of L-endoglin, this region is composed by 47 amino acids with a high frequency of serine and threonine residues susceptible to be phosphorylated. Also, the sequence serine-methionine-alanine, SMA, in the C-terminal end is a docking site for proteins with a PDZ domain and is involved in the cytoskeleton organization (Koleva et al., 2006). By contrast, the sequence of the S-endoglin cytoplasmic tail is 14 amino acids long and contains only one serine and threonine residues; also the last 7 residues are specific for this isoform (Figure 1B). These data suggest that L-endoglin and S-endoglin may elicit different functional effects on the endothelial cell.

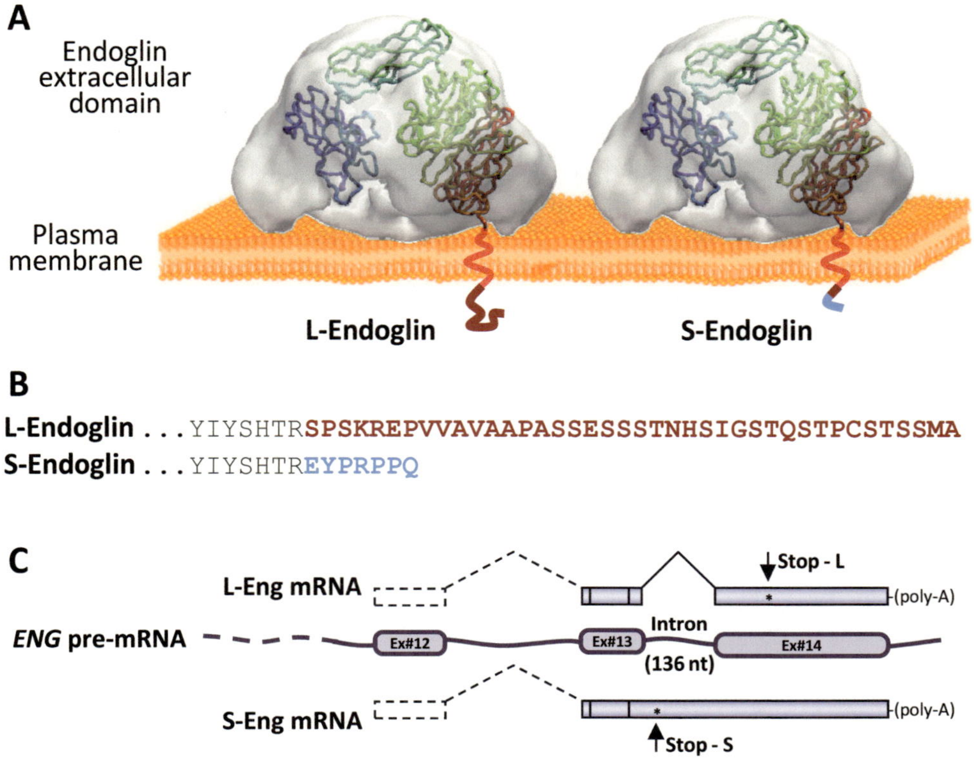

Fig. 1. The two endoglin isoforms. (A) The electron microscopy density map (grey) of the endoglin extracellular region shows the overall structure. The backbone of a theoretical atomic model of the endoglin monomer is fitted inside (adapted from Llorca et al., 2007). This structure is common to both endoglin variants. The transmembrane domain (red) and cytoplasmic tails (brown, L; blue, S) are schematized. (B) The amino acid sequence of the cytoplasmic domain is detailed for both isoforms. (C) The endoglin pre-mRNA is represented in the middle of the mature transcripts that originate each isoform. The retention of the final intron by an alternative splicing process leads to S-endoglin expression.

S-endoglin arises as the result of an alternative splicing mechanism by which the last intron, between exons #13 and #14, is retained in the mature mRNA (Figure 1C). Consequently, an early stop codon appears in the open reading frame and truncates the mature protein in the cytoplasmic region. Although this mechanism of intron retention normally involves a rapid degradation by the nonsense-mediated decay machinery (Lareau et al., 2004; Nott et al., 2003), under certain conditions it may also lead to a biologically active isoform (Sakabe & de Souza, 2007); and this is the case of endoglin. Thus, when endothelial cells become senescent during the ageing process, they show an up-regulation of S-endoglin (Blanco et al., 2008). At this senescent stage, both endoglin isoforms are co-expressed likely forming heterodimers, as it occurs in mice (Perez-Gomez et al., 2005), and some of the cellular responses to TGF-β are oppositely regulated by each isoform. Indeed, the S-endoglin increase has an antiangiogenic role in the blood vessels and contributes to vascular pathology (Blanco et al., 2008; Perez-Gomez et al., 2005; Velasco et al., 2008).

3. Endothelial senescence and TGF-β

It is well known that ageing *per se* is the major risk factor for the development of cardiovascular diseases. Thus, senescence has been widely and mainly analyzed in *in vitro* studies but there are also evidences that this process takes place *in vivo* (Erusalimsky & Kurz, 2005; Minamino & Komuro, 2007). The first evidence of cellular senescence in primary cultures *in vitro* is the deceleration in the proliferation, that is, an increase in the doubling time of the cell population. In parallel, cells experience morphological changes along theses passages that involve the augment of the cellular size and shape. However, these observations are usually complemented with a useful tool based on the abnormal behaviour associated with senescent cells of the lysosomal hydrolase β-galactosidase. Thus, the senescence-associated β-galactosidase (SA β-gal) activity at pH 6 is widely accepted as an easily detectable senescence histochemical marker (Dimri et al., 1995).

Endothelial senescence is a cellular process that is clearly linked to both ageing and the development of vascular pathologies as well (Brandes et al., 2005; Erusalimsky, 2009; Minamino & Komuro, 2007). Basically, senescence constitutes a stress and damage response phenomenon that involves a permanent growth arrest (Campisi & d'Adda di Fagagna, 2007). Consequently, senescent cells undergo diverse changes in gene and protein expression that lead to an impairment of cellular functions (Foreman & Tang, 2003; Young & Narita, 2009). Thus, these changes usually affect to the endothelial phenotype favouring a pro-inflammatory, pro-atherosclerotic, or a prothrombotic state (Erusalimsky, 2009).

Here, TGF-β plays an important role owing to its ability to prompt senescence in a variety of cell types (Cipriano et al., 2011; Kordon et al., 1995; Tremain et al., 2000; van der Kraan et al., 2011; Wu et al., 2009). In the vascular context, it has been reported, e. g., elevated levels of TGF-β in the aging varicose veins that likely favour the fibrous process and the consequent venous insufficiency (Pascual et al., 2007). In this sense, the profibrotic effect of TGF-β is mediated by the stimulation via Smad3 signalling of the plasminogen activator inhibitor (PAI)-1 expression, a key regulator of the synthesis and deposition of the extracellular matrix in the tissue homeostasis (Ghosh & Vaughan, 2011). Thus, the increase of TGF-β up-regulates PAI-1 expression, which contributes to the accumulation of collagen and other extracellular matrix components. This PAI-1 increase is also in line with the decrease of the antithrombogenic properties of a senescent endothelium due to the inhibition of the urokinase- and tissue-type plasminogen activator (uPA and tPA, respectively)/plasmin axis (Comi et al., 1995; Schneiderman et al., 1992).

3.1 Replicative senescence

Senescence was initially considered to reflect the finite capacity for division that normal diploid cells exhibit when propagated in culture. This statement is based on the successive rounds of cell division that imply the progressively shortening and eventual dysfunction of telomeres, the physical ends of chromosomes, in a phenomenon known as Hayflick's limit (Hayflick, 2003; Shay & Wright, 2007). Thus, the down-regulation of telomerase, the enzyme responsible for maintaining the telomeres length, is clue for the senescence program. Besides, because telomerase is re-activated in the majority of neoplastic processes, it is postulated that inhibiting telomerase activity should result in senescence induction by telomere shortening which can cause the death of cancer cells (Folini et al., 2011). Interestingly, the senescence inducer TGF-β down-regulates the telomerase activity. Thus, upon TGF-β treatment, Smad3 is able to interact with the transcription factor c-myc, so repressing the promoter of the hTERT gene, encoding the catalytic subunit of telomerase (Figure 2). Thus, the c-myc activity is blocked in the Smad3 complexes which negatively affects to the cell cycle (Li & Liu, 2007; Li et al., 2006). In addition, this repression of the hTERT promoter mediated by TGF-β can be alternatively reinforced by the activation of the TGF-β activated kinase (TAK)-1 pathway that abrogates the transcriptional activity of Sp1 on the hTERT promoter (Fujiki et al., 2007).

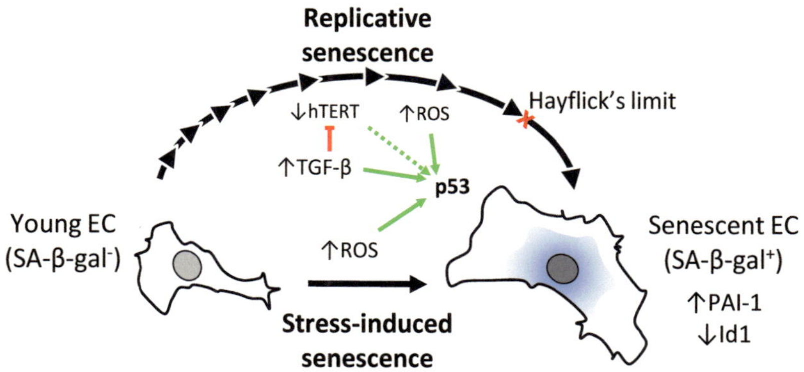

Fig. 2. The endothelial senescence. Endothelial cells extensively cultured *in vitro* enlarge their size and shape, showing a positive blue staining for the SA-β-gal activity. Endothelial senescence is reached by, at least, two different routes, including replicative or oxidative stress-induced. Both pathways involve the activation of p53 and are characterized by an increase in PAI-1 expression and the repression of Id1.

The characteristic and irreversible growth arrest observed in senescent cells occurs in the transition from phase G1 to phase S of the cell cycle and is dependent on the retinoblastoma family proteins, playing the tumour suppressor p53 a key role which senses the telomeric DNA damage (Wesierska-Gadek et al., 2005). In this transition, the abolition of p53 expression interferes with the senescence process that would be related to the low levels of PAI-1, one of the p53 target genes (Kortlever et al., 2008). Conversely, it is well known that the p53 overexpression or activation is able to arrest the cell cycle and launch the senescence program, suggesting that this process could be useful in cancer therapy (Chen & Goligorsky, 2006; Ewald et al., 2010; Rosso et al., 2006; Sugrue et al., 1997). Furthermore, it was demonstrated that the prolonged treatment with interferon (IFN)-γ induces cellular senescence in endothelial cells, involving cell cycle arrest and an up-regulation of p53 and p21 proteins cells (Kim et al., 2009).

Another TGF-β target protein that is associated with endothelial senescence is the helix-loop-helix (HLH) transcription factor Id1, or inhibitor of DNA binding 1. Id1 lacks a basic DNA-binding domain, but is able to form heterodimers with other HLH proteins, thereby inhibiting DNA binding, a process that is essential for cellular proliferation (Benezra et al., 1990). In epithelial cells, TGF-β induces the formation of a Smad3/ATF3 heteromeric complex that represses the Id1 expression and negatively regulates the cell cycle (Kang et al., 2003). Hence, the decrease in the Id1 expression is considered a biomarker of endothelial senescent cells (Tang et al., 2002).

3.2 Oxidative stress-induced senescence

Endothelial senescence can also be triggered by telomere-independent events that in general involve damages in the DNA. In this sense, the oxidative stress is a major stimulus for the induction of this type of senescence, which is due to the generation of reactive oxygen species (ROS, including oxygen ions and peroxides) in the mitochondria (Collins & Tzima, 2011; Erusalimsky & Skene, 2009). Thus, the cellular metabolism is the central source of ROS, but often they have an extracellular origin such as the one induced by radiation. In any case, ROS can either provoke or accelerate the development of senescence by damaging the DNA (Figure 2), which triggers multiple response mechanisms that usually act through the retinoblastoma protein family pathways, the final effectors of the senescence program (Campisi & d'Adda di Fagagna, 2007; Erusalimsky, 2009).

In cell culture, ROS induce an acute form of senescence termed stress-induced premature senescence, which does not require extensive cell culture but which resembles somehow the replicative one (Toussaint et al., 2000). This type of senescence is relatively easy to analyze in *in vitro* assays because the sole treatment with hydrogen peroxide (H_2O_2) for a short lapse of time is enough to prompt this type of senescence (Chen et al., 1998). By contrast, using antioxidant agents such as the grape stilbenoid resveratrol protect from the oxidative stress-induced premature senescence (Kao et al., 2010). Also, several lines of evidence show that ROS can interact and deplete the nitric oxide (NO) generated by the endothelium in the vasodilator responses, so contributing to the endothelial dysfunction associated to ageing (Grisham et al., 1998; Steiner et al., 2002). This is in line with the availability of NO-donors to inhibit endothelial cell senescence (Hayashi et al., 2006). In fact, comparing elderly with young adults one can find that the NO levels, or its bioavailability, are decreased in the first group but, interestingly, without any difference regarding to the expression levels or activation state of the endothelial nitric oxide synthase (eNOS), the enzyme responsible of the NO generation (Sun et al., 2004; Taddei et al., 2001). In parallel, this decrease in the NO levels attenuates the negative interference that it exerts on the TGF-β signalling pathway (Saura et al., 2005), which contributes to prompt the senescence program.

On the other hand, radiation is an exogenous trigger for ROS. In human skin fibroblasts, repeated exposure to ultraviolet-B light at subcytotoxic level is able to prompt premature senescence. Interestingly, this effect is mediated by the increase in the TGF-β expression and consequently by its downstream signalling pathway (Debacq-Chainiaux et al., 2005). In the vascular context, this source of ROS has been poorly studied beyond the methodological interest to induce premature senescence because endothelial cells enter rapidly in apoptosis due to their high sensitivity to radiation (Paris et al., 2001). In this regard, a recent study has demonstrated that ionizing radiation suppresses angiogenesis in mice and this effect is mediated through the TGF-β/ALK5-dependent inhibition of endothelial cell sprouting (Imaizumi et al., 2010).

4. Induction of S-endoglin and its role in endothelial senescence

The molecular changes involved or associated to the senescent program not only concern to the induction or repression of a specific set of genes. Many of the changes described in the literature report post-translational modifications, e. g., the advanced glycation endproducts

(AGEs) which have been implicated in age-related disease and aging itself; as well as the p53 acetylation in stress-induced senescence (Furukawa et al., 2007). In addition, a growing body of evidence supports the involvement of the post-transcriptional modifications that occur in senescence, i. e., the alternative splicing processes associated with senescence (Harries et al., 2011; Meshorer & Soreq, 2002). Thus, alterations in the splicing pattern have been described for several age-related diseases, such as the Hutchison Gilford progeria syndrome (Eriksson et al., 2003), or the Alzheimer's disease-related tauopathies (Chen et al., 2010).

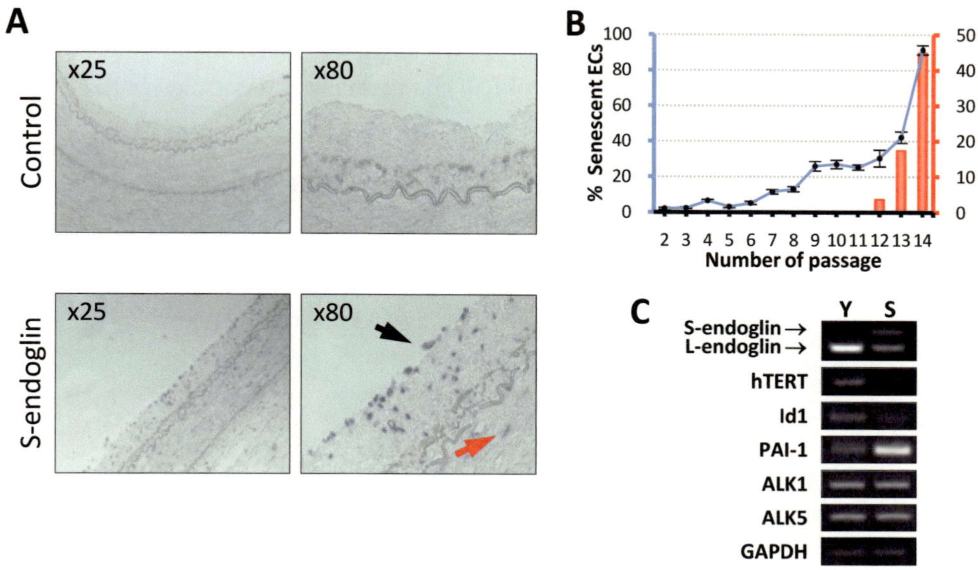

Fig. 3. S-endoglin expression in senescence. (A) The expression of S-endoglin in blood vessels can be revealed by *in situ* hybridization in the endothelium of human coronary artery (black arrow) and in some smooth muscle cells (red arrow). (B) The increase in the percentage of senescent endothelial cells *in vitro* (blue graph) is concomitant with the induction of S-endoglin (red graph). (C) Primary cultures of human umbilical vein endothelial cells (HUVECs) maintained *in vitro* along passages co-express both endoglin isoforms comparing young (Y) versus senescent (S) cells in RT-PCR assays. In parallel, PAI-1 is increased, while Id1 and telomerase (hTERT) are down-regulated in senescent cell. As a control, the expression levels of the TGF-β type I receptors ALK1 and ALK5 are not altered. (Figure adapted from Blanco et al., 2008).

Nonetheless, little is known about the role of splicing in the vascular context during senescence. A recent study demonstrates that TGF-β induces the distal splice-site selection leading to an antiangiogenic variant of the vascular endothelial growth factor (VEGF) (Nowak et al., 2008), and this could be one of the reasons why there is a reduced capability to form tubular-like structure by senescent endothelial *in vitro* (Chang et al., 2005).

As described above, the role of TGF-β in senescence has been clearly established, modulating specific intracellular effectors and leading to the cell growth arrest. In a first step, TGF-β binds to the specific receptor complex at the endothelial cell surface. Then, the signal is transmitted into the cytoplasm by different pathways depending on the type I receptor present in the complex. Thus, ALK5 signals via Smad2 and Smad3, whereas ALK1 mainly activates Smad1 and Smad5. In the TGF-β receptor complex, the presence of the predominantly expressed isoform, L-endoglin, favours the ALK1/Smad1 pathway and is related to the activation phase of the angiogenesis (Blanco et al., 2005; Lebrin et al., 2004). However, a post-transcriptional change during endothelial senescence, such as the retention of the last and small intron in the endoglin mRNA, has important consequences. Thus, the up-regulation of S-endoglin *in vitro* and *in vivo* is clearly associated with the ageing (Figures 3A and 3B). The co-expression of S- and L-endoglin in the senescent endothelial cells is able to tilt the angiogenic balance toward the resolution phase (ALK5/Smad3 pathway) in detriment of the ALK1/Smad1 route (Blanco et al., 2008). Also, S-endoglin induces the up-regulation of the PAI-1 and the repression of Id1, changes clearly associated to the cell cycle arrest in senescence (Figure 3C and 4).

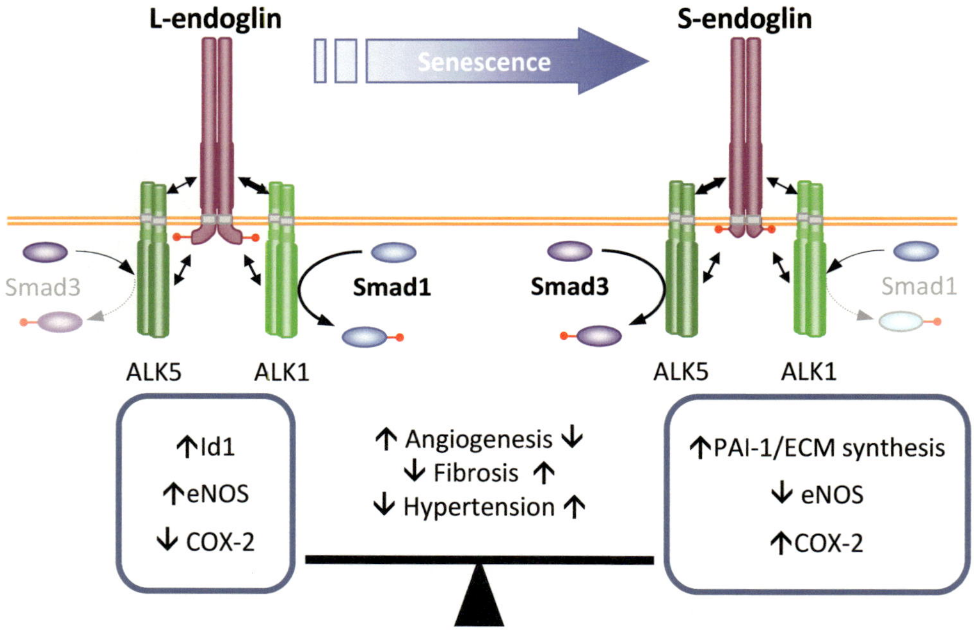

Fig. 4. Functional effects of S-endoglin in endothelial senescence. The S-endoglin up-regulation in aged endothelial cells promotes the ALK5/Smad3 signalling pathway. As a consequent, the vascular physiology is affected decreasing the angiogenesis, increasing the fibrosis and unbalancing the eNOS/COX-2 system which is related to hypertension. (Figure adapted from Blanco et al., 2008)

Furthermore, transgenic mice that overexpress the human S-endoglin isoform (*S-Eng*$^{+}$) experience a significant increase in the mean arterial pressure and a failure in the control on the NO-dependent vascular homeostasis, similarly to what happens in the endoglin deficient mouse model (*Eng*$^{+/-}$) that resembles the HHT disease (Blanco et al., 2008; Santibanez et al., 2007). Supporting this, a common compensatory mechanism takes place in *S-Eng*$^{+}$ and *Eng*$^{+/-}$ mice involving the up-regulation of the cyclooxigenase (COX)-2 enzyme

(Blanco et al., 2008; Jerkic et al., 2006). Taken together, the induction of S-endoglin during endothelial senescence might be at the basis of the development of cardiovascular pathologies associated with ageing, including atherosclerosis and hypertension (Figure 4).

4.1 Regulation of endoglin alternative splicing in senescence

Briefly, the alternative splicing is a molecular process by which organisms notably increase the diversity and functionality of their proteome from a finite number of genes. This process is carried out by the spliceosome, a huge ribonucleoprotein complex that works with amazing fidelity: i) skipping or shuffling exons; ii) selecting alternative splice sites; or iii) retaining introns (Graveley, 2001; Kwan et al., 2007). In humans, there are two distinct spliceosome complexes, named the major (M-Sp) and the minor (m-Sp) spliceosome. The M-Sp is involved in the vast majority of the splicing events and comprises five snRNPs named U1, U2, U4, U5, and U6 and a multitude of non-snRNP splicing factors (Jurica & Moore, 2003; Matlin et al., 2005; Zhou et al., 2002). Likewise, the m-Sp is composed by four unique snRNPs, U11, U12, U4atac, and U6atac, besides the U5 snRNP shared by both spliceosomes (Hall & Padgett, 1996; Tarn & Steitz, 1996). The m-Sp was first associated with the maturation of the so-called non-canonical introns but its role on standard splicing has been recently reported (Sheth et al., 2006; Will & Luhrmann, 2005). Interestingly, the difference between the major spliceosome and the minor spliceosome is their spatial segregation. While the M-Sp is in the nucleus, the m-Sp can be detected in the cytosol (Caceres & Misteli, 2007; Konig et al., 2007). In both cases, the spliceosome assembly is driven by a set of snRNPs that sequentially recognize the 5′ and 3′ splice sites, as well as the branch point element in between them (Burge et al., 1999). These snRNPs constitute the basal machinery of the spliceosome, besides a number of essential proteins that takes part in the spliceosome assembly. Moreover, there are several groups of auxiliary proteins that may regulate the alternative splicing. These splicing factors, or *trans*-elements, recognize binding sites, or *cis*-elements, spatially distributed inside the introns or exons and act as silencers or enhancers (Moore & Silver, 2008; Singh & Valcarcel, 2005; Sperling et al., 2008; Wang et al., 2006). Unfortunately, the alternative splicing during endothelial senescence has been poorly studied so far, but its importance has been suggested by the lifespan extension provoked by the overexpression of the splicing factor SNEV (Voglauer et al., 2006).

One of the best characterized groups of splicing factors is the serine/arginine (SR) protein family, from which the alternative splicing factor/splicing factor 2 (ASF/SF2) is the prototypical member (Graveley, 2000). ASF/SF2 is involved in both constitutive and alternative splicing processes. Although ASF/SF2 is mainly found in the nuclear speckles, it continuously shuttles between the nucleus and the cytoplasm depending on the phosphorylation and/or methylation states, which in turn determines its activity (Sanford et al., 2008; Sanford et al., 2005; Sinha et al., 2010). In this context, it has been recently reported the role of ASF/SF2 in the regulation of the S-endoglin intron retention during endothelial senescence (Blanco & Bernabeu, 2011). In endothelial senescent cells, the subcellular pattern of ASF/SF2 is mainly cytoplasmic, where ASF/SF2 interferes with the minor spliceosome inhibiting the elimination of the last intron of endoglin mRNA. The role of cytoplasmic ASF/SF2 as a senescent inductor is supported by its antiangiogenic properties, because the inhibition of the ASF/SF2 phosphorylation promotes its cytoplasmic localization and this is associated with increased expression levels of the antiangiogenic isoform VEGF165b (Nowak et al., 2010).

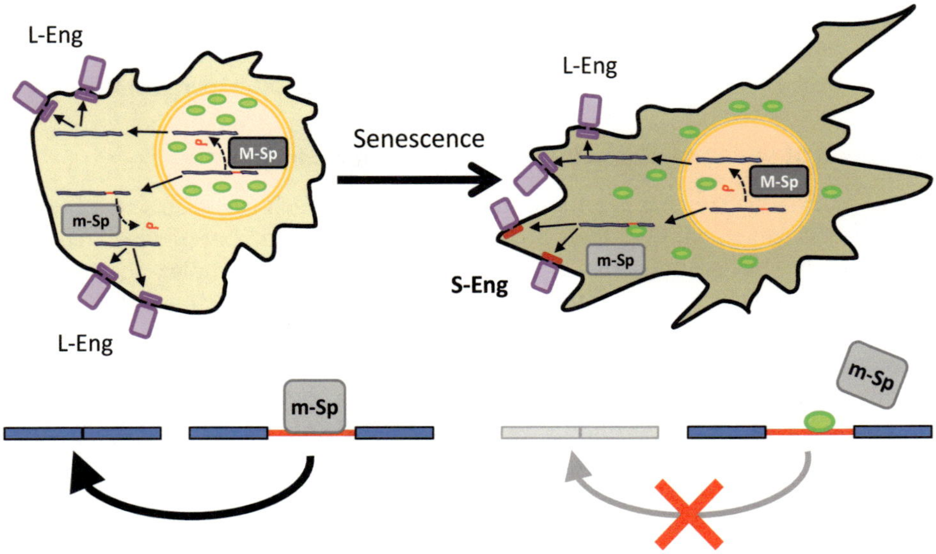

Fig. 5. Regulation of the alternative splicing of endoglin in senescent endothelial cells. In this hypothetical model, the last intron of the *ENG* gene is eliminated in the mature mRNA, so that L-endoglin is the predominantly expressed isoform. In this mRNA processing, both spliceosomes (nuclear M-Sp and cytoplasmic m-Sp) can be involved. However, in senescent endothelial cells, the splicing factor ASF/SF2 (green) is translocated to the cytoplasm, stabilizing the S-endoglin mRNA and interfering with the m-Sp activity. Consequently, ASF/SF2 promotes the intron retention, thus up-regulating the levels of S-endoglin mRNA (adapted from Blanco & Bernabeu, 2011).

5. Conclusions

Vascular physiology progressively declines with age due to multiple factors including an increase in oxidative stress, DNA damage, and advanced cellular replication involving telomere attrition. All these events converge in the key molecule p53, which acts typically arresting the cell cycle and triggering the endothelial senescence. At this stage, the expression of many specific genes is modulated, regarding not only to their expression levels but also the post-translational modifications and alternative processing of their premature mRNA molecules, which give rise to interesting protein variants. Nowadays, it can be postulated that this phenomenon is at the cellular basis of several age-associated cardiovascular pathologies, such as hypertension or atherosclerosis.

TGF-β is able to induce endothelial senescence via a cell surface receptor complex that includes the type I (ALK1 and ALK5) and the type II signalling receptors as well as endoglin. Endoglin is a TGF-β co-receptor highly expressed as L-(long)-endoglin by endothelial cells which is associated with active angiogenesis foci and vascular remodelling processes. Conversely, an alternative spliced and shorter isoform (S-endoglin) with opposite effects to those of L-endoglin in the context of the TGF-β system has been described. Usually, S-endoglin is almost undetectable in endothelial cells, but is induced during senescence. In this up-regulation, the senescence-induced cytoplasmic localization of the splicing factor ASF/SF2 plays a key role favouring the retention of the intron between exons

#13 and #14. Thus, the up-regulated expression of S-endoglin is considered to be part of the endothelial senescence program. Moreover, *in vitro* and *in vivo* studies suggest that S-endoglin contributes to vascular pathology associated with ageing. In this regard, mutations in the human *ENG* gene are responsible for HHT-1, an autosomic dominant vascular disease whose symptoms increase and become worse with age. Currently, the haploinsufficiency of the predominantly expressed L-endoglin isoform is widely accepted as the pathogenic mechanism of the disease. Because S-endoglin is up-regulated in aged mice as well as during senescence of endothelial cells and S-endoglin counteracts the function of L-endoglin, the increased S-endoglin expression during ageing would increase the functional L-endoglin haploinsufficiency in HHT-1 and could explain why the symptoms become worse with ageing. Therefore, one could predict that the age-dependent penetrance of the HHT-1 is due, at least in part, to the S-endoglin induction mediated by ASF/SF2.

In summary, these data suggest an important role for the TGF-β co-receptor endoglin as a modulator of the vascular pathology associated with endothelial senescence.

6. Acknowledgments

This work was supported by grants of the Spanish Ministry of Science and Innovation to CB (SAF2010-19222) and *Genoma España* (MEICA). FJB is a post-doctoral researcher of the *Centro de Investigación Biomédica en Red* (CIBER) *de Enfermedades Raras*, ISCIII, Spain. CB is a research professor in the *Centro de Investigaciones Biológicas*, CSIC, Spain.

7. References

Bellon, T.; Corbi, A.; Lastres, P.; Cales, C.; Cebrian, M.; Vera, S.; Cheifetz, S.; Massague, J.; Letarte, M. & Bernabeu, C. (1993). Identification and expression of two forms of the human transforming growth factor-beta-binding protein endoglin with distinct cytoplasmic regions. *European Journal of Immunology*, Vol. 23, No. 9, (September 1993), pp. 2340-2345, ISSN 0014-2980.

Benezra, R.; Davis, R.L.; Lockshon, D.; Turner, D.L. & Weintraub, H. (1990). The protein Id: a negative regulator of helix-loop-helix DNA binding proteins. *Cell*, Vol. 61, No. 1, (April 1990), pp. 49-59, ISSN 0092-8674.

Bernabeu, C.; Lopez-Novoa, J.M. & Quintanilla, M. (2009). The emerging role of TGF-beta superfamily coreceptors in cancer. *Biochimica et Biophysica Acta*, Vol. 1792, No. 10, (July 2009), pp. 954-973, ISSN 0006-3002.

Blanco, F.J. & Bernabeu, C. (2011). Alternative splicing factor or splicing factor-2 plays a key role in intron retention of the endoglin gene during endothelial senescence. *Aging Cell*, Vol. 10, No. 5, (June 2011), pp. 896-907, ISSN 1474-9726.

Blanco, F.J.; Grande, M.T.; Langa, C.; Oujo, B.; Velasco, S.; Rodriguez-Barbero, A.; Perez-Gomez, E.; Quintanilla, M.; Lopez-Novoa, J.M. & Bernabeu, C. (2008). S-endoglin expression is induced in senescent endothelial cells and contributes to vascular pathology. *Circulation Research*, Vol. 103, No. 12, (November 2008), pp. 1383-1392, ISSN 1524-4571.

Blanco, F.J.; Santibanez, J.F.; Guerrero-Esteo, M.; Langa, C.; Vary, C.P. & Bernabeu, C. (2005). Interaction and functional interplay between endoglin and ALK-1, two components of the endothelial transforming growth factor-beta receptor complex. *Journal of Cellular Physiology*, Vol. 204, No. 2, (February 2005), pp. 574-584, ISSN 0021-9541.

Brandes, R.P.; Fleming, I. & Busse, R. (2005). Endothelial aging. *Cardiovascular Research*, Vol. 66, No. 2, (May 2005), pp. 286-294, ISSN 0008-6363.

Burge, C.; Tuschl, T. & Sharp, P. (1999). Splicing of precursors to mRNAs by the spliceosoomes, In: *The RNA World*. R. Gesteland, T. Cech, and J. Atkins (eds.), pp. 525-560. Cold Spring Harbor Laboratory Press, ISBN 0-87969-589-7, Plainview, NY, United States of America.

Caceres, J.F. & Misteli, T. (2007). Division of labor: minor splicing in the cytoplasm. *Cell*, Vol. 131, No. 4, (November 2007), pp. 645-647, ISSN 0092-8674.

Campisi, J. & d'Adda di Fagagna, F. (2007). Cellular senescence: when bad things happen to good cells. *Nature Reviews Molecular Cell Biology*, Vol. 8, No. 9, (August 2007), pp. 729-740, ISSN 1471-0080.

Carmeliet, P. & Jain, R.K. (2011). Molecular mechanisms and clinical applications of angiogenesis. *Nature*, Vol. 473, No. 7347, (May 2011), pp. 298-307, ISSN 1476-4687.

Cipriano, R.; Kan, C.E.; Graham, J.; Danielpour, D.; Stampfer, M. & Jackson, M.W. (2011). TGF-beta signaling engages an ATM-CHK2-p53-independent RAS-induced senescence and prevents malignant transformation in human mammary epithelial cells. *Proceedings of the National Academy of Sciences of the United States of America*, Vol. 108, No. 21, (May 2011), pp. 8668-8673, ISSN 1091-6490.

Collins, C. & Tzima, E. (2011). Hemodynamic forces in endothelial dysfunction and vascular aging. *Experimental Gerontology*, Vol. 46, No. 2-3, (October 2010), pp. 185-188, ISSN 1873-6815.

Comi, P.; Chiaramonte, R. & Maier, J.A. (1995). Senescence-dependent regulation of type 1 plasminogen activator inhibitor in human vascular endothelial cells. *Experimental Cell Research*, Vol. 219, No. 1, (July 1995), pp. 304-308, ISSN 0014-4827.

Conway, E.M. & Carmeliet, P. (2004). The diversity of endothelial cells: a challenge for therapeutic angiogenesis. *Genome Biology*, Vol. 5, No. 2, (January 2004), pp. 207, ISSN 1465-6914.

Chang, M.W.; Grillari, J.; Mayrhofer, C.; Fortschegger, K.; Allmaier, G.; Marzban, G.; Katinger, H. & Voglauer, R. (2005). Comparison of early passage, senescent and hTERT immortalized endothelial cells. *Experimental Cell Research*, Vol. 309, No. 1, (June 2005), pp. 121-136, ISSN 0014-4827.

Chen, J. & Goligorsky, M.S. (2006). Premature senescence of endothelial cells: Methusaleh's dilemma. *American Journal of Physiology. Heart and Circulatory Physiology*, Vol. 290, No. 5, (April 2006), pp. H1729-1739, ISSN 0363-6135.

Chen, Q.M.; Bartholomew, J.C.; Campisi, J.; Acosta, M.; Reagan, J.D. & Ames, B.N. (1998). Molecular analysis of H2O2-induced senescent-like growth arrest in normal human fibroblasts: p53 and Rb control G1 arrest but not cell replication. *Biochemical Journal*, Vol. 332 (Pt 1), (May 1998), pp. 43-50, ISSN 0264-6021.

Chen, S.; Townsend, K.; Goldberg, T.E.; Davies, P. & Conejero-Goldberg, C. (2010). MAPT isoforms: differential transcriptional profiles related to 3R and 4R splice variants. *Journal of Alzheimer's Disease*, Vol. 22, No. 4, (October 2010), pp. 1313-1329, ISSN 1875-8908.

Debacq-Chainiaux, F.; Borlon, C.; Pascal, T.; Royer, V.; Eliaers, F.; Ninane, N.; Carrard, G.; Friguet, B.; de Longueville, F.; Boffe, S.; Remacle, J. & Toussaint, O. (2005).

Repeated exposure of human skin fibroblasts to UVB at subcytotoxic level triggers premature senescence through the TGF-beta1 signaling pathway. *Journal of Cell Science*, Vol. 118, No. 4, (January 2005), pp. 743-758, ISSN 0021-9533.

Dimri, G.P.; Lee, X.; Basile, G.; Acosta, M.; Scott, G.; Roskelley, C.; Medrano, E.E.; Linskens, M.; Rubelj, I.; Pereira-Smith, O. & et al. (1995). A biomarker that identifies senescent human cells in culture and in aging skin in vivo. *Proceedings of the National Academy of Sciences of the United States of America*, Vol. 92, No. 20, (September 1995), pp. 9363-9367, ISSN 0027-8424.

Eriksson, M.; Brown, W.T.; Gordon, L.B.; Glynn, M.W.; Singer, J.; Scott, L.; Erdos, M.R.; Robbins, C.M.; Moses, T.Y.; Berglund, P.; Dutra, A.; Pak, E.; Durkin, S.; Csoka, A.B.; Boehnke, M.; Glover, T.W. & Collins, F.S. (2003). Recurrent de novo point mutations in lamin A cause Hutchinson-Gilford progeria syndrome. *Nature*, Vol. 423, No. 6937, (April 2003), pp. 293-298, ISSN 0028-0836.

Erusalimsky, J.D. (2009). Vascular endothelial senescence: from mechanisms to pathophysiology. *Journal of Applied Physiology*, Vol. 106, No. 1, (November 2008), pp. 326-332, ISSN 8750-7587.

Erusalimsky, J.D. & Kurz, D.J. (2005). Cellular senescence in vivo: its relevance in ageing and cardiovascular disease. *Experimental Gerontology*, Vol. 40, No. 8-9, (June 2005), pp. 634-642, ISSN 0531-5565.

Erusalimsky, J.D. & Skene, C. (2009). Mechanisms of endothelial senescence. *Experimental Physiology*, Vol. 94, No. 3, (October 2008), pp. 299-304, ISSN 1469-445X.

Ewald, J.A.; Desotelle, J.A.; Wilding, G. & Jarrard, D.F. (2010). Therapy-induced senescence in cancer. *Journal of the National Cancer Institute*, Vol. 102, No. 20, (September 2010), pp. 1536-1546, ISSN 1460-2105.

Ferrari, A.U.; Radaelli, A. & Centola, M. (2003). Invited review: aging and the cardiovascular system. *Journal of Applied Physiology*, Vol. 95, No. 6, (December 2003), pp. 2591-2597, ISSN 8750-7587.

Folini, M.; Venturini, L.; Cimino-Reale, G. & Zaffaroni, N. (2011). Telomeres as targets for anticancer therapies. *Expert Opinion on Therapeutic Targets*, Vol. 15, No. 5, (February 2011), pp. 579-593, ISSN 1744-7631.

Foreman, K.E. & Tang, J. (2003). Molecular mechanisms of replicative senescence in endothelial cells. *Experimental Gerontology*, Vol. 38, No. 11-12, (November 2003), pp. 1251-1257, ISSN 0531-5565.

Foteinos, G.; Hu, Y.; Xiao, Q.; Metzler, B. & Xu, Q. (2008). Rapid endothelial turnover in atherosclerosis-prone areas coincides with stem cell repair in apolipoprotein E-deficient mice. *Circulation*, Vol. 117, No. 14, (April 2008), pp. 1856-1863, ISSN 1524-4539.

Fraisl, P.; Mazzone, M.; Schmidt, T. & Carmeliet, P. (2009). Regulation of angiogenesis by oxygen and metabolism. *Developmental Cell*, Vol. 16, No. 2, (February 2009), pp. 167-179, ISSN 1878-1551.

Fujiki, T.; Miura, T.; Maura, M.; Shiraishi, H.; Nishimura, S.; Imada, Y.; Uehara, N.; Tashiro, K.; Shirahata, S. & Katakura, Y. (2007). TAK1 represses transcription of the human telomerase reverse transcriptase gene. *Oncogene*, Vol. 26, No. 36, (February 2007), pp. 5258-5266, ISSN 0950-9232.

Furukawa, A.; Tada-Oikawa, S.; Kawanishi, S. & Oikawa, S. (2007). H2O2 accelerates cellular senescence by accumulation of acetylated p53 via decrease in the function of SIRT1 by NAD+ depletion. *Cellular Physiology and Biochemistry*, Vol. 20, No. 1-4, (June 2007), pp. 45-54, ISSN 1015-8987.

Ghosh, A.K. & Vaughan, D.E. (2011). PAI-1 in Tissue Fibrosis. *Journal of Cellular Physiology*, (April 2011), DOI: 10.1002/jcp.22783, ISSN 1097-4652.

Graveley, B.R. (2000). Sorting out the complexity of SR protein functions. *RNA*, Vol. 6, No. 9, (September 2000), pp. 1197-1211, ISSN 1355-8382.

Graveley, B.R. (2001). Alternative splicing: increasing diversity in the proteomic world. *Trends in Genetics*, Vol. 17, No. 2, (February 2001), pp. 100-107, ISSN 0168-9525.

Grisham, M.B.; Granger, D.N. & Lefer, D.J. (1998). Modulation of leukocyte-endothelial interactions by reactive metabolites of oxygen and nitrogen: relevance to ischemic heart disease. *Free Radical Biology & Medicine*, Vol. 25, No. 4-5, (September 1998), pp. 404-433, ISSN 0891-5849.

Hall, S.L. & Padgett, R.A. (1996). Requirement of U12 snRNA for in vivo splicing of a minor class of eukaryotic nuclear pre-mRNA introns. *Science*, Vol. 271, No. 5256, (March 1996), pp. 1716-1718, ISSN 0036-8075.

Harries, L.W.; Hernandez, D.; Henley, W.; Wood, A.R.; Holly, A.C.; Bradley-Smith, R.M.; Yaghootkar, H.; Dutta, A.; Murray, A.; Frayling, T.M.; Guralnik, J.M.; Bandinelli, S.; Singleton, A.; Ferrucci, L. & Melzer, D. (2011). Human aging is characterized by focused changes in gene expression and deregulation of alternative splicing. *Aging Cell*, Vol. 10, No. 5, (June 2011), pp. 868-878, ISSN 1474-9726.

Hayashi, T.; Matsui-Hirai, H.; Miyazaki-Akita, A.; Fukatsu, A.; Funami, J.; Ding, Q.F.; Kamalanathan, S.; Hattori, Y.; Ignarro, L.J. & Iguchi, A. (2006). Endothelial cellular senescence is inhibited by nitric oxide: implications in atherosclerosis associated with menopause and diabetes. *Proceedings of the National Academy of Sciences of the United States of America*, Vol. 103, No. 45, (November 2006), pp. 17018-17023, ISSN 0027-8424.

Hayflick, L. (2003). Living forever and dying in the attempt. *Experimental Gerontology*, Vol. 38, No. 11-12, (December 2003), pp. 1231-1241, ISSN 0531-5565.

Imaizumi, N.; Monnier, Y.; Hegi, M.; Mirimanoff, R.O. & Ruegg, C. (2010). Radiotherapy suppresses angiogenesis in mice through TGF-betaRI/ALK5-dependent inhibition of endothelial cell sprouting. *PLoS One*, Vol. 5, No. 6, (June 2010), pp. e11084, ISSN 1932-6203.

Jerkic, M.; Rivas-Elena, J.V.; Santibanez, J.F.; Prieto, M.; Rodriguez-Barbero, A.; Perez-Barriocanal, F.; Pericacho, M.; Arevalo, M.; Vary, C.P.; Letarte, M.; Bernabeu, C. & Lopez-Novoa, J.M. (2006). Endoglin regulates cyclooxygenase-2 expression and activity. *Circulation Research*, Vol. 99, No. 3, (July 2006), pp. 248-256, ISSN 1524-4571.

Jurica, M.S. & Moore, M.J. (2003). Pre-mRNA splicing: awash in a sea of proteins. *Molecular Cell*, Vol. 12, No. 1, (July 2003), pp. 5-14, ISSN 1097-2765.

Kang, J.S.; Liu, C. & Derynck, R. (2009). New regulatory mechanisms of TGF-beta receptor function. *Trends in Cell Biology*, Vol. 19, No. 8, (August 2009), pp. 385-394, ISSN 1879-3088.

Kang, Y.; Chen, C.R. & Massague, J. (2003). A self-enabling TGFbeta response coupled to stress signaling: Smad engages stress response factor ATF3 for Id1 repression in epithelial cells. *Molecular Cell*, Vol. 11, No. 4, (April 2003), pp. 915-926, ISSN 1097-2765.

Kao, C.L.; Chen, L.K.; Chang, Y.L.; Yung, M.C.; Hsu, C.C.; Chen, Y.C.; Lo, W.L.; Chen, S.J.; Ku, H.H. & Hwang, S.J. (2010). Resveratrol protects human endothelium from H(2)O(2)-induced oxidative stress and senescence via SirT1 activation. *Journal of Atherosclerosis and Thrombosis*, Vol. 17, No. 9, (July 2010), pp. 970-979, ISSN 1880-3873.

Kim, K.S.; Kang, K.W.; Seu, Y.B.; Baek, S.H. & Kim, J.R. (2009). Interferon-gamma induces cellular senescence through p53-dependent DNA damage signaling in human endothelial cells. *Mechanisms of Ageing and Development*, Vol. 130, No. 3, (December 2008), pp. 179-188, ISSN 0047-6374.

Koleva, R.I.; Conley, B.A.; Romero, D.; Riley, K.S.; Marto, J.A.; Lux, A. & Vary, C.P. (2006). Endoglin structure and function: Determinants of endoglin phosphorylation by transforming growth factor-beta receptors. *Journal of Biological Chemistry*, Vol. 281, No. 35, (June 2006), pp. 25110-25123, ISSN 0021-9258.

Konig, H.; Matter, N.; Bader, R.; Thiele, W. & Muller, F. (2007). Splicing segregation: the minor spliceosome acts outside the nucleus and controls cell proliferation. *Cell*, Vol. 131, No. 4, (November 2007), pp. 718-729, ISSN 0092-8674.

Kordon, E.C.; McKnight, R.A.; Jhappan, C.; Hennighausen, L.; Merlino, G. & Smith, G.H. (1995). Ectopic TGF beta 1 expression in the secretory mammary epithelium induces early senescence of the epithelial stem cell population. *Developmental Biology*, Vol. 168, No. 1, (March 1995), pp. 47-61, ISSN 0012-1606.

Kortlever, R.M.; Nijwening, J.H. & Bernards, R. (2008). Transforming growth factor-beta requires its target plasminogen activator inhibitor-1 for cytostatic activity. *Journal of Biological Chemistry*, Vol. 283, No. 36, (July 2008), pp. 24308-24313, ISSN 0021-9258.

Kwan, T.; Benovoy, D.; Dias, C.; Gurd, S.; Serre, D.; Zuzan, H.; Clark, T.A.; Schweitzer, A.; Staples, M.K.; Wang, H.; Blume, J.E.; Hudson, T.J.; Sladek, R. & Majewski, J. (2007). Heritability of alternative splicing in the human genome. *Genome Research*, Vol. 17, No. 8, (August 2007), pp. 1210-1218, ISSN 1088-9051.

Lareau, L.F.; Green, R.E.; Bhatnagar, R.S. & Brenner, S.E. (2004). The evolving roles of alternative splicing. *Current Opinion in Structural Biology*, Vol. 14, No. 3, (June 2004), pp. 273-282, ISSN 0959-440X.

Lebrin, F.; Goumans, M.J.; Jonker, L.; Carvalho, R.L.; Valdimarsdottir, G.; Thorikay, M.; Mummery, C.; Arthur, H.M. & ten Dijke, P. (2004). Endoglin promotes endothelial cell proliferation and TGF-beta/ALK1 signal transduction. *The EMBO Journal*, Vol. 23, No. 20, (September 2004), pp. 4018-4028, ISSN 0261-4189.

Li, H. & Liu, J.P. (2007). Mechanisms of action of TGF-beta in cancer: evidence for Smad3 as a repressor of the hTERT gene. *Annals of the New York Academy of Sciences*, Vol. 1114, (October 2007), pp. 56-68, ISSN 0077-8923.

Li, H.; Xu, D.; Li, J.; Berndt, M.C. & Liu, J.P. (2006). Transforming growth factor beta suppresses human telomerase reverse transcriptase (hTERT) by Smad3 interactions with c-Myc and the hTERT gene. *Journal of Biological Chemistry*, Vol. 281, No. 35, (June 2006), pp. 25588-25600, ISSN 0021-9258.

Lopez-Novoa, J.M. & Bernabeu, C. (2010). The physiological role of endoglin in the cardiovascular system. *American Journal of Physiology. Heart and Circulatory Physiology*, Vol. 299, No. 4, (July 2010), pp. H959-974, ISSN 1522-1539.

Llorca, O.; Trujillo, A.; Blanco, F.J. & Bernabeu, C. (2007). Structural model of human endoglin, a transmembrane receptor responsible for hereditary hemorrhagic telangiectasia. *Journal of Molecular Biology,* Vol. 365, No. 3, (November 2006), pp. 694-705, ISSN 0022-2836.

Mahmoud, M.; Allinson, K.R.; Zhai, Z.; Oakenfull, R.; Ghandi, P.; Adams, R.H.; Fruttiger, M. & Arthur, H.M. (2010). Pathogenesis of arteriovenous malformations in the absence of endoglin. *Circulation Research,* Vol. 106, No. 8, (March 2010), pp. 1425-1433, ISSN 1524-4571.

Massague, J.; Seoane, J. & Wotton, D. (2005). Smad transcription factors. *Genes & Development,* Vol. 19, No. 23, (December 2005), pp. 2783-2810, ISSN 0890-9369.

Matlin, A.J.; Clark, F. & Smith, C.W. (2005). Understanding alternative splicing: towards a cellular code. *Nature Reviews Molecular Cell Biology,* Vol. 6, No. 5, (June 2005), pp. 386-398, ISSN 1471-0072.

McAllister, K.A.; Grogg, K.M.; Johnson, D.W.; Gallione, C.J.; Baldwin, M.A.; Jackson, C.E.; Helmbold, E.A.; Markel, D.S.; McKinnon, W.C.; Murrell, J. & et al. (1994). Endoglin, a TGF-beta binding protein of endothelial cells, is the gene for hereditary haemorrhagic telangiectasia type 1. *Nature Genetics,* Vol. 8, No. 4, (December 1994), pp. 345-351, ISSN 1061-4036.

Meshorer, E. & Soreq, H. (2002). Pre-mRNA splicing modulations in senescence. *Aging Cell,* Vol. 1, No. 1, (October 2002), pp. 10-16, ISSN 1474-9718.

Meurer, S.K.; Tihaa, L.; Borkham-Kamphorst, E. & Weiskirchen, R. (2011). Expression and functional analysis of endoglin in isolated liver cells and its involvement in fibrogenic Smad signalling. *Cellular Signalling,* Vol. 23, No. 4, (December 2010), pp. 683-699, ISSN 1873-3913.

Minamino, T. & Komuro, I. (2007). Vascular cell senescence: contribution to atherosclerosis. *Circulation Research,* Vol. 100, No. 1, (January 2007), pp. 15-26, ISSN 1524-4571.

Minamino, T. & Komuro, I. (2008). Role of telomeres in vascular senescence. *Frontiers in Bioscience,* Vol. 13, (January 2008), pp. 2971-2979, ISSN 1093-4715.

Minamino, T.; Miyauchi, H.; Yoshida, T.; Tateno, K.; Kunieda, T. & Komuro, I. (2004). Vascular cell senescence and vascular aging. *Journal of Molecular and Cellular Cardiology,* Vol. 36, No. 2, (February 2004), pp. 175-183, ISSN 0022-2828.

Moore, M.J. & Silver, P.A. (2008). Global analysis of mRNA splicing. *RNA,* Vol. 14, No. 2, (December 2007), pp. 197-203, ISSN 1469-9001.

Nott, A.; Meislin, S.H. & Moore, M.J. (2003). A quantitative analysis of intron effects on mammalian gene expression. *RNA,* Vol. 9, No. 5, (April 2003), pp. 607-617, ISSN 1355-8382.

Nowak, D.G.; Amin, E.M.; Rennel, E.S.; Hoareau-Aveilla, C.; Gammons, M.; Damodoran, G.; Hagiwara, M.; Harper, S.J.; Woolard, J.; Ladomery, M.R. & Bates, D.O. (2010). Regulation of vascular endothelial growth factor (VEGF) splicing from pro-angiogenic to anti-angiogenic isoforms: a novel therapeutic strategy for angiogenesis. *Journal of Biological Chemistry,* Vol. 285, No. 8, (November 2009), pp. 5532-5540, ISSN 1083-351X.

Nowak, D.G.; Woolard, J.; Amin, E.M.; Konopatskaya, O.; Saleem, M.A.; Churchill, A.J.; Ladomery, M.R.; Harper, S.J. & Bates, D.O. (2008). Expression of pro- and anti-angiogenic isoforms of VEGF is differentially regulated by splicing and growth factors. *Journal of Cell Science,* Vol. 121, No. Pt 20, (October 2008), pp. 3487-3495, ISSN 0021-9533.

Pardali, E.; Goumans, M.J. & ten Dijke, P. (2010). Signaling by members of the TGF-beta family in vascular morphogenesis and disease. *Trends in Cell Biology*, Vol. 20, No. 9, (September 2010), pp. 556-567, ISSN 1879-3088.

Paris, F.; Fuks, Z.; Kang, A.; Capodieci, P.; Juan, G.; Ehleiter, D.; Haimovitz-Friedman, A.; Cordon-Cardo, C. & Kolesnick, R. (2001). Endothelial apoptosis as the primary lesion initiating intestinal radiation damage in mice. *Science*, Vol. 293, No. 5528, (July 2001), pp. 293-297, ISSN 0036-8075.

Pascual, G.; Mendieta, C.; Garcia-Honduvilla, N.; Corrales, C.; Bellon, J.M. & Bujan, J. (2007). TGF-beta1 upregulation in the aging varicose vein. *Journal of Vascular Research*, Vol. 44, No. 3, (March 2007), pp. 192-201, ISSN 1018-1172.

Perez-Gomez, E.; Del Castillo, G.; Santibanez, J.F.; Lopez-Novoa, J.M.; Bernabeu, C. & Quintanilla, M. (2010). The role of the TGF-beta coreceptor endoglin in cancer. *The Scientific World Journal*, Vol. 10, (December 2010), pp. 2367-2384, ISSN 1537-744X.

Perez-Gomez, E.; Eleno, N.; Lopez-Novoa, J.M.; Ramirez, J.R.; Velasco, B.; Letarte, M.; Bernabeu, C. & Quintanilla, M. (2005). Characterization of murine S-endoglin isoform and its effects on tumor development. *Oncogene*, Vol. 24, No. 27, (April 2005), pp. 4450-4461, ISSN 0950-9232.

Rivard, A.; Fabre, J.E.; Silver, M.; Chen, D.; Murohara, T.; Kearney, M.; Magner, M.; Asahara, T. & Isner, J.M. (1999). Age-dependent impairment of angiogenesis. *Circulation*, Vol. 99, No. 1, (January 1999), pp. 111-120, ISSN 0009-7322.

Rodríguez-Mañas, L.; El-Assar, M.; Vallejo, S.; López-Dóriga, P.; Solís, J.; Petidier, R.; Montes, M.; Nevado, J.; Castro, M.; Gómez-Guerrero, C.; Peiró, C. & Sánchez-Ferrer, C.F. (2009). Endothelial dysfunction in aged humans is related with oxidative stress and vascular inflammation. *Aging Cell*, Vol. 8, No. 3, (June 2009), pp. 226-238, ISSN 1474-9726.

Rosso, A.; Balsamo, A.; Gambino, R.; Dentelli, P.; Falcioni, R.; Cassader, M.; Pegoraro, L.; Pagano, G. & Brizzi, M.F. (2006). p53 Mediates the accelerated onset of senescence of endothelial progenitor cells in diabetes. *Journal of Biological Chemistry*, Vol. 281, No. 7, (December 2005), pp. 4339-4347, ISSN 0021-9258.

Sakabe, N.J. & de Souza, S.J. (2007). Sequence features responsible for intron retention in human. *BMC Genomics*, Vol. 8, (February 2007), pp. 59, ISSN 1471-2164.

Sanford, J.R.; Coutinho, P.; Hackett, J.A.; Wang, X.; Ranahan, W. & Caceres, J.F. (2008). Identification of nuclear and cytoplasmic mRNA targets for the shuttling protein SF2/ASF. *PLoS One*, Vol. 3, No. 10, (October 2008), pp. e3369, ISSN 1932-6203.

Sanford, J.R.; Ellis, J.D.; Cazalla, D. & Caceres, J.F. (2005). Reversible phosphorylation differentially affects nuclear and cytoplasmic functions of splicing factor 2/alternative splicing factor. *Proceedings of the National Academy of Sciences of the United States of America*, Vol. 102, No. 42, (October 2005), pp. 15042-15047, ISSN 0027-8424.

Santibanez, J.F.; Letamendia, A.; Perez-Barriocanal, F.; Silvestri, C.; Saura, M.; Vary, C.P.; Lopez-Novoa, J.M.; Attisano, L. & Bernabeu, C. (2007). Endoglin increases eNOS expression by modulating Smad2 protein levels and Smad2-dependent TGF-beta signaling. *Journal of Cellular Physiology*, Vol. 210, No. 2, (October 2006), pp. 456-468, ISSN 0021-9541.

Saura, M.; Zaragoza, C.; Herranz, B.; Griera, M.; Diez-Marques, L.; Rodriguez-Puyol, D. & Rodriguez-Puyol, M. (2005). Nitric oxide regulates transforming growth factor-beta signaling in endothelial cells. *Circulation Research*, Vol. 97, No. 11, (October 2005), pp. 1115-1123, ISSN 1524-4571.

Schneiderman, J.; Sawdey, M.S.; Keeton, M.R.; Bordin, G.M.; Bernstein, E.F.; Dilley, R.B. & Loskutoff, D.J. (1992). Increased type 1 plasminogen activator inhibitor gene expression in atherosclerotic human arteries. *Proceedings of the National Academy of Sciences of the United States of America*, Vol. 89, No. 15, (August 1992), pp. 6998-7002, ISSN 0027-8424.

Shay, J.W. & Wright, W.E. (2007). Hallmarks of telomeres in ageing research. *Journal of Pathology*, Vol. 211, No. 2, (January 2007), pp. 114-123, ISSN 0022-3417.

Sheth, N.; Roca, X.; Hastings, M.L.; Roeder, T.; Krainer, A.R. & Sachidanandam, R. (2006). Comprehensive splice-site analysis using comparative genomics. *Nucleic Acids Research*, Vol. 34, No. 14, (August 2006), pp. 3955-3967, ISSN 1362-4962.

Shovlin, C.L. (2010). Hereditary haemorrhagic telangiectasia: pathophysiology, diagnosis and treatment. *Blood Reviews*, Vol. 24, No. 6, (September 2010), pp. 203-219, ISSN 1532-1681.

Singh, R. & Valcarcel, J. (2005). Building specificity with nonspecific RNA-binding proteins. *Nature Structure Molecular Biology*, Vol. 12, No. 8, (August 2005), pp. 645-653, ISSN 1545-9993.

Sinha, R.; Allemand, E.; Zhang, Z.; Karni, R.; Myers, M.P. & Krainer, A.R. (2010). Arginine methylation controls the subcellular localization and functions of the oncoprotein splicing factor SF2/ASF. *Molecular Cell Biology*, Vol. 30, No. 11, (March 2010), pp. 2762-2774, ISSN 1098-5549.

Sperling, J.; Azubel, M. & Sperling, R. (2008). Structure and function of the Pre-mRNA splicing machine. *Structure*, Vol. 16, No. 11, (November 2008), pp. 1605-1615, ISSN 0969-2126.

Steiner, D.R.; Gonzalez, N.C. & Wood, J.G. (2002). Interaction between reactive oxygen species and nitric oxide in the microvascular response to systemic hypoxia. *Journal of Applied Physiology*, Vol. 93, No. 4, (September 2002), pp. 1411-1418, ISSN 8750-7587.

Sugrue, M.M.; Shin, D.Y.; Lee, S.W. & Aaronson, S.A. (1997). Wild-type p53 triggers a rapid senescence program in human tumor cells lacking functional p53. *Proceedings of the National Academy of Sciences of the United States of America*, Vol. 94, No. 18, (September 1997), pp. 9648-9653, ISSN 0027-8424.

Sun, D.; Huang, A.; Yan, E.H.; Wu, Z.; Yan, C.; Kaminski, P.M.; Oury, T.D.; Wolin, M.S. & Kaley, G. (2004). Reduced release of nitric oxide to shear stress in mesenteric arteries of aged rats. *American Journal of Physiology. Heart and Circulatory Physiology*, Vol. 286, No. 6, (January 2004), pp. H2249-2256, ISSN 0363-6135.

Taddei, S.; Virdis, A.; Ghiadoni, L.; Salvetti, G.; Bernini, G.; Magagna, A. & Salvetti, A. (2001). Age-related reduction of NO availability and oxidative stress in humans. *Hypertension*, Vol. 38, No. 2, (August 2001), pp. 274-279, ISSN 1524-4563.

Tang, J.; Gordon, G.M.; Nickoloff, B.J. & Foreman, K.E. (2002). The helix-loop-helix protein id-1 delays onset of replicative senescence in human endothelial cells. *Laboratory Investigation*, Vol. 82, No. 8, (August 2002), pp. 1073-1079, ISSN 0023-6837.

Tang, Y.; Yang, X.; Friesel, R.E.; Vary, C.P. & Liaw, L. (2011). Mechanisms of TGF-beta-Induced Differentiation in Human Vascular Smooth Muscle Cells. *Journal of Vascular Research*, Vol. 48, No. 6, (August 2011), pp. 485-494, ISSN 1423-0135.

Tarn, W.Y. & Steitz, J.A. (1996). Highly diverged U4 and U6 small nuclear RNAs required for splicing rare AT-AC introns. *Science*, Vol. 273, No. 5283, (September 1996), pp. 1824-1832, ISSN 0036-8075.

ten Dijke, P.; Goumans, M.J. & Pardali, E. (2008). Endoglin in angiogenesis and vascular diseases. *Angiogenesis*, Vol. 11, No. 1, (February 2008), pp. 79-89, ISSN 0969-6970.

Toussaint, O.; Medrano, E.E. & von Zglinicki, T. (2000). Cellular and molecular mechanisms of stress-induced premature senescence (SIPS) of human diploid fibroblasts and melanocytes. *Experimental Gerontology*, Vol. 35, No. 8, (December 2000), pp. 927-945, ISSN 0531-5565.

Tremain, R.; Marko, M.; Kinnimulki, V.; Ueno, H.; Bottinger, E. & Glick, A. (2000). Defects in TGF-beta signaling overcome senescence of mouse keratinocytes expressing v-Ha-ras. *Oncogene*, Vol. 19, No. 13, (April 2000), pp. 1698-1709, ISSN 0950-9232.

van der Kraan, P.M.; Goumans, M.J.; Blaney Davidson, E. & Ten Dijke, P. (2011). Age-dependent alteration of TGF-beta signalling in osteoarthritis. *Cell and Tissue Research*, DOI: 10.1007/s00441-011-1194-6, (June 2011), ISSN 1432-0878.

Velasco, S.; Alvarez-Munoz, P.; Pericacho, M.; Dijke, P.T.; Bernabeu, C.; Lopez-Novoa, J.M. & Rodriguez-Barbero, A. (2008). L- and S-endoglin differentially modulate TGFbeta1 signaling mediated by ALK1 and ALK5 in L6E9 myoblasts. *Journal of Cell Science*, Vol. 121, No. Pt 6, (February 2008), pp. 913-919, ISSN 0021-9533.

Venkatesha, S.; Toporsian, M.; Lam, C.; Hanai, J.; Mammoto, T.; Kim, Y.M.; Bdolah, Y.; Lim, K.H.; Yuan, H.T.; Libermann, T.A.; Stillman, I.E.; Roberts, D.; D'Amore, P.A.; Epstein, F.H.; Sellke, F.W.; Romero, R.; Sukhatme, V.P.; Letarte, M. & Karumanchi, S.A. (2006). Soluble endoglin contributes to the pathogenesis of preeclampsia. *Nature Medicine*, Vol. 12, No. 6, (June 2006), pp. 642-649, ISSN 1078-8956.

Voglauer, R.; Chang, M.W.; Dampier, B.; Wieser, M.; Baumann, K.; Sterovsky, T.; Schreiber, M.; Katinger, H. & Grillari, J. (2006). SNEV overexpression extends the life span of human endothelial cells. *Experimental Cell Research*, Vol. 312, No. 6, (January 2006), pp. 746-759, ISSN 0014-4827.

Wang, Z.; Xiao, X.; Van Nostrand, E. & Burge, C.B. (2006). General and specific functions of exonic splicing silencers in splicing control. *Molecular Cell*, Vol. 23, No. 1, (June 2006), pp. 61-70, ISSN 1097-2765.

Wesierska-Gadek, J.; Wojciechowski, J.; Ranftler, C. & Schmid, G. (2005). Role of p53 tumor suppressor in ageing: regulation of transient cell cycle arrest and terminal senescence. *Journal of Physiology and Pharmacology*, Vol. 56, No. 1, (March 2005), pp. 15-28, ISSN 0867-5910.

Will, C.L. & Luhrmann, R. (2005). Splicing of a rare class of introns by the U12-dependent spliceosome. *Biological Chemistry*, Vol. 386, No. 8, (October 2005), pp. 713-724, ISSN 1431-6730.

Wu, S.; Hultquist, A.; Hydbring, P.; Cetinkaya, C.; Oberg, F. & Larsson, L.G. (2009). TGF-beta enforces senescence in Myc-transformed hematopoietic tumor cells through induction of Mad1 and repression of Myc activity. *Experimental Cell Research*, Vol. 315, No. 18, (September 2009), pp. 3099-3111, ISSN 1090-2422.

Young, A.R. & Narita, M. (2009). SASP reflects senescence. *EMBO Reports*, Vol. 10, No. 3, (February 2009), pp. 228-230, ISSN 1469-3178.

Zhou, Z.; Licklider, L.J.; Gygi, S.P. & Reed, R. (2002). Comprehensive proteomic analysis of the human spliceosome. *Nature*, Vol. 419, No. 6903, (September 2002), pp. 182-185, ISSN 0028-0836.

21

Quantification of Elastin, Collagen and Advanced Glycation End Products as Functions of Age and Hypertension

Milena Atanasova[1], Aneliya Dimitrova[2], Boryana Ruseva[3], Angelina Stoyanova[4], Miglena Georgieva[5] and Emiliana Konova[5,6]
[1]*Department of Biology, Medical University of Pleven, Pleven,*
[2]*Department of Pathophysiology, Medical University of Pleven, Pleven,*
[3]*Department of Physiology, Medical University of Pleven, Pleven,*
[4]*Department of Chemistry, Medical University of Pleven, Pleven,*
[5]*Medical Center "Clinical Institute for Reproductive Medicine", Pleven,*
[6]*Center for Reproductive Health; Medical University of Pleven, Pleven,*
Bulgaria

1. Introduction

Elastin and collagen are the major extracellular matrix (ECM) proteins that make up the framework of the elastic arteries structure. These two fibrous proteins are the main structural components of arterial walls, and they provide the strength and resilience needed by the aorta to accommodate the pressure and volume variations during each heartbeat (Coquand et al., 2011). Elastin is a polymer of linear polypeptide chains and constituting more than 50% of the dry weight of the proximal parts of the aorta. It is the main provider of tissue elasticity, while collagen acts to stiffen the wall and to limit its extensibility (Samila & Carter, 1981). During aging the aorta diameter and stiffness increases because of degenerative changes in elastin, resulting in a transfer of stress to less extensible collagenous components of the aorta (Coquand et al., 2011).

Elastin production takes place during late gestation and before the end of childhood, but expression in very low rate persists in adulthood. The turnover rate for collagen and elastin is low in healthy arteries, but vascular pathology upsets the regulatory pathways that maintain this balance. In response to hypertension, the overexpression of both proinflammatory and proteinase-inhibitory molecules dramatically increases arterial ECM synthesis (Arribas et al., 2006; Jacob et al., 2001; Jacob, 2003). Elastin and elastic fibers are progressively degraded by enzymatic processes involving an age-related imbalance between anti-proteases and proteases. In particular, elastin degrading enzymes, i.e. elastases, include several matrix metalloproteases (MMP), such as MMP-2 and MMP-9 (Jacob, 2003; McNulty et al., 2005). Imbalance in matrix metalloproteinase/tissue inhibitors of metalloproteinases may contribute to alteration in collagen turnover and extracellular matrix remodelling. However, the ECM proteins synthesized in response to hypertension have a three-dimensional architecture that is functionally less optimal than those deposited during fetal development and may play an important role in determining the modulus of pathological elastin tissue (Arribas et al., 2006; Jacob et al., 2001; Jacob, 2003). The increase of aortic stiffness is not only because of enzymatic degradation of elastin, but also is due to other mechanisms mainly including age-dependent increase in the collagen content and arterial wall thickening, non-enzymatic glycation of proteins (elastin and collagens), leading to the formation of deleterious advanced glycation end-products (AGEs) and related molecular cross-links which modify the tissue mechanical properties (Gibbons & Dzau, 1994; Corman et al., 1998; Lakatta, 2003; O'Routke, 2007).

Advanced glycation is a major pathway for the posttranslational modifications of tissue proteins and begins with non-enzymatic addition of sugars to the primary amino groups of proteins. These early glucose-derived Schiff bases and Amadori products undergo a series of inter- and intramolecular rearrangement, dehydration, and oxidation-reduction reactions and produce the late products termed advanced glycation end products (AGEs). Excessive accumulation of AGE on tissue proteins has been implicated in the pathogenesis of many of the sequels of diabetes and normal aging. Protein-linked AGEs act to crosslink connective tissue proteins and to chemically inactive nitric oxide activity and thus are associated with endothelial dysfunction. They also act as a recognition signals for AGE receptor systems that are present on diverse cell types (Yang et al.,1991; Vlassara, 1994). Accumulation of AGEs in vascular walls increases intimal medial thickening, collagen is impaired, more cross-linked and elastin fibrils are broken. Large arteries are stiffen and mechanical stress increases, leading to hypertension and all its deleterious consequences (Dart & Kingwell, 2001; Zieman & Kass, 2004)

Excessive accumulation of AGEs on tissue proteins changes their structure and respectively functions, reduces their susceptibility to degradation and none of the last place immunogenicity. Specifically, the interaction of AGEs with vessel wall components increases vascular permeability, the expression of procoagulant activity and the generation of ROS (Yan et al., 1994). Glycated proteins form common immunological epitopes which raise formation of population of anti-AGE autoantibodies (AGEAb). These antibodies recognize and react with AGE-epitopes regardless of the proteins they have been formed on. Assessment of the levels of these antibodies shows that they are present at low titres even in sera of healthy subjects, perhaps as a part of homeostatic mechanism which clears glycated structures via *in situ* destruction or via opsonization of the gflycated proteins and products of their degradation (Baydanoff et al., 1996). However, in the conditions of increased non-enzymatic glycation the homeostatic control is inefficient and the generation of these antibodies increases (Baydanoff et al., 1996).

The aim of our study was to investigate the effects of age and hypertension on quantity and quality of elastin and collagen in the aortic wall of the rats. In order to reach this aim we used the spontaneously hypertensive rats (SHR), that are appropriate genetical model for studying essential hypertension compared to normotensive Wistar-Kyoto rats (WKR) at 2-, 4- and 8-months of age.

2. Materials and methods

2.1 Animals

Female and male Spontaneously Hypertensive Rats (SHR, n=30) and Wistar Kyoto Rats (WKY, n=33) were used. Animals were born and raised under conventional conditions in the animal facility of the Medical University of Pleven and were allowed free access to tap water and a standard laboratory chow. Animals were housed and kept under a normal 12 h light/dark cycle at 22 °± 2°C. They were divided into 6 groups: 2-month-old SHR (2mSHR, n=7, 4 female and 3 male); 4-month-old SHR (4m SHR, n=9, 5/4); 8-month-old SHR (8mSHR, n=14, 9/5); 2-month-old WKY (2mWKY, n=12, 5/7); 4-month-old SHR (4mWKY, n=9, 5/4); 8-month-old WKY (8mWKY, n=12, 5/7). Our experimental design was approved by the Animal Care and Use of Laboratory Animals group of the Ethical Committee of the University, based on the principles described in the Guide for the Care and Use of Laboratory Animals (Bayne, 1996).

2.2 Blood collection

At the end of the 2nd, 4th and 8th month, following overnight fasting, the abdominal cavity of rats was opened under pentobarbitone sodium anesthesia (26 mg/kg body weight, i.p.). Blood was collected from the bifurcation of the aorta and put at 37 ˚C to clot. After separation 0.02% NaN_3 was added to each serum sample and stored at - 20 ˚C prior to use.

2.3 Quantification of elastin in the thoracic aorta

The quantity of elastin was measured after dissection of the descending thoracic aorta and cleaning of blood and surrounding adipose tissue. Length and width (both sides) of the vessels were recorded by using a grid in the eyepiece, after opening of the vessel in length.

Elastin was then quantified by using a protocol deriving from a previously described method (Wolinski, 1972) with small modifications. Briefly, after delipidation in acetone/diethyl ether (1:1, vol/vol) and drying, the dry weight was recorded by using a Kern ALS 120-4 balance (precision: 0.01 mg). Cell proteins were extracted by gentle agitation in 0.3% SDS for 24 h and then 3 times in 5 M guanidinium chloride with preservative 0.02% sodium azide for 2 h. After washing 3 times in distilled water the extracellular proteins, other than elastin remaining in the aortic segments, were solubilized by three 15-minute extractions in 1 ml of 0.1 M NaOH in a boiling water bath. Elastin was quantified by determining the dry weight of the residue as percent dry weight of the aorta or mg/cm.

2.4 Quantification of collagen in the thoracic aorta

The content of the aortic collagen was assayed by determination the hydroxyproline presented in NaOH solution. The solution was evaporated to dryness and hydrolyzed in 6N HCl under vacuum conditions for 24 hours at 110 °C. A colorimetric assay according Woessner (1961) was applied for determination of the hydroxyproline. Assuming that collagen contains 12.77% hydroxyproline by weight its quantity was presented as mg collagen per cm aorta (Keeley et al., 1984).

2.5 Direct determination of advanced glycation end-products (AGEs) formed *in vivo*

Soluble α-elastin was obtained from the descending thoracic aorta by the method of Partridge (1955). Insoluble elastin was hydrolyzed 5 times in 0.25 M oxalic acid in boiling water bath, and then dialyzed against phosphate buffered saline (PBS). Protein content of each sample was determined by measurement of the absorption of UV light at 280 nm wavelength and calculated according to a standard curve, constructed on the basis of different dilutions of rat α-elastin (EPC, St. Louis, USA).

Maillard reaction-related fluorescence (FC), representative of AGEs formed *in vivo*, was measured as an index of advanced glycation in 360/450 nm excitation/emission (Baydanoff et al., 1994; Monnier et al., 1984) with Corning-EEL fluorimeter. Quinine sulfate 1 µM in 0.1N H_2SO_4 was used as a standard. The levels of AGEs were expressed as arbitrary fluorescence units (AU) per mg protein.

2.6 Measurement of circulating AGEAb

2.6.1 Glycation of KLH

Keyhole Limpets Hemocyanin (KLH) (Sigma) - 20mg/ml was glycated *in vitro* with 3.33 M glucose in 0.4 M phosphate buffer, pH 7.5 with preservative 0.04% NaN_3, at 37°C, for 12 weeks. The formation of advanced glycated end product of KLH (AGE-KLH) was determined via measuring the fluorescence at 360/440 nm excitation/emission. After dialyzing against phosphate buffer, the obtained AGE-KLH was used as antigen in home-made ELISA.

2.6.2 ELISA for determination of circulating anti-AGE antibodies

AGEAb were assessed by home-made ELISA, as described in Dimitrova et al. (2009). The assay was performed as follows: Microtiter 96 well plates (Greiner Microlon) were coated with 100 µl of AGE-KLH per well in carbonate buffer (pH 9.6) with concentration 5 µg/ml. The plates were incubated 2 hours at 37 °C and then overnight at 4 °C to complete binding. Then the plates were washed three times with PBS with 0.05 % Tween 20 (PBS-Tween) before their blocking with 0.1 % BSA and incubation for 1 h at 37 °C. The next step was addition of 100 µl of tested rat serum, diluted 1:10 with PBS-Tween. Bound antibodies were reacted with anti-mouse IgG peroxidase conjugate, diluted 1:3200 in 1% human serum albumin for 1 h at 37 °C (BulBio - Sofia, Bulgaria). Ortho-phenyene diamine was used as colorimetric substrate. The reaction was terminated by 50 µl 8N H_2SO_4 and the absorbance (A) was read at 492 nm on automatic micro-ELISA plate reader. Serum samples were analyzed in triplicate and the average calculated.

2.7 Statistics

Comparisons of SHR and control rats were assessed using one- or two-way ANOVA followed when necessary by Fisher's least significant difference test (LSD) for paired value comparisons. The results are presented as mean values ±SEM, and p values ≤0.05 were considered as statistically significant. The correlations between investigated parameters were tested by the method of Pearson. The statistical package used was SPSS v. 15.

3. Results

3.1 Elastin content in the thoracic aorta

Figure 1 shows elastin content in the thoracic aortas of both rat strains aged 2, 4 and 8 months. When the elastin quantity was presented as percentage of the dry weight of the aorta (fig. 1A) SHR at different ages did not differ significantly, whereas in the WKR groups factor "age" was found to have a significant effect ($p<0.05$) - elastin quantity decreased with age. Elastin content was significantly larger ($p<0.032$) in 8-month-old hypertensive animals compared to age matched normotensive group. When the elastin quantity was presented as milligrams per centimeter of aorta (fig. 1B) the absolute amount of elastin in SHR at different ages did not differ from age matched WKR.

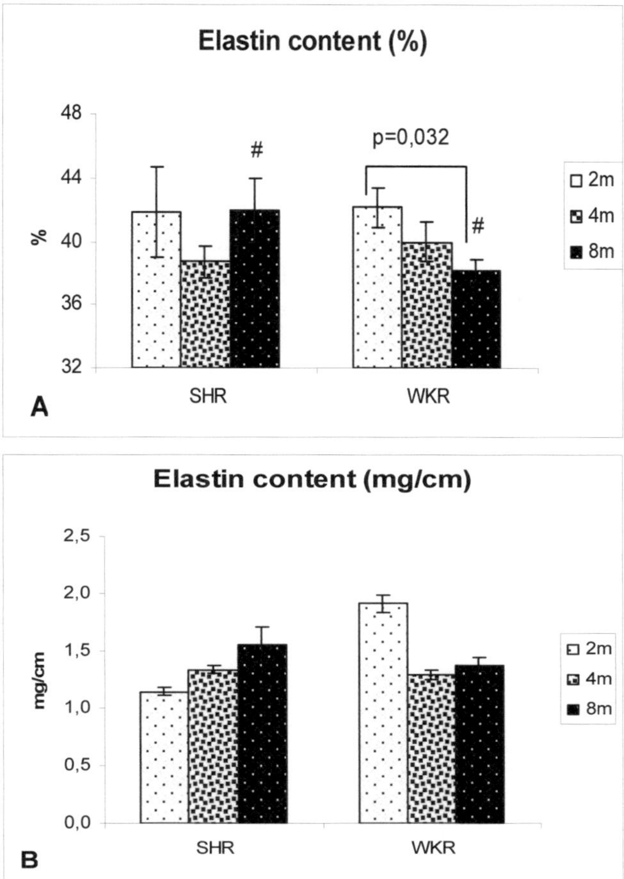

Fig. 1. Quantity of elastin in the thoracic aorta of SHR and WKR at three different ages, expressed as (A) percent dry weight of the aorta and (B) mg elastin per cm aorta.
Significant difference between 8-months-old SHR and WKR (p = 0.032).

3.2 Collagen content in the thoracic aorta

The collagen quantity showed a trend towards increase with age, but without reaching the statistically significant threshold (fig. 2). SHR at 2 and 4 months of age had significantly larger collagen content then age matched WKR. The groups of 8-month-old animals did not differ significantly. Hypertension was found to have significant effect ($p=0.019$) on the collagen content of the thoracic aorta of the investigated rats, but age was not.

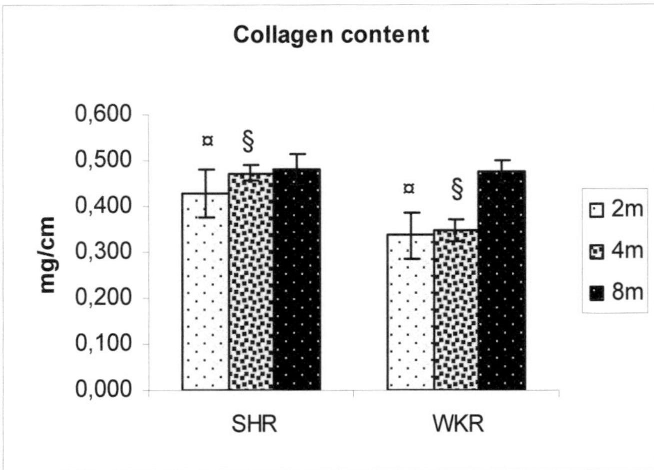

Fig. 2. Quantity of collagen in the thoracic aorta of SHR and WKR at three different ages, expressed as mg collagen per cm aorta. ¤ - Significant difference between 2-months-old SHR and WKR (p = 0.056); § - Significant difference between 4-months-old SHR and WKR (p = 0.007).

3.3 Direct determination of AGEs formed *in vivo*

Results obtained by direct determination of AGEs formed *in vivo* are presented in AU per mg elastin (fig. 3). The direct measurement of Maillard reaction-related fluorescence of obtained aortic α-elastin was found to increase with age in both strains and to be significantly higher (p=0.036) in elastin obtained by 8-month-old SHR samples compared to WKR at the same age.

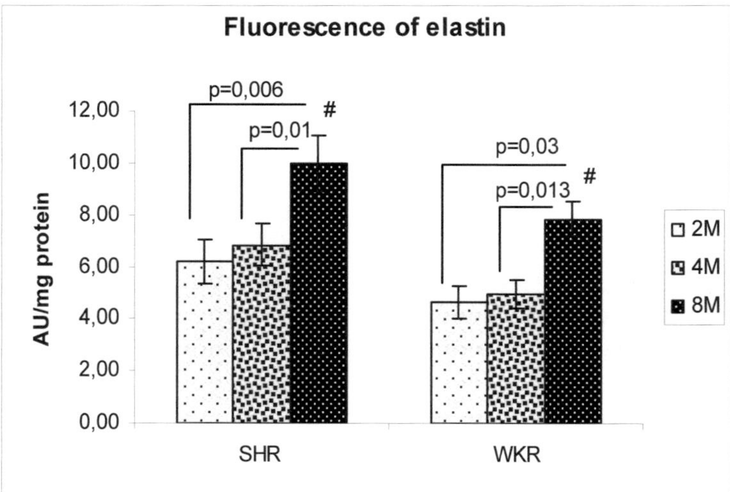

Fig. 3. Direct determination of AGEs formed *in vivo*. Maillard reaction-related fluorescence, measured for the soluble α-elastin obtained from the three aged groups of SHR and WKR. #- Significant difference between 8-months-old SHR and WKR (p = 0.036). AU – arbitrary units

ANOVA analysis showed that fluorescence of the purified elastin was influenced significantly by the age and hypertension (p=0.001 and p=0.0026).

3.4 Circulating anti-AGE antibodies

AGEAb were presented in all the sera tested. The serum levels of these antibodies (fig.4) in SHR substantially increased with age. Their mean values in WKR showed a trend towards increase with age, but without being significant. The youngest animals group from the two strains did not differ in contrast with the other two age groups in which antibody levels were significantly higher in hypertensive animals, compared to normotensive ones. The correlation (Pearson coefficient) between the serum levels of anti-AGEAb and the age and hypertension was highly significant (r = 0.553, p = 0.001 for age and r = - 0.440, p = 0.009 for hypertension).

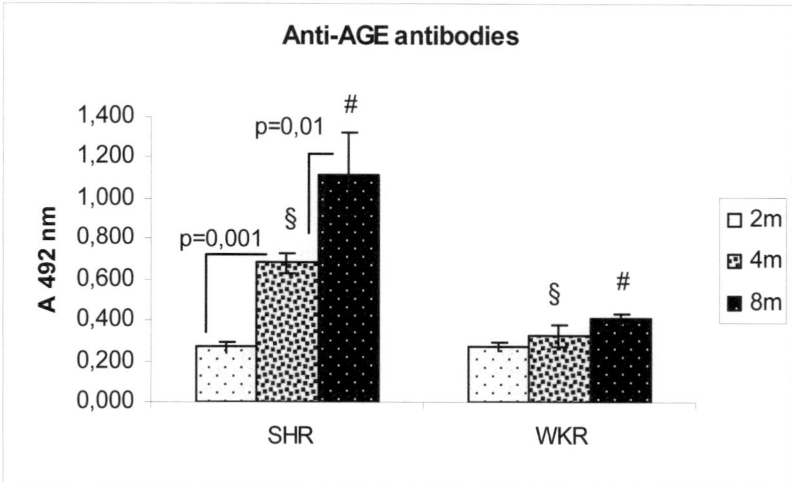

Fig. 4. Serum levels of AGEAb, measured by indirect home-made ELISA. § - Significant difference between 4-months-old SHR and WKR (p = 0.012). #- Significant difference between 8-months-old SHR and WKR (p = 0.001).

4. Discussion

Elastin and collagen fibrils are the structures that endow the vascular wall with elasticity and strength. But similarly to most of the connective tissue proteins they are proved to be pliable of cross-linking and thus their physiological turnover is changed and they become resistant to hydrolytic degradation (Zieman 2003). Altered by non-enzymatic glycation they accumulate in the vessel matrix in unorganized and non-functional pattern (Bailey 2001). This structural disorganization affects mainly the media and leads to mechanical alteration of the aortic wall especially in the condition of hypertension (Laurent, 1995; Bezie et al.,1998). Marque et al., (1999) explained age-linked aortic stiffening in SHR with more rapid increase with age of the aortic collagen content in and accelerated accumulation of advanced glycation end products on elastin and collagen fibers.

In the present study, we compared the elastin and collagen content of thoracic aortas from Wistar-Kyoto rats (WKR) and spontaneously hypertensive rats (SHR) at three different ages. In addition, glycation of purified aortic elastin and antibodies against AGEs were determined. The investigated parameters were compared as functions of age and hypertension.

Elastin production was investigated at the protein level, through the measurement of aortic elastin content. The relative elastin content (expressed as a percentage of dry weight) was significantly lower in the 8-month-old WKR, compared to the 2-month-old WKR and 8-month-old SHR. However, no significant differences were observed when the elastin content in the aorta was expressed as weight per aorta length (mg/cm). This can be explained with variations in body size and, thus, aortic dry weight among individual rats from both sexes, the absolute amount of elastin varied widely (Sauvage et al., 1999). The expression of elastin content relative to dry weight eliminates considerations of these large individual variations in aortic dry weight. It appeared that age had no general significant effect on the joint distribution of elastin content ($p>0.05$), but there is a slight decrease with age in aortic elastin content (-9%) in the oldest WKR (Fig. 1).

In the literature there is not clear age-related trend of decrease or increase of both elastin and collagen quantity and during hypertension development. Tsoporis et al., (1998) followed the biosynthesis of collagen and elastin during the development of spontaneous hypertension in SHR. They found that both collagen and elastin synthesis (as revealed by specific hydroxyproline activity) exceeded WKR control levels in the prehypertensive period (at the age of 4 weeks), decreased in the development of hypertension (to the age of 14-16 weeks), and increased again in the period of the established hypertensive state (beyond the age of 16 weeks). Several studies showed that this second increase in connective tissue proteins may be prevented, depending on the choice of antihypertensive therapy (Tsoporis et al., 1998; Han et al., 2009).

From the two main collagen types present, synthesis of collagen type III exceeded that of type I in the prehypertensive period (at the age of 4 weeks) and this relation was reversed during the period of established hypertension. They suggested that the vascular connective tissue metabolism in SHR differs from that in strain-matched controls, and the reverse rate of collagen type III to collagen type I synthesis during hypertension development may be considered an adaptive response to the increasing pressure load which may alter the mechanical properties of the vessel wall (Deil et al., 1987).

Han et al (2009) investigated medial and adventitial layers of the thoracic aorta 4- and 8-month-old SHR and WKR. They discovered that compared with WKR, SHR exhibited greater collagen and elastin content in the media, but decreased collagen and elastin content in the adventitial layer. Both medial and adventitial collagen and elastin content increased significantly with age in both strains and was greater in 8-month-old rats compared to 4-month-old rats (Han 2009).

It has been shown that the elastin network plays a major role in the maintenance of aortic elastic properties in adult SHR, not through variations of its total amount but through increases of the extent of its anchorage to the smooth muscle cells (Laurent, 1995, Bezieet al., 1998). Our data also supported the finding that quantity of elastin is not generally changed in the conditions of hypertension that is why we tested the Maillard reaction-related fluorescence to check the index of advanced glycation.

Hypertension is characterized by insulin resistance, and a number of studies have suggested that it plays a major role in its etiology (DeLano & Schmidt-Schonbein, 2007).

Other study of DeLano & Schmid-Schönbein (2008) states emphatically that in hypertensive rats, proteases cleave extracellular portions of several protein receptors, such as the insulin receptor, so that insulin can no longer bind and facilitate normal metabolism of glucose. In insulin resistance, alterations in glucose and lipid turnover lead to the production of excess AGEs (Vasdev et al.,2007; Potenza et al., 2005). AGEs are complex group of compounds, and the structure of a lot of them is identified - N-carboxymethil-lysine (CML), pentosidine, imidasolones, pirraline, etc. Although the chemistry of AGEs is not fully discovered, increased levels of circulating and tissue AGEs have been demonstrated in both animal and human studies in pathologies and aging (Brüel & Oxlund, 1996; Zieman & Kass, 2004). Increase of non-enzymatic glycation with aging is due to the life-long exposure to glucose even in normoglycemia. In pathology or aging conditions, when non-enzymatic glycation of proteins is increased, the capacity of normal homeostasis seems to be inefficient. This way AGEs are accumulated and contribute to the development of long-term aging process especially in long-lived proteins (Konova et al., 2004). Our results from the fluorescence studies of obtained aortic α-elastin showed increase with age especially in the hypertensive animals. The highest fluorescence was measured in the group of 8-month-old SHR which was significantly higher ($p=0.036$) in comparison to WKR at the same age. These results suggest an increase of non-enzymatic glycation with aging, even in normoglycemic animals and are in agreement with our previous investigations of age-dependent glycation of human aortic elastin (Konova et al., 2004). Moreover, we demonstrated the accelerating role of hypertension for the increase of formation of irreversible late advanced glycation end products in long-lived connective tissue proteins.

We did not find significant differences in AGEAb levels between SHR and WKR rats at 2 months of age. At about two months of age in arterial walls of SHR occur alterations that are consequences of developed hypertension. Observed vascular wall hypertrophy also plays an important role in hypertension by reducing tissue flexibility and elasticity (Mecham & Davis, 1994). During the early phases of hypertension development, wall distensibility might even be augmented in the SHR rats but long-term hypertension decreases arterial distensibility (Zanchi et al., 1997). Formed AGEs affect the biochemical and physical properties of proteins and ECM, including the charge, hydrophobicity, turnover and elasticity of collagen and elastin (Baydanov et al, 1994), and the cell adhesion, permeability and pro-inflammatory properties of the ECM (Baines, 2001). These structural and functional changes alter the antigenicity and immunogenicity of vascular elements. This provokes the immune system to react by producing different types of antibodies including AGEAb, directed to their own but altered structures. In our study AGEAb were presented in all the investigated rat sera but their levels were in positive correlation to the increasing age only in hypertensive animals. We observed significantly higher levels of AGE Abs in 8-month-old SHR compared to other age groups and age matched WKR. Our previous studies in patients with occupational vegetative polyneuropathy of upper limbs and in male SHR demonstrated similar results (Dimitrova et al., 2009, 2010).

5. Conclusion

In general, there were not clearly drawn age-related differences in the elastin and collagen quantity of the thoracic aortas of the investigated rats. But there were significant differences in the late products of glycation of the purified elastin and serum levels of antibodies against them. The quantity of obtained elastin did not change but the quality did. It appeared that the investigated factors had a generally significant effect and we observed a substantial increase of AGEs and AGEAb with age especially in the condition of hypertension.

Although AGEs in proteins are probably correlative, rather than causative, with respect to aging, they accumulate to high levels in tissues in age-related chronic diseases, such as atherosclerosis, diabetes, arthritis and neurodegenerative diseases. Inhibition of AGE formation in these diseases may limit oxidative and inflammatory damage in tissues, retarding the progression of pathophysiology and improve the quality of life during aging. It is necessary to investigate genetic, pharmacologic, and nutritional factors, which could decrease the levels of AGEs, to break cross-links in the glycated structures of ECM and to restore the turnover balance in order to improve the functionality of the vessel walls.

6. References

Arribas, S. Hinek, A. & Gonzalez, M. (2006). Elastic Fibres and Vascular Structure in Hypertension. *Pharmacol Ther* No.111, pp. 771–791

Atanasova, M. Konova, E. Georgieva, M. Dimitrova, A. Coquand-Gandit, M. Faury, G, & Baydanoff, S. (2010). Age-related Changes of Anti-elastin Antibodies in Senescence-Accelerated Mice. *Gerontology,* No. 56, pp. 310-318 DOI: 10.1007/BF00731464

Bailey, A. (2001). Molecular Mechanisms of Aging in Connective Tissues. *Mech Ageing Dev,* No. 122, pp. 735-757

Baydanoff, S. Konova, E. & Ivanova, N. (1996). Determination of Anti-AGE antibodies in Human Serum. *Glycoconj J,* No.13, pp. 335-339

Baydanoff, S. Konova, E. Dosheva, I. & Dorovski, P. (1994). Non-enzymatic glycation of elastin. *Glycosylation Dis.* No. 1, pp. 53-58

Bayne, K. (1996). Revised guide for the care and use of laboratory animals available. *Physiologist,* Vol. 39, No. 199, pp., 208–11, ISSN

Baynes, J. (2001). The Role of AGEs in Aging: *Causation or Correlation Experimental Gerontology* Vol. 36, Issue 9, pp. 1527-1537

Bezie, Y Lacolley, P. Laurent, S. & Gabella, G. (1998). Connection of Smooth Muscle Cells to Elastic Lamellae in Aorta of Spontaneously Hypertensive Rats. *Hypertension,* No.32, pp. 166 -169

Cattell, M. Anderson, J. & Hasleton, P. (1996). Age-related Changes in Amounts and Concentrations of Collagen and Elastin in Normotensive Human Thoracic Aorta. *Clin Chim Acta,* No.245, pp.73-84

Coquand-Gandit, M. Jakob, MP. Romero, B. Georgieva, M. Andrieu, JP. Bouilot, S. Garsia-Honduvilla, N. Starcher, B. Atanasova, M. Bujan, J. & Faury, G. (2011). Large Vessels of SAM-P8 and SAM-R1 Mice Exhibit Structural and Functional Differencses Related to implementation of Cardiovascular Therapies. *In Press*

Corman B, Duriez, M. Poitevin, P. Heudes, D. Bruneval, P. Tedgui, A. & Levy, B. (1998). Aminoguanidine Prevents Age-related Arterial Stiffening and Cardiac Hypertrophy. *Proc Natl Acad Sci USA,* No.95, pp. 1301-1306

Dart, A. & Kingwell, B. (2001). Pulse Pressure – a Review of Mechanisms and Clinical Relevance. *J Am Coll Cardiol* No. 37, pp. 975-984

Deil, Z. Jelínek, J. Macek, K. Chaldakov, G. & Vankov, V. (1987). Collagen and Elastin Synthesis in the Aorta of Spontaneously Hypertensive Rats. *Blood Vessels*, Vol. 24, No.6, pp. 313-320

DeLano, F. & Schmid-Schonbein, G. (2007). Proteinase Activity In The Spontaneously Hypertensive Rat: Free Radical Production, Receptor Cleavage, and Insulin Resistance. *FASEB J*, No.21,pp. 422

DeLano, F. & Schmid-Schönbein, G. (2008). Proteinase Activity and Receptor Cleavage. Mechanism for Insulin Resistance in the Spontaneously Hypertensive Rat. *Hypertension*, No.52, pp. 415-423

Dimitrova, A. Stoilova, I. Atanasova, M. Georgieva, M. Russeva, A. Strashimirov, D. & Tzachev, K. (2009). Anti-AGE Antibodies and Serum Concentration of Zinc, Copper and Selenium in Patients with Occupational Vegetative Polyneuropathy of Upper Limbs. *J Biomed Clin Res.* No.2, pp. 31-35

Dimitrova, A. Atanasova, M. Georgieva, M. Ruseva, A. Strashimirov, D. & Baydanoff, S. (2010). Anti-AGE Antibodies and Markers of Oxidative Stress in Spontaneously Hipertensive Rats at Different Ages. *J Biomed Clin Rec.* Vol.3, No.1, pp. 33-39

Gibbons, G. & Dzau V. (1994).The Emerging Concept of Vascular Remodeling. *N Engl J Med;* 330:1431-1438

Han, W. Wu, L. Zhou, H. Zhang, J. Che, Z. Wu, Y. Liu, J. Zhu, D. & Gao, P. (2009). Changes in the Composition of the Thoracic Aortic Wall in Spontaneously Hypertensive Rats Treated with Losartan or Spironolactone. *Clin Exp Pharmacol Physiol.* May;36(5-6), pp. 583-538

Jacob, MP. Badier-Commander, C. Fontaine, V. Benazzoug, Y. Feldman, L. & Michel, JB. (2001). Extracellular Matrix Remodeling in the Vascular Wall. *Pathol Biol (Paris)*, No.49, pp. 326–332

Jacob, MP. (2003). Extracellular Matrix Remodeling and Matrix Metalloproteinases in the Vascular Wall During Aging and in Pathological Conditions. *BiomedPharmacother*, No.57, pp. 195–202

Jacob, MP. (2006). Extracellular Matrix and Vascular Ageing. *Med Sci* (Paris); No. 22, pp. 273-278

Keeley, F. Morin, J. &Vesely, S. (1984). Characterization of Collagen from Normal Human Sclera. *Exp Eye Res*, No.39, pp. 533-542

Konova, E. Baydanoff, S. Atanasova, M. and Velkova, A. (2004). Age-related changes in the glycation of human aortric elastin. *Exp Gerontol*, Vol. 39, No.2, pp. 249-254

Lakatta, E. (2003). Arterial and Cardiac Aging: Major Shareholders in Cardiovascular Disease Enterprises. Part III: Cellular and Molecular Clues to Heart and Arterial Aging. *Circulation*, No.107, pp. 490-497.

Laurent, S. (1995). Arterial Wall Hypertrophy and Stiffness in Essential Hypertensive patients. *Hypertension*, No.26, pp. 355–362

Marque, V. Kieffer, P. Atkinson, J. Lartaud-Idjouadiene, I. (1999). Elastic Properties and Composition of the Aortic Wall in Old Spontaneously Hypertensive Rats. *Hypertension*. No.34, pp. 415-422

McNulty, M. Spiers, P. McGovern, E., Feely, J. (2005). Aging is Associated with Increased Matrix Metalloproteinase-2 Activity in the Human Aorta. *Am J Hypertens*, No.18, pp. 504-509

Mecham, R. & Davis, E. (1994). Elastic Fiber Structure and Assembly. In: *Extracellular Matrix Assembly and Structure.* Yurchenko, P. Birk, D. Mecham, R. Ed. Academic Press, pp. 281-310

Monnier, V. Kohn, R. & Cerami, A. (1984). Accelerated Age-Related Browning of Human Collagen in Diabetes Mellitus. *Proc Natl Acad Sci,* USA, No. 81, pp. 583-587

O'Rourke, M. (2007). Arterial Aging: Pathophysiological Principles. *Vasc Med,* No.12, pp. 329-341

Partridge, S. Davis, H. & Adair, G. (1955). The chemistry of connective tissues soluble proteins derived from partial hydrolysis of elastin. *Biochem J,* Vol.61, pp. 11-15

Potenza, M. Marasciulo, F. Chieppa, D. Brigiani, G. Formoso, G. Quon, M. Montagnani, M. (2005). Insulin Resistance in Spontaneously Hypertensive Rats (SHR) Is Associated With Endothelial Dysfunction Characterized by Imbalance Between NO and ET-1. *Am J Physiol Heart Circ Physiol* , No.289, pp. H813-H822

Samila, Z. & Carter, S. (1981). The Effect of Age on the Unfolding of Elastin Lamellae and Collagen Fibers with Stretch in Human Carotid Arteries. *Can J Physiol Pharmacol,* No.59, pp. 1050-1057

Sauvage, M. Osborne-Pellegrin, M. Deslandes-Le Flohic, F. & Jacob, MP. (1999). Influence of Elastin Gene Polymorphism on the Elastin content of the Aorta. *Arterioscler Thromb Vasc Biol.* No.19 pp. 2308-2315

Tsoporis, J. Keeley, F. Lee, W. & Leenen, H. (1998). Arterial Vasodilatation and Vascular Connective Tissue Changes in Spontaneously Hypertensive Rats. *Journal of cardiovascular pharmacology,* Vol.31, No.6, pp. 960-62

Vasdev, S. Gill, V. Singal, P. (2007). Role of Advanced Glycation End Products in Hypertension and Atherosclerosis: Therapeutic Implications. *Cell Biochem Biophys,* Vol.49, No.1, pp. 148-63

Vlassara, H. (1994). AGE-receptors and in vivo biological effects of AGEs. In: Labuza T., Reineccius, G. Monnier, V. O'Brien, J. Baynes, J. (eds). Maillard Reactions in Chemistry, Food and Health. *The Royal Society of Chemistry,* UK. Vol.151, pp. 254-261

Woessner, J. (1961).The Determination of hydroxyproline in Tissue and Protein Samples Containing Small Proportions of This Amino Acid. *Arch Biochem Biophys.* No. 93, pp. 440-447

Wolinsky, H. (1972). Effects of Androgen Treatment on the Male Rat Aorta. *J Clin Invest,* No.51, pp. 2552-2555

Yan, S. Schmidt, A. Anderson, G. et al. (1994). Enhanced Cellular Oxidant Stress by the Interaction of Advanced Glycation End Products with Their Receptors. *J Biol Chem.* No. 269, pp. 9889-9897

Yang, Z. Makita, Z. Horii, Y. et al. (1991). Two Novel Rat Liver Membrane Proteins that Bind Glycosylation End Products: Relationship to Macrophage Receptor for Glucose-Modified Proteins. *J Exp Med,* No.174, pp. 515-524

Zanchi, A. Brunner, H. & Hayoz, D. (1997). Age-related Changes of the Mechanical Properties of the Carotid Artery in Spontaneously Hypertensive Rats. *J Hypertens,* No.15, pp. 1415–1422

Zieman, S. & Kass, D. (2003). Advanced Glycation end Products Cross-Linking: Pathophysiologic Role and Therapeutic Target in Cardiovascular Disease. *Congestive Heart Failure* , No. 10, pp. 144-151, ISSN 1751-7133

22

Calcium Regulation in Neuronal Function with Advancing Age: Limits of Homeostasis

John N. Buchholz[1], William J. Pottorf[2], Conwin K. Vanterpool[3], Erik J. Behringer[4] and Sue P. Duckles[5]
[1]*Department of Physiology and Pharmcology, Loma Linda University, School of Medicine, Loma Linda, California*
[2]*Department of Medical Affairs, Aztra Zeneca, Wilmington, Deleware*
[3]*Department of Biological Sciences, Alabama A&M, Normal, Alabama*
[4]*Department of Medical Pharmacology and Physiology, University of Columbia, Columbia, Missouri*
[5]*Department of Pharmacology, College of Medicine, University of California, Irvine, California*
USA

1. Introduction

Neurons are specialized excitable cells that transmit information to other neurons or to end effector cells such as skeletal muscle, heart muscle and blood vessel smooth muscle cells, maintaining posture, locomotion and cardiovascular function. Transmission of information from neurons to effector cells usually involves secretion of neurotransmitters contained in clustered pools of synaptic vesicles. This unique anatomical arrangement allows for rapid response to the stimulus of calcium influx and sustained release of neurotransmitters under low and higher frequency conditions (Peirbone *et al.*, 1995; Siksou *et al.*, 2011).

Calcium is hypothesized to act as a universal second messenger in excitable cells; a large volume of literature spanning more than 30 years supports this idea. Calcium integrates multiple neuronal cell functions including initiation of neurotransmitter release, regulation of gene expression, proliferation, excitability and plasticity, and activation of cell death pathways in apoptosis (Malenka *et al.*, 1989; Choi, 1992; Berridge, 1995, 1998; Clapham, 1995; Ginty, 1997; Wuytack *et al.*, 2002; Cavazzini *et al.*, 2005).

In resting neurons a large electrochemical gradient of approximately 10,000-fold exists between the extracellular environment and the cytosol; this physical arrangement allows for rapid activation of transmitter release via mobilization of release vesicles. In peripheral neurons including sympathetic neurons, calcium signaling begins with rapid opening of voltage-gated L, N and some R type calcium channels allowing calcium to enter the cytosol (Kostyuk, 1989; Kostyuk *et al.*, 1993; Trouslard *et al.*, 1993; Vanterpool *et al.*, 2005). More recently the nomenclature of L, N and R type channels has taken on increased complexity due to definition of differences in their activation voltages, coding genes and hence amino acid sequences of the α_1-subunits that comprise the channel pore (Catterall *et al.*, 2005). For example L and N type channels have been divided into five groups: $Ca_v1.1$. Ca_v 1.2, Ca_v 1.3 and Ca_v 1.4 (L-type) and Ca_v 2.2 (N-type). R type channels, originally termed "residual" because they are resistant to dihidropyridines, which block L-type channels and omega conotoxin, which blocks N-type channels (Catteral *et al.*, 2005), are now denoted as Ca_v 2.3. Given the importance of precise neuronal signaling and the need for regulatory mechanisms to sustain efficient signaling, a number of additional cellular mechanisms play a critical role in modulating cellular calcium. These complex calcium regulatory mechanisms are illustrated in figure 1(A). Following the activation of calcium influx through voltage-gated calcium channels, much of the calcium increase is immediately dampened by multiple calcium buffering proteins (Dove *et al.*, 2000). Despite this rapid calcium buffering, functional signaling is sustained by rapid release of calcium from smooth endoplasmic reticulum (SER) stores. This process has been termed calcium-induced calcium release (CICR) and is mediated by calcium activation of ryanodine receptor (RyR) channels (Belan *et al.*, 1993; Verkhratsky & Shmigol, 1996; Usachev & Thayer, 1997, 1999a,b; Verkhratsky & Petersen, 1998; Akita & Kuba, 2000; Berridge 2002; Behringer et al., 2009[a]).

A variety of additional calcium buffering systems can be activated by a rise in intracellular calcium ($[Ca^{2+}]i$), depending on both the magnitude and duration of the $[Ca^{2+}]i$ transient. Buffering systems include calcium-buffering proteins, energy dependent SER Ca^{2+} ATPases (SERCA), plasmalemmal Ca^{2+}-ATPases (PMCA), mitochondrial Ca^{2+}/H^+ symporters and Na^+/Ca^{2+}-exchangers. All of these calcium buffering systems act to modulate the shape and magnitude of stimulus-evoked $[Ca^{2+}]i$ transients and contribute to restoration of $[Ca^{2+}]i$ levels (Werth & Thayer, 1994; Buchholz *et al.*, 1996; Werth*et al.*, 1996; Usachev & Thayer, 1999a; Pottorf *et al* ., 2000[a,c], 2002; Wuytack *et al.*, 2002). Furthermore, the SERCA function and the CICR process are interdependent, as SERCA pumps not only buffer $[Ca^{2+}]i$ transients but also refill SER calcium stores. This interdependence maintains CICR during repeated neuronal activation (Vanterpool *et al.*, 2005). Disruption of any of these mechanisms with advancing age may result in altered function and health of peripheral neurons. This chapter will focus on the impact of advancing age, from young adult to senescence, on the function of adrenergic nerves and the mechanisms by which alterations in function may be related to age-related changes in modulation of $[Ca^{2+}]i$ with ongoing neuronal activity. Data from seminal studies on function of peripheral sensory and central neurons will also be included as important background for understanding the impact of age on adrenergic nerves.

2. Adrenergic neurons arising from the Superior Cervical Ganglion as an important study model

The superior cervical ganglion (SCG) is a peripheral neuroendocrine center, as many tissues receive adrenergic input from the SCG (Cardinali et al., 1981). For example, cardiac output, a function of heart rate and stroke volume, is modulated via the SCG. The SCG relays cardioregulatory signals from the central nervous system (CNS) via the SCG axons terminating in the heart. These nerves release noradrenaline (NA) and increase heart rate and contractile tension through β_1-adrenergic receptors (Wingerd *et al.*, 2004). Furthermore, these nerves are implicated in sudden cardiac death following myocardial infarction (MI), as the density of adrenergic innervation increases after MI resulting in severe arrhythmias (Chen *et al.*, 2001). Adrenergic nerve density within the SCG is maintained by neuronal growth factor (NGF); thus this trophic factor ensures proper function of these nerves in target tissues innervated by the SCG. Indeed, there is an age-related decline in NGF; however, the trophic response of aged peripheral adrenergic nerves to added NGF is maintained (Cowen & Gavazzi, 1998; Isaacson & Crutcher, 1998; Dickason & Isaacson, 2002). Loss of NGF during the aging process may have implications for the function of target organs innervated by the SCG. Nevertheless, peripheral neurons can still respond to trophic influences later in life.

Within the rat cerebrovasculature, sensory and adrenergic innervation of blood vessels is complete within the first 30 days of life (Tsai et al., 1989). In addition, adrenergic innervation of cerebral blood vessels influences vascular development and motor function, and the presence of a functional innervation is critical for maintenance of angiogenesis and the modulation of contractile function. For example, in rabbits aged 3–20 weeks, removal of the SCG results in loss of vascular smooth muscle mass, reduced wall thickness and attenuated contractile responses to NA (Bevan & Tsuru, 1981).

Hemorrhagic stroke is a major issue in human health in terms of morbidity, mortality, and health care costs, accounting for about 10% of cerebrovascular disease. Risk factors include low birth weight, premature birth, maternal hypertension and age over 60 years. (Martyn *et. al.*, 1996; Abbott *et. al.*, 2003; Zhang *et. al.*, 2003; Lawes *et. al.*, 2004; Hermes-Desantis and Clyman, 2006; Barker 2008). Constriction or dilation of cerebral blood vessels in response to changing pressure is termed autoregulation and serves to maintain cerebral blood flow (CBF) constant over a normal systolic pressure range of 60-120 mmHg (Faraci and Heisted, 1998; Zhang *et al.*, 2003). Sympathetic nerves arising from the SCG provide a short-term mechanism to increase the upper limit of autoregulation of cerebral blood flow. When systolic pressures exceed ~140 mmHg, activation of sympathetic nerves is important in activating further constriction of cerebral blood vessels to further protect from forced dilation and rupture (Faraci and Heisted 1998; Furuichi *et al.*, 1999; vanLieshout and Secher, 2008). In humans, acute hypercapnia elevates arterial pressure and CBF, which is attenuated by sympathetic nerve activity (Jordan *et al.*, 2000). In lambs with elevated systolic pressures above 140 mmHg or elevated systolic pressure during REM sleep, sympathetic discharge from the SCG significantly increases (Cassaglia *et. al.*, 2008, 2009). Thus, increased activity of the SCG in response to elevated blood pressure helps to protect cerebral blood vessels from rupture.

Studies on how neural input regulates cerebrovascular tone and blood flow have underscored the importance of the "neurovascular unit" in brain function. The combination of neuronal input to vascular smooth muscle and the inherent contractile properties of smooth muscle provide for the optimum function of cerebral blood vessels (reviewed by Hamel, 2006). Given that adrenergic nerves arising from the SCG innervate numerous organs including cerebral blood vessels and the importance of the homeostatic modulatory function of blood vessels in the brain, our group has chosen to focus our aging studies on this neuronal model.

3. General overview of calcium regulation in aging neurons

The 20th century brought extraordinary gains in public health, medicine and food production. These gains have resulted in increased life span with a progressive decline in the ratio of people less than 20 years old to those aged 65 and older (Gems, 2011). Aging is a natural and progressive process and has been suggested to involve a combination of factors including genetic and environmental influences, altered hormonal levels and an inborn aging process. Exquisite studies have shown that the rate of the aging process in animal models can be altered by genetic manipulations resulting in reduction of insulin growth factor 1 signaling and reduced oxidative stress. (Harman, 1998; Guarente & Kenyon, 2000; Clancy *et al.*, 2001; Tatar *et al.*, 2001; Troen, 2003). More recently androgen replacement has been shown to reverse age-related cognitive declines in male rats (Frye *et al.*, 2010). These data suggest that androgenic hormones play a role in modulating neuronal function, and hormone replacement may attenuate and/or restore changes in cognition that occur with advancing age. Caloric restriction in animal models has also been shown to prolong lifespan and reduce age-related morbidity and organ pathology via reduced oxidative stress that accompanies metabolism (Bodkin *et al.*, 2003; Forster *et al.*, 2003). However, these outstanding studies on caloric restriction, hormone replacement, reduced oxidative stress, and lifespan do not fully explain age-related changes in the function of critical organ and neuronal systems or the vulnerability of particular physiological processes to advancing age.

As discussed above, ionized free calcium is a ubiquitous second messenger in neurons serving as both a charge carrier and chemical intermediate linking physiological stimuli to intracellular effectors (Friel and Chiel, 2008). Subtle age-related declines in mechanisms that modulate stimulation-evoked increases in $[Ca^{2+}]i$ have been hypothesized to contribute to age-related neuronal dysfunction and degeneration; this has became known as the "calcium hypothesis" of neuronal aging (Khachaturian, 1987; Landfield, 1987). Indeed subtle declines in mechanisms that modulate $[Ca^{2+}]i$ levels may be responsible for the elevated resting cytosolic $[Ca^{2+}]i$ that has been seen in several types of peripheral and central neurons in tissue culture, as well as in acutely isolated tissue slices or neurons (Kirischuk & Verkhratsky, 1996; Verkhratsky & Toescu, 1998; Raza *et al.*, 2007). One potential consequence of an age-related decline in regulation of intracellular calcium is that calcium overload increases mitochondrial calcium uptake, in turn activating caspases that mediate neuronal cell apoptosis, reducing neuronal survival with age (Ichas & Mazat, 1998; Thibault *et al .*, 1998; Begley *et al .*, 1999; Toescu, and Verkhratsky, 2007).

As the population ages there is an increased incidence of age-related pathology, leading to a tendency to assume a general age-related deterioration in cellular function, including calcium regulatory processes, leading to increased susceptibility to pathology and cell death (Porter *et al.*, 1997). However, this common assumption does not take into account that human populations in developed countries are living longer and healthier than at any point within history (Gems, 2011). Thus, with regards to the function of cellular mechanisms that regulate $[Ca^{2+}]i$ homeostasis, a change in the function of one system may actuate compensatory calcium regulatory mechanisms maintaining some degree of neuronal function in senescent neurons or during acute insults such as stroke (Murchinson & Griffith, 1998; Verkhratsky & Toescu, 1998; Lee *et al.*, 1999; Griffith *et al.*, 2000; Pottorf *et al.*, 2000[a], 2002; Buchholz *et al.*, 2007). Studying normal aging in the absence of pathology, healthy aging, offers the most promise in trying to understand fundamental aging processes.

4. Aging alters function of adrenergic neurons via multiple mechanisms

There is a correlation between risk of stroke and advancing age, which is associated with an age-related increase in systolic blood pressure (Faraci & Heisted, 1998; Abbott *et al.*, 2003;

Zhang *et al.*, 2003; Lawes *et al.*, 2004). Systolic blood pressure rises with age in both F344-rats and humans; this is correlated with rising plasma catecholamine levels. Thus there may be fundamental age-related changes in the function of peripheral adrenergic nerves, vascular responses to NA and ability to modulate circulating levels of NA (Palmer *et al.*, 1978; Esler *et al.*, 1981[a,b]; Barnes *et al.*, 1982; Yu *et al.*, 1985; Insel, 1993). The concept of altered function of peripheral adrenergic nerves with advancing age is supported by our *in vitro* studies showing that stimulation-evoked fractional NA release increases with age in the rat tail and superior mesenteric arteries (Buchholz & Duckles, 1990; Buchholz *et al.*, 1998). In addition, this age-related increase in NA release occurs over a wide range of stimulation frequencies from 0.5 - 8 Hz (Tsai *et al.*, 1995). An explanation for the observed age-related change in function of vascular adrenergic neurons is complex, involving multiple mechanisms such as changes in density of adrenergic neurons, NA content, re-uptake, function of prejunctional inhibitory α_2-autoreceptors, and calcium regulation (Pottorf *et al.*, 2000[b]). In addition, other mechanisms may also modulate the function of adrenergic nerves, and these complicating factors must also be addressed. For example, our studies and others have shown that the SCG (Dun *et al.*, 1995; Wu *et al.*, 1997) and the cerebral vasculature contain adrenergic and neuronal nitric oxide (nNOS) containing nerves; NO released from nNOS neurons facilitates stimulation-evoked NA release in both blood vessels and the CNS (Montague *et al.*, 1994; Yamamoto *et al.*, 1997; Zhang *et al.*, 1998; Lee *et al.*, 2000; Mbaku *et al.*, 2000, 2003). Facilitated function of adrenergic nerves via nNOS nerves may occur through enhancement of Ca^{2+} influx and/or Ca^{2+}release from internal stores. These mechanisms may also be altered with age and cannot be discounted in future discussions on the impact of age on function of adrenergic nerves.

4.1 Neurotransmitter content and density of adrenergic nerves with advancing age

In peripheral organs and blood vessels NA content serves as an index of adrenergic density. In the rat heart, NA content decreases with age (Martinez *et al.*, 1981; Dawson & Meldrum, 1992), while in blood vessels the story is more opaque. NA content in rat renal, femoral, and saphenous arteries increases with age, while in renal, femoral, and saphenous veins there is no change, and a decline in tail arteries (Handa & Duckles, 1987). Consistent with measurements of NA content in rat arteries, catecholamine histofluorescence, another measure of adrenergic nerve density, increases with age in rat superior mesenteric and renal arteries and portal vein (Mione *et al.*, 1988). In contrast spinal cord blood vessels show no age-related change in adrenergic nerve density (Amenta *et al.*, 1990). In two studies by the same group sympathetic innervation in the internal carotid artery and anterior cerebral arteries was found to decline with age. Interestingly after intracerebral infusion of NGF, the number of sympathetic axons, NA content and numbers of tyrosine hydroxylase-containing nerve fibers increased in these same arteries from aged animals (Isaacson & Crutcher, 1998; Dickason & Isaacson, 2002). These studies would suggest that there is an innate age-related ability to maintain a critical number of functioning sympathetic neurons. The NGF studies cited above open up possibilities for therapeutic interventions to maintain cardiovascular homeostasis with advancing age. However, there is no clear relationship between age-related changes in adrenergic nerve density, increases in circulating plasma NA levels reported by others and increased stimulation-evoked NA release in our earlier studies; age-related changes in NA content appear to be species or vascular bed dependent.

4.2 Transmitter uptake and function of inhibitory prejunctional α_2-adrenoceptors

NA concentration in the synaptic cleft is modulated by NA re-uptake and activation of prejunctional α_2-adrenceptors. The latter mechanism has been shown to attenuate NA release by decreasing stimulation-evoked calcium influx in adrenergic neurons by reducing the open probability of voltage-gated calcium channels (Schofield, 1990; Delcour & Tsien, 1993). These mechanisms control the moment-to-moment biophase concentrations of NA with ongoing vascular adrenergic nerve activity (Illes, 1986; Langer & Arbilla, 1990; Buchholz *et al.*, 1992; Insel, 1993; Esler *et al.*, 1995).

Chemical agents such as cocaine and deoxycorticosterone that block the neuronal and extraneuronal uptake of NA, respectively, are used to estimate the function of these systems. Neuronal and extraneuronal uptake of NA has been shown to be reduced with age in the atria and vas deferens in the pithed rat (Borton & Docherty, 1989; De Avellar *et al.*, 1990). These studies suggest that NA uptake declines with age in peripheral adrenergic nerves. In contrast, direct measurement of ^{3}H-NA uptake supports the idea that the function of NA uptake transporters does not change with age in peripheral adrenergic nerves (Duckles *et al.*, 1985). In other studies in the rat heart (Limas, 1975) and tail artery (Buchholz & Duckles, 1990), the effect of cocaine and deoxycorticosterone on NA uptake increased with advancing age. Reconciling these contrasting studies would appear difficult. However, in the tail artery model, when the measured release of NA in the presence of uptake blockers was corrected for total NA release in the absence of uptake blockers, there was no change with age (Buchholz & Duckles, 1990). Thus, age-related changes in the effectiveness of uptake blockers on NA may merely reflect age-related differences in NA concentrations within the junctional cleft of the model under study. If there is less or more NA released with age in a particular model, then the observed effectiveness of the uptake blockers may only reflect the concentration of NA in the synaptic cleft. Therefore, data in the tail artery model would suggest that NA uptake with advancing age remains as a constant fraction of the amount of NA released.

If the age-related increase in stimulation-evoked fractional NA release in peripheral adrenergic nerves cannot be explained by an age-related change in the function of NA transporters, an explanation must lie elsewhere, such as possible age-related changes in presynaptic inhibition of NA release. There are a number of studies aimed at measuring changes in the feedback function of prejunctional α_2-adrenoceptors. Measurements of NA overflow have shown an age-related decline in the effect of prejunctional α_2 -adrenoceptor antagonists in pithed rats, rat vas deferens, heart, and tail artery (Hyland & Docherty, 1985; Docherty & Hyland, 1986; Daly *et al.*, 1989; Buchholz & Duckles, 1990). On the surface these studies seem to offer support for the idea of a general age-related decline in the function of prejunctional α_2-adrenoceptors. However, the issue appears to be more complicated as the studies cited above used only single concentrations of competitive α_2-antagonists. In the rat tail artery, we measured NA overflow over a full concentration range of the competitive α_2-antagonist, idazoxan. We found that the sensitivity of the prejunctional α_2-adrenoceptors to idazoxan declined with advancing age; however, the maximal response to this drug was not altered with advancing age (Buchholz *et al.*, 1992). As fractional stimulation-evoked NA release increases with age, there would be more NA in the junctional cleft interacting with the α_2-adrenoceptor and increased competition between higher NA levels and an antagonist. Chemical competition between NA and the α_2-adrenoceptor antagonists may possibly reduce the apparent sensitivity of the applied antagonist and account for the decrease in the potency of α_2-adrenoceptor antagonists with age (Pottorf *et al.*, 2000b). In light of the studies cited above, age-related changes in NA release are not adequately explained in terms of age-related alterations in the function of NA uptake mechanisms or α_2-adrenoceptor function. Therefore, we looked at other mechanisms that may account for age-related changes in adrenergic nerve activity, including studies of stimulation-evoked NA release with altered extracellular calcium, calcium influx and altered calcium buffering capacity.

4.3 Role of calcium influx in transmitter release and the effect of altering buffering capacity on transmitter release in aged peripheral neurons

Our studies of the rat tail artery cited above showed that stimulation-evoked NA release increased with advancing age. However, altered function of NA uptake or prejunctional α_2-adrenoceptors appears to reflect increased concentrations of NA in the junctional cleft as opposed to real changes in function of these two systems. Thus, our attention was directed toward the possibility that age-related changes in stimulation-evoked NA release are due to changes in calcium regulation in the nerve endings. Calcium entry through voltage-gated calcium channels provides the secretory potential that initiates NA release in sympathetic neurons. Thus we carried out experiments to examine the effects of increased or lowered extracellular calcium, which alters the chemical driving force of calcium, on stimulation-evoked NA release in tail arteries of young and old rats using short or long stimulation protocols (Buchholz *et al.*, 1994). When extracellular calcium was reduced or elevated, stimulation-evoked fractional NA release declined or increased, respectively in tail arteries from both young and old animals. However, in senescent animals the reduction in extracellular calcium reduced stimulation-evoked NA release to a lesser degree while elevated extracellular calcium increased NA release to a greater degree than in the young animals. In addition, at the highest elevated extracellular calcium concentration, 7.5 mM, the increase in stimulation-evoked NA release was maintained in tail arteries from young animals but declined in tail arteries from senescent animals. The explanation for these results may be attributable a variety of possible functional changes, including altered calcium influx, buffering capacity, or sensitivity of the NA release mechanisms to stimulation-evoked increases in $[Ca^{2+}]i$. Indeed higher extracellular calcium significantly elevated NA release by a greater magnitude in old as compared to young tail arteries suggesting that stimulation-evoked $[Ca^{2+}]i$ transients may be greater and more sustained in adrenergic nerves in senescent animals. The significant decline in stimulation-evoked NA release from adrenergic nerves in tail arteries from old animals at the highest extracellular calcium concentrations suggests that older nerves no longer possess the ability to modulate high $[Ca^{2+}]i$ loads which may then become toxic.

Studies on the impact of age on calcium influx are mixed; calcium influx has been reported to increase with age in central neurons (Landfield & Pitler, 1984; Pitler & Landfield, 1990), decrease in peripheral neurons (Kostyuk *et al.*, 1993), or remain unchanged in central neurons (Murchinson & Griffith, 1996). Thus, we measured the impact of age on stimulation-evoked NA release employing three protocols, two of which involved calcium influx through calcium channels and a third where calcium channels were bypassed using the calcium ionophore, ionomycin (Tsai *et al.*, 1997). When we measured NA release from rat-tail arteries via transmural nerve stimulation or depolarization of nerves with high KCl,

NA release was greater in tail arteries from old as compared to young animals. These data could be explained in part by an age-related increase in calcium influx with age. However, when we bypassed voltage-gated calcium channels using the calcium ionophore, ionomycin, we found that the age-related increase in NA release persisted (Tsai *et al.*, 1997). In these experiments $[Ca^{2+}]i$ is elevated via an ionophore, so that $[Ca^{2+}]i$ buffering systems would be the primary mechanisms modulating the magnitude and duration of $[Ca^{2+}]i$ transients and hence transmitter release. While these data do not rule out the possibility that stimulation-evoked calcium increases with age in the rat tail artery model, these data also suggest that other mechanisms, such as $[Ca^{2+}]i$ buffering systems and/or the sensitivity of NA release to calcium, may also be altered with age.

We continued to test the hypothesis that an alteration in the function of $[Ca^{2+}]i$ buffering systems may contribute to the increase in NA release from rat tail arteries (Tsai *et al.*, 1997). In this set of experiments we measured stimulation-evoked NA release before and after the addition of a membrane permeant, non-endogenous $[Ca^{2+}]i$ chelator, 1,2-bis(o-aminophenoxy)ethane-N,N,N',N'-tetraacetic acid acetomethoxy ester (BAPTA). In the presence of BAPTA, stimulation-evoked NA release was attenuated to a greater extent in old arteries as compared to young, suggesting that age-related changes in NA release are in part due to altered calcium-buffering capacity. Overall, these studies suggest that age-related changes in NA release from peripheral adrenergic neurons appear to be due in part to altered $[Ca^{2+}]i$ handling mechanisms. However, age-related alterations in the sensitivity of NA release mechanisms per se have not been ruled out.

5. Alterations in neuronal calcium buffering and extrusion during aging in peripheral neurons

The magnitude and temporal properties of calcium signals are critical, and sustained high levels of $[Ca^{2+}]i$ can be toxic. Thus, calcium is tightly regulated by channels, pumps, exchangers and protein buffers that control the shape and duration of stimulation-evoked $[Ca^{2+}]i$ transients (Fig. 1A; Friel and Chiel 2008). Age-related changes in the function of any one or a combination of the components of this $[Ca^{2+}]i$ control system may alter the function of neurons and/or contribute to neuronal degeneration (Meldrum & Garthwait, 1990; Peterson, 1992; Verkhratsky *et al.*, 1994; Pottorf *et al.*, 2000b, 2002). Given the complex interplay between calcium influx and numerous buffering systems, declining function of one or more systems may possibly be compensated for by increased function of other mechanisms (Pottorf *et al.*, 2000b). Thus, in aging studies investigators cannot assume that a decline in one or more buffering systems automatically leads to cellular dysfunction, as other systems may be able to compensate for decline in a particular calcium buffering system. In this sense, senescent neurons may still maintain a degree of homeostasis even though the limits of that ability are narrower as compared to younger neurons.

The advent in the last 25 years of cell permeable dyes capable of rapid and reversible binding to calcium as $[Ca^{2+}]i$ levels change has contributed greatly to understanding the dynamics of cellular $[Ca^{2+}]i$ signaling. Quantification of dynamic $[Ca^{2+}]i$ transients is possible because the emission fluorescence intensity of these dyes is altered by reversible binding of calcium (Tsien *et al.*, 1985; Roe *et al.*, 1990; Thayer & Miller, 1990; Neher, 1995; Baylor and Hollingworth, 2000; Friel and Chiel, 2008). Microfluorometry coupled with calcium sensitive dyes has allowed investigators to measure the impact of advancing age on the mechanisms that modulate stimulation-evoked [Ca^{2+}]i transients and overall calcium homeostasis (Kirischuk *et al.*, 1992; Kirischuk & Verkhratsky, 1996; Neher, 1998; Baylor & Hollingworth, 2000; Pottorf *et al.*, 2002).

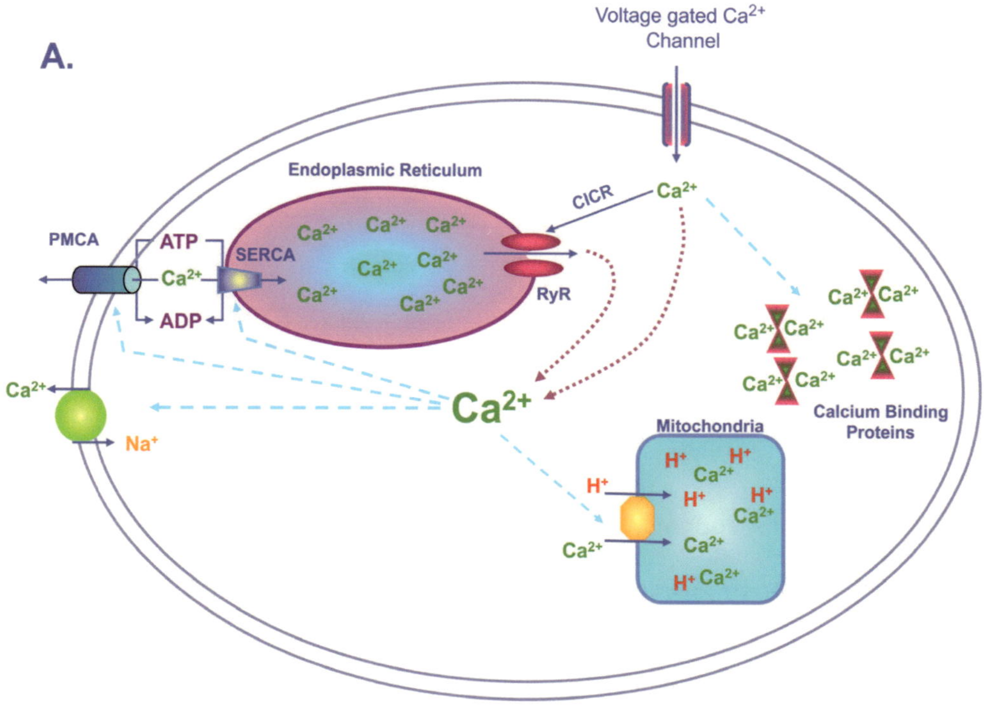

Fig. 1. (A) Representation of mechanisms that modulate stimulation-evoked [Ca^{2+}]i transients in peripheral adrenergic nerves. Depolarization elevates [Ca^{2+}]i via calcium influx through voltage-gated calcium channels. The calcium influx is immediately attenuated via calcium-binding proteins; however, the residual elevated calcium exceeding particular threshold will act on ryanodine receptors (RyR) to evoke "all or none" release of calcium from the endoplasmic reticulum known as calcium-induced calcium release (CICR). The elevation in [Ca^{2+}] is controlled by a dynamic interplay of multiple buffering systems, including: (1) smooth endoplasmic reticulum calcium ATPases (SERCA) sequestration of calcium into the ER that serves to buffer and refill ER calcium stores thus maintaining the ability of the neuron to undergo repetitive CICR; (2) mitochondrial calcium uptake by a H^+/Ca^{2+} uniporter; (3) removal of calcium via plasma membrane calcium ATPase (PMCA) pumps and the Na^+/Ca^{2+} exchanger. Plum dotted lines represent calcium influx and release pathways that elevate [Ca^{2+}]i. Light blue dashed lines represent calcium-buffering pathways that control increases in [Ca^{2+}]i and restoration to basal levels.

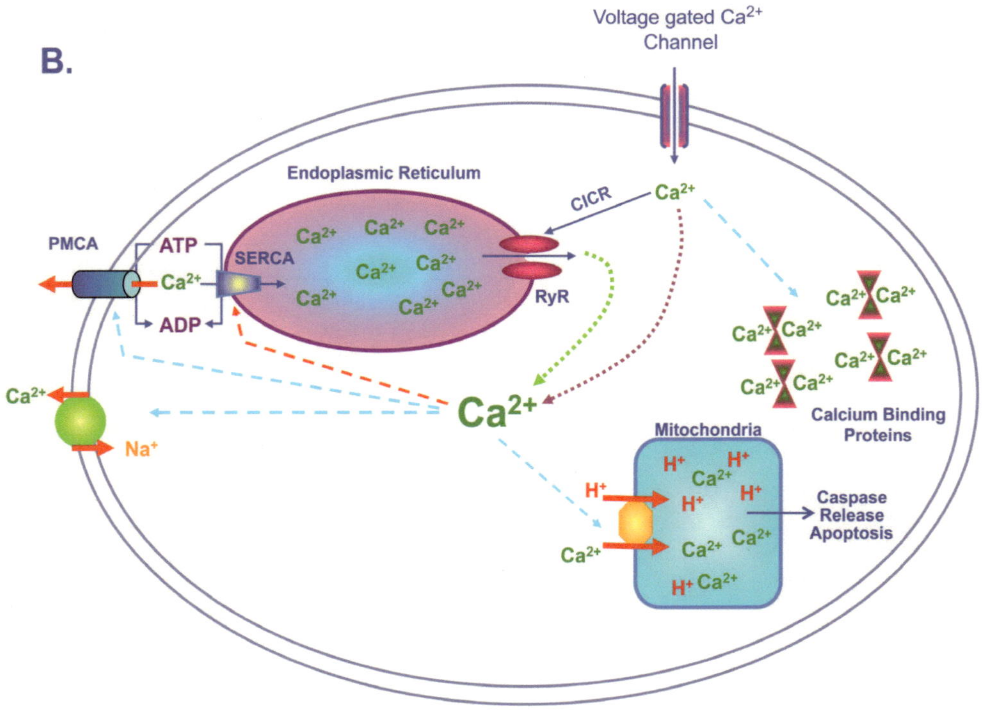

Fig. 1. (B) A model of the current hypothesis that advancing age, in the absence of pathology, results in a subtle decline in the control of $[Ca^{2+}]I$ in peripheral adrenergic neurons. Compensation by other control mechanisms may allow neurons to adapt to an age-related decline in control of $[Ca^{2+}]i$. This model illustrates the mechanisms that lead to elevated $[Ca^{2+}]i$ in aged peripheral adrenergic neurons. The rise in $[Ca^{2+}]i$ mediated via calcium influx and release from the SER is buffered by SERCA whose function declines with age (broken red line). In response to the decline in SERCA function, mitochondria, PMCA and Na^+/Ca^{2+} exchangers compensate (thick red solid lines) by increasing Ca^{2+} uptake and removal so as to preserve neuronal viability. However, increased mitochondrial calcium uptake may also reduce long-term neuronal survival by activation of caspases leading to apoptosis. Another feature of this model is that the decline in SERCA function in senescent neurons reduces ER Ca^{2+} filling levels and reduces CICR (bright green line).

5.1 Age-related changes in SERCA function in peripheral and central neurons

It has been suggested that an age-related decline in SERCA function contributes to calcium dysregulation in peripheral sympathetic and sensory neurons (Kirischuk *et al.*, 1992; Kirischuk & Verkhratsky, 1996; Pottorf *et al.*, 2002). Such a decline in SERCA function with age may also have additional consequences with regards to calcium signaling in neurons. The SER serves as a source of calcium that can be released by a process called CICR. SERCA buffer $[Ca^{2+}]i$ transients and reload the SER calcium stores with ongoing neuronal activity. Thus an age-related decline in SERCA function may possibly also cause alterations in CICR from the SER (Murchinson & Griffith, 1999; Usachev & Thayer, 1999a; Behringer *et al.*, 2009).

Studies of stimulation-evoked NA release in rat tail artery sympathetic neurons suggested age-related changes in SERCA function (Tsai *et al.*, 1998). When SERCA were blocked with the irreversible or reversible SERCA antagonists, thapsigargin or CPA respectively, stimulation-evoked NA release from sympathetic nerves increased only in tail arteries from young animals with no change in arteries from old animals. These data suggest that in sympathetic neurons from young animals SERCA-mediated calcium buffering modulates depolarization-induced $[Ca^{2+}]i$ transients and hence transmitter release. In contrast, in old animals, SERCA-mediated calcium buffering does not appear to affect transmitter release. To further explore this hypothesis, we measured intracellular calcium in isolated SCG cells and quantified the function of SERCA using reversible or irreversible SERCA blockers, cyclopiazonic acid and thapsigargin, respectively. Each of these agents caused a decline in the rate of recovery of high K^+-evoked $[Ca^{2+}]i$ transients only in cells from young animals with no significant change in old cells (Tsai *et al.*, 1998), supporting our conclusion that SERCA function is lost in sympathetic nerves of old animals.

In a more complex study using SCG cells, we blocked the contribution of PMCA's, mitochondria and the Na^+/Ca^{2+} exchanger and measured $[Ca^{2+}]i$ transients evoked by high K^+. To block PMCA and mitochondrial calcium buffering we utilized low concentrations of vanadate and dinitrophenol (DNP), respectively. To block the Na^+/Ca^{2+} exchanger we replaced Na^+ with the charge carrier tetra-ethyl ammonium. Under these conditions, neurons must rely on SERCA to modulate the rate of recovery of high K^+- evoked transients. Remarkably, with the loss of three calcium buffering systems, SERCA were still able to control the magnitude of $[Ca^{2+}]i$ transients and return elevated $[Ca^{2+}]i$ to resting levels. However, the rate of recovery of high $[Ca^{2+}]i$ transients was significantly slowed in SCG cells from both young and old animals with a significantly greater slowing in SCG cells from old animals (Pottorf *et al.*, 2000c). Thus one important mechanism that can account for a decline in $[Ca^{2+}]i$ homeostasis in aged peripheral neurons is a loss of SERCA function. One possible explanation for a decline in SERCA function is a decline in the genetic expression of SERCA isoforms. Indeed myocardial SERCA-mediated $^{45}Ca^{2+}$ uptake declines with age and there is a decline in genetic expression of SERCA isoforms (Maciel *et al.*, 1990). However, paradoxically, SERCA protein levels remain stable. This study suggests that, even if the genetic expression of SERCA may decline with age, changes in translation of mRNA coding for SERCA or alterations in mRNA stability may be able to compensate for the age-related decline in SERCA gene expression. Alternatively, alterations in mechanisms that modulate on-going SERCA activity, such as phosphorylation, may offer an explanation for the decline in SERCA function (Gafni & Yuh, 1989; Xu & Narayanan, 1998). Indeed, more in-depth studies using a wider range of excitable cell models will be necessary to uncover the mechanisms that account for an age-related alteration in SERCA function.

5.2 Age and mitochondrial calcium buffering

The role of mitochondria in modulation of $[Ca^{2+}]i$ has been an area of intense study. Mitochondria can sequester calcium and act as a buffer using the energy contained in the proton motive force and a Ca^{2+}/H^+ symporter to transport cytosolic calcium into the mitochondria. Early studies suggested that mitochondria only buffer $[Ca^{2+}]i$ transients in excess of 2 μM which may occur only under excessive stimulation or pathological conditions (Nicholls, 1978, 1985). In contrast to this view, however, mitochondrial calcium uptake has been shown to produce a clear "mitochondrial set point" or shoulder in the shape of depolarization evoked $[Ca^{2+}]i$, transients in central and peripheral sensory neurons (Thayer *et al.*, 1994; Murchison *et al.*, 2004). Furthermore, proton motive force disruptors such as dinitrophenol (DNP) and carbonyl cyanide *m*-chlorophenyl hydrazone (CCCP) demonstrate the role of mitochondria in buffering normal $[Ca^{2+}]i$ transients (Thayer & Miller, 1990; Miller, 1991; Werth and Thayer, 1994; Buchholz *et al.*, 1996; Murchinson & Griffith, 1999; Colegrove *et al.*, 2000, Murchison *et al.*, 2004). Thus, it is clear that mitochondria play a role in shaping stimulation-evoked $[Ca^{2+}]i$ transients in central and peripheral sensory and sympathetic neurons under normal $[Ca^{2+}]i$ concentrations in the mid to high nanomolar ranges. Since mitochondria are an integral part of neuronal cellular calcium buffering mechanisms, either a decrease in mitochondrial calcium uptake or an increased reliance on mitochondria to control $[Ca^{2+}]i$ levels could potentially disrupt mitochondrial function leading to calcium overload and apoptosis.

There are studies in central neurons supporting an age-related decline in mitochondrial calcium uptake (Vitorica & Satrustegui, 1985; Villalba *et al.*, 1995; Satrustegui *et al.*, 1996). In a more recent study using basal forebrain neurons the addition of CCCP to dissipate the mitochondrial proton motive force significantly elevated both high K^+ and caffeine-evoked $[Ca^{2+}]i$ transients in neurons from 1-7 month-old rats with little effect in neurons from 24-27 month-old (Murchison *et al.*, 2004). These studies suggest a general decline in mitochondrial calcium buffering capacity accompanying the process of advancing age in CNS neurons.

However, the picture is quite different in peripheral neurons, such as those from the SCG or adrenergic nerve endings in blood vessels, where we have shown that mitochondrial calcium uptake actively participates in buffering high-K^+ evoked $[Ca^{2+}]i$ transients in neurons from old animals. Our studies suggest that, in peripheral neurons, the function of mitochondrial calcium uptake is preserved with advancing age. We first measured stimulation-evoked NA release from adrenergic nerve endings in tail arteries and blocked mitochondrial calcium uptake with DNP. In this case, stimulation-evoked NA release increased in arteries from old animals with no significant effect in young arteries (Tsai *et al.*, 1995). To follow up, SCG neurons were exposed to DNP to block mitochondrial calcium uptake, and $[Ca^{2+}]i$ transients were measured. The peak and rate of rise of high K^+-evoked $[Ca^{2+}]i$ transients were both increased in neurons from old animals with no significant effect in young neurons (Buchholz *et al.*, 1996). In another study we blocked PMCA, SERCA, and Na^+/Ca^{2+} exchangers from participating in calcium buffering in SCG neurons. Under these conditions the neurons must rely primarily on mitochondrial calcium uptake to regulate high K^+-evoked $[Ca^{2+}]i$ transients (Pottorf *et al.*, 2000a). A remarkable aspect is that, despite compromising multiple calcium modulatory systems, mitochondria were still capable of controlling $[Ca^{2+}]i$ transients in SCG neurons, and mitochondrial calcium uptake appeared to be preserved with advancing age. Overall, our studies in the SCG and adrenergic nerve endings suggest that mitochondrial calcium buffering is maintained with advancing age, and there is an increased tendency with age to rely on mitochondria to control $[Ca^{2+}]i$ transients. This increased reliance on mitochondria to modulate elevated $[Ca^{2+}]i$ may possibly place an added stress on aged neurons. Indeed in experiments using brain slices from mice, mitochondrial depolarization served as an index of mitochondrial calcium uptake in response to high K^+-evoked $[Ca^{2+}]i$ transients. Mitochondrial depolarization was observed in brain slices from both young and old mice; however, in old animals the rate of mitochondrial repolarization was significantly slower corresponding to slowed recovery of high K^+-evoked $[Ca^{2+}]i$ transients (Xiong *et al.*, 2002). Thus, increased reliance on mitochondrial calcium uptake with advancing age has a downside in the case of high neuronal activity in CNS neurons. As mitochondrial repolarization is slowed with advancing age, over time the ability of the mitochondria to sustain its buffering of repeated $[Ca^{2+}]i$ transients may be compromised.

All of the studies cited above are consistent in suggesting that mitochondrial calcium uptake is essential for modulation of $[Ca^{2+}]i$ transients with advancing age. However, as more stress is placed on mitochondria to control stimulation-evoked increases in $[Ca^{2+}]i$, the 'polarization state' which maintains the ability of the mitochondria to produce vital cellular energy and modulate $[Ca^{2+}]i$ transients may subtly decline over the lifespan (Toescu and Verkhratsky, 2007). Overall, with advancing age mitochondrial calcium uptake may become more central to controlling neuronal $[Ca^{2+}]i$ transients. Maintenance of mitochondrial function is critical to healthy aging as altered mitochondrial function is thought to play a role in the progression of age related diseases (Miller, 2005). Maintaining mitochondrial function with improved diet and exercise as humans age may reduce the burden of health-related costs that comes with an aging population (Duckles *et al.*, 2006).

5.3 Aging and the potential for PMCA to compensate for age-related declines in SERCA function

The PMCA and Na^+/Ca^{2+} exchange systems are two vital plasma membrane calcium-pumping mechanisms in peripheral and central neurons; each of these plays a role in buffering $[Ca^{2+}]i$ transients via extrusion of calcium from the cytosol. PMCA, like SERCA, requires energy and pumps calcium against the chemical gradient from the cytosol to the extracellular fluid. The Na^+/Ca^{2+} exchanger utilizes energy stored in the Na^+ gradient to pump calcium out of the cellular cytosol (Werth *et al.*, 1996; Blaustein & Lederer, 1999; Pottorf & Thayer, 2002; Pottorf *et al.*, 2006). A noted feature of the PMCA is that its activity can be elevated by a priming stimulus which induces prolonged elevated $[Ca^{2+}]i$ transients. Following prolonged elevation of $[Ca^{2+}]i$, the PMCA-mediated rate of recovery of depolarization-evoked $[Ca^{2+}]i$ is accelerated, and this elevated function can be retained for up to 40 min after the priming stimulus (Pottorf and Thayer, 2002). These studies suggest that some buffering systems are flexible and can elevate their function during times of high neuronal activity to protect the cell from $[Ca^{2+}]i$ overload. There are at least two mechanisms that can account for increased function of PMCA with sustained $[Ca^{2+}]i$ loads: induction of PMCA gene expression and interaction with calmodulin. Blocking SERCA function with SERCA antagonists combined with prolonged $[Ca^{2+}]i$ transients has been shown to induce PMCA gene expression (Kuo et al., 1997). Furthermore, accelerated function of PMCA with prolonged $[Ca^{2+}]i$ transients increased the interaction of calmodulin with PMCA (Pottorf & Thayer, 2002). Thus redundant calcium buffering components, along with functional alteration of some components mediated by molecular modulators, can compensate for a reduction in function of one or more calcium buffering components as illustrated by the case of prolonged $[Ca^{2+}]i$ transients. Further support for this proposition comes from studies showing that, in the failing myocardium, Na^+/Ca^{2+} exchanger levels increase as SERCA levels decline (Hasenfuss *et al.*, 1991).

Our studies of isolated SCG neurons lend direct support to the idea that multiple components of the calcium buffering system can compensate for a loss of SERCA function. As discussed above we found that, with advancing age, SCG neurons become more reliant on mitochondria to control high K^+-evoked $[Ca^{2+}]i$ transients. In a study with isolated SCG neurons, when both SERCA and mitochondrial calcium uptake were blocked with thapsigargin and DNP respectively, PMCA and Na^+/Ca^{2+} exchangers are required to control high K^+-evoked $[Ca^{2+}]i$ transients. In this case SCG neurons from both young and old animals were able to recover from high K^+-evoked $[Ca^{2+}]i$ transients (Tsai *et al.*, 1998). These data suggest that, in peripheral adrenergic neurons, plasma membrane calcium extrusion systems can by themselves control $[Ca^{2+}]i$, and their function is maintained with advancing age. In support of this study, we used a unique ATPase antagonist, vanadate, a compound that, at low concentrations (0.25 µM), selectively blocks PMCA function but does not significantly alter SERCA function. Under these conditions, the rate of recovery of $[Ca^{2+}]i$ transients was diminished to a greater extent in SCG neurons from old as compared to young animals (Pottorf *et al.*, 2000a). This shows again that PMCA function may be elevated to meet the calcium buffering demands that occur as SERCA function declines with advancing age. Although PMCA function has been reported to decline with age in synaptosomes derived from neurons in the CNS (Qin *et al.*, 1998), our studies suggest that during normal aging PMCA function in peripheral adrenergic neurons is maintained with age.

6. Consequences of age-related changes in SERCA function: Aging and SER calcium levels and the role of CICR in neuronal function

Neuronal function depends in part on release of calcium from the SER in response to $[Ca^{2+}]i$ elevation (Usachev & Thayer, 1997, 1999a,b; Behringer *et al.*, 2009). Rapid calcium buffers immediately dampen much of the calcium influx through voltage-gated calcium channels while rapid release of calcium from the SER sustains depolarization-evoked increases in $[Ca^{2+}]i$. This process has been termed CICR, is mediated by RyR channels and has been shown to be relevant in modulating release of neurotransmitters and hormones. For example, when RyR are blocked and hence CICR, excitatory or inhibitory post synaptic currents, indices of presynaptic transmitter release, significantly decline (Emptage *et al.*, 2001; Galante and Marty, 2003).

A unique feature of the CICR process, the "all or none" release of calcium from the SER, has been observed in peripheral sensory neurons (Usachev and Thayer, 1997). Using a combination of patch clamp and microfluorometry, $[Ca^{2+}]i$ was elevated with graded step depolarizations of varied time length. This method produces small graded elevations in $[Ca^{2+}]i$ until a "threshold" of $[Ca^{2+}]i$ is reached, and the full $[Ca^{2+}]i$ transient due to combined calcium influx and CICR is achieved. As CICR is mediated via the opening of RyR channels, agents such as caffeine, which sensitize RyR to calcium, reduce the threshold of $[Ca^{2+}]$ necessary to evoke CICR (Usachev and Thayer, 1997; reviewed by Usachev and Thayer, 1999a,b). In addition, ryanodine, which blocks RyR channel function can ablate CICR so that stimulation-evoked $[Ca^{2+}]i$ transients reflect calcium influx through calcium channels only (Usachev and Thayer, 1997; Behringer *et al.*, 2009).

As CICR is a regenerative process it is sustained during ongoing neuronal activity via refilling of the SER calcium stores through calcium influx and subsequent uptake into the

SER via SERCA pumps (Kostyuk & Verkhratsky, 1994; Verkhratsky *et al.*, 1994; Shmigol *et al.*, 1996). Therefore, it is clear that calcium pumps such as SERCA serve at least two functions, buffering of elevated $[Ca^{2+}]i$ and refilling $[Ca^{2+}]i$ stores to maintain calcium signaling via CICR. In CNS, SCG, and sensory neurons, SER calcium stores can be rapidly refilled by activation of voltage gated calcium channels or following depletion with caffeine they can spontaneously refill within 3–10 min via activation of store operated calcium channels (SOCC) (Friel & Tsien, 1992; Shmigol *et al.*, 1994, 1996; Usachev & Thayer, 1999b; Baba *et al.*, 2003; Vanterpool *et al.*, 2005).

SOCC channels have received much attention recently, and their function and modulation is an ongoing topic in excitable cell models (Cahalan, 2009). SOCC channels on the plasmalemma mediate a process called "store operated calcium entry." This is a complex process involving calcium-sensing proteins within the SER, STIM1 and STIM2, that activate SOCC. The STIM proteins contain calcium-binding sites, the "EF-hand domain", within the SER lumen and act as "sensors" of SER calcium levels. When SER calcium levels are high, STIM proteins form dimers, but when SER calcium levels fall calcium dissociates from the EF-hand domain, and the STIM proteins form oligomers and aggregate in puncta in the SER. STIM oligomers then interact with SOCC dimers to form SOCC tetramers, which conduct calcium (Cahalan, 2009). Calcium influx through SOCC coupled with SERCA-mediated calcium uptake allows for refilling of SER calcium stores.

Our work with adrenergic nerve endings and isolated SCG cells has consistently shown that SERCA-mediated calcium uptake is compromised in senescent animals. As SERCA function declines with age in the SCG, we studied the impact of advancing age on refilling and release of calcium from the SER. Two protocols were used to measure rapid depolarization-evoked refilling of SER calcium stores and spontaneous refilling following caffeine-evoked depletion of SER calcium stores in isolated Fura-2 loaded SCG neurons from rats aged 6-24 months. Following caffeine-evoked depletion of SER calcium stores, rapid high K^+-evoked refilling of these stores markedly declined in SCG cells from 20 and 24 month-old animals but not in 6 and 12 month-old animals. Next we measured spontaneous refilling of SER via the opening of SOCC channels and subsequent SERCA-mediated uptake of calcium into the SER following selective caffeine-evoked depletion of SER calcium stores. To ensure that the rising $[Ca^{2+}]i$ following caffeine-evoked depletion of SER calcium stores was mediated via activated SOCC, we used the SOCC blocker lanthanum which, indeed, abolished the influx of calcium. Spontaneous refilling of SER calcium stores significantly declined in SCG cells from 20 and 24 month-old animals. Overall, these data suggest that a functional consequence of reduced SERCA activity with advancing age is a compromise in the ability of SCG neurons to sustain release of $[Ca^{2+}]i$ during ongoing neuronal activity (Vanterpool *et al.*, 2005).

In a more recent series of experiments we tested the hypothesis that reduced refilling of SER calcium stores with advancing age would reduce the contribution of CICR to electrical field stimulation (EFS)-evoked $[Ca^{2+}]i$ transients in isolated SCG cells from 6, 12 and 24 month-old rats (Behringer et al., 2009). We used small, graded increases of applied EFS current at a constant stimulation train length. With this protocol and measuring the peak and rate of rise of $[Ca^{2+}]i$ we were able to estimate the contribution of CICR to EFS-evoked elevations in $[Ca^{2+}]i$. In the presence of ryanodine to block the contribution of CICR, peak and rate of rise of EFS-evoked $[Ca^{2+}]i$ transients were significantly reduced in SCG cells from both 6 and 12 month-old animals. In contrast, in SCG cells from 24 month-old animals ryanodine had no effect on peak or rate of rise of EFS-evoked $[Ca^{2+}]i$ transients. These data suggest that the contribution of CICR to calcium signaling in senescent SCG neurons is virtually absent, and function of calcium signaling in senescent SCG neurons is maintained only by calcium influx through voltage gated calcium channels (Behringer *et al.*, 2009). There are at least two possible mechanisms accounting for this precipitous loss of CICR in senescent neurons. The first is our demonstration of an age-related decline in SERCA function, which would result in depleted SER calcium levels with age. The second mechanism is that the function of RyR channels may also decline with age. Indeed caffeine is a ryanodine agonist and has been used to sensitize CICR to EFS-evoked $[Ca^{2+}]i$ transients (Usachev and Thayer, 1997). Thus, we tested the hypothesis that CICR may still possibly contribute to EFS-evoked $[Ca^{2+}]i$ transients in senescent neurons in the presence of the RyR agonist caffeine. Indeed, caffeine significantly increased EFS-evoked $[Ca^{2+}]i$ transients with short stimulation train lengths in SCG cells from 6, 12 and 24 month-old animals (Behringer *et al.*, 2009). These data suggest that although CICR from the SER may not contribute to calcium signaling in senescent SCG neurons, possibly due to a combination of reduced SERCA and RyR function, senescent neurons still retain some capacity for CICR in the presence of a RyR agonist.

7. Altered expression of ryanodine receptors (RyR) and modulators of CICR with advancing age

We have shown that the contribution of CICR to EFS-evoked $[Ca^{2+}]i$ transients is abolished with advancing age in SCG neurons; this may be a consequence of reduced SERCA and/or RyR function (Behringer et al., 2009). In this section we will discuss RyR function in more depth so as to illuminate possible age-related changes. As discussed above, release of calcium from the SER is mediated via RyR ion channels. RyR function is controlled both by gene expression and by secondary molecular modulators, which regulate the sensitivity of RyR to $[Ca^{2+}]i$ levels. For example, regulators of RyR play an important role in other excitable cells such as in the heart, and altered regulation of RyR appears to be a root cause of cardiac arrhythmias that occur in the elderly as well as in other pathological states (Marx and Marks, 2002). Thus, RyR are an important clinical target for therapeutic intervention in cardiovascular challenges faced by aging populations.

Modulators of RyR include FK506 binding protein, phosphorylation and intracellular molecules including cyclic adenosine diphosphate ribose (cADPr). FK506 inhibits the channel when bound to RyR, while phosphorylation of RyR reduces the binding of FK506, activating RyR by increasing its open probability (Danila and Hamilton, 2004). In the case of cADPr, in excitable cells including sympathetic neurons, this modulator can mobilize calcium from SER calcium stores and sensitize the RyR to elevated $[Ca^{2+}]i$, thus reducing the threshold of elevated $[Ca^{2+}]i$ necessary to evoke CICR (Galione, 1993; Hua *et al.*, 1994; Ogawa *et al.*, 2000; Hagashida et al., 2001; Marx & Marks, 2002). Furthermore, there are reports that RyR function is influenced by neuronal nitric oxide synthase (nNOS), via nitosylation of RyR by NO itself and modulation of cADPr levels (Galione, 1993; Eu *et al.*, 1999; Hagashida *et al.*, 2001; Balshaw *et al.*, 2002; Meissner, 2002).

Three isoforms of RyR are known; these are RyR1 (skeletal muscle), RyR2 (cardiac muscle and neurons), and RyR3 (neurons and other tissue types). All three have been shown to participate as calcium release channels responsible for CICR (Ogawa et al., 2000). Because RyR are integral components in [Ca^{2+}]i signaling in SCG neurons, we tested the hypothesis that, with advancing age, expression of the predominant RyR isoform(s) in adult rat SCG, along with selective modulators, is altered (Vanterpool *et al.*, 2006). For this study we used F-344 rats aged 6, 12 and 24 months and molecular techniques of reverse transcription polymerase chain reaction and enzyme-linked immunosorbent assays (ELISA). ELISA was used to measure RyR protein levels as these proteins are larger than 500 kDa, limiting the accuracy of Western blots.

Much to our surprise we found that RyR1 mRNA was undetectable in the rat SCG, in direct contrast with other studies demonstrating that RyR1 mRNA is expressed in excitable cells, including neurons (Fill & Copello, 2002). Thus, RyR1 does not appear to play a role in mediating CICR from SER calcium stores in the SCG, regardless of animal age. However, RyR2 and RyR3 mRNA are amply present in rat SCG, appearing to be the major receptor isoforms regulating calcium release from RyR-sensitive stores in all age groups. Furthermore, RyR3 mRNA and protein levels increased from 6 to 12 months and then decreased in senescent (24 month) animals, while RyR2 mRNA and protein levels remained constant with advancing age (Vanterpool *et al.*, 2006). From these data showing the impact of age on mRNA and protein levels of RyR3 it is difficult to make a straightforward conclusion. However, as discussed above, protein levels are not the only important measure of RyR function, as activity of these channels is be regulated by several factors.

Therefore, we extended our studies to investigate possible age-related changes in selected modulators of the RyR, including phosphorylation and nNOS levels which are known to modulate levels of cADPr (Vanterpool *et al.*, 2006). We found that total phosphorylation of RyR channels was not altered with age, suggesting that steady state phosphorylation of RyR and hence regulation by this mechanism does not necessarily change with advancing age. In contrast, however, nNOS protein levels increased from 6 to 12 months and significantly declined from 12 to 24 months. Since nNOS function modulates cADPr levels a reasonable inference is that cADPr levels may also decline with age. In the SCG, as there appear to be only two RyR contributing to calcium release, it is possible that the decline in RyR3 coupled with a decline in nNOS levels resulting in reduced cADPr may account in part for a decline in RyR function with age.

We have shown that caffeine-evoked release of calcium declines with age suggesting that the capacity of RyR to release calcium from the SER declines with advancing age. In addition, the contribution of CICR to EFS-evoked [Ca^{2+}]i transients is abolished in SCG cells from senescent animals (Vanterpool *et al.*, 2005; Behringer et al., 2009). Both agonist-mediated release of calcium from the SER and CICR activated via calcium influx depend on SER calcium filling levels, as well as modulation of RYR. Indeed, we have shown that SERCA function declines in the SCG (Tsai *et al.*, 1998; Pottorf *et al.*, 2000c). In light of these former studies a reasonable inference is that filling levels of the SER may be compromised, altering both agonist-mediated capacity of calcium release and activation of CICR from the SER.

8. Proposed model for age-related changes in [Ca2+]i regulation in peripheral adrenergic neurons

We have cited various reports and reviews suggesting that advancing age leads to [Ca^{2+}]i dysregulation and neuronal loss (Choi, 1992; Kirischuk & Verkhratsky, 1996; Ichas & Mazat,

1998; Thibault *et al.*, 1998; Begley *et al.*, 1999; Toescu and Verkhratsky, 2007). However, this hypothesis may be more applicable to pathological conditions as opposed to normal aging. For example, in our studies of peripheral adrenergic neurons, despite age-related changes in $[Ca^{2+}]i$ buffering which in turn alter $[Ca^{2+}]i$ signaling, the cells remain both viable and functional within reasonable limits. Thus, we pose another hypothesis: In the absence of any visible pathology, advancing age leads to subtle changes in the control of $[Ca^{2+}]i$ that may lead to altered neuronal function, but adjustments of other $[Ca^{2+}]i$ control mechanisms may allow neurons to adapt. This model is summarized in Fig. 1(B), emphasizing that loss of SERCA function may be compensated for by increased mitochondrial calcium uptake and plasma membrane calcium extrusion, so as to preserve some degree of cell viability in the face of advancing age. However, increased reliance on mitochondrial calcium buffering may have consequences for long-term viability as increased mitochondrial calcium may increase the chance of mitochondrial dysfunction and release of the apoptotic signals, caspases. This model also suggests that decline with age in SERCA function reduces SER calcium levels, thus reducing the contribution of CICR to overall calcium signaling in aging peripheral neurons.

9. Summary and conclusions

These data from our laboratory and supporting studies from others suggest that, in peripheral autonomic neurons in the absence of recognizable pathology, advancing age is a subtle and complex process that does necessarily lead to dramatic deterioration. Moreover, it is clear that advancing age does not alter the function of excitable neurons in a uniform manner, as we point out differences in the function of peripheral and central neurons with advancing age. With regards to age-related changes in $[Ca^{2+}]i$ regulation, we presented the idea that cell viability of peripheral neurons is maintained as they compensate for an age related decline in the function of at least one calcium-buffering system, SERCA, by increased function of other calcium-buffering systems, namely, the mitochondria and plasmalemmal calcium extrusion. Increased mitochondrial calcium uptake as a compensatory mechanism may leave the cell more susceptible to apoptosis which contributes to cell death (Ichas & Mazat, 1998; Thibault *et al.*,1998; Begley *et al.*, 1999; Toescu and Verkhratsky, 2007). This review summarizes the major findings in our work on the dynamics of $[Ca^{2+}]i$ regulation and possible consequences for autonomic nerve function with advancing age.

Based on results of our most current studies and reviews (Vanterpool *et al.*, 2005, 2006; Buchholz *et al.*, 2007; Behringer *et al.*, 2009) and our previous work and that of others we propose the following: With advancing age an alteration in $[Ca^{2+}]i$ signaling and function of peripheral adrenergic neurons results from a complex interplay of mechanisms, including increased sensitivity of the NA release mechanism to calcium, decline in SERCA function that alters calcium buffering and refilling of SER calcium stores, reduced RyR3 and decline in nNOS levels, which in turn modulates cADPr levels. This combination ultimately reduces the capacity of the SER to release calcium and abolishes the CICR process. With respect to the loss of CICR, this apparently leaves calcium influx as the primary mechanism to elevate $[Ca^{2+}]i$ in response to nerve activation, allowing some function to continue in senescent neurons. In addition, despite loss in the contribution of CICR to EFS-evoked $[Ca^{2+}]i$ transients, some residual CICR capacity is still retained if RyR are sensitized to elevated $[Ca^{2+}]i$ with an agonist. This latter observation offers some intriguing clinical possibilities to treat an age-related alteration in calcium signaling and hence peripheral neuronal function.

10. Future directions

Given advances in molecular techniques, including the explosion of knowledge of the function of micro RNA as inhibitors of mRNA translation and hence gene function (Saugstad, 2010), future studies are limitless. These may include investigations on the impact of advancing age on the genetic expression and protein levels of multiple buffering systems, including soluble calcium-buffering proteins, SERCA, mitochondrial calcium pumps, PMCA, and the Na^+/Ca^{2+} exchanger. Our work also strongly suggests that calcium influx through store operated calcium channels is compromised with age. Thus, genetic expression and function with advancing age of store operated channels may provide another fruitful avenue of research. Finally, all of our studies suggest that SER calcium levels decline with age, compromising CICR. New calcium indicators are now available to directly study SER calcium levels; this approach may allow more in depth studies of the impact of advancing age on SER calcium levels. These types of future studies and many more may be expected to provide more direct insight on how CICR may be altered with advancing age, potentially leading to novel therapeutic modalities to prevent and/or treat age- and disease-related alterations in neuronal and cardiovascular function.

11. References

Abbott RD, Curb JD, Rodriguez BL, Masaki KH, Popper JS, Ross GW and Petrovitch H (2003) Age-related changes in risk factor effects on the incidence of thromboembolic and hemorrhagic stroke. *J Clin Epidemiol* 56: 479-486.

Akita T and Kuba K. (2000) Functional triads consisting of ryanodine receptors, Ca^{2+} channels, and Ca^{2+}-activated K^+ channels in bullfrog sympathetic neurons: plastic modulation action potential. *J. Gen. Physiol.* 116: 697–720.

Amenta F, Bronzetti E, Ferrante F, Ricci A (1990) The noradrenergic innervation of spinal cord blood vessels in old rats. *Neurobiol. Aging* 11: 47–50.

Balshaw DM, Yamaguchi N, Meissner G (2002) Modulation of intracellular calcium-release channels by calmodulin. *J. Membr. Biol.* 185: 1–8.

Barker DJ (2008) Human growth and cardiovascular disease. *Nestle Nutr Workshop Ser Pediatr Program* 61:21-38.

Barnes RF, Rashkind M, Gumbrecht G, Halter JB (1982) The effects of age on the plasma catecholamine response to mental stress in man. *J. Clin. Endocrinol. Metab.* 54: 64–69.

Baylor SM and Hollingworth S (2000) Measurement and Interpretation of Cytoplasmic $[Ca^{2+}]i$ Signals From Calcium-Indicator Dyes. *News Physiol. Sci.* 15: 19-26.

Begley JG, Duan W, Chan S, Duff K, Mattson MP (1999) Altered calcium homeostasis and mitochondrial dysfunction in cortical synaptic compartments of presinilin-1 mutant mice. *J. Neurochem.* 72: 1030–1039. *Physiol.* 107: 1223-1234.

Behringer EJ, Leite LD, Buchholz NE, Keeney MG, Pearce WJ, Vanterpool CK, Wilson SM and Buchholz JN (2009[a]) Maturation and long-term hypoxia alters Ca^{2+}-induced Ca^{2+} release in sheep cerbrovascular sympathetic neurons. *J. Appl. Pysiol.* 107(4): 1223-1234.

Behringer EJ, Vanterpool CK, Pearce WJ, Wilson SM and Buchholz JN (2009[b]) Advancing age alters the contribution of calcium release from smooth endoplasmic reticulum stores in superior cervical ganglion cells. J. *Gerontol. A Biol. Sci. Med. Sci.* 64A(1): 34-44.

Belan P, Kostyuk P, Snitsarev V, Tepikin A (1993) Calcium clamp in isolated neurons of the snail *Helix pomatia. J. Physiol. (Lond.)* 462: 47–58.

Berridge MJ (1995) Calcium signaling and cell proliferation. *Bioessays* 17: 491-500.

Berridge MJ (1998) Neuronal calcium signaling. *Neuron* 21: 13-26.

Berridge MJ (2002) The endoplasmic reticulum: a multifunctional signaling organelle. *Cell Calcium* 32(5-6): 235-249, 2002.

Bevan RD, Tsuru H (1981) Functional and structural changes in the rabbit ear artery after sympathetic denervation. *Circ. Res.* 48: 478–485.

Blaustein MP, Lederer WJ (1999) Sodium/calcium exchange: its physiological implications. *Physiol. Rev.* 79: 763–854.

Bodkin NL, Alexander TM, Ortmeyer HK, Johnson E, Hansen BC (2003) Mortality and morbidity in laboratory-maintained Rhesus monkeys and effects of long-term dietary restriction. *J. Gerontol. A Biol. Sci. Med. Sci.* 58: 212–219.

Borton M, Docherty JR (1989) The effects of ageing on neuronal uptake of noradrenaline in the rat. *Naunyn Schmiedebergs Arch. Pharmacol.* 340: 139–143.

Buchholz JN, Behringer EJ, Pottorf WJ, Pearce WJ, Vanterpool CK (2007) Age-dependent changes in Ca^{2+} homeostasis in peripheral neurones: implications for changes in function. *Aging Cell* 6: 285-296

Buchholz J, Duckles SP (1990) Effect of age on prejunctional modulation of NE release. *J. Pharmacol. Exp. Ther.* 252, 159–164.

Buchholz J, Nikkah L, Duckles SP (1994) Age-related changes in the sensitivity of sympathetic nerves to altered extracellular calcium in tail arteries of F-344 rats. *Neurobiol. Aging* 15: 197–201.

Buchholz J, Sexton P, Hewitt W (1998) Impact of age on modulation of norepinephrine release from sympathetic nerves in the rat superior mesentery artery. *Life Sci.* 62: 679–686.

Buchholz J, Tsai H, Foucart S, Duckles SP (1996) Advancing age alters intracellular calcium buffering in rat adrenergic nerves. *Neurobiol. Aging* 17: 885–892.

Buchholz J, Tsai H, Friedman D, Duckles SP (1992) Influence of age on control of norepinephrine release from the rat tail artery. *J. Pharmacol. Exp. Ther.* 260: 722–727.

Cahalan MD (2009) STIMulating store-operated Ca^{2+} entry. *Nat. Cell Biol.* 11(6): 669-677.

Cardinali DP, Vacas MI, Gejman PV (1981) The sympathetic superior cervical ganglia as peripheral neuroendocrine centers. *J. Neural Transm.* 52, 1–21.

Cassaglia PA, Griffiths RI, Walker AM (2008) Sympathetic nerve activity in the superior cervical ganglia increases in response to imposed increases in arterial pressure. *Am J Physiol Regul Integr Comp Physiol* 294:R1255-1261.

Cassaglia PA, Griffiths RI, Walker AM (2009) Cerebral sympathetic nerve activity has a major regulatory role in the cerebral circulation in REM sleep. *J Appl Physiol.* 106:1050-1056.

Catterall WA, Perez-Reyes E, Snutch TP, Striessnig J (2005) International union of pharmacology. XLVII. Nomenclature and structure-function relationships of voltage-gated calcium channels. *Pharmacol. Rev.* 54(4): 411-425.

Cavazzini M, Bliss T, Emptage N (2005) Ca^{2+} and synaptic plasticity. *Cell Calcium* 38: 355-367.

Chen PS, Chen LS, Cao JM, Sharifi B, Karagueuzian HS, Fishbein MC (2001) Sympathetic nerve sprouting, electrical remodeling and the mechanisms of sudden cardiac death. *Cardiovasc. Res.* 50, 409–416.

Choi DW (1992) Excitotoxic cell death. *J. Neurobiol.* 23: 1261-1276.

Clancy DJ, Gems D, Harshman LG, Oldham S, Stocker H, Hafen E, Leevers SJ, Partridge L (2001) Extension of life-span by loss of CHICO, a drosphila insulin receptor substrate protein. *Science* 292, 104–106.

Clapham DE (1995) Calcium signaling. *Cell* 80: 259-268.

Colegrove SL, Albrecht MA, Friel DD (2000) Quantitative analysis of mitochondrial Ca^{2+} uptake and release pathways in sympathetic neurons. *J. Gen. Physiol.* 115: 371–388.

Cowen T, Gavazzi I (1998) Plasticity in adult and aging sympathetic neruons. *Prog. Neurobiol.* 54: 249–288.

Daly RN, Goldberg PB, Roberts J (1989) The effect of age on presynaptic α_2-adrenoceptor auto regulation of norepinephrine release. *J. Gerontol.* 44: B59–B66.

Danila CI, Hamilton SL (2004) Phosphorylation of ryanodine receptors. *Biol. Res.* 37: 521–525.

Dawson R Jr, Meldrum MJ (1992) Norepinephrine content in cardiovascular tissues from the aged Fischer 344 rat. *Gerontology* 38: 185–191.

De Avellar MCW, Kobashi YL, Markus RP (1990) Age-related changes in neuronal uptake of noradrenaline. *Naunyn Schmiedebergs Arch. Pharmacol.* 341: 295–300.

Delcour AH, Tsien RW (1993) Altered prevalence of gating modes in neurotransmitter inhibition of N-type calcium channels. *Science* 259: 980–983.

Dickason AK, Isaacson LG (2002) Plasticity of aged perivascular axons following exogenous NGF: analysis of catecholamines. *Neurobiol. Aging* 23: 125–134.

Docherty JR, Hyland L (1986) Alpha-adrenoceptor responsiveness in the aged rat. *Eur. J. Pharmacol.* 126: 75–80.

Dove LS, Nahm SS, Murchison D, Abbott LC and Griffith WH (2000) Altered calcium homeostasis in cerebellar Purkinje cells of leaner mutant mice. *J Neurophysiol* 84: 513–524.

Duckles SP, Carter BJ, Williams CL (1985) Vascular adrenergic neuroeffector function does not decline in aged rats. *Circ. Res.* 56: 109–116.

Duckles SP, Krause DN, Stirone C, Procaccio V (2006) Estrogen and mitochondria: a new paradigm for vascular protection. *Mol. Interv.* 6: 26–35.

Dun NJ, Dun SL, Chiba T, Forsterman U (1995) Nitric oxide synthase immunoreactive vagal afferent fibers in rat superior cervical ganglia. *Neuroscience* 65: 231–239.

Emptage NJ, Reid CA, Fine A (2001) Calcium Stores in Hippocampal Synaptic Boutons Mediate Short-Term Plasticity, Store-Operated Ca^{2+} Entry, and Spontaneous Transmitter Release. *Neuron* 29: 197-208.

Esler M, Jackman G, Bobik A, Leonard P, Kelleher LD, Skews H, Jennings G, Korner P (1981[a]) Norepinephrine kinetics in essential hypertension. Defective neuronal uptake of norepinephrine in some patients. *Hypertension* 3: 149-156.

Esler M, Skews H, Lionard P, Jackman G, Bobik A, Korner P (1981[b]) Age-dependence of noradrenaline kinetics in normal subjects. *Clin. Sci.* (*Lond*) 60: 217–219.

Esler MD, Thompson JM, Kaye DM, Turner AG, Jennings GL, Cox HS, Lambert GW, Seals DR (1995) Effects of ageing on the responsiveness of human cardiac sympathetic nerves to stressors. *Circulation* 91: 351–358.

Eu JP, Xu L, Stamler JS, Meissner G (1999) Regulation of ryanodine receptors by reactive nitrogen species. *Biochem. Pharmacol.* 57: 1079–1084.

Faraci FM and Heistad DD (1998) Regulation of the cerebral circulation: role of endothelium and potassium channels. *Physiol Rev* 78:53-97.

Fill M, Copello JA (2002) Ryanodine receptor calcium release channels. *Physiol. Rev.* 82: 893–922.

Forster MJ, Morris P, Sohal RS (2003) Genotype and age influence the effect of caloric intake on mortality in mice. *FASEB J.* 17: 690–692.A

Friel DD, and Chiel HJ (2008) Calcium dynamics: analyzing the Ca^{2+} regulatory network in intact cells. Trends Neurosci 31(1): 8-19.

Frye CA, Edinger KL, Edwin D. Lephart ED, Walf AA (2010) 3α-androstanediol, but not testosterone, attenuates age-related decrements in cognitive, anxiety, and depressive behavior of male rats. *Front. Aging Neurosci.* 15(2): 1-21.

Furuichi S, Endo S, Haji A, Takeda R, Nisijima M and Takaku A (1999) Related changes in sympathetic activity, cerebral blood flow and intracranial pressure, and effect of an alpha-blocker in experimental subarachnoid haemorrhage. *Acta Neurochir (Wien)* 141: 415-423; discussion 423-414.

Gafni A, Yuh KC (1989) A comparative study of the Ca^{2+}–Mg^{2+} dependent ATPase from skeletal muscles of young, adult and old rats. *Mech. Ageing Dev.* 49: 105–117.

Galante M, Marty A (2003) Presynaptic Ryanodine-Sensitive Calcium Stores Contribute to Evoked Neurotransmitter Release at the Basket Cell–Purkinje Cell Synapse. *J Neurosci.* 23(35): 11229-11234.

Galione A (1993) Cyclic ADP-ribose: a new way to control calcium. *Science* 259, 325–326.

Gems D (2011) Aging: To treat or not to treat. *Amer. Scientist* 99: 178-280.

Ginty DD (1997) Calcium regulation of gene expression: isn't that spatial? *Neuron* 18: 183-186.

Griffith WH, Jasek MC, Bain SH, Murchison D (2000) Modification of ion channels and calcium homeostasis of basal forebrain neurons during aging. *Behav. Brain Res.* 115: 219–233.

Guarente L, Kenyon C (2000) Genetic pathways that regulate ageing in model organisms. *Nature* 408: 255–262.

Hagashida H, Hashii, M Yokoyama S, Hoshi N, Chen XL, Egorova A, Noda M, Zhang JS (2001) Cyclic ADP-ribose as a second messenger revisited from a new aspect of signal transduction from receptors to ADP-ribosyl cyclase. *Pharmacol. & Therap.* 90: 283- 296

Handa RK, Duckles SP (1987) Influence of age on norepinephrine content in arteries and veins of Fischer 344 rats. *Neurobiol. Aging* 8: 511–516.

Hamel E (2006) Perivascular nerves and the regulation of cerebrovascular tone. *J Appl Physiol* 100:1059-1064.

Harman D (1998) Aging and oxidative stress. *J. Int. Fed. Clin. Chem.* 10: 24–27.

Hasenfuss G, Schillinger W, Lehnart SE, Preuss M, Pieske B, Maier LS, Prestle J, Minami K, Heizmann CW, Hunziker W (1991) Intracellular calcium-binding proteins: more sites than insights. *Trends Biochem. Sci.* 16: 98–103.

Hermes-DeSantis ER and Clyman RI (2006) Patent ductus arteriosus: pathophysiology and management. *J Perinatol* 26 Suppl 1: S14-18; discussion S22-23.

Hua SY, Tokimasa T, Takasawa S, Furuya Y, Nohmi M, Okamoto H, Kuba K (1994) Cyclic ADP-ribose modulates Ca^{2+} release channels for activation by physiological Ca^{2+} entry in bullfrog sympathetic neurons. *Neuron* 12: 1073–1079.

Hyland L, Docherty JR (1985) Further examination of the effects of ageing on the adrenoceptor responsiveness of the rat vas deferens. *Eur. J. Pharmacol.* 110: 241–246.

Ichas F, Mazat JP (1998) From signaling to cell death: two conformations for the mitochondrial permeability transition pore. Switchin from low- to high-conductance state. *Biocim. Biophys. Acta* 1366: 33–50.

Illes P (1986) Mechanisms of receptor-mediated modulation of transmitter release in noradrenergic, cholinergic and sensory neurones. *Neuroscience* 17: 909–928.

Insel PA (1993) Adrenergic receptors, G proteins, and cell regulation: implications for aging research. *Exp. Gerontol.* 28: 341–348.

Isaacson LG, Crutcher KA (1998) Uninjured aged sympathetic neurons response to exogenous NGF. *Neurobiol. Aging* 19: 333–339.

Jordan J, Shannon JR, Diedrich A, Black B, Costa F, Robertson D and Biaggioni I (2000) Interaction of carbon dioxide and sympathetic nervous system activity in the regulation of cerebral perfusion in humans. *Hypertension* 36: 383-388.

Khachaturian ZS (1987) Hypothesis on the regulation of cytosol calcium concentration and the aging brain. *Neurobiol. Aging* 8: 345–346.

Kirischuk S, Pronchuk N, Verkhratsky A (1992) Measurements of intracellular calcium in sensory neurons of adult and old rats. *Neurosci.* 50: 957–951.

Kirischuk S, Verkhratsky A (1996) Calcium homeostasis in aged neurones. *Life Sci.* 59: 451–459.

Kostyuk PG (1989) Diversity of calcium ion channels in cellular membranes. *Neuroscience* 28: 253-261.

Kostyuk PG, Pronchuk N, Savchenko A, Verkhratsky A (1993) Calcium currents in aged rat dorsal root ganglion neurones. *J. Phsyiol. (Lond.)* 461: 467-483.

Kuo TH, Liu BF, Yu Y, Wuytack F, Raeymaekers L, Tsang W (1997) Coordinated regulation of the plasma membrane calcium pump and sarco (endo) plasmic reticular calcium pump gene expression by Ca^{2+}. *Cell Calcium* 21: 399–408

Landfield PW (1987) 'Increased calcium-current' hypothesis of brain aging. *Neurobiol. Aging* 8: 346–347.

Landfield PW, Pitler TA (1984) Prolonged Ca^{2+}-dependent after hyperpolarizations in hippocampal neurons of aged rats. *Science* 226: 1089–1092.

Langer SZ, Arbilla S (1990) Presynaptic receptors on peripheral adrenergic neurons. *Ann. N. Y. Acad. Sci.* 604: 7–16.

Lawes CM, Bennett DA, Feigin VL and Rodgers A (2004) Blood pressure and stroke: an overview of published reviews. *Stroke* 35: 776-785.

Lee TJF, Zhang W, Sarwinski S (2000) Pre-synaptic β2-adrenoceptors mediate nicotine-induced NOergic neurogenic dilation in porcine basilar arteries. *Am. J. Physiol. Heart Circ. Physiol.* 279: H808–H816.

Lee JM, Zipfel GJ, Choi DW (1999) The changing landscape of ischemic brain injury mechanisms. *Nature* 399: A7–A14.

Limas CJ (1975) Comparison of the handling of norepinephrine in the myocardium of adult and old rats. *Cardiovasc. Res.* 9: 664–668.

Maciel LM, Polikar R, Rohrer D, Popovich BK, Dillmann WH (1990) Age induced decreases in the messenger RNA coding for the sarcoplasmic reticulum Ca^{2+}-ATPase of the rat heart. *Circ. Res.* 67: 230–234.

Martinez JL, Vasquez BJ, messing RB, Jennsen RA, Liang KC, McCaugh JL (1981) Age related changes in catecholamine content of peripheral organs in male and female F-344 rats. *J. Gerontol.* 36: 280–284.

Martyn CN, Barker DJ and Osmond C (1996) Mothers' pelvic size, fetal growth, and death from stroke and coronary heart disease in men in the UK. *Lancet* 348: 1264-1268.

Marx SO, Marks AR (2002) Regulation of the ryanodine receptor in heart failure. *Basic Res. Cardiol.* 97 (Suppl. 1): I49–I51.

Mbaku EN, Zhang L, Duckles SP, Buchholz JN (2000) Nitric oxide synthase containing nerves facilitate adrenergic transmitter release in sheep middle cerebral arteries. *J. Pharmacol. Exp. Ther.* 293: 397–402.

Mbaku EN, Zhang L, Pearce WJ, Duckles SP, Buchholz J (2003) Chronic hypoxia alters the function of NOS nerves in cerebral arteries of near term fetal and adult sheep. *J. Appl. Physiol.* 94: 724–732.

Meissner G (2002) Regulation of mammalian ryanodine receptors. *Front. Biosci.* 7: d2072–d2080.

Meldrum B, Garthwaite J (1990) Excitatory amino acid neurotoxicity and neurodegenerative disease. *Trends Pharmac. Sci.* 11: 379–387.

Miller RA (2005)The anti-aging sweepstakes: Catalase runs for the ROSes. *Science* 308: 1875–1876.

Miller, RJ (1991) The control of neuronal Ca^{2+} homeostasis. *Prog Neurobiol.* 37: 255-285.

Mione MC, Erdo SL, Kiss B, Ricci A, Amenta F (1988) Age-related changes of noradrenergic innervation of rat splanchnic blood vessels: a histofluorescence and neurochemical study. *J. Auton. Nerv. Syst.* 25: 27–33.

Montague PR, Gancayco CD, Winn MJ, Marchase RB, Friedlander MJ (1994) Role of NO production in NMDA receptor-mediated neurotransmitter release in cerebral cortex. *Science* 263: 973–977.

Murchinson D, Griffith WH (1996) High-voltage-activated calcium currents in basal forebrain neurons during ageing. *J. Neurophysiol.* 76: 158–174.

Murchinson D, Griffith WH (1998) Increased calcium buffering in basal forebrain neurons during aging. *J. Neurophysiol.* 80: 350–364.

Murchinson D, Griffith WH (1999) Age-related alterations in caffeine sensitive calcium stores and mitochondrial buffering in rat basal forebrain. *Cell Calcium* 25: 439–452.

Murchison D, Zawieja DC, Griffith WH (2004) Reduced mitochondrial buffering of voltage-gated calcium influx in aged rat basal forebrain neurons. *Cell Calcium* 36: 62-75.

Neher E (1995) The use of Fura-2 for estimating Ca buffers and Ca fluxes. *Neuropharmacology* 34: 1423–1442.

Nicholls DG (1978) The regulation of extramitochondrial free calcium ion concentration by rat liver mitochondria. *Biochem. J.* 176: 463-474.

Nicholls DG (1985) A role for the mitochondrion in the protection of cells against calcium overload? *Prog. Brain Res.* 63: 97-106.

Ogawa Y, Kurebayashi N, Murayama T (2000) Putative roles of type 3 ryanodine receptor isoforms (RyR3). *Trends Cardiovasc. Med.* 10: 65–70.

Palmer GJ, Ziegler MG, Lake CR (1978) Response to NE and blood pressure to stress increases with age. *J. Gerontol.* 33: 482–
487.

Peterson C (1992) Changes in calcium's role as a messenger during aging in neuronal and non-neuronal cells. *Ann. N. Y. Acad. Sci.* 663: 279–293.

Pieribone, VA, Shupliakov O, Brodin L, Hilfiker-Rothenfluh S, Czernik AJ and Greengard P (1995) Distinct pools of synaptic vesicles in neurotransmitter release. *Lett. to Nature* 375: 493-496.

Pitler TA, Landfield PW (1990) Aging-related prolongation of calcium spike duration in rat hippocampal slice neurons. *Brain Res.* 508: 1–6.

Porter NM, Thibault O, Thibault V, Chen KY, Landfield PW (1997) Calcium channel density and hippocampal cell death with age in long-term culture. *J. Neurosci.* 17: 5629–5639.

Pottorf WJ, Duckles SP, Buchholz JN (2000[a]) Adrenergic nerves compensate for a decline in calcium buffering during ageing. *J. Auton.Pharmacol.* 20: 1–13.

Pottorf WJ, Duckles SP, Buchholz JN (2000[b]) Mechanisms of calcium buffering in adrenergic neurones and effects of aging: testing the limits of homeostasis. *J. Auton. Pharmacol.* 20: 63–75.

Pottorf WJ, Duckles SP, Buchholz JN (2000[c]) SERCA function declines with age in adrenergic nerves from the superior cervical ganglion. *J. Auton. Pharmacol.* 20: 281–290.

Pottorf WJ, Duckles SP, Buchholz JN (2002) Aging and calcium buffering in adrenergic neurons. *Auton. Neurosci.* 96: 2–7.

Pottorf WJ, Johanns TM, Derrington SM, Strehler EE, Enyedi A, Thayer SA (2006) Glutamate-induced protease-mediated loss of plasma membrane Ca^{2+} pump activity in rat hippocampal neurons. *J. Neurochem.* 98: 1646–1656.

Pottorf WJ, Thayer SA (2002) Transient rise in intracellular calcium produces long lasting increase in plasma membrane calcium pump activity in rat sensory neurons. *J. Neurochem.* 83: 1002–1008.

Qin Z, Zaidi A, Gao J, Krainev AG, Michaelis ML, Squier TC, Bigelow DJ (1998) Decrease in Ca-ATPase activity in age synaptosomal membranes is not associated with changes in fatty acyl chain dynamics. *Mech. Aging Dev.* 105, 291–300.

Raza M, Deshpande LS, Blair RE, Carter DS, Robert J. DeLorenzo RJ (2007) Aging is associated with elevated intracellular calcium levels and altered calcium homeostatic mechanisms in hippocampal neurons. *Neurosci. Letters* 418: 77-81.

Roe MW, Lemasters JJ, Herman B (1990) Assessment of Fura-2 for measurements of cytosolic free calcium. *Cell Calcium* 11: 63–73.

Satrustegui J, Villalba M, Pereira R, Bogonez E, Martinez-Serrano A (1996) Cytosolic and mitochondrial calcium in synaptosomes during ageing. *Life Sci.* 59: 429–434.

Saugstad JA (2010) MicroRNAs as effectors of brain function with roles in ischemia and injury, neuroprotection, and neurodegeneration. J. Cereb. Blood Flow Metab. 30: 1564–1576.

Schofield GG (1990) Norepinephrine blocks a calcium current of adult rat sympathetic neurons via an α2-adrenoceptor. *Eur. J. Pharmacol.* 180: 37–47.

Siksou L, Triller A and Marty S. Ultrastructural organization of presynaptic terminals (2011) *Curr. Opinion in Neurobiol.* 21: 1-8.

Tatar M, Kopelman A, Epstein D, Tu MP, Yin CM, Garofalo RS (2001) A mutant drosophila insulin receptor homolog that extends life span and impairs neuroendocrine function. *Science* 292: 107–110.

Thayer SA, Miller RJ (1990) Regulation of the intracellular free calcium concentration in single rat dorsal root ganglion neurones *in vitro*. *J. Physiol.* 425: 85–115.

Thibault O, Porter NM, Chen KC, Blalock EM, Kaminker PG, Clodfelter GV, Brewer LD, Landfield PW (1998) Calcium dysregulation in neuronal aging and Alzheimers disease: history and new directions. *Cell Calcium* 24: 417–433.

Toescu EC, Verkhratsky A (2007) The importance of being subtle: small changes in calcium homeostasis control cognitive decline in normal aging. *Aging Cell* 6: 267-273.

Troen BR (2003) The biology of aging. *Mt. Sinai J. Med.* 70, 3–22.

Trouslard J, Marsh SJ, Brown DA (1993) Calcium entry through nicotinic receptor channels and calcium channels in cultured rat superior cervical ganglion cells. *J. Physiol. (Lond.)* 468: 53-71.

Tsai H, Hewitt CW, Buchholz JN, Duckles SP (1997) Intracellular calcium buffering declines in ageing adrenergic nerves. *Neurobiol. Aging* 18: 229–233.

Tsai H, Pottorf WJ, Buchholz JN, Duckles SP (1998) Adrenergic nerve smooth endoplasmic reticulum calcium buffering declines with age. *Neurobiol. Aging* 19: 89–96.

Tsai SH, Tew JM, Shipley MT (1989) Cerebral arterial innervation II. Development of calcitonin gene-related peptide and norepinephrine in the rat. *J. Comp. Neurol.* 27:, 1–12.

Tsien RY, Rink TJ, Poenie M (1985) Measurement of cytosolic free Ca^{2+} in individual small cells using fluorescent microscopy with dual excitation wavelengths. *Cell Calcium* 6: 145–157.

Usachev YM, Thayer SA (1997) All-or-none Ca^{2+} release from intracellular stores triggered by Ca^{2+} influx through voltage-gated Ca^{2+} channels in rat sensory neurons. *J. Neurosci.* 17: 7404–7414.

Usachev YM and Thayer SA (1999[a]). Controlling the urge to surge: all or none Ca^{2+} release in neurons. *Bioessays* 21: 743–750.

Usachev YM and Thayer SA (1999[b]) Ca^{2+} influx in resting rat sensory neurones that regulates and is regulated by ryanodine-sensitive Ca^{2+}stores. *J. Physiol.* 519 (Part 1), 115–130.

van Lieshout JJ and Secher NH (2008) Point:Counterpoint: Sympathetic activity does/does not influence cerebral blood flow. Point: Sympathetic activity does influence cerebral blood flow. *J Appl Physiol* 105: 1364-1366.

Vanterpool CK, Pearce WJ, Buchholz JN (2005) Advancing age alters rapid and spontaneous refilling of caffeine-sensitive calcium stores in sympathetic superior cervical ganglion cells. *J. Appl. Physiol.* 99: 963-971.

Vanterpool CK, Vanterpool EA, Pearce WJ, Buchholz JN (2006) Advancing age alters the expression of the ryanodine receptor 3 isoform in adult rat superior cervical ganglia. *J. Appl. Physiol.* 101: 392-400.

Verkhratsky AJ and Petersen OH (1998) Neuronal calcium stores. *Cell Calcium* 24: 333–343.

Verkhratsky AJ and Shmigol A (1996) Calcium-induced calcium release in neurones. *Cell Calcium* 19: 1–14.

Verkhratsky A, Shmigol A, Kirischuk S, Pronchuk N, Kostyuk P (1994) Age-dependent changes in calcium currents and calcium homeostasis in mammalian neurons. *Ann. N. Y. Acad. Sci.* 747: 365–381.

Verkhratsky A, Toescu EC (1998) Calcium and neuronal ageing. *TINS* 21: 2–7.

Vitorica J, Satrustegui J (1985) Impairment of glutamate uptake and absence of alterations in the energy-transducing ability of old rat brain mitochondria. *Mech. Ageing Dev.* 29: 255–266.

Villalba M, Pereira R, Martinez-Serrano A, Satrustegui J (1995) Altered cell calcium regulation in synaptosomes and brain cells of the 30-month-old rat prominent effects in hippocampus. *Neurobiol. Aging* 16: 809–816.

Werth JL, Thayer SA (1994) Mitochondria buffer physiological calcium loads in cultured rat dorsal root ganglion neurons. *J. Neurosci.* 14: 348–356.

Werth JL, Usachev YM, Thayer SA (1996) Modulation of Ca^{2+} efflux from rat dorsal root ganglion neurons. *J. Neurosci.* 16: 1008–1015.

Wingerd KL, Goodman NL, Leu ST, Clegg DO (2004) Expression and function of integrin alpha4beta1 and vascular cell adhesion molecule- 1 (VCAM-1) during sympathetic innervation of the heart. *Dev. Dyn.* 231: 359–369.

Wu SY, Dun SL, Forstermann U, Dun NJ (1997) Nitric oxide and excitatory postsynaptic currents in immature rat sympathetic preganglionic neurons *in vitro*. *Neuroscience* 79: 237–245

Wuytack F, Raeymaekers L, Missiaen L (2002) Molecular physiology of the SERCA and SPCA pumps. *Cell Calcium* 32: 279–305.

Xiong J, Verkhratsky A, Toescu E (2002) Changes in mitochondrial status associated with altered Ca^{2+} homeostasis in aged cerebellar granule neurons in brain slices. *J. Neurosci.* 22: 10761–10771.

Xu A, Narayanan N (1998) Effects of aging on sarcoplasmic reticulum Ca^{2+}-cycling proteins and their phosphorylation in rat myocardium. *Am. J. Physiol. Heart Circ. Physiol.* 275: H2087–H2094.

Yamamoto R, Wada A, Asada Y, Toshihiko Y, Tomoaki Y, Niina H, Sumiyoshi A, Kobayashi H, Lee TJF (1997) Nitric oxide-dependent and independent norepinephrine release in rat mesenteric arteries. *Am. J. Physiol. Heart Circ. Physiol.* 272, H207–H210.

Yu BP, Masoro EJ, McMahan A (1985) Nutritional influences on aging of F-344 rats. *J. Gerontol.* 40: 657–670.

Zhang W, Edvinsson L, Lee TJF (1998) Mechanism of nicotine-induced relaxation in the porcine basilar artery. *J. Pharmacol. Exp. Ther.* 284: 790–797.

Zhang B, Fugleholm K, Day LB, Ye S, Weller RO and Day IN (2003) Molecular pathogenesis of subarachnoid haemorrhage. *Int J Biochem Cell Biol* 35: 1341-1360.

23

All Your Eggs in One Basket: Mechanisms of Xenobiotic Induced Female Reproductive Senescence

Alexander P. Sobinoff, Ilana R. Bernstein and Eileen A. McLaughlin
Priority Research Centre in Chemical Biology,
University of Newcastle
Australia

1. Introduction

The irreplaceable mammalian primordial follicle represents the basic unit of female fertility, serving as the primary source of all developing oocytes in the ovary. These primordial follicles remain quiescent, often for decades, until recruited into the growing pool throughout a woman's adult reproductive years. Once recruited, <1% will reach ovulation, with the remainder undergoing an apoptotic process known as atresia (Hirshfield, 1991). Menopause, or ovarian senescence, occurs when the pool of primordial follicles becomes exhausted.

Pre-mature ovarian failure (POF; or early menopause) is an ovarian defect characterised by the premature loss of menstrual cyclicity before the age of 40, well below the median age of natural menopause (51 years). Approximately 1-4% of the female population suffers from this condition, making POF a significant contributor of female infertility (Coulam et al., 1986). There is now a growing body of evidence which suggests that foreign synthetic chemicals, also known as xenobiotics, are capable of causing POF by inducing premature follicular depletion. Indeed, exposure to pesticides, workplace chemicals, chemotherapeutic agents and cigarette smoke have all been associated with primordial follicle reduction resulting in premature ovarian senescence (Hoyer and Devine, 2001; Mattison et al., 1983a, 1983b; Sobinoff et al., 2010, 2011).

In addition to infertility, the loss of ovarian hormones which accompanies POF has been connected with an increased risk of early morbidity and mortality (Shuster et al., 2010). With current statistics indicating an increasing trend in western women opting to delay childbirth, xenobiotic exposure could have long lasting repercussions for both the fertility and long term health of these women. In this review we discuss the susceptible nature of primordial follicles and the consequences of xenobiotic induced POF. We then examine the mechanisms of ovotoxicity for environmental toxicants and xenobiotics known to target immature follicles, and discuss the development of novel methods of wildlife fertility control utilizing these ovotoxicants.

2. The primordial follicle: Precious and vulnerable

Oocyte development and maturation occurs within ovarian follicles. These follicles assemble when primary oocytes (arrested at meiosis prophase I) are enveloped by a single layer of flattened granulosa cells, forming the most immature stage of follicular development, the primordial follicle. The timing of this event is species-specific, but generally occurs in the primitive ovary during foetal development (McNatty et al., 2000). Due to the nature of follicular formation, the number of oocytes established around the time of birth is finite, and represents the total number of germ cells available to the mammalian female throughout her entire life (Edson et al., 2009). It is therefore the size and persistence of this primordial follicle pool which determines the female reproductive lifespan (Fig. 1).

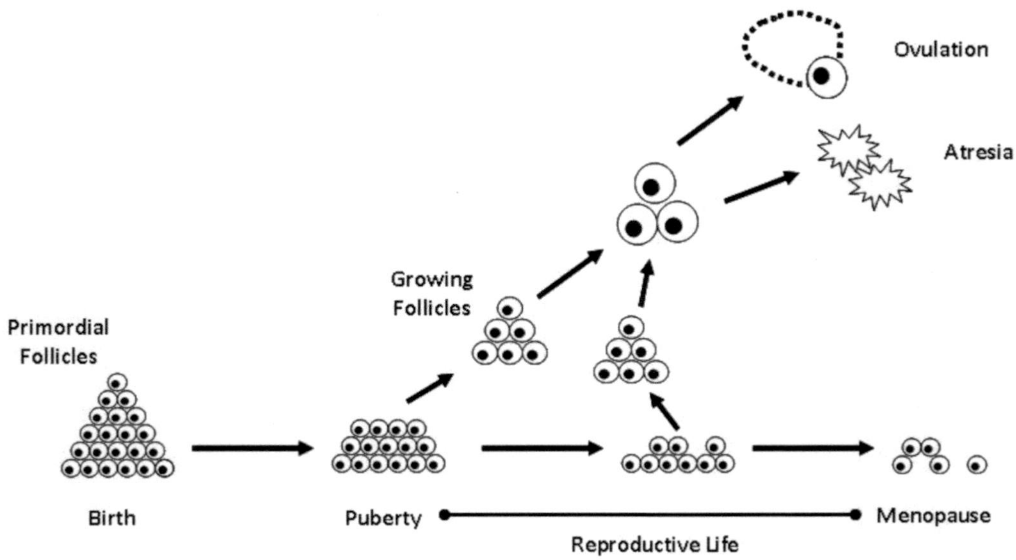

Fig. 1. Simple mechanistic diagram of the human female reproductive lifespan.

The first stage of folliculogenesis involves the recruitment of selected primordial follicles into the growing population. To prolong the length of the female reproductive lifespan, only a few primordial follicles are chosen for recruitment at any one time, with some follicles remaining in a quiescent (non-proliferative) state for months or years (Fig 1). This event occurs in regular waves, and is continuous from birth until ovarian senescence (McGee and Hsueh, 2000). Overall, only a few hundred of all the recruited follicles will complete folliculogenesis and undergo ovulation, with the vast majority being lost to atresia (Hirshfield, 1991). Atresia is thought to be an apoptotic process which selects the healthiest follicles for ovulation, although its mechanism of action is poorly understood. As virtually all follicles are lost during optimal follicular development, it is important that primordial follicles not only survive but also are maintained in a healthy state. Over-stimulation of primordial follicle activation and premature atresia results in the extensive depletion of the primordial follicle pool, resulting in premature ovarian senescence (Reddy et al., 2008).

There is now an increasing volume of studies which link primordial follicle depletion with xenobiotic exposure, suggesting that these irreplaceable follicles are highly sensitive to cytotoxic insult (Hoyer and Devine, 2001; Mattison et al., 1983a, 1983b; Sobinoff et al., 2010, 2011). It is thought that this sensitivity may stem from the primordial follicles quiescent nature. For example, somatic cells which undergo regular rounds of proliferation constantly renew macromolecules and organelles by virtue of mitosis. However, the oocyte and granulosa cells of the primordial follicle are non-proliferative, and do not benefit from mitotic renewal, perhaps making them excessively vulnerable to xenobiotics which cause sub-lethal damage to mitochondria and other structures over time (Tarin, 1996). Similarly the location of the primordial follicle population within a poorly vascularised region of the ovarian cortex also makes them highly susceptible to toxins which damage ovarian blood vessels, with the resulting cortexual fibrosis destroying primordial follicle rich segments of the ovary (Guraya, 1985; Meirow et al., 2007; van Wezel and Rodgers, 1996).

In addition to direct primordial follicle injury, certain xenobiotics which target developing follicles have been shown to cause excessive primordial follicle activation (Keating, 2009; Sobinoff et al., 2010, 2011). This may be due to a homeostatic mechanism of follicular replacement, in which destroyed developing follicles result in primordial follicle activation to replace the developing pool. If the offending xenobiotic is not removed, this could potentially lead to a vicious cycle of primordial follicle depletion.

3. Consequences of xenobiotic induced primordial follicle depletion

The overall impact of xenobiotic induced follicular depletion on female reproduction depends on the type of follicle targeted for destruction, dose, and duration of exposure (Hoyer and Sipes, 1996). For example, xenobiotics which target large developing follicles have an immediately noticeable effect on female fertility. Antral follicles are the primary producers of ovarian estrogen, and therefore play an important role in the FSH-LH negative feedback loop responsible for ovulation. Xenobiotics which selectively target antral follicles consequently have harmful effects on ovarian cyclicity, effectively acting as endocrine disruptors (Jarrell et al., 1991; Mattison and Schulman, 1980). Fortunately, both prolonged and acute exposure to these ovotoxic agents only causes temporary infertility, as these follicles can be replaced by the primordial follicle pool once the harmful xenobiotic is removed from the immediate environment.

Conversely, xenobiotics which target small pre-antral follicles have more permanent effects on female fertility which could potentially go unrecognised for years. Due to the non-renewing nature of primordial follicles, these xenobiotics are particularly damaging to female fertility, causing permanent infertility and premature ovarian senescence. What makes this type of ovotoxicity concerning is that it has a delayed effect on reproduction which is not made apparent until such a time that follicular recruitment cannot be supported (Hooser et al., 1994). Thus this extended period of time between cause and effect means that the detrimental action of xenobiotic contact often goes unnoticed, and consequently steps are not taken to minimise exposure until it is too late. Thus even a systemic low dose of xenobiotics may produce cumulative effects over time, resulting in the same consequences on female fertility as a large single exposure. With current statistics suggesting an increasing trend in developed countries of women opting to delay childbirth until late in their reproductive life (>30 years), accelerated follicle loss resulting from xenobiotic exposure can deprive these women of the chance to start a family in the conventional manner (Martin et al., 2003).

In addition to permanent infertility, the loss of ovarian hormones which accompanies early menopause has been associated with an increased risk for a variety of health problems. For example, estrogen deficiency (a consequence of menopause) is the most common cause of osteoporosis in humans (Cenci et al., 2003). Bone loss results from the absence of estrogen production by maturing ovarian follicles, which leads to a subsequent increase in FSH production due to the negative feedback of estrogen on pituitary gonadotropin secretion. In terms of bone remodelling, increased FSH production stimulates tumor necrosis factor (TNF) secretion, which in turn increases osteoclast formation and bone reabsorption (Cenci et al., 2003). Menopause induced estrogen withdrawal has also been associated with an increase in many traditional cardiovascular risk factors, including body fat redistribution, insulin resistance and high blood pressure, increased plasma triglyceride levels and high-density lipid cholesterol absorption (Bilianou, 2008; Rosano et al., 2007). Increased risk for Alzheimer's disease is also associated with the menopause induced loss of sex steroid hormones as evidenced by various epidemiological and experimental studies, although some clinical findings refute this evidence (Pike et al., 2009).

Over the course of the 20th century, the average life expectancy for women in the developing world has increased by ~40%, resulting in women now living up to a third of their lives in post menopausal years. Unfortunately, this means that women are now spending a larger proportion of their life with increased health risks brought about by the onset of menopause. In addition, increased risk resulting from xenobiotic induced premature menopause means an enhanced chance for problems. It is therefore important to understand the mechanisms behind xenobiotic induced primordial follicle depletion.

4. Mechanisms of xenobiotic induced primordial follicle depletion

4.1 The Aryl Hydrocarbon Receptor

The Aryl Hydrocarbon Receptor (Ahr) is a ligand activated transcription factor implicated in the regulation of a variety of physiological and developmental effects, including xenobiotic metabolism, cell cycle progression, apoptosis and oxidative stress (Denison and Heath-Pagliuso, 1998; Nebert et al., 2000). In its inactivated state, Ahr is found in the cytoplasm bound to a number of molecular chaperones including hsp90, Xap2, and p23 (Carlson and Perdew, 2002; Petrulis and Perdew, 2002). Ligand binding causes conformational changes which expose a nuclear import signal on the Ahr, resulting in its translocation into the nucleus (Pollenz et al., 1994). Once imported the Ahr-ligand receptor complex disassociates with its chaperones and dimerizes with the aryl hydrocarbon receptor nuclear translocator (ARNT) to form an active transcription factor with high affinity to specific DNA sequences known as xenobiotic-response elements (XRE) within the promoter region of a variety of genes, inducing transcription (Fig.2) (Reyes et al., 1992).

The Ahr-ARNT ligand activated transcription factor is known to regulate the toxicity of various xenobiotic compounds such as polycyclic aromatic hydrocarbons, polychlorinated dibenzofurans and polychlorinated biphenyls which are found ubiquitously in the environment and are highly resistant to metabolic breakdown (Nguyen and Bradfield, 2007; Stapleton and Baker, 2003). In an adaptive response to their accumulation in the cell, Ahr induces the expression of a number of xenobiotic metabolising enzymes, including members of the cytochrome P450 A and B families which oxygenate the intruding xenobiotic as part of a three tiered enzymatic detoxification mechanism (Conney, 1982). Unfortunately, this oxygenation often results in the bioactivation of the parent xenobiotic into a more reactive and therefore toxic metabolite (Harrigan et al., 2004; Melendez-Colon et al., 1999). Indeed, many of Ahr's known xenobiotic ligands, such as the polycyclic aromatic hydrocarbons benzo[a]pyrene (BaP), 9:10-dimethyl-1:2-benzanthracene (DMBA), and 3-methylcholanthrene (3-MC), cause primordial follicle destruction through Ahr initiated cytochrome P450 induced bioactivation (Borman et al., 2000; Mattison and Thorgeirsson, 1979). For example, BaP is initially metabolised by Ahr regulated cyp1A1 and cyp1B1 enzymes resulting in its biotransformation into 7,8-diol, and 9,10-diol macromolecular-adduct forming metabolites within the ovary. Inhibition of Ahr by α-naphthoflavone nullifies its effects on primordial follicle destruction (Bengtsson et al., 1983; Mattison et al., 1983a).

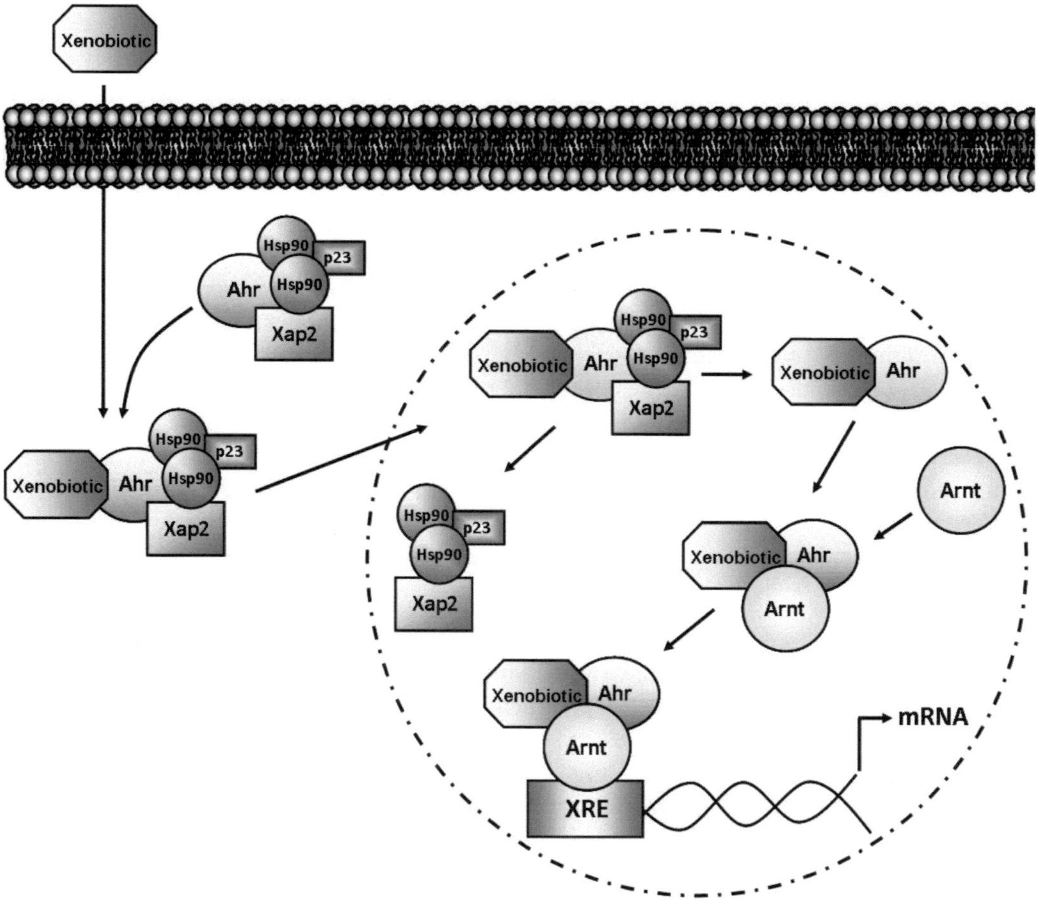

Fig. 2. Molecular mechanism of Arh-Arnt directed gene expression in response to xenobiotic exposure.

In addition to detoxification, the development of Ahr-deficient mice has revealed a physiological role for Ahr in regulating reproduction, growth and development (Benedict et al., 2000, 2003; Nebert et al., 1984; Robles et al., 2000; Schmidt et al., 1996). Benedict et al.

(2000) demonstrated that ovaries from mice deficient for Ahr expression contained significantly more fully formed primordial follicles compared to wild type mice on PND2-3. Robles et al (2000) found similar results, identifying more than a two-fold significant increase in the primordial follicle pool of Ahr deficient PND4 mice compared to wild type mice. These results suggest a developmental role for Ahr in regulating primordial follicle formation and atresia in the mouse. Although the exact details of Ahr role in the regulation of the primordial follicle pool have yet to be determined, given that Ahr xenobiotic ligands cause primordial follicle depletion, we hypothesise that part of these ovotoxic compounds method of ovotoxicity may involve perturbed AhR developmental signalling, inducing premature primordial follicle atresia.

4.2 Bioactivation

Humans come into contact with a variety of xenobiotics over the course of their lifetime, and have evolved a number of physiological mechanisms designed to remove their harmful influence from within the body. Hydrophilic xenobiotics tend to be less toxic, as the body is able to directly excrete them relatively unchanged. However, if the xenobiotic is lipophilic, it will need to be modified by a series of biochemical reactions before it can be eliminated (Pavek and Dvorak, 2008). This series of biochemical reactions is termed biotransformation, and can be divided into two phases. Phase I metabolism involves the introduction or exposure of a reactive polar group on the xenobiotic via oxidation, resulting in a more reactive/water soluble metabolite to facilitate excretion and/or the induction of phase II metabolism. The cytochrome p450 super family of oxidases catalyse the majority of these reactions, although other oxidases, esterases, amidases, and monooxygenases can also be involved (Schroer et al., 2010). Phase II metabolism involves the conjugation of charged species such as glutathione, sulphate, glycine or glucuronic acid to the phase I metabolite to increase its water solubility (Kohalmy and Vrzal, 2011). The addition of these large anionic groups detoxifies reactive electrophiles, resulting in a more polar metabolite which can be actively transported out of the cell. These reactions are carried out by a broad range of transferases, such as glutathione S-transferase, UDP-glucuronosyltransferases, sulfotransferases, N-acetyltransferases, and methyltransferases (Jancovaa et al., 2010).

Unfortunately, phase I metabolism of xenobiotics by the liver and other tissues occasionally results in the production of a more cytotoxic metabolite, a process known as bioactivation (Dekant, 2009). These highly reactive metabolites are electrophilic, and are capable of forming covalent bonds (or adducts) with the nucleophilic centers of cellular macromolecules, such as proteins, DNA, and RNA. Cellular toxicity occurs when these adducts disrupt the normal structure and/or function of these macromolecules, resulting in apoptosis, necrosis or carcinogenesis. The main site of xenobiotic biotransformation within the body is the liver, although the ovary is capable of both phase I and phase II metabolism (Igawa et al., 2009; Rajapaksa et al., 2007a, 2007b; Shimada et al., 2003). Therefore, there is potential for the vulnerable primordial follicle to come into contact with bioactivated ovotoxic metabolites via several routes of exposure. Bioactivated metabolites produced by the liver maybe stable enough to diffuse back into the venous circulatory system, resulting in direct ovarian exposure. Additionally, as the primordial follicle is capable of expressing xenobiotic metabolising enzymes itself, oocytes may be exposed to localised bioactivation. Finally, the xenobiotic may be bioactivated locally into its ovotoxic metabolite by neighbouring somatic ovarian cells and taken up by the primordial oocyte, contributing to localised bioactivation.

A number of studies performed *in vitro* have revealed that the ovary is capable of the localised bioactivation of a number of xenobiotics into ovotoxic intermediates which target primordial follicles for destruction (Rajapaksa et al., 2007a, 2007b). An example of this localised bioactivation is the reported metabolism of the polycyclic aromatic hydrocarbon DMBA (Fig.3). Ovarian exposure to DMBA disrupts folliculogenesis, resulting in the destruction of all follicle populations leading to POF in rodents, although recent evidence suggests an alternate mechanism of ovotoxicity resulting in primordial follicle depletion in the mouse (Mattison and Schulman, 1980; Sobinoff et al., 2011). This toxicity has been attributed to the bioactivation of DMBA into its ultimate DNA-adduct forming intermediate DMBA-3,4-diol-1,2-epoxide (Shiromizu and Mattison, 1985). DMBA is bioactivated by Cyp1B1 to a 3,4-epoxide which is then converted into a 3,4-diol by the microsomal epoxide hydrolase (MeH) phase II enzyme. This intermediate is then further modified by either Cyp1A1 or Cyp1B1 to form the ultimate ovotoxicant DMBA-3,4-diol-1,2-epoxide (Shimada and Fujii Kuriyama, 2004; Shimada et al., 2001). These three enzymes required for DMBA's biotransformation are all expressed and induced by DMBA exposure in the murine ovary (Igawa et al., 2009; Rajapaksa et al., 2007b; Shimada et al., 2003). In further support of localised DMBA bioactivation, inhibition of MeH in cultured rat ovaries inhibited DMBA induced ovotoxicity, while ovarian culture in the presence of DMBA-3,4-diol induced significantly more primordial follicle depletion than DMBA alone (Igawa et al., 2009; Rajapaksa et al., 2007b).

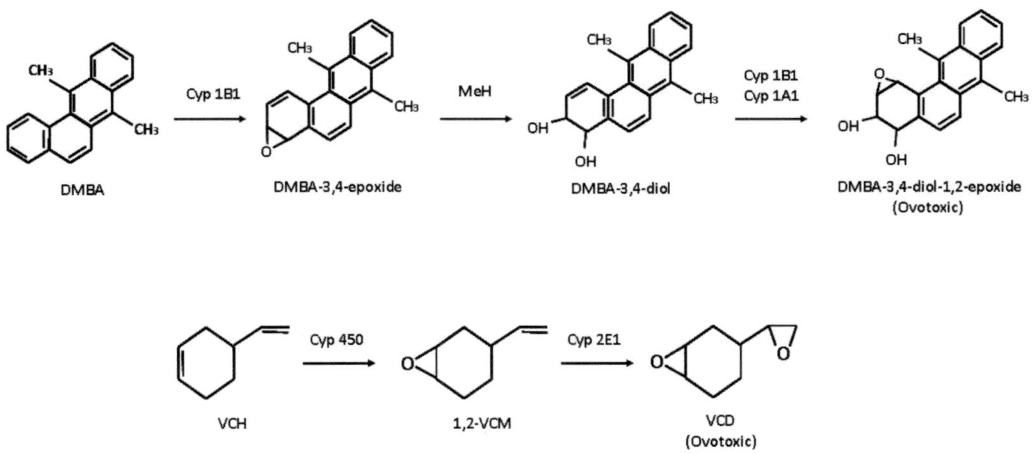

Fig. 3. Metabolism of DMBA and VCD into their ovotoxic metabolites.

Another example of localised bioactivation is the conversion of the industrial chemical 4-Vinylcyclohexene (VCH) into VCH diepoxide (VCD) (Fig. 3). VCH is metabolised by cytochrome P450 phase I enzymes to form VCM-monoepoxide (VCM), which is then converted into VCD. Studies have shown VCD to be the ultimate ovotoxicant, targeting both primordial and primary follicles for depletion (Hu et al., 2001; Smith et al., 1990; Sobinoff et al., 2010). As demonstrated *in vivo* and *in vitro* via knockout studies, VCH/VCM is bioactivated into VCD exclusively by the cyp2e1 isoform in the ovary (Rajapaksa et al.,

2007a). Rajapaksa et al (2007a) cultured neonatal ovaries from both cyp2e1$^{+/+}$ and cyp2e1$^{-/-}$ neonatal mice in VCM and VCD containing media. Both VCH metabolites caused primordial follicle depletion in cyp2e1$^{+/+}$ cultured ovaries. However, unlike VCD, VCM did not produce an ovotoxic affect in cyp2e1$^{-/-}$ cultured ovaries, thus demonstrating its role in VCH induced bioactivation.

4.3 Xenobiotic induced reactive oxygen species generation

Reactive oxygen species (ROS), such as superoxide anion, hydrogen peroxide and the highly toxic hydroxyl free radical, are highly reactive oxygen-containing molecules which are produced naturally as a consequence of oxidative energy metabolism (Valko et al., 2007). These short lived ROS play an important role in regulating signal transduction, selectively oxidizing cysteine residues on proteins resulting in a variety of reversible molecular interactions (Janssen-Heininger et al., 2008). However, in excess these highly unstable molecules may lead to perturbed signal transduction and/or oxidative damage to cellular macromolecules, inducing DNA mutations, lipid peroxidation and premature protein degradation. These molecular lesions coupled with perturbed signal transduction can ultimately result in abnormal cellular function, apoptosis and necrosis (Valko et al., 2006, 2007; Wells et al., 2009).

The ovary is a highly redox sensitive organ, with oocytes themselves being particularly vulnerable to excess ROS exposure due to the low rates of oxidative repair in post-mitotic cells (Cadenas and Davies, 2000; Terman et al., 2006). According to the free radical hypothesis of ageing, non-renewing primordial follicles, which can remain quiescent for many years, gradually produce ROS through electron leakage from the mitochondrial electron transport chain (Tarin, 1996). Over time this excess ROS damages the mitochondrial membranes, leading to more electron leakage and further ROS production. Given the redox sensitive nature of primordial follicles, it is reasonable to assume that the generation of xenobiotic induced ROS formed through detoxification may exacerbate this process, contributing to primordial follicle loss (Bondy and Naderi, 1994; Danielson, 2002; Wells et al., 2009).

Xenobiotic enhanced ROS formation may occur via several mechanisms in the primordial follicle (Fig.4). If the ovotoxic xenobiotic contains a quinone-like structure, it may undergo redox cycling with the corresponding semiquinone radical to produce superoxide anions. Further enzymatic and/or spontaneous dismutation of the superoxide anions produces hydrogen peroxide, which can further react with trace amounts of iron or other transition metals to form hydroxyl free radicals (Bolton et al., 2000). Given the futile cyclical nature of redox cycling, this would allow a relatively small concentration of quinone-like xenobiotics to generate an amplified production of ROS in the ovary (Park et al., 2005). For example, menadione (MEN), a synthetic vitamin K with a quinone-like structure, is a potent toxicant which exerts its cytotoxic affect via quinone cycling (Thor et al., 1982). Recently, we examined the effects of MEN on folliculogenesis in neonatal mouse ovaries *in vitro* (Sobinoff et al., 2010). This study found that MEN caused wide spread oxidative stress and DNA damage resulting in primordial and small developing follicle destruction, as evidenced by the detection of increased levels of the hydroxyl radical–induced mutagenic DNA lesion 8-

hydroxyguanine, and Terminal deoxynucleotidyl transferase dUTP nick end labelling (TUNEL) analysis (Klaunig and Kamendulis, 2004).

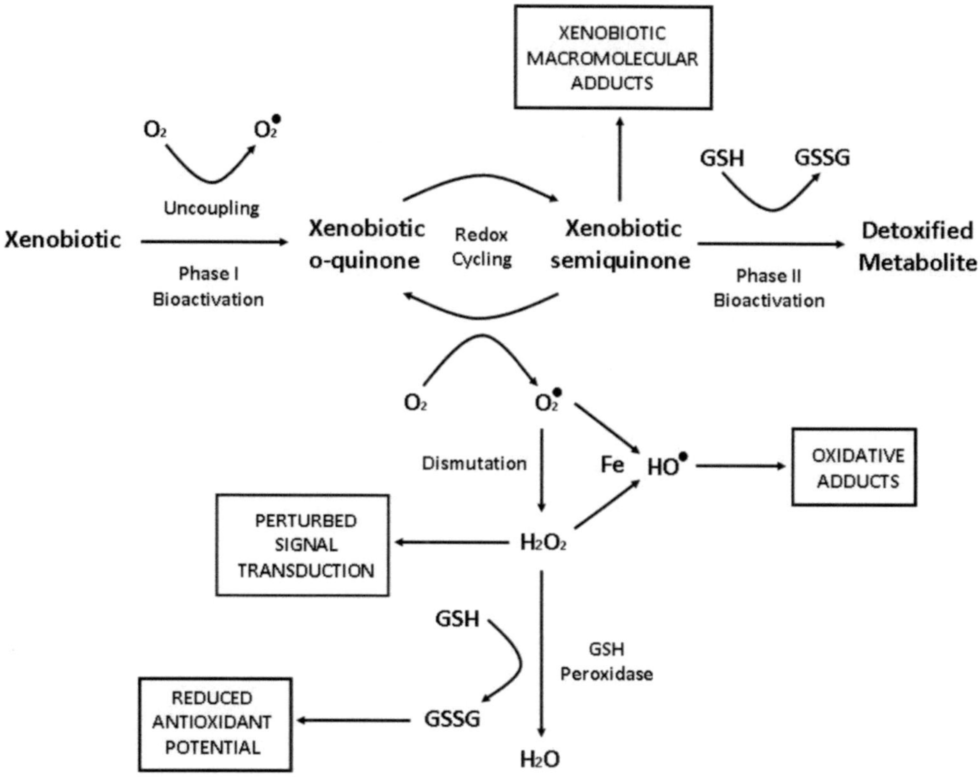

Fig. 4. Biochemical pathways outlining the mechanisms of xenobiotic induced ROS production which may contribute to primordial follicle depletion. Abbreviations: Fe, iron; $O_2^{\bullet}$, superoxide; H_2O_2, hydrogen peroxide; $HO^{\bullet}$, hydroxyl radical.

Another mechanism of xenobiotic induced ROS formation is the phase I bioactivation of the offending xenobiotic into reactive and redox active o-quinone metabolites. As mentioned previously, the PAH BaP is converted into 7,8-diol, and 9,10-diol by Ahr induced cyp1A1 and cyp1B1 enzymes in the ovary (Bengtsson et al., 1983). Studies have also shown that cyp1A1 is also capable of converting BaP into the BaP o-quinones benzo[a]pyrene-3,6-dione and benzo[a]pyrene-6,12-dion (Schwarz et al., 2001). Additionally, cyp 1A1 bioactivated BaP 7,8-diol can be further metabolised via NAD(P)$^+$-dependent oxidation by the phase I dihydrodiol dehydrogenase Akr1c1 enzyme, resulting in the formation of a ketol. This ketol then undergoes tautomerisation to form catechol 7,8-dihydroxybenzo[a]pyrene. Two subsequent 1-electron auto-oxidation events produce a *o*-semiquinone anion, followed by the formation of the o-quinone benzo[a]pyrene-7,8-dione (Trevor et al., 1996). Given the increases observed in cyp 1A1 expression in the ovary in response to BaP exposure, and the relatively high level of dihydrodiol dehydrogenase expression in the ovary compared to the liver, it is reasonable to assume BaP may be exerting part of its ovotoxic affect through o-quinone formation (Hou et al., 1994). Indeed, both benzo[a]pyrene-3,6-dione and benzo[a]pyrene-6,12-dion were detected in rat ovaries after a single dose exposure of BaP in rodents (Ramesh et al., 2010).

The un-natural "uncoupling" of phase I cytochrome P450 enzymes may also contribute to xenobiotic induced ovotoxicity via ROS production. Cytochrome P450 enzymes use H^+ obtained from NADPH to reduce O_2, which leads to the production of hydrogen peroxide and/or superoxide anion radicals as part of phase I oxygenation. Unfortunately, the P450 catalytic cycle can be uncoupled, resulting in the release of the reactive hydrogen peroxide and/or superoxide anion radical from the enzyme substrate complex (Meunier et al., 2004). Although all cytochrome P450 enzymes experience uncoupling, cyp 2E1 experiences a high rate of the phenomenon (Caro and Cederbaum, 2004). Even in the absence of substrate, cyp 2E1 undergoes un-natural "uncoupling" due to its NADPH oxidase activity independent of phase I metabolism (Ekstrom and Ingelman-Sundberg, 1989). As described previously, VCH is exclusively bioactivated by cyp 2E1 to produce the ovotoxic metabolite VCD. It is therefore possible that VCH may partially cause primordial follicle depletion via excess ROS production. Indeed, studies conducted in our laboratory have demonstrated VCD itself, along with the pesticide methoxychlor (MXC) and MEN, is capable of inducing cyp 2E1 expression and oxidative stress in the form of 8-hydroxyguanine adduct formation in primordial follicles (Sobinoff et al., 2010).

Another mechanism by which ovotoxic xenobiotics may cause oxidative stress is through the depletion of glutathione peroxidase (GSH) via detoxification. GSH is the body's most abundant antioxidant, providing protection against all forms of oxidative stress by scavenging ROS by virtue of its reducing thiol group, forming oxidised glutathione disulfide (GSSG) (Kidd, 1997). The glutathione system (GSH/GSSG ratio) acts as a homoeostatic redox buffer that contributes to maintenance of the cellular redox balance, with a reduction in the GSH/GSSG ratio indicating oxidative stress (Schafer and Buettner, 2001). In addition to its function as a ROS scavenger, GSH is also employed in the phase II metabolism of many ovotoxic xenobiotics (Keating et al., 2010; Tsai-Turton et al., 2007; Wu and Berger, 2008). For example, VCD is conjugated to GSH by the glutathione S-transferase Gst isoform pi (Gstp) as part of phase II detoxification in the ovary (Keating et al., 2010).

The mammalian ovary itself is highly redox sensitive, with maturing oocytes containing the highest concentration of GSH compared to any other cell type in the body (Calvin et al., 1986; Clague et al., 1992; Luderer et al., 2001). It is therefore likely that ovarian somatic and germ cell GSH plays an important role in protecting ovarian follicles from damage by ovotoxic xenobiotics. This is especially evident in primordial follicles, where a natural decrease in the GSH/GSSG ratio with advancing reproductive age increases primordial follicle susceptibility to xenobiotic induced destruction (Mattison et al., 1983b). Therefore, we hypothesise that the detoxification of ovotoxic xenobiotics via GSH conjugation reduces the GSH/GSSG ratio in primordial follicles, leaving them vulnerable to oxidative stress and primordial follicle depletion. Indeed, DMBA detoxification involves GSH conjugation, and its ovotoxic ROS production can be reduced through the addition of GSH, curbing its ovotoxicity (Tsai-Turton et al., 2007). There is controversial evidence for this mechanism of ovotoxicity in VCD induced primordial follicle loss. Rodent exposure to VCD was shown to reduce GSH concentrations by 25% and 55% in rat and mouse ovaries 2 hours after VCD administration (Bhattacharya and Keating, 2011). Additionally, rodents given the same dose of VCD over a period of several days caused specific primordial follicle depletion only after 15 days of continual dosing (Springer et al., 1996). The significant decrease in GSH concentrations almost immediately after exposure, coupled with the delayed loss of follicles following chronic exposure suggest that GSH reduction over time due to VCD detoxification could leave the susceptible primordial follicle vulnerable to increasing concentrations of xenobiotic induced ROS, resulting in primordial follicle destruction. It is pertinent that a single dose of a higher concentration of VCD (320 mg/kg) causes significant primordial follicle depletion 6 days after exposure, but is not specific to the primordial follicle pool (Devine et al., 2004). Additionally, VCD *in vitro* culture assays have linked an increase in Gstp expression with the first signs of primordial follicle loss after 6 days of exposure in neonatal rat ovaries (Bhattacharya and Keating, 2011; Keating et al., 2010). As Gstp catalyses VCD-GSH conjugation, the increase in enzymatic expression and therefore activity could have contributed to the observed primordial follicle loss due to a reduction in GSH/GSSG oxidative buffer. Conversely, substituting VCD culture media with antioxidant such as GSH does not prevent primordial follicle depletion, suggesting it is not the ultimate cause of depletion (Devine et al., 2004).

4.4 Xenobiotic induced primordial follicle activation

Traditionally, studies attempting to identify the molecular mechanisms behind xenobiotic induced POF have focused on premature follicular atresia as the main source of primordial follicle depletion. However, there is now a growing body of evidence which suggests that xenobiotics cause primordial follicle depletion through accelerated primordial follicle activation (Keating, 2009, 2011; Sobinoff et al., 2010, 2011). A study of VCD and MXC induced primordial follicle depletion has revealed a selective mechanism of pre-antral ovotoxicity involving small developing follicle atresia and primordial follicle activation both *in vitro* and *in vivo* (Sobinoff et al., 2010). Extracted neonatal mouse ovaries cultured in either VCD or MXC were immunopositive for the apoptotic markers caspase 2, caspase 3, and TUNEL in small developing follicles from the primary stage onward, but were absent in primordial follicles (Fig.5). In addition, the primordial follicles in VCD and MXC cultured ovaries expressed proliferating cell nuclear antigen (PCNA), a marker of primordial follicle activation (Picut et al., 2008; Tománek and Chronowska, 2006). VCD and MXC exposure also induces primordial follicle activation and developing follicle atresia *in vivo* as evidenced by increased primordial follicle PCNA expression and histomorphological analysis (Sobinoff et al., 2010). Microarray analysis confirmed via qPCR also showed VCD and MXC up-regulated PI3K/Akt and mTOR signalling, two synergistic pathways intimately associated with primordial follicle activation (Reddy et al., 2010). Further evidence for PI3K/Akt signalling in VCD induced primordial follicle activation comes from a study conducted by Hoyer et al (2009), in which LY294002, an inhibitor of PI3K, prevented primordial follicle depletion in cultured rat ovaries (Vlahos et al., 1994).

The polycyclic aromatic hydrocarbon DMBA, which was previously thought to cause indiscriminate follicular destruction, has also been shown to cause pre-antral ovotoxicity through selective immature follicle destruction and primordial follicle activation (Mattison and Schulman, 1980; Sobinoff et al., 2011). In addition to showing signs of maturing follicle atresia (caspase 2, caspase 3, TUNEL) and primordial follicle activation (PCNA), DMBA induced Akt1 phosphorylation, mTOR activation, and decreased FOXO3a expression in DMBA cultured primordial oocytes. All of these events occur downstream of the PI3K/Akt and mTOR signalling pathways, providing evidence for these pathways involvement in xenobiotic induced primordial follicle depletion (Reddy et al., 2010). Unlike VCD however, PI3K/Akt inhibitor studies utilising LY294002 in DMBA cultured rat ovaries caused accelerated primordial follicle depletion (Keating, 2009). In addition to its role in primordial follicle activation, PI3k/Akt signalling is also responsible for augmenting cellular survival by inhibiting the activation of proapoptotic proteins and transcription factors (Blume-Jensen et al., 1998; Testa and Bellacosa, 2001). Therefore, in addition to acting synergistically with mTOR signalling to cause primordial follicle activation, PI3k/Akt signalling may help preserve the primordial follicle pool in times of cytotoxic stress. Interestingly however, mTOR signalling does not require PI3k/Akt signalling to induce primordial follicle activation, and in fact may be the sole driver of DMBA induced primordial follicle activation (Adhikari et al., 2010).

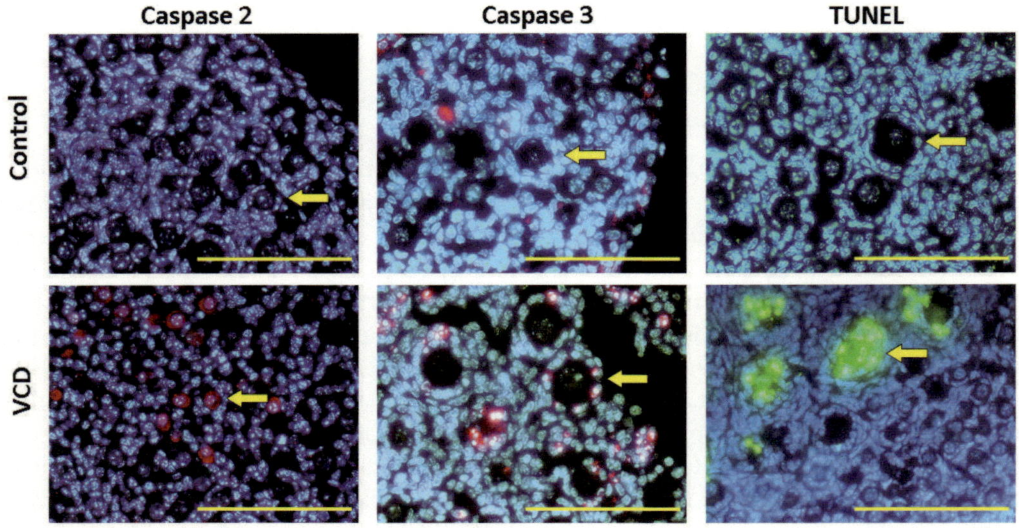

Fig. 5. Immunohistological staining of apoptotic markers in VCD exposed neonatal mouse ovaries. Blue staining (DAPI) represents nuclear staining; red staining (Cy-5) represents specific staining for the protein of interest; green staining (Fluorescein) represents specific staining for degraded DNA (TUNEL). Thin arrow=developing follicle; scale bar is equal to 50μm.

As xenobiotic induced primordial follicle activation is reportedly accompanied by small pre-antral follicular destruction, it has been hypothesised that xenobiotic induced primordial follicle depletion is the result of a homeostatic mechanism of follicular replacement (Keating, 2009; Sobinoff et al., 2010). In this hypothesis, the ovotoxic xenobiotic targets and destroys developing follicles, leading to increased primordial follicle recruitment to maintain the developing pool (Fig. 6). Although the developing pool may be maintained for some time, eventually the rate of developing follicle destruction will exceed the dwindling primordial follicle pools rate of replacement, resulting in POF. Indeed, it is well known that rapidly dividing cells, such as the granulosa cells of developing follicles, are highly susceptible to the action of cytotoxic xenobiotics (Blumenfeld and Haim, 1997; Hirshfield, 1991). Therefore, if the xenobiotic targeted these proliferating granulosa cells for destruction, the entire follicular structure would demise (Hughes and Gorospe, 1991). Even given the vulnerable nature of the primordial follicle explained earlier in this review, the primordial follicles quiescent nature may reduce their susceptibility to certain xenobiotics, and are only destroyed once a commitment to activation/recruitment has been made.

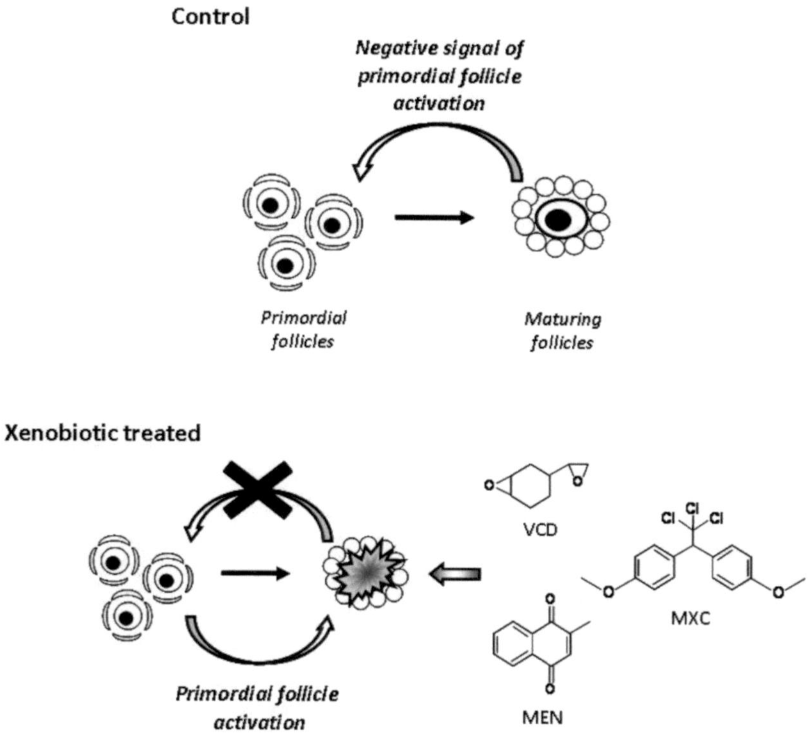

Fig. 6. Homeostatic mechanism of follicular replacement hypothesis. Under control conditions, premature primordial follicle activation is prevented by negative cytokine signals excreted from the developing pool of follicles. Xenobiotic exposure results in the destruction of this developing pool, removing these negative signals causing primordial follicle activation.

Another proposed mechanism of xenobiotic induced primordial follicle activation may involve perturbed signal transduction caused by oxidative stress. As described previously, ROS play a physiological role in regulating signal transduction by selectively oxidising cysteine residues on proteins resulting in a variety of reversible molecular interactions (Wells et al., 2009). It is therefore conceivable that increased levels of xenobiotic induced ROS could lead to abnormal cysteine oxidation and consequently dysregulated signal transduction. For example, the PI3K/Akt signalling pathway has been shown to be up-regulated by increased levels of ROS through the H_2O_2 oxidation of phosphatases which negatively regulate the pathway (Kim et al., 2005; Naughton et al., 2009). Given the PI3K/Akt pathway's role in the regulation of primordial follicle recruitment, increased ROS production could potentially cause primordial follicle activation in xenobiotic treated ovaries. Indeed, all three xenobiotics which have thus far been reported to induce primordial follicle activation also cause oxidative stress and induce the expression/activation of members of the PI3K/Akt signalling pathway in the ovary (Sobinoff et al., 2010, 2011; Tsai-Turton et al., 2007).

Xenobiotic induced primordial follicle activation may also be the result of abnormal cross-talk between signalling pathways. For example, DMBA exposure was shown to induce *Dnajb6* expression, a heat shock protein whose expression is normally induced by Nrf2 and Hsf1 in response to oxidative stress (Sobinoff et al., 2011; Thimmulappa et al., 2002; Wang, K. et al., 2009). Dnajb6 responds to stress by inhibiting nuclear factor of activated T cells (NFAT) transcriptional activity through the recruitment of class II histone deacetylase (Dai et al., 2005). In turn NFAT positively regulates PTEN expression, a known inhibitor of Akt1 phosphorylation. Therefore DMBA induced Dnajb6 expression may inhibit NFAT transcriptional activity, reducing PTEN expression and stimulating Akt1 phosphorylation, resulting in primordial follicle activation (Baksh et al., 2002; Reddy et al., 2010; Wang, Q. et al.).

4.5 Xenobiotic induced cell death

Ovarian follicles undergo physiological cell death via the apoptotic process of atresia, which is thought to select dysfunctional follicles and thus reserving the healthiest follicles for ovulation (Tilly et al., 1991). A number of studies have concluded that ovotoxic xenobiotics which target primordial follicles for destruction do so by inducing premature follicular atresia (Hu et al., 2001; Matikainen et al., 2001; Tilly and Robles, 1999). In this review we have already discussed the mechanisms by which ovotoxic xenobiotics may induce follicular atresia in primordial follicles (Ahr activation, Bioactivation, and ROS generation). However, other forms of cell death have been reportedly induced by xenobiotic exposure. Cell death by necrosis usually occurs in response to tissue injury, and elicits an inflammatory response in the surrounding tissue. Necrosis can be distinguished from apoptosis via histomorphological and ultrastructural analysis (Gobe and Harmon, 2001). In a study by Mattison (1980), the three PAHs BaP, 3-MC, and DMBA were shown to cause morphological changes in mouse primordial follicle oocytes which were consistent with necrosis (Mattison, 1980). The alkylating chemotherapeutic agent cyclophosphamide was also shown to cause necrotic damage in mouse primordial follicle oocytes three days after a single i.p injection (Plowchalk and Mattison, 1992). However, lower doses of cyclophosphamide produced atretic changes in primordial follicle oocytes, suggesting the type of cell death (apoptosis/necrosis) caused by xenobiotic exposure depends upon the dose given, and the duration of exposure. Therefore, concentrations of xenobiotic which cause mild cellular damage may result in active cell death, or apoptosis, while concentration which result in severe damage will result in passive cell death, or necrosis (Raffray and Gerald, 1997).

Autophagy or "self eating" is another possible non-apoptotic mechanism of cell death which may result in primordial follicle depletion. This conserved catabolic process involves the lysosomal-dependant turnover of cytoplasmic organelles and proteins during times of starvation or nutrient deficiency, allowing the regeneration of metabolic precursor molecules to ensure survival (Levine and Klionsky, 2004). Increased incidences of autophagy have also been observed in response to other environmental stresses, including hypoxia, oxidative stress, and xenobiotic exposure (Kiffin et al., 2006; Kondo et al., 2005). Under these conditions autophagy may renew damaged or dysfunctional organelles, thereby maintaining a healthy cell population. Although the activation of autophagy in response to cell stress may be a cellular adaptation to promote survival, excessive activation beyond a key threshold may result in cellular collapse and atrophy, a process known as autophagic cell death (Galluzzi et al., 2008). While debatable whether autophagic cell death is independent from apoptosis, it has been almost universally accepted that excess autophagy can induce apoptosis (Levine and Yuan, 2005; Maiuri et al., 2007). Recent studies have suggested autophagy as an alternate form of programmed cell death in the ovary, with evidence indicating it is the main mechanism by which oogonia are lost prior to primordial follicle formation (Duerrschmidt et al., 2006; Lobascio et al., 2007; Rodrigues et al., 2009). Thus prolonged xenobiotic exposure resulting in organelle damage may induce autophagic cell death in primordial follicles, resulting in depletion. Indeed, proteins responsible for regulating apoptosis, such as members of the Bcl2 family, have also been found to regulate autophagy (Maiuri et al., 2007; Shimizu et al., 2004). Therefore, gene expression studies in which these pathways have been thought to induce xenobiotic atresia could be inducing primordial follicle destruction by apoptotic independent or dependent autophagy (Flaws et al., 2006).

5. Ovotoxic xenobiotics as agents for wildlife fertility control

Population control of native and exotic pest species is necessary to prevent environmental degradation, competition and predation of native wildlife, the spread of pathogenic diseases, and conflicts with humans over food production. Traditionally, population control has involved the elimination of the target species through poisoning, trapping and shooting (McAlpine et al., 2007). Although effective immediately, these methods are seen as inhuman, unsustainable, and ineffective over the long term. Manipulating the reproductive rate, particularly in females, instead of increasing the mortality rate is potentially more humane, species specific, and effective at curtailing populations (Kirkpatrick, 2007). The use of ovotoxic xenobiotics as agents of contraception/sterilisation represents a novel approach to fertility control. Of particular interest are xenobiotics which have been shown to cause POF by specifically targeting the primordial follicle population for degradation (Hoyer and Devine, 2001; Sobinoff et al., 2010), thus causing permanent sterility.

To achieve widespread efficacy ovotoxic xenobiotics in fertility control must be delivered via single or minimal oral administration. To be successful an oral agent must also have permanent or very long lasting effects, be specific for the target pest species and be humane/environmentally safe (Castle and Dean, 1996). Rodents such as the rice-field rat represent a serious pest in cereal agriculture, accounting for an average annual loss of between 5-10% of rice crops in Asia, 17% of rice crops in Indonesia, between 15-100% of maize in Africa, and between 5-90% of total crop production in South America (Geddes, 1992; Mwanjabe and Leirs, 1997; Rodríguez and Jaime, 1993; Singleton, 2003; Taylor, 1968).

VCD represents an ideal fertility control agent due to its ability to induce rapid small follicle depletion resulting in POF in rodents at concentrations which do not cause widespread cytotoxicity (Springer et al., 1996). Additionally, VCD metabolism in the liver and hepatic tissue of rodents results in the production and excretion of the inert compound from the body, potentially reducing its effects on predators and its bioaccumulation in the environment (Flaws et al., 1994; Keating et al., 2010; Rajapaksa et al., 2007a). However, VCD does have disadvantages which make it fall short of the ideal fertility control agent. As described previously, VCD requires multiple doses to cause complete infertility in the rodent model (Springer et al., 1996). In addition, a VCD containing bait would need to be both attractive and palatable to the pest species, but not palatable or accessible to non-pest species. Currently, VCD is being trialled as an oral fertility control agent in the rice-field rat *Rattus argentiventer*. Registered by SenesTech Inc. as ContraPest®, the company website suggests the formulated bait is palatable, causes complete sterility within one month's ingestion, and does not adversely affect the animal's health and well being (http://www.senestech.com/). The use of other ovotoxicants as oral fertility control agents has been less successful. In a study by Sanders et al (2011) ERL-4221, a less toxic diepoxide, cycloaliphatic epoxide resin, which recently replaced VCD in industry, was investigated as a possible fertility control agent for pigs. A 20 day treatment period using palatable bait containing 16.0 mg ERL-4221 kg–1 bodyweight failed to produce any difference in follicular composition compared to control treated animals (Sanders et al., 2011). In summary, ovotoxicants represent potential fertility control agents, provided the xenobiotic delivers significant follicle depletion without side effects, and does not adversely affect the environment or food chain.

6. Conclusions

Ovotoxic xenobiotics cause primordial follicle depletion via several mechanisms which ultimately lead to their destruction or activation. These chemicals are rarely ovotoxic by themselves, and require hepatic or ovarian metabolism to exert their destructive effects on reproduction. This type of ovotoxicity is insidious in its nature, and is not usually detected until the primordial follicle pool has become severely depleted, resulting in premature reproductive senescence. Besides a loss in fertility, reproductive senescence is also associated with an increased incidence of a variety of health problems. Despite the negatives associated with ovotoxic xenobiotics, there is potential to use their destructive nature for wildlife control and agricultural gain. It is a form of poetic justice that ovotoxic xenobiotics which prevent women from conceiving may be used to combat one of the biggest causes of death in the third world, starvation. Future research should be aimed at further elaborating the specific mechanisms of primordial follicle ovotoxicity, improving our ability to predict/detect human risk from environmental exposure, and investigating the possibility of using these ovotoxicants for the environmental control of pest species.

7. Acknowledgments

The authors gratefully acknowledge the financial assistance to EAM by the Australian Research Council, Hunter Medical Research Institute and the Newcastle Permanent Building Society Charitable Trust. APS is the recipient of an Australian Postgraduate Award PhD scholarship. This work was supported by National Health and Medical Research Council (Project grant #510735) to EAM.

8. References

Adhikari, D., W. Zheng, Y. Shen, N. Gorre, T. Hämäläinen, A. J. Cooney, I. Huhtaniemi, Z. J. Lan and K. Liu (2010). "Tsc/mTORC1 signaling in oocytes governs the quiescence and activation of primordial follicles." *Human molecular genetics* 19(3): pp. 397-410, ISSN 0964-6906.

Baksh, S., H. R. Widlund, A. A. Frazer-Abel, J. Du, S. Fosmire, D. E. Fisher, J. A. DeCaprio, J. F. Modiano and S. J. Burakoff (2002). "NFATc2-mediated repression of cyclin-dependent kinase 4 expression." *Molecular cell* 10(5): pp. 1071-1081, 1097-2765.

Benedict, J. C., T. M. Lin, I. K. Loeffler, R. E. Peterson and J. A. Flaws (2000). "Physiological role of the aryl hydrocarbon receptor in mouse ovary development." *Toxicological Sciences* 56(2): pp. 382-388, ISSN 1096-6080.

Benedict, J. C., K. P. Miller, T. M. Lin, C. Greenfeld, J. K. Babus, R. E. Peterson and J. A. Flaws (2003). "Aryl hydrocarbon receptor regulates growth, but not atresia, of mouse preantral and antral follicles." *Biology of reproduction* 68(5): pp. 1511-1517, ISSN 0006-3363.

Bengtsson, M., J. Montelius, L. Mankowitz and J. Rydström (1983). "Metabolism of polycyclic aromatic hydrocarbons in the rat ovary comparison with metabolism in adrenal and liver tissues." *Biochemical Pharmacology* 32(1): pp. 129-136, ISSN 0006-2952.

Bhattacharya, P. and A. F. Keating (2011). "Ovarian metabolism of xenobiotics." *Experimental Biology and Medicine* 236(7): pp. 765-771, ISSN 1535-3702.

Blume-Jensen, P., R. Janknecht and T. Hunter (1998). "The kit receptor promotes cell survival via activation of PI 3-kinase and subsequent Akt-mediated phosphorylation of Bad on Ser136." *Current biology* 8(13): pp. 779-785, ISSN 0960-9822.

Blumenfeld, Z. and N. Haim (1997). "Prevention of gonadal damage during cytotoxic therapy." *Annals of medicine* 29(3): pp. 199-206, ISSN 0785-3890.

Bolton, J. L., M. A. Trush, M. Trevor, G. Dryhurst and T. J. Monks (2000). "Role of quinones in toxicology." *Chemical Research in Toxicology* 13(3): pp. 135-160, ISSN 0893-228X.

Bondy, S. C. and S. Naderi (1994). "Contribution of hepatic cytochrome P450 systems to the generation of reactive oxygen species." *Biochemical pharmacology* 48(1): pp. 155-159, ISSN 0006-2952.

Borman, S. M., P. J. Christian, I. G. Sipes and P. B. Hoyer (2000). "Ovotoxicity in female Fischer rats and B6 mice induced by low-dose exposure to three polycyclic aromatic hydrocarbons: comparison through calculation of an ovotoxic index." *Toxicology and applied pharmacology* 167(3): pp. 191-198, ISSN 0041-008X.

Cadenas, E. and K. J. A. Davies (2000). "Mitochondrial free radical generation, oxidative stress, and aging." *Free Radical Biology and Medicine* 29(3-4): pp. 222-230, ISSN 0891-5849.

Calvin, H. I., K. Grosshans and E. J. Blake (1986). "Estimation and manipulation of glutathione levels in prepuberal mouse ovaries and ova: relevance to sperm nucleus transformation in the fertilized egg." *Gamete research* 14(3): pp. 265-275, ISSN 1554-3919.

Carlson, D. B. and G. H. Perdew (2002). "A dynamic role for the Ah receptor in cell signaling? Insights from a diverse group of Ah receptor interacting proteins." *Journal of biochemical and molecular toxicology* 16(6): pp. 317-325, ISSN 1099-0461.

Caro, A. A. and A. I. Cederbaum (2004). "Oxidative Stress, Toxicology, and Pharmacology of CYP2E1*." *Annu. Rev. Pharmacol. Toxicol.* 44: pp. 27-42, ISSN 0066-4170.

Castle, P. E. and J. Dean (1996). "Molecular genetics of the zona pellucida: implications for immunocontraceptive strategies." *Journal of reproduction and fertility. Supplement* 50: pp. 1-8, ISSN 0449-3087.

Cenci, S., G. Toraldo, M. N. Weitzmann, C. Roggia, Y. Gao, W. P. Qian, O. Sierra and R. Pacifici (2003). "Estrogen deficiency induces bone loss by increasing T cell proliferation and lifespan through IFN- -induced class II transactivator." *Proceedings of the National Academy of Sciences of the United States of America* 100(18): pp. 10405-10410, ISSN 0027-8424.

Clague, N., M. Sevcik, G. Stuart, M. Brännström, P. O. Janson and J. F. Jarrell (1992). "The effect of estrous cycle and buthionine sulfoximine on glutathione release from the in vitro perfused rat ovary." *Reproductive Toxicology* 6(6): pp. 533-539, ISSN 0890-6238.

Conney, A. H. (1982). "Induction of microsomal enzymes by foreign chemicals and carcinogenesis by polycyclic aromatic hydrocarbons: GHA Clowes Memorial Lecture." *Cancer research* 42(12): pp. 4875-4917, ISSN 0008-5472.

Coulam, C. B., S. C. Adamson and J. F. Annegers (1986). "Incidence of premature ovarian failure." *Obstetrics & Gynecology* 67(4): pp. 604-606, ISSN 0029-7844.

Dai, Y. S., J. Xu and J. D. Molkentin (2005). "The DnaJ-related factor Mrj interacts with nuclear factor of activated T cells c3 and mediates transcriptional repression through class II histone deacetylase recruitment." *Molecular and cellular biology* 25(22): pp. 9936, 0270-7306.

Danielson, P. B. (2002). "The cytochrome P450 superfamily: biochemistry, evolution and drug metabolism in humans." *Current Drug Metabolism* 3(6): pp. 561-597, ISSN 1389-2002.

Dekant, W. (2009). "The role of biotransformation and bioactivation in toxicity." *Molecular, Clinical and Environmental Toxicology* 99: pp. 57-86, ISSN 1023-294X.

Denison, M. S. and S. Heath-Pagliuso (1998). "The Ah receptor: a regulator of the biochemical and toxicological actions of structurally diverse chemicals." *Bulletin of environmental contamination and toxicology* 61(5): pp. 557-568, ISSN 0007-4861.

Devine, P. J., I. G. Sipes and P. B. Hoyer (2004). "Initiation of delayed ovotoxicity by in vitro and in vivo exposures of rat ovaries to 4-vinylcyclohexene diepoxide." *Reproductive Toxicology* 19(1): pp. 71-77, ISSN 0890-6238.

Duerrschmidt, N., O. Zabirnyk, M. Nowicki, A. Ricken, F. A. Hmeidan, V. Blumenauer, J. Borlak and K. Spanel-Borowski (2006). "Lectin-like oxidized low-density lipoprotein receptor-1-mediated autophagy in human granulosa cells as an alternative of programmed cell death." *Endocrinology* 147(8): pp. 3851-3860, ISSN 0013-7227.

Edson, M. A., A. K. Nagaraja and M. M. Matzuk (2009). "The mammalian ovary from genesis to revelation." *Endocrine reviews* 30(6): pp. 624-712, ISSN 1945-7189.

Ekstrom, G. and M. Ingelman-Sundberg (1989). "Rat liver microsomal NADPH-supported oxidase activity and lipid peroxidation dependent on ethanol-inducible cytochrome P-450 (P-450IIE1)." *Biochemical pharmacology* 38(8): pp. 1313-1319, ISSN 0006-2952.

Flaws, J. A., S. L. Marion, K. P. Miller, P. J. Christian, J. K. Babus and P. B. Hoyer (2006). "Effect of bcl-2 overexpression in mice on ovotoxicity caused by 4-vinylcyclohexene." *Toxicology and applied pharmacology* 215(1): pp. 51-56, ISSN 0041-008X.

Flaws, J. A., K. L. Salyers, I. G. Sipes and P. B. Hoyer (1994). "Reduced ability of rat preantral ovarian follicles to metabolize 4-vinyl-1-cyclohexene diepoxide in vitro." *Toxicology and applied pharmacology* 126(2): pp. 286-294, ISSN 0041-008X.

Galluzzi, L., J. M. Vicencio, O. Kepp, E. Tasdemir, M. C. Maiuri and G. Kroemer (2008). "To die or not to die: that is the autophagic question." *Curr Mol Med* 8(2): pp. 78-91, ISSN 1566-5240.

Geddes, A. M. W. (1992). The relative importance of pre-harvest crop pests in Indonesia, *Natural Resources Institute Bulletin (United Kingdom)*, A. M. W. Geddes, pp. 1-70, Natural Resources Institute, ISBN 0-85954-295-5. Chatham, UK.

Gobe, G. and B. Harmon (2001). Apoptosis: Morphological Criteria and Other Assays, *Encyclopedia of Life Sciences*, Y. Zheng, <http://dx.doi.org/10.1002/9780470015902.a0002569.pub3 >

Guraya, S. S. (1985). Primordial follicle, *Biology of Ovarian Follicles in Mammals*, pp. 3-14, Springer-Verlag, ISBN 9783540150220. Berlin, Germany.

Harrigan, J. A., C. M. Vezina, B. P. McGarrigle, N. Ersing, H. C. Box, A. E. Maccubbin and J. R. Olson (2004). "DNA adduct formation in precision-cut rat liver and lung slices exposed to benzo [a] pyrene." *Toxicological Sciences* 77(2): pp. 307-314, ISSN 1096-6080.

Hirshfield, A. N. (1991). "Development of follicles in the mammalian ovary." *International review of cytology* 124: pp. 43-101, ISSN 0074-7696.

Hooser, S. B., D. P. Douds, D. G. DeMerell, P. B. Hoyer and I. G. Sipes (1994). "Long-term ovarian and gonadotropin changes in mice exposed to 4-vinylcyclohexene." *Reproductive Toxicology* 8(4): pp. 315-323, ISSN 0890-6238.

Hou, Y. T., W. Xia, J. E. Pawlowski and T. M. Penning (1994). "Rat dihydrodiol dehydrogenase: complexity of gene structure and tissue-specific and sexually dimorphic gene expression." *Cancer research* 54(1): pp. 247-255, ISSN 0008-5472.

Hoyer, P. B. and P. J. Devine (2001). "Ovarian toxicity of 4-vinylcyclohexene diepoxide: a mechanistic model." *Toxicologic pathology* 29(1): pp. 91-99, ISSN 0192-6233.

Hoyer, P. B. and I. G. Sipes (1996). "Assessment of follicle destruction in chemical-induced ovarian toxicity." *Annual review of pharmacology and toxicology* 36(1): pp. 307-331, ISSN 0362-1642.

Hu, X., P. J. Christian, K. E. Thompson, I. Glenn Sipes and P. B. Hoyer (2001). "Apoptosis induced in rats by 4-vinylcyclohexene diepoxide is associated with activation of the caspase cascades." *Biology of reproduction* 65(1): pp. 87-93, ISSN 0006-3363.

Hughes, F. M. and W. C. Gorospe (1991). "Biochemical identification of apoptosis (programmed cell death) in granulosa cells: evidence for a potential mechanism underlying follicular atresia." *Endocrinology* 129(5): pp. 2415-2422, ISSN 0013-7227.

Igawa, Y., A. F. Keating, K. S. Rajapaksa, I. G. Sipes and P. B. Hoyer (2009). "Evaluation of ovotoxicity induced by 7, 12-dimethylbenz [a] anthracene and its 3, 4-diol metabolite utilizing a rat in vitro ovarian culture system." *Toxicology and applied pharmacology* 234(3): pp. 361-369, ISSN 0041-008X.

Jancovaa, P., P. Anzenbacherb and E. Anzenbacherovaa (2010). "Phase II drug metabolizing enzymes." *Biomed Pap Med Fac Univ Palacky Olomouc Czech Repub* 154(2): pp. 103-116, ISSN 1213-8118.

Janssen-Heininger, Y. M. W., B. T. Mossman, N. H. Heintz, H. J. Forman, B. Kalyanaraman, T. Finkel, J. S. Stamler, S. G. Rhee and A. van der Vliet (2008). "Redox-based regulation of signal transduction: principles, pitfalls, and promises." *Free Radical Biology and Medicine* 45(1): pp. 1-17, ISSN 0891-5849.

Jarrell, J. F., L. Bodo, E. V. Younglai, R. D. Barr and G. J. O'Connell (1991). "The short-term reproductive toxicity of cyclophosphamide in the female rat." *Reproductive Toxicology* 5(6): pp. 481-485, ISSN 0890-6238.

Keating, A. F. (2009). "Effect of phosphatidylinositol-3 kinase inhibition on ovotoxicity caused by 4-vinylcyclohexene diepoxide and 7, 12-dimethylbenz [a] anthracene in neonatal rat ovaries." *Toxicology and applied pharmacology* 241(2): pp. 127-134, ISSN 0041-008X.

Keating, A. F., S. M. Fernandez, C. J. Mark-Kappeler, N. Sen, I. G. Sipes and P. B. Hoyer (2011). "Inhibition of PIK3 Signaling Pathway Members by the Ovotoxicant 4-Vinylcyclohexene Diepoxide in Rats." *Biology of reproduction* 84(4): pp. 743-751, ISSN 0006-3363.

Keating, A. F., N. Sen, I. G. Sipes and P. B. Hoyer (2010). "Dual protective role for Glutathione S-transferase class pi against VCD-induced ovotoxicity in the rat ovary." *Toxicology and applied pharmacology* 247(2): pp. 71-75, ISSN 0041-008X.

Kidd, P. M. (1997). "Glutathione: systemic protectant against oxidative and free radical damage." *Alternative Medicine Review* 2(3): pp. 155-176, ISSN 1089-5159.

Kiffin, R., U. Bandyopadhyay and A. M. Cuervo (2006). "Oxidative stress and autophagy." *Antioxidants & redox signaling* 8(1-2): pp. 152-162, ISSN 1523-0864.

Kirkpatrick, J. F. (2007). "Measuring the effects of wildlife contraception: the argument for comparing apples with oranges." *Reproduction, Fertility and Development* 19(4): pp. 548-552, ISSN 1448-5990.

Klaunig, J. E. and L. M. Kamendulis (2004). "The role of oxidative stress in carcinogenesis." *Annu. Rev. Pharmacol. Toxicol.* 44: pp. 239-267, ISSN 0066-4170.

Kohalmy, K. and R. Vrzal (2011). "Regulation of Phase II Biotransformation Enzymes by Steroid Hormones." *Current Drug Metabolism* 12(2): pp. 104-123, ISSN 1389-2002.

Kondo, Y., T. Kanzawa, R. Sawaya and S. Kondo (2005). "Role of autophagy in cancer development and response to therapy." *Nature Reviews Cancer* 5(9): pp. 726-734, ISSN 1474-175X.

Levine, B. and D. J. Klionsky (2004). "Development by Self-Digestion:: Molecular Mechanisms and Biological Functions of Autophagy." *Developmental cell* 6(4): pp. 463-477, ISSN 1534-5807.

Levine, B. and J. Yuan (2005). "Autophagy in cell death: an innocent convict?" *Journal of Clinical Investigation* 115(10): pp. 2679-2688, ISSN 0021-9738.

Lobascio, A. M., F. G. Klinger, M. L. Scaldaferri, D. Farini and M. De Felici (2007). "Analysis of programmed cell death in mouse fetal oocytes." *Reproduction* 134(2): pp. 241-252, ISSN 1470-1626.

Luderer, U., T. J. Kavanagh, C. C. White and E. M. Faustman (2001). "Gonadotropin regulation of glutathione synthesis in the rat ovary." *Reproductive Toxicology* 15(5): pp. 495-504, ISSN 0890-6238.

Maiuri, M. C., E. Zalckvar, A. Kimchi and G. Kroemer (2007). "Self-eating and self-killing: crosstalk between autophagy and apoptosis." *Nature Reviews Molecular Cell Biology* 8(9): pp. 741-752, ISSN 1471-0072.

Martin, J. A., B. E. Hamilton, P. D. Sutton, S. J. Ventura, F. Menacker and M. L. Munson (2003). "Births: final data for 2002." *National vital statistics reports* 52(10): pp. 1-113, ISSN 1551-8930.

Matikainen, T., G. I. Perez, A. Jurisicova, J. K. Pru, J. J. Schlezinger, H. Y. Ryu, J. Laine, T. Sakai, S. J. Korsmeyer and R. F. Casper (2001). "Aromatic hydrocarbon receptor-driven Bax gene expression is required for premature ovarian failure caused by biohazardous environmental chemicals." *Nature Genetics* 28(4): pp. 355-360, ISSN 1061-4036.

Mattison, D. R. (1980). "Morphology of oocyte and follicle destruction by polycyclic aromatic hydrocarbons in mice." *Toxicology and Applied Pharmacology* 53(2): pp. 249-259, ISSN 0041-008X.

Mattison, D. R. and J. D. Schulman (1980). "How xenobiotic chemicals can destroy oocytes." *Contemp Obstet Gynecol* 15: pp. 157-169, ISSN 1471-8359.

Mattison, D. R., K. Shiromizu and M. S. Nightingale (1983a). "Oocyte destruction by polycyclic aromatic hydrocarbons." *American journal of industrial medicine* 4(1-2): pp. 191-202, ISSN 0271-3586.

Mattison, D. R., K. Shiromizu, J. A. Pendergrass and S. S. Thorgeirsson (1983b). "Ontogeny of ovarian glutathione and sensitivity to primordial oocyte destruction by cyclophosphamide." *Pediatric pharmacology (New York, NY)* 3(1): pp. 49-55, ISSN 0270-322X.

Mattison, D. R. and S. S. Thorgeirsson (1979). "Ovarian aryl hydrocarbon hydroxylase activity and primordial oocyte toxicity of polycyclic aromatic hydrocarbons in mice." *Cancer Research* 39(9): pp. 3471-3475, ISSN 0008-5472.

McAlpine, C. A., S. Heyenga, B. Taylor, A. N. N. Peterson and G. McDonald (2007). "Regional planning in Queensland's rangelands: challenges and prospects for biodiversity conservation." *Geographical Research* 45(1): pp. 27-42, ISSN 1745-5871.

McGee, E. A. and A. J. W. Hsueh (2000). "Initial and cyclic recruitment of ovarian follicles." *Endocrine reviews* 21(2): pp. 200-214, ISSN 1945-7189.

McNatty, K. P., A. E. Fidler, J. L. Juengel, L. D. Quirke, P. R. Smith, D. A. Heath, T. Lundy, A. O'Connell and D. J. Tisdall (2000). "Growth and paracrine factors regulating follicular formation and cellular function." *Molecular and Cellular Endocrinology* 163(1-2): pp. 11-20, ISSN 0303-7207.

Meirow, D., J. Dor, B. Kaufman, A. Shrim, J. Rabinovici, E. Schiff, H. Raanani, J. Levron and E. Fridman (2007). "Cortical fibrosis and blood-vessels damage in human ovaries exposed to chemotherapy. Potential mechanisms of ovarian injury." *Human reproduction* 22(6): pp. 1626-1633, ISSN 0268-1161.

Melendez-Colon, V. J., A. Luch, A. Seidel and W. M. Baird (1999). "Cancer initiation by polycyclic aromatic hydrocarbons results from formation of stable DNA adducts rather than apurinic sites." *Carcinogenesis* 20(10): pp. 1885-1891, ISSN 0143-3334.

Meunier, B., S. P. De Visser and S. Shaik (2004). "Mechanism of oxidation reactions catalyzed by cytochrome P450 enzymes." *Chemical reviews* 104(9): pp. 3947-3980, ISSN 0009-2665.

Mwanjabe, P. S. and H. Leirs (1997). "An early warning system for IPM-based rodent control in smallholder farming systems in Tanzania." *Belgian Journal of Zoology* 127: pp. 49-58, ISSN 0777-6276.

Nebert, D. W., D. D. Brown, D. W. Towne and H. J. Eisen (1984). "Association of fertility, fitness and longevity with the murine Ah locus among (C57BL/6N)(C3H/HeN) recombinant inbred lines." *Biology of reproduction* 30(2): pp. 363-373, ISSN 0006-3363.

Nebert, D. W., A. L. Roe, M. Z. Dieter, W. A. Solis, Y. I. Yang and T. P. Dalton (2000). "Role of the aromatic hydrocarbon receptor and [Ah] gene battery in the oxidative stress response, cell cycle control, and apoptosis." *Biochemical pharmacology* 59(1): pp. 65-85, ISSN 0006-2952.

Nguyen, L. P. and C. A. Bradfield (2007). "The search for endogenous activators of the aryl hydrocarbon receptor." *Chemical research in toxicology* 21(1): pp. 102-116, ISSN 0893-228X.

Park, J. H., S. Gopishetty, L. M. Szewczuk, A. B. Troxel, R. G. Harvey and M. Trevor (2005). "Formation of 8-oxo-7, 8-dihydro-2'-deoxyguanosine (8-oxo-dGuo) by PAH o-quinones: involvement of reactive oxygen species and copper (II)/copper (I) redox cycling." *Chemical research in toxicology* 18(6): pp. 1026-1037, ISSN 0893-228X.

Pavek, P. and Z. Dvorak (2008). "Xenobiotic-induced transcriptional regulation of xenobiotic metabolizing enzymes of the cytochrome P450 superfamily in human extrahepatic tissues." *Current drug metabolism* 9(2): pp. 129-143, ISSN 1389-2002.

Petrulis, J. R. and G. H. Perdew (2002). "The role of chaperone proteins in the aryl hydrocarbon receptor core complex." *Chemico-biological interactions* 141(1-2): pp. 25-40, ISSN 0009-2797.

Picut, C. A., C. L. Swanson, K. L. Scully, V. C. Roseman, R. F. Parker and A. K. Remick (2008). "Ovarian follicle counts using proliferating cell nuclear antigen (PCNA) and semi-automated image analysis in rats." *Toxicologic pathology* 36(5): pp. 674-679, ISSN 0192-6233.

Plowchalk, D. R. and D. R. Mattison (1992). "Reproductive toxicity of cyclophosphamide in the C57BL/6N mouse: 1. Effects on ovarian structure and function." *Reproductive Toxicology* 6(5): pp. 411-421, ISSN 0890-6238.

Pollenz, R. S., C. A. Sattler and A. Poland (1994). "The aryl hydrocarbon receptor and aryl hydrocarbon receptor nuclear translocator protein show distinct subcellular localizations in Hepa 1c1c7 cells by immunofluorescence microscopy." *Molecular pharmacology* 45(3): pp. 428-438, ISSN 0026-895X.

Raffray, M. and M. C. Gerald (1997). "Apoptosis and necrosis in toxicology: a continuum or distinct modes of cell death?" *Pharmacology & therapeutics* 75(3): pp. 153-177, ISSN 0163-7258.

Rajapaksa, K. S., E. A. Cannady, I. G. Sipes and P. B. Hoyer (2007a). "Involvement of CYP 2E1 enzyme in ovotoxicity caused by 4-vinylcyclohexene and its metabolites." *Toxicology and applied pharmacology* 221(2): pp. 215-221, ISSN 0041-008X.

Rajapaksa, K. S., I. G. Sipes and P. B. Hoyer (2007b). "Involvement of microsomal epoxide hydrolase enzyme in ovotoxicity caused by 7, 12-dimethylbenz [a] anthracene." *Toxicological sciences* 96(2): pp. 327-334, ISSN 1096-6080.

Ramesh, A., A. E. Archibong and M. S. Niaz (2010). "Ovarian Susceptibility to Benzo [a] Pyrene: Tissue Burden of Metabolites and DNA Adducts in F-344 Rats." *Journal of toxicology and environmental health. Part A* 73(23): pp. 1611-1625, ISSN 1528-7394.

Reddy, P., L. Liu, D. Adhikari, K. Jagarlamudi, S. Rajareddy, Y. Shen, C. Du, W. Tang, T. Hämäläinen and S. L. Peng (2008). "Oocyte-specific deletion of Pten causes premature activation of the primordial follicle pool." *Science* 319(5863): pp. 611-613, ISSN 0036-8075.

Reddy, P., W. Zheng and K. Liu (2010). "Mechanisms maintaining the dormancy and survival of mammalian primordial follicles." *Trends in Endocrinology & Metabolism* 21(2): pp. 96-103, ISSN 1043-2760.

Reyes, H., S. Reisz-Porszasz and O. Hankinson (1992). "Identification of the Ah receptor nuclear translocator protein (Arnt) as a component of the DNA binding form of the Ah receptor." *Science* 256(5060): pp. 1193-1195, ISSN 0036-8075.

Robles, R., Y. Morita, K. K. Mann, G. I. Perez, S. Yang, T. Matikainen, D. H. Sherr and J. L. Tilly (2000). "The aryl hydrocarbon receptor, a basic helix-loop-helix transcription factor of the PAS gene family, is required for normal ovarian germ cell dynamics in the mouse." *Endocrinology* 141(1): pp. 450-453, ISSN 0013-7227.

Rodrigues, P., D. Limback, L. K. McGinnis, C. E. Plancha and D. F. Albertini (2009). "Multiple mechanisms of germ cell loss in the perinatal mouse ovary." *Reproduction* 137(4): pp. 709-720, ISSN 1470-1626.

Rodríguez, M. and A. Jaime (1993). Rodent plague: a continuing problem in Latin America and the Caribbean. *Latin American Conference on Rodent Biology and Control of Plague*, ISBN 9718709053, Santa Cruz, Bolivia, October 1991.

Sanders, D. L., F. Xie, R. E. Mauldin, J. C. Hurley, L. A. Miller, M. R. Garcia, R. W. DeYoung, D. B. Long and T. A. Campbell (2011). "Efficacy of ERL-4221 as an ovotoxin for feral pigs (Sus scrofa)." *Wildlife Research* 38(2): pp. 168-172, ISSN 1448-5494.

Schafer, F. Q. and G. R. Buettner (2001). "Redox environment of the cell as viewed through the redox state of the glutathione disulfide/glutathione couple." *Free Radical Biology and Medicine* 30(11): pp. 1191-1212, ISSN 0891-5849.

Schmidt, J. V., G. H. Su, J. K. Reddy, M. C. Simon and C. A. Bradfield (1996). "Characterization of a murine Ahr null allele: involvement of the Ah receptor in hepatic growth and development." *Proceedings of the National Academy of Sciences* 93(13): pp. 6731-6736, ISSN 0027-8424.

Schroer, K., M. Kittelmann and S. Lütz (2010). "Recombinant human cytochrome P450 monooxygenases for drug metabolite synthesis." *Biotechnology and bioengineering* 106(5): pp. 699-706, ISSN 1097-0290.

Schwarz, D., P. Kisselev, I. Cascorbi, W. H. Schunck and I. Roots (2001). "Differential metabolism of benzo [a] pyrene and benzo [a] pyrene-7, 8-dihydrodiol by human CYP1A1 variants." *Carcinogenesis* 22(3): pp. 453-459, ISSN 0143-3334.

Shimada, T. and Y. Fujii Kuriyama (2004). "Metabolic activation of polycyclic aromatic hydrocarbons to carcinogens by cytochromes P450 1A1 and1B1." *Cancer science* 95(1): pp. 1-6, ISSN 1349-7006.

Shimada, T., Y. Oda, E. M. J. Gillam, F. P. Guengerich and K. Inoue (2001). "Metabolic activation of polycyclic aromatic hydrocarbons and other procarcinogens by cytochromes P450 1A1 and P450 1B1 allelic variants and other human cytochromes P450 in Salmonella typhimurium NM2009." *Drug metabolism and disposition* 29(9): pp. 1176-1182, ISSN 0090-9556.

Shimada, T., A. Sugie, M. Shindo, T. Nakajima, E. Azuma, M. Hashimoto and K. Inoue (2003). "Tissue-specific induction of cytochromes P450 1A1 and 1B1 by polycyclic aromatic hydrocarbons and polychlorinated biphenyls in engineered C57BL/6J mice of arylhydrocarbon receptor gene." *Toxicology and applied pharmacology* 187(1): pp. 1-10, ISSN 0041-008X.

Shimizu, S., T. Kanaseki, N. Mizushima, T. Mizuta, S. Arakawa-Kobayashi, C. B. Thompson and Y. Tsujimoto (2004). "Role of Bcl-2 family proteins in a non-apoptotic programmed cell death dependent on autophagy genes." *Nature cell biology* 6(12): pp. 1221-1228, ISSN 1465-7392.

Shiromizu, K. and D. R. Mattison (1985). "Murine oocyte destruction following intraovarian treatment with 3 methylcholanthrene or 7, 12 dimethylbenz (a) anthracene: Protection by alpha naphthoflavone." *Teratogenesis, carcinogenesis, and mutagenesis* 5(6): pp. 463-472, ISSN 1520-6866.

Shuster, L. T., D. J. Rhodes, B. S. Gostout, B. R. Grossardt and W. A. Rocca (2010). "Premature menopause or early menopause: long-term health consequences." *Maturitas* 65(2): pp. 161-166, ISSN 0378-5122.

Singleton, G. R. (2003). "Impacts of rodents on rice production in Asia." *IRRI Discuss. Pap. Ser* 45: pp. 1-30, ISSN 0115-3862.

Smith, B. J., D. R. Mattison and I. G. Sipes (1990). "The role of epoxidation in 4-vinylcyclohexene-induced ovarian toxicity." *Toxicology and applied pharmacology* 105(3): pp. 372-381, ISSN 0041-008X.

Sobinoff, A. P., M. Mahony, B. Nixon, S. D. Roman and E. A. McLaughlin (2011). "Understanding the villain: DMBA induced pre-antral ovotoxicity involves selective follicular destruction and primordial follicle activation through PI3K/Akt and mTOR signalling." *Toxicological Sciences*: pp. kfr195v1-kfr195, ISSN 1096-6080.

Sobinoff, A. P., V. Pye, B. Nixon, S. D. Roman and E. A. McLaughlin (2010). "Adding Insult to Injury: Effects of Xenobiotic-Induced Preantral Ovotoxicity on Ovarian Development and Oocyte Fusibility." *Toxicological Sciences* 118(2): pp. 653-666, ISSN 1096-6080.

Springer, L. N., M. E. McAsey, J. A. Flaws, J. L. Tilly, I. G. Sipes and P. B. Hoyer (1996). "Involvement of apoptosis in 4-vinylcyclohexene diepoxide-induced ovotoxicity in rats." *Toxicology and applied pharmacology* 139(2): pp. 394-401, ISSN 0041-008X.

Stapleton, H. M. and J. E. Baker (2003). "Comparing polybrominated diphenyl ether and polychlorinated biphenyl bioaccumulation in a food web in Grand Traverse Bay, Lake Michigan." *Archives of environmental contamination and toxicology* 45(2): pp. 227-234, ISSN 0090-4341.

Tarin, J. J. (1996). "Potential effects of age-associated oxidative stress on mammalian oocytes/embryos." *Molecular human reproduction* 2(10): pp. 717-724, ISSN 1360-9947.

Taylor, K. D. (1968). "An outbreak of rats in agricultural areas of Kenya in 1962." *East African Agricultural and Forestry Journal* 34(1): pp. 66-77, ISSN 0012-8325.

Terman, A., B. Gustafsson and U. T. Brunk (2006). "The lysosomal-mitochondrial axis theory of postmitotic aging and cell death." *Chemico-biological interactions* 163(1-2): pp. 29-37, ISSN 0009-2797.

Testa, J. R. and A. Bellacosa (2001). "AKT plays a central role in tumorigenesis." *Proceedings of the National Academy of Sciences* 98(20): pp. 10983-10985, ISSN 0027-8424.

Thimmulappa, R. K., K. H. Mai, S. Srisuma, T. W. Kensler, M. Yamamoto and S. Biswal (2002). "Identification of Nrf2-regulated genes induced by the chemopreventive agent sulforaphane by oligonucleotide microarray." *Cancer research* 62(18): pp. 5196-5203, ISSN 0008-5472.

Thor, H., M. T. Smith, P. Hartzell, G. Bellomo, S. A. Jewell and S. Orrenius (1982). "The metabolism of menadione (2-methyl-1, 4-naphthoquinone) by isolated hepatocytes. A study of the implications of oxidative stress in intact cells." *Journal of Biological Chemistry* 257(20): pp. 12419-12425, ISSN 0021-9258.

Tilly, J. L., K. I. Kowalski, A. L. Johnson and A. J. W. Hsueh (1991). "Involvement of apoptosis in ovarian follicular atresia and postovulatory regression." *Endocrinology* 129(5): pp. 2799-2801, ISSN 0013-7227.

Tilly, J. L. and R. Robles (1999). Apoptosis and its impact in clinical reproductive medicine, *Molecular biology in reproductive medicine,* B. C. J. M. Fauser, A. J. Rutherford, J. F. Strauss and A. Van Steirteghem, pp. 79–101, ISBN 1850709947. New York, USA.

Tománek, M. and E. Chronowska (2006). "Immunohistochemical localization of proliferating cell nuclear antigen (PCNA) in the pig ovary." *Folia histochemica et Cytobiologica* 44(4): pp. 269-274, ISSN 0239-8508.

Trevor, M., S. T. Ohnishi, T. Ohnishi and R. G. Harvey (1996). "Generation of reactive oxygen species during the enzymatic oxidation of polycyclic aromatic hydrocarbon trans-dihydrodiols catalyzed by dihydrodiol dehydrogenase." *Chemical research in toxicology* 9(1): pp. 84-92, ISSN 0893-228X.

Tsai-Turton, M., B. N. Nakamura and U. Luderer (2007). "Induction of apoptosis by 9, 10-dimethyl-1, 2-benzanthracene in cultured preovulatory rat follicles is preceded by a rise in reactive oxygen species and is prevented by glutathione." *Biology of Reproduction* 77(3): pp. 442-451, ISSN 0006-3363.

Valko, M., D. Leibfritz, J. Moncol, M. T. D. Cronin, M. Mazur and J. Telser (2007). "Free radicals and antioxidants in normal physiological functions and human disease." *The international journal of biochemistry & cell biology* 39(1): pp. 44-84, ISSN 1357-2725.

Valko, M., C. J. Rhodes, J. Moncol, M. Izakovic and M. Mazur (2006). "Free radicals, metals and antioxidants in oxidative stress-induced cancer." *Chemico-biological interactions* 160(1): pp. 1-40, ISSN 0009-2797.

van Wezel, I. L. and R. J. Rodgers (1996). "Morphological characterization of bovine primordial follicles and their environment in vivo." *Biology of reproduction* 55(5): pp. 1003-1011, ISSN 0006-3363.

Vlahos, C. J., W. F. Matter, K. Y. Hui and R. F. Brown (1994). "A specific inhibitor of phosphatidylinositol 3-kinase, 2-(4-morpholinyl)-8-phenyl-4H-1-benzopyran-4-one (LY294002)." *Journal of Biological Chemistry* 269(7): pp. 5241-5248, ISSN 0021-9258.

Wang, K., H. Fang, D. Xiao, X. Zhu, M. He, X. Pan, J. Shi, H. Zhang, X. Jia and Y. Du (2009). "Converting redox signaling to apoptotic activities by stress-responsive regulators

HSF1 and NRF2 in fenretinide treated cancer cells." *PLoS One* 4(10): pp. e7538, ISSN 1932-6203.

Wang, Q., Y. Zhou, L. N. Jackson, S. M. Johnson, C. W. Chow and B. M. Evers "Nuclear factor of activated T cells (NFAT) signaling regulates PTEN expression and intestinal cell differentiation." *Molecular Biology of the Cell* 22(3): pp. 412,

Wells, P. G., G. P. McCallum, C. S. Chen, J. T. Henderson, C. J. J. Lee, J. Perstin, T. J. Preston, M. J. Wiley and A. W. Wong (2009). "Oxidative stress in developmental origins of disease: teratogenesis, neurodevelopmental deficits, and cancer." *Toxicological sciences* 108(1): pp. 4-18, ISSN 1096-6080.

Wu, K. L. and T. Berger (2008). "Reduction in rat oocyte fertilizability mediated by S-(1, 2-dichlorovinyl)-L-cysteine: a trichloroethylene metabolite produced by the glutathione conjugation pathway." *Bulletin of environmental contamination and toxicology* 81(5): pp. 490-493, ISSN 0007-4861.

Part 3

Human

24

Parkinson's Disease: Insights from the Laboratory and Clinical Therapeutics

Jing-ye Zhou, Yong Yu, Xian-Lun Zhu,
Chi-Ping Ng, Gang Lu* and Wai-Sang Poon
*Division of Neurosurgery, Department of Surgery,
The Chinese University of Hong Kong, Hong Kong,
China*

1. Introduction

Parkinson's disease (PD), a neurodegenerative disorder that was first described by James Parkinson (1755-1824) in 1817, is characterized partly by a progressive loss of dopaminergic neurons in the substantia nigra pars compact. It affects approximately 1.5% of the global population over 65 years of age. PD is the type of Parkinsonism that is defined as any combination of six specific and independent motoric features: bradykinesia, resting tremor, rigidity, loss of postural reflexes, flexed posture and the freezing phenomenon. Current dopamine replacement strategies, which include levodopa (L-DOPA, the precursor of dopamine) and dopamine receptor agonists, as well as monoamine oxidase B and catechol O-methyltransferase inhibitors, can effectively improve these symptoms. Many reviews of this field are available elsewhere; therefore we focus here on the most recent outcomes regarding the identification of key biomedical progress in PD, describe the most promising biological research targets that are currently being assessed to find ideal treatments, and provide insights from progress in laboratory research and clinical therapeutics.

2. The pathogenesis of Parkinson's disease

Decades of research have not found a single cause for PD and therefore a single factor is unlikely to emerge. Current research is mainly carried out on animal models of PD induced by intoxication with 1-methyl-4-phenyl-1,2,3,6-tetrahydropyridine (MPTP) and models of postencephalitic parkinsonism, neither of which has fully reproduced the clinical and pathological features of true PD. However, it is believed that PD is a multifactorial disease caused by both environmental factors and genetic susceptibility. Aging is an obvious factor because PD mainly targets elderly people. Studies have shown that the incidence of PD is around 10-15 cases per 100 000 person–years (1), but this figure increased to 93.1 in people aged between 70 and 90 years (2). Male sex appeared to be another risk factor, because the incidence of PD in men was 1.5 times higher than that in women (3). Geographically, China has a similar prevalence of PD to western countries (4), whereas Africans have a lower rate compared with African Americans (5).

---

* Corresponding Author

2.1 Environmental factors

Many environmental factors may increase the risk of developing PD. Priyadarshi et al. (6-7) showed the association between PD and farming, professional pesticide use, and drinking well-water in a meta-analysis. Other environmental factors, such as metals, solvents, electromagnetic fields and lifestyles, have also been determined as possible risk factors (8). Studies over the past two to three decades have provided more supportive findings. Tanner and Goldman (9) linked the consumption of well-water to the occurrence of PD. Living in rural areas was associated with farming and pesticide use, which led to an increased incidence of PD patients (10-11). This was association was clarified by another study that demonstrated that the effect of pesticide use was independent from that of farming (12). A lifestyle study found similar evidence of increased herbicide exposure in patients with PD (13). The discovery that exposure to MPTP induced parkinsonian syndromes initiated a new field in PD research - the study of exposure to pesticides (14-15). Many different pesticides have been investigated. MPTP has a similar structure to paraquat, a herbicide that is widely used in many countries. Paraquat was found to be associated with PD based on a 20-year exposure study (16). In a study in Germany, organochlorine pesticides were identified as risk factors for PD (17). Dithiocarbamates, which have been shown to enhance MPTP toxicity (18), were considered to be another risk factor for PD (19). Manganese, a constituent of several pesticides and herbicides, induced parkinsonism in humans following chronic exposure (20). Pesticides and herbicides may be used in combination, which results in a higher level of toxicity. One study showed that exposure to paraquat plus manganese ethylenebis-dithiocarbamate (maneb) resulted in 4.17-fold greater risk for PD compared with unexposed populations (21).

In addition to the above agricultural risk factors, industrial factors also play an important role in the development of PD. Chronic exposure to copper, manganese, and lead was associated with the risk for PD (22) and PD patients who had worked in factories that used chemicals, iron or copper had higher death rates (23). A German study also reported an association between exposure to lead and PD (17). Furthermore, the relationship between PD and head trauma has been investigated: a history of head trauma was associated with onset of PD at an earlier age (24-25).

As discussed above, many risk factors are involved in the development of PD; however, two environmental factors could lower this risk: cigarette smoking (26) and coffee drinking (27), although their mechanisms are unknown. Studies of twins showed an inverse association between cigarette smoking and PD (28-29), and similar results were reported by a study that compared PD cases with their unaffected siblings (30). A meta-analysis reported an inverse association between PD and coffee drinking which was independent of smoking (31). However, this was seen in men but not in women (27).

2.2 Genetic susceptibility

Most cases of PD are sporadic, but some patients (10-15%) show a positive familial history of the disease (32). Although the cause of PD is still unknown, both environmental and genetic factors are considered to be important. The discovery of several causative mutations and genes (33) has allowed a better understanding of PD.

2.2.1 α-Synuclein (PARK1)

α-Synuclein, also called PARK1, was the first gene to be linked to PD (34), and mutations in α-synuclein gene have been linked to rare cases of familial PD (35-37). Genomic multiplications have been reported and both mRNA and protein levels of α-synuclein were increased in the brain (38). However, a large screening study has shown that α-synuclein multiplication is a rare cause of parkinsonism (39). Nevertheless, there is a link between α-synuclein level and age at onset and severity: when α-synuclein duplication causes the disease at an earlier age, then PD has a more aggressive form (39-40). α-Synuclein is a small neuronal protein that is involved in neurotransmitter release and synaptic vesicle recycling. Without genetic changes, α-synuclein is an abundant protein and a major component of Lewy bodies (LBs) in idiopathic, apparently sporadic PD (41-42). This supports the role of α-synuclein in the pathogenesis of PD.

2.2.2 Parkin (PARK2)

The PARK2 gene was identified as parkin in autosomal recessive forms of familial juvenileparkinsonism (AR-JP) (43). AR-JP is most commonly seen in Japanese populations and typically has an onset before the age of 40 years (44-45). Interestingly, no LBs have been found in parkin-positive brains. Parkin was reported to act as an E3-ubiquitin ligase that targets cytoplasmic proteins for proteasomal degradation and plays a role in receptor trafficking (46-47). A wide variety of parkin mutations have been found including large homozygous deletions in exons (43); frame-shift mutations, point mutations, duplications and triplications of exons (48); and deletions in the promoter (49). Parkin mutations were identified in nearly 50% of familial cases with disease onset before the age of 45 years (50) and in 15% of sporadic young-onset cases (51). In the subset of cases with onset before the age of 20 years, this proportion increased to 70% (51).

2.2.3 Ubiquitin carboxyl-terminal hydrolase L1 (UCH-L1; PARK5)

UCH-L1 is an enzyme that hydrolyzes the C-terminus of ubiquitin to generate ubiquitin monomers that can be recycled to clear other proteins. A single missense mutation in UCH-L1 was reported in two siblings with typical PD in a German family (52). A second rare mutation was reported in French families but was not restricted to PD (53). No other carriers of this mutation and no other mutations in UCH-L1 have been identified (54-55), which has raised doubts about the relevance of UCH-L1 to PD.

2.2.4 PTEN-induced kinase 1 (PINK1; PARK6)

PINK1 encodes a widely expressed protein kinase that is localized in mitochondria. PINK1 is the second most common cause of AR-JP (56) and may play an important role in sporadic PD (57). Several mutations have been identified including transitions (56), single heterozygous mutations (57), and heterozygous deletion of the PINK1 gene plus a splice site mutation on the remaining copy (58). One study suggested that heterozygous mutations are a significant risk factor in the development of PD (59). Briefly, PINK1 mutations may cause loss of function in patients with recessively inherited forms of PD because most mutations fall in the kinase domain (60).

2.2.5 Oncogene DJ-1 (PARK7)

The DJ-1 gene encodes a ubiquitous and highly conserved protein, and has been identified as a causative gene for early-onset autosomal recessive PD (61). A couple of mutations have been reported but these were found in only a few patients with early-onset PD (61-62). DJ-1 protein is not an essential component of LBs but is localized in mitochondria that protect against neuronal death (63).

2.2.6 Leucine-rich repeat kinase 2 (LRRK2; PARK8)

LRRK2 mutations are the most common mutations identified in either familial or sporadic PD. Although other LRRK2 mutations have been described, the G2019S mutation has been found to be the most common pathogenic cause of PD, and has been reported in 5–6.6% of cases of autosomal dominant PD (64-65) and 2–8% of sporadic cases (66-67). Penetrance in G2019S patients was age dependent, and increased from 17% at the age of 50 years to 85% at the age of 70 years (68). Nigral neuron loss and LB formation have been observed in the brains of sporadic PD patients with G2019S mutations (66).

2.2.7 Adenosine triphosphatase type 13A2 (ATP13A2; PARK9)

ATP13A2 has been identified as the causative gene in Kufor-Rakeb syndrome (69), a rare form of juvenile-onset parkinsonism caused by autosomal recessive neurodegeneration. Studies in PD patients have reported mutations of 22bp duplication in exon 16 (70) and missense mutation in exon 15 (71), indicating that they are possible causes of PD.

2.2.8 OMI/HTRA serine peptidase 2 (OMI/HTRA2; PARK13)

A missense mutation in the OMI/HTRA2 gene has been found in sporadic PD patients (72). The OMI/HTRA2 gene is located within the PARK3 linkage region, but its role in PD is unknown.

Other genetic factors, such as glucocerebrosidase (73), microtubule-associated protein tau (74) and progranulin (75), have shown an association with PD but their causality has yet to be elucidated.

3. Experimental models in PD research

3.1 Neurotoxin models

The development of experimental models is essential for a better understanding of the etiopathogenesis of PD and to provide effective therapeutic agents. Neurotoxins that target the dopamine (DA) system, such as 6-hydroxydopamine (6-OHDA) and MPTP were used in early animal models for PD research and are still widely in current use (76).

3.1.1 6-OHDA

6-OHDA was the first agent used in an animal model of PD (77). Because of its structural similarity to DA and norepinephrine, 6-OHDA can enter and accumulate in both dopaminergic and noradrenergic neurons. Catecholaminergic structures are destroyed by 6-

OHDA through reactive oxygen species (ROS) and quinines (78-79). Because 6-OHDA crosses the blood-brain barrier (BBB) poorly, it is usually injected directly into the brain stereotaxically. Intraventricular and intracisternal administrations of 6-OHDA to rats produce a bilateral loss of DA and motor abnormalities that can be partially corrected by dopaminergic receptor agonists (80). However, the motor deficits induced are caused by considerable depletion of DA that requires high doses of 6-OHDA. Thus, animals often die due to aphagia and adipsia from severe stress (77, 81). In contrast, a unilateral intracerebral injection is more practical and useful. This model provides an approach to measure asymmetrical turning behavior in response to DA agonists with an internal control - the unlesioned contralateral side of the brain. To induce unilateral lesions, 6-OHDA is typically injected into the striatum, substantia nigra or the median forebrain bundle. Striatal injection of 6-OHDA produces slow retrograde degeneration of the nigrostriatal system over 1 month (82) and apoptotic morphology in the neurons that die (83-84). After injection of 6-OHDA into the substantia nigra or the medial forebrain bundle, dopaminergic neurons die more quickly than after striatal injection and no apoptotic morphology is seen (85). It should be noted that no typical LB formation has been demonstrated in this model (86). Unilateral lesions produce typical asymmetric circling motor behavior, especially after injection into the substantia nigra or the medial forebrain bundle which leads to more readily detectable behavioral deficits. The quantification of this circling behavior has been applied widely to evaluate new anti-parkinsonian drugs, and stem-cell and gene therapies (86).

6-OHDA has mainly been used in small animals, such as rodents, but has also been administered to non-human primates (86) and has been applied *in vitro* in various different models (87). The unilateral lesion induced by 6-OHDA in rats is one of the most popular models of PD (88-89). This model has advantages for testing cell replacement therapies and investigating regenerative therapies (90). However, 6-OHDA models demonstrate only one dimension of a complex illness: one type of cell loss and cellular stress. Moreover, 6-OHDA causes an acute model and cannot replicate many features of PD (90).

3.1.2 MPTP

MPTP was discovered in the early 1980s (14). Unlike 6-OHDA, MPTP is highly lipophilic and can cross the BBB easily after systemic administration. In the brain, it is metabolized to the 1-methyl-4-phenylpyridinium ion (MPP^+), which can enter dopaminergic neurons via the DA transporter (DAT) (91), and results in mitochondrial complex I inhibition and ROS formation (92). No LBs have been observed in MPTP-induced parkinsonism in either human or animal models (93-94).

Systemic administration of MPTP to many different species satisfies most of the requirements for an ideal parkinsonian model (90). The most commonly used PD model is the MPTP mouse model cause of the relatively low cost and acceptable timing for research. Acute administration of MPTP caused depletion in striatal DA (95), whereas the subacute model showed striatal DA depletion and cell loss in the substantia nigra (96-97). However, the acute model showed a greater loss of striatal DA than the subacute model. Moreover, the mechanism of cell death appears to differ in these two models: non-apoptotic mechanisms after acute (98) versus apoptotic mechanisms after subacute administration of MPTP (99). In addition, Acute treatment of animals with MPTP induced clear microglial activation in the striatum and the substantia nigra (100-101) and over-expression of inducible nitric oxide synthase (102), whereas the subacute model showed only minimal microglial activation (101). Consequently, anti-inflammatory and anti-microglial compounds could be potential neuroprotective agents for PD and have been investigated using the acute MPTP model.

Although the mouse model has been used extensively in PD research, the non-human primate model is considered to be the "gold standard" for assessment before clinical trials because it reproduces the main pathological defect of PD, and the parkinsonian symptoms induced match many clinical features of PD. Acute and chronic non-human primate models are available, and both show similar motor symptoms of parkinsonism, although the mechanisms differ. Schneider et al. reported that the acute MPTP monkey model inuced increased binding to striatal DA D1 and D2 receptors and increased striatal prepronkephalin mRNA expression. In contrast to these findings, striatal preprotachykinin mRNA expression was decreased in both acute and chronic MPTP monkey models. Notablely, chronic administration of MPTP to animals with cognitive but no motor deficits induced no changes in preprotachykinin expression in the striaturn (103).

MPTP has been used to produce the best-characterized model of PD (104) in many different species, including non-human primates, small vertebrates, such as mice, and even invertebrates, such as worms (105-107). However, rats are relatively resistant to MPTP-induced neurotoxicity compared with mice (108-109) and primates are the most sensitive model (110). MPTP models develop pathological and neurochemical changes similar to those of PD patients (111) and produce an irreversible and severe parkinsonian syndrome that includes rigidity, tremor, bradykinesia, posture abnormalities and even freezing (86, 112). PD is a slowly progressive illness but the MPTP mouse model is an acute or subacute process. The chronic administration of MPTP to primates induced the slow development of a parkinsonian syndrome (113).

3.1.3 Rotenone

Rotenone is one of the most recent neurotoxins to be used in PD models (114). It is widely used as an insecticide throughout the world, and the rotenone model was the first to use an environmental toxin. Rotenone is highly lipophilic and can thus move freely and rapidly across cellular membranes without transporters. In mitochondria, it interferes with the electron transport chain, resulting in mitochondrial complex I inhibition (115). Furthermore, it also inhibits the formation of microtubules from tubulin (116) and the excess of tubulin monomers may be toxic to cells (117). The complex I inhibition induced by rotenone led to increased levels of oxidative stress which occurred predominantly in dopaminergic regions including the striatum, ventral midbrain and the olfactory bulb (118). Rotenone is a mitochondrial complex I inhibitor and acts evenly throughout the brain (119), which indicates that dopaminergic neurons are uniquely sensitive to mitochondrial complex I inhibition. Sherer et al (120) detected microglial activation in the striatum and substantia nigra of rotenone-infused rats. In the same model, the hallmark of PD pathology - LBs - were observed (114, 121) in the ventral midbrain regions (122). Exposure of animals to rotenone caused selective nigrostriatal dopaminergic neurodegeneration but had minimal effects on neurons of other brain regions (114, 121). It has been reported that parkinsonian symptoms in humans, such as rigidity and bradykinesia, are caused by reduced striatal dopaminergic activity (123); this change in motor behavior has also been reported in rotenone-exposed rats (114, 121). Rats treated with rotenone displayed a significant increase in abnormal motor behavior and decline in locomotor activities (124).

Rotenone-treated animal models reproduce all the pathological and behavioral features of typical human PD. Rotenone has been used successfully in a variety of species, including non-human primates, mice, and snails. However, there is some variation between the models and not all treated rats displayed these features. Briefly, this model provides very similar clinical features to typical PD but the low reproducibility and high mortality rate (88) may limit its practical use (117). Interestingly, rotenone was found to be involved in a multisystem disorder (125): enteric nervous system dysfunction (126) and loss of myenteric neurons in rats (127).

3.1.4 Other neurotoxins

Other neurotoxins used in PD models include paraquat and maneb. Paraquat is a common herbicide, has a similar chemical structure to MPP^+, the oxidized metabolite that mediates MPTP neurotoxicity, and has been suggested to be a risk factor for PD (128). Epidemiological studies have also indicated that exposure to paraquat may play an important role in the development of PD (16). After crossing the BBB, paraquat inhibits mitochondrial complex I in dopaminergic neurons (129). The treatment of mice with paraquat caused destruction of dopamine neurons in the substantia nigra (130). The paraquat-induced neurodegeneration is probably triggered by c-Jun N-terminal kinase signaling pathways (131). In this model, microglial activation has been identified and may act as a risk factor for dopaminergic cell death (132). Further investigations showed that the activated microglia produce potentially harmful molecules, such as superoxide anion and nitric oxide, resulting in redox cycling reactions and ROS formation which enhance tissue vulnerability in the paraquat model (133-135). In addition, oxidative stress plays an important role in nigrostriatal degeneration (136-137). The paraquat model demonstrated α-synuclein up-regulation and aggregation associated with dopaminergic cell death in the substantia nigra pars compacta in mice (138).

Maneb is a fungicide that is always used in combination with paraquat in agriculture. In PD research, maneb potentiates the DA toxicity of paraquat in mice (139). Maneb alone inhibits mitochondrial complex III and causes selective dopaminergic neurodegeneration (140). The combination of maneb and paraquat induced more pronounced behavioral and pathological changes than paraquat alone (141-142). Barlow et al. (143) explained that this effect could be due to the ability of maneb to modify the biodisposition and thus increase the concentration of paraquat. Findings in co-exposure models have important implications for the risk of PD in humans because they are liable to be exposed to the synergistic mixtures in agricultural or residential areas where both agents are applied jointly (139).

As a model of environmental exposure, administration of paraquat/maneb reproduces neurodegenerative changes and is useful for the investigation and understanding of the neurotoxic mechanisms of risk factors for PD. Although this model cannot achieve the severe nigrostriatal neurodegeneration induced by MPTP and 6-OHDA, it is a good complement for the comprehensive understanding of PD.

3.2 Genetic models

The majority of PD cases are sporadic but several causative genes and mutations have been discovered and have led to new approaches in the investigation of the mechanisms involve in PD. Several genetic animal models of PD reported in recent years are discussed below.

3.2.1 α-Synuclein

Many different transgenic mice models that over-express human α-synuclein have been generated and applied to pathogenesis and drug research. Transgenic mice induced by the tyrosine hydroxylase promoter expressed α-synuclein containing A30P and A53T mutations and showed a progressive decline in locomotor activity and loss of substantia nigra neurons and striatal DA content (144-145). When transgenic mice were induced by the neuron-specific platelet-derived growth factor β promoter, α-synuclein over-expression was observed, together with reduced tyrosine hydroxylase immunoreactivity and DA content in the striatum and impaired motor performance (146). Mice that over-expressed A53T mutant α-synuclein under the mouse prion promoter (PrP) developed an adult-onset progressive neurodegenerative disorder (147-148). Another neuron-specific promoter, thymocyte differentiation antigen 1 (Thy1), was used in mice to induce a high level of widespread expression of α-synuclein in most neuronal populations (149-150). Both Thy-1 and PrP mice are the only models that have intraneuronal inclusions, degeneration and mitochondrial DNA damage in the neurons (151).

A rat model that over-expresses wild-type or mutant α-synuclein induced by adenoassociated viruses in substantia nigra neurons, displayed progressive age-dependent loss of DA neurons, motor impairment, and α-synuclein-positive cytoplasmic inclusions (152). In Drosophila, α-synuclein over-expression led to age-dependent loss of dorsomedial dopaminergic neurons, accumulation of LB-like inclusions with α-synuclein immunoreactivity and compromised locomotor activity (153). α-Synuclein over-expression in Caenorhabditis elegans caused accelerated dopaminergic neuronal loss and motor impairment (154-155).

PC12 cells have been widely used in PD research to understand the regulation of the neuronal level of α-synuclein. α-Synuclein expression in PC12 cells was low but could be greatly increased by treatment with nerve growth factor (NGF) (156). NGF signal transduction was indicated via the MAP/ERK and PI3 kinase pathways (157). Another study with PC12 cells reported that wild-type α-synuclein was selectively translocated into lysosomes and degraded by the chaperone-mediated autophagy pathway (158). However, the mutant α-synuclein bound to the receptor on the lysosomal membrane inhibited both its own degradation and that of other substrates (158). PC12 cells over-expressing mutant α-synuclein showed impaired proteasomal activity and enhanced sensitivity to proteasomal inhibitors (159). Endoplasmic reticulum stress and mitochondrial dysfunction played important roles in increased cell death (160). The same model in another study showed impairment in both proteasomal and lysosomal functions, a high level of autophagic cell death and loss of chromaffin granules (161).

Yeast has been widely used to investigate the role of α-synuclein toxicity in human diseases, including PD. When expressed in yeast, α-synuclein became cytotoxic in a concentration-dependent manner (162). α-Synuclein in yeast was highly selectively associated with the plasma membrane and formed cytoplasmic inclusions (162). The growth inhibition induced by α-synuclein was accompanied by cellular consequences, such as proteasome impairment, heat-shock and oxidative stress, formation of ubiquitin-positive α-synuclein inclusion bodies, and emergence of apoptotic markers (162-164). Because the molecules that inhibit α-synuclein toxicity are potential therapeutic agents, α-synuclein toxicity in the yeast model has been used for genetic screening to identify genetic modifiers (165-166) and for small molecule or chemical screening to identify novel compounds.

Studies of α-synuclein in cell-free systems have focused on its aggregation pathway, post-translational modification, self-assembly and structure characterization. Test-tube models are critical for the investigation of PD-related protein α-synuclein and its related molecules as they provide more detailed information than any other approaches. However, some findings may not fully account for the biological complexity of α-synuclein *in vivo*. Therefore, further validation in cell cultures or *in vivo* is required.

3.2.2 Parkin

Parkin mutations have been found in a number of cases with recessive juvenile onset (167) and are the second genetic cause of PD. In a rat model, over-expression of parkin protected against the toxicity of mutant α-synuclein as demonstrated by a reduction in α-synuclein-induced neuropathology (168). In addition, parkin over-expression through viral transduction protected mice from mild MPTP-induced lesions (169). However, parkin knockout mice showed no impairment in the dopaminergic system (170-171). A parkin knockout Drosophila model exhibited locomotor defects and male sterility (172). These tissue-specific phenotypes were due to mitochondrial dysfunction. Further studies showed that oxidative stress components and genes involved in innate immunity were induced in parkin mutants, which indicated that oxidative stress and/or inflammation may play a fundamental role in the etiology of AR-JP (173). Another study showed that the expression of mutant human parkin in Drosophila caused age-dependent, selective degeneration of dopaminergic neurons accompanied by progressive motor impairment (174). Both the loss of function and toxicity of parkin have been demonstrated in the Drosophila model.

In experiments using cell-free models, mutant forms of parkin associated with AR-JP were reported to have reduced ubiquitin ligase activity (175-176). Catechol-modified parkin in the substantia nigra - a vulnerability of parkin to modification by dopamine - suggested a mechanism for the progressive loss of parkin function in dopaminergic neurons (177). Another modification - phosphorylation by cyclin-dependent kinase 5 - may contribute to the accumulation of toxic parkin substrates and decrease the ability of dopaminergic cells to cope with toxic insults in PD (178).

3.2.3 PINK1

PINK1 knockout mice had no dramatic abnormalities in the dopaminergic system (179). In Drosophila models, compared with the loss of parkin, the loss of PINK1 showed a strong similarity in phenotype: shortened lifespan, infertility and wing postural defect; in addition, identical loss of mitochondrial integrity was found in both cases (180-182). However, one difference was also observed: up-regulation of parkin rescued PINK1 mutants, whereas PINK1 up-regulation could not rescue parkin mutation (180-182). Cell-free models have been used to investigate the enzymatic function of PINK1 and the effects of mutations.

PINK1 was shown to phosphorylate downstream effector tumor necrosis factor receptor-associated protein 1 directly and prevent oxidative stress-induced apoptosis (183). It was also reported that the PINK1 kinase domain catalyzed the phosphorylation of artificial protein substrates, including α-casein (184) and histone H1 (60). Kinase assays suggested that multiple PINK1 mutants associated with autosomal recessive PD have reduced kinase activity (60, 183-185).

3.2.4 DJ-1

DJ-1 knockout mice exhibited a deficit in scavenging mitochondrial hydrogen peroxide due to its function of atypical peroxiredoxin-like peroxidase (186). Further studies have been carried out using Drosophila. DJ-1 knockout caused selective sensitivity to the oxidative toxins, paraquat and rotenone (187-189). DJ-1 protein undergoes oxidative modification on cysteine residue, which was also seen in Drosophila (189), and the oxidative modification occurred with aging and after exposure to paraquat (190). Cell-free models have helped researchers to characterize the crystal structure of DJ-1, investigate its function and activity, and reveal the effect of oxidative modifications on the stability and function of DJ-1.

3.2.5 LRRK2

In cell models, LRRK2 mutations significantly increased autophosphorylation activity (191-194). Over-expression of mutant LRRK2 caused condensed and fragmented nuclei, resulting in increased cellular toxicity (191). Because the cellular toxicity induced by mutant LRRK2 can be prevented by inactivation of the kinase domain in cell models, the kinase domain could be a therapeutic target for LRRK2-associated PD. Cell-free systems have been used to investigate the kinase function and how it is affected by pathogenic mutations. Reports indicated that LRRK2 catalyzed its autophosphorylation or the phosphorylation of artificial substrates (191-192, 195). This suggested that LRRK2-mediated phosphorylation was regulated by the binding of guanine triphosphate (GTP); in addition, both GTP binding and protein kinase activity are necessary for LRRK2 neurotoxicity (192, 196).

4. Clinical therapeutic insights

From the traditional view, PD is considered to be a single clinical entity, but this is currently under scrutiny (197-198). Clinically, the subtypes of this heterogeneous disease can be recognized on the basis of age at onset, predominant clinical features and progression rate. There are two major clinical subtypes: the tremor-predominant form which is often observed in younger people, and generally leads to a slow decline in motor function; in the other type, known as "postural imbalance and gait disorder" that is often observed in older people (>70 years old), motor function declines more rapidly, and is characterized by akinesia, rigidity, and gait and balance impairment. (198).

4.1 Dopamine replacement therapies

During the years of disease progression, the treatment of PD has to be adapted to alternating periods of reduced mobility and abnormal involuntary movements and is complicated by the onset of motor fluctuations and dyskinesia (199). PD was essentially an untreated motor disorder before L-DOPA was developed as a treatment. For the next two decades, the symptoms of hallucinations and delirium or other motor complications and psychiatric manifestations became the prevailing clinical problems in PD after treatment with L-DOPA. However, bradykinesia, resting tremors and rigidity which are the major symptoms of PD (200) can be controlled by long-term use of L-DOPA and other dopaminergic agents. Although the dopamine precursor, L-DOPA, and dopamine agonists are very effective in treating motor symptoms, they can cause substantial motor and behavioural adverse effects. Many reports have claimed that some patients treated with dopaminergic drugs develop impulse control disorders, a dopamine dysregulation syndrome or other abnormal behaviors (201). Because of these flaws, new treatments for PD should be developed to tackle two unresolved problems: the alternation between therapies that alleviate symptoms and those that modify the disease; and reduction of the real causes of disability in long-term PD, which include autonomic dysfunction, balance loss, cognitive impairment and the growing prevalence of other non-motor symptoms.

Peak-dose dyskinesia, diphasic dyskinesia and off-period dystonia are the three forms of dyskinesias that commonly occur with L-DOPA use and negatively affect the quality of life of patients in the advanced stages of the disease (202). Peak-dose dyskinesia occurs when plasma L-DOPA levels are highest; diphasic dyskinesia refers to the abnormal involuntary movements that occur transiently at the onset and end of L-DOPA efficacy; and off-period dystonia occurs when a patient receives subtherapeutic levels of L-DOPA. Recent advances in the treatment of severe disabling dyskinesias have lessened but not entirely eliminated their effects. Specific examples of such advances include deep brain stimulation (DBS) of the subthalamic nucleus, continuous subcutaneous infusion of apomorphine and continuous duodenal infusion of L-DOPA. Currently, a major focus of drug development is the identification of agents that can acutely suppress existing disabling dyskinesias and of agents that do not induce dyskinesias.

More than 80% of patients who have had PD for 20 years develop dementia. Once this occurs, irrespective of their age or the duration of the disease, death follows shortly (203). From an anatomopathological point of view, PD dementia is believed to be due to a combination of the extension of Lewy bodies into limbic and cortical structures with concomitant Alzheimer's disease(AD)-related neurofibrillary tangles and amyloid-β plaque pathology (203-204). The recent observation that lower levels of amyloid-β_{1-42} in the cerebral spinal fluid may predict a more rapid cognitive decline supports the contribution of AD-related pathologies to the cognitive impairment that is seen in patients with PD (205). Relief from neuropsychiatric cognitive and behavioral symptoms without worsening motor impairment or altering the relief of symptoms that is provided by L-DOPA are the goals of current treatment in PD dementia. To achieve these goals, reliance is placed on fine-tuning the balance between dopaminergic and non-dopaminergic (prominently cholinergic) neurotransmission strategies.

4.2 Surgical treatment and deep brain stimulation (DBS)

In recent years, DBS has become an established treatment for the advanced stages of PD. It is efficacious and is approved by the US Food and Drug Administration for the treatment of advanced, L-DOPA-responsive PD and medically refractory essential tremor. New anatomical targets for DBS, such as the pedunculopontine nucleus, are currently being explored in patients with PD who have gait disorders. In the search for new targets, smart DBS techniques such as coordinated reset stimulation are currently under development (206).

Many reports have enlarged described the long-term outcome of DBS in PD, but, as with L-DOPS treatment, flaws still remain. Subthalamic nucleus DBS (STN DBS) can substantially improve motor function and quality of life in some patients with PD; however, a minority of patients experience cognitive and emotional difficulties after surgery. Better controlled randomized trials that compared STN DBS with the best medical therapy failed to substantiate the findings of widespread or marked cognitive deterioration (207-208).

Smeding and colleagues (209) reported on predictors of the cognitive and psychosocial effects of STN DBS in patients with PD. Varied mood outcomes were observed: 16 patients treated with STN DBS (15%) showed improvements, but the same percentage showed deterioration. Strutt and colleagues (210) have shown that mood (depression) changes cannot be attributed solely to symptoms of somatic depression that overlap with those of PD.

The pre-operative selection of patients who are suitable for STN DBS is critical; response to L-DOPA is considered to be not only a predictor of motor outcomes, but perhaps also of neurocognitive and quality of life outcomes. As pre-operative impairments can predict neuropsychological outcomes after therapy, neuropsychological evaluation should be undertaken before surgery. Mood states should also be evaluated, but reliance on self-reported questionnaires should be discouraged (211).

Although aging is suggested to be a prognostic factor of neurosurgical outcome (212-213), studies that trace the long-term clinical evolution among subgroups of patients with early-onset versus late-onset PD after STN DBS are still lacking. The latest study of a cohort of 19 subjects treated with subthalamic nucleus DBS after more than 20 years of disease reported clinical and neuropsychological data up to a mean of 30 years after disease onset (214). A higher prevalence of axial and non-L-DOPA-responsive symptoms was observed during long-term evaluations compared with other STN DBS follow-up studies. This confirms that, even in patients with an early onset of disease and a previous long-lasting response to dopaminergic therapies, several complex aspects underlie the development of non-motor symptoms and other features of the progression of PD. Therefore, the surgical option of STN DBS should be proposed earlier, since the progression of PD might not follow a single direction, and it is possible that age might affect the development of non-motor features more than the duration of the disease.

4.3 Transplantation treatment

Pharmacological agents that increase DA can alleviate motor symptoms as mentioned above; however, patients develop severe effects with long-term use. Cell transplantation therapy has therefore been investigated as an alternative treatment in recent years. Since only one cell type is affected in a distinct location of the brain, cell replacement therapy is liable to be successful for PD, and has already been used in many other diseases. Transplantation treatment is considered to be an on-going alternative strategy for an effective cure for PD.

Stem-cell replacement therapy has been suggested as a treatment for neurodegenerative diseases caused by the degeneration of DA neurons in the substantia nigra of the brain, and especially for PD (215). Stem cell-derived DA neurons can replace endogenous degenerated neurons. Clinical studies using fetal midbrain tissue proved the principle that cell transplantation could be a feasible treatment for PD(216).

Although it has shown promise for the treatment of PD, the safety and efficacy of transplanted stem cells induced by different methods are variable. Fetal-tissue transplants have gained some success, but their availability is limited. Human induced pluripotent stem cells (hiPSCs) are a promising alternative for personalized therapy; many cells can be generated and the chances of immunorejection are low. Several reprograming methods can generate hiPSCs, the most common of which are lentiviral and retroviral methods, but these can generate mutations and lead to chromosomal aberrations.

Recently, Rhee and colleagues (217) compared the safety of several types of hiPSCs, and found that they were able to generate healthy DA neurons. Neural precursor cells from protein-based hiPSCs were transplanted into a rat model of PD. The transplanted tissue not only survived well but also was able to rescue motor deficits in the model animals. These findings suggest that protein-based hiPSCs can be considered as a safe, viable alternative to virus-induced cells; moreover, they could potentially be used for transplantation and treatment in patients with PD (218).

4.4 Neuroprotective effects

DA substitution therapy and DBS do not completely relieve the symptoms of PD. Hence, there is still a need to identify neuroprotective agents that can modify the progression of the underlying disease processes.

Due to its robust effects in preventing degeneration of the nigrostriatal system in commonly used neurotoxin-based pre-clinical models of the disease, glial cell line-derived neurotrophic factor (GDNF) has gained most attention as a candidate neuroprotective molecule in PD. GDNF may be used in two ways to afford substantial neuroprotection in rodent and primate models of PD induced by either 6-OHDA or MPTP: infusion and viral-mediated delivery of GDNF, and transplantation of GDNF-producing cells (219-222).

Because of these promising pre-clinical results, more clinical trials to evaluate the efficacy of GDNF and neurturin in patients with PD are now in progress. However, the results obtained from these trials to date remain inconclusive (223-225).

Another recent study demonstrated that viral vector-mediated delivery of GDNF is unable to prevent the degeneration of the nigrostriatal DA neurons induced by over-expression of human wild-type α-synuclein at levels that have been shown to be efficient in the toxin models; this highlights the importance of performing pre-clinical tests on potential therapeutic compounds in mechanistically different models of PD (226).

5. Conclusions

As is the case for many other diseases that humans have been fighting for decades, there is a common gap between laboratory research and the ideal clinical therapy: how to ensure that products derived from laboratory experiments are both efficacious and safe. Although various studies have made progress towards a definitive solution for PD, several unresolved areas still remain. A better understanding of its biochemical pathogenesis is the best method to develop new disease-modifying therapies. However, through novel therapies and the refinement of old treatments, the management of this disease has been considerably up-graded over the past 20 years. Clinical experience shows that most patients who have accepted treatment now have a relatively good quality of life despite having suffered the effects of PD for many years. We should be confident that all these new developments will provide advances for PD treatment, and give us a hope of a final triumph in fighting the disease.

6. References

[1] Twelves D, Perkins KS, Counsell C. Systematic review of incidence studies of Parkinson's disease. Movement disorders : official journal of the Movement Disorder Society. 2003;18(1):19-31. doi: 10.1002/mds.10305.

[2] Bower JH, Maraganore DM, McDonnell SK, Rocca WA. Incidence and distribution of parkinsonism in Olmsted County, Minnesota, 1976-1990. Neurology. 1999;52(6):1214-20.

[3] Elbaz A, Bower JH, Maraganore DM, McDonnell SK, Peterson BJ, Ahlskog JE, et al. Risk tables for parkinsonism and Parkinson's disease. Journal of clinical epidemiology. 2002;55(1):25-31.

[4] Zhang ZX, Roman GC, Hong Z, Wu CB, Qu QM, Huang JB, et al. Parkinson's disease in China: prevalence in Beijing, Xian, and Shanghai. Lancet. 2005;365(9459):595-7. doi: 10.1016/S0140-6736(05)17909-4.

[5] Schoenberg BS, Osuntokun BO, Adeuja AO, Bademosi O, Nottidge V, Anderson DW, et al. Comparison of the prevalence of Parkinson's disease in black populations in the rural United States and in rural Nigeria: door-to-door community studies. Neurology. 1988;38(4):645-6.

[6] Priyadarshi A, Khuder SA, Schaub EA, Priyadarshi SS. Environmental risk factors and Parkinson's disease: a metaanalysis. Environmental research. 2001;86(2):122-7. doi: 10.1006/enrs.2001.4264.

[7] Priyadarshi A, Khuder SA, Schaub EA, Shrivastava S. A meta-analysis of Parkinson's disease and exposure to pesticides. Neurotoxicology. 2000;21(4):435-40.

[8] Migliore L, Coppede F. Genetics, environmental factors and the emerging role of epigenetics in neurodegenerative diseases. Mutation research. 2009;667(1-2):82-97. doi: 10.1016/j.mrfmmm.2008.10.011.

[9] Tanner CM, Goldman SM. Epidemiology of Parkinson's disease. Neurologic clinics. 1996;14(2):317-35.

[10] Barbeau A, Roy M, Bernier G, Campanella G, Paris S. Ecogenetics of Parkinson's disease: prevalence and environmental aspects in rural areas. The Canadian journal of neurological sciences Le journal canadien des sciences neurologiques. 1987;14(1):36-41.

[11] Gorrell JM, DiMonte D, Graham D. The role of the environment in Parkinson's disease. Environmental health perspectives. 1996;104(6):652-4.

[12] Gorell JM, Johnson CC, Rybicki BA, Peterson EL, Richardson RJ. The risk of Parkinson's disease with exposure to pesticides, farming, well water, and rural living. Neurology. 1998;50(5):1346-50.

[13] Semchuk KM, Love EJ, Lee RG. Parkinson's disease and exposure to agricultural work and pesticide chemicals. Neurology. 1992;42(7):1328-35.

[14] Langston JW, Ballard P, Tetrud JW, Irwin I. Chronic Parkinsonism in humans due to a product of meperidine-analog synthesis. Science. 1983;219(4587):979-80.

[15] Langston JW. The etiology of Parkinson's disease with emphasis on the MPTP story. Neurology. 1996;47(6 Suppl 3):S153-60.

[16] Liou HH, Tsai MC, Chen CJ, Jeng JS, Chang YC, Chen SY, et al. Environmental risk factors and Parkinson's disease: a case-control study in Taiwan. Neurology. 1997;48(6):1583-8.
[17] Seidler A, Hellenbrand W, Robra BP, Vieregge P, Nischan P, Joerg J, et al. Possible environmental, occupational, and other etiologic factors for Parkinson's disease: a case-control study in Germany. Neurology. 1996;46(5):1275-84.
[18] Corsini GU, Pintus S, Chiueh CC, Weiss JF, Kopin IJ. 1-Methyl-4-phenyl-1,2,3,6-tetrahydropyridine (MPTP) neurotoxicity in mice is enhanced by pretreatment with diethyldithiocarbamate. European journal of pharmacology. 1985;119(1-2):127-8.
[19] Semchuk KM, Love EJ, Lee RG. Parkinson's disease and exposure to rural environmental factors: a population based case-control study. The Canadian journal of neurological sciences Le journal canadien des sciences neurologiques. 1991;18(3):279-86.
[20] Huang CC, Lu CS, Chu NS, Hochberg F, Lilienfeld D, Olanow W, et al. Progression after chronic manganese exposure. Neurology. 1993;43(8):1479-83.
[21] Costello S, Cockburn M, Bronstein J, Zhang X, Ritz B. Parkinson's disease and residential exposure to maneb and paraquat from agricultural applications in the central valley of California. American journal of epidemiology. 2009;169(8):919-26. doi: 10.1093/aje/kwp006.
[22] Gorell JM, Johnson CC, Rybicki BA, Peterson EL, Kortsha GX, Brown GG, et al. Occupational exposures to metals as risk factors for Parkinson's disease. Neurology. 1997;48(3):650-8.
[23] Rybicki BA, Johnson CC, Uman J, Gorell JM. Parkinson's disease mortality and the industrial use of heavy metals in Michigan. Movement disorders : official journal of the Movement Disorder Society. 1993;8(1):87-92. doi: 10.1002/mds.870080116.
[24] Maher NE, Golbe LI, Lazzarini AM, Mark MH, Currie LJ, Wooten GF, et al. Epidemiologic study of 203 sibling pairs with Parkinson's disease: the GenePD study. Neurology. 2002;58(1):79-84.
[25] Goldman SM, Tanner CM, Oakes D, Bhudhikanok GS, Gupta A, Langston JW. Head injury and Parkinson's disease risk in twins. Annals of neurology. 2006;60(1):65-72. doi: 10.1002/ana.20882.
[26] Baron JA. Cigarette smoking and Parkinson's disease. Neurology. 1986;36(11):1490-6.
[27] Ascherio A, Zhang SM, Hernan MA, Kawachi I, Colditz GA, Speizer FE, et al. Prospective study of caffeine consumption and risk of Parkinson's disease in men and women. Annals of neurology. 2001;50(1):56-63.
[28] Wirdefeldt K, Gatz M, Pawitan Y, Pedersen NL. Risk and protective factors for Parkinson's disease: a study in Swedish twins. Annals of neurology. 2005;57(1):27-33. doi: 10.1002/ana.20307.
[29] Tanner CM, Goldman SM, Aston DA, Ottman R, Ellenberg J, Mayeux R, et al. Smoking and Parkinson's disease in twins. Neurology. 2002;58(4):581-8.
[30] Scott WK, Zhang F, Stajich JM, Scott BL, Stacy MA, Vance JM. Family-based case-control study of cigarette smoking and Parkinson disease. Neurology. 2005;64(3):442-7. doi: 10.1212/01.WNL.0000150905.93241.B2.
[31] Hernan MA, Takkouche B, Caamano-Isorna F, Gestal-Otero JJ. A meta-analysis of coffee drinking, cigarette smoking, and the risk of Parkinson's disease. Annals of neurology. 2002;52(3):276-84. doi: 10.1002/ana.10277.

[32] Elbaz A, McDonnell SK, Maraganore DM, Strain KJ, Schaid DJ, Bower JH, et al. Validity of family history data on PD: evidence for a family information bias. Neurology. 2003;61(1):11-7.
[33] Farrer MJ. Genetics of Parkinson disease: paradigm shifts and future prospects. Nature reviews Genetics. 2006;7(4):306-18. doi: 10.1038/nrg1831.
[34] Polymeropoulos MH, Higgins JJ, Golbe LI, Johnson WG, Ide SE, Di Iorio G, et al. Mapping of a gene for Parkinson's disease to chromosome 4q21-q23. Science. 1996;274(5290):1197-9.
[35] Polymeropoulos MH, Lavedan C, Leroy E, Ide SE, Dehejia A, Dutra A, et al. Mutation in the alpha-synuclein gene identified in families with Parkinson's disease. Science. 1997;276(5321):2045-7.
[36] Kruger R, Kuhn W, Muller T, Woitalla D, Graeber M, Kosel S, et al. Ala30Pro mutation in the gene encoding alpha-synuclein in Parkinson's disease. Nature genetics. 1998;18(2):106-8. doi: 10.1038/ng0298-106.
[37] Zarranz JJ, Alegre J, Gomez-Esteban JC, Lezcano E, Ros R, Ampuero I, et al. The new mutation, E46K, of alpha-synuclein causes Parkinson and Lewy body dementia. Annals of neurology. 2004;55(2):164-73. doi: 10.1002/ana.10795.
[38] Farrer M, Kachergus J, Forno L, Lincoln S, Wang DS, Hulihan M, et al. Comparison of kindreds with parkinsonism and alpha-synuclein genomic multiplications. Annals of neurology. 2004;55(2):174-9. doi: 10.1002/ana.10846.
[39] Lockhart PJ, Kachergus J, Lincoln S, Hulihan M, Bisceglio G, Thomas N, et al. Multiplication of the alpha-synuclein gene is not a common disease mechanism in Lewy body disease. Journal of molecular neuroscience : MN. 2004;24(3):337-42. doi: 10.1385/JMN:24:3:337.
[40] Fuchs J, Nilsson C, Kachergus J, Munz M, Larsson EM, Schule B, et al. Phenotypic variation in a large Swedish pedigree due to SNCA duplication and triplication. Neurology. 2007;68(12):916-22. doi: 10.1212/01.wnl.0000254458.17630.c5.
[41] Spillantini MG, Schmidt ML, Lee VM, Trojanowski JQ, Jakes R, Goedert M. Alpha-synuclein in Lewy bodies. Nature. 1997;388(6645):839-40. doi: 10.1038/42166.
[42] Spillantini MG, Crowther RA, Jakes R, Hasegawa M, Goedert M. alpha-Synuclein in filamentous inclusions of Lewy bodies from Parkinson's disease and dementia with lewy bodies. Proceedings of the National Academy of Sciences of the United States of America. 1998;95(11):6469-73.
[43] Kitada T, Asakawa S, Hattori N, Matsumine H, Yamamura Y, Minoshima S, et al. Mutations in the parkin gene cause autosomal recessive juvenile parkinsonism. Nature. 1998;392(6676):605-8. doi: 10.1038/33416.
[44] Takahashi H, Ohama E, Suzuki S, Horikawa Y, Ishikawa A, Morita T, et al. Familial juvenile parkinsonism: clinical and pathologic study in a family. Neurology. 1994;44(3 Pt 1):437-41.
[45] Ishikawa A, Tsuji S. Clinical analysis of 17 patients in 12 Japanese families with autosomal-recessive type juvenile parkinsonism. Neurology. 1996;47(1):160-6.
[46] Shimura H, Hattori N, Kubo S, Mizuno Y, Asakawa S, Minoshima S, et al. Familial Parkinson disease gene product, parkin, is a ubiquitin-protein ligase. Nature genetics. 2000;25(3):302-5. doi: 10.1038/77060.
[47] Fallon L, Belanger CM, Corera AT, Kontogiannea M, Regan-Klapisz E, Moreau F, et al. A regulated interaction with the UIM protein Eps15 implicates parkin in EGF

receptor trafficking and PI(3)K-Akt signalling. Nature cell biology. 2006;8(8):834-42. doi: 10.1038/ncb1441.
[48] Mata IF, Lockhart PJ, Farrer MJ. Parkin genetics: one model for Parkinson's disease. Human molecular genetics. 2004;13 Spec No 1:R127-33. doi: 10.1093/hmg/ddh089.
[49] Lesage S, Magali P, Lohmann E, Lacomblez L, Teive H, Janin S, et al. Deletion of the parkin and PACRG gene promoter in early-onset parkinsonism. Human mutation. 2007;28(1):27-32. doi: 10.1002/humu.20436.
[50] Lucking CB, Durr A, Bonifati V, Vaughan J, De Michele G, Gasser T, et al. Association between early-onset Parkinson's disease and mutations in the parkin gene. The New England journal of medicine. 2000;342(21):1560-7. doi: 10.1056/NEJM200005253422103.
[51] Periquet M, Latouche M, Lohmann E, Rawal N, De Michele G, Ricard S, et al. Parkin mutations are frequent in patients with isolated early-onset parkinsonism. Brain : a journal of neurology. 2003;126(Pt 6):1271-8.
[52] Leroy E, Boyer R, Auburger G, Leube B, Ulm G, Mezey E, et al. The ubiquitin pathway in Parkinson's disease. Nature. 1998;395(6701):451-2. doi: 10.1038/26652.
[53] Farrer M, Destee T, Becquet E, Wavrant-De Vrieze F, Mouroux V, Richard F, et al. Linkage exclusion in French families with probable Parkinson' s disease. Movement disorders : official journal of the Movement Disorder Society. 2000;15(6):1075-83.
[54] Harhangi BS, Farrer MJ, Lincoln S, Bonifati V, Meco G, De Michele G, et al. The Ile93Met mutation in the ubiquitin carboxy-terminal-hydrolase-L1 gene is not observed in European cases with familial Parkinson's disease. Neuroscience letters. 1999;270(1):1-4.
[55] Lincoln S, Vaughan J, Wood N, Baker M, Adamson J, Gwinn-Hardy K, et al. Low frequency of pathogenic mutations in the ubiquitin carboxy-terminal hydrolase gene in familial Parkinson's disease. Neuroreport. 1999;10(2):427-9.
[56] Valente EM, Abou-Sleiman PM, Caputo V, Muqit MM, Harvey K, Gispert S, et al. Hereditary early-onset Parkinson's disease caused by mutations in PINK1. Science. 2004;304(5674):1158-60. doi: 10.1126/science.1096284.
[57] Valente EM, Salvi S, Ialongo T, Marongiu R, Elia AE, Caputo V, et al. PINK1 mutations are associated with sporadic early-onset parkinsonism. Annals of neurology. 2004;56(3):336-41. doi: 10.1002/ana.20256.
[58] Marongiu R, Brancati F, Antonini A, Ialongo T, Ceccarini C, Scarciolla O, et al. Whole gene deletion and splicing mutations expand the PINK1 genotypic spectrum. Human mutation. 2007;28(1):98. doi: 10.1002/humu.9472.
[59] Abou-Sleiman PM, Muqit MM, McDonald NQ, Yang YX, Gandhi S, Healy DG, et al. A heterozygous effect for PINK1 mutations in Parkinson's disease? Annals of neurology. 2006;60(4):414-9. doi: 10.1002/ana.20960.
[60] Sim CH, Lio DS, Mok SS, Masters CL, Hill AF, Culvenor JG, et al. C-terminal truncation and Parkinson's disease-associated mutations down-regulate the protein serine/threonine kinase activity of PTEN-induced kinase-1. Human molecular genetics. 2006;15(21):3251-62. doi: 10.1093/hmg/ddl398.
[61] Bonifati V, Rizzu P, van Baren MJ, Schaap O, Breedveld GJ, Krieger E, et al. Mutations in the DJ-1 gene associated with autosomal recessive early-onset parkinsonism. Science. 2003;299(5604):256-9. doi: 10.1126/science.1077209.

[62] Pankratz N, Pauciulo MW, Elsaesser VE, Marek DK, Halter CA, Wojcieszek J, et al. Mutations in DJ-1 are rare in familial Parkinson disease. Neuroscience letters. 2006;408(3):209-13. doi: 10.1016/j.neulet.2006.09.003.

[63] Miller DW, Ahmad R, Hague S, Baptista MJ, Canet-Aviles R, McLendon C, et al. L166P mutant DJ-1, causative for recessive Parkinson's disease, is degraded through the ubiquitin-proteasome system. The Journal of biological chemistry. 2003;278(38):36588-95. doi: 10.1074/jbc.M304272200.

[64] Di Fonzo A, Rohe CF, Ferreira J, Chien HF, Vacca L, Stocchi F, et al. A frequent LRRK2 gene mutation associated with autosomal dominant Parkinson's disease. Lancet. 2005;365(9457):412-5. doi: 10.1016/S0140-6736(05)17829-5.

[65] Nichols WC, Pankratz N, Hernandez D, Paisan-Ruiz C, Jain S, Halter CA, et al. Genetic screening for a single common LRRK2 mutation in familial Parkinson's disease. Lancet. 2005;365(9457):410-2. doi: 10.1016/S0140-6736(05)17828-3.

[66] Gilks WP, Abou-Sleiman PM, Gandhi S, Jain S, Singleton A, Lees AJ, et al. A common LRRK2 mutation in idiopathic Parkinson's disease. Lancet. 2005;365(9457):415-6. doi: 10.1016/S0140-6736(05)17830-1.

[67] Zabetian CP, Samii A, Mosley AD, Roberts JW, Leis BC, Yearout D, et al. A clinic-based study of the LRRK2 gene in Parkinson disease yields new mutations. Neurology. 2005;65(5):741-4. doi: 10.1212/01.wnl.0000172630.22804.73.

[68] Kachergus J, Mata IF, Hulihan M, Taylor JP, Lincoln S, Aasly J, et al. Identification of a novel LRRK2 mutation linked to autosomal dominant parkinsonism: evidence of a common founder across European populations. American journal of human genetics. 2005;76(4):672-80. doi: 10.1086/429256.

[69] Hampshire DJ, Roberts E, Crow Y, Bond J, Mubaidin A, Wriekat AL, et al. Kufor-Rakeb syndrome, pallido-pyramidal degeneration with supranuclear upgaze paresis and dementia, maps to 1p36. Journal of medical genetics. 2001;38(10):680-2.

[70] Ramirez A, Heimbach A, Grundemann J, Stiller B, Hampshire D, Cid LP, et al. Hereditary parkinsonism with dementia is caused by mutations in ATP13A2, encoding a lysosomal type 5 P-type ATPase. Nature genetics. 2006;38(10):1184-91. doi: 10.1038/ng1884.

[71] Di Fonzo A, Chien HF, Socal M, Giraudo S, Tassorelli C, Iliceto G, et al. ATP13A2 missense mutations in juvenile parkinsonism and young onset Parkinson disease. Neurology. 2007;68(19):1557-62. doi: 10.1212/01.wnl.0000260963.08711.08.

[72] Strauss KM, Martins LM, Plun-Favreau H, Marx FP, Kautzmann S, Berg D, et al. Loss of function mutations in the gene encoding Omi/HtrA2 in Parkinson's disease. Human molecular genetics. 2005;14(15):2099-111. doi: 10.1093/hmg/ddi215.

[73] Sidransky E, Nalls MA, Aasly JO, Aharon-Peretz J, Annesi G, Barbosa ER, et al. Multicenter analysis of glucocerebrosidase mutations in Parkinson's disease. The New England journal of medicine. 2009;361(17):1651-61. doi: 10.1056/NEJMoa0901281.

[74] Zabetian CP, Hutter CM, Factor SA, Nutt JG, Higgins DS, Griffith A, et al. Association analysis of MAPT H1 haplotype and subhaplotypes in Parkinson's disease. Annals of neurology. 2007;62(2):137-44. doi: 10.1002/ana.21157.

[75] Baker M, Mackenzie IR, Pickering-Brown SM, Gass J, Rademakers R, Lindholm C, et al. Mutations in progranulin cause tau-negative frontotemporal dementia linked to chromosome 17. Nature. 2006;442(7105):916-9. doi: 10.1038/nature05016.

[76] Schober A. Classic toxin-induced animal models of Parkinson's disease: 6-OHDA and MPTP. Cell and tissue research. 2004;318(1):215-24. doi: 10.1007/s00441-004-0938-y.

[77] Ungerstedt U. Postsynaptic supersensitivity after 6-hydroxy-dopamine induced degeneration of the nigro-striatal dopamine system. Acta physiologica Scandinavica Supplementum. 1971;367:69-93.

[78] Saner A, Thoenen H. Model experiments on the molecular mechanism of action of 6-hydroxydopamine. Molecular pharmacology. 1971;7(2):147-54.

[79] Cohen G. Oxy-radical toxicity in catecholamine neurons. Neurotoxicology. 1984;5(1):77-82.

[80] Rodriguez Diaz M, Abdala P, Barroso-Chinea P, Obeso J, Gonzalez-Hernandez T. Motor behavioural changes after intracerebroventricular injection of 6-hydroxydopamine in the rat: an animal model of Parkinson's disease. Behavioural brain research. 2001;122(1):79-92.

[81] Zigmond MJ, Stricker EM. Recovery of feeding and drinking by rats after intraventricular 6-hydroxydopamine or lateral hypothalamic lesions. Science. 1973;182(113):717-20.

[82] Sauer H, Oertel WH. Progressive degeneration of nigrostriatal dopamine neurons following intrastriatal terminal lesions with 6-hydroxydopamine: a combined retrograde tracing and immunocytochemical study in the rat. Neuroscience. 1994;59(2):401-15.

[83] Marti MJ, James CJ, Oo TF, Kelly WJ, Burke RE. Early developmental destruction of terminals in the striatal target induces apoptosis in dopamine neurons of the substantia nigra. The Journal of neuroscience : the official journal of the Society for Neuroscience. 1997;17(6):2030-9.

[84] Marti MJ, Saura J, Burke RE, Jackson-Lewis V, Jimenez A, Bonastre M, et al. Striatal 6-hydroxydopamine induces apoptosis of nigral neurons in the adult rat. Brain research. 2002;958(1):185-91.

[85] Jeon BS, Jackson-Lewis V, Burke RE. 6-Hydroxydopamine lesion of the rat substantia nigra: time course and morphology of cell death. Neurodegeneration : a journal for neurodegenerative disorders, neuroprotection, and neuroregeneration. 1995;4(2):131-7.

[86] Bove J, Prou D, Perier C, Przedborski S. Toxin-induced models of Parkinson's disease. NeuroRx : the journal of the American Society for Experimental NeuroTherapeutics. 2005;2(3):484-94.

[87] Falkenburger BH, Schulz JB. Limitations of cellular models in Parkinson's disease research. Journal of neural transmission Supplementum. 2006;(70):261-8.

[88] Terzioglu M, Galter D. Parkinson's disease: genetic versus toxin-induced rodent models. The FEBS journal. 2008;275(7):1384-91. doi: 10.1111/j.1742-4658.2008.06302.x.

[89] Hisahara S, Shimohama S. Toxin-induced and genetic animal models of Parkinson's disease. Parkinson's disease. 2010;2011:951709. doi: 10.4061/2011/951709.

[90] Dawson T, Mandir A, Lee M. Animal models of PD: pieces of the same puzzle? Neuron. 2002;35(2):219-22.

[91] Bezard E, Gross CE, Fournier MC, Dovero S, Bloch B, Jaber M. Absence of MPTP-induced neuronal death in mice lacking the dopamine transporter. Experimental neurology. 1999;155(2):268-73. doi: 10.1006/exnr.1998.6995.

[92] Ramsay RR, Singer TP. Energy-dependent uptake of N-methyl-4-phenylpyridinium, the neurotoxic metabolite of 1-methyl-4-phenyl-1,2,3,6-tetrahydropyridine, by mitochondria. The Journal of biological chemistry. 1986;261(17):7585-7.

[93] Langston JW, Forno LS, Tetrud J, Reeves AG, Kaplan JA, Karluk D. Evidence of active nerve cell degeneration in the substantia nigra of humans years after 1-methyl-4-phenyl-1,2,3,6-tetrahydropyridine exposure. Annals of neurology. 1999;46(4):598-605.

[94] Forno LS, DeLanney LE, Irwin I, Langston JW. Similarities and differences between MPTP-induced parkinsonsim and Parkinson's disease. Neuropathologic considerations. Advances in neurology. 1993;60:600-8.

[95] Sonsalla PK, Heikkila RE. The influence of dose and dosing interval on MPTP-induced dopaminergic neurotoxicity in mice. European journal of pharmacology. 1986;129(3):339-45.

[96] Ricaurte GA, Langston JW, Delanney LE, Irwin I, Peroutka SJ, Forno LS. Fate of nigrostriatal neurons in young mature mice given 1-methyl-4-phenyl-1,2,3,6-tetrahydropyridine: a neurochemical and morphological reassessment. Brain research. 1986;376(1):117-24.

[97] Schneider JS, Denaro FJ. Astrocytic responses to the dopaminergic neurotoxin 1-methyl-4-phenyl-1,2,3,6-tetrahydropyridine (MPTP) in cat and mouse brain. Journal of neuropathology and experimental neurology. 1988;47(4):452-8.

[98] Jackson-Lewis V, Jakowec M, Burke RE, Przedborski S. Time course and morphology of dopaminergic neuronal death caused by the neurotoxin 1-methyl-4-phenyl-1,2,3,6-tetrahydropyridine. Neurodegeneration : a journal for neurodegenerative disorders, neuroprotection, and neuroregeneration. 1995;4(3):257-69.

[99] Tatton NA, Kish SJ. In situ detection of apoptotic nuclei in the substantia nigra compacta of 1-methyl-4-phenyl-1,2,3,6-tetrahydropyridine-treated mice using terminal deoxynucleotidyl transferase labelling and acridine orange staining. Neuroscience. 1997;77(4):1037-48.

[100] Kurkowska-Jastrzebska I, Wronska A, Kohutnicka M, Czlonkowski A, Czlonkowska A. The inflammatory reaction following 1-methyl-4-phenyl-1,2,3, 6-tetrahydropyridine intoxication in mouse. Experimental neurology. 1999;156(1):50-61. doi: 10.1006/exnr.1998.6993.

[101] Furuya T, Hayakawa H, Yamada M, Yoshimi K, Hisahara S, Miura M, et al. Caspase-11 mediates inflammatory dopaminergic cell death in the 1-methyl-4-phenyl-1,2,3,6-tetrahydropyridine mouse model of Parkinson's disease. The Journal of neuroscience : the official journal of the Society for Neuroscience. 2004;24(8):1865-72. doi: 10.1523/JNEUROSCI.3309-03.2004.

[102] Liberatore GT, Jackson-Lewis V, Vukosavic S, Mandir AS, Vila M, McAuliffe WG, et al. Inducible nitric oxide synthase stimulates dopaminergic neurodegeneration in the MPTP model of Parkinson disease. Nature medicine. 1999;5(12):1403-9. doi: 10.1038/70978.

[103] Wade TV, Schneider JS. Expression of striatal preprotachykinin mRNA in symptomatic and asymptomatic 1-methyl-4-phenyl-1,2,3,6-tetrahydropyridine-exposed monkeys is related to parkinsonian motor signs. The Journal of neuroscience : the official journal of the Society for Neuroscience. 2001;21(13):4901-7.

[104] Bloem BR, Irwin I, Buruma OJ, Haan J, Roos RA, Tetrud JW, et al. The MPTP model: versatile contributions to the treatment of idiopathic Parkinson's disease. Journal of the neurological sciences. 1990;97(2-3):273-93.
[105] Zigmond MJ, Stricker EM. Animal models of parkinsonism using selective neurotoxins: clinical and basic implications. International review of neurobiology. 1989;31:1-79.
[106] Kopin IJ. MPTP: an industrial chemical and contaminant of illicit narcotics stimulates a new era in research on Parkinson's disease. Environmental health perspectives. 1987;75:45-51.
[107] Kitamura Y, Kakimura J, Taniguchi T. Protective effect of talipexole on MPTP-treated planarian, a unique parkinsonian worm model. Japanese journal of pharmacology. 1998;78(1):23-9.
[108] Giovanni A, Sieber BA, Heikkila RE, Sonsalla PK. Studies on species sensitivity to the dopaminergic neurotoxin 1-methyl-4-phenyl-1,2,3,6-tetrahydropyridine. Part 1: Systemic administration. The Journal of pharmacology and experimental therapeutics. 1994;270(3):1000-7.
[109] Giovanni A, Sonsalla PK, Heikkila RE. Studies on species sensitivity to the dopaminergic neurotoxin 1-methyl-4-phenyl-1,2,3,6-tetrahydropyridine. Part 2: Central administration of 1-methyl-4-phenylpyridinium. The Journal of pharmacology and experimental therapeutics. 1994;270(3):1008-14.
[110] Przedborski S, Jackson-Lewis V, Naini AB, Jakowec M, Petzinger G, Miller R, et al. The parkinsonian toxin 1-methyl-4-phenyl-1,2,3,6-tetrahydropyridine (MPTP): a technical review of its utility and safety. Journal of neurochemistry. 2001;76(5):1265-74.
[111] Tolwani RJ, Jakowec MW, Petzinger GM, Green S, Waggie K. Experimental models of Parkinson's disease: insights from many models. Laboratory animal science. 1999;49(4):363-71.
[112] Sedelis M, Hofele K, Auburger GW, Morgan S, Huston JP, Schwarting RK. MPTP susceptibility in the mouse: behavioral, neurochemical, and histological analysis of gender and strain differences. Behavior genetics. 2000;30(3):171-82.
[113] Jenner P. The contribution of the MPTP-treated primate model to the development of new treatment strategies for Parkinson's disease. Parkinsonism & related disorders. 2003;9(3):131-7.
[114] Betarbet R, Sherer TB, MacKenzie G, Garcia-Osuna M, Panov AV, Greenamyre JT. Chronic systemic pesticide exposure reproduces features of Parkinson's disease. Nature neuroscience. 2000;3(12):1301-6. doi: 10.1038/81834.
[115] Schuler F, Casida JE. Functional coupling of PSST and ND1 subunits in NADH:ubiquinone oxidoreductase established by photoaffinity labeling. Biochimica et biophysica acta. 2001;1506(1):79-87.
[116] Marshall LE, Himes RH. Rotenone inhibition of tubulin self-assembly. Biochimica et biophysica acta. 1978;543(4):590-4.
[117] Burke D, Gasdaska P, Hartwell L. Dominant effects of tubulin overexpression in Saccharomyces cerevisiae. Molecular and cellular biology. 1989;9(3):1049-59.
[118] Sherer TB, Betarbet R, Testa CM, Seo BB, Richardson JR, Kim JH, et al. Mechanism of toxicity in rotenone models of Parkinson's disease. The Journal of neuroscience : the official journal of the Society for Neuroscience. 2003;23(34):10756-64.

[119] Uversky VN. Neurotoxicant-induced animal models of Parkinson's disease: understanding the role of rotenone, maneb and paraquat in neurodegeneration. Cell and tissue research. 2004;318(1):225-41. doi: 10.1007/s00441-004-0937-z.

[120] Sherer TB, Betarbet R, Kim JH, Greenamyre JT. Selective microglial activation in the rat rotenone model of Parkinson's disease. Neuroscience letters. 2003;341(2):87-90.

[121] Sherer TB, Kim JH, Betarbet R, Greenamyre JT. Subcutaneous rotenone exposure causes highly selective dopaminergic degeneration and alpha-synuclein aggregation. Experimental neurology. 2003;179(1):9-16.

[122] Betarbet R, Canet-Aviles RM, Sherer TB, Mastroberardino PG, McLendon C, Kim JH, et al. Intersecting pathways to neurodegeneration in Parkinson's disease: effects of the pesticide rotenone on DJ-1, alpha-synuclein, and the ubiquitin-proteasome system. Neurobiology of disease. 2006;22(2):404-20. doi: 10.1016/j.nbd.2005.12.003.

[123] Klockgether T. Parkinson's disease: clinical aspects. Cell and tissue research. 2004;318(1):115-20. doi: 10.1007/s00441-004-0975-6.

[124] Alam M, Schmidt WJ. Rotenone destroys dopaminergic neurons and induces parkinsonian symptoms in rats. Behavioural brain research. 2002;136(1):317-24.

[125] Hely MA, Morris JG, Reid WG, Trafficante R. Sydney Multicenter Study of Parkinson's disease: non-L-dopa-responsive problems dominate at 15 years. Movement disorders : official journal of the Movement Disorder Society. 2005;20(2):190-9. doi: 10.1002/mds.20324.

[126] Greene JG, Noorian AR, Srinivasan S. Delayed gastric emptying and enteric nervous system dysfunction in the rotenone model of Parkinson's disease. Experimental neurology. 2009;218(1):154-61. doi: 10.1016/j.expneurol.2009.04.023.

[127] Drolet RE, Cannon JR, Montero L, Greenamyre JT. Chronic rotenone exposure reproduces Parkinson's disease gastrointestinal neuropathology. Neurobiology of disease. 2009;36(1):96-102. doi: 10.1016/j.nbd.2009.06.017.

[128] Di Monte D, Sandy MS, Ekstrom G, Smith MT. Comparative studies on the mechanisms of paraquat and 1-methyl-4-phenylpyridine (MPP+) cytotoxicity. Biochemical and biophysical research communications. 1986;137(1):303-9.

[129] Shimizu K, Matsubara K, Ohtaki K, Fujimaru S, Saito O, Shiono H. Paraquat induces long-lasting dopamine overflow through the excitotoxic pathway in the striatum of freely moving rats. Brain research. 2003;976(2):243-52.

[130] Brooks AI, Chadwick CA, Gelbard HA, Cory-Slechta DA, Federoff HJ. Paraquat elicited neurobehavioral syndrome caused by dopaminergic neuron loss. Brain research. 1999;823(1-2):1-10.

[131] Peng J, Mao XO, Stevenson FF, Hsu M, Andersen JK. The herbicide paraquat induces dopaminergic nigral apoptosis through sustained activation of the JNK pathway. The Journal of biological chemistry. 2004;279(31):32626-32. doi: 10.1074/jbc.M404596200.

[132] Purisai MG, McCormack AL, Cumine S, Li J, Isla MZ, Di Monte DA. Microglial activation as a priming event leading to paraquat-induced dopaminergic cell degeneration. Neurobiology of disease. 2007;25(2):392-400. doi: 10.1016/j.nbd.2006.10.008.

[133] Dringen R. Oxidative and antioxidative potential of brain microglial cells. Antioxidants & redox signaling. 2005;7(9-10):1223-33. doi: 10.1089/ars.2005.7.1223.

[134] Bonneh-Barkay D, Langston WJ, Di Monte DA. Toxicity of redox cycling pesticides in primary mesencephalic cultures. Antioxidants & redox signaling. 2005;7(5-6):649-53. doi: 10.1089/ars.2005.7.649.
[135] Bonneh-Barkay D, Reaney SH, Langston WJ, Di Monte DA. Redox cycling of the herbicide paraquat in microglial cultures. Brain research Molecular brain research. 2005;134(1):52-6. doi: 10.1016/j.molbrainres.2004.11.005.
[136] McCormack AL, Atienza JG, Langston JW, Di Monte DA. Decreased susceptibility to oxidative stress underlies the resistance of specific dopaminergic cell populations to paraquat-induced degeneration. Neuroscience. 2006;141(2):929-37. doi: 10.1016/j.neuroscience.2006.03.069.
[137] Peng J, Stevenson FF, Doctrow SR, Andersen JK. Superoxide dismutase/catalase mimetics are neuroprotective against selective paraquat-mediated dopaminergic neuron death in the substantial nigra: implications for Parkinson disease. The Journal of biological chemistry. 2005;280(32):29194-8. doi: 10.1074/jbc.M500984200.
[138] Manning-Bog AB, McCormack AL, Li J, Uversky VN, Fink AL, Di Monte DA. The herbicide paraquat causes up-regulation and aggregation of alpha-synuclein in mice: paraquat and alpha-synuclein. The Journal of biological chemistry. 2002;277(3):1641-4. doi: 10.1074/jbc.C100560200.
[139] Thiruchelvam M, Brockel BJ, Richfield EK, Baggs RB, Cory-Slechta DA. Potentiated and preferential effects of combined paraquat and maneb on nigrostriatal dopamine systems: environmental risk factors for Parkinson's disease? Brain research. 2000;873(2):225-34.
[140] Zhang J, Fitsanakis VA, Gu G, Jing D, Ao M, Amarnath V, et al. Manganese ethylene-bis-dithiocarbamate and selective dopaminergic neurodegeneration in rat: a link through mitochondrial dysfunction. Journal of neurochemistry. 2003;84(2):336-46.
[141] Thiruchelvam M, Richfield EK, Baggs RB, Tank AW, Cory-Slechta DA. The nigrostriatal dopaminergic system as a preferential target of repeated exposures to combined paraquat and maneb: implications for Parkinson's disease. The Journal of neuroscience : the official journal of the Society for Neuroscience. 2000;20(24):9207-14.
[142] Thiruchelvam M, McCormack A, Richfield EK, Baggs RB, Tank AW, Di Monte DA, et al. Age-related irreversible progressive nigrostriatal dopaminergic neurotoxicity in the paraquat and maneb model of the Parkinson's disease phenotype. The European journal of neuroscience. 2003;18(3):589-600.
[143] Barlow BK, Thiruchelvam MJ, Bennice L, Cory-Slechta DA, Ballatori N, Richfield EK. Increased synaptosomal dopamine content and brain concentration of paraquat produced by selective dithiocarbamates. Journal of neurochemistry. 2003;85(4):1075-86.
[144] Richfield EK, Thiruchelvam MJ, Cory-Slechta DA, Wuertzer C, Gainetdinov RR, Caron MG, et al. Behavioral and neurochemical effects of wild-type and mutated human alpha-synuclein in transgenic mice. Experimental neurology. 2002;175(1):35-48. doi: 10.1006/exnr.2002.7882.
[145] Thiruchelvam MJ, Powers JM, Cory-Slechta DA, Richfield EK. Risk factors for dopaminergic neuron loss in human alpha-synuclein transgenic mice. The European journal of neuroscience. 2004;19(4):845-54.

[146] Masliah E, Rockenstein E, Veinbergs I, Mallory M, Hashimoto M, Takeda A, et al. Dopaminergic loss and inclusion body formation in alpha-synuclein mice: implications for neurodegenerative disorders. Science. 2000;287(5456):1265-9.

[147] Giasson BI, Duda JE, Quinn SM, Zhang B, Trojanowski JQ, Lee VM. Neuronal alpha-synucleinopathy with severe movement disorder in mice expressing A53T human alpha-synuclein. Neuron. 2002;34(4):521-33.

[148] Lee MK, Stirling W, Xu Y, Xu X, Qui D, Mandir AS, et al. Human alpha-synuclein-harboring familial Parkinson's disease-linked Ala-53 --> Thr mutation causes neurodegenerative disease with alpha-synuclein aggregation in transgenic mice. Proceedings of the National Academy of Sciences of the United States of America. 2002;99(13):8968-73. doi: 10.1073/pnas.132197599.

[149] Rockenstein E, Mallory M, Hashimoto M, Song D, Shults CW, Lang I, et al. Differential neuropathological alterations in transgenic mice expressing alpha-synuclein from the platelet-derived growth factor and Thy-1 promoters. Journal of neuroscience research. 2002;68(5):568-78. doi: 10.1002/jnr.10231.

[150] Song DD, Shults CW, Sisk A, Rockenstein E, Masliah E. Enhanced substantia nigra mitochondrial pathology in human alpha-synuclein transgenic mice after treatment with MPTP. Experimental neurology. 2004;186(2):158-72. doi: 10.1016/S0014-4886(03)00342-X.

[151] Martin LJ, Pan Y, Price AC, Sterling W, Copeland NG, Jenkins NA, et al. Parkinson's disease alpha-synuclein transgenic mice develop neuronal mitochondrial degeneration and cell death. The Journal of neuroscience : the official journal of the Society for Neuroscience. 2006;26(1):41-50. doi: 10.1523/JNEUROSCI.4308-05.2006.

[152] Kirik D, Rosenblad C, Burger C, Lundberg C, Johansen TE, Muzyczka N, et al. Parkinson-like neurodegeneration induced by targeted overexpression of alpha-synuclein in the nigrostriatal system. The Journal of neuroscience : the official journal of the Society for Neuroscience. 2002;22(7):2780-91. doi: 20026246.

[153] Feany MB, Bender WW. A Drosophila model of Parkinson's disease. Nature. 2000;404(6776):394-8. doi: 10.1038/35006074.

[154] Lakso M, Vartiainen S, Moilanen AM, Sirvio J, Thomas JH, Nass R, et al. Dopaminergic neuronal loss and motor deficits in Caenorhabditis elegans overexpressing human alpha-synuclein. Journal of neurochemistry. 2003;86(1):165-72.

[155] Kuwahara T, Koyama A, Gengyo-Ando K, Masuda M, Kowa H, Tsunoda M, et al. Familial Parkinson mutant alpha-synuclein causes dopamine neuron dysfunction in transgenic Caenorhabditis elegans. The Journal of biological chemistry. 2006;281(1):334-40. doi: 10.1074/jbc.M504860200.

[156] Stefanis L, Kholodilov N, Rideout HJ, Burke RE, Greene LA. Synuclein-1 is selectively up-regulated in response to nerve growth factor treatment in PC12 cells. Journal of neurochemistry. 2001;76(4):1165-76.

[157] Clough RL, Stefanis L. A novel pathway for transcriptional regulation of alpha-synuclein. The FASEB journal : official publication of the Federation of American Societies for Experimental Biology. 2007;21(2):596-607. doi: 10.1096/fj.06-7111com.

[158] Cuervo AM, Stefanis L, Fredenburg R, Lansbury PT, Sulzer D. Impaired degradation of mutant alpha-synuclein by chaperone-mediated autophagy. Science. 2004;305(5688):1292-5. doi: 10.1126/science.1101738.

[159] Tanaka Y, Engelender S, Igarashi S, Rao RK, Wanner T, Tanzi RE, et al. Inducible expression of mutant alpha-synuclein decreases proteasome activity and increases sensitivity to mitochondria-dependent apoptosis. Human molecular genetics. 2001;10(9):919-26.
[160] Smith WW, Jiang H, Pei Z, Tanaka Y, Morita H, Sawa A, et al. Endoplasmic reticulum stress and mitochondrial cell death pathways mediate A53T mutant alpha-synuclein-induced toxicity. Human molecular genetics. 2005;14(24):3801-11. doi: 10.1093/hmg/ddi396.
[161] Stefanis L, Larsen KE, Rideout HJ, Sulzer D, Greene LA. Expression of A53T mutant but not wild-type alpha-synuclein in PC12 cells induces alterations of the ubiquitin-dependent degradation system, loss of dopamine release, and autophagic cell death. The Journal of neuroscience : the official journal of the Society for Neuroscience. 2001;21(24):9549-60.
[162] Outeiro TF, Lindquist S. Yeast cells provide insight into alpha-synuclein biology and pathobiology. Science. 2003;302(5651):1772-5. doi: 10.1126/science.1090439.
[163] Dixon C, Mathias N, Zweig RM, Davis DA, Gross DS. Alpha-synuclein targets the plasma membrane via the secretory pathway and induces toxicity in yeast. Genetics. 2005;170(1):47-59. doi: 10.1534/genetics.104.035493.
[164] Flower TR, Chesnokova LS, Froelich CA, Dixon C, Witt SN. Heat shock prevents alpha-synuclein-induced apoptosis in a yeast model of Parkinson's disease. Journal of molecular biology. 2005;351(5):1081-100. doi: 10.1016/j.jmb.2005.06.060.
[165] Cooper AA, Gitler AD, Cashikar A, Haynes CM, Hill KJ, Bhullar B, et al. Alpha-synuclein blocks ER-Golgi traffic and Rab1 rescues neuron loss in Parkinson's models. Science. 2006;313(5785):324-8. doi: 10.1126/science.1129462.
[166] Willingham S, Outeiro TF, DeVit MJ, Lindquist SL, Muchowski PJ. Yeast genes that enhance the toxicity of a mutant huntingtin fragment or alpha-synuclein. Science. 2003;302(5651):1769-72. doi: 10.1126/science.1090389.
[167] Douglas MR, Lewthwaite AJ, Nicholl DJ. Genetics of Parkinson's disease and parkinsonism. Expert review of neurotherapeutics. 2007;7(6):657-66. doi: 10.1586/14737175.7.6.657.
[168] Lo Bianco C, Schneider BL, Bauer M, Sajadi A, Brice A, Iwatsubo T, et al. Lentiviral vector delivery of parkin prevents dopaminergic degeneration in an alpha-synuclein rat model of Parkinson's disease. Proceedings of the National Academy of Sciences of the United States of America. 2004;101(50):17510-5. doi: 10.1073/pnas.0405313101.
[169] Paterna JC, Leng A, Weber E, Feldon J, Bueler H. DJ-1 and Parkin modulate dopamine-dependent behavior and inhibit MPTP-induced nigral dopamine neuron loss in mice. Molecular therapy : the journal of the American Society of Gene Therapy. 2007;15(4):698-704. doi: 10.1038/sj.mt.6300067.
[170] Von Coelln R, Thomas B, Savitt JM, Lim KL, Sasaki M, Hess EJ, et al. Loss of locus coeruleus neurons and reduced startle in parkin null mice. Proceedings of the National Academy of Sciences of the United States of America. 2004;101(29):10744-9. doi: 10.1073/pnas.0401297101.
[171] Goldberg MS, Fleming SM, Palacino JJ, Cepeda C, Lam HA, Bhatnagar A, et al. Parkin-deficient mice exhibit nigrostriatal deficits but not loss of dopaminergic neurons.

The Journal of biological chemistry. 2003;278(44):43628-35. doi: 10.1074/jbc.M308947200.

[172] Greene JC, Whitworth AJ, Kuo I, Andrews LA, Feany MB, Pallanck LJ. Mitochondrial pathology and apoptotic muscle degeneration in Drosophila parkin mutants. Proceedings of the National Academy of Sciences of the United States of America. 2003;100(7):4078-83. doi: 10.1073/pnas.0737556100.

[173] Greene JC, Whitworth AJ, Andrews LA, Parker TJ, Pallanck LJ. Genetic and genomic studies of Drosophila parkin mutants implicate oxidative stress and innate immune responses in pathogenesis. Human molecular genetics. 2005;14(6):799-811. doi: 10.1093/hmg/ddi074.

[174] Sang TK, Chang HY, Lawless GM, Ratnaparkhi A, Mee L, Ackerson LC, et al. A Drosophila model of mutant human parkin-induced toxicity demonstrates selective loss of dopaminergic neurons and dependence on cellular dopamine. The Journal of neuroscience : the official journal of the Society for Neuroscience. 2007;27(5):981-92. doi: 10.1523/JNEUROSCI.4810-06.2007.

[175] Imai Y, Soda M, Inoue H, Hattori N, Mizuno Y, Takahashi R. An unfolded putative transmembrane polypeptide, which can lead to endoplasmic reticulum stress, is a substrate of Parkin. Cell. 2001;105(7):891-902.

[176] Shimura H, Schlossmacher MG, Hattori N, Frosch MP, Trockenbacher A, Schneider R, et al. Ubiquitination of a new form of alpha-synuclein by parkin from human brain: implications for Parkinson's disease. Science. 2001;293(5528):263-9. doi: 10.1126/science.1060627.

[177] LaVoie MJ, Ostaszewski BL, Weihofen A, Schlossmacher MG, Selkoe DJ. Dopamine covalently modifies and functionally inactivates parkin. Nature medicine. 2005;11(11):1214-21. doi: 10.1038/nm1314.

[178] Avraham E, Rott R, Liani E, Szargel R, Engelender S. Phosphorylation of Parkin by the cyclin-dependent kinase 5 at the linker region modulates its ubiquitin-ligase activity and aggregation. The Journal of biological chemistry. 2007;282(17):12842-50. doi: 10.1074/jbc.M608243200.

[179] Kitada T, Pisani A, Porter DR, Yamaguchi H, Tscherter A, Martella G, et al. Impaired dopamine release and synaptic plasticity in the striatum of PINK1-deficient mice. Proceedings of the National Academy of Sciences of the United States of America. 2007;104(27):11441-6. doi: 10.1073/pnas.0702717104.

[180] Clark IE, Dodson MW, Jiang C, Cao JH, Huh JR, Seol JH, et al. Drosophila pink1 is required for mitochondrial function and interacts genetically with parkin. Nature. 2006;441(7097):1162-6. doi: 10.1038/nature04779.

[181] Park J, Lee SB, Lee S, Kim Y, Song S, Kim S, et al. Mitochondrial dysfunction in Drosophila PINK1 mutants is complemented by parkin. Nature. 2006;441(7097):1157-61. doi: 10.1038/nature04788.

[182] Yang Y, Gehrke S, Imai Y, Huang Z, Ouyang Y, Wang JW, et al. Mitochondrial pathology and muscle and dopaminergic neuron degeneration caused by inactivation of Drosophila Pink1 is rescued by Parkin. Proceedings of the National Academy of Sciences of the United States of America. 2006;103(28):10793-8. doi: 10.1073/pnas.0602493103.

[183] Pridgeon JW, Olzmann JA, Chin LS, Li L. PINK1 protects against oxidative stress by phosphorylating mitochondrial chaperone TRAP1. PLoS biology. 2007;5(7):e172. doi: 10.1371/journal.pbio.0050172.

[184] Silvestri L, Caputo V, Bellacchio E, Atorino L, Dallapiccola B, Valente EM, et al. Mitochondrial import and enzymatic activity of PINK1 mutants associated to recessive parkinsonism. Human molecular genetics. 2005;14(22):3477-92. doi: 10.1093/hmg/ddi377.

[185] Beilina A, Van Der Brug M, Ahmad R, Kesavapany S, Miller DW, Petsko GA, et al. Mutations in PTEN-induced putative kinase 1 associated with recessive parkinsonism have differential effects on protein stability. Proceedings of the National Academy of Sciences of the United States of America. 2005;102(16):5703-8. doi: 10.1073/pnas.0500617102.

[186] Andres-Mateos E, Perier C, Zhang L, Blanchard-Fillion B, Greco TM, Thomas B, et al. DJ-1 gene deletion reveals that DJ-1 is an atypical peroxiredoxin-like peroxidase. Proceedings of the National Academy of Sciences of the United States of America. 2007;104(37):14807-12. doi: 10.1073/pnas.0703219104.

[187] Park J, Kim SY, Cha GH, Lee SB, Kim S, Chung J. Drosophila DJ-1 mutants show oxidative stress-sensitive locomotive dysfunction. Gene. 2005;361:133-9. doi: 10.1016/j.gene.2005.06.040.

[188] Menzies FM, Yenisetti SC, Min KT. Roles of Drosophila DJ-1 in survival of dopaminergic neurons and oxidative stress. Current biology : CB. 2005;15(17):1578-82. doi: 10.1016/j.cub.2005.07.036.

[189] Meulener M, Whitworth AJ, Armstrong-Gold CE, Rizzu P, Heutink P, Wes PD, et al. Drosophila DJ-1 mutants are selectively sensitive to environmental toxins associated with Parkinson's disease. Current biology : CB. 2005;15(17):1572-7. doi: 10.1016/j.cub.2005.07.064.

[190] Meulener MC, Xu K, Thomson L, Ischiropoulos H, Bonini NM. Mutational analysis of DJ-1 in Drosophila implicates functional inactivation by oxidative damage and aging. Proceedings of the National Academy of Sciences of the United States of America. 2006;103(33):12517-22. doi: 10.1073/pnas.0601891103.

[191] West AB, Moore DJ, Biskup S, Bugayenko A, Smith WW, Ross CA, et al. Parkinson's disease-associated mutations in leucine-rich repeat kinase 2 augment kinase activity. Proceedings of the National Academy of Sciences of the United States of America. 2005;102(46):16842-7. doi: 10.1073/pnas.0507360102.

[192] West AB, Moore DJ, Choi C, Andrabi SA, Li X, Dikeman D, et al. Parkinson's disease-associated mutations in LRRK2 link enhanced GTP-binding and kinase activities to neuronal toxicity. Human molecular genetics. 2007;16(2):223-32. doi: 10.1093/hmg/ddl471.

[193] Greggio E, Lewis PA, van der Brug MP, Ahmad R, Kaganovich A, Ding J, et al. Mutations in LRRK2/dardarin associated with Parkinson disease are more toxic than equivalent mutations in the homologous kinase LRRK1. Journal of neurochemistry. 2007;102(1):93-102. doi: 10.1111/j.1471-4159.2007.04523.x.

[194] MacLeod D, Dowman J, Hammond R, Leete T, Inoue K, Abeliovich A. The familial Parkinsonism gene LRRK2 regulates neurite process morphology. Neuron. 2006;52(4):587-93. doi: 10.1016/j.neuron.2006.10.008.

[195] Ito G, Okai T, Fujino G, Takeda K, Ichijo H, Katada T, et al. GTP binding is essential to the protein kinase activity of LRRK2, a causative gene product for familial Parkinson's disease. Biochemistry. 2007;46(5):1380-8. doi: 10.1021/bi061960m.

[196] Smith WW, Pei Z, Jiang H, Dawson VL, Dawson TM, Ross CA. Kinase activity of mutant LRRK2 mediates neuronal toxicity. Nature neuroscience. 2006;9(10):1231-3. doi: 10.1038/nn1776.

[197] Langston JW. The Parkinson's complex: parkinsonism is just the tip of the iceberg. Ann Neurol. 2006;59(4):591-6. doi: 10.1002/ana.20834.

[198] Selikhova M, Williams DR, Kempster PA, Holton JL, Revesz T, Lees AJ. A clinico-pathological study of subtypes in Parkinson's disease. Brain. 2009;132(Pt 11):2947-57. doi: awp234 [pii] 10.1093/brain/awp234.

[199] Marsden CD. Studies on the normal and disordered human motor cortex. Electroencephalogr Clin Neurophysiol Suppl. 1982;36:430-4.

[200] Jankovic J. Parkinson's disease and movement disorders: moving forward. Lancet Neurol. 2008;7(1):9-11. doi: S1474-4422(07)70302-2 [pii] 10.1016/S1474-4422(07)70302-2.

[201] Voon V, Krack P, Lang AE, Lozano AM, Dujardin K, Schupbach M, et al. A multicentre study on suicide outcomes following subthalamic stimulation for Parkinson's disease. Brain. 2008;131(Pt 10):2720-8. doi: awn214 [pii] 10.1093/brain/awn214.

[202] Pechevis M, Clarke CE, Vieregge P, Khoshnood B, Deschaseaux-Voinet C, Berdeaux G, et al. Effects of dyskinesias in Parkinson's disease on quality of life and health-related costs: a prospective European study. Eur J Neurol. 2005;12(12):956-63. doi: ENE1096 [pii] 10.1111/j.1468-1331.2005.01096.x.

[203] Kempster PA, O'Sullivan SS, Holton JL, Revesz T, Lees AJ. Relationships between age and late progression of Parkinson's disease: a clinico-pathological study. Brain. 2010;133(Pt 6):1755-62. doi: awq059 [pii] 10.1093/brain/awq059.

[204] Emre M, Aarsland D, Brown R, Burn DJ, Duyckaerts C, Mizuno Y, et al. Clinical diagnostic criteria for dementia associated with Parkinson's disease. Mov Disord. 2007;22(12):1689-707; quiz 837. doi: 10.1002/mds.21507.

[205] Siderowf A, Xie SX, Hurtig H, Weintraub D, Duda J, Chen-Plotkin A, et al. CSF amyloid {beta} 1-42 predicts cognitive decline in Parkinson disease. Neurology. 2010;75(12):1055-61. doi: WNL.0b013e3181f39a78 [pii] 10.1212/WNL.0b013e3181f39a78.

[206] Hauptmann C, Tass PA. Therapeutic rewiring by means of desynchronizing brain stimulation. Biosystems. 2007;89(1-3):173-81. doi: S0303-2647(06)00256-5 [pii] 10.1016/j.biosystems.2006.04.015.

[207] Weaver FM, Follett K, Stern M, Hur K, Harris C, Marks WJ, Jr., et al. Bilateral deep brain stimulation vs best medical therapy for patients with advanced Parkinson disease: a randomized controlled trial. JAMA. 2009;301(1):63-73. doi: 301/1/63 [pii] 10.1001/jama.2008.929.

[208] Williams A, Gill S, Varma T, Jenkinson C, Quinn N, Mitchell R, et al. Deep brain stimulation plus best medical therapy versus best medical therapy alone for advanced Parkinson's disease (PD SURG trial): a randomised, open-label trial. Lancet Neurol. 2010;9(6):581-91. doi: S1474-4422(10)70093-4 [pii] 10.1016/S1474-4422(10)70093-4.

[209] Smeding HM, Speelman JD, Huizenga HM, Schuurman PR, Schmand B. Predictors of cognitive and psychosocial outcome after STN DBS in Parkinson's Disease. J Neurol Neurosurg Psychiatry. 2011;82(7):754-60. doi: jnnp.2007.140012 [pii] 10.1136/jnnp.2007.140012.

[210] Strutt AM, Simpson R, Jankovic J, York MK. Changes in cognitive-emotional and physiological symptoms of depression following STN-DBS for the treatment of Parkinson's disease. Eur J Neurol. 2011. doi: 10.1111/j.1468-1331.2011.03447.x.

[211] Voon V, Saint-Cyr J, Lozano AM, Moro E, Poon YY, Lang AE. Psychiatric symptoms in patients with Parkinson disease presenting for deep brain stimulation surgery. J Neurosurg. 2005;103(2):246-51. doi: 10.3171/jns.2005.103.2.0246.

[212] Ory-Magne F, Brefel-Courbon C, Simonetta-Moreau M, Fabre N, Lotterie JA, Chaynes P, et al. Does ageing influence deep brain stimulation outcomes in Parkinson's disease? Mov Disord. 2007;22(10):1457-63. doi: 10.1002/mds.21547.

[213] Parent BA, Cho SW, Buck DG, Nalesnik MA, Gamblin TC. Spontaneous rupture of hepatic artery aneurysm associated with polyarteritis nodosa. Am Surg. 2010;76(12):1416-9.

[214] Merola A, Zibetti M, Angrisano S, Rizzi L, Lanotte M, Lopiano L. Comparison of subthalamic nucleus deep brain stimulation and Duodopa in the treatment of advanced Parkinson's disease. Mov Disord. 2011;26(4):664-70. doi: 10.1002/mds.23524.

[215] Lindvall O, Kokaia Z, Martinez-Serrano A. Stem cell therapy for human neurodegenerative disorders-how to make it work. Nat Med. 2004;10 Suppl:S42-50. doi: 10.1038/nm1064 nm1064 [pii].

[216] Freed WJ, Vawter MP. Microarrays: applications in neuroscience to disease, development, and repair. Restor Neurol Neurosci. 2001;18(2-3):53-6.

[217] Rhee YH, Ko JY, Chang MY, Yi SH, Kim D, Kim CH, et al. Protein-based human iPS cells efficiently generate functional dopamine neurons and can treat a rat model of Parkinson disease. J Clin Invest. 2011;121(6):2326-35. doi: 45794 [pii] 10.1172/JCI45794.

[218] Merola A, Zibetti M, Angrisano S, Rizzi L, Ricchi V, Artusi CA, et al. Parkinson's disease progression at 30 years: a study of subthalamic deep brain-stimulated patients. Brain. 2011;134(Pt 7):2074-84. doi: awr121 [pii] 10.1093/brain/awr121.

[219] Bjorklund A, Lindvall O. Parkinson disease gene therapy moves toward the clinic. Nat Med. 2000;6(11):1207-8. doi: 10.1038/81291.

[220] Kirik D, Georgievska B, Bjorklund A. Localized striatal delivery of GDNF as a treatment for Parkinson disease. Nat Neurosci. 2004;7(2):105-10. doi: 10.1038/nn1175 nn1175 [pii].

[221] Ramaswamy S, Soderstrom KE, Kordower JH. Trophic factors therapy in Parkinson's disease. Prog Brain Res. 2009;175:201-16. doi: S0079-6123(09)17514-3 [pii] 10.1016/S0079-6123(09)17514-3.

[222] Klein AA, Arrowsmith JE. Should routine pre-operative testing be abandoned? Anaesthesia. 2010;65(10):974-6. doi: 10.1111/j.1365-2044.2010.06503.x.

[223] Gill SS, Patel NK, Hotton GR, O'Sullivan K, McCarter R, Bunnage M, et al. Direct brain infusion of glial cell line-derived neurotrophic factor in Parkinson disease. Nat Med. 2003;9(5):589-95. doi: 10.1038/nm850 nm850 [pii].

[224] Lang AE, Gill S, Patel NK, Lozano A, Nutt JG, Penn R, et al. Randomized controlled trial of intraputamenal glial cell line-derived neurotrophic factor infusion in Parkinson disease. Ann Neurol. 2006;59(3):459-66. doi: 10.1002/ana.20737.

[225] Bartus RT, Herzog CD, Chu Y, Wilson A, Brown L, Siffert J, et al. Bioactivity of AAV2-neurturin gene therapy (CERE-120): differences between Parkinson's disease and nonhuman primate brains. Mov Disord. 2011;26(1):27-36. doi: 10.1002/mds.23442.

[226] Decressac M, Ulusoy A, Mattsson B, Georgievska B, Romero-Ramos M, Kirik D, et al. GDNF fails to exert neuroprotection in a rat {alpha}-synuclein model of Parkinson's disease. Brain. 2011;134(Pt 8):2302-11. doi: awr149 [pii] 10.1093/brain/awr149.

25

The Emerging Role of Centromere/Kinetochore Proteins in Cellular Senescence

Kayoko Maehara
Department of Maternal-Fetal Biology
National Research Institute for Child Health and Development, Tokyo, Japan

1. Introduction

Cellular senescence is an irreversible growth arrest triggered by several types of stress, including DNA damage, oxidative stress, telomere shortening, and oncogene activation (Ben-Porath & Weinberg, 2005; Collado et al., 2007; Deng et al., 2008; Hayflick & Moorhead, 1961; Serrano et al., 1997). Although how senescence is initiated remains to be determined, it has been shown to be triggered by certain defects in chromosome integrity, such as telomere shortening (Ben-Porath & Weinberg, 2005; Deng et al., 2008). In contrast to telomere shortening, the roles of which in senescence have been studied extensively, alterations in the centromere/kinetochore structure involved in senescence program remain to be elucidated. This chapter presents a discussion of the emerging roles of centromere/kinetochore proteins, particularly Centromere protein A (CENP-A, the centromere-specific variant of histone H3), in senescence.

2. Crucial roles of centromere/kinetochore proteins in mitosis

The genome of a cell is duplicated and segregated into two daughter cells during cell division (Fig. 1). Accurate chromosome segregation during cell division is essential for genome integrity and this process is mainly achieved by the structural/functional integrity of the microtubule spindle apparatus (kinetochore-microtubule interactions) and spindle assembly checkpoint (SAC) signaling (Cleveland et al., 2003; Musacchio, & Salmon, 2007; Tanaka, 2010). Spindle microtubules emanating from spindle pole bodies (centrosomes) attach to chromosomes via specialized structures called kinetochores where more than 100 proteins assemble at the centromeric region of each chromosome during mitosis. This interaction is monitored by the SAC signaling pathway to ensure high-fidelity chromosome segregation (Musacchio, & Salmon, 2007). Chromosome missegregation arising from defects in the structural integrity of the microtubule spindle apparatus and the SAC signaling pathway leads to aneuploidy, i.e., chromosome gain or loss (Compton, 2011). Aneuploidy is thought to be a major cause of congenital disorders. High rates of aneuploidy have been observed in various cancers and aneuploidy is speculated to be involved in tumorigenesis.

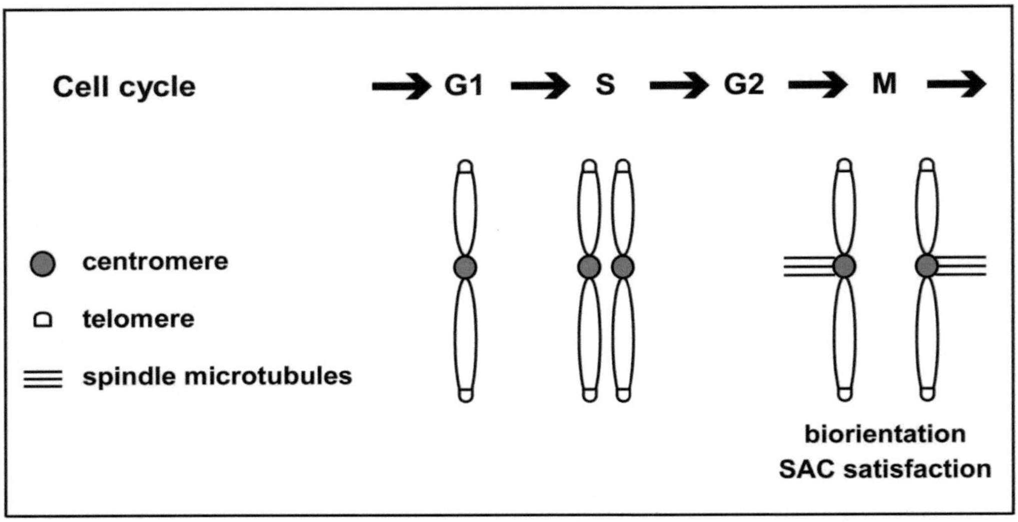

Fig. 1. Chromosome cycle and cell cycle (Adapted from Maehara, 2011)

In higher eukaryotes, the DNA sequence does not generally determine the functional centromeres except in the budding yeast *Saccharomyces cerevisiae*, in which the centromere, a 125-bp DNA element, is specified by its sequence. Centromeres in other organisms lack sequence specificity, but many of the proteins localizing at centromeres are well conserved across species (Fig. 2).

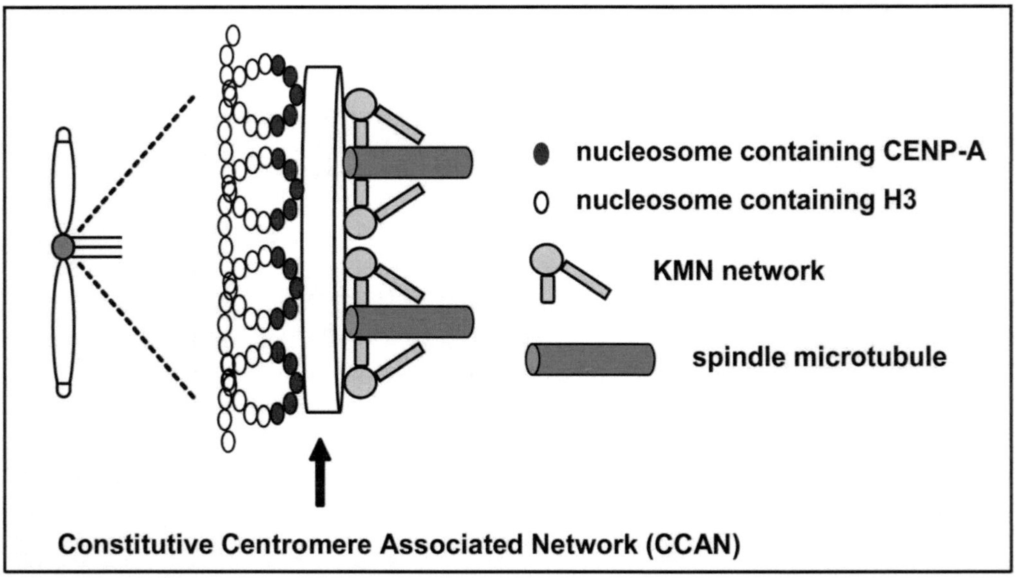

Fig. 2. Schematic representation of the kinetochore (Adapted from Maehara, 2011)

Among the numerous kinetochore-associated proteins identified to date, CENP-A represents an excellent candidate as an epigenetic marker of functional centromeres for several reasons. First, CENP-A is an evolutionarily conserved centromere-specific histone H3 variant (Blower & Karpen, 2001; Buchwitz et al, 1999; Earnshaw & Rothfield, 1985; Meluh et al., 1998; Palmer et al., 1987; Stoler et al., 1995; Takahashi et al., 2000). Canonical nucleosomes in chromosome arms consist of 146 bp of DNA wrapped around a histone octamer comprised of two subunits of each of H2A, H2B, H3, and H4. H3 is replaced with the H3 variant CENP-A at the centromeres. Second, many centromere-associated proteins are recruited to the centromere in a CENP-A-dependent manner (Foltz et al., 2006; Izuta et al., 2006; Obuse et al., 2004a, Okada et al., 2006). Third, neocentromeres, which are established as functional centromeres at ectopic chromosomal loci devoid of alpha satellite repeats, have been shown to contain CENP-A (Marshall et al., 2008). Thus, CENP-A seems to be an identifier of the functional centromere. Studies in a variety of organisms have indicated that CENP-A plays a crucial role in organizing kinetochore chromatin for precise chromosome segregation. Another conserved centromere protein, CENP-B, binds to a specific centromeric DNA sequence, the 17-bp "CENP-B box" in type I alpha satellite repeats in mammals (alphoid DNA in humans) (Earnshaw et al., 1987; Masumoto et al., 1989). CENP-B is essential for heterochromatin formation of pericentromeres and is thought to be important for the proper organization of kinetochore chromatin (Nakagawa et al., 2002; Nakano et al., 2008; Okada et al., 2007), although CENP-B is not essential for viability in higher eukaryotes (Hudson et al., 1998; Kapoor et al., 1998; Perez-Castro et al., 1998). In addition to the above proteins, several studies using proteomic approaches have identified 15 proteins known as the **C**onstitutive **C**entromere **A**ssociated **N**etwork (CCAN) (Foltz et al., 2006; Izuta et al., 2006; Okada et al., 2006). Several of these proteins have DNA binding activity or associate directly with CENP-A. The KMN network (KNL1, Mis12 complex, and Ndc80 complex) is also important as it forms the interface for kinetochore-microtubule attachment (Cheeseman et al., 2006; Obuse et al., 2004b; Ruchaud et al., 2007). SAC is a surveillance mechanism that is capable of delaying anaphase if not all chromosomes have established biorientation within the spindle (Musacchio & Salmon, 2007). It should be noted that many other centromere/kinetochore-associated proteins not mentioned in this chapter also have crucial roles in mitosis. Thus, multiple biological processes including kinetochore, microtubule functions, the mitotic spindle apparatus, and SAC signaling pathway ensure high-fidelity chromosome segregation during cell division.

3. The emerging roles of centromere/kinetochore proteins in senescence

The importance of kinetochore in regulating proper chromosome segregation has been well established. Next, I highlight some recent work on the roles of centromere/kinetochore proteins in senescence in mammals.

3.1 SAC proteins are involved in the senescence program

The SAC signaling pathway monitors the attachment of spindle microtubules to kinetochores. Core components of SAC include Mad1, Mad2, Bub1, Bub3, and BubR1, and many other proteins are also involved in this checkpoint. The onset of anaphase is triggered by activation of the anaphase-promoting complex/cyclosome (APC/C), which degrades cyclin B and securin. SAC generates an inhibitory signal to block APC/C in the presence of unaligned chromosomes and stalls for time to establish biorientation. Mouse models have been generated with manipulation of the genes encoding SAC proteins. Complete loss of SAC proteins, including Mad2, Bub1, BubR1, Bub3, and Rae1, caused early embryonic lethality (Baker et al., 2004; Baker et al., 2006; Dobles et al., 2000; Jeganathan et al., 2007; Wang et al., 2004). These gene knockout studies revealed the essential nature of mammalian mitotic checkpoint proteins for viability. Intriguingly BubR1-insufficient (*Bub 1b*$^{H/H}$) mice, in which the levels of BubR1 are about 10% those in normal animals, develop progressive aneuploidy along with a variety of progeroid features, including short lifespan, cachectic dwarfism, lordokyphosis, cataracts, loss of subcutaneous fat, and impaired wound healing (Baker et al., 2004). Consistent with the features of premature aging of *Bub 1b*$^{H/H}$ mice, mouse embryonic fibroblasts derived from *Bub 1b*$^{H/H}$ mice show rapid senescence. Both premature aging and cellular senescence observed in *Bub 1b*$^{H/H}$ mice are attenuated by inactivation of p16, a tumor suppressor and an effector of senescence (Baker et al., 2008). In humans, biallelic mutations in *BUB1B* encoding BubR1 cause mosaic variegated aneuploidy (MVA) (Hanks et al., 2004). MVA is a rare recessive condition characterized by constitutional mosaic aneuploidy, growth retardation, microcephaly, and predisposition to cancers such as rhabdomyosarcoma, Wilms tumor, and leukemia. Although aneuploidy and cataracts are common features detected in both *Bub 1b*$^{H/H}$ mice and individuals with MVA, MVA patients do not have typical features of premature aging. The difference in phenotype between *Bub 1b*$^{H/H}$ mice and individuals with MVA may be explained by the degree of BubR1 defects. A recent study indicated that mutations in *CEP57* also cause MVA (Snape et al., 2011). CEP57 is a centrosomal protein and is involved in nucleating and stabilizing microtubules. This suggests that *BUB1B* mutations underlie only a proportion of MVA, and other genes involved in regulating chromosome segregation may cause the disease. Bub3/Rae1-haploinsufficient mice have been reported to display an array of early aging-associated phenotypes (Baker et al., 2006) and Bub1 suppression in human fibroblasts activates a p53-dependent premature senescence response (Gjoerup et al., 2007). These studies involving the manipulation of SAC genes demonstrated that low levels of several SAC proteins play crucial roles in regulating commitment to the senescent state, although it remains to be determined how individual components of this checkpoint control cell viability and cell fate.

3.2 The roles of constitutively centromere-localized proteins in senescence

In contrast to SAC proteins, which localize to the kinetochore during mitosis, CENP-A localizes to the centromere throughout cell cycle and provides a structural and functional foundation for the kinetochore. I detail the role of CENP-A in senescence.

3.2.1 CENP-A has an impact on cell proliferation

Despite extensive studies of centromere-associated proteins, it remains unclear whether these proteins are involved in the control of cell proliferation; previous studies focused on the roles of centromere proteins in chromosome segregation, and were mainly conducted in immortalized cell lines, such as HeLa (Goshima et al., 2003). With regard to CENP-A, studies in a variety of organisms have indicated that the effects of CENP-A loss on proliferation vary widely according to the species, cell type, and methods used to delete or deplete CENP-A. *Cenpa* null mice fail to survive (Howman et al., 2000). Disruption of CID by antibody injection into *Drosophila* embryos and RNAi in cells in tissue culture exhibits a range of phenotypes affecting both cell cycle progression and mitotic chromosome segregation (Blower & Karpen, 2001). CENP-A-depleted chicken DT40 cells exhibit defects in kinetochore function and stop proliferating, although the apparent cessation of cell proliferation is caused by extensive cell death and the cells are still cycling (Régnier et al., 2005). CENP-A-depleted HeLa cells proliferate but exhibit misalignment and lagging of chromosomes during mitosis (Goshima et al., 2003). In HeLa cells, two tumor suppressor molecules, p53 and retinoblastoma protein (Rb), which have been shown to play crucial roles in cell cycle arrest in primary human cells, are inactivated due to the integration of the human papillomavirus that leads to their immortalization. Although it is essential to use primary human cells to uncover the regulatory roles of centromere proteins in cell proliferation, no such studies have yet been reported. To address whether CENP-A has an impact on cell proliferation, we examined the effects of CENP-A depletion in human primary somatic cells with functional p53 and Rb (Maehara et al., 2010). The reduction of CENP-A by retrovirally transducing CENP-A shRNA did not show growth arrest in HeLa cells, consistent with the previous results in CENP-A RNAi-mediated HeLa cells (Goshima et al., 2003). However, depletion of CENP-A in primary human TIG3 fibroblasts resulted in the immediate cessation of proliferation accompanied by increased levels of p16 and p21 expression, upregulated SAHF formation, and increased SA-β-gal activity, all of which are common markers of cellular senescence (Alcorta et al., 1996; Dimri et al., 1995; Hara et al., 1996; Narita et al., 2003; Zhang et al., 2005). Inactivation of p53 in CENP-A-depleted TIG3 cells restores proliferation leading to an increase in number of cells exhibiting aberrant chromosome behavior. These results indicate that the reduction of CENP-A drives normal human diploid fibroblasts into a senescent state in a p53-dependent manner. The senescence that arises from CENP-A depletion may be a self-defense mechanism to suppress the otherwise catastrophic impact upon genome integrity that would arise from kinetochore dysfunction following certain types of stress. It should be noted that reduction of CENP-A does not result in irreversible growth arrest in human pluripotent stem cells (Ambartsumyan et al., 2010). Ambartsumyan et al. demonstrated that CENP-A-depleted undifferentiated human pluripotent stem cells were capable of maintaining a functional centromere marks and showed no changes in morphology or proliferation rate relative to control cells, whereas CENP-A-depleted BJ fibroblasts showed arrest in G2/M and underwent apoptosis. Although the pluripotent state may cause the different phenotypes in response to CENP-A depletion, CENP-A has an impact on cell proliferation in human primary somatic cells.

3.2.2 CENP-A is downregulated in senescent human cells

Model systems with manipulation of gene expression/deletion have clearly revealed that some centromere/kinetochore-associated proteins play crucial roles in regulating commitment to the senescent state. However, the mechanisms of senescence and individual aging are presumed to be complex. To gain insights into the mechanisms that control lifespan and age-related phenotypes, Ly et al. examined mRNA abundance of more than

6000 known genes in dermal fibroblasts derived from elderly human subjects and from those with Hutchinson–Gilford Progeria Syndrome (HGPS), a rare genetic disorder characterized by accelerated aging (Ly et al., 2000). They found that genes involved in cell cycle progression, spindle assembly, and chromosome segregation, such as cyclins A, B, polo kinase, CENP-A, CENP-F, and kinesin-related proteins, were downregulated in elderly individuals and those with HGPS. We showed that CENP-A mRNA expression was reduced in both replicative and *ras*-induced senescent human TIG3 cells (Maehara et al., 2010). Another group reported a reduction in the levels of CENP-A transcripts in senescent human IMR90 fibroblasts (Narita et al., 2006). Therefore, the reduction of CENP-A mRNA levels appears to be a common feature of cellular senescence and individual aging. However, this reduction is not specific to senescence; we observed a marked reduction of CENP-A mRNA level in quiescent cells that had transiently exited from the cell cycle (Maehara et al., 2010). As CENP-A transcription is regulated by the cell cycle and occurs in G2 phase in human cells (Shelby et al., 1997), the transcription of CENP-A ceases immediately when cells are arrested regardless of whether the arrest is promoted by senescence or quiescence, even though reduction in CENP-A transcript level shows a strong association with the reduced proliferation potential of senescent cells.

In contrast to the levels of CENP-A transcript, which are reduced in both senescent and quiescent cells, CENP-A protein levels are markedly reduced in senescent cells, while quiescent cells retain similar levels of CENP-A protein to their actively growing counterparts (Maehara et al., 2010). These observations suggest that both transcriptional and posttranslational regulation are involved in the senescence-associated reduction of CENP-A protein level. CENP-A protein may be degraded via the ubiquitin - proteasome-dependent pathway in these cells. A previous study demonstrated that cullin-4A, human ring finger protein 2, and hypothetical protein FLJ23109, which have been reported or assumed to possess ubiquitin ligase activity, were coimmunoprecipitated with anti-CENP-A antibody from HeLa interphase nuclear extract (Obuse et al., 2004a). It is noteworthy that CENP-A also undergoes destruction when human cells are infected with herpes simplex virus type 1 protein ICP0 (Lomonte et al., 2001). Ubiquitin-dependent proteolysis of the yeast Cse4/CENP-A incorporated at non-centromeric regions has been reported (Collins et al., 2004). In addition to CENP-A, linker histone H1 protein level is decreased in senescent human WI38 cells, presumably because of posttranslational regulation (Funayama et al., 2006). A mitotic exit network kinase, WARTS/LATS1, was also reported to be reduced in senescent human cells (Takahashi et al., 2006). The reduction of this kinase was attenuated by addition of MG132. These results imply the presence of a senescence-associated proteolysis pathway in primary human cells. The senescence-associated proteolysis pathway may contribute to maintenance of metabolism and biosynthesis in senescent cells by recycling proteins that are no longer required for non-dividing cells and to ensure irreversible growth arrest by destruction of proteins essential for proliferation. Although the molecular mechanism of CENP-A reduction remains to be clarified, reduced levels of CENP-A protein seem to be common to cellular senescence and individual aging.

3.2.3 CENP-A reduction enhances centromeric heterochromatin formation

In our exploration of senescence-associated alterations in nuclear structure using primary human cells, we found that CENP-A levels were markedly reduced in senescent cells. In contrast to CENP-A, the levels of the other centromere proteins, CENP-B and hMis12, increased gradually, as the cells became senescent (Maehara et al., 2010). In addition, increased HP1 proteins, which are essential components of the pericentric heterochromatin region, were enriched on centromeres alongside CENP-B. These changes in the levels of centromere proteins alter the centromere chromatin structure, and are thought to represent physiologically significant phenomena associated with cellular senescence. Forced reduction of CENP-A alters the distributions of CENP-B and HP1 proteins, which are similar to those observed in replicative and *ras*-induced senescent cells, suggesting that this centromere alteration is triggered, at least in part, by the reduction of CENP-A protein level. Recent studies have demonstrated the remarkable role of CENP-B in heterochromatin formation in the centromere. In fission yeast, the disruption of CENP-B homologs, Abp1 and Cbh1, causes a reduction of Swi6, a homolog of HP1, at centromeric chromatin and a decrease in heterochromatin-specific modifications of histone H3 (Nakagawa et al., 2002). Using human artificial chromosomes (HAC) and alpha-satellite arrays integrated into chromosomal arms as models, Okada et al. demonstrated a dual role of CENP-B in CENP-A assembly and heterochromatin formation (Okada et al., 2007). Although CENP-B is required for de novo CENP-A assembly on HAC, CENP-B enhances histone H3K9 trimethylation and DNA methylation in chromosomally integrated alphoid DNA and suppresses centromere formation. Furthermore, Nakano et al. generated HAC containing both integrated alpha satellite and tet operator (tetO) sequences and tethered tet repressor (tetR) chromatin-modifying protein fusions to the HAC centromere (Nakano et al., 2008). Stimulation of the formation of a heterochromatin state by forced binding of silencers or targeted nucleation of HP1 resulted in the inactivation of a functional HAC centromere. Depletion of dimethylated histone H3K4 (H3K4me2) by tethering the lysine-specific demethylase 1 (LSD1) causes CENP-A loss from HAC kinetochores and ultimately results in inactivation of the kinetochore (Bergmann et al., 2011). These observations suggest that inactivation of the centromere occurs through epigenetic mechanisms. Thus, the loss of CENP-A and the extended heterochromatinization mediated by CENP-B and HP1 proteins on the centromere in senescent cells are assumed to promote centromere inactivation. During senescence, primary human cells alter their centromere states from a functional centromere, which is required for faithful segregation of chromosomes, to an inactivated centromere, which is likely to contribute to the establishment of the senescent state. Further qualitative and quantitative studies are needed to understand the structural and the functional changes that occur in the centromere during the senescence process.

3.2.4 How do primary human somatic cells sense centromere/kinetochore dysfunction and undergo senescence?

Forced depletion of CENP-A induces senescence-like phenotypes in the primary cells and CENP-A appears to be actively degraded in the senescent cells. This raises the question of whether CENP-A reduction is a cause or a consequence of cellular senescence. As cellular senescence is a complex trait, it is not possible to provide a clear answer to this question. There may be a positive feedback circuit between CENP-A degradation and induction of cellular senescence during senescence. I hypothesize that primary human somatic cells possess a mechanism for monitoring centromere/kinetochore integrity, which activates the p53-dependent senescence pathway in response to centromere/kinetochore defects, such as insufficient incorporation of CENP-A at the centromere (Fig. 3).

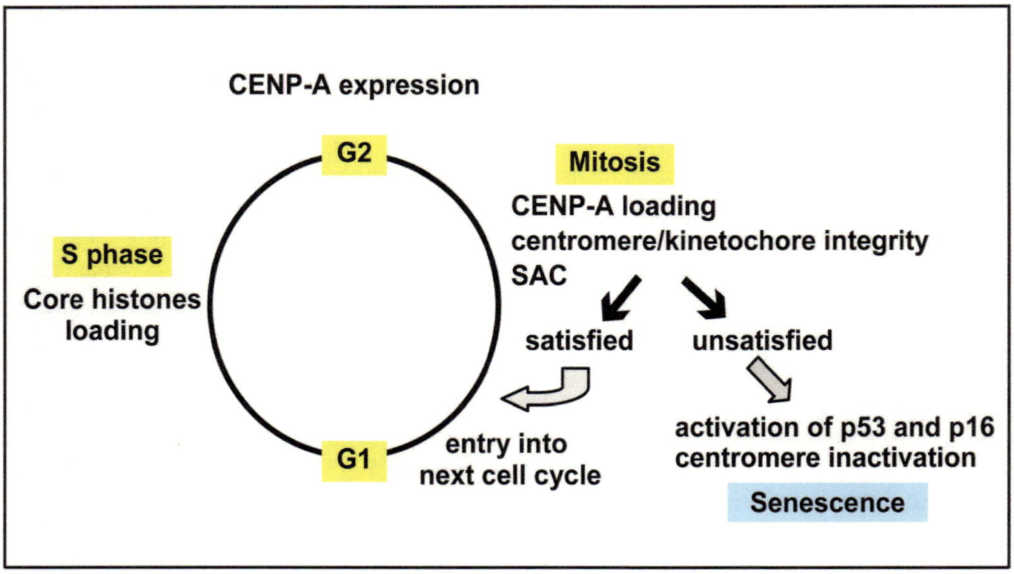

Fig. 3. A model of the roles of centromere/kinetochore proteins in senescence

How do the primary cells sense centromere/kinetochore dysfunction?

Telomere shortening triggers the DNA damage response (DDR), which is a major intrinsic factor to induce cellular senescence. Previous studies clearly demonstrated that p53 activation in oncogene-induced senescence is due to activation of the DDR (Bartkova et al., 2006; Di Micco et al., 2006; Mallette et al., 2007). We examined whether DDR plays a crucial role in activation of p53 in response to a reduction of CENP-A level. The presence of DNA damage foci (phosphorylated histone H2A.X, γ-H2AX), chk2 phosphorylated on threonine 68 and chk1 phosphorylated on serine 345, which are associated with DDR, were not detected in CENP-A-depleted-senescent cells (Maehara et al., 2010), suggesting that CENP-A depletion is not causally linked to DDR. Excess growth signals produced by oncogenes and telomere shortening seem to be sensed as DNA replication stresses, while CENP-A reduction is not. This may explain the unconventional type of senescence that does not require the activation of DNA damage signaling.

Unlike canonical core histones that are loaded into chromatin during DNA replication, newly synthesized CENP-A is incorporated into centromeric chromatin in telophase and early G1 phase (Fig. 3). Mis18 complex and HJURP/Smc3 have been implicated in the centromeric loading of CENP-A (Barnhart et al., 2011; Dunleavy et al., 2009; Foltz et al., 2009; Fujita et al., 2007; Hayashi et al, 2004). Primary cells may monitor CENP-A loading and centromere/kinetochore integrity during M and early G1 phases and immediately cease proliferation before entry into the next cell cycle in response to fatal centromere/kinetochore dysfunction under conditions in which some key centromere proteins and/or the SAC are not functioning properly. Under these conditions, senescence seems to not only prevent the cells from producing abnormal chromosomes, but also protects the organism from the potentially hazardous consequences of proliferation of cells harboring chromosomal abnormalities that arose as a consequence of defective mitosis.

4. Conclusion

Recent studies have revealed novel roles of centromere/kinetochore-associated proteins in the senescence program mainly using model systems in which target genes were manipulated. As highlighted in this chapter, while low levels of several centromere/kinetochore-associated proteins play crucial roles in regulating commitment to the senescent state, the interactions between centromere/kinetochore proteins and components of the senescence pathway remains to be determined. Further studies are required to determine the epigenetic mechanisms of centromere inactivation, particularly histone modification, and components involved in regulating the ratio of CENP-A to heterochromatin during senescence.

5. Acknowledgments

I thank Hiroshi Masumoto (Kazusa DNA Research Institute) for discussions concerning the centromere inactivation. I apologize to authors whose work could not be cited here due to space limitation. This work was supported by a Grant-in-Aid for Scientific Research (C) from the Japan Society for the Promotion of Science and Takeda Science Foundation.

6. References

Alcorta, D.A., Xiong, Y., Phelps, D., Hannon, G., Beach, D., & Barrett, J.C. (1996) Involvement of the cyclin-dependent kinase inhibitor p16 (INK4a) in replicative senescence of normal human fibroblasts. *Proc Natl Acad Sci U S A* Vol.93, No.24, (November 1996), pp. 13742-13747, ISSN 1091-6490

Ambartsumyan, G., Gill, R.K., Perez, S.D., Conway, D., Vincent, J., Dalal, Y., & Clark, A.T. (2010) Centromere protein A dynamics in human pluripotent stem cell self-renewal, differentiation and DNA damage. *Hum Mol Genet* Vol.19, No.20, (October 2010), pp. 3970-3982, ISSN 0964-6906

Baker, D.J., Jeganathan, K.B., Cameron, J.D., Thompson, M., Juneja, S., Kopecka, A., Kumar, R., Jenkins, R.B., de Groen, P.C., Roche, P., & van Deursen, J.M. (2004) BubR1 insufficiency causes early onset of aging-associated phenotypes and infertility in mice. *Nat Genet* Vol.36, No.7, (July 2004), pp. 744-749, ISSN 1061-4036

Baker, D.J., Jeganathan, K.B., Malureanu, L., Perez-Terzic, C., Terzic, A,, & van Deursen, J.M. (2006) Early aging-associated phenotypes in Bub3/Rae1 haploinsufficient mice. *J Cell Biol* Vol.172, No.4, (February 2006), pp. 529-540, ISSN 0021-9525

Baker, D.J., Perez-Terzic, C., Jin, F., Pitel, K., Niederländer, N.J., Jeganathan, K., Yamada, S., Reyes, S., Rowe, L., Hiddinga, H.J., Eberhardt, N.L., Terzic, A., & van Deursen, J.M. (2008) Opposing roles for p16Ink4a and p19Arf in senescence and ageing caused by BubR1 insufficiency. *Nat Cell Biol* Vol.10, No.7, (July 2008), pp. 825-836, ISSN 1465-7392

Barnhart, M.C., Kuich, P.H.J.L., Stellfox, M.S., Ward, J.A., Bassett, E.A., Black, B.E., & Foltz, D.R. (2011) HJURP is a CENP-A chromatin assembly factor sufficient to form a functional de novo kinetochore. *J Cell Biol* Vol.194, No.2, (July 2011), pp. 229-243, ISSN 0021-9525

Bartkova, J., Rezaei, N., Liontos, M., Karakaidos, P., Kletsas, D., Issaeva, N., Vassiliou, L.V., Kolettas, E., Niforou, K., Zoumpourlis, V.C., Takaoka, M., Nakagawa, H., Tort, F.,

Fugger, K., Johansson, F., Sehested, M., Andersen, C.L., Dyrskjot, L., Ørntoft, T., Lukas, J., Kittas, C., Helleday, T., Halazonetis, T.D., Bartek, J., & Gorgoulis, V.G. (2006) Oncogene-induced senescence is part of the tumorigenesis barrier imposed by DNA damage checkpoints. *Nature* Vol.444, No.7119, (November 2006), pp. 633-637, ISSN 0028-0836

Ben-Porath, I., & Weinberg, R.A. (2005) The signals and pathways activating cellular senescence. *Int J Biochem Cell Biol* Vol.37, No.5, (May 2005), pp. 961-976, ISSN 1357-2725

Bergmann, J.H., Rodríguez, M.G., Martins, N.M.C., Kimura, H., Kelly, D.A., Masumoto, H., Larionov, V., Lansen, L.E.T., & Earnshaw, W.C. (2011) Epigenetic engineering shows H3K4me2 is required for HJURP targeting and CENP-A assembly on a synthetic human kinetochore. *EMBO J* Vol.30, No.2, (January 2011), pp. 328-340, ISSN 0261-4189

Blower, M.D., & Karpen, G.H. (2001) The role of Drosophila CID in kinetochore formation, cell-cycle progression and heterochromatin interactions. *Nat Cell Biol* Vol.3, No.8, (August 2001), pp. 730-739, ISSN 1465-7392

Buchwitz, B.J., Ahmad, K., Moore, L.L., Roth, M.B., & Henikoff, S. (1999) A histone-H3-like protein in *C. elegans. Nature* Vol.401, No.6753, (October 1999), pp. 547-548, ISSN 0028-0836

Cheeseman, I.M., Chappie, J.S., Wilson-Kubalek, E.M., & Desai, A. (2006) The conserved KMN network constitutes the core microtubule-binding site of the kinetochore. *Cell* Vol.127, No.5, (December 2006), pp. 983-997, ISSN 0092-8674

Cleveland, D.W., Mao, Y., & Sullivan, K.F. (2003) Centromeres and kinetochores: from epigenetics to mitotic checkpoint signaling. *Cell* Vol.112, No.4, (February 2003), pp. 407-421, ISSN 0092-8674

Collado, M., Blasco, M.A., & Serrano, M. (2007) Cellular senescence in cancer and aging. *Cell* Vol.130, No.2, (July 2007), pp. 223-233, ISSN 0092-8674

Collins, K.A., Furuyama, S., & Biggins, S. (2004) Proteolysis contributes to the exclusive centromere localization of the yeast Cse4/CENP-A histone H3 variant. *Curr Biol* Vol.14, No.21, (November 2004), pp. 1968-1972, ISSN 0960-9822

Compton, D.A. (2011) Mechanisms of aneuploidy. *Curr Opin Cell Biol* Vol.23, No.1, (February 2011), pp. 109-113, ISSN 0955-0674

Deng, Y., Chan, S.S., & Chang, S. (2008) Telomere dysfunction and tumour suppression: the senescence connection. *Nat Rev Cancer* Vol.8, No.6, (June 2008), pp. 450-458, ISSN 1474-1768

Di Micco, R., Fumagalli, M., Cicalese, A., Piccinin, S., Gasparini, P., Luise, C., Schurra, C., Garré, M., Nuciforo, P.G., Bensimon, A., Maestro, R., Pelicci, P.G., & d'Adda di Fagagna, F. (2006) Oncogene-induced senescence is a DNA damage response triggered by DNA hyper-replication. *Nature* Vol.444, No.7119, (November 2006), pp. 638-642, ISSN 0028-0836

Dimri, G.P., Lee, X., Basile, G., Acosta, M., Scott, G., Roskelley, C., Medrano, E.E., Linskens, M., Rubelj, I., Pereira-Smith, O., Peacocke, M., & Campisi, J. (1995) A biomarker that identifies senescent human cells in culture and in aging skin in vivo. *Proc Natl Acad Sci U S A* Vol.92, No.20, (September 1995), pp. 9363-9367, ISSN 1091-6490

Dobles, M., Liberal, V., Scott, M.L., Benezra, R., & Sorger, P.K. (2000) Chromosome missegregation and apoptosis in mice lacking the mitotic checkpoint protein Mad2. *Cell* Vol.101, No.6, (June 2000), pp. 635-645, ISSN 0092-8674

Dunleavy, E.M., Roche, D., Tagami, H., Lacoste, N., Ray-Gallet, D., Nakamura, Y., Daigo, Y., Nakatani, Y., & Almouzni-Pettinotti, G. (2009) HJURP is a cell-cycle-dependent maintenance and deposition factor of CENP-A at centromeres. *Cell* Vol.137, No.3, (May 2009), pp. 485-497, ISSN 0092-8674

Earnshaw, W.C., & Rothfield, N. (1985) Identification of a family of human centromere proteins using autoimmune sera from patients with scleroderma. *Chromosoma* vol.91, No.3-4, (January 1985), pp. 313-321, ISSN 0009-5915

Earnshaw, W.C., Sullivan, K.F., Machlin, P.S., Cooke, C.A., Kaiser, D.A., Pollard, T.D., Rothfield, N.F., & Cleveland, D.W. (1987) Molecular cloning of cDNA for CENP-B, the major human centromere autoantigen. *J Cell Biol* Vol.104, No.4, (January 1987), pp. 817-829, ISSN 0021-9525

Foltz, D.R., Jansen, L.E.T., Black, B.E., Bailey, A.O., Yates, JR, 3rd, & Cleveland, D.W. (2006) The human CENP-A centromeric nucleosome-associated complex. *Nat Cell Biol* Vol.8, No.5, (May 2006), pp. 458-469, ISSN 1465-7392

Foltz, D.R., Jansen, L.E.T., Bailey, A.O., Yates, JR, 3rd, Bassett, E.A., Wood, S., Black, B.E., & Cleveland, D.W. (2009) Centromere-specific assembly of CENP-A nucleosomes is mediated by HJURP. *Cell* Vol.137, No.3, (May 2009), pp. 472-484, ISSN 0092-8674

Fujita, Y., Hayashi, T., Kiyomitsu, T., Toyoda, Y., Kokubo, A., Obuse, C., & Yanagida, M. (2007) Priming of centromere for CENP-A recruitment by human hMis18α, hMis18β, and M18BP1. *Dev Cell* Vol.12, No.1, (January 2007), pp. 17-30, ISSN 1534-5807

Funayama, R., Saito, M., Tanobe, H., & Ishikawa, F. (2006) Loss of linker histone H1 in cellular senescence. *J Cell Biol* Vol.175, No.6, (December 2006), pp. 869-880, ISSN 0021-9525

Gjoerup, O.V., Wu, J., Chandler-Militello, D., Williams, G.L., Zhao, J., Schaffhausen, B., Jat, P.S., & Roberts, T.M. (2007) Surveillance mechanism linking Bub1 loss to the p53 pathway. *Proc Natl Acad Sci U S A* Vol.104, No.20, (May 2007), pp. 8334-8339, ISSN 1091-6490

Goshima, G., Kiyomitsu, T., Yoda, K., & Yanagida, M. (2003) Human centromere chromatin protein hMis12, essential for equal segregation, is independent of CENP-A loading pathway. *J Cell Biol* Vol.160, No.1, (January 2003), pp. 25-39, ISSN 0021-9525

Hanks, S., Coleman, K., Reid, S., Plaja, A., Firth, H., FitzPatrick, D., Kidd, A., Méhes, K., Nash, R., Robin, N., Shannon, N, Tolmie, J., Swansbury, J., Irrthum, A., Douglas, J., & Rahman, N. (2004) Constitutional aneuploidy and cancer predisposition caused by biallelic mutations in *BUB1B*. *Nat Genet* Vol.36, No.11, (November 2004), pp. 1159-1161, ISSN 1061-4036

Hara, E., Smith, R., Parry, D., Tahara, H., Stone, S., & Peters, G. (1996) Regulation of p16CDKN2 expression and its implications for cell immortalization and senescence. *Mol Cell Biol* Vol.16, No.3, (March 1996), pp. 859-867, ISSN 0270-7306

Hayashi, T., Fujita, Y., Iwasaki, O., Adachi, Y., Takahashi, K., & Yanagida, M. (2004) Mis16 and Mis18 are required for CENP-A loading and histone deacetylation at centromeres. *Cell* Vol.118, No.6, (September 2004), pp. 715-729, ISSN 0092-8674

Hayflick, L., & Moorhead, P.S. (1961) The serial cultivation of human diploid cell strains. *Exp Cell Res* Vol.25, No.3, (December 1961), pp. 585-621, ISSN 0014-4827

Howman, E.V., Fowler, K.J., Newson, A.J., Redward, S., MacDonald, A.C., Kalitsis, P., & Choo, K.H.A. (2000) Early disruption of centromeric chromatin organization in centromere protein A (Cenpa) null mice. *Proc Natl Acad Sci U S A* Vol.97, No.3, (February 2000), pp. 1148-1153, ISSN 1091-6490

Hudson, D.F., Fowler, K.J., Earle, E., Saffery, R., Kalitsis, P., Trowell, H., Hill, J., Wreford, N.G., de Kretser, D.M., Cancilla, M.R., Howman, E., Hii, L., Cutts, S.M., Irvine, D.V., & Choo, K.H.A. (1998) Centromere protein B null mice are mitotically and meiotically normal but have lower body and testis weights. *J Cell Biol* Vol.141, No.2, (April 1998), pp. 309-319, ISSN 0021-9525

Izuta, H., Ikeno, M., Suzuki, N., Tomonaga, T., Nozaki, N., Obuse, C., Kisu, Y., Goshima, N., Nomura, F., Nomura, N., & Yoda, K. (2006) Comprehensive analysis of the ICEN (Interphase Centromere Complex) components enriched in the CENP-A chromatin of human cells. *Genes Cells* Vol.11, No.6, (June 2006), pp. 673-684, ISSN 1356-9597

Jeganathan, K., Malureanu, L., Baker, D.J., Abraham, S.C., & van Deursen, J.M. (2007) Bub1 mediates cell death in response to chromosome missegregation and acts to suppress spontaneous tumorigenesis. *J Cell Biol* Vol.179, No.2, (October 2007), pp. 255-267, ISSN 0021-9525

Kapoor, M., Montes, de Oca, Luna, R., Liu, G., Lozano, G., Cummings, C., Mancini, M., Ouspenski, I., Brinkley, B.R., May, G.S. (1998) The *cenpB* gene is not essential in mice. *Chromosoma* Vol.107, No.8, (December 1998), pp. 570-576, ISSN 0009-5915

Lomonte, P., Sullivan, K.F., & Everett, R.D. (2001) Degradation of nucleosome-associated centromeric histone H3-like protein CENP-A induced by herpes simplex virus type 1 protein ICP0. *J Biol Chem* Vol.276, No.8, (February 2001), pp. 5829-5835, ISSN 0021-9258

Ly, D.H., Lockhart, D.J., Lerner, R.A., & Schultz, P.G. (2000) Mitotic misregulation and human aging. *Science* Vol.287, No.5462, (March 2000), pp. 2486-2492, ISSN 0036-8075

Maehara, K., Takahashi, K., & Saitoh, S. (2010) CENP-A reduction induces a p53-dependent cellular senescence response to protect cells from executing defective mitoses. *Mol Cell Biol* Vol.30, No.9, (May 2010), pp. 2090-2104, ISSN 0270-7306

Maehara, K. (2011) Cellular senescence as a self-defense mechanism against centromere dysfunction. *Biomed Gerontol* Vol.35, No.1, (February 2011), pp. 17-23, ISSN 0912-8921

Mallette, F.A., Gaumont-Leclerc, M.F., & Ferbeyre, G. (2007) The DNA damage signaling pathway is a critical mediator of oncogene-induced senescence. *Genes Dev* Vol.21, No.1, (January 2007), pp. 43-48, ISSN 0890-9369

Marshall, O.J., Chueh, A.C., Wong, L.H., & Choo, K.H. (2008) Neocentromere: new insights into centromere structure, disease development, and karyotype evolution. *Am J Hum Genet* Vol.82, No.2, (February 2008), pp. 261-282, ISSN 0002-9297

Masumoto, H., Masukata, H., Muro, Y., Nozaki, N., & Okazaki, T. (1989) A human centromere antigen (CENP-B) interacts with a short specific sequence in alphoid DNA, a human centromeric satellite. *J Cell Biol* Vol.109, No.5, (November 1989), pp. 1963-1973, ISSN 0021-9525

Meluh, P.B., Yang, P., Glowczewski, L., Koshland, D., & Smith, M.M. (1998) Cse4p is a component of the core centromere of Saccharomyces cerevisiae. *Cell* Vol.94, No.5, (September 1998), pp. 607-613, ISSN 0092-8674

Musacchio, A., & Salmon, E.D. (2007) The spindle-assembly checkpoint in space and time. *Nat Rev Mol Cell Biol* Vol.8, No.5, (May 2007), pp. 379-393, ISSN 1471-0072

Nakagawa, H., Lee, J.K., Hurwitz, J., Allshire, R.C., Nakayama, J., Grewal, S.I., Tanaka, K., & Murakami, Y. (2002) Fission yeast CENP-B homologs nucleate centromeric heterochromatin by promoting heterochromatin-specific histone tail modifications. *Genes Dev* Vol.16, No.14, (July 2002), pp.1766-1778, ISSN 0890-9369

Nakano, M., Cardinale, S., Noskov, V.N., Gassmann, R., Vagnarelli, P., Kandels-Lewis, S., Larionov, V., Earnshaw, W.C., & Masumoto, H. (2008) Inactivation of a human kinetochore by specific targeting of chromatin modifiers. *Dev Cell* Vol.14, No.4, (April 2008), pp. 507-522, ISSN 1534-5807

Narita, M., Nuñez, S., Heard, E., Narita, M., Lin, A.W., Hearn, S.A., Spector, D.L., Hannon, G.J., & Lowe, S.W. (2003) Rb-mediated heterochromatin formation and silencing of E2F target genes during cellular senescence. *Cell* Vol.113, No.6, (June 2003), pp. 703-716, ISSN 0092-8674

Narita, M., Narita, M., Krizhanovsky, V., Nuñez, S., Chicas, A., Hearn, S.A., Myers, M.P., & Lowe, S.W. (2006) A novel role for High-Mobility Group A proteins in cellular senescence and heterochromatin formation. *Cell* Vol.126, No.3, (August 2006), pp. 503-514, ISSN 0092-8674

Obuse, C., Yang, H., Nozaki, N., Goto, S., Okazaki, T., & Yoda, K. (2004a) Proteomics analysis of the centromere complex from HeLa interphase cells: UV-damaged DNA binding protein 1 (DDB-1) is a component of the CEN-complex, while BMI-1 is transiently co-localized with the centromeric region in interphase. *Genes Cells* Vol.9, No.2, (February 2004), pp. 105-120, ISSN 1356-9597

Obuse, C., Iwasaki, O., Kiyomitsu, T., Goshima, G., Toyoda, Y., & Yanagida, M. (2004b) A conserved Mis12 centromere complex is linked to heterochromatic HP1 and outer kinetochore protein Zwint-1. *Nat Cell Biol* Vol.6, No.11, (November 2004), pp. 1135-1141, ISSN 1465-7392

Okada, M., Cheeseman, I.M., Hori, T., Okawa, K., McLeod, I.X., Yates, JR, 3rd, Desai, A., & Fukagawa, T. (2006) The CENP-H-I complex is required for the efficient incorporation of newly synthesized CENP-A into centromeres. *Nat Cell Biol* Vol.8, No.5, (May 2006), pp. 446-457, ISSN 1465-7392

Okada, T., Ohzeki, J., Nakano, M., Yoda, K., Brinkley, W.R., Larionov, V., & Masumoto, H. (2007) CENP-B controls centromere formation depending on the chromatin context. *Cell* Vol.131, No.7, (December 2007), pp. 1287-1300, ISSN 0092-8674

Palmer, D.K., O'Day, K., Wener, M.H., Andrews, B.S., & Margolis, R.L. (1987) A 17-kD centromere protein (CENP-A) copurifies with nucleosome core particles and with histones. *J Cell Biol* Vol.104, No.4, (January 1987), pp. 805-815, ISSN 0021-9525

Perez-Castro, A.V., Shamanski, F.L., Meneses, J.J., Lovato, T.L., Vogel, K.G., Moyzis, R.K., & Pedersen, R. (1998) Centromeric protein B null mice are viable with no apparent abnormalities. *Dev Biol* Vol.201, No.2, (September 1998), pp. 135-143, ISSN 0012-1606

Régnier, V., Vagnarelli, P., Fukagawa, T., Zerjal, T., Burns, E., Trouche, D., Earnshaw, W., & Brown, W. (2005) CENP-A is required for accurate chromosome segregation and sustained kinetochore association of BubR1. *Mol Cell Biol* Vol.25, No.10, (May 2005), pp. 3967-3981, ISSN 0270-7306

Ruchaud, S., Carmena, M., & Earnshaw, W.C. (2007) Chromosomal passengers: conducting cell division. *Nat Rev Mol Cell Biol* Vol.8, No.10, (October 2007), pp. 798-812, ISSN 1471-0072

Serrano, M., Lin, A.W., McCurrach, M.E., Beach, D., & Lowe, S.W. (1997) Oncogenic *ras* provokes premature cell senescence associated with accumulation of p53 and $p16^{INK4a}$. *Cell* Vol.88, No.5, (March 1997), pp. 593-602, ISSN 0092-8674

Shelby, R.D., Vafa, O., & Sullivan, K.F. (1997) Assembly of CENP-A into centromeric chromatin requires a cooperative array of nucleosomal DNA contact sites. *J Cell Biol* Vol.136, No.3, (February 1997), pp. 501-513, ISSN 0021-9525

Snape, K., Hanks, S., Ruark, E., Barros-Nuñez, P., Elliott, A., Murray, A., Lane, A.H., Shannon N., Callier, P., Chitayat, D., Clayton-Smith, J., FitzPatrick, D., Gisselsson, D., Jacquemont, S., Asakura-Hay, K., Micale, M.A., Tolmie, J., Turnpenny, P.D., Wright, M., Douglas, J., & Rahman, N. (2011) Mutations in *CEP57* cause mosaic variegated aneuploidy syndrome. *Nat Genet* Vol.43, No.6, (June 2011), pp. 527-529, ISSN 1061-4036

Stoler, S., Keith, K.C., Curnick, K.E., & Fitzgerald-Hayes, M. (1995) A mutation in CSE4, an essential gene encoding a novel chromatin-associated protein in yeast, causes chromosome nondisjunction and cell cycle arrest at mitosis. *Genes Dev* Vol.9, No.5, (March 1995), pp. 573-586, ISSN 0890-9369

Takahashi, A., Ohtani, N., Yamakoshi, K., Iida, S., Tahara, H., Nakayama, K., Nakayama, K.I., Ide, T., Saya, H., & Hara, E. (2006) Mitogenic signalling and the p16INK4a-Rb pathway cooperate to enforce irreversible cellular senescence. *Nat Cell Biol* Vol.8, No.11, (November 2006), pp. 1291-1297, ISSN 1465-7392

Takahashi, K., Chen, E.S., & Yanagida, M. (2000) Requirement of Mis6 centromere connector for localizing a CENP-A-like protein in fission yeast. *Science* Vol.288, No.5474, (June 2000), pp. 2215-2219, ISSN 0036-8075

Tanaka, T.U. (2010) Kinetochore-microtubule interactions: steps towards bi-orientation. *EMBO J* Vol.29, No.24, (December 2010), pp. 4070-4082, ISSN 0261-4189

Wang, Q., Liu, T., Fang, Y., Xie, S., Huang, X., Mahmood, R., Ramaswamy, G., Sakamoto, K.M., Darzynkiewicz, Z., Xu, M., & Dai, W. (2004) BUBR1 deficiency results in abnormal megakaryopoiesis. *Blood* Vol.103, No.4, (February 2004), pp. 1278-1285, ISSN 0006-4971

Zhang, R., Poustovoitov, M.V., Ye, X., Santos, H.A., Chen, W., Daganzo, S.M., Erzberger, J.P., Serebriiskii, I.G., Canutescu, A.A., Dunbrack, R.L., Pehrson, J.R., Berger, J.M., Kaufman, P.D., & Adams, P.D. (2005) Formation of MacroH2A-containing senescence-associated heterochromatin foci and senescence driven by ASF1a and HIRA. *Dev Cell* Vol.8, No.1, (January 2005), pp. 19-30, ISSN 1534-5807

26

The Functioning of "Aged" Heterochromatin

Teimuraz A. Lezhava, Tinatin A. Jokhadze and Jamlet R. Monaselidze
Department of Genetics, Iv.Javakhishvili Tbilisi State University, Tbilisi, Georgia

1. Introduction

1.1 Heterochromatin – Substratum of aging

The aging process is programmed in the genome of each organism and is manifested late in life. Any change in normal homeostasis, particularly any further loss of the cell function with aging, occurs in the functional units of the chromatin domains.

Modification of the chromatin structure and function by hetero- or deheterochromatinization occurs throughout life and plays a pivotal role in the irreversible process in aging by affecting gene expression, replication, recombination, mutation, repair, and programming (Gilson and Magdinier, 2009; Elcock and Bridger, 2010). Among chromatin modifications, methylation and acetilation of lysine residues in histones H3 and H4 are critical to the regulation of chromatin structure and gene expression. Compacted heterochromatin regions are generally hypoacetylated and methylated in a discrete combination of lysine methylated marks such as H3K9me2 and 3 (its recognition by specific structural proteins such as HP1 is required for heterochromatin assembly and spreading) and H4K20me1 (Trojer and Reinberg, 2007; Vaquero, 2009). Hypermethylation may cause heterochromatinization and thus would result in gene silencing (Mazin, 1994, 2009). It was found that HP1 is associated with transcripts of more than one hundred euchromatic genes. All these proteins are in fact involved both in RNA transcript processing and in heterochromatin formation. Loss of HP1 proteins causes chromosome segregation defects and lethality in some organisms; a reduction in levels of HP1 family members is associated with cancer progression in humans (Dialynas et al., 2008). This suggests that, in general, similar epigenetic mechanisms have a significant role on both RNA and heterochromatin metabolisms (Piacentini et al., 2009).

Current evidence suggests that SirT1-7 (NAD-dependent deacetylase activity proteins), now called "sirtuins," have been emerging as a critical epigenetic regulator for aging (Imai, 2009). The first event, arrival of and SirT1 at chromatin, results in deacetylation of H4K 16 and H3K9Ac, and direct recruitment of the linker histone H1, in the formation of heterochromatin, a key factor in the formation of the 30 nm fiber (Vaquero, 2004; Michishita *et al.*, 2005). The fact that such histones modifications are reversible (Dialynas *et al.*, 2008; Kouzarides, 2007) offers the potential for therapy (Dialynas *et al.*, 2008). The first level of chromatin organization, the 10 nm fiber, corresponds to a nucleosome array. This fiber is accessible to the transcriptional machinery and is associated with transcriptionally active regions, which are also known as active chromatin or euchromatin (Trojer and Reinberg, 2007).

Heterochromatin is divided into two main forms according to their distinct structural functional dynamics: constitutive heterochromatin (CH) and facultative heterochromatin (FH). CH refers to the regions that are always maintained as heterochromatin; these span large portions of the chromosome and have a structural role. CH regions contain few genes and are located primarily in pericentromeric regions and telomeres. FH refers to those regions that can be formed as heterochromatin in a certain situation but can revert to euchromatin once required. FH can span from a few kilobases to a whole chromosome and generally includes regions with a high density of genes. SirT1 contains both forms of heterochromatin (Prokofieva-Belgobskaya, 1986; Vaquero, 2004, 2009). Heterochromatin composed of distinct life-important functional domains, includes: 1. constitutive heterochromatin, almost entirely composed of non-coding sequences (satellite DNA) that are mostly localized at or are adjacent to the centromeric and telomeric regions; 2. NOR-satellite stalk heterochromatin reflecting the activity of synthetic processes (Ag-positive - coding chromatin and Ag-negative – non-coding chromatin) and 3. facultative heterochromatin (heterochromatinization - condensed euchromatic regions) that mainly consist of "closed" transcribe genes.

According to this view, we discuss of the levels of: 1) total heterochromatin; 2) constitutive (structural) heterochromatin; 3) nucleolus organizer regions (NORs) heterochromatin and 4) facultative heterochromatin in lymphocytes cultured from individuals at the age of 80 and over.

2. Facultative heterochromatin (condensation of eu- and heterochromatin regions)

We have used differential scanning microcalorimetry to produce a calorimetric curve in cultured human lymphocytes over the temperature range 38–130°C. It was determined that the clearly expressed shoulder of the heat absorption curve in the temperature interval from 40°C to 50°C with Tm(I)=45+1°C corresponds to melting of membranes and some cytoplasm proteins, maxima at Tm(II)=55+1°C correspond to melting (denaturation) of non-histone nuclei proteins, maxima at Tm(IV)70+1°C corresponds to the ribonucleoprotein complex, and maxima at Tm(III)=63+1°C and Tm(V)=83+1°C correspond to cytoplasm proteins. Other clearly expressed peaks at Tm(VI)=96+1°C and Tm(VII)=104+1°C correspond to the chromatin denaturation (Monaselidz et al.,2006,2008). The heating process produced clear and reproducible endothermic heat absorption peaks. We found that an endothermic peak at T_m=104±1°C corresponds to melting of 30 nm-thick fibers, which represents the most condensed state of chromatin in interphase nuclei (heterochromatin), and that an endothermic peak at 96±1°C corresponds to melting of 11 nm-thick filaments.

The chromatin heat absorption peaks VI and VII changed significantly with age. In particular, in the shifted endotherms VI and VII, the temperatures increased by 2°C and 3°C accordingly in old age (80-86 years). Additional condensation of the eu- and heterochromatin was demonstrated by an increase in T_m by 2°C and 3°C in comparison with the meddle age (25-40 years) (Fig.1). These prominent changes in chromatin stability indicated transformation of eu- and heterochromatin in condensed chromatin (heterochromatinization).

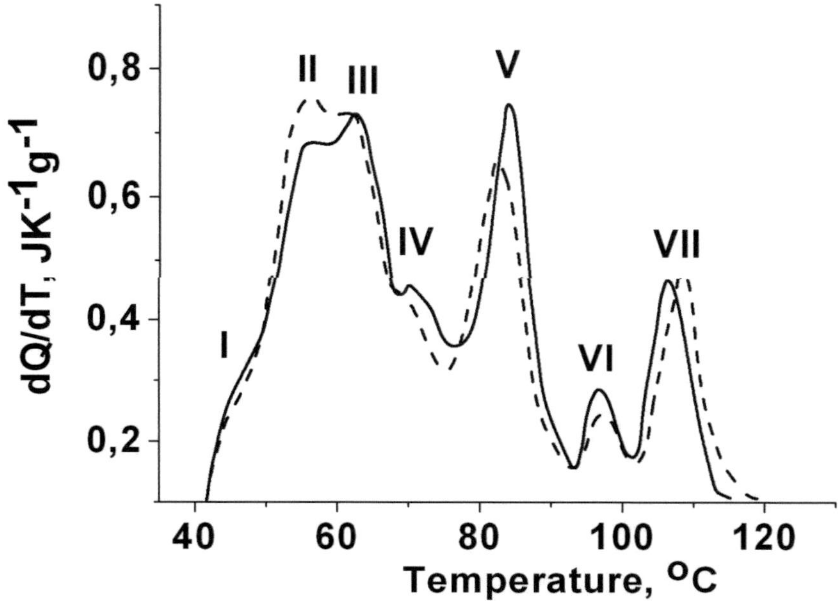

Fig. 1. The excess of heat capacity (ΔC_p=dQ/dT) as function of temperature for lymphocytes cultures from young donors (------) and old donors (— —) (48 -hour cell culture), dry biomass (------) - 8.5 mg and 87 µg DNA, dry biomass (— —) 8.8mg and 90 µg DNA

One of the potential epigenetic mechanisms is heterochromatinization of chromatin within the region of the genome containing a gene sequence, which inhibits any further molecular interactions with that underlying gene sequence and effectively inactivates that gene (Ellen *et al.,* 2009). The chromatin peak behavior described above shows progressive heterochromatinization of lymphocyte chromosomes from old individuals and confirms previously reported data (Lezhava, 1984, 2001, 2006; Vaquero, 2004).

These significant changes in chromatin stability in old age indicate that the aging process involves transformation of the eu- and heterochromatin into condensed forms and that further compaction or progressive heterochromatinization occurs during aging.

3. Constitutive heterochromatin (pericentromeric and telomeric heterochromatin)

Centromeric and telomeric heterochromatin differs from each other by structure and sensitivity to exogenous factors. Centromeric heterochromatin showed increased H3-K27 trimethilation in the absence of SUV39h1 and Suv39h2HMTases. Such modification was not detectable at telomeric heterochromatin. Despite the differences between the two heterochromatin domains and the distinction of functions, they have much in common (Blasco, 2004; Lam *et al.,* 2006).

3.1 Pericentromeric heterochromatin

The heterochromatin regions of human chromosomes near the centromere vary and the degree of variability is related to the amount and molecular organization of DNA, which contains only a fraction of satellite DNA. The amount and function of heterochromatin regions have a close relationship with the organization and functioning of the entire genome.

Satellite DNA (tandemly repeated noncoding DNA sequences) stretch over almost all native centromeres and surrounding pericentromeric heterochromatin. Satellite DNA was considered to be an inert by-product of genome dynamics in heterochromatic regions. However, recent studies have shown that the evolution of satellite DNA involved an interplay of stochastic events and selective pressure. This points to the functional significance of satellite sequences, which in (peri) centromeres may play some fundamental roles. First, specific interactions between satellite sequences and DNA-binding proteins are proposed to complement sequence-independent epigenetic processes. Second, transcripts of satellite DNA sequences initialize heterochromatin formation through an RNAi mechanism. In addition, satellite DNAs in (peri)centromeric regions affect chromosomal dynamics and genome plasticity (Mehta *et al.*, 2007; Plohl *et al.*, 2008). Satellite DNA is localized in human (peri) centromeres heterochromatin chromosomes 1,9, 16 and Y.

The data on comparative of (peri) centromeric heterochromatin (C-segment) were provided for all three chromosome pairs (1, 9 and 16) indicating that the variants of large C-segments (d and e) were registered more often in old individuals than in the cells of the younger ones: for chromosome 1 – X^2_4 =21.9, ($p<0.001$); for chromosome 9 – X^2_4 =10,6 ($p<0.001$); for chromosome 16 – X^2_4 =18.7, ($p<0.001$). The increased size of the C-segments were also found in the Y- chromosomes of the family : the father and the grandfather (59 and 88 years, respectively), compared with the 30 year old son (Lezhava, 2006).

Thus, the (peri) centromeric heterochromatin on three chromosome pairs (1, 9 and 16) and the C-segments of the Y chromosome increase in size in old age, pointing to the heterochromatinization of these heterochromatin regions of chromosomes.

In some cases, without pretreatment metaphases from old individuals, blocks of centromeric heterochromatin were common on homologous chromosomes 1qh C-band locations were similar to those seen after an alkaline or thermal pretreatment or staining with buffered Giemsa.

In a percentage without pretreatment of metaphases, the heterochromatin-positive 1qh chromosomes displayed some packing impairment. Sizes and distribution of centromeric heterochromatin on the 1qh homologous varied in some metaphases of 6 from 24 individuals aged 81 to 114 years and was absents in control group ranging in age from 13 to 34 years.

Of interest was a sample from a 114-year-old man whose 1qh showed dark-stained heterochromatin sites sized 1.5-fold greater than counterpart sites in other individuals samples. However, intrahomologous variability was often related to sizes and the absents of heterochromatin blocks in one of the homologous chromosome 1 (Fig.2).

The control of cellular senescence by specific human chromosomes was examined in interspecies cell hybrids between diploid human fibroblasts and an immortal, Syrian hamster cell line. Most such hybrids exhibited a limited life span comparable to that of the human fibroblasts, indicating that cellular senescence is dominant in these hybrids. Karyotypic analyses of the hybrid clones that did not senesce revealed that all these clones had lost both copies of human chromosome 1, whereas all other human chromosomes were observed in at least some of the immortal hybrids. The application of selective pressure for retention of human chromosome 1 to the cell hybrids resulted in an increased percentage of hybrids that senesced. Further, the introduction of a single copy of human chromosome 1 to the hamster cells by microcell fusion caused typical signs of cellular senescence. These findings indicate that human chromosome 1 may participate in the control of cellular senescence and further support a genetic basis for cellular senescence (Sugawara et al., 1990).

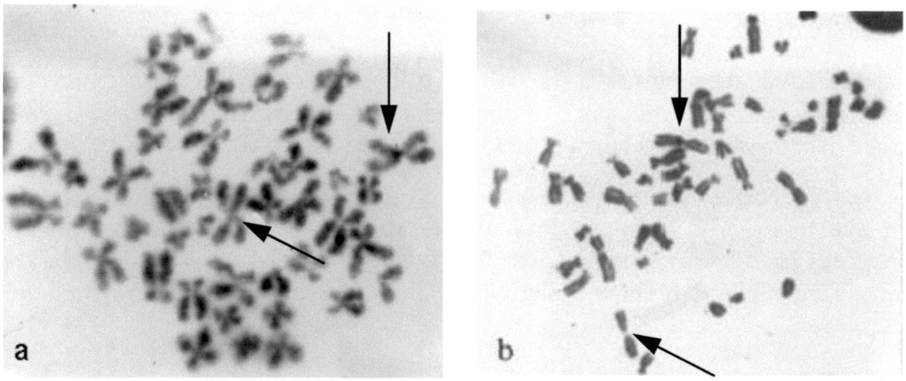

Fig. 2. Distribution of C-bands on one of the homologous of the 1qh chromosomes without preparation pretreatment and unbuffered Unna blue staining. Metaphases: from 114-year-old man (a) and from 83-year-old man (b). Arrows indicate: homologous chromosomes 1 with and without bands

3.2 Telomeric heterochromatin

Telomeres are specialized DNA-protein structures that form loops at the ends of chromosomes (Boukamp et al., 2005). In human cells they contain short DNA repeat sequences $(TTAGGG)_n$ added to the ends of chromosomes by telomerase. Telomere heterochromatin in most human somatic cells loses 50–200 bp per cell division (lansdorp, 2000; Geserick and Blasco, 2006). Telomeres serve multiple functions, including the protection of chromosome ends and prevention of chromosome fusions. They are essential for maintaining individuality and genome stability (Lo *et al.*, 2002; Murnane, 2006). A major mechanism of cellular senescence involves telomere shortening (Horikawa and Barrett, 2003; Opresko et al., 2005), which is directly associated with many DNA damage-response proteins that induce a response similar to that observed with DNA breaks (Bradshow et al., 2005; Wright and Shay, 2005).

Terminal telomere structures consist of tandemly repeated DNA sequences, which vary in length from 5 to 15 kb in humans. Several proteins are attached to this telomeric DNA, including PARP-1, Ku70/80, DNA-PKcs, Mre11, XRCC4, ATM, NBS and BLM, some of which are also involved in different DNA damage response (repair) pathways. Mutations in the genes coding for these proteins cause a number of rare genetic syndromes characterized by chromosome and/or genetic instability and cancer predisposition (Callen and Surralles, 2004; Hande, 2004; Bradshow et al., 2005).

Based on the presented data, we concluded that telomeric chromatin undergoes progressive heterochromatinization (condensation) with aging that determines: (a) inactivation of the gene coding for the catalytic subunit of telomerase, hTERT; and (b) switching off the genes for Ku80, Mre11, NBS, BLM, etc causing chromosome disorders related to chromosome syndromes. Telomere shortening is another consequence of age-related.

Heterochromatinization that is reportedly due to unrepaired single-strand breaks of DNA in telomere regions resulting in unequal interchromatid and interchromosome exchanges and inactivation of the telomerase-coding gene-determining telomere length (Golubev,2001; Gonzalo et al., 2006).

Our experimental data showed that the number of cell with end-to-and telomere associations and the total frequency of aberrant telomeres were considerably increased at the old age in comparison with those at middle age (lezhava,2006).

The higher frequency of chromosome end-to-and telomere associations in extreme old age may be due to the loss of heterochromatin telomere regions (Fig.3). Mouse embryonic fibroblast cells lacking Suv39h1 and Suv39h2 exhibit reduced levels of H3K9me and HP1 (deheterochromatinization).These alterations in chromatin correlate with telomere elongation (Garcia-Cao et al., 2004).

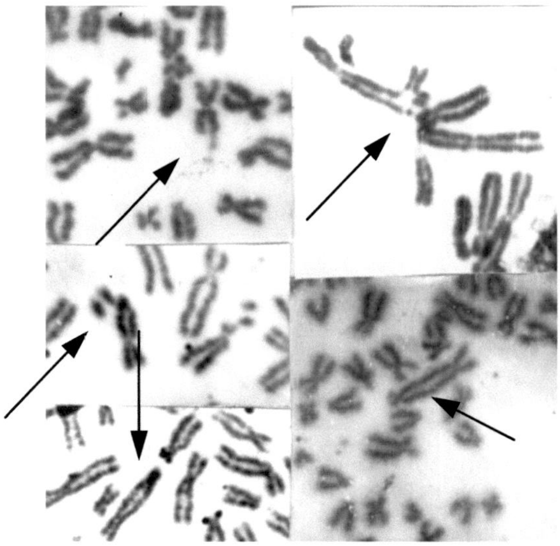

Fig. 3. Telomeres aberrations and end-to-end associations of chromosomes from elderly are shown by arrows.

According to previous publications (Prokofieva-Belgovskaya, 1986; Hawley and Arbe, 1993) sister chromosome exchanges (SCEs) do not occur or are less frequent in heterochromatin or heterochromatinized regions. The evaluation of SCE in individuals aged 80 years and more has revealed that single-cell SCE counts appear to be lower than in middle age (lezhava, 2006), that is, exchanges between sister chromatids mostly take place in euchromatic regions.

In old age, $CoCl_2$ alone and in combination with the tetrapeptide bioregulator Livagen enhanced the distribution of SCE; that is, pericentromeric heterochromatin appeared to be more sensitive to the $CoCl_2$ effect alone (15.4 ± 1.8% SCE), whereas SCE was mostly observed in telomere heterochromatin when $CoCl_2$ in combination with livagen was used (12 ± 1.2% SCE) (control, 2.8 ± 0.5% SCE, respectively).Because exchanges occur in euchromatic uncondensated regions, the obvious effect of $CoCl_2$ alone and in combination with Livagen could be attributed to its decondensing deheterochromatinization effect on pericentromeric and telomeric heterochromatin, which would elevate the possibility of SCE ((lezhava and Jokhadze, 2007). At the same time, the deheterochromatinization of telomeric heterochromatin contributes to activation of DNA repair. That is, the intensity of unscheduled DNA synthesis increases (lezhava and Jokhadze, 2004) and creates a basis for activation of inactivated genes during aging and development of diseases.

4. Nucleolus Organizer Regions (NOR) heterochromatin

The heterochromatic regions of secondary constrictions (NORs) in human D (13, 14, 15) and G (21, 22) group acrocentric chromosomes contain genes coding for 18S and 28 ribosomal RNA. It has been established that genetically active NORs can appear with nucleolar form of DNA-dependent RNA-polymerase and selectively stain with silver (Ag-stained). It has also been found that association between Ag-stained satellite stalks of acrocentric chromosomes in metaphase cells (Fig.4) are determined primarily by their function as nucleolar organizers.

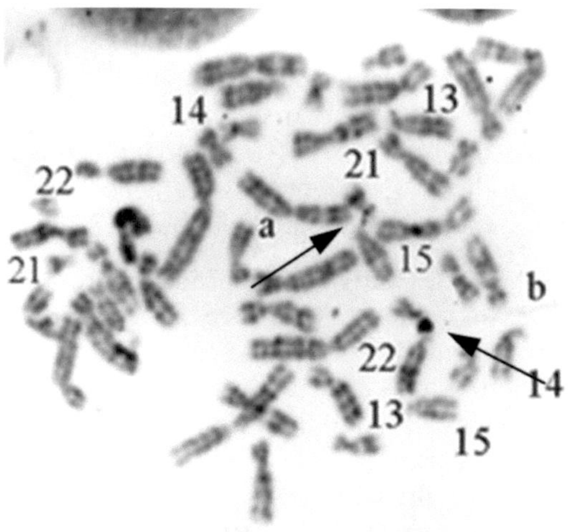

Fig. 4. Metaphases with variable sizes of Ag-positive nucleolar organizer regions. Arrows indicate a - "open" satellite stalks association; b - "closed" satellite stalks association.

The acrocentric association phenomenon may induce acrocentric nondisjunction during the meiosis or early zygote division, and chromosome rearrangements. Chromosomes can associate when two chromatid satellites are available, and so they are defined as associated, when their satellites make up a pair. Therefore, prematurely condensed silver-stained acrocentrics have similar rates of interphase and metaphase association. It was shown (Lezhava,1984; Verma and Rodriguez, 1985) that the likelihood of acrocentric chromosome associations is related to an extent of satellite stalk heterochromatinization.

Heterochromatinization of stalks - NORs has been studied by association frequencies in lymphocytes. In humans of a very old age (80–93 years), the estimated number of Ag-positive nucleolus organizer regions (NORs) for all chromosomes per cell, both associated and nonassociated, was significantly lower (6.10 in individuals 80–93 years old) in comparison with that in young individuals (7.05; $p < 0.01$). The frequency of acrocentric chromatid association in individuals aged 80 years and over was significantly decreased in comparison with those in a control group.

Increase of associations frequency was parallel to the growth of Ag segment size. At the same time, chromosomes containing NORs of grade 2 frequently formed associations among the middle-aged individuals, rather than in the older group.

Moreover, the transcriptional activity of ribosomal cistrons, which determine activity of a nucleolar form of DNA-dependent RNA polymerase - were from 668–721 imp/min in old individuals. They were significantly decreased in comparison with the control: from 1020 to 1120 imp/min.

The above considerations imply that a decreased number of chromosomes with Ag-positive NORs, a lower frequency of association of acrocentric chromatids, and a decrease in endogenic RNA-polymerase activity of ribosomal cistrons, result in alterations in the length of chromosomal satellite stalks that is caused by heterochromatinization in the process of aging (Lezhava and Dvalishvili,1992).

4.1 Cis- and trans-types of chromatid association

Most of acrocentric chromosome associations (85 percent) are formed by single chromatid satellite stalks (Lezhava et al., 1972; Verma et al., 1983). The exposure of lymphocyte cultures to 5-bromodeoxyuridine (BrDU) during two replication cycles revealed two-acrocentric associations that were either at a cis-position (differentially stained acrocentric chromatids with a dark-to-dark or light-to-light association) or a trans-position (chromatids with a dark-to-light or light-to-dark association) (Chemitiganti et al., 1984).

Frequencies of the cis- and trans-orientation of acrocentric chromatid association have been studied in old individuals. Lymphocyte cultures were prepared with a conventional methodology. The study examined 173 metaphases from 9 individuals aged 80 to 89 years and 124 metaphases from 6 individuals aged 20 to 48 years. For differential staining of sister chromatids BrDU (7.7 μg/ml) was added to the cultures immediately on their initiation. The lymphocytes were incubated in darkness for 96 h at 37°C. Giemsa stain was employed after DNA thymine was substituted by BrDU. In DNA thymine was totally substituted in one of second-mitosis sister chromatids which stained light and was denoted chromatid 1; only half of DNA thymine was substituted in the other chromatid which stained dark and was defined as chromatid 2 (Fig. 5). According to association criteria of cis-1 position was the term adopted for the light-to-light association, cis-2 position for the dark-to-dark association, and trans-position for the light-to-dark association (Fig. 5).

Statistical analysis of association frequencies proceeded from the assumption that the cis-1 and cis-2 associations have similar chances to occur, and the chances make half of the probability of the trans-oriented association, that is

$$P_{\text{cis-1}}(DD) = P_{\text{cis-2}}(DD) = 1/2\, P_{\text{trans}}(DD) \qquad (1)$$

$$P_{\text{cis-1}}(GG) = P_{\text{cis-2}}(GG) = 1/2\, P_{\text{trans}}(GG) \qquad (2)$$

$$P_{\text{cis-1}}(DG) = P_{\text{cis-2}}(DG) = 1/2\, P_{\text{trans}}(DG) \qquad (3)$$

These equalities represent the hypothesis that chromatids-1 and chromatids-2 participated in the association with the same probability.

The data of the middle-aged group fitted the hypotheses (2) and (3). The statistics

$$X^2(GG) = \frac{\left(V_{cis-1}(GG) - V(GG)/4\right)^2}{(1/4)V(GG)} + \frac{\left(V_{cis-2}(GG)) - V(GG)/4\right)^2}{(1/4)V(GG)} + \frac{(V_{trans}GG) - V\left(GG/2\right)^2}{(1/2)V(GG)}$$

should be almost $X^2(2)$-distributed if (3) is true; they yielded the value of 0.69. Similar statistics X^2(DG) for testing (3) gave the value of 1.54. Equalities (1) proved less supportive: the verifying statistics X^2(DD) gave 5.14 while the presumptive value was 0.08.

A different pattern was seen in the old individuals group. While the data fitted equalities (2), (1) and (3) had to be rejected since the statistics were X^2(DD) = 5.76 and X^2(DG) = 18.

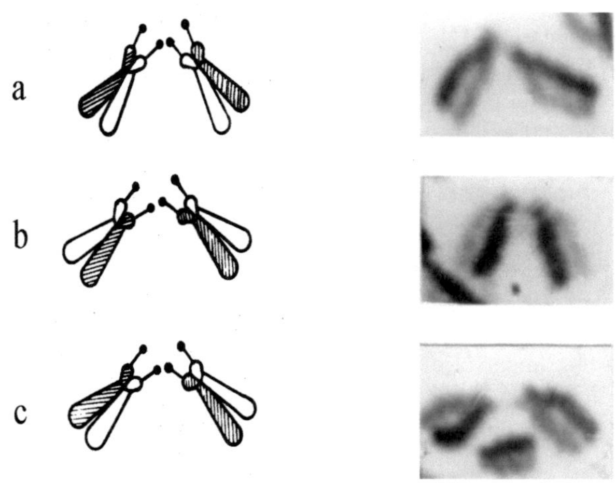

Fig. 5. Associations of acrocentric chromatid satellite stalks. a - cis-1 position (light -to-light chromatid association); b - cis -2 position (dark-to dark association); c - trans-position (dark-to-light association).

An important consideration is deviation of the data from the hypotheses (1)-(3). The deviation suggested that chromatids 1 and 2 of D chromosomes had different associative activities, unlike G-chromosome chromatids. Indeed, if D-chromosome chromatid 2 were more active than chromatid 1, probabilities should be

$$P_{\text{cis-1}}(DD) < 1/2\, P_{\text{trans}}(DD) < P_{\text{cis-2}}(DD) \quad (4)$$

$$P_{\text{cis-1}}(DG) < 1/2\, P_{\text{trans}}(DG) < P_{\text{cis-2}}(DG) \quad (5)$$

and these agreed well with the actual findings.

In conclusion, sister chromatids of acrocentric chromosomes show a functional heterogeneity in very old individuals (Lezhava, 1987, 2006).

5. Correlation between mutation, repair and hetheterochromatinization of chromosomes in aging

Progressive heterochromatinization of chromosome regions observed during aging correlates with the greater frequency of chromosome aberrations and the reduced intensity of reparative events. Chromosome alterations have been studied in 70 individuals aged 80–114 years (30 women and 40 men). In these samples, the percentages of aberrant metaphase and chromosomal aberrations were 4.08±0.41% in women and 5.15±0.45% in men; these values are significantly higher than the published control levels (aged 25–40 years)of 1.8±0.42% and 2.15±0.35%, respectively (Lezhava, 2001, 2006).

The incidence of cell with chromosome aberrations in 80- to 90-year-old individuals was 4.75±0.71% for 25 women and 3.06±0.54% for 31 men; these means were also above those of 20-to 48-year-old individuals. The incidence of aberrant cells in men aged 91 to 114 years (5.62±1.45%) was higher than that in women aged 91 to 108 years and control individuals (Fig. 6, 7).

Our studies have also demonstrated a marked decline in the unscheduled DNA synthesis (repair) rates in 80-90 year- old individuals in response to UV irradiation at a dose of 10–15 J/mm^2 compared with the middle-aged individuals ($P < 0.03$, $P < 0.01$ respectively). These data suggest that human lymphocytes from older people have a significantly reduced capacity for unscheduled DNA synthesis–excision repair (Lezhava, 1984, 2001).

Progressive heterochromatinization of chromosome regions observed during senescence correlates with the lowered intensity of reparative events and the increases frequency of chromosome aberrations. To explain the prevalence of the accumulation of damage in heterochromatin and in the heterochromatinization regions, it has been assumed that the repair of lesions capable of causing aberrations is possible only in those areas of DNA that are actively involved in transcription and that are within physically accessible of reparative enzymes, i.e. in euchromatin areas (Yeilding, 1971). Assuming that heterochromatinized regions are inaccessible to reparative enzymes and therefore number of cells with chromosome aberrations profoundly affects the functioning of the genome in old age (Fig.8).

Our results indicate that decreases in the repair processes and increases in the frequency of chromosomal aberrations in aging are secondary to the progressive heterochromatinization and that chromosome heterochromatinization is a key factor in aging.

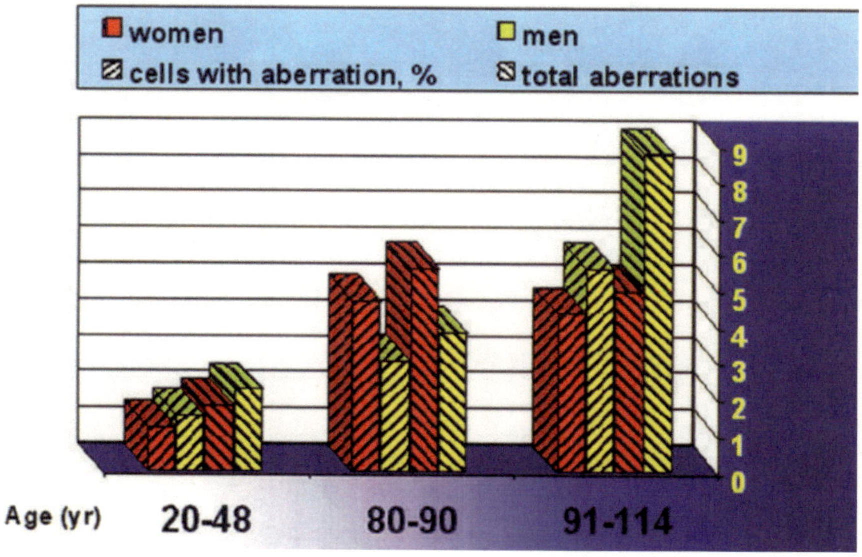

Fig. 6. Spontaneously structural chromosome aberration at 80 years and over

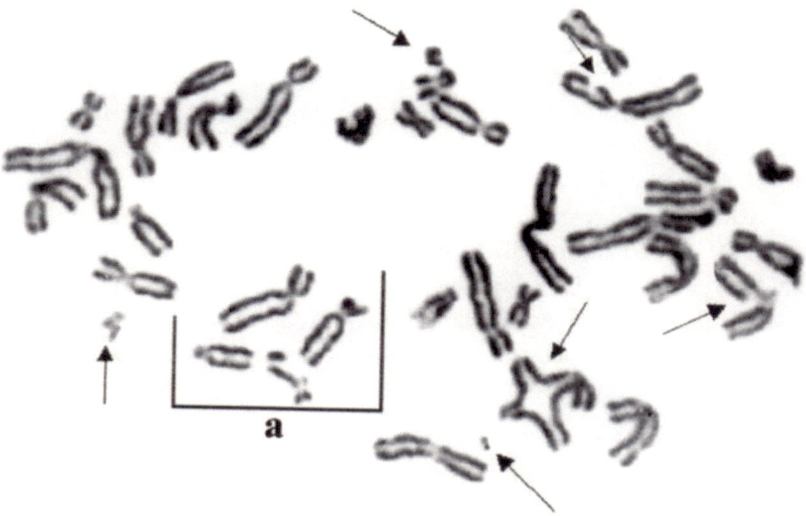

Fig. 7. 114-year-old man's metaphase with aberrant chromosomes. a – association of telomeric regions

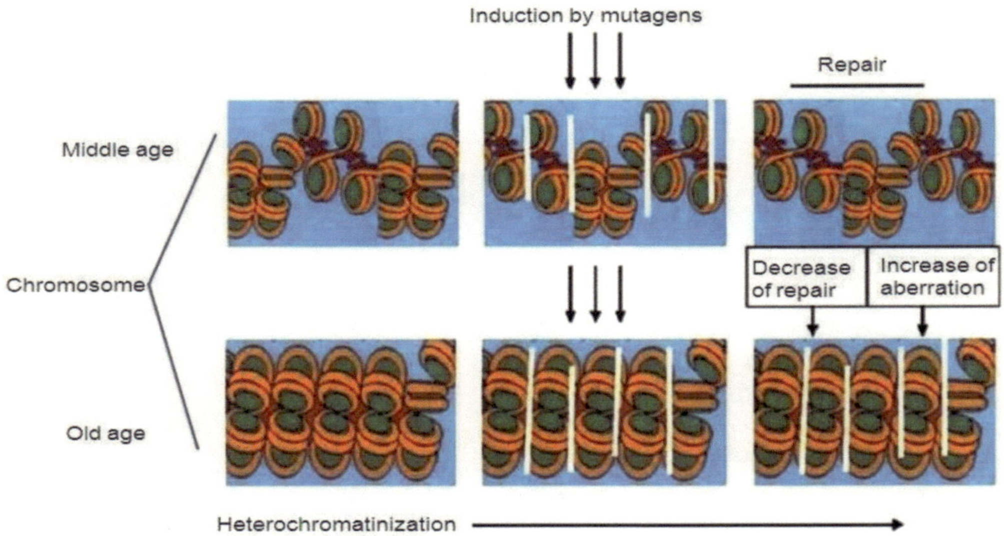

Fig. 8. Heterochromatinized regions inaccessible to reparative enzymes and therefore the number of cells with chromosome aberrations profoundly affects the functioning of the genome in old age.

6. Heterochromatin and pathology

Heterochromatinization progresses with aging and can deactivate many previously functioning active genes. It blocks certain stages of normal metabolic processes of the cell, which inhibits many specific enzymes and leads to aging pathologies. The action of genetic systems reveals general rules in the behavior of such systems, such as the connection between the structural and functional interrelationships between the "directing" and "directed" structures. In the respect, it should be noted that heterochromatinized regions in chromosomes can reverse. Many physical and chemical agents, hormones and peptide bioregulators (Epitalon - Ala-Glu-Asp-Gly; Livagen - Lys-Glu-Asp-Ala; Vilon - Lys-Glu) (Khavinson *et al.*, 2003; Lezhava and Bablishvili, 2003; Lezhava *et al.*, 2004, 2008) cause deheterochromatinization (decondensation) releasing the inactive (once being active)genes that seems to favour purposive treatment of diseases of aging.

We have demonstrated also that Co^{2+} ions alone and in combination with the bioregulator Livagen can reverse the deheterochromatinization of precentromeric and telomeric heterochromatin (Fig.9), to normalize the telomere length in cells from old individuals (Lezhava and Jokhadze, 2007; Lezhava *et al.*,2008). Blood cholesterol levels in an animal model (rabbit) for atherosclerosis was reduced (41% on the average) by pretreatment with combination of livagen and $CoCl_2$ - normalization of telomere length (unpublished data of research – STCU 4307- grants in 2007-2009) (Lezhava *et al.*, 2007-2009).

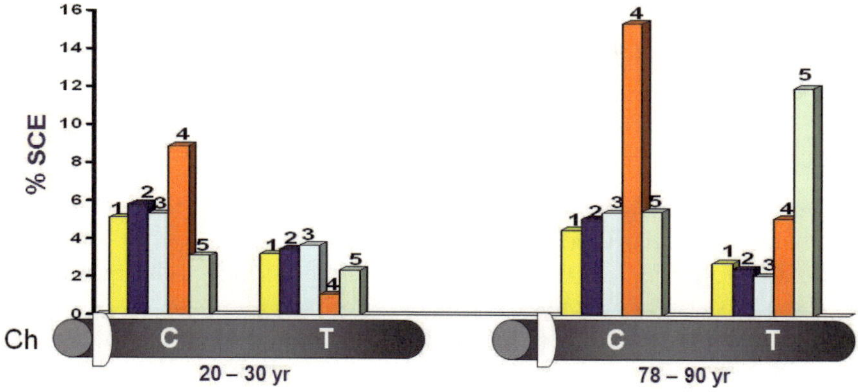

1. Control	5,1 ± 0,64	3,2 ± 0,51	4,5 ± 0,60	2,8 ± 0,48
2. Epitalon	5,2 ± 0,99	3,0 ± 0,76	5,1 ± 0,98	2,5 ± 0,70
3. Livagen	5,3 ± 1,01	3,7 ± 0,85	5,4 ± 0,80	2,1 ± 0,42
4. CoCl2	8,9 ± 1,44	1,1 ± 0,52	15,4 ± 1,8	5,1 ± 1,11
5. Livagen+CoCl2	3,1 ± 0,89	2,4 ± 0,98	5,5 ± 1,15	12,0 ± 1,2

Ch – chromosome C – centromere T - telomere

Fig. 9. The effect of Co^{2+} ions separate and with peptide bioregulators Epitalon (Ala-Glu-Asp-Gly) and Livagen (Lys -Glu-Asp-Ala) distribution of SCE among centromer and telomer heterochromatin regions.

7. Conclusion

In the present investigation, we assessed the modification of total, constitutive (pericentromeric, telomeric and nucleolus organizer region (NOR) heterochromatin) and facultative heterochromatin in cultured lymphocytes exposed to the influence of heavy metal and bioregulators from individuals aged 80 years and over.

The results showed that: (1) progressive heterochromatinization of total, constitutive (pericentromeric, telomeric and NOR heterochromatin) and facultative heterochromatin occurred with aging; (2) a decrease in repair processes and an increase in frequency of chromosome aberrations with aging is secondary to the progressive heterochromatinization of chromosomes; (3) peptide bioregulators induce deheterochromatinization of chromosomes in old age and (4) Co^{2+} ions alone and in combination with the tetrapeptide bioregulator, Livagen (Lys-Glu-Asp-Ala), have different chromosomal target regions; that is, deheterochromatinization of pericentromeric (Co^{2+} ions) and telomeric (Co^{2+} ions in combination with livagen) heterochromatin regions in lymphocytes of olderaged individuals.

The proposed genetic mechanism responsible for constitutive (pericentromeric, telomeric and nucleolus organizer region (NOR) heterochromatin) and facultative heterochromatin remodeling (hetero- and deheterochromatinization) of senile pathogenesis highlights the importance of external and internal factors in the development of diseases and may lead to the development of therapeutic treat.

8. Acknowledgements

This article is dedicated to the memory of professor **A.A. Prokofieva-Belgovskaya** from her greatful students.

9. References

Blasco, M. (2004). Telomere epigenetics: a higher-order control of telomere length in mammalian cells. *Carcinogenesis,* Vol.25, pp. 1083-1087

Boukamp, P.; Popp, S. & Krunic, D. (2005). Telomere-dependent chromosomal instability. *J Investig Dermatol Sym Proc,* Vol.10, pp. 89-94

Bradshow, P.; Stavropoulos, P. & Mey, M. (2005). Human telomeric protein TRF2 associates with genomic double-strand breaks as an early response to DNA damage. *Nat Genet,* Vol.37, pp. 116-118

Callen, E. & Surralles, J. (2004). Telomere dysfunction in genome instability syndromes. *Mutat Res,* Vol.567, pp. 85-104

Chemitiganti, S.; Verma, R.; Ved Brat, S.; Dosik, H.(1984).Random single chromatid type segregation of human acrocentric chromosomes in BrdU-labeled mitosis. *Can J Genet and Cytol,* Vol.26, pp. 137-140

Dialynas, G.; Vitalini, M. & Wallrath, L. (2008). Linking heterovhromatin protein 1 (HP1) to cancer progression. *Mutat Res,* Vol. 647, pp. 13-28

Elcock, L. & Bridger, J. (2010). Exploring the relationship between interphase gene positioning, transcriptional regulation and the nuclear matrix.*Biochem Soc Trans,* Vol. 38, pp. 263-267

Ellen, T.; Kluz, T.; Harder, M.; Xiong, J. & Costa, M. (2009). Heterochromatinization as a potential mechanism on nickel-induced carcinogenesis. *Biochemistry,* Vol.48, pp. 4626-4632

Garcia-Cao, M.; O'Sullivan, R.; Peters, A. et al. (2004). Epigenetic regulation of telomere length in mammalian cells by the Suv39h1 and Suv39h2 histone methyltransferases. *Nat Genet,* Vol.36, pp. 94-99

Geserick, C. & Blasco, M. (2006). Novel roles for telomerase in aging. *Mech Ageing Dev,* Vol.127, pp. 579-583

Gilson, E. & Magdinier, F. (2009). Chromosomal position effect and aging. In Epigenetics and aging. *Springer New York,* Vol.2, pp. 151-175

Golubev, A. (2001). The natural history of telomeres. *Adv.Gerontol* , Vol.7, pp. 95-104

Gonzalo, S.; Jaco, I.; Fraga, M. et al. (2006). DNA methyltransferases control telomere length and telomere recombination in mammalian cells. *Nat Cell Biol,* Vol.8, pp. 416-424

Hande,M.(2004).DNA repair factors and telomere-chromosome intergrity in mammalian cells. *Cytogenet Genome Res.* Vol.104, pp.116-122.

Hawley, R. & Arbel, T. (1993). Yeast genetics and the fall of classical view of meiosis. *Cell,* Vol. 72, pp. 301-303

Horikawa, I. & Barrett, J. (2003). Transcriptional regulation of the telomeraze hTERT gene as a target for cellular and viral oncogenic mechanisms. *Carcinogenesis,* Vol.24, pp. 1167-1176

Imai, S. (2009). From heterochromatin islands to the NAD World: a hierarchical view of aging through the functions of mammalian Sirt1 and systemic NAD biosynthesis. *Biochim Biophys Acta,* Vol.1790, pp. 997-1004

Khavinson, V.; Lezhava, T.; Monaselidze, J. et al. (2003). Peptide Epitalon activates chromatin at the old age. *Neuroendocrinol letters,* Vol.24, pp. 329-333
Kouzarides, U. (2007). Chromatin modifications and their function. *Cell,* Vol.128, pp. 693-705
Lam, A.; Bovin, C.; Bonney, C. et al. (2006). Human centromeric is a dynamic chromosomal domain that can spread over noncentromeric DNA. *Proc Natl Acad Sci USA,* Vol.103, pp. 4186-4191
Lansdorp, P. (2000). Repair of telomeric DNA prior to replicative. *Mech Ageing Dev,* Vol.118, pp. 23-34
Lezhava, T. hitashvili, R.; Khmaladze E.(1972).Use of mathematical"satellite model" for association of acrocentric chromosomes depending on human age. *Bio-medical Computing,* Vol.3, pp. 101-199
Lezhava, T. (1984). Heterochromatinization as a key factor of aging. *Mech Ageing and Dev,* Vol.28, pp. 279-288
Lezhava, T. (1987).Sister chromatidexchange in human lymphocyte in extreme age. *Proc Japan Acad,* Vol.63, pp. 369-372
Lezhava, T. (2001). Chromosome and aging:genetic conception of aging. *Biogerontology,* Vol.2, pp. 253-260
Lezhava, T. (2006). Human chromosomes and aging. From 80 to 114 years. *Nova biomedical, ISBN 1-60021-043-0,* New York, USA
Lezhava, T. & Bablishvili, N. (2003). Reactivation of heterochromatin induced by sodium hydrophospate at the old age. *Proc Georg Acad Sci, Biol Ser B* Vol.1, pp. 1-5
Lezhava, T. & Dvalishvili, N. (1992). Cytogenetic and biochemical studies on the nucleolus organizing regions of chromosomes in vivo and in vitro aging. *Age,* Vol.15, pp. 41-43
Lezhava, T. & Jokhadze, T. (2004). Variability of unscheduled DNA synthesis induced by nikel ions and peptide bioregulator epitalon in old people. *Proc Georg Acad Sci,* Vol.2, pp. 65-70
Lezhava, T. & Jokhadze, T. (2007). Activation of pericentromeric and telomeric heterochromatin in cultured lymphocytes from old individuals. *Ann N Y Acad Sci,* Vol.1100, pp. 387-399
Lezhava, T.; Khavinson, V.; Monaselidze, J. et al. (2004). Bioregulator Vion-induced reactivation of chromatin in cultured lymphocytes from old people. *Biogerontology,* Vol.4, pp. 73-79
Lezhava, T.; Monaselidze, J. & Jokhadze, T. (2008). Decondensation of chromosmes heterochromatinization regions by effect of heavy metals and bioregulators in cultured lymphocytes from old individuals. *Proceeding of the 10th International Symposium of Metal Ions in Biology and Medicine, Bastia France May 19-22 Edited by Philippe Collery,* 10, pp. 569- 576
Lezhava, T.; Monaselidze, J.; Jokhadze, T.; Kakauridze, N. & Kordeli, N. (2007-2009). Decondensation of telomeric heterochromatin as a protective means from Atherosclerosis. *Project Proposal, STCU* 4307
Lo, A.; Sprung, C.; Fouladi, B.; Pedram, M. et al. (2002). Chromosome instability as a result of double - strend breaks near telomeres in mouse embryonic stem cells. *Mol Cell Biol,* Vol.22, pp. 4836-4850
Kouzarides, U. (2007). Chromatin modifications and their function. *Cell,* Vol.128, pp. 693-705

Mazin, A. (1994). Enzimatic DNA methylation as an aging mechanism. *Mol Biol Mosc,* Vol.28, pp. 21-51

Mazin, A. (2009). Suicidal function of DNA methylation in age-related genome disintegration. *Ageing Res Rev,* Vol. 8, pp. 314-327

Mehta, I.; Figgitt, M.; Clements, C. et al. (2007). Alterations to nuclear architecture and genome and genome behavior in senescent cells. *Ann NY Acad Sci,* Vol.1100 pp. 250-263

Michishita, E.; Park, J.; Burneskis, J. et al. (2005). Etvolutionarily conserved and nonconserved cellular localizations and functions of human SIRT proteins. *Mol Biol,* Vol.16, pp. 4623-4635

Monaselidze, J.; Abuladze, M.; Asatiani, N. et al. (2006). Characterization of Chromium-induced Apoptosis in Cultured Mammalian Cells. A Different Scanning Calolorimetry Study. *Thermochemia Acta,* Vol.441, pp. 8–15

Monaselidze, J.; Bregadze, V.; Barbakadze, Sh. et al. (2008). Influence of metal ions of thermodina stability of leukemic DNA in vivo. Microcalorimetri investigation. *Proceeding of the 10th International Symposium of Metal Ions in Biology and Medicine, Bastia France May 19-22 Edited by Philippe Collery,* 10, pp. 451-457

Murnane, J. (2006). Telomeres and chromosome instability. *DNA Repair, (Amst)* Vol.8, pp. 1082-1092

Opresko, P.; Fan, J.; Danzy, S. et al. (2005). Oxidative damage in telomeric DNA disrupts recognition by TRF1 and TRF2. *Nucleic Acids Res,* Vol.33, pp. 1230-1239

Piacentini, L.; Fanti, L.; Negri, R. at al. (2009). Heterochromatin protein 1 (HP1a) positively regulates euchromatic gene expression through RNA transcript association and interaction with hnRNPs in Drosophila. *PloS Genet,* 10, e1000670

Plohl, M.; Luchetti, A.; Metrovic, N.; Mantovani, B. (2008). Satellite DNAs between selfishness andfunctionality: structure, genomics and evolution of tandem repeats in centromer (hetero) chromatin. *Gene,* Vol.409, pp. 72-82

Prokofieva-Belgovskaya, A. (1986). *Heterochromatin regions of chromosomes.* M Nauka, ISBN 575.113+576.316

Sugawara, O.; Oshimura, M.; Koi, M. et al. (1990) Induction of cellular senescence in immortalized cells by human chromosome. *Science,* Vol.247, pp. 707-710

Trojer, P. & Reinberg, D. (2007). Facultative Heterochromatin. Is There a Distinctive Molecular Signature? *Mol Cell,* Vol.28, pp. 1-13

Vaquero, A. (2009). The conserved role of sirtuims in chromatin regulation. *Int J De Biol,* Vol.53, pp. 303-322

Vaquero, A.; Scher, M.; Lee, D. et al. (2004). Human SirT1interacts with histone H1 and promotes formation of facultative heterochromatin. *Mol Cell,* Vol.16, pp. 93-105

Verma, R.; Shah ,J.; Dosic H. (1983). Frequencies of chromosome and chromatid types of associations of nucleolar human chromosomes demonstrated by the N-banding technique. *Cytobios,* Vol.36, pp. 25-29

Verma, R. & Rodriguez, J. (1985) Structural organization of ribosomal cistrons in human nucleolar organizing chromosomes. Cytobios, Vol.44, pp. 25-28

Wright, W. & Shay, J. (2005). Telomera-binding factors and general DNA repair. *Nat Genet,* Vol.37, pp. 193-197

Yelding, K. (1974). Model for aging based on differential of somatic mutational damage. *Perspect Biol Med,* Vol.17, pp. 201-208

27

New Targets for the Identification of an Anti-Inflammatory Anti-Senescence Activity

Patrizia d'Alessio[1], Annelise Bennaceur-Griscelli[2], Rita Ostan[3] and Claudio Franceschi[3]
[1]*University Paris Sud-11 ESTEAM Stem Cell Core Facility and AISA Therapeutics, Evry,*
[2]*University Paris Sud-11 ESTEAM Stem Cell Core Facility and Inserm U935, Villejuif,*
[3]*Department of Experimental Pathology, University of Bologna, Bologna,*
[1,2]*France*
[3]*Italy*

"L'esprit étant précisément une force qui peut tirer d'elle même plus qu'elle ne contient, rendre plus qu'elle ne reçoit, donner plus qu'elle n'a."

Henri Bergson (1911)
La conscience et la vie

1. Introduction

Aging is necessarily associated to cell senescence, but is it its sole motor or phenomenon? Replicative cell senescence can be accelerated by stress, inflammation and uneven life conditions. We talk about stress-induced premature senescence when cell metabolism is exposed to a systemic profile of cortisol and catecholamines and inflammation is maintained by a high profile of cytokines. These latter are detrimental for cells and stem-cells, accelerating the senescence of both.

Aging is increasingly an issue in developed countries as life expectancy increases and birth rate decreases. These demographic trends have led to a strong increase of age-related pathologies, and an understanding of immune senescence promises to limit the development and progression of these diseases. Thus, "immunosenescence" is the term coined for the age-associated decrease in immune competence that renders individuals more susceptible to disease and increases morbidity and mortality due to infectious diseases in the elderly compared with the young (Franceschi et al., 2000). The main observed result at old age is a decrease in adaptive immunity and an increase of low-grade chronic inflammatory status, which has been referred to as "inflammaging" (De Martinis et al., 2005).

Inflammaging is pivotal in many ways and determines whether an individual will become either a healthy centenarian or will have to face sickness and depression for much of his/her life. It is well known that major age related pathologies such as cardiovascular disease, metabolic syndrome and frailty are associated with a progressive low grade inflammation process. While these diseases are thoroughly investigated, the role of the inflammatory process in other important age-related diseases involving the CNS such as depression and dementia, is relatively neglected. The importance of this topic is reinforced by the hypothesis that inflammation likely plays a major role also in CNS diseases such as chronic mood disorders and schizophrenia (Franceschi et al., 2001).

Ever-increasing longevity has produced the ambition for a personalized lifestyle and consequently the introduction of new standards of health. In this context, the aging population is comparable to a new subject, to which science and society will have to bring up new responses and solutions. Mainly based on prevention and maintenance, several indicators have been identified as preventing degenerative issues, aimed at healthy aging. Environmental quality and the role of nutrition are important elements of this strategy.

The importance of microbiome (Biagi et al., 2010) in the maintenance of host health has been recognized for years. Recent studies suggest an association between inflammation status and the presence of chronic disease in the elderly. They also indicate that an altered host-gut microbiota might contribute to maintaining a low systemic inflammatory status in the elderly. Nevertheless, the aging process and longevity in particular also depend on genetic and metabolic stability, as well as resistance to stress. However, if stress persists, it may lead to chronic disease, thus accelerating aging. Moderate stress, independent of conventional risk factors, can also induce a potent alteration in health as stressful life conditions induce a systemic pro-inflammatory status, consequently shortening life quality and lifespan.

In the present work, we would like to focus on the relationship between cell senescence at a daily scale and long-term consequence such as the loss of performance of organs, tissues and cells, and aging as it appears with osteoporosis, memory loss and immune-senescence (Ostan et al., 2008).

Inflammation is a critical defense mechanism, that, uncontrolled, contributes to chronic conditions with inflammatory pathogenesis. Markers of inflammation indicate vascular endothelial activation and dysfunction (d'Alessio, 2004; AISA Patent Family n°1).

Chronic inflammation appears to be determinant, in that it also affects functional aspects of stem cells, which are crucial to the maintenance of long term homeostasis of organs and tissues during lifetime. In fact, as reports from mice models and more recently from humans including centenarians (Bagnara et al., 2000) have confirmed, stem cells also undergo aging, as do somatic differentiated cells (Chambers et al., 2007; Ergen & Goodell, 2009). Most of the results have shown that the stem cell compartment becomes compromised, not by a quantitative loss, but by the progressive loss of function. These age-related changes have been suggested to be due to factors intrinsic to the stem cell (SC) including epigenetic changes and expression of transcription factors.

Aging can also be due to extrinsic (Rossi, 2008) environmental factors including the microenvironment of the SC local context (Bagnara et al., 2000). Very recent evidence has shown that there is a dialogue between the niche and the stem cell compartment leading to the maintenance of cellular homeostasis (Rossi et al., 2005). One of the key factors of the degeneration of the stem cell within its niche is certainly the inflammatory challenge (Chambers et al., 2007). Moreover, the dysfunction of stem cells is probably the result of epigenetic events. We consider the usefulness of studying strategies that could partially reverse it. An indirect evidence linking stress and lifespan comes from the studies of Linda Buck showing that human anti-depressant drug mianserin and serotonin receptor antagonists ser-3 and ser-4 were able to increase lifespan in *C. elegans* (Petrascheck et al., 2007). Other natural substances (such as curcumin) that have been characterized for their anti-inflammatory activity could be of the same value. AISA terpens have shown their incidence on replicative senescence in cells, as well as anti-inflammatory and anti-stress effects in pre-clinical and clinical studies (Bisson et al., 2008).

2. Current theories

2.1 "Inflammaging" and "SIPS"

The concept based on observations in immunology, linking inflammation with aging was proposed by Claudio Franceschi (Franceschi et al., 2000; Franceschi et al., 2007), whereas the concept based on proteomic analysis, linking stress to the appearance of premature senescence (SIPS, abbreviation of Stress Induced Premature Senescence) was proposed by Olivier Toussaint. These two researchers were showing that *aging stands in a biologically relevant link to inflammation*. According to the stochastic theories of aging, damage that accumulates with time in the cellular components is responsible for cellular aging. Some sort of premature senescence would appear when the damage level is artificially increased due to the presence of stressing agents at sub-cytotoxic level. Several models have shown that after sub-cytotoxic long-term stresses, human diploid fibroblasts (HDFs) display biomarkers of replicative senescence (RS), which led to the concept of SIPS (Dierick et al., 2002) as compared to telomere-dependent RS, changes accounting for "molecular scars" of sub-cytotoxic stresses.

2.2 Judith Campisi and her double-edged sword theory of cellular senescence

Pr. Campisi is internationally known for the work she has performed on cellular aging, genome stability and tumor suppressor genes during the last 20 years. After 11 years at the Lawrence Berkeley National Laboratory, she now works closely with several laboratories at the Buck Institute to understand and manipulate the cell phenotypes of characteristic of aging, cancer and age-related degeneration (Campisi, 2011). Trying to understand the cellular and molecular biology of aging, she has studied the importance of the cellular senescence, cell death and the effects of DNA damage regarding premature aging and cancer. Campisi's recent work indicates an interesting new insight on cell aging (senescence/death) and both cancer (hyper-proliferation) and degenerative diseases (Bazarov et al., 2010; de Keizer et al., 2010).

2.3 ROS, mitochondria decline and DNA damage

2.3.1 Harmann's theory on free radical damage

Harmann's theory on free radical damage formulated in 1956 has generated several important insights and further raised the importance of DNA damage and DNA repair for aging and longevity respectively (reparosome dependent mechanisms).

2.3.2 Miroslav Radman's vaccination

Radman's work accounts for several mechanisms of DNA repair that *E. coli* have extrapolated, ex. gr. the exceptional resistance of *D. radiodurans* to DNA damaging agents (radiations and chemicals) and to desiccation (Zahradka et al., 2006). He described the global mechanism of DNA fragment reassembly as a two-stage process, which involves mutually dependent DNA replication and recombination events (Babic et al., 2008), and defined key steps in this most efficient and precise DNA repair process, assigned gene and protein function to critical repair steps, and showed the kinetics of the key steps.

2.4 Tom Kirkwood's systems-biology approach

Starting from the damage theory published in *Cell* in 2005, the extent of investment of organism's genome in survival stands at the heart of the 'disposable soma' theory, formulated in early 1977 in *Nature*. What is possible instead, according to this scientist, is to slow the rate at which damage accumulates, given the malleability of the aging process (Kirkwood, 2008). *Here we are conceptually very close to a putative concept of 'reversibility' that has nothing to do with repair and that we claim to be able to demonstrate.* As Kirkwood says 'the devil is in the details', i.e. where should the critical point be situated when random damage becomes damage oriented to the development of frailty? Indeed the concept of 'robustness' as opposed to 'vulnerability' is at the heart of systems biology (Kitano, 2007). In spite of numerous affecting defects in cells, tissues and molecules, none of them contributes to characterize the senescent phenotype. Moreover the systematic stochasticity of all events with resulting variability and increasing multiplicity, impairs the identification of a unifying element for a true explanation of the increasing lifespan phenomenon in humans, described as "healthy aging".

2.5 Linda B. Buck's (2004 Nobel Prize) bio-products targeting mechanisms of olfaction and lifespan in *C. elegans*

Determinants of aging and lifespan by Buck's laboratory on the short-lived nematode *Caenorhabditis elegans* (*C. elegans*) have identified a number of genes that can influence the lifespan of this organism (Petrascheck et al., 2007). Looking for the identification of chemicals that would increase *C. elegans* lifespan, studies on the endogenous targets of Buck's chemicals provided additional insights into the underlying mechanisms of aging. By conducting a high-throughput screening, she identified 100 compounds that increase *C. elegans* lifespan when given only during adulthood. The animal's lifespan can be increased about 30 percent by mianserin, a drug used as an antidepressant in humans. This effect requires a specific serotonin receptor, SER-3 or SER-4, a receptor for another neurotransmitter, octopamine. ***The drug increases lifespan via mechanisms linked to dietary restriction.*** Curiously, the drug does not appear to reduce food intake. One possible explanation for these findings is that the inhibitory effect of mianserin on SER-3 and SER-4 mimics a reduction in food intake and thereby triggers anti-aging mechanisms associated with dietary restriction. This approach is particularly interesting because of the concomitant effects on senescence and mood - via the management of the inflammatory reaction - such as observed for bio-products identified by us.

2.6 Sirtuins anti-inflammatory action

Sirtuins (Dali-Youcef et al., 2007) (LP Guarente laboratory) exhibit protection of DNA from metabolic damage and are therefore thought to affect regulatory systems of longevity (Donmez

& Guarente, 2010). The idea that sirtuins can affect inflammation comes from the evidence that they are able to inactivate NF-κB, which is not according to us, a sufficient element to claim for an anti-inflammatory and thus potentially anti-aging activity. These results, shown into a variety of lower organisms, have been transferred into a transgenic mice model by M. Serrano (Spanish National Cancer Center, Madrid) who confirmed that Sir-1 improves healthy aging concluding about a consequent anti-aging activity. We think that sirtuins may protect from metabolic syndrome (Herranz et al., 2009) and decrease spontaneous cancer.

2.7 Interaction of biological and social factors

There is increasing recognition that intra-uterine life can influence the health of the newborn well into his/hers adult years, although the mechanisms through which these occur are, as yet, unclear. These evidences form the basis of the Barker Hypothesis, formulated on human aging (de Kretser, 2010), which links under-nutrition in utero, leading to low birth weight, with an increased risk of hypertension, coronary artery disease, stroke, diabetes and the metabolic syndrome in adulthood. All these syndromes may be the result of impaired nephrogenesis and a greater susceptibility to renal disease, impaired development of the endothelium and increased sensitivity to glucocorticoid hormones (Froy & Miskin, 2010; Kolokotrones et al., 2010). Given that the *in utero* 'environmental status' affects the organ function many years later, there is a strong possibility that the mechanism will involve imprinting of genes. But also, concerning the social impact on aging, the psychological stress in adult life has shown its risk for development of psychiatric diseases, based on the recognition of molecular makers of aging (von Zglinicki et al., 2001). In women aged 20–50 years, those with the highest levels of psychological stress had the shortest telomeres and the lowest telomerase activity in peripheral blood leukocytes, and showed the highest levels of oxidative stress with consequent impairment of SC repair capacity and generation of metabolic syndrome diseases (Mathieu et al., 2010; Ingram & Mussolino, 2010).

2.8 Stem cell based approach to the study of intrinsic senescence

2.8.1 Telomere shortening and its implication for SC niches' aging

Telomeres are specialized structures that adorn the ends of human chromosomes, essential for the integrity of chromosomes. These nucleoprotein caps are maintained by the enzyme telomerase. The importance of adequate telomerase activity and maintenance of telomere length for both replicative potential in culture and aging in organisms was initially inferred from studies of primary human fibroblasts. In culture, division of fibroblasts results in progressive telomere attrition, culminating in a state of proliferative arrest — or cellular senescence — after a finite number of cell divisions, a barrier known as the Hayflick limit. Moreover, enforced expression of TERT, the catalytic subunit of telomerase, in cultured human fibroblasts stabilized telomere length and endowed the cells with unlimited replicative potential without engendering malignant properties. The remarkable capacity of experimentally induced telomerase activity to circumvent senescence and allow indefinite growth has been documented in many other human cell types. Telomere dynamics bear relevance to the processes of aging, and human population studies have correlated decreased telomere length in peripheral blood leukocytes with higher mortality rates in individuals who are more than 60 years old; a recent large cohort study did report a positive link between telomere length and years of healthy life (Sahin & DePinho, 2010); another recent study on centenarians and their offspring found a positive link between telomere length and longevity; in particular, those with longer telomeres had an overall improved health profile (with decreased age-associated disease and better cognitive function and lipid profiles) with respect to controls (Atzmon et al., 2010).

2.8.2 SC's aging is relevant to cell senescence

De Pinho's lab at Boston Harvard Medical School has established that we age, in part, because our self-renewing stem cells grow old as a result of heritable intrinsic events, such as DNA damage, as well as extrinsic forces, such as changes in their supporting niches. Mechanisms that suppress the development of cancer, such as senescence and apoptosis, which rely on telomere shortening and the activities of p53 and p16 (INK4a), may also induce an unwanted consequence: a decline in the replicative function of certain stem-cell types with advancing age. This decreased regenerative capacity appears to contribute to some aspects of mammalian aging, with new findings pointing to a *'stem-cell hypothesis' for human age-associated conditions such as frailty, atherosclerosis and type 2 diabetes*. This approach is of particular interest for us, because of the possibility to look at the role of reprogrammed SC in the identification of cell/tissue signature of characterized by increased repair activity.

2.8.3 Epigenetic deregulation responsible for SC decline

Goodell M, Texas and Scadden D, have characterized inflammatory stress responsible for niche component degeneration (Chambers et al., 2007). In the continuity of this work, organ specific targets have been looked at. Muscle and adipose tissue are concerned with age-related muscle dysfunction (Degens, 2007). Stem cell reprogramming, as well as the adipocyte role in promoting accelerated cell senescence and aging on the base of its capacity to stock pro-inflammatory cytokines, have to be taken into account (Naveiras et al., 2009).

3. Our approach: Cell senescence as multi-factorial process

Cell senescence is a pleiotropic process, initially determined by genetic and environmental conditions. In the experimental work presented here, we focus on replicative senescence phenomena in a nearly non dividing human cell type, the endothelial cell lining the vascular wall. Among its numerous functions, endothelium is also implicated in the regulation of several steps of the inflammatory process. Two scenarios are prone to accelerate senescence in inflammation.

1. One is the tissue repair sequence that follows the primary neutralization of the microbial or traumatic agent. In this case intense neo-angiogenesis of low quality as well as tissue replacement take place.
2. On the other hand, it is possible that the incoming *noxa* will not be neutralized (here the stress model is extremely useful to illustrate endogenous cell senescence) and the pro-inflammatory stimulation persists.

Thereby, a high concentration of pro-inflammatory cytokines occurring during the inflammatory response, will promote the appearance of premature senescence of endothelial cells, independently of the age of the subject. When chronic inflammatory disease develops, it contributes to the deterioration of endothelial cell function, further increasing their premature senescence. This ancient if not universal mechanism is conserved in stem cell, niches undergoing senescence by the same (pro-inflammatory) mechanisms. In fact, the cytokine TNF-α (Tumor Necrosis Factor-α) is mainly responsible for the major cell modifications of the senescent cell that we have identified in three categories:

1. loss of contact inhibition;
2. overexpression of cell adhesion molecules (d'Alessio, 2004);
3. modification of cell morphology sustained by the development of stress fibers into a large mono-directional fiber system (AISA Patent Family n°1).

Based on this "senescent" phenotype, we have launched a bio-guided research aiming at the reversibility of these characteristics. We have characterized a family of molecules able to inhibit the expression of inflammatory markers and, in particular, of adhesion molecule expression in endothelial cells following TNF-α stimulation. We have named these molecules "AISA" (Anti Inflammatory Senescence Actives), because not only a change in cell shape occurred but also the consequences of replicative senescence were reversed (*in vitro* studies). Moreover, *in vivo* studies with one of these compounds ("AISA 5203-L") showed an exceptional capacity to restore both the colon's enterocytes and dermis from pro-inflammatory agonists and toxic substances (AISA Patent Family n°3). Most probably the protective effect is due to the capacity of AISA 5203-L to inhibit circulating Tumor Necrosis Factor- α (TNF- α), Interlukin-6 (IL-6) and Interlukin-1 (IL-1), most relevant to the inflammatory reaction in relationship to the aging process by *inflammaging.* AISA 5203-L was used as treatment (oral administration) in an rat model for non-pathologic stress (defined by anxiety situations such as isolation or separation). It showed a compelling anti-stress activity, as measured by a FOB (Functional Observation Battery), whereby analgesic effects were associated to enhanced motility and less irritability.

4. Relevance of chronic inflammation

As humans grow older, systemic inflammation can inflict devastating degenerative effects throughout the body. Chronic inflammation is an underlying cause of many apparently unrelated, age-related diseases. This fact is often overlooked, yet persuasive scientific evidence exists that correcting a chronic inflammatory disorder will enable many of the infirmities of aging to be prevented or reversed.

When we envisage a link between aging and recurrent or chronic inflammation, we refer to pathological consequences of inflammation in well-documented medical literature. Regrettably, the origins as well as the consequences of systemic inflammation continue to be ignored. By following specific prevention protocols (such as weight loss), the inflammatory stimulation could be significantly reduced. An important role in preventing the onset of a chronic inflammatory condition has been attributed either to the practice of a physical activity or to the prescription of a personalized diet, or both. In the frame of the EU Capacities study RISTOMED (www.ristomed.eu), AISA Therapeutics treatment associated as dietary supplementation to a controlled diet in a cohort of elderly otherwise healthy individuals (65-85 years) was validated as anti-inflammatory medical food.

5. Low grade inflammation and cell degeneration

The immune function also is affected in aging. As lymphocyte function decreases, macrophages take over concomitantly with an enhanced secretion of inflammatory cytokines, such as TNF-α and IL-6. This mechanism is of vital importance for tissue defense from microorganisms (and anti-infectious defense is crucial in the elderly), but it also contributes to the progression of many degenerative diseases. Rheumatoid arthritis is a classic autoimmune disorder in which exceeding levels of cytokines such as IL-6, IL-1β and/or IL-8 are known to cause or contribute to the inflammatory syndrome.

Chronic inflammation is also involved in diseases associated to the metabolic syndrome resulting in atherosclerosis, heart valve dysfunction, obesity, diabetes, congestive heart failure, and digestive system diseases. Cancer and Alzheimer's disease have both been shown to benefit from a systemic inflammation for their progression. In aged people with multiple degenerative diseases, the inflammatory marker C-reactive protein is often elevated, indicating the presence of an underlying inflammatory condition. Moreover, when a cytokine blood profile is conducted on people in a weakened condition, an excess level of one or more of the inflammatory cytokines, e.g., TNF- α , IL-6, IL-1 β , as well as IL-8, are usually found.

6. Systemic markers of cell senescence

In 2000 the New England Journal of Medicine published several studies showing that the blood indicators of inflammation are strong predictive factors for determining susceptibility to undergo a heart attack. Many international studies subsequently validated this first communication (Ridker et al., 1997; Harris et al., 1999; Walston et al., 2002; Ziccardi et al., 2002; Clément et al., 2004).

Again, C-reactive protein represents a critical inflammatory marker. This marker indicates an increased risk for destabilized atherosclerotic plaque (here we are beyond senescence) and abnormal arterial clotting, which can lead to an acute heart attack. One of these studies (Ridker et al., 1997) showed that people with high levels of C-reactive protein were almost three times as likely to die from a heart attack. This also implicates that elevated C-reactive protein, IL-6 and other inflammatory cytokines indicate significantly greater risks of contracting or dying from specific diseases (heart attack, stroke, Alzheimer's disease).

Moreover, C-reactive protein and IL-6 could also predict the risk of all-cause mortality as addressed by a study conducted on a sample of 1,293 healthy elderly people (Harris et al., 1999) followed for a period of 4.6 years. Higher IL-6 levels were associated with a twofold greater risk of death. Higher C-reactive protein was also associated with a greater risk of death, but to a lesser extent than elevated IL-6. Subjects with both high C-reactive protein and IL-6 were 2.6 times more likely to die during follow up than those with low levels of both of these measurements of inflammation.

Thus it would seem that C-reactive protein and IL-6 may be useful for identification of high-risk subgroups for anti-inflammatory interventions. Indeed, in 2003, the American Heart Association and Centers for Disease Control & Prevention (CDC) jointly endorsed the C-reactive protein test and screen for coronary-artery inflammation to identify patients at risk for heart attack. Interestingly, together with other relevant markers, C-reactive protein has been importantly diminished by AISA treatment.

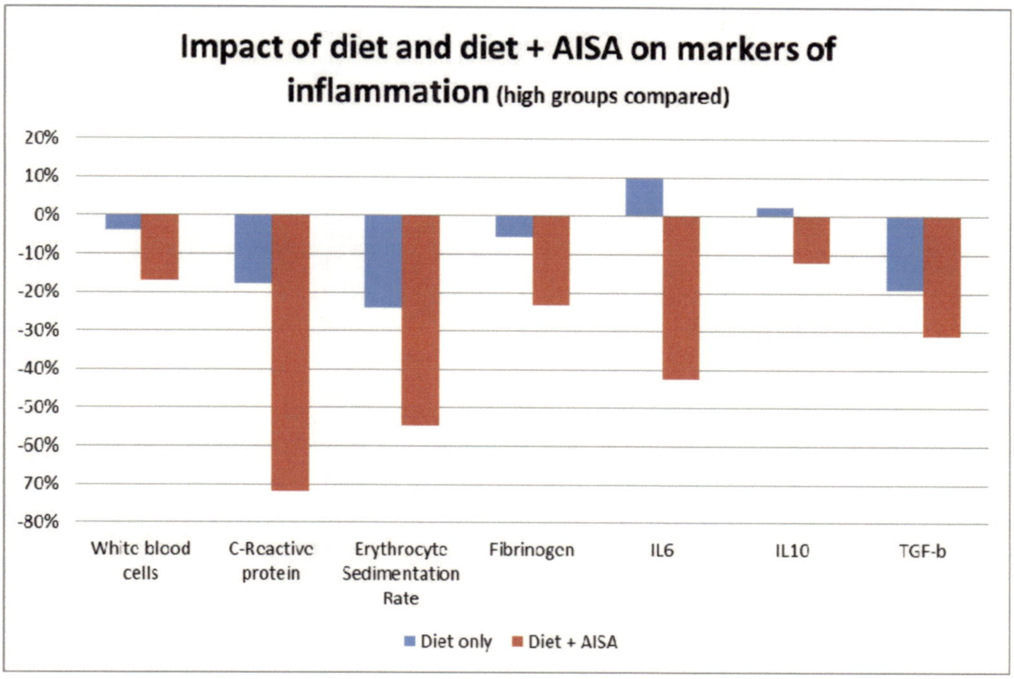

Fig. 1. In the aforementioned RISTOMED study, relevant pro-inflammatory markers characterizing the specific degree of the inflammatory reaction in the studied population, as well as the capacity by AISA compounds to lower them, have been measured. In particular, CRP (aspecific marker) and IL-6 (specific marker, relevant in arthritis) were significantly lowered. (For each inflammatory marker the T1 data were taken as baseline and the difference T56-T1 was expressed as a % of T1).

7. Frailty and inflammatory profiles

Results addressing the role of inflammation during aging were further developed by a new study on almost 5,000 elderly people (Walston et al., 2002) that have compared frail seniors to their healthier counterparts for the presence of increased inflammation markers. Associated to the elevated blood inflammatory markers, these frail seniors also tended to show an enhanced clotting activity, muscle weakness, fatigue and disability when compared to the not frail elderly people. For the moment, we are not able to document to what extent these clinical outcomes are the origin or the consequence of inflammatory status, but once we recognize that they are interdependent, we can address them by prevention and treatment.

Collectively, these studies should motivate public health policies as well as conscious individuals to monitor their inflammatory status. If C-reactive protein is elevated, then the Inflammatory Cytokine Test Panel would be also highly recommended. Secondly, all those who suffer from any type of chronic disease may also consider to access to the Inflammatory Cytokine Test Panel in order to identify the specific inflammatory mediator that is causing or contributing to their health problem.

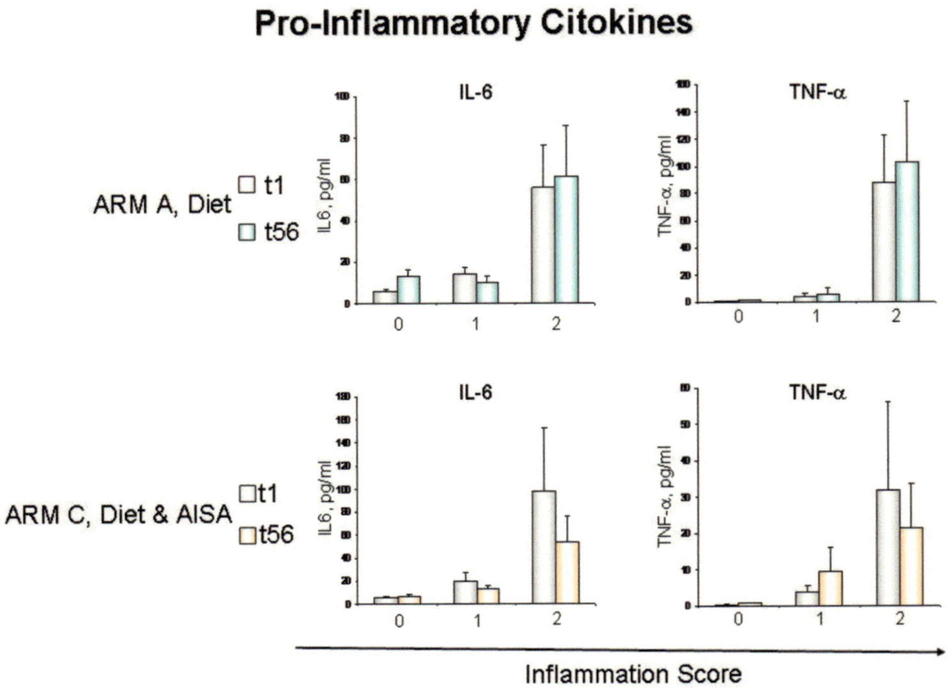

Fig. 2. The histograms show the levels of IL-6 and TNF-α in two arms of Ristomed project: the diet (Arm A) and of the diet with AISA (Arm C). Subjects were clustered on the basis of the inflammation score. Considering "low" and "medium" inflamed subjects (IS=0 and IS=1, the left and centre pairs in each chart), diet (arm A) and diet with AISA (Arm C) seems to have no effect on IL-6 and TNF-α levels. Considering "high inflamed" subjects (IS=2, the right hand pair in each chart) Arm A seems to slightly increase IL-6 and TNF-α whereas arm C (terpens) lowers them.

8. Anti-inflammation to decrease cell senescence

For a long time the identification and production of anti-inflammatory drugs has concentrated on symptom remission, ignoring vascular mechanisms of inflammation and their consequences in the long term, such as increased cell replicative senescence, promoting degenerative disease. Now we know that the presence of pro-inflammatory markers in blood may be in part responsible for degenerative diseases, characteristic of aging and reposing on accelerated cell senescence. Through their clinical relevance, inflammatory markers can witness, via endothelial dysfunction, their implication in the occurring of disease (Edelman, 1993; Vanier, 2005; Farhadi et al., 2003; Garcìa-Cardena & Gimbrone, 2006; Ingber, 2003; Marconi et al., 2003).

In the past, monoterpens, sesquiterpenes, diterpens and triterpens (Zhang et al., 2006) have been characterized by several authors (Vigushin et al., 1998; Crowell et al., 1992; Hardcastle et al., 1999) as potential anti-cancer drugs on the basis of *in vitro* and *in vivo* studies, but their role as anti-inflammatory drugs has remained elusive.

In 2002, following our bio-guided selection, performed by means of our *in vitro* cell biology screening platform, we were able to identify 4 molecules out of 2000 as able to reverse inflammatory markers in senescent endothelial cells. Focusing on functional criteria, we were aiming at the identification of non-toxic molecules able to inhibit *in vitro* the hallmarks of the inflammatory response, such as the expression of adhesion molecules (ICAM-1, VCAM-1, selectins), as well as the concomitant actin polymerization in endothelial cells. The four monoterpens were contained in plants extracts (kindly provided by the University of Hanoi) originating from regional medicinal plants.

9. Pre-clinical studies

After an acute toxicity study and several dose-response studies aiming at the appreciation of the therapeutic window, pre-clinical studies were performed on a female rat TNBS induced colitis model and a murine SHK TPA model. These studies showed that the inhibition of adhesion molecules were comparable in the *in vitro / in vivo* experiments (Yamada et al., 1992; Medeiros et al., 2007; AISA Patent Family n°3).

Our studies also allowed us to establish that the therapeutic window corresponded to the *in vivo* pharmacological active dose of 10 mg/kg given either *per os* or applied topically. Moreover, our *in vivo* data showed that plasma concentration of TNF-α is greatly reduced by the administration of AISA 5203-L and the score of post-lesional tissue regeneration was comparable with that of ibuprofen. Unlike ibuprofen, AISA 5203-L also importantly contributes to mood matching. Finally, on the quite differentiated capacity to elicit adhesion molecule expression following TNF stimulation by different steroid and non steroid anti-inflammatory drugs (Zhang et al., 2006), AISA molecules do persistently inhibit their expression.

10. AISA pertinence for combating cell senescence

Monoterpenes are a class of isoprenoid molecules derived from the anabolism of acetate by the mevalonic acid branch biosynthetic pathways of plants. *d*-Limonene for example, a major component of orange peel oil, is formed by the cyclization of the 10-carbon isoprene intermediate geranylpyrophosphate. Interest in *d*-Limonene came from the ability of the compound to inhibit carcinogenesis in the murine benzo(*a*)pyrene-induced skin tumor model and inhibition of dibenzopyrene-induced s.c. sarcomas. The mechanisms by which *d*-Limonene and other cyclic monoterpenes inhibit tumor growth have not been firmly established. Geranylpyrophosphate, the isoprene intermediate from which these compounds are derived, is required for synthesis of cholesterol, coenzyme Q (ubiquinone), and substrates used in the isoprenylation of several cellular proteins. Crowell *et al.* found that *d*-Limonene and other monoterpenes inhibited isoprenylation of M_r 21,000–26,000 proteins, including $p21^{ras}$ and other members of the ras family of GTP-binding proteins involved in signal transduction and growth regulation. The post-translational isoprenylation of these and other proteins is an essential covalent modification required for protein localization and function. For example, farnesylation is required for plasma membrane association and signaling function of $p21^{ras}$. Other intracellular proteins require isoprenylation by addition of a farnesyl (15-carbon) or geranylgeranyl (20-carbon) group to the COOH terminus for localization to a cellular compartment or for interaction with other proteins. The four molecules, identified by the AISA Therapeutics cell biology platform for their specific anti-inflammatory activity, following an *in vitro* screening on endothelial targets associating cyto - protective and adhesion inhibiting activities, turned out to be monoterpens: more, geraniol, geranyl acetate, d-Limonene and iso-menthone are intimately linked by a metabolic loop.

Although data available emphasized the anti-cancer activities of geraniol and *d*-Limonene, we were tempted to find out about the *in vitro / in vivo* consistency of our data in models adapted to the study of acute and chronic inflammation. In confirmation to our *in vitro* results, the capacity of geraniol (AISA 5202-G) to inhibit the adhesion of leukocytes following TNF-α stimulation had already been established. As for *d*-Limonene, in consideration of the efficacy of its metabolite, perillyl alcohol (POH), already tested in clinical trials in patients with refractory solid malignancies (Miller et al., 2011), it seems plausible that it plays the role of a precursor. In conclusion, the complex sequence of events of the inflammatory response including endothelial adhesion molecule expression for the vascular recruitment of leukocytes to the site of injury, concomitant with actin polymerization challenges the signaling pathway of the rho GTPase family (Xu et al., 2009; Burridge & Wennerberg, 2004; Millan & Ridley, 2005; Dillon & Goda, 2005). The activation of these proteins requires a post-translational iso-prenylation. *We think that the same mechanisms of action of the anti-cancer effects reported for geraniol and d-Limonene could equally be at the origin of their anti-inflammatory properties, here reported.* This shared mechanism between cancer and inflammation again suggests the existence of a mechanism connecting stem cell biology and cancer proliferation.

11. Why stress is relevant for cell senescence

Important effects on mood in presence of stress situations had been documented by us in a rodent model thus motivating our choice to explore more in detail this unexpected effect (AISA Patent Family n°2; MacPhail, 1987; Shibeshi et al., 2007; Esler et al., 2008; Querè et al., 2009; May et al., 2009; Chandola et al., 2008).

As established by our Functional Observation Battery (FOB), *d*-Limonene was able to substantially contribute to pain tolerance and mood stabilization. However, the most intriguing result, was the fact that the stressed animal (by a so-called non-pathological stress stimulating anxiety, comparable to maternal deprivation), instead of developing a freezing attitude, following oral administration of *d*-Limonene, developed a "ludic" activity, starting to play with the wheel next to it. This is particularly interesting when compared to other mood or anxiety treating molecules, displaying substantially a hypnotic effect. Moreover the Ristomed study results obtained for quality of life assessment, SF-36v2™ Health Survey, *Summary* (PCS) *Mental Component Summary* (MCS), General Health Questionnarie-12 (GHQ-12) and mood by the State-Trait Anxiety Inventory-X (STAI-X) and Center for Epidemiologic Studies Depression Scale (CES-D) by use of questionnaires were interestingly confirming our findings on mood modulation, especially in females.

Arm		N	FEMALES - CES-D	mean	SD	differences in pairs		
						mean	SD	Sig. (2-code)
A	Diet	17	CES-D (T1)	8,94	7,267	3,06	5,080	*0,025*
		17	CES-D (T56)	5,88	5,183			
B	Diet & Probiotic	16	CES-D (T1)	8,19	5,671	2,06	5,579	*0,160*
		16	CES-D (T56)	6,13	5,620			
C	Diet & Terpene	16	CES-D (T1)	14,94	11,457	6,13	9,069	*0,016*
		16	CES-D (T56)	8,81	7,035			
D	Diet & Argan Oil	18	CES-D (T1)	8,06	8,335	2,06	3,208	*0,015*
		18	CES-D (T56)	6,00	7,507			

Arm		N	CES-D	mean	SD	differences in pairs		
						mean	SD	Sig. (2-code)
A	Diet	31	CES-D (T1)	6,71	6,659	2,55	4,280	*0,002*
		31	CES-D (T56)	4,16	4,670			
B	Diet & Probiotic	31	CES-D (T1)	6,74	5,416	2,13	4,924	*0,022*
		31	CES-D (T56)	4,61	5,149			
C	Diet & Terpene	29	CES-D (T1)	10,41	10,304	4,03	7,351	*0,006*
		29	CES-D (T56)	6,38	6,264			
D	Diet & Argan Oil	32	CES-D (T1)	8,28	7,809	1,66	5,033	*1,66*
		32	CES-D (T56)	6,63	7,487			

Fig. 3. CES-D evaluation showed (the analysis stratified by arm of study), that the significant differences between T1-T56 were in the arm "A" (p = 0,002), "B" (p = 0,022) and "C" (P = 0,006) but not in arm "D"; analyzing separately male and female, the significant statistical difference was confirmed for males only in the arm "A" (p = 0,38) and for females in the arm "A" (p = 0,025), "C" (p = 0,016) and "D" (P = 0,015) but not in arm "B", but by far the **highest score difference was observed in arm "C" (mean difference score T1-T56 = 6,13 ± 9,069) that show the greatest improvement of how the subject feels and behaves in the preceding week.**

12. Discussion

In summary, we claim that links between inflammation, senescence and stress so far addressed in a fragmentary way should be considered by an integrated approach to better elucidate the senescence process. Therefore the identification of molecules able to prove anti- inflammatory effective on replicative senescence having a subtle but tangible effect on mood became a way to put this link in evidence. In this regard, at the end of this chapter, I would evoke the historical and almost anecdotal properties of such molecules in food and recipes throughout the ages.

12.1 How inflammation takes advantage from ongoing cell senescence

Inflammatory diseases are numerous and systemic inflammation is a silent companion of stress and age. On the other hand, psychological stress in response to pain appears as an important customer of inflammation. Pharmacological strategies trying to inhibit inflammatory symptoms and related clinical episodes have gone far, and when properly prescribed can be considered successful despite recent side effects reported for several of them. But disease is, independently from its etio-pathology, a stressing agent by itself, able to anticipate inflammation by not yet totally unraveled mechanisms. Unfortunately, a sustained anti-inflammatory treatment is inevitably associated with adverse effects, thus opening a field of research and development for new, less or non-toxic and better tolerated anti-inflammatory strategies. In particular, we could provide evidence that the expression of vascular adhesion molecules is challenged by the most frequently-used anti-inflammatory steroid and non-steroid drugs when compared to the effect of a triterpen contained in an edible plant used by Chinese populations since centuries to prevent rheumatoid arthritis (Zhang et al., 2006).

12.2 How inflammation and stress define the senescent phenotype

Recently, much attention has been given to stress as promoter of disease and syndromes implied in health decline and we have addressed this issue in a review and a research article (d'Alessio, 2004; Bisson et al., 2008).

Indeed, compounds found in natural substances, mostly plants, have acquired a new status as valid pharmacological candidates for the development of new drugs preventing, maintaining and curing on the basis of body integrity and substantially addressing wellness more than health. We think that if the aging process depends on genetic stability, metabolic control, and resistance to stress, longevity in particular seems related to the latter. If responses to stress anticipate adaptation to an unacceptable disparity between real or imagined personal experience and expectation, they include adaptive stress, anxiety, and depression. However, if stress persists, it may lead to chronic diseases, ranging from inflammation and cancer to degenerative diseases. If in the past only extreme stress was acknowledged to induce immune and vascular alterations, such as infection or hypertension, now it is known that also moderate stress independent of conventional risk factors can induce a potent alteration of health conditions and consequently shorten life quality and lifespan. If inflammation is a critical defense mechanism, that, uncontrolled, contributes to chronic conditions with inflammatory pathogenesis, stressful life conditions turn out to induce a diffuse (systemic) pro-inflammatory status. Moreover, if sub-clinical chronic inflammation is an important pathogenic factor in the development of metabolic syndrome, a cluster of common pathologies, including cardiovascular disease, will include markers associated with endothelial activation and dysfunction.

13. Perspectives

In fact, the comprehension of the mechanisms underlying inflammation and neuro-inflammation in aging and age-related disease is of particular importance as far as public health is concerned, since these diseases are characterized by a high rate of prevalence in the western countries and have a great impact in terms of social and economic costs. A better understanding of the mechanisms that cause such diseases will help to design new therapeutic approaches, particularly useful in the early phases of the diseases.

In particular, the correlation of data from the analysis of inflammatory mechanisms and new treatments based on iPSC (induced Pluripotent Stem Cells), will provide potentially useful markers to researchers and clinicians for possible new targets for treatments based upon lowering of pro-inflammatory status in age-related diseases.

Tissue stem cells' fate and age-related phenomena are quite related. The anatomical and physiological changes associated with advancing age emerge with variable onset, pace and severity in individuals, and affect organs and tissue types both with highly mitotic and quiescent profiles. In the whole organism, the hallmarks of aging include loss of muscle mass (sarcopenia), decreased musculoskeletal mobility, reduction in bone mass (osteoporosis), thinning and reduced elasticity of skin (wrinkling). The aging haematopoietic system exhibits progressive altered immune profiles. During lifetime, our bodies possess a remarkable ability for extensive and sustained tissue renewal. This continuous self-renewal capacity is maintained by reservoirs of somatic tissue stem cells (Sharpless & DePinho, 2007). These tissue stem cells have garnered increasing attention in aging and regenerative research given accumulating evidence that age-associated physiological decline, particularly in highly proliferative organs, parallels blunted proliferative responses and misdirected differentiation of resident tissue stem cells.

By a multidisciplinary approach using reprogrammed stem cell lines new bioassays for the identification of specific cell signatures, both genetic and epi-genetic, could be designed. For example, crossing cell lines from dementia-free healthy centenarians with Down syndrome's would allow to identify intrinsic or extrinsic maintenance mechanisms. Advanced post-genomic techniques may also be aimed to the definition of a signature of response of cells to different challenges (e.g: inflammation effectors, pathogens). In particular :

We need to validate of the hypothesis of "inflammaging" : characterization of the contribution of inflammation of the acceleration of senescence within biobank cell collections (dementia free centenarians vs. Down syndrome) and its consequences for phenotype stability.

We need to add new evidences linking inflammation and aging ("extrinsic aging") which does encompass the stem cell compartment as well, contributing to new insight on the "intrinsic" cell senescence mechanisms as they may depend on whole organisms compliance.

In addition, we need to validate the relevance of bio-products as cyto-protectants on engineered differentiated cells from patients specific iPSC : can they enhance their maintenance contributing to the inhibition of the "intrinsic" aging mechanism and / or the accelerated replicative senescence due to inflammatory challenge ("extrinsic" aging) ?

Finally, validate the possibility that *ex vivo* cell collections from dementia-free centenarians, as well as Down's syndrome could be characterized at the biologic, genetic and epigenetic level, characterizing their inflammatory phenotype (by system biology approach).

Coming towards an end, the reader should be alerted to a few conclusive remarks (Galeno, 1973; Issuree et al., 2009; Atzei, 2004).

Today our study contributes to enhance evidence for the relevance of a specific class of molecules contained in substances which may have been used either in the domesticated fruit and vegetable environment as food, such as the oleocantal ibuprofen-like molecule contained in olive oil (Beauchamp et al., 2005), or as ritual substances, such as the incense and myrrh (Nomicos, 2007) containing anti-inflammatory and mood modulating terpens. We presume that for centuries these raw materials were integrated in sacred recipes devoted to the maintenance of health and the prevention of aging, because of their content in biological active molecules, displaying their curing properties, either as anti-inflammatory remedies or inducing mood modulation allowing an enhanced perception of life.

But the question we will not be able to avoid is, if cell senescence can be moderated by plant molecules, we eat and drink (caffeine), drugs as potent as man ever has known, raising the problem of a new pharmaco-vigilance and a global change in our assumption on what is healthy and what is not, regardless of the elasticity of our lifespan.

14. References

AISA Patent Family n°1, "Composition for treating or preventing cell degeneration using at least one molecule capable of maintaining adhesion molecule expression reversibility and inhibit vascular endothelium actin fiber polymerization" (FR 2 869 230, WO 2005/105074, EP1748771, US-2009-0012162-A1).

AISA Patent Family n°2 « Use of a monoterpen to treat or prevent stress » (EP1990047, WO 2008/138905).

AISA Patent Family n°3 « Use of a monoterpene to increase tissue repair » (EP2042167, WO 2009/040420).

Atzei, A.D. (2004) « Le piante nella tradizione popolare della Sardegna » (Plants of the popular tradition in Sardinia) *Carlo Delfino ed.*, Sassari, Italy.

Atzmon, G., Cho, M., Cawthon, R.M., Budagov, T., Katz, M., Yang, X., Siegel, G., Bergman, A., Huffman, D.M., Schechter, C.B., Wright, W.E., Shay, J.W., Barzilai, N., Govindaraju, D.R., and Suh, Y. (2010) Evolution in health and medicine Sackler colloquium: Genetic variation in human telomerase is associated with telomere length in Ashkenazi centenarians. *Proc Natl Acad Sci U S A.* 107 Suppl 1, pp. 1710-7.

Babic, A., Linder, A.B., Vulic, M., Stewart, E.J., & Radman, M. (2008) Direct visualization of horizontal gene transfer. *Science*, 319(5869), pp. 1533-6.

Bagnara, G.P., Bonsi, L., Strippoli, P., Bonifazi, F., Tonelli, R., D'Addato, S., Paganelli, R., Scala, E., Fagiolo, U., Monti, D., Cossarizza, A., and, Bonafè, M., & Franceschi, C. (2000) Hemopoiesis in healthy old people and centenarians: well-maintained responsiveness of $CD34^+$ cells to hemopoietic growth factors and remodeling of cytokine network. *J Gerontol A Biol Sci Med Sci.* , 55, pp. B61-6.

Bazarov, A., Van Sluis, M., Hines, W.C., Bassett, E., Beliveau, A., Campeau, E., Mukhopadhyay, R., Lee, W.J., Melodyev, S., Zaslavsky, Y., Lee, L., Rodier, F., Chicas, A., Lowe, S.W., Benhattar, J., Ren, B., Campisi, J., & Yaswen, P. (2010) p16 (INK4a)-mediated suppression of telomerase in normal and malignant human breast cells. *Aging Cell*, 9, pp. 736-46.

Beauchamp, G.K., Keast, R.S., Morel, D., Lin, J., Pika, J., Han, Q., Lee, C.H., Smith, A.B., & Breslin, P.A. (2005) Phytochemistry: ibuprofen-like activity in extra-virgin olive oil. *Nature*, 437, pp. 45-6.

Biagi, E., Nylund, L., Candela, M., Ostan, R., Bucci, L., Pini, E., Nikkïla, J., Monti, D., Satokari, R., Franceschi, C., Brigidi, P., & De Vos, W. (2010) Through Ageing, and Beyond: Gut Microbiota and Inflammatory Status in Seniors and Centenarians. *PLoS ONE* 5, e10667 *PLoS One*, 17;5(5): e10667. Erratum in: PLoS One. 2010;5(6).

Bisson, J.F., Menut, C., & d'Alessio, P. (2008) New pharmaceutical interventions in aging. *Rejuvenation Research*, 11, 399-407.

Burridge, K., & Wennerberg, K. (2004) Rho and Rac take center stage. *Cell*, 116, pp. 167–179.

Campisi, J. (2011) Cellular senescence: putting the paradoxes in perspective. *Current opinion in genetics & development*, 21(1), pp. 107-12Epub ahead of print.

Chambers, S.M., Shaw, C.A., Gatza, C., Fisk, C.J., Donehower, L.A., & Goodell, M.A. (2007) Aging Hematopoietic stem Cells decline in Function and Exhibit Epigenetic Dysregulation. *PLOS Biology*, 5, pp. 1750-62.

Chandola, T., Britton, A., Brunner, E., Hemingway, H., Malik, M., Kumari, M., Badrick, E., Kivimaki, M., & Marmot, M. (2008) Work stress and coronary heart disease: what are the mechanisms? *European Heart Journal*, 29, pp. 640-8.

Clément, K., Viguerie, N., Poitou, C., Carette, C., Pelloux, V., Curat, C.A., Sicard, A., Rome, S., Benis, A., Zucker, J.D., Vidal, H., Laville, M., Barsh, G.S., Basdevant, A., Stich, V., Cancello, R., & Langin, D. (2004) Weight loss regulates inflammation-related genes in white adipose tissue of obese subjects. *FASEB J*,. 18, pp. 1657-69.

Crowell, P.L., Lin, S., Vedejs, E., & Gould, M.N. (1992) Identification of metabolites of the anti-tumor agent *d*-Limonene capable of inhibiting protein isoprenylation and cell growth. *Cancer Chemother Pharmacol*, 31, pp. 205–212.

d'Alessio, P. (2004) Aging and the endothelium. *Journal of Experimental Gerontology*, 39, pp.165-171.

Dali-Youcef, N., Lagouge, M., Froelich, S., Koehl, C., Schoojans, K., & Auwerx, J. (2007) Sirtuins: The "magnificient seven", function, metabolism and longevity. *Annals of Medicine*, 39, pp. 335-45.

de Keizer, P.L.J., Laberge, R.M., & Campisi, J. (2010) p53: Pro-aging or pro-longevity? " *Aging (Albany NY)*, 2, pp. 377-9.

de Kretser, D.M. (2010) Determinants of male health: the interaction of biological and social factors. *Asian Journal of Andrology*, 12, pp. 291-7.

De Martinis, M., Franceschi, C., Monti, D., & Ginaldi, L. (2005) Inflamm-ageing and lifelong antigenic load as major determinants of ageing rate and longevity. *FEBS Lett.* , 579, pp. 2035-9.

Degens, H. (2007) Age-related skeletal muscle dysfunction: causes and mechanisms. *J. Musculoskelet Neuronal Interact*, 7, pp. 246-52.

Dierick, J.F., Eliaers, F., Remacle, J., Raes, M., Fey, S.J., Larsen, P.M., & Toussaint, O. (2002) Stress-induced premature senescence and replicative senescence are different phenotypes, proteomic evidence. *Biochemical Pharmacology*, 64, pp. 1011-7.

Dillon, C., & Goda, Y. (2005) The actin cytoskeleton: integrating form and function at the synapse. *Annu Rev Neurosci.*, 28, pp. 25-55.

Donmez, G., & Guarente, L. (2010) Aging and disease: connections to sirtuins. *Aging Cell*, 9, pp. 285-90.

Edelman, G. (1993) The golden age for adhesion. Cell Adhes Commun., 1, pp. 1-7.

Ergen, A.V.V, & Goodell, M.A. (2009) Mechanisms of hematopoietic stem cell aging. *Experimental Gerontology*, 45, pp. 286-90.

Esler, M., Eikelis, N., Schlaich, M., Lambert, G., Alvarenga, M., Dawood, T., Kaye, D., Barton, D., Pier, C., Guo, L., Brenchley, C., Jennings, G., & Lambert, E. (2008) Chronic mental stress is a cause of essential hypertension: presence of biological markers of stress. *Clinical and Experimental Pharmacology and Physiology*, 35, pp. 498-502.

Farhadi, A., Banan, A., & Keshavarzian, A. (2003) Role of cytoskeletal structure in modulation of intestinal permeability. In : *Archives Iranian Medicine*, 6, pp. 49-53.

Franceschi, C., Bonafè, M., Valensin, S., Olivieri, F., De Luca, M., Ottaviani, E., & De Benedictis, G. (2000) An evolutionary perspective on immunosenescence. *Ann N Y Acad Sci*, 908, pp. 244-54.

Franceschi, C., Valensin, S., Lescai, F., Olivieri, F., Licastro, F., Grimaldi, L.M., Monti, D., De Benedictis, G., & Bonafe, M. (2001) Neuroinflammation and the genetics of Alzheimer's disease: the search for a pro-inflammatory phenotype. *Aging (Milano)*, 13, pp. 163-70.

Franceschi, C., Capri, .M., Monti, D., Giunta, S., Olivieri,i F., Sevini, F., Panourgia, M.P., Invidia, L., Celani, L., Scurti, M., Cevenini, E., Castellani, G.C, & Salvioli, S. (2007) Inflammaging and anti-inflammaging: a systemic perspective on aging and longevity emerged from studies in humans. *Mech Ageing Dev.*, 128, pp. 92-105.

Froy, O., & Miskin, R. (2010) Effect of fedding feeding regiments on circadian rhythms: Implications for aging and longevity. *Aging*, 2, pp. 7-27.

Galeno (Galen) *La dieta dimagrante* (The thinning diet), pp. 45-47 Paravia ed., 1973, Torino, Italy.

García-Cardeña, G., & Gimbrone, M.A. Jr. (2006) Biomechanical modulation of endothelial phenotype: implications for health and disease. *Handb Exp Pharmacol*, 2, pp. 79-95.

Hardcastle, I.R., Rowlands, M.G., Barber, A.M., Grimshaw, R.M., Mohan, M.K., Nutley, B.P., & Jarman, M. (1999) Inhibition of protein prenylation by metabolites of limonene. *Biochem Pharmacol*, 57, pp. 801- 809.

Harris, T.B., Ferrucci, L., Tracy, R.P., Corti, M.C., Wacholder, S., Ettinger, W.H. Jr, Heimovitz, H., Cohen, H.J., & Wallace, R. (1999) Associations of elevated interleukin-6 and C-reactive protein levels with mortality in the elderly. *Am J Med*, 106(5), pp. 506-12.

Herranz, D., Munos-Martin, M., Canamero, M., Mulero, F., Martinez-Pastor, B., Fernandez-Capetillo, O., & Serrano, M. (2009) Sirt1 improves healthy ageing and protects from metabolic syndrome-associated cancer. *Nature Communications*, 1, pp. 1-8.

Ingber, D.E. (2003) Mechanobiology and diseases of mechanotransduction. *Ann Med*,. 35, pp. 564-77.

Ingram, D.D., & Mussolino, M.E. (2010) Weight loss from maximum body weight and mortality: the Third National Health and Nutrition Examination Survey Linked Mortality File. *International Journal of Obesity*, 34, pp. 1044-50.

Issuree, P.D., Pushparaj, P.N., Pervaiz, S., & Melendez, A.J. (2009) Resveratrol attenuates C5a-induced inflammatory responses *in vitro* and *in vivo* by inhibiting phospholipase D and sphingosine kinase activities. *FASEB J*, 23, pp. 2412-2424.

Kirkwood, T.B.L. (2008) Healthy old age. *Nature*, 455, pp. 739-40.

Kitano, H. (2007) Towards a theory of biological robustness. *Mol Syst Biol*, 3:137.

Kolokotrones, T., Savage, V., Deeds, E.J., & Fontana, W. (2010) Curvature in metabolic scaling. *Nature*, 464, pp. 753-6.

MacPhail, R.C., (1987) Observational batteries and motor activity. *Zentralbl Bakteriol Mikrobiol Hyg B.*, 185, pp. 21-7.

Marconi, A., Darquenne, S., Boulmerka, A., Mosnier, M., & d'Alessio, P. (2003) Naftidrofuryl-driven regulation of endothelial ICAM-1 involves Nitric Oxide. *Free Rad Biol Med*, 34, pp. 616-625.

Mathieu, P., Lemieux, I.I., & Després, J.P. (2010) Obesity, Inflammation, and Cardiovascular Risk. *Clinical Pharmacology & Therapeutics*, 87, pp. 407-16.

May, L., van den Biggelaar, A.H., van Bodegom, D., Meij, H.J., de Craen, A.J., Amankwa, J., Frölich, M., Kuningas, M., & Westendorp, R.G. (2009) Adverse environmental conditions influence age-related innate immune responsiveness. *Immun Ageing,* 30, pp. 6-7.

Medeiros, R., Otuki, M.F., Avellar, M.C., & Calixto, J.B. (2007) Mechanisms underlying the inhibitory actions of the pentacyclic triterpene alpha-amyrin in the mouse skin inflammation induced by phorbol ester 12-O- tetradecanoylphorbol-13-acetate. *Eur J Pharmacol,* 559, pp. 227-35.

Millan, J., & Ridley, A.J. (2005) Rho GTPases and leucocyte-induced endothelial remodelling. *Biochem J,* 385, pp. 329–337.

Miller, J.A., Thompson, P.A., Hakim, I.A., Sherry Chow, H.H., & Thomson, C.A. (2011) d-Limonene: a bioactive food component from citrus and evidence for a potential role in breast cancer prevention and treatment. *Oncol Rev,* 5, pp. :31–42.

Naveiras, O., Nardi, V., Wenzel, P.L., Hauschka, P.V., Fahey, F., & Daley, G.Q. (2009) Bone-Marrow adipocytes as negative regulators of the haematopoietic microenvironment. *Nature,* 460, pp. 259-63.

Nomicos, E.Y. (2007) Myrrh: medical marvel or myth of the Magi? *Holist Nurs Pract,*. 21, pp. 308-23.

Ostan, R. , Bucci, L., Capri, M., Salvioli, S., Scurti, M., Pini, E., Monti, D., & Franceschi, C. (2008) Immunosenescence and immunogenetics of human longevity. et al. (2008) Immunosenescence and immunogenetics of human longevity. *Neuroimmunomodulation,* 15, pp. 224-40.

Petrascheck, M., Ye, X., & Buck, L.B. (2007) An antidepressant that extends lifespan in adult *Caenorhabditis elegans. Nature* 450, pp. 553-7.

Queré, N., Noël, E., Lieutaud, A. & d'Alessio, P., (2009) Fasciatherapy combined with Pulsology induces changes in blood turbulence potentially beneficial for the Endothelium. *J Bodyw Mov Ther.*, 3, pp. 239-45.

Ridker, P.M., Cushman, M., Stampfer, M.J., Tracy, R.P., & Hennekens, C.H. (1997) Inflammation, aspirin, and the risk of cardiovascular disease in apparently healthy men. *N Engl J Med,* 336(14) pp. 973-9. Erratum in: *N Engl J Med* 1997; 337(5): 356.

Rossi, D.J., D Bryder, D., Zahn, J.M., Ahlenius, H., Sonu, R., Wagers, A.J., & Weissman, I.L. (2005) Intrinsic alterations underlie hematopoietic stem cell aging. *Proc Natl Acad Sci U S A,* 102, pp. 9194-99.

Rossi, D.J., Jamieson, C.H., & Weissman, I.L. (2008) Stems cells and the pathways to aging and cancer. *Cell,* 132, pp. 681-96.

Sahin, E., & DePinho, R.A. (2010) Linking functional decline of telomeres, mitochondria and stem cells during ageing. *Nature,* 464, pp. 520-8.

Sharpless, N.E., & DePinho, R.A. (2007) How stem cells age and why this makes us grow old. *Nature,* 8, pp. 703-13.

Shibeshi, W.A., Young-Xu, Y., & Blatt, C.M. (2007) Anxiety worsens prognosis in patients with coronary artery disease. *Journal of American College of Cardiology,* 49, pp. 2021–2027.

Toussaint, O., Royer, V., Salmon, M., & Remacle, J. (2002) Stress-induced premature senescence and tissue ageing. *Biological Pharmacology,* 64, pp. 1007-9.

Vanier, B. (2005) Intercellular adhesion molecule-1 (ICAM-1) in ulcerative colitis. *Digestive Diseases Sciences,* 54, 313-327.

Vigushin, D.M., Poon, G.K., Boddy, A., English, J., Halbert, G.W., Pagonis, C., Jarman, M., & Coombes, R.C. (1998) Phase I and pharmacokinetic study of *d*-limonene in patients with advanced cancer. Cancer Research Campaign Phase I/II Clinical Trials Committee. *Cancer Chemother Pharmacol,* 42, pp. 111–117.

von Zglinicki, T., Bürkle, A., & Kirkwood, T.B.L. (2001) Stress, DNA damage and ageing - an integrative approach. *Experimental Gerontology,* 36, pp. 1049-62.

Walston, J., McBurnie, M.A., Newman, A., Tracy, R.P., Kop, W.J., Hirsch, C.H., Gottdiener, J., & Fried, L.P. (2002) Cardiovascular Health Study. Frailty and activation of the inflammation and coagulation systems with and without clinical comorbidities: results from the Cardiovascular Health Study. *Arch Intern Med,* 162(20), pp. 2333-41.

Xu, Y., Li, J., Ferguson, G.D., Mercurio, F., Khambatta, G., Morrison, L., Lopez-Girona, A., Corral, L.G., Webb, D.R., Bennett, B.L., & Xie, W. (2009) Immunomodulatory drugs reorganize cytoskeleton by modulating Rho GTPases. *Blood,* 114, pp. 338-45.

Yamada, Y., Marshall, S., Specian, R.D., & Grisham, M.B. (1992) A comparative analysis of two models of colitis in rats. *Gastroenterology,* 102, pp. 1524-34.

Zahradka, K., Slade, D., Bailone, A., Sommer, S., Averbeck, D., Petranovic, M., Linder, A.B., & Radman, M. (2006) Reassembly of shattered chromosomes in *Deinococcus radiodurans. Nature,* 443(7111), pp. 569-73.

Zhang, D.H., Marconi, A., Xu, L.M., Yang, C.X., Sun, G.W., Feng, X.L., Ling, C.Q., Qin, W.Z., Uzan, G., & d'Alessio, P. (2006) Tripterine inhibits the expression of adhesion molecules in activated endothelial cells. *Journ Leuko Biol,* 80, pp. 309-319.

Ziccardi, P., Nappo, F., Giugliano, G., Esposito, K., Marfella, R., Cioffi, M., D'Andrea, F., Molinari, A.M., & Giugliano, D. (2002) Reduction of inflammatory cytokine concentrations after weight loss over one year. *Circulation,* 105, pp. 804-9.

28

Molecular Biomarkers of Aging

Sergio Davinelli[1], Sonya Vasto[2], Calogero Caruso[2], Davide Zella[3] and Giovanni Scapagnini[1]
[1]Department of Health Sciences, University of Molise, Campobasso,
[2]Department of Pathobiology and Biomedical Methodologies, Immunosenescence Unit, University of Palermo, Palermo,
[3]Department of Biochemistry and Molecular Biology, Institute of Human Virology-School of Medicine, University of Maryland, Baltimore, MD,
[1,2]Italy
[3]USA

1. Introduction

In the Western World, the public perception of advanced aging involves the inability to survive due to chronic diseases and the combined loss of mobility, sensory functions, and cognition with an exponential growth of health costs. Therefore, biomarkers of human aging are urgently needed to assess the health state of elderly and the possible therapeutic interventions. Aging is considered a process that changes the performances of most physiological systems and increases susceptibility to diseases and death. The aging phenotype is a complex interaction of stochastic, environmental, genetic and epigenetic variables. However, these variables do not create the aging phenotype but favour the lost of molecular fidelity and therefore as the random accumulation of damages in the human organism's cells, tissues, or whole organism during life increases, the probability of disease and death also augments in proportion (Candore et al., 2008). What a biomarker for aging should be or predict is quite broadly defined. A biomarker should not only (i) reflect some basic property of aging, but also (ii) be reproducible in cross-species comparison, (iii) change independently of the passage of chronological time (so that the biomarker indicates biological rather than chronological age), (iv) be obtainable by non invasive means, and (v) be measurable during a short interval of life span. A biomarker should reflect the underlying aging process rather than disease (Warner et al., 2004). In addition, a set of biomarkers should be based on mechanisms described by major theories of aging. A sustained number of biomarkers are currently under investigation, such as inflammatory markers, markers of oxidative stress or markers of telomere shorthening but the definition of biomarker is strictly related to the understanding of the mechanisms of aging and we might not be able to define an ideal biomarker yet. Moreover, the biomarkers of aging discussed in literature, are associated not only to age but also to diseases Accordingly, it is crucial to monitor basic mechanisms that underlies the aging process. Noteworthy, a recent study reported that biomarkers of cardiovascular diseases (CVD) and diabetes are useful predictors of healthy aging (Crimmins et al., 2008).

Another problem, which is probably even more challenging, is to understand if a biomarker validated for rodents could be applied equally to humans.

Notably, it should be highlighted that mammalian cells have developed highly refined inducible systems against a variety of stressful conditions; upon stimulation, each one of these systems can be engaged concertedly to alleviate and hinder the manifestation of a distinctive age-related disorder. In this context, increasing scientific evidence supports a pivotal role for the heat shock proteins in the protection against oxidative stress and inflammation. Heat shock response is a fundamental cellular survival pathway, involving both transcriptional and post-trascriptional regulation. The impairment of this regulatory mechanism might directly contribute to the defective cellular stress response to oxidative stress and deregulation of inflammatory processes, which characterizes senescence.

In the present chapter, we will focus on the importance of biomarkers involved in inflammatory responses, oxidative stress but also markers based on immunosenescence. Additionally, we will describe the major experimental methods that are available in biogerontology for the interpretation of the aging phenotypes. In summary, we will present an overview on the current knowledge of the complex molecular and biological events leading to cellular senescence and how we can measure this progression to possibly improve our quality of life.

2. Aging and the immune system

Aging is accompanied by a general dysregulation in immune system function, commonly referred to as immunosenescence. This progressive deterioration affects both innate and adaptive immunity, although accumulating evidence indicates that the adaptive arm of the immune system may exhibit more profound changes. Most of our current understanding of immune senescence stems from clinical and rodent studies. Studies have suggested that aging is associated with increase permeability of mucosal barriers, decreased phagocytic activity of macrophages and dendritic cells (DCs), reduced natural killer (NK) cell cytotoxicity, and dysregulated production of soluble mediators such as cytokines and chemokines (Weiskopf et al., 2009). These alterations could lead to increased pathogen invasion and poor activation of the adaptive immune response mediated by T and B-lymphocytes. The age-related changes which occur in the adaptive and innate immune response are summarized in Table 1.

Aging, is also associated with quantitative and qualitative changes within the naive CD4+T-cell compartment (Aspinall & Andrew, 2000; Fulop et al., 2006; Kilpatrick et al., 2008). Decreased numbers of recent thymic emigrants (RTE), shortened telomeres, hyporesponsiveness to stimulation, decreased proliferative capacity, reduced IL-2 production, alterations in signal transduction and changes in cell surface phenotype (Whisler et al, 1996; Fulop et al., 2006; Kilpatrick et al., 2008) have all been reported. These changes likely contribute to the poor response to vaccines and increased susceptibility to infectious diseases and neoplasms reported for older adults (Webster, 2000; Effros, 2000; Herndler-Brandstetter et al., 2006).

Aging causes a shift in the ratio of naive to memory T-cells, with associated changes in the cytokine profile that favor increases in pro-inflammatory interleukin-1β (IL-1β), interleukin-6 (IL-6), interferon γ (IFNγ), tumor necrosis factor (TNFα), and transforming growth factor

(TGFβ) (Sansoni et al., 2008). The production of IL-6, but not IL-1β or TNF-α, by peripheral blood mononuclear cells increases in the elderly (Roubenoff et al., 1998), and IL-1β production increases in peripheral blood mononuclear cells in older animals (Chung et al., 2006). In contrast, IL-1β levels are higher and IL-6 levels lower in the livers of old rats than young rats (Rikans et al., 1999).

As the hematopoietic system ages, the immune function deteriorates, the lymphoid potential diminishes, and the incidence of myeloid leukemia increases (Rossi et al., 2005). Aging leads to increased stem cell dysfunction, and as a result leukemia can develop in failed attempts by the bone marrow to return to a homeostatic condition after stress or injury. Stem cells leave the hibernation state and undergo self-renewal and expansion to prevent premature hematopoietic stem cell (HSC) exhaustion under conditions of hematopoietic stress (Walkey et al., 2005). HSCs in older mice produce a decreased number of progenitors per cell, decreased self-renewal and increased apoptosis with stress (Janzen et al., 2006).

The remaining stem cells divided more rapidly as if to compensate for those that were lost. Stimulating old stem cells to grow more rapidly, perhaps by stress such as infrared (IR), puts stem cells at greater risk of becoming cancer cells because of acquired DNA damage.

Metabolically active senescent cells, identified by the biomarkers of cellular aging, such as the *γ-H2AX* foci and perhaps the senescence-associated β-galactosidase (SA-β-gal) enzyme, accumulate in aging primates (Herbig et al., 2006). Cellular senescence can be induced in one of two ways. Firstly, reactive oxygen species (ROS) may contribute to the plentiful single-strand breaks (SSBs) and double-strand breaks (DSBs) present in senescent cells (Sedelnikova et al., 2004); this is a form of telomere-independent stress-induced senescence. Alternatively, telomere-dependent uncapping of telomere DNA causes replicative senescence. An increase in oxidative stress is a more probable cause of HSC senescence than telomere erosion (Beauséjour et al., 2007). High doses of IR lead to apoptosis of HSCs, while lower doses cause HSCs to senesce and lose the ability to clone themselves (Wang et al., 2006). Furthermore, irradiated normal human fibroblasts and tumor cell lines can also lose their clonogenic potential and undergo to accelerated senescence (Mirzayans et al., 2005). The inhibition of tumorigenesis by cellular senescence is oncogene-induced and linked to increased expression of tumor suppressor genes cyclin-dependent kinase inhibitor 2A (*p16INK4a* or *CDKN2A*) and tumor protein 53 (*TP53*) via the DNA damage response (Bartkova et al., 2006). Recent research points to the p16INK4a protein being an important aging biomarker as its concentrations in peripheral blood exponentially increase with chronological age, reducing stem cell self-renewal (Liu et al., 2009). The few articles published to date linking radiation's health effects and p16INK4a can be paradoxical with regard to aging. A Chinese study showed the cumulative radiation dose of radon gas among uranium miners to be positively associated with the aberrant promoter methylation and inactivation of the *p16INK4a* and *O6-methylguanine-DNA methyltransferase* (MGMT) genes in sputum, perhaps indicating the early DNA damage and a greater susceptibility to lung cancer (Su et al., 2006).

The number and proliferation potential of stem cell populations, including those of the intestinal crypt and muscle, decrease with age, leading to a progressive deterioration of tissue and organ maintenance and function (Schultz et al., 1982; Martin et al., 1998). Macromolecular damage in general and DNA damage in particular, accumulate in HSCs with age (Rossi et al., 2007). The reduced ability to repair DNA DSBs leads to a progressive loss of HSCs and bone marrow cellularity during aging (Nijnik et al., 2007). In addition, high radiation dose (>12.5 Gy) from 45Ca, a bone-targeting beta-ray emitter (Barranco et al., 1969), resulted in marked reduction in marrow cellularity, similar to the one observed in normal aging indicating a possible contribution of the DNA-repair mechanisms to the aging process.

	IMMUNE BIOMARKERS	AGE-RELATED INCREASE	AGE-RELATED DECREASE
INNATE IMMUNE SYSTEM	Cytokines and Chemokines	Serum levels of IL6, IL1β and TNFα	
	NK cells	Total number of cells	Proliferative response
	Dendritic cells		Capacity to stimulate antigen specific T-cells
	Neutrophils		Bactericidal activity; Oxidative burst
	Macrophages		Phagocytic capacity
ADAPTIVE IMMUNE SYSTEM	T-lymphocytes	Release of proinflammatory cytokines	Number of naive T-cells; Diversity of the T-cell repertoire
	B-lymphocytes	Autoreactive serum antibodies	Number of naive B-cells; Antibody affinity; Generation of B-cell precursors

Table 1. Age-related changes in the innate and adaptive immune system.

3. Oxidative stress and inflammation as causes of aging

To date, there are several theories which attempt to explain the process of aging, such as telomere theory, caloric restriction, and evolutionary theory. The oxidative stress hypothesis/free radical theory of aging, updated by Harman in 2006 (Harman, 2006) offers a possible biological explanation of the entire aging process. In a biological context, a condition of oxidative stress occurs when there is an imbalance between oxidant molecules and antioxidant defensive molecules. Such critical balance is disrupted when antioxidants are depleted or if the formation of ROS increases beyond the ability of the antioxidative systems. Additionally, the free radical theory proposed that the production of intracellular ROS is the major determinant of life span.

However, the most critical problem is to find a correlation between oxidative biomarkers amounts and human health. Nevertheless, according to the free radical theory of aging, oxidative stress increases with increasing age resulting in oxidative DNA damage, protein oxidation and lipid peroxidation.

One of major risk markers of oxidative damage of nucleic acids is the 8-hydroxy-29-deoxyguanosine (8-OHdG). So far, 8-OHdG is the most studied oxidative DNA lesion and it is formed when ROS act on deoxyguanine in DNA (Ravanat et al., 2000). 8-OHdG can alter gene expression, inhibits methylation and its mutagenic potential leads to GC → AT conversion. The formation of 8-OHdG in leukocyte DNA and the excretion of 8-OHdG into urine have been frequently measured to assess oxidative stress in humans. However, even though interesting results have been obtained with 8-OHdG, several studies have associated aging with a progressive loss of antioxydant defence.

Recently, several findings have emphasized the importance of lipid peroxidation in relation to the role of caloric restriction and the extension of longevity (Sanz et al., 2006). Lipid peroxidation products have also been shown to be mutagenic and carcinogenic and has been implicated as the underlying mechanisms in numerous disorders including aging. Notably, lipid oxidation not only causes membrane disruption but also produces aldehydic species, such as malondialdehyde (MDA), able to perpetrate further damage by binding to and modifying proteins. Although producing contradictory results, the measure of lipid peroxidation is an example of biomarkers of oxidative stress. The measurement of MDA is very easy to perform, fast and not expensive. MDA is often utilized to evaluate human aging and in numerous studies MDA was significantly higher in healthy elderly, confirming the presence of increased lipoperoxidation in old age.

Another important product generated by lipid peroxidation is 4-hydroxy-2-nonenal (HNE) that reacts with nucleic acids, proteins, and phospholipids inducing many cytotoxic, mutagenic, and genotoxic effects (Uchida, 2003). Low-density lipoproteins (LDL) seems to be another good marker because oxidised LDL appears to be involved in the development of various pathological conditions aging related. Measurements of LDL could be obtained *in vivo* by measuring oxidised LDL particles in blood using immunological methods with appropriate specificity.

In addition, phosphatidylcholine hydroperoxides (PCOOH) measured in blood or tissue is also an acceptable marker of lipid peroxidation.

Recently, isoprostanes (IsoPs), compounds that are produced *in vivo* by free radical-induced peroxidation of arachidonic acid, have been also proposed to assess the oxidative stress status but we have only few experimental evidence and convincing outcomes have not emerged yet (Montuschi et al., 2007). Particularly, the analysis of F2-isoprostanes has revealed a role for free radicals and oxidant injury in a wide variety of human diseases. However, it must be taking into account that the measurement of F2-isoprostanes represents a snapshot of oxidant stress at a discrete point in time. Indeed, F2-isoprostanes are cleared rapidly from the circulation. However, such molecules that are stable isomers of prostaglandin F2, seems to be the best reliable marker and it has been proposed as most affidable index of systemic or " whole body" oxidative stress over time.

Closely related to oxidative stress is the protein oxidation. The main molecular characteristic of aging is the progressive accumulation of damages in macromolecules and age related damage in proteins have been reported in cells, tissues and organs (Rattan, 2006). The measurement of the protein oxidation is a clinically important factor for the prediction of the aging process and age-related diseases. The most widely studied oxidative stress-induced modification to proteins is the formation of carbonyl derivatives. Carbonyl formation can occur through a variety of mechanisms including direct oxidation of certain amino-acid side chains and oxidation-induced peptide cleavage. Furthermore, advanced oxidation protein products considered as biomarkers to estimate the degree of oxidative modifications of proteins and carbonyl groups may be introduced into proteins by reactions with aldehydes, reactive carbonyl derivatives or through their oxidation products with lysine residues of proteins. Although all organs and all proteins can potentially be modified by oxidative stress, certain tissues and specific protein may be especially sensitive. For istance, recent studies characterized oxidatively modified proteins in the brain and identified specific proteins that are oxidatively modified in Alzheimer' s disease (Butterfield & Sultana, 2007).

Aging is accompanied by chronic low-grade inflammation status and inflammatory mediators may be usefull to monitor aging processes. Molecular activation of pro-inflammatory genes by altered redox signaling pathways will eventually lead to inflamed tissues and organs. Accordingly, molecular inflammation is an important biological component of aging. In this perspective, nuclear factor of kappa light polypeptide gene enhancer in B-cells (NF-kβ) is a transcription factor that plays a pivotal role in modulating cellular signaling of oxidative stress-induced molecular inflammation. For example, stimulus-mediated phosphorylation and the subsequent proteolytic degradation of nuclear factor of kappa light polypeptide gene enhancer in B-cells inhibitor (Ikβ) allows the release and nuclear translocation of NF-κB, where transactivates several target genes such as forkhead box (*FOXO*), *IL-lβ*, *IL-6*, *TNFa*, adhesion molecules, cyclooxygenase-2 (*COX-2*) and nitric oxide synthases inducible (*iNOS*), all key players in inflammation.

Aging is associated with activation of both the innate and the adaptive immune system. As mentioned above, during aging increased blood levels of proinflammatory cytokines such as IL-6 and TNFa can be observed. In healthy elderly populations, high circulating levels of TNFa and IL-6 predict mortality, in a manner independent from comorbidity (Bruunsgaard & Pedersen, 2003).

Addionally, an inflammatory response appears to be the prevalent triggering mechanism driving tissue damage associated with different age-related diseases and the definition of "inflamm-aging" has been coined to explain the underlining inflammatory changes common to most age-associated diseases (Licastro et al. 2005).

Finally, reduced glutathione (GSH) is a major intracellular non-protein -SH compound and is accepted as the most important intracellular hydrophilic antioxidant (Melov, 2002). Glutathione system is the most important endogenous defense system against oxidative stress in body. Under oxidative conditions GSH is reversibly oxidized to glutathione disulfide (GSSG). A recent study on age-related changes in GSH in rat brain suggests a significant age-related reduction in the GSH level in all regions of the brain, associated with an increase in GSH oxidation to GSSG and decrease in the GSH/GSSG ratio (Zhu et al., 2006).

4. Methods for analysis of biological aging

The aging research requires multi- and transdisciplinary approaches and new high-throughput technologies are continually in development, increasing exponentially the amount of biological informations in aging research and elucidating complex unknown mechanisms. Although there have been extraordinary advances in study related to gene expression, proteomic and functional data, one challenge in aging research is to bring together this large variety of data that are still fragmented. Here, we provide a brief description of the main technological approaches for biomarkers discovery and for analyzing the molecular and cellular changes involved in aging cells. We also describe the major databases, computational tools and bioinformatics methods that are available in biogerontology for data interpretation of the aging phenotypes.

Analysis of gene-expression data has led to remarkable progress in many biomedical disciplines, including gerontology. Numerous methods have been developed for this analysis, but the emergence of high-throughput expression profiling and sequencing, such as microarray technology (Blalock et al., 2003) or more recently next-generation sequencing RNA-Seq have become diffusely used leading to breakthroughs in the investigations of aging (Twine et al., 2011). The application of microarray technology to gerontological studies has improved our understanding of mechanisms of aging (Golden & Melov, 2007) allowing to elucidate molecular differences associated with aging and to scan the entire genome for genes that change expression with age. The core principle of a microarray experiment is the hybridization of RNA/DNA strands of at least two different conditions, such as normal and disease or different ages, with a microarray chip. Briefly, the data collection is followed by bioinformatics analysis that require background noise subtraction, normalization and identification of statistically significant changes with dedicated software packages that calculate through multiple statistical measurements the significance for each gene. Ultimately, an application of transcriptomic microarray reported the first assessment of age-related alterations in gene expression in a large population-based cohort suggesting that modification of messenger RNA (mRNA) processing may comprise an important feature of human aging (Harries et al., 2011). In addition, an example of differential expression analysis in aging is the comparison of Ames dwarf mice *Prop1*$^{df/df}$ versus *Prop1*$^{+/+}$and Little mice *Ghrhr*$^{lit/lit}$ versus *Ghrhr*$^{+/lit}$ (Amador-Noguez et al., 2004). In both cases, the mutants show delayed aging with significantly increased lifespan and the authors found 1125 and 1152 differentially expressed genes in these mutants, respectively, using analysis of variance (ANOVA). There is a growing number of age-related molecular repositories and one database of gene expression profiles during aging is the Gene Aging Nexus, which features a compilation of aging microarray data and microarray datasets across different platforms and species (http://gan.usc.edu/) (Pan et al., 2007).

The genomic convergence approach is a new powerful method alternative to genome-wide association studies that combines trascriptional profiling, expression of quantitative trait mapping and gene association. Briefly, microarray technology are used to identify genes that show age-related changes in expression. In the next step single nucleotide polymorphisms (SNPs) are tested for association with the expression of age-regulated genes and finally the expression of quantitative trait loci (eQTLs) are tested for association with a phenotype of aging (Wheeler et al., 2009).

Currently, basic methods to understand biological processes and to identify possible candidate biomarkers for a specific pathology are shifted toward "omics" approaches, where all classes of biological compounds can be analyzed by respective "omic" techniques. To date, proteomic investigations have special relevance to aging-related research since altered protein interactions may have a key role in aging-related diseases. Different proteomic technology platforms were applied to define the proteomes and conventional techniques as two-dimensional gel electrophoresis (2DE), surface-enhanced laser desorption/ionization (SELDI), liquid chromatography-mass spectrometry (LC-MS), capillary electrophoresis (CE) coupled to mass spectrometry (CE-MS) and protein arrays are also associated to aging related studies. The proteomic analysis require adequate tools for data analysis and there are several bioinformatic approaches in proteomics. Many algorithms have now been designed to handle the increasing amount of data that are available thanks to proteomic analysis and numerous computational approaches and software tools have been developed to automatically assign candidate peptide sequences to fragment ion spectra, for example, SEQUEST, MASCOT or ProteinProspector. In addition, quantitative proteomics based on stable isotope labeling, such as isotope-coded affinity tags (ICAT) or stable isotope labeling by amino acids in cell culture (SILAC) represents a promising approach for aging studies providing important information to interpret protein biomarkers of age-related disease (Zhang et al., 2005). The investigation of changes in metabolite fluxes or the analysis of all metabolites in high-throughput fashion, called metabolomics (or metabonomics), is an attractive and expanding field in aging research. One goal of the metabolomics is to assess the impact of metabolite concentrations on aging phenotyope. Several studies have emerged with metabolomics approach traditionally using nuclear magnetic resonance (NMR) and recently MS techniques. An example of the application of MS-based metabolomics in aging research is given by Lawton et al. which analyzed the plasma of 269 individuals and discovered that age significantly altered the concentrations of over 100 metabolites (Lawton et al., 2008).

In addition, there are available for metabolomics researchers interested in aging databases for metabolite identification, such as METLIN that contains information on metabolites, as well as MS data (http://metlin.scripps.edu/) or The Human Metabolome Database (http://www.hmdb.ca/) with information on small molecule human metabolites.

Taking into account that the human aging phenotype is a highly polygenic trait which involves changes in genes involved in multiple processes and results from a combination of different factors, systems biology approach is particularly powerful in studies of aging. To date it seems to be the only method able to define and connect the large volumes of experimental data generated by "omics" fields. The final aim of the systems biology of aging is to generate an integrative approach which elucidates the molecular mechanisms of aging and to characterize this phenotype at systemic/organism level. In addition to quantify and integrate data produced by high-throughput technologies, the systems biology approach combines data-driven modelling and hypothesis-driven experimental studies in order to link aging phenotypes and its causes. One area in which sistems biology can be applied to aging research is the generation of a conceptual whole cell model that considers the dynamic behaviors of cellular metabolism. The whole cell representation is structured into subcellular entities not only connected by protein-protein interactions but also by process related to metabolism, oxidative stress or trascriptional regulation. The goal of aging cell modelling is to build a conceptual framework through the simulation of dynamic system and to make predictions about the aging phenotype. The systems biology community has developed tools and modeling platforms to facilitate the representation of metabolic and signaling pathways among biological processes and allowing the understanding of complex phenomena such as aging. Systems Biology Markup Language (SBML) is the main language for coding biological models and currently there are two softwares that support construction of models in SMBL, CellDesigner and JDesigner (Oda et al., 2005). Recently, by using SBML, McAuley et al. generated an *in silico* brain aging model which may help to predict aging-related brain changes in older people (McAuley et al., 2009). Most of genes and proteins exert their functions within a complex network of interactions and another applications of systems biolgy is the assemblage of interactomes. The building of interaction networks allow to define changes in interaction of proteins implicated in aging process that are involved in maintaining the integrity of the human genome. In the protein-protein interaction (PPI) networks, each protein is a node and each interaction an edge and the first attempt towards constructing a "human longevity network" via analysis of human PPIs was made by Budovsky et al. in 2007 (Budovsky et al., 2007). According to the BioGrid database, the authors constructed a "core longevity network" that comprises 153 longevity-associated proteins and 33 non-longevity-associated proteins that have connections with at least five longevity-associated proteins or more. Therefore, network-based approaches are notably valuable for deciphering complex biological systems providing insights about aging, longevity and age-related disease. In addition, there are several collections of online resources available for biogerontologists that can also serve for the visualization of protein-protein interactions. Databases focused on genes related to aging and/or longevity include GeneAge and AnAge featured by the Human Aging Genomic Resources (http://genomics.senescence.info/) that is a collection of databases and tools designed for understanding the genetics of human aging. GeneAge is a curated reference database of different searchable data sets of genes associated with the human aging phenotype. One possible approach of GeneAge is the visualizzation of protein-protein interactions with one or more genes as query but additional ways can be used to build genes and protein interaction networks in conjunction with data stored in interaction databases such as IntAct (Kerrien et al., 2007). There is an expanding number of age-related repositories, such as NetAge (http://netage-project.org/) which provides information on microRNA-regulated protein-protein interaction networks that are involved in aging and related processes. Furthermore, one gene expression database is AGEMAP (Zahn et al., 2007), which allows to analize multiple genes and mechanisms affect aging decribing changes in expression levels in different mouse tissues. Finally, one database on human aging which will be available to the public is MARK-AGE (http://www.mark-age.eu/), a large-scale integrated project supported by the European Community. The aim of this project is to conduct a population study in order to identify a set o biomarkers of aging.

The coordinate assessment of genotypes, trascriptional and proteomic profiles in association with system and computational biology strategies will be able to reach a comprehensive model for the study of human aging and longevity but also for healthy aging.

5. Conclusion

Biomarkers of aging are an hot topic and have the ability to improve our life. Various parameters are directly affected and altered during aging and several indicators are being used to evaluate the aging process. However, not all can be used as biomarker of aging because many of them are influenced by different factors such as diet, enviroment or type of tissue. In addition, some biomarkers are dependent by the methods used to measure them. Accordingly, there is not yet a "pure" biomarkers of aging and the markers discussed are related not only to age but also to disease.

Furthermore, it is a subject of debate whether the determination of biological age markers is really addressing aging itself, or if it indicates stress induced acceleration of the age process by exogenic factors.

Aging is a multi-dimensional process and these biomarkers could be used to monitor and identify the development of age-associated disease providing new anti-aging strategies.

6. Acknowledgment

The authors would like to thank all their collegues for helpful comments regarding this manuscript and the respective departments for the support.

7. Abbreviations

The abbreviations used are: CVD, cardiovascular diseases; DCs, dendritic cells; NK, natural killer; RTE, thymic emigrants; IL-1β, Interleukin-1β; IL-6, Interleukin-6; IFNγ, interferon γ; TNFα, tumor necrosis factor α; HSC, hematopoietic stem cell; SA-β-gal, Senescence-Associated β-galactosidase; ROS, reactive oxygen species; SSBs, single-strand breaks; DSBs, double-strand breaks; IR, infrared; *p16INK4a* or CDKN2A, cyclin-dependent kinase inhibitor 2A; TP53, tumor protein 53;MGMT,O6-methylguanine-DNAmethyltransferase;8-OHdG,8-hydroxy-29 deoxyguanosine; MDA, malondialdehyde; HNE, 4-hydroxy-2-nonenal; LDL, low-density lipoproteins; PCOOH, phosphatidylcholine hydroperoxides; IsoPs, isoprostanes; NF-kβ, nuclear factor of kappa light polypeptide gene enhancer in B-cells; Ikβ, nuclear factor of kappa light polypeptide gene enhancer in B-cells inhibitor; FOXO, forkhead box; COX-2, cyclooxygenase-2; GSH, reduced glutathione; GSSG, glutathione disulfide; mRNA, messenger RNA; SNPs, single nucleotide polymorphisms; eQTLs, expression of quantitative trait loci; 2DE, two-dimensional gel electrophoresis; SELDI, surface-enhanced laser desorption/ionization; MS, mass spectrometry; LC, liquid chromatography; CE, capillary electrophoresis; NMR, nuclear magnetic resonance; SBML, Systems Biology Markup Language; PPI, protein-protein interaction.

8. References

Amador-Noguez D, Yagi, K, Venable S., Darlington G. (2004). Gene expression profile of long-lived Ames dwarf mice and Little mice. *Aging Cell* 3(6):423-41.

Aspinall R. & Andrew D. (2000). Thymic involution in aging. *J Clin Immunol* 20(4): 250–256.

Barranco SC., Beers RF. Jr., Merz T. (1969). Marrow cell injury following Ca45 uptake in bone: changes in marrow and peripheral blood cellularity. *Am J Roetgenol Radium Ther Nucl Med* 106(4):794-801.

Bartkova J., Rezaei N., Liontos M., Karakaidos P., Kletsas D., Issaeva N., Vassiliou LV., Kolettas E., Niforou K., Zoumpourlis VC., Takaoka M., Nakagawa H., Tort F., Fugger K., Johansson F., Sehested M., Andersen CL., Dyrskjot L., Ørntoft T., Lukas J., Kittas C., Helleday T., Halazonetis TD., Bartek J., Gorgoulis VG. (2006). Oncogene-induced senescence is part of the tumorigenesis barrier imposed by DNA damage checkpoints. *Nature* 444(7119):633-637.

Beauséjour C. (2007). Bone marrow-derived cells: the influence of aging and cellular senescence. *Handb Exp Pharmacol* 180:67-88.

Blalock EM., Chen KC., Sharrow K, Herman JP., Porter NM., Foster TC., Landfield PW. (2003). Gene microarrays in hippocampal aging: statistical profiling identifies novel processes correlated with cognitive impairment. *J Neurosci* 23(9):3807-19.

Bruunsgaard H. & Pedersen BK. (2003). Age-related inflammatory cytokines and disease. *Immunol Allergy Clin North Am* 23(1):15-39.

Budovsky A, Abramovich A, Cohen R, Chalifa-Caspi V, Fraifeld V. (2007). Longevity network: construction and implications. *Mech Ageing Dev* 128(1):117-24.

Butterfield DA. & Sultana R. (2007). Redox proteomics identification of oxidatively modified brain proteins in Alzheimer's disease and mild cognitive impairment: insights into the progression of this dementing disorder. *J Alzheimers Dis* 12(1):61–72.

Candore G., Balistreri C.R., Listì F., Grimaldi M.P., Vasto S., Colonna-Romano G., Franceschi C., Lio D., Caselli G., Caruso G. (2006). Immunogenetics, gender, and longevity. *Ann N Y Acad Sci.* 1089:516-37.

Chung HY., Cesari M., Anton S., Marzetti E., Giovannini S., Seo AY., Carter C., Yu BP., Leeuwenburgh C. (2009). Molecular inflammation: underpinnings of aging and agerelated diseases. *Ageing Res Rev* 8(1):18-30.

Crimmins E., Vasunilashorn S., Kim J.K., Alley D. (2008). Biomarkers related to aging in human populations. *Adv Clin Chem* 46:161-216.

Effros RB. (2000). Long-term immunological memory against viruses. *Mech Aging Dev* 121 (1-3):161–171.

Fulop T., Larbi A., Douziech N., Levesque I., Varin A., Herbein G. (2006). Cytokine receptor signalling and aging. *Mech Ageing Dev* 127(6):526-37.

Golden TR., Melov S. (2007). Gene expression changes associated with aging in C. elegans. *WormBook* 12:1-12.

Harman D. (2006). Free radical theory of aging: An update. *Ann N Y Acad Sci* 1067: 1–12.

Harries LW., Hernandez D., Henley W., Wood AR., Holly AC., Bradley-Smith RM., Yaghootkar H., Dutta A., Murray A., Frayling TM., Guralnik JM., Bandinelli S., Singleton A., Ferrucci L., Melzer D. (2011). Human aging is characterized by focused changes in gene expression and deregulation of alternative splicing. *Aging Cell* doi: 10.1111/j.1474-9726.2011.00726.x.

Herbig U., Ferreira M., Condel L., Carey D., Sedivy JM. (2006). Cellular senescence in aging primates. *Science* 311(5765):1257.

Herndler-Brandstetter D., Cioca DP., Grubeck-Loebenstein B. (2006). Immunizations in the elderly: do they live up to their promise? *Wien med Wochenschr* 156(5-6): 130–141.

http://gan.usc.edu/

http://metlin.scripps.edu/

http://www.hmdb.ca/

http://genomics.senescence.info/

http://netage-project.org/

http://www.mark-age.eu/

Janzen V., Forkert R., Fleming HE., Saito Y., Waring MT., Dombkowski DM., Cheng T., DePinho RA., Sharpless NE., Scadden DT. (2006). Stem-cell ageing modified by the cyclin-dependent kinase inhibitor p16INK4a. *Nature* 443(7110):421-426.

Kerrien S., Alam-Faruque Y., Aranda B., Bancarz I., Bridge A., Derow C., Dimmer E., Feuermann M., Friedrichsen A., Huntley R., Kohler C., Khadake J., Leroy C., Liban A., Lieftink C., Montecchi-Palazzi L., Orchard S., Risse J., Robbe K., Roechert B., Thorneycroft D., Zhang Y., Apweiler R., Hermjakob H. (2007). IntAct open source resource for molecular interaction data. *Nucleic Acids Res* 35:D561–D565.

Kilpatrick RD., Rickabaugh T., Hultin LE., Hultin P., Hausner MA., Detels R., Phair J., Jamieson BD. (2008). Homeostasis of the naive CD4+ T cell compartment during aging. *J Immunol* 180(3):1499–1507.

Lawton KA., Berger A., Mitchell M., Milgram KE., Evans AM., Guo L., Hanson RW., Kalhan SC., Ryals JA., Milburn MV. (2008). Analysis of the adult human plasma metabolome. *Pharmacogenomics* 9(4):383-97.

Licastro F., Candore G., Lio D., Porcellini E., Colonna-Romano G., Franceschi C., Caruso C. (2005). Innate immunity and inflammation in Aging: a key for understanding age-related diseases. *Immun Aging* 18;2:8.

Liu Y., Sanoff HK., Cho H., Burd CE., Torrice C., Ibrahim JG., Thomas NE., Sharpless NE. (2009). Expression of *p16INK4a* in peripheral blood T-cells is a biomarker of human aging. *Aging Cell* 8(4):439 448.

Martin K., Kirkwood TB., Potten CS. (1998). Age changes in stem cells of murine small intestinal crypts. *Exp Cell Res* 241(2):316-323.

McAuley MT., Kenny RA., Kirkwood TB., Wilkinson DJ., Jones JJ., Miller VM. (2009). A mathematical model of aging-related and cortisol induced hippocampal dysfunction. *BMC Neurosci* 10:26.

Melov S. (2002). Animal models of oxidative stress, aging and therapeutic antioxidant interventions. *Int J Biochem Cell Biol* 34(11):1395–1400.

Mirzayans R., Scott A., Cameron M., Murray D. (2005). Induction of accelerated senescence by gamma radiation in human solid tumor-derived cell lines expressing wild-type *TP53*. *Radiat Res* 163(1):53-62.

Montuschi P., Barnes P., Roberts LJ 2nd. (2007). Insights into oxidative stress: the isoprostanes. *Curr Med Chem* 14(6):703-17.

Nijnik A., Woodbine L., Marchetti C., Dawson S., Lambe T., Liu C., Rodrigues NP., Crockford TL., Cabuy E., Vindigni A., Enver T., Bell JI., Slijepcevic P., Goodnow CC., Jeggo PA., Cornall RJ. (2007). DNA repair is limiting for haematopoietic stem cells during ageing. *Nature* 447(7145):686-690.

Oda K., Matsuoka Y., Funahashi A., Kitano H. (2005). A comprehensive pathway map of epidermal growth factor receptor signaling. *Mol Syst Biol* 1:2005.0010.

Pan F., Chiu CH., Pulapura S., Mehan MR., Nunez-Iglesias J., Zhang K., Kamath K., Waterman MS., Finch CE., Zhou XJ. (2007). Gene aging nexus: a web database and data mining platform for microarray data on aging. *Nucleic Acids Res* 35: D756-D9.

Rattan SI. (2006). Theories of biological aging: Genes, proteins and free radicals. *Free Radic Res* 40(12):10–12.

Ravanat JL., Di Mascio P., Martinez GR., Medeiros MH., Cadet J. (2000). Singlet oxygen induces oxidation of cellular DNA. *J Biol Chem 275*(51): 40601–40604.

Rikans LE., DeCicco LA., Hornbrook KR., Yamano T. (1999). Effect of age and carbon tetrachloride on cytokine concentrations in rat liver. *Mech Ageing Dev* 108(2):173-182.

Rossi DJ., Bryder D., Seita J., Nussenzweig A., Hoeijmakers J., Weissman IL. (2007) Deficiencies in DNA damage repair limit the function of haematopoietic stem cells with age. *Nature* 447(7145):725 729.

Rossi DJ., Bryder D., Zahn JM., Ahlenius H., Sonu R., Wagers AJ., Weissman IL. (2005). Cell intrinsic alterations underlie hematopoietic stem cell aging. *Proc Natl Acad Sci U S A* 102(26):9194-9199.

Roubenoff R., Harris TB., Abad LW., Wilson PW., Dallal GE., Dinarello CA. (1998). Monocyte cytokine production in an elderly population: effect of age and inflammation. *J Gerontol A Biol Sci Med Sci* 53(1):M20-6.

Sansoni P., Vescovini R., Fagnoni F., Biasini C., Zanni F., Zanlari L., Telera A., Lucchini G., Passeri G., Monti D., Franceschi C., Passeri M. (2008). The immune system in extreme longevity. *Exp Gerontol* 43(2):61-65.

Sanz A., Pamplona R., Barja G. (2006). Is the mitochondrial free radical theory of aging intact? *Antioxid Redox Signal* 8(3-4):582–599

Schultz E. & Lipton BH. (1982). Skeletal muscle satellite cells: changes in proliferative potential as function of age. *Mech Ageing Dev* 20(4):377-383.

Sedelnikova OA., Horikawa I., Zimonjic DB., Popescu NC., Bonner WM., Barrett JC. (2004). Senescing human cells and ageing mice accumulate DNA lesions with unrepairable double-strand breaks. *Nat Cell Biol* 6(2):168-170.

Su S., Jin Y., Zhang W., Yang L., Shen Y., Cao Y., Tong J. (2006). Aberrant promoter methylation of *p16INK4a* and *O6-methylguanine-DNA methyltransferase* genes in workers at a Chinese uranium mine. *J Occup Health* 48(4):261 266.

Twine NA., Janitz K., Wilkins MR., Janitz M. (2011). Whole transcriptome sequencing reveals gene expression and splicing differences in brain regions affected by Alzheimer's disease. *PLoS One* 6(1):e16266.

Uchida K. (2003). 4-Hydroxy-2-nonenal: a product and mediator of oxidative stress. *Prog Lipid Res* 42(4):318–343.

Walkley CR., Fero ML., Chien WM., Purton LE., McArthur GA. (2005). Negative cell-cycle regulators cooperatively control self-renewal and differentiation of haematopoietic stem cells. *Nat Cell Biol* 7(2):172-178.

Wang Y., Schulte BA., LaRue AC., Ogawa M., Zhou D. (2006). Total body irradiation selectively induces murine hematopoietic stem cell senescence. *Blood* 107(1):358-366.

Warner HR. (2004) Current status of efforts to measure and modulate the biological rate of aging. *J Gerontol A Biol Sci Med Sci* 59(7):692-6.

Webster RG. (2000). Immunity to influenza in the elderly. *Vaccine* 18(16): 1686–1689.

Weiskopf D., Weinberger B., Grubeck-Loebenstein B. (2009). The aging of the immune system. *Transpl Int* 22(11):1041–1050.

Wheeler HE., Metter EJ., Tanaka T., Absher D., Higgins J., Zahn JM., Wilhelmy J., Davis RW., Singleton A., Myers RM., Ferrucci L., Kim SK. (2009). Sequential use of transcriptional profiling, expression quantitative trait mapping, and gene association implicates MMP20 in human kidney aging. *PLoS Genet* 5(10):e1000685.

Whisler RL., Newhouse YG., Bagenstose SE. (1996). Age-related reductions in the activation of mitogen-activated protein kinases p44mapk/ERK1 and p42mapk/ ERK2 in human T cells stimulated via ligation of the T cell receptor complex. *Cell Immunol* 168(2): 201–210.

Zahn JM., Poosala S., Owen AB., Ingram DK., Lustig A., Carter A., Weeraratna AT., Taub DD., Gorospe M., Mazan-Mamczarz K., Lakatta EG., Boheler KR., Xu X., Mattson

MP., Falco G., Ko MS., Schlessinger D., Firman J., Kummerfeld SK., Wood WH 3rd., Zonderman AB., Kim SK., Becker KG. (2007). AGEMAP: a gene expression database for aging in mice. *PLoS Genet* 3(11):e201.

Zhang J., Goodlett DR., Peskind ER., Quinn JF., Zhou Y., Wang Q., Pan C., Yi E., Eng J., Aebersold RH., Montine TJ. (2005). Quantitative proteomic analysis of age-related changes in human cerebrospinal fluid. *Neurobiol Aging* 26(2):207-27.

Zhu Y., Carvey PM., Ling Z. (2006). Age-related changes in glutathione and glutathione-related enzymes in rat brain. *Brain Res* 1090(11):35–44.

29

Female Vascular Senescence

Susana Novella[1], Ana Paula Dantas[2], Gloria Segarra[1], Carlos Hermenegildo[1] and Pascual Medina[1]
[1]*Departamento de Fisiología, Universitat de València, Instituto de Investigación Sanitaria INCLIVA, Hospital Clínico Universitario, Valencia,*
[2]*Institut d'Investigacions Biomèdiques August Pi i Sunyer (IDIBAPS) Institut Clinic de Tòrax, Hospital Clinic Barcelona*
Spain

1. Introduction

Long before the existence of cardiovascular imaging, Sir William Osler axiom that *"man is as old as his arteries"*. Followed by several physicians for decades, this aphorism has been widely confirmed by studies demonstrating that risk factors for cardiovascular disease increase as we age (Cooper et al., 1994; Lakatta & Levy, 2003). Nevertheless, a flaw in this statement is the generalization that men and women age similarly. Much data from clinical and basic research have established that vascular aging in women does not follow the same chronology as in men (Shaw et al., 2006; Pereira et al., 2010; Takenouchi et al., 2009). If known risk factors that influence cardiovascular aging are excluded (e.g. smoking, cholesterol, hypertension), men display a pattern of progressive vascular aging, while timing for vascular aging in women presents a clear hallmark, i.e. menopause (Taddei et al., 1996; Bucciarelli & Mannucci, 2009). Until menopause women are considered "hemodynamically younger" than men, based on epidemiological studies showing that the incidence of cardiovascular diseases in premenopausal women is markedly low compared to age-matched men (Messerli et al., 1987; Bairey Merz et al., 2006; Shaw et al., 2006). After menopause, however, these numbers rise to values that are close, or even higher, to those found in men (Lerner & Kannel, 1986; Eaker et al., 1993; Eaker et al., 1994). And so it one could say that *"man is as old as his arteries, although the arteries of a woman are as young as her hormones"*.

Cardiovascular disease is the primary cause of death among women after menopause (55%), compared to men (43%) even above all cancers combined (Rosamond et al., 2008). With increasing recognition of the importance of cardiovascular disease in women, the interest and emphasis on research concerning women and cardiovascular disease have grown substantially (Bairey Merz et al., 2006; Shaw et al., 2006). Despite this, there is still a concerning gap in the knowledge, understanding, and general awareness of mechanisms for cardiovascular aging in women. In this review, we will discuss clinical and experimental data that document the effects of aging, estrogens and hormonal replacement therapy on vascular function of females.

2. Effects of aging on vascular function

Vascular aging is a natural phenomenon that could be simply described as a consequence of physical stress. Arteries are elastic tissues, and as such are predisposed to fatigue and fracture with time, as a consequence of extension-relaxation cycles during heartbeats (Avolio et al., 1983; Avolio et al., 1985; O'Rourke & Hashimoto, 2007). In fact, fracture of elastic lamellae is observed with aging in aorta, and can account for the major physical changes seen in elder: dilation (after fracture of load-bearing material) and stiffening (by transfer of stress to the more rigid collagenous component of the arterial wall) (Lakatta, 2003).

There is growing evidence that vascular aging begins early in life, with evidence for alteration in vascular matrix proteins as early as the third decade in health individuals (Wallace, 2005; Tracy, 2006; Redheuil et al., 2010). This theory is mathematically supported by engineering studies establishing that fatigue and fracture of 10% of natural rubber occurs at $8x10^8$ extension-relaxation cycles, which is equivalent to 30 years at a heart rate of 70 beats/min (O'Rourke & Hashimoto, 2007). Biologically, a combination of imaging and histology studies have described age-associated increase in arterial thickening and a progressive reduction in aortic strain and distensibility, and have linked those changes to increased risk for cardiovascular disease (Lakatta & Levy, 2003; Lakatta, 2003; O'Rourke & Nichols, 2005; Redheuil et al., 2010). Although age-associated remodeling of arterial wall has been mostly described in patients with established risk for cardiovascular disease, few recent studies have shown similar age-related changes in healthy asymptomatic individuals (Redheuil et al., 2010). Similar age-related effects on arterial remodeling have been described in rodents and non-human primate without risk factors for cardiovascular disease, strengthening the hypothesis that aging *per se* can cause a series of alterations on mechanical properties that affect vascular function and lead to subsequent increased risk of cardiovascular disease.

Besides mechanical modifications, aging is also associated with several biochemical changes that are also implicated on the development and progression of cardiovascular disease. Dysfunction of both endothelial and smooth muscle molecular signaling appear to occur during aging process and favors vasospasm, thrombosis, inflammation and abnormal cell migration and proliferation (Lakatta, 2003; Briones et al., 2005; Barton, 2010; Herrera et al., 2010). The presence of endothelial dysfunction in the elder has been largely associated with malfunctioning of vascular tissue resulting, in turn, into cardiovascular disease (including atherosclerosis, hypertension or coronary artery disease) (Lakatta, 2003; Herrera et al., 2010), as well as renal dysfunction (Schmidt et al., 2001; Erdely et al., 2003), Alzheimer (Price et al., 2004) and erectile dysfunction (Burnett, 2006).

The mechanisms for age-associated endothelial dysfunction are multiple, though they are mostly associated to a decrease on nitric oxide (NO) bioavailability (Hayashi et al., 2008; Santhanam et al., 2008; Erusalimsky, 2009; Kim et al., 2009). NO is the major vascular messenger molecule involved in many physiological processes, including vasodilation and inhibition of thrombosis, cell migration and proliferation (Dudzinski & Michel, 2007; Lamas et al., 2007; Michel & Vanhoutte, 2010). Reduced endothelium-dependent and NO-mediated vasodilation has been described during aging in both human and animal models (Kim et al., 2009; Virdis et al., 2010).

A lower NO production in elderly may be based in either decreased NO synthesis or increased NO degradation. Several mechanisms to explain a reduction on NO production have been pointed out and include: 1) a decrease on the expression of endothelial NO synthase (eNOS) (Briones et al., 2005; Yoon et al., 2010); 2) a deficiency on NO precursor (L-arginine) (Santhanam et al., 2008) and eNOS cofactor (tetrahydrobiopterin - BH_4) (Yoshida et al., 2000; Eskurza et al., 2005); or 3) an increase of endogenous eNOS inhibitors (asymmetric dimethylarginine - ADMA) (Xiong et al., 2001; Kielstein et al., 2003). On the other hand, strong evidences support the hypothesis that age-associated increase in oxidative stress, and consequent production of superoxide anion (O_2^-) is a potent contributor to lowering NO bioavailability and increasing endothelial dysfunction (Jacobson et al., 2007; Rodriguez-Manas et al., 2009).

Despite the decline in NO bioavailability could sufficiently explain most of the changes in the functioning of vascular cells, other molecules that are crucial to control vascular function have also been described to be modified by aging. In the regulation of vasomotion, cyclooxygenase (COX)-derived factors are of particular importance as they control both vascular relaxation and contraction. Under normal condition, COX-derived relaxing (PGI_2) and contracting (TXA_2 and PGH_2) are in perfect balance, and few studies have reported a prevalence in the production of relaxing COX factors in the vasculature of young and healthy individuals. During aging, however, a swap in this balance favoring to the release of contracting factors occurs, leading to an increase of vascular contraction. Moreover, activation of inflammatory pathways in the vascular wall plays a central role in the process of vascular aging. Several studies have created an important link between arterial aging and a pro-inflammatory endothelial phenotype, even in the absence of traditional risk factors for atherosclerosis. An age-associated shift to a pro-inflammatory gene expression profile, known as endothelial activation, induces up-regulation of cellular adhesion molecules and cytokines which increases endothelial-leukocyte interactions and permeability, mechanisms considered crucial on the initial steps for the development of atherosclerosis (Herrera et al., 2010; Seals et al., 2011).

Even though endothelial function is undoubtedly impaired in the elderly, how aging affects molecular biochemistry of vascular cells is largely unknown. Going back to the observation that vascular aging is a consequence of mechanical fatigue, one might speculate that the mechanical forces on the vascular wall could contribute to the damage on endothelial cell functioning. In fact, it is well known that blood vessels are under constant mechanical loading from flowing blood which cause internal stresses, known as endothelial shear stress (caused by flow) and circumferential stretch (caused by pressure). These mechanical forces not only cause morphological changes of endothelium and blood vessel wall, but also trigger a myriad of intracellular events in endothelial cells and activate biochemical and biological events (Lu & Kassab, 2011). The triggering of endothelial signaling by mechanic forces seems to be mostly determined by the cytoskeleton, which represents a highly dynamic network that constantly assembles and disassembles, playing an active role in responding to mechanical stimuli (Wong et al., 1983). The cytoskeleton rearranges upon changes on stress and stretch and activates signaling molecules, such as NO production, that are capable to regulate vascular tone in order to keep homeostasis (Su et al., 2005; Su et al., 2007). An increase in arterial wall stiffening by aging could alter the impact of a mechanical stimulus, and therefore induce a significant reduction or dysfunction in the signaling pathways activated by shear stress (Kliche et al., 2011). In this regard, the chronically stiffed cells will lead to a decrease of NO, which will eventually lead to endothelial dysfunction.

Continuous damage to the endothelium from the daily pounding of the cycling pressure can also activate maintenance repair systems. When maintenance system is efficient (as in young individuals), endothelial cells likely correct the defect and keep going. On the other hand, when an irreversible damage occur or when endothelial cells are senescent, those inefficient cells are eventually eliminated by a mechanism yet to be described, while a "sister" circulating progenitor endothelial cells assume some repair function and will divide to fill up the gap (Thorin & Thorin-Trescases, 2009). Recent findings on progenitor stem cell research suggest that continuous division of progenitor endothelial cells for maintenance is likely the main response of an injured endothelium (Hill et al., 2003; Van Craenenbroeck & Conraads, 2010). Continuous cell division during life causes shortening in telomeres, a region of repetitive DNA sequences at the end of a chromosome, which protects the chromosomes from deterioration (Allsopp et al., 1995). Increasing evidence have support a role for reduction on telomere length with changes on cellular function and cellular senescence that may contribute to increased risk of vascular damage. In the long term, therefore, the regenerated endothelium may become dysfunctional as senescent endothelial cells start to express a pro-inflammatory, pro-oxidative, and pro-atherogenic phenotype (Chang & Harley, 1995; Bekaert et al., 2007; De Meyer T. et al., 2011).

In addition to mechanical fatigue, the vascular endothelium also undergoes important oxidative damage. The free-radical theory of aging states that organisms age because cells accumulate oxidative stress damage over time (de Grey, 2006; Camici et al., 2011). In other words, one can say that the body literally *"rusts"* with time. Growing evidence from research studies have supported this theory and have described an intimate relationship of increased oxidative stress with vascular dysfunction and increased risk for cardiovascular disease (Touyz, 2003; Griendling & Alexander, 1997; Harrison, 1997). Numerous studies underscore the importance of dysregulated oxidant and antioxidant balance in advancing age (Moon et al., 2001) and in the development and progression of atherosclerosis (Wassmann et al., 2004). Aging-associated increase in reactive oxygen species (ROS) are common to many species and despite decades of investigation, the mechanisms for the aging-related increase in ROS and how they affect vascular function have yet to be defined.

The main ROS proposed to be implicated on vascular aging process is the O_2^-. Increased O_2^- in the vessel wall has been well associated with decrease of NO bioavailability due to its rapid interaction and inactivation by O_2^-. In this regard, an increase of oxidative stress, and more specifically O_2^-, during aging could cause vascular damage simply by reducing the protective effect of NO in the vessel wall (Squadrito & Pryor, 1998; Harrison, 1997). However, increased oxidative stress has been implicated in more complex modulatory mechanisms that may affect vascular function by aging. Numerous studies have demonstrated that increase of oxidative stress contributes to the activation of transcriptional factors (such as NF-κB) that are key regulators of endothelial activation. By this way, aging-associated increase of ROS could favor endothelial cells to express a pro-inflammatory phenotype and increase the risk for cardiovascular disease (Herrera et al., 2010).

But proper vascular function does not lean on endothelium only. Vascular smooth muscle cells comprised by medial layer of blood vessels represent a dynamic component of the vasculature, and thus may also be affected by aging. In fact, vascular smooth muscle cells degenerate and decrease in number when subjects reach middle or advanced age. Smooth muscle cells are intercalated between the elastic lamina and the elastic fibers that also undergo a process of degeneration, thinning, sectioning, fracture and decrease in volume with aging. In parallel, there is a marked increase on collagen fibers, mucinous substrate, and calcification of the intercellular substrates begins (Toda et al., 1980).

Biochemical studies have shown that the content of elastin in human aorta decreases with age (Spina et al., 1983). Large amounts of elastin are produced during the fetal or neonatal period but not later (Godfrey et al., 1993). An age-related decrease in the cross-links in elastin contributes significantly to the reduction in arterial elasticity (Watanabe et al., 1996). As the turnover of elastin and collagen requires a very long period of time (lasting more than 10 years), these molecules are likely to undergo the addition of a sugar or a glycooxidative reaction. Thus, advanced glycation end-products accumulate in the arteries with age and partially contribute to age-related arterial stiffness (Konova et al., 2004; Semba et al., 2009). Type I, III, and V collagens are the major components of the collagen fibers of large conductance vessels such as aorta. During infancy or early childhood, collagen fibers are absent in the aorta and begin to accumulate with age; this process is known as fibrosis or sclerosis. Most studies have shown an age-related increase in the collagen content in the aorta (Spina et al., 1983) and increase in the number of collagen cross-links (Watanabe et al., 1996). Both an increase in the collagen content and the number of cross-links contributes significantly to the stiffening of the elastic arteries, namely atherosclerosis.

Senescent vascular smooth muscle cells have been shown to exhibit a pro-calcificatory/osteoblastic phenotype (Reid & Andersen, 1993; Burton, 2009; Nakano-Kurimoto et al., 2009), that could play a major role in the pathophysiology of age-related vascular calcification, a well-known major risk factor for the development of cardiovascular diseases (Adragao et al., 2004; Thompson & Partridge, 2004). Calcification in tunica media (medial calcification) increases throughout ageing, and accumulation of calcium in the elastin-rich layer of the media is ≥30-times more in the thoracic aorta at 90 years of age than that at 20 years of age (Elliott & McGrath, 1994). The underlying mechanisms that lead to the development of vascular calcification currently remain elusive. Calcification in the media usually occurs in the absence of macrophages and lipids, and is associated with α-smooth muscle actin-positive vascular smooth muscle cells, suggesting that vascular smooth muscle cells are the main key player in medial calcification (Luo et al., 1997). Alternatively, ROS may have some involvement in the osteoblastic transition of vascular smooth muscle cells (Byon et al., 2008).

Researchers have examined the role of the redox state in vascular smooth muscle cells in the pathogenesis of vascular disease (Clempus & Griendling, 2006; Lyle & Griendling, 2006). Vascular smooth muscle cells present in atherosclerotic lesions proliferate more rapidly and show increased expression of genes for growth factors and other molecules involved in extracellular matrix remodeling (Schwartz, 1997; Newby, 2006). Proliferation of vascular smooth muscle cells is part of the initiation and the progression of atherosclerosis (Ross, 1993) and may occur in response to injury or as a result of aberrant apoptosis (Clarke et al., 2006). Besides, vascular smooth muscle cells appear to undergo an age-associated phenotypic modulation toward a dedifferentiated and synthetic state. Smooth muscle cell migration from the medial to the intimal compartment is a plausible mechanism for the increased number of vascular smooth muscle cells within the diffusely thickened intima of central arteries as animals age (Miller et al., 2007).

In general, growth factors and hormones are the most potent activators that stimulate vascular smooth muscle growth, migration, and extracellular matrix synthesis. For instance, angiotensin II (Ang II) signaling has been widely linked to an age-associated increase in the migratory capacity of vascular smooth muscle cells and to the proinflammatory features of arterial aging. Ang II increases within the aged arterial wall and activates matrix metalloproteinase type II (MMP2) (Wang et al., 2003; Jiang et al., 2008). Ang II appears to initiate growth-promoting signal transduction through ROS-sensitive tyrosine kinases (Frank & Eguchi, 2003; Touyz et al., 2003).

3. Gender differences on vascular aging

Although arteries from females are so exposed to mechanical and oxidative damage as arteries from males, they seem do not follow the same time course for vascular aging, or at least, they do not age in the same way. Experimental and clinical studies support the hypothesis that men are hemodynamically older than age-matched, premenopausal women (Messerli et al., 1987; Bairey Merz et al., 2006; Shaw et al., 2006). With aging, the progression of cardiovascular disease occurs at an earlier age and become more severe in males compared to age-matched premenopausal females (Taddei et al., 1996; Virdis et al., 2010).

Arterial stiffening and distensibility are established markers for vascular aging and have been found to progressively increase with aging in both men and women. Studies in rodents indicate that there are gender differences in aging vessels, with stiffness increasing more in male than in females (Ruiz-Feria et al., 2009; Chan et al., 2011). Also in nonhuman primates, aortic stiffness has shown to be increased more in old male monkeys than in old females (Qiu et al., 2007). However, gender-associated relationship with those markers in humans remains unclear and currently limited studies have addressed to the evaluation of age-related vascular changes in man and women separately. Even though, many studies have performed their analysis on aging correlation with arterial stiffness and distensibility in men and women separately, their statistical models generally mask the gender differences in the influence of these variables (Breithaupt-Grogler & Belz, 1999; Segers et al., 2007; Redheuil et al., 2010; Miyoshi et al., 2011). In most clinical studies using small population group, the data do not provide sufficient power to detect significant gender-related differences in the rate of age-dependent change in vascular wall structure. The field still misses a large multi-centric populational study to identify whether aging-related effects are modulated by gender.

When it comes to the endothelium, sexual dimorphism on endothelial dysfunction and the progression of cardiovascular disease has also been well documented in various animal models (Ouchi et al., 1987; Ashton & Balment, 1991; Dantas et al., 2004a). With aging, males exhibit signals of impairment on endothelium-dependent relaxation at earlier age than do females (Kauser & Rubanyi, 1995; Huang et al., 1997). Thus far, the mechanisms better established to explain the gender- and aging-associated differences involve: 1) increased NO production by females (Huang et al., 1997); and 2) increased oxidative stress in male blood vessels (Dantas et al., 2004a). In this area of age-associated effects, a translation of animal models to humans can be performed. Early clinical studies on gender- and aging-related effects on endothelium-dependent relaxation in forearm blood flow have identified a constant age-related decline in maximal vasodilation to acetylcholine per year (Taddei et al., 1996). In contrast, women were found to show a slight decrease per year in vasodilation to acetylcholine up to middle-age (around 50's). After that, the vascular decline in the responses to the endothelium-dependent vasodilator hasten, and even decline more quickly in comparison with men (Taddei et al., 1996).

Gender modulation of vascular tone is also observed in functional studies. Contractile responses are greater in the aorta of male than female rats (Stallone et al., 1991; Crews et al., 1999; Tostes et al., 2000). These differences may be related to the vasodilatory effects of estrogens (Crews et al., 1999; Kanashiro & Khalil, 2001) through a direct action on vascular smooth muscle (Jiang et al., 1992; Mugge et al., 1993; Gerhard & Ganz, 1995; Crews & Khalil, 1999). Expression of estrogen receptors in smooth muscle may vary depending on the gender and the gonadal status (Tamaya et al., 1993). The decreased vascular responses to constrictors may be related to 1) the higher relative abundance of estrogen receptors in females arteries (Collins et al., 1995), 2) estrogen-induced down-regulation of gene expression of vasoconstrictor receptors, such as Ang II (Nickenig et al., 2000), and 3) signaling mechanisms of vascular smooth muscle contraction downstream from receptor activation.

As intracellular free Ca^{2+} concentration ($[Ca^{2+}]i$) is important for the initiation of smooth muscle contraction (Horowitz et al., 1996), several studies have used isolated vascular preparations and smooth muscle cells from control and gonadectomized male and female animals to investigate the effect of estrogen on $[Ca^{2+}]i$ and the Ca^{2+}-mobilization mechanisms (i.e. Ca^{2+} release from the intracellular stores and Ca^{2+} entry from the extracellular space) (Zhang et al., 1994; Crews & Khalil, 1999; Crews et al., 1999; Murphy & Khalil, 1999; Murphy & Khalil, 2000; Novella et al., 2010).

Taken together those studies can suggest that, with aging, women are more protected against its deleterious consequences in the cardiovascular system than men. After menopause, however, this protection seems to be lost, since the incidence of cardiovascular disease increases considerably to levels similar (or higher) to those found in men. Because the onset of menopause is marked by the loss of endogenous estrogen production from the ovaries, estrogen is felt to confer the premenopausal protection.

4. Vascular aging in females: Effects of estrogen on vascular function and aging

In women, arterial aging includes an aggravating risk factor in comparison to men. The decrease in estrogen production by menopause is thought to contribute to increased cardiovascular risk. Although aging *per se* has detrimental effects in the vasculature of middle aged female, these effects seem to be potentiated by the lack of estrogen with menopause, and restored by estrogen replacement (Harman, 2004; Stice et al., 2009; Novella et al., 2010). For this reason it is particularly difficult to distinguish what would be the contribution of aging and the lack of estrogen in the control of vascular function in menopausal women.

Epidemiological observations and extensive basic laboratory research has shown that female sex hormones, and more specifically estrogen, has direct beneficial effects in the cardiovascular system (Staessen et al., 1989; Dantas et al., 1999; Tostes et al., 2003; Dantas et al., 2004b; Hinojosa-Laborde et al., 2004). Estrogen has been described to display a myriad of metabolic, hemodynamic, and vascular effects, which have been largely associated to cardiovascular protection in females. For instance, estrogen can promote cardiovascular protection by indirectly influence on the metabolism of lipoproteins or directly by acting on the modulation of molecular pathways in the vessel wall (Miller & Duckles, 2008). Receptors for estrogen have been identified biochemically and show a plentiful expression in both vascular smooth muscle and endothelium, reinforcing the idea that estrogen play a key role in the control of vascular function (Couse et al., 1997; Pau et al., 1998; Arnal et al., 2010).

When considering the major structural changes caused by aging, cross-sectional studies have shown that postmenopausal females taking hormone replacement therapy present lower arterial stiffness compared with their peers not taken estrogen (Moreau et al., 2003; Sumino et al., 2005; Sumino et al., 2006). Besides, radial artery distensibility fluctuates in accordance with estrogen levels during menstrual cycles (Giannattasio et al., 1999). Basic research using animal models for estrogen withdrawn and aging have proposed that estrogen play a modulatory role in the molecular mechanisms to prevent stiffening of arterial wall. As mentioned above, content of collagen and elastin into arterial wall is a key factor that contributes to arterial wall thickening and stiffening, and is mostly regulated by the activity of matrix metalloproteinases (MMP), a family of enzymes capable of degrading components of the extracellular matrix. During aging there is a marked decrease of MMP activity which results in increase of collagen accumulation and consequent stiffening. Data from studies in female rodents have found that estrogen replacement in ovariectomized animals increases MMP activity and restores structural properties of aged arteries similar to that of the young group (Zhang et al., 2000). Altogether these studies suggest that estrogen can exert a favorable modulatory effect on arterial stiffness with aging in females.

Endothelial dysfunction secondary to estrogen deprivation has been largely described and has been mostly associated with reductions in NO availability. Estrogen is known to increases NO bioavailability by mechanisms that involve either increase of NO generation directly or by decreasing O_2^- concentration, and thereby attenuating O_2^- mediated inactivation of NO. The mechanisms involved in estrogen-induced increases in NO availability include: 1) transcriptional stimulation of endothelial NO synthase (eNOS) gene expression (Huang et al., 1997; Sumi & Ignarro, 2003); 2) non-genomic activation of enzyme activity via a phosphatidylinositol-3-OH kinase (PI3-kinase)/phosphokinase B (PKB/AKT) mediated signaling pathway (Hisamoto et al., 2001); 3) increased $[Ca^{2+}]_i$ in endothelial cells (Rubio-Gayosso et al., 2000); 4) decreased production of eNOS endogenous inhibitor, ADMA (Monsalve et al., 2007), and 5) attenuated O_2^- concentrations (Wassmann et al., 2001; Dantas et al., 2002; Ospina et al., 2002).

In addition to NO, actions of estrogen in the vasculature also influence the metabolism of other endothelium-derived factors (EDF). Estrogen has been described to positively up-regulate the production of endothelium-derived relaxing factors (EDRF), such as PGI_2 (Sobrino et al., 2009; Sobrino et al., 2010) and the endothelium-derived hyperpolarizing factors (EDHF) (Golding & Kepler, 2001), both of which are important mediators of vascular relaxation in resistance-sized arteries. Concomitantly, a modulating role of estrogen on constrictor factors (EDCF) is observed. Studies have shown that the beneficial effects of estrogen on the endothelium can be partially explained by an inhibitory effect on the production or action of the COX-derived vasoconstrictor agents (PGH_2 and TXA_2) (Davidge & Zhang, 1998; Dantas et al., 1999; Novella et al., 2010) and endothelin- 1 (ET-1) (David et al., 2001).

Estrogen has been shown to be a modulator of contractile responses by directly interfering with Ca^{2+} into the vascular smooth muscle cells. Although some studies have shown that estrogen does not inhibit Ca^{2+} release from the intracellular stores (Crews & Khalil, 1999; Murphy & Khalil, 1999), others have described that, supraphysiological concentrations of estrogen inhibit Ca^{2+} influx from the extracellular space (Han et al., 1995; Crews & Khalil, 1999; Murphy & Khalil, 1999) by inhibiting Ca^{2+} entry through voltage-gated Ca^{2+} channels (Freay et al., 1997; Kitazawa et al., 1997; Crews & Khalil, 1999; Murphy & Khalil, 1999). The expression of the L-type Ca^{2+} channels in cardiac muscle is substantially increased in estrogen receptor-deficient mice (Johnson et al., 1997), suggesting that estrogen may regulate Ca^{2+} mobilization by a receptor-mediated system.

Although a genomic action of physiological concentrations of estrogen on the expression of the Ca^{2+} channels may underlie the reduced cell contraction and $[Ca^{2+}]i$ observed in vascular smooth muscle cells of females, it is less likely to account for the acute inhibitory effects of 17β-estradiol on cell contraction and $[Ca^{2+}]i$ *in vitro*. The acute nature of the vasorelaxant effects of exogenous estrogen may represent additional non-genomic effects of estrogen on the mechanisms of Ca^{2+} entry into vascular smooth muscle (Kitazawa et al., 1997; Crews & Khalil, 1999; Murphy & Khalil, 1999). Whether estrogen inhibits Ca^{2+} entry by a direct or indirect action on plasmalemmal Ca^{2+} channels remains unclear. Some studies have shown that estrogen blocks Ca^{2+} channels in smooth muscle cells (Zhang et al., 1994; Nakajima et al., 1995) and others have shown that estrogen activates large conductance Ca^{2+}-activated K^+ channels, which could lead to hyperpolarization and decreased Ca^{2+} entry through voltage-gated channels (White et al., 1995; Wellman et al., 1996). Estrogen may also decrease $[Ca^{2+}]i$ by stimulating Ca^{2+} extrusion via the plasmalemmal Ca^{2+} pump (Prakash et al., 1999). However, this mechanism seems less likely because the rate of decay of $[Ca^{2+}]i$ transients in smooth muscle incubated in Ca^{2+}-free solution are not affected by estrogen (Crews & Khalil, 1999; Murphy & Khalil, 1999).

Other systems critically involved in the control of vascular function are also known to undergo estrogen modulation. For example, estrogen has been described to exert direct modulation on the components of renin-angiotensin system (RAS), which is a key regulator of blood pressure and smooth muscle cell growth. Estrogen reduces production of the active hormone of the RAS, Ang II in part, by inhibiting angiotensin-converting enzyme (ACE) expression. ACE activity in the circulation and in tissues, including the kidney and aorta, is reduced upon chronic estrogen replacement in animal models of menopause as well as in postmenopausal women (Brosnihan et al., 1999; Seely et al., 2004). Furthermore, estrogen attenuates the expression and tissue response to type 1 (AT_1) angiotensin receptor in several cardiovascular tissues including the aorta, heart and kidney (Silva-Antonialli et al., 2000; Wu et al., 2003).

Because increased oxidative stress play a crucial role on aging-associated vascular damage, numerous studies have assessed the antioxidant potential of estrogens. Basic research in human cultured endothelial cells revealed an antioxidant effect of estradiol (Hermenegildo et al., 2002a). In addition, clinical experimental studies have shown that different estrogens are capable of reducing oxidation of LDL- cholesterol and consequently the development of atherosclerosis (Keaney, Jr. et al., 1994; Shwaery et al., 1998; Hermenegildo et al., 2001; Hermenegildo et al., 2002b). In addition to its antioxidant role, estradiol exerts a direct effect by restoring the ADMA levels rise induced by oxidized LDL in human cultured endothelial cells acting through estrogen receptor α. Estrogen also attenuates the deleterious effects induced by increased generation of ROS follow ischemia/reperfusion in distinct research models (Kim et al., 1996; Kim et al., 2006; Guo et al., 2010).

As a result of their phenolic molecular structure, several estrogens, such as 17β-estradiol, estrone or estriol, have been described to act as ROS scavengers by virtue of the hydrogen-donating capacity of their phenolic groups (Halliwell & Grootveld, 1987; Dubey & Jackson, 2001). However, in these studies the direct effect of estrogens as scavenger can only be observed at concentrations above 1 micromolar (Arnal et al., 1996; Kim et al., 1996). Considering that plasma concentrations of estrogen in physiological conditions are in the nanomolar range is likely that the direct action as a scavenger is not the main anti-oxidant mechanism by estrogen. In fact, studies have established that estrogen modulates ROS concentration a mechanism that involves interaction with its nuclear receptor to decrease oxidative proteins and/or increase antioxidant enzymes expression. Many studies have shown that changes in estrogen levels are associated with altered levels of anti-oxidant enzymes including glutathione peroxidase, catalase and superoxide dismutase (Capel et al., 1981; Robb & Stuart, 2011; Sivritas et al., 2011). Moreover, recent studies have shown a modulatory effect of estrogen on O_2^-, via modulation of NADH/NADPH oxidases and AT_1 receptor gene expression (major sources of O_2^- production) (Wassmann et al., 2001; Dantas et al., 2002).

Among all research on cellular aging process and its complication, there is a growing interest on mechanisms to delay or decrease telomere shortening by aging, and therefore, keeping cellular integrity and function (Allsopp et al., 1995). In this sense, few studies have explored the effects of estrogen on telomere shortening, and even fewer have addressed this issue in association with vascular aging. Mechanistic studies have found that estrogen treatment up-regulates transcription of hTERT, the catalytic subunit of human telomerase, in distinct cell lines, including endothelial cells (Farsetti et al., 2009). Intriguingly, activation of hTERT by NO signaling has also been reported (Vasa et al., 2000). Considering that estrogen augments NO production, one can suggest that estrogens doubly prevent vascular senescence: by directly interacting with its receptor and by increasing NO.

Although estrogen modulates several mechanisms that are closely associated with vascular aging, assuming that estrogen put a break on vascular aging in females would be rather speculative. There is no sufficient data available to correlate estrogen levels with a delay on progression of vascular aging and recent clinical trials have questioned the value of estrogen replacement therapy in protecting vascular function. The benefits of hormone replacement therapy on the life expectancy and vascular health of women have dramatically lost consensus since publication of the results of the Women's Health Initiative study (WHI) (Rossouw et al., 2002). The WHI trial did not find any cardiovascular benefit from estrogen in postmenopausal women and in fact, showed hormone replacement therapy was associated with increased risk to the cardiovascular system (Rossouw et al., 2002).

There is much controversy over the interpretation of WHI. Concerns raised include that the estrogens used in those trials are not naturally occurring and thus would not act identically to natural estrogens. Most importantly was the fact that the WHI, as well as the majority of clinical trial on hormone replacement therapy, studied a population of women that were estrogen deficient for, on average, 10 years before hormone replacement was initiated. Currently, it is not known if the vascular effects of estrogen are modified by aging in females. These observations, together with observational studies, have led scientists to create the so-called "timing hypothesis". This theory states that estrogen-mediated benefits to prevent cardiovascular disease only occur when treatment is initiated before the detrimental effects of aging are established on vascular wall (Harman, 2006). In this regard, few recent basic studies have shown that aging is associated with significant reductions in the direct estrogen-mediated mechanisms of vascular relaxation (Wynne et al., 2004; LeBlanc et al., 2009; Lekontseva et al., 2010). The lack of estrogen responses in those animals was not related to age-associated changes in the plasma levels of estrogen or activity of estrogen receptors, but rather by possible age-related changes in estrogen-mediated signaling pathways in the vasculature.

Moreover, recent clinical studies have revealed that different risk factors for cardiovascular disease in postmenopausal women were lower among women 50 to 59 years old at enrolment for estrogen replacement therapy (Manson et al., 2007; Sherwood et al., 2007). Nevertheless, the field lacks detailed research on the long-term effects by estrogen and how it modulates cardiovascular function during aging. It remains unclear to what extent the protective effects of estrogen replacement well described in young females can be extrapolated to older ones. The aging issue still needs to be addressed in both experimental and clinical studies, and together, these studies demonstrate that estrogen has complex biologic effects and may influence the risk of cardiovascular events and other outcomes through multiple pathways. Therefore aging of a giving organism should always be taken into account when the pharmacological and physiological responses by estrogens are determined.

5. Conclusion

We live in an aging society, with life expectancy far greater today than a century ago. The increasing incidence of older-age people in our society represents the culmination of centuries of medical, scientific, and social accomplishments. The challenge for modern medicine is how to increase the number of disease-free years in elderly people and improve quality of life in later years. However, a disproportionate number of people who reach old age suffer from cardiovascular diseases.

Clinical and basic studies have established that vascular aging in women does not follow the same chronology as in men. Men display a pattern of progressive vascular aging, while timing for vascular aging in women presents a clear hallmark, i.e. menopause. Several studies have shown that the incidence of cardiovascular diseases in premenopausal women is markedly low compared to age-matched men. After menopause, however, these figures increase to values that are close, or even higher, to those found in men. Cardiovascular disease is the primary cause of death among women after menopause. Despite this, there is still a concerning gap in the knowledge, understanding, and general awareness of mechanisms for cardiovascular aging in women.

It has become apparent that to improve diagnosis and treatment of vascular aging, the gender differences in cardiovascular control must be addressed. The impact of the menstrual cycle and hormonal replacement therapy on vascular function of females should also be taken into consideration. Different strategies have shown benefit in preventing, delaying or attenuating vascular aging. Nevertheless, it yet remains to be fully demonstrated whether vascular aging can be pharmacologically prevented. Further research efforts are needed to understand the causes and consequences of female vascular aging and propose new therapeutic strategies for the management of vascular senescence in women.

6. Acknowledgment

This work was supported by the Spanish Ministerio de Ciencia e Innovación, Instituto de Salud Carlos III - FEDER-ERDF (grants FIS PI10/00518, FIS PI080176 and Red HERACLES RD06/0009), Consellería de Sanidad, Generalitat Valenciana (grants AP 097/2011, AP 104/2011 and GE 027/2011), and Spanish Society of Cardiology (DN040480).

7. References

Adragao, T.; Pires, A.; Lucas, C.; Birne, R.; Magalhaes, L.; Goncalves, M., & Negrao, A.P. (2004). A simple vascular calcification score predicts cardiovascular risk in haemodialysis patients. *Nephrol Dial Transplant*, 19, 1480-1488.

Allsopp, R.C.; Chang, E.; Kashefi-Aazam, M.; Rogaev, E.I.; Piatyszek, M.A.; Shay, J.W., & Harley, C.B. (1995). Telomere shortening is associated with cell division in vitro and in vivo. *Exp Cell Res*, 220, 194-200.

Arnal, J.F.; Clamens, S.; Pechet, C.; Negre-Salvayre, A.; Allera, C.; Girolami, J.P.; Salvayre, R., & Bayard, F. (1996). Ethinylestradiol does not enhance the expression of nitric oxide synthase in bovine endothelial cells but increases the release of bioactive nitric oxide by inhibiting superoxide anion production. *Proc Natl Acad Sci U S A*, 93, 4108-4113.

Arnal, J.F.; Fontaine, C.; Billon-Gales, A.; Favre, J.; Laurell, H.; Lenfant, F., & Gourdy, P. (2010). Estrogen receptors and endothelium. *Arterioscler Thromb Vasc Biol*, 30, 1506-1512.

Ashton, N., & Balment, R.J. (1991). Sexual dimorphism in renal function and hormonal status of New Zealand genetically hypertensive rats. *Acta Endocrinol (Copenh)*, 124, 91-97.

Avolio, A.P.; Chen, S.G.; Wang, R.P.; Zhang, C.L.; Li, M.F., & O'Rourke, M.F. (1983). Effects of aging on changing arterial compliance and left ventricular load in a northern Chinese urban community. *Circulation*, 68, 50-58.

Avolio, A.P.; Deng, F.Q.; Li, W.Q.; Luo, Y.F.; Huang, Z.D.; Xing, L.F., & O'Rourke, M.F. (1985). Effects of aging on arterial distensibility in populations with high and low prevalence of hypertension: comparison between urban and rural communities in China. *Circulation*, 71, 202-210.

Bairey Merz, C.N.; Shaw, L.J.; Reis, S.E.; Bittner, V.; Kelsey, S.F.; Olson, M.; Johnson, B.D.; Pepine, C.J.; Mankad, S.; Sharaf, B.L.; Rogers, W.J.; Pohost, G.M.; Lerman, A.; Quyyumi, A.A., & Sopko, G. (2006). Insights from the NHLBI-Sponsored Women's Ischemia Syndrome Evaluation (WISE) Study: Part II: gender differences in presentation, diagnosis, and outcome with regard to gender-based pathophysiology of atherosclerosis and macrovascular and microvascular coronary disease. *J Am Coll Cardiol*, 47, S21-S29.

Barton, M. (2010). Obesity and aging: determinants of endothelial cell dysfunction and atherosclerosis. *Pflugers Arch*, 460, 825-837.

Bekaert, S.; De Meyer T.; Rietzschel, E.R.; De Buyzere, M.L.; De Bacquer D.; Langlois, M.; Segers, P.; Cooman, L.; Van Damme P.; Cassiman, P.; Van Criekinge W.; Verdonck, P.; De Backer, G.G.; Gillebert, T.C., & Van Oostveldt P. (2007). Telomere length and cardiovascular risk factors in a middle-aged population free of overt cardiovascular disease. *Aging Cell*, 6, 639-647.

Breithaupt-Grogler, K., & Belz, G.G. (1999). Epidemiology of the arterial stiffness. *Pathol Biol (Paris)*, 47, 604-613.

Briones, A.M.; Montoya, N.; Giraldo, J., & Vila, E. (2005). Ageing affects nitric oxide synthase, cyclooxygenase and oxidative stress enzymes expression differently in mesenteric resistance arteries. *Auton Autacoid Pharmacol*, 25, 155-162.

Brosnihan, K.B.; Senanayake, P.S.; Li, P., & Ferrario, C.M. (1999). Bi-directional actions of estrogen on the renin-angiotensin system. *Braz J Med Biol Res*, 32, 373-381.

Bucciarelli, P., & Mannucci, P.M. (2009). The hemostatic system through aging and menopause. *Climacteric*, 12 Suppl 1, 47-51.

Burnett, A.L. (2006). The role of nitric oxide in erectile dysfunction: implications for medical therapy. *J Clin Hypertens (Greenwich)*, 8, 53-62.

Burton, D.G. (2009). Cellular senescence, ageing and disease. *Age (Dordr)*, 31, 1-9.

Byon, C.H.; Javed, A.; Dai, Q.; Kappes, J.C.; Clemens, T.L.; Darley-Usmar, V.M.; McDonald, J.M., & Chen, Y. (2008). Oxidative stress induces vascular calcification through modulation of the osteogenic transcription factor Runx2 by AKT signaling. *J Biol Chem*, 283, 15319-15327.

Camici, G.G.; Shi, Y.; Cosentino, F.; Francia, P., & Luscher, T.F. (2011). Anti-aging medicine: molecular basis for endothelial cell-targeted strategies - a mini-review. *Gerontology*, 57, 101-108.

Capel, I.D.; Jenner, M.; Williams, D.C.; Donaldson, D., & Nath, A. (1981). The effect of prolonged oral contraceptive steroid use on erythrocyte glutathione peroxidase activity. *J Steroid Biochem*, 14, 729-732.

Chan, V.; Fenning, A.; Levick, S.P.; Loch, D.; Chunduri, P.; Iyer, A.; Teo, Y.L.; Hoey, A.; Wilson, K.; Burstow, D., & Brown, L. (2011). Cardiovascular changes during maturation and ageing in male and female spontaneously hypertensive rats. *J Cardiovasc Pharmacol*, 57, 469-478.

Chang, E., & Harley, C.B. (1995). Telomere length and replicative aging in human vascular tissues. *Proc Natl Acad Sci U S A*, 92, 11190-11194.

Clarke, M.C.; Figg, N.; Maguire, J.J.; Davenport, A.P.; Goddard, M.; Littlewood, T.D., & Bennett, M.R. (2006). Apoptosis of vascular smooth muscle cells induces features of plaque vulnerability in atherosclerosis. *Nat Med*, 12, 1075-1080.

Clempus, R.E., & Griendling, K.K. (2006). Reactive oxygen species signaling in vascular smooth muscle cells. *Cardiovasc Res*, 71, 216-225.

Collins, P.; Rosano, G.M.; Sarrel, P.M.; Ulrich, L.; Adamopoulos, S.; Beale, C.M.; McNeill, J.G., & Poole-Wilson, P.A. (1995). 17β-Estradiol attenuates acetylcholine-induced coronary arterial constriction in women but not men with coronary heart disease. *Circulation*, 92, 24-30.

Cooper, L.T.; Cooke, J.P., & Dzau, V.J. (1994). The vasculopathy of aging. *J Gerontol*, 49, B191-B196.

Couse, J.F.; Lindzey, J.; Grandien, K.; Gustafsson, J.A., & Korach, K.S. (1997). Tissue distribution and quantitative analysis of estrogen receptor-alpha (ERα) and estrogen receptor-beta (ERβ) messenger ribonucleic acid in the wild-type and ERα-knockout mouse. *Endocrinology*, 138, 4613-4621.

Crews, J.K., & Khalil, R.A. (1999). Antagonistic effects of 17β-estradiol, progesterone, and testosterone on Ca^{2+} entry mechanisms of coronary vasoconstriction. *Arterioscler Thromb Vasc Biol*, 19, 1034-1040.

Crews, J.K.; Murphy, J.G., & Khalil, R.A. (1999). Gender differences in Ca^{2+} entry mechanisms of vasoconstriction in Wistar-Kyoto and spontaneously hypertensive rats. *Hypertension*, 34, 931-936.

Dantas, A.P.; Franco, M.C.; Silva-Antonialli, M.M.; Tostes, R.C.; Fortes, Z.B.; Nigro, D., & Carvalho, M.H. (2004a). Gender differences in superoxide generation in microvessels of hypertensive rats: role of NAD(P)H-oxidase. *Cardiovasc Res*, 61, 22-29.

Dantas, A.P.; Franco, M.C.; Tostes, R.C.; Fortes, Z.B.; Costa, S.G.; Nigro, D., & Carvalho, M.H. (2004b). Relative contribution of estrogen withdrawal and gonadotropins increase secondary to ovariectomy on prostaglandin generation in mesenteric microvessels. *J Cardiovasc Pharmacol*, 43, 48-55.

Dantas, A.P.; Scivoletto, R.; Fortes, Z.B.; Nigro, D., & Carvalho, M.H. (1999). Influence of female sex hormones on endothelium-derived vasoconstrictor prostanoid generation in microvessels of spontaneously hypertensive rats. *Hypertension*, 34, 914-919.

Dantas, A.P.; Tostes, R.C.; Fortes, Z.B.; Costa, S.G.; Nigro, D., & Carvalho, M.H. (2002). In vivo evidence for antioxidant potential of estrogen in microvessels of female spontaneously hypertensive rats. *Hypertension*, 39, 405-411.

David, F.L.; Carvalho, M.H.; Cobra, A.L.; Nigro, D.; Fortes, Z.B.; Reboucas, N.A., & Tostes, R.C. (2001). Ovarian hormones modulate endothelin-1 vascular reactivity and mRNA expression in DOCA-salt hypertensive rats. *Hypertension*, 38, 692-696.

Davidge, S.T., & Zhang, Y. (1998). Estrogen replacement suppresses a prostaglandin H synthase-dependent vasoconstrictor in rat mesenteric arteries. *Circ Res*, 83, 388-395.

de Grey, A.D. (2006). Free radicals in aging: causal complexity and its biomedical implications. *Free Radic Res*, 40, 1244-1249.

De Meyer T.; Rietzschel, E.R.; De Buyzere, M.L.; Van Criekinge W., & Bekaert, S. (2011). Telomere length and cardiovascular aging: the means to the ends? *Ageing Res Rev*, 10, 297-303.

Dubey, R.K., & Jackson, E.K. (2001). Estrogen-induced cardiorenal protection: potential cellular, biochemical, and molecular mechanisms. *Am J Physiol Renal Physiol*, 280, F365-F388.

Dudzinski, D.M., & Michel, T. (2007). Life history of eNOS: partners and pathways. *Cardiovasc Res*, 75, 247-260.

Eaker, E.; Chesebro, J.H.; Sacks, F.M.; Wenger, N.K.; Whisnant, J.P., & Winston, M. (1994). Special report: cardiovascular disease in women. Special writing group. *Heart Dis Stroke*, 3, 114-119.

Eaker, E.D.; Chesebro, J.H.; Sacks, F.M.; Wenger, N.K.; Whisnant, J.P., & Winston, M. (1993). Cardiovascular disease in women. *Circulation*, 88, 1999-2009.

Elliott, R.J., & McGrath, L.T. (1994). Calcification of the human thoracic aorta during aging. *Calcif Tissue Int*, 54, 268-273.

Erdely, A.; Greenfeld, Z.; Wagner, L., & Baylis, C. (2003). Sexual dimorphism in the aging kidney: Effects on injury and nitric oxide system. *Kidney Int*, 63, 1021-1026.

Erusalimsky, J.D. (2009). Vascular endothelial senescence: from mechanisms to pathophysiology. *J Appl Physiol*, 106, 326-332.

Eskurza, I.; Myerburgh, L.A.; Kahn, Z.D., & Seals, D.R. (2005). Tetrahydrobiopterin augments endothelium-dependent dilatation in sedentary but not in habitually exercising older adults. *J Physiol*, 568, 1057-1065.

Farsetti, A.; Grasselli, A.; Bacchetti, S.; Gaetano, C., & Capogrossi, M.C. (2009). The telomerase tale in vascular aging: regulation by estrogens and nitric oxide signaling. *J Appl Physiol*, 106, 333-337.

Frank, G.D., & Eguchi, S. (2003). Activation of tyrosine kinases by reactive oxygen species in vascular smooth muscle cells: significance and involvement of EGF receptor transactivation by angiotensin II. *Antioxid Redox Signal*, 5, 771-780.

Freay, A.D.; Curtis, S.W.; Korach, K.S., & Rubanyi, G.M. (1997). Mechanism of vascular smooth muscle relaxation by estrogen in depolarized rat and mouse aorta. Role of nuclear estrogen receptor and Ca^{2+} uptake. *Circ Res*, 81, 242-248.

Gerhard, M., & Ganz, P. (1995). How do we explain the clinical benefits of estrogen? From bedside to bench. *Circulation*, 92, 5-8.

Giannattasio, C.; Failla, M.; Grappiolo, A.; Stella, M.L.; Del, B.A.; Colombo, M., & Mancia, G. (1999). Fluctuations of radial artery distensibility throughout the menstrual cycle. *Arterioscler Thromb Vasc Biol*, 19, 1925-1929.

Godfrey, M.; Nejezchleb, P.A.; Schaefer, G.B.; Minion, D.J.; Wang, Y., & Baxter, B.T. (1993). Elastin and fibrillin mRNA and protein levels in the ontogeny of normal human aorta. *Connect Tissue Res*, 29, 61-69.

Golding, E.M., & Kepler, T.E. (2001). Role of estrogen in modulating EDHF-mediated dilations in the female rat middle cerebral artery. *Am J Physiol Heart Circ Physiol*, 280, H2417-H2423.

Griendling, K.K., & Alexander, R.W. (1997). Oxidative stress and cardiovascular disease. *Circulation*, 96, 3264-3265.

Guo, J.; Krause, D.N.; Horne, J.; Weiss, J.H.; Li, X., & Duckles, S.P. (2010). Estrogen-receptor-mediated protection of cerebral endothelial cell viability and mitochondrial function after ischemic insult in vitro. *J Cereb Blood Flow Metab*, 30, 545-554.

Halliwell, B., & Grootveld, M. (1987). The measurement of free radical reactions in humans. Some thoughts for future experimentation. *FEBS Lett*, 213, 9-14.

Han, S.Z.; Karaki, H.; Ouchi, Y.; Akishita, M., & Orimo, H. (1995). 17β-Estradiol inhibits Ca^{2+} influx and Ca^{2+} release induced by thromboxane A_2 in porcine coronary artery. *Circulation*, 91, 2619-2626.

Harman, S.M. (2004). What do hormones have to do with aging? What does aging have to do with hormones? *Ann N Y Acad Sci*, 1019, 299-308.

Harman, S.M. (2006). Estrogen replacement in menopausal women: recent and current prospective studies, the WHI and the KEEPS. *Gend Med*, 3, 254-269.

Harrison, D.G. (1997). Endothelial function and oxidant stress. *Clin Cardiol*, 20, II-7.

Hayashi, T.; Yano, K.; Matsui-Hirai, H.; Yokoo, H.; Hattori, Y., & Iguchi, A. (2008). Nitric oxide and endothelial cellular senescence. *Pharmacol Ther*, 120, 333-339.

Hermenegildo, C.; Garcia-Martinez, M.C.; Tarin, J.J., & Cano, A. (2002a). Estradiol reduces $F_{2\alpha}$-isoprostane production in cultured human endothelial cells. *Am J Physiol Heart Circ Physiol*, 283, H2644-H2649.

Hermenegildo, C.; Garcia-Martinez, M.C.; Tarin, J.J.; Llacer, A., & Cano, A. (2001). The effect of oral hormone replacement therapy on lipoprotein profile, resistance of LDL to oxidation and LDL particle size. *Maturitas*, 38, 287-295.

Hermenegildo, C.; Garcia-Martinez, M.C.; Valldecabres, C.; Tarin, J.J., & Cano, A. (2002b). Transdermal estradiol reduces plasma myeloperoxidase levels without affecting the LDL resistance to oxidation or the LDL particle size. *Menopause*, 9, 102-109.

Herrera, M.D.; Mingorance, C.; Rodriguez-Rodriguez, R., & Alvarez de Sotomayor M. (2010). Endothelial dysfunction and aging: an update. *Ageing Res Rev*, 9, 142-152.

Hill, J.M.; Zalos, G.; Halcox, J.P.; Schenke, W.H.; Waclawiw, M.A.; Quyyumi, A.A., & Finkel, T. (2003). Circulating endothelial progenitor cells, vascular function, and cardiovascular risk. *N Engl J Med*, 348, 593-600.

Hinojosa-Laborde, C.; Craig, T.; Zheng, W.; Ji, H.; Haywood, J.R., & Sandberg, K. (2004). Ovariectomy augments hypertension in aging female Dahl salt-sensitive rats. *Hypertension*, 44, 405-409.

Hisamoto, K.; Ohmichi, M.; Kurachi, H.; Hayakawa, J.; Kanda, Y.; Nishio, Y.; Adachi, K.; Tasaka, K.; Miyoshi, E.; Fujiwara, N.; Taniguchi, N., & Murata, Y. (2001). Estrogen induces the Akt-dependent activation of endothelial nitric-oxide synthase in vascular endothelial cells. *J Biol Chem*, 276, 3459-3467.

Horowitz, A.; Menice, C.B.; Laporte, R., & Morgan, K.G. (1996). Mechanisms of smooth muscle contraction. *Physiol Rev*, 76, 967-1003.

Huang, A.; Sun, D.; Kaley, G., & Koller, A. (1997). Estrogen maintains nitric oxide synthesis in arterioles of female hypertensive rats. *Hypertension*, 29, 1351-1356.

Jacobson, A.; Yan, C.; Gao, Q.; Rincon-Skinner, T.; Rivera, A.; Edwards, J.; Huang, A.; Kaley, G., & Sun, D. (2007). Aging enhances pressure-induced arterial superoxide formation. *Am J Physiol Heart Circ Physiol*, 293, H1344-H1350.

Jiang, C.; Sarrel, P.M.; Poole-Wilson, P.A., & Collins, P. (1992). Acute effect of 17β-estradiol on rabbit coronary artery contractile responses to endothelin-1. *Am J Physiol*, 263, H271-H275.

Jiang, L.; Wang, M.; Zhang, J.; Monticone, R.E.; Telljohann, R.; Spinetti, G.; Pintus, G., & Lakatta, E.G. (2008). Increased aortic calpain-1 activity mediates age-associated angiotensin II signaling of vascular smooth muscle cells. *PLoS One*, 3, e2231.

Johnson, B.D.; Zheng, W.; Korach, K.S.; Scheuer, T.; Catterall, W.A., & Rubanyi, G.M. (1997). Increased expression of the cardiac L-type calcium channel in estrogen receptor-deficient mice. *J Gen Physiol*, 110, 135-140.

Kanashiro, C.A., & Khalil, R.A. (2001). Gender-related distinctions in protein kinase C activity in rat vascular smooth muscle. *Am J Physiol Cell Physiol*, 280, C34-C45.

Kauser, K., & Rubanyi, G.M. (1995). Gender difference in endothelial dysfunction in the aorta of spontaneously hypertensive rats. *Hypertension*, 25, 517-523.

Keaney, J.F., Jr.; Shwaery, G.T.; Xu, A.; Nicolosi, R.J.; Loscalzo, J.; Foxall, T.L., & Vita, J.A. (1994). 17β-estradiol preserves endothelial vasodilator function and limits low-density lipoprotein oxidation in hypercholesterolemic swine. *Circulation*, 89, 2251-2259.

Kielstein, J.T.; Bode-Boger, S.M.; Frolich, J.C.; Ritz, E.; Haller, H., & Fliser, D. (2003). Asymmetric dimethylarginine, blood pressure, and renal perfusion in elderly subjects. *Circulation*, 107, 1891-1895.

Kim, J.; Kil, I.S.; Seok, Y.M.; Yang, E.S.; Kim, D.K.; Lim, D.G.; Park, J.W.; Bonventre, J.V., & Park, K.M. (2006). Orchiectomy attenuates post-ischemic oxidative stress and ischemia/reperfusion injury in mice. A role for manganese superoxide dismutase. *J Biol Chem*, 281, 20349-20356.

Kim, J.H.; Bugaj, L.J.; Oh, Y.J.; Bivalacqua, T.J.; Ryoo, S.; Soucy, K.G.; Santhanam, L.; Webb, A.; Camara, A.; Sikka, G.; Nyhan, D.; Shoukas, A.A.; Ilies, M.; Christianson, D.W.; Champion, H.C., & Berkowitz, D.E. (2009). Arginase inhibition restores NOS coupling and reverses endothelial dysfunction and vascular stiffness in old rats. *J Appl Physiol*, 107, 1249-1257.

Kim, Y.D.; Chen, B.; Beauregard, J.; Kouretas, P.; Thomas, G.; Farhat, M.Y.; Myers, A.K., & Lees, D.E. (1996). 17 beta-Estradiol prevents dysfunction of canine coronary endothelium and myocardium and reperfusion arrhythmias after brief ischemia/reperfusion. *Circulation*, 94, 2901-2908.

Kitazawa, T.; Hamada, E.; Kitazawa, K., & Gaznabi, A.K. (1997). Non-genomic mechanism of 17β-oestradiol-induced inhibition of contraction in mammalian vascular smooth muscle. *J Physiol*, 499 (Pt 2), 497-511.

Kliche, K.; Jeggle, P.; Pavenstadt, H., & Oberleithner, H. (2011). Role of cellular mechanics in the function and life span of vascular endothelium. *Pflugers Arch*, 462, 209-217.

Konova, E.; Baydanoff, S.; Atanasova, M., & Velkova, A. (2004). Age-related changes in the glycation of human aortic elastin. *Exp Gerontol*, 39, 249-254.

Lakatta, E.G. (2003). Arterial and cardiac aging: major shareholders in cardiovascular disease enterprises: Part III: cellular and molecular clues to heart and arterial aging. *Circulation*, 107, 490-497.

Lakatta, E.G., & Levy, D. (2003). Arterial and cardiac aging: major shareholders in cardiovascular disease enterprises: Part I: aging arteries: a "set up" for vascular disease. *Circulation*, 107, 139-146.

Lamas, S.; Lowenstein, C.J., & Michel, T. (2007). Nitric oxide signaling comes of age: 20 years and thriving. *Cardiovasc Res*, 75, 207-209.

LeBlanc, A.J.; Reyes, R.; Kang, L.S.; Dailey, R.A.; Stallone, J.N.; Moningka, N.C., & Muller-Delp, J.M. (2009). Estrogen replacement restores flow-induced vasodilation in coronary arterioles of aged and ovariectomized rats. *Am J Physiol Regul Integr Comp Physiol*, 297, R1713-R1723.

Lekontseva, O.N.; Rueda-Clausen, C.F.; Morton, J.S., & Davidge, S.T. (2010). Ovariectomy in aged versus young rats augments matrix metalloproteinase-mediated vasoconstriction in mesenteric arteries. *Menopause*, 17, 516-523.

Lerner, D.J., & Kannel, W.B. (1986). Patterns of coronary heart disease morbidity and mortality in the sexes: a 26-year follow-up of the Framingham population. *Am Heart J*, 111, 383-390.

Lu, D., & Kassab, G.S. (2011). Role of shear stress and stretch in vascular mechanobiology. *J R Soc Interface*, 8, 1379-1385.

Luo, G.; Ducy, P.; McKee, M.D.; Pinero, G.J.; Loyer, E.; Behringer, R.R., & Karsenty, G. (1997). Spontaneous calcification of arteries and cartilage in mice lacking matrix GLA protein. *Nature*, 386, 78-81.

Lyle, A.N., & Griendling, K.K. (2006). Modulation of vascular smooth muscle signaling by reactive oxygen species. *Physiology (Bethesda)*, 21, 269-280.

Manson, J.E.; Allison, M.A.; Rossouw, J.E.; Carr, J.J.; Langer, R.D.; Hsia, J.; Kuller, L.H.; Cochrane, B.B.; Hunt, J.R.; Ludlam, S.E.; Pettinger, M.B.; Gass, M.; Margolis, K.L.; Nathan, L.; Ockene, J.K.; Prentice, R.L.; Robbins, J., & Stefanick, M.L. (2007). Estrogen therapy and coronary-artery calcification. *N Engl J Med*, 356, 2591-2602.

Messerli, F.H.; Garavaglia, G.E.; Schmieder, R.E.; Sundgaard-Riise, K.; Nunez, B.D., & Amodeo, C. (1987). Disparate cardiovascular findings in men and women with essential hypertension. *Ann Intern Med*, 107, 158-161.

Michel, T., & Vanhoutte, P.M. (2010). Cellular signaling and NO production. *Pflugers Arch*, 459, 807-816.

Miller, S.J.; Watson, W.C.; Kerr, K.A.; Labarrere, C.A.; Chen, N.X.; Deeg, M.A., & Unthank, J.L. (2007). Development of progressive aortic vasculopathy in a rat model of aging. *Am J Physiol Heart Circ Physiol*, 293, H2634-H2643.

Miller, V.M., & Duckles, S.P. (2008). Vascular actions of estrogens: functional implications. *Pharmacol Rev*, 60, 210-241.

Miyoshi, H.; Mizuguchi, Y.; Oishi, Y.; Iuchi, A.; Nagase, N.; Ara, N., & Oki, T. (2011). Early detection of abnormal left atrial-left ventricular-arterial coupling in preclinical patients with cardiovascular risk factors: evaluation by two-dimensional speckle-tracking echocardiography. *Eur J Echocardiogr*, 12, 431-439.

Monsalve, E.; Oviedo, P.J.; Garcia-Perez, M.A.; Tarin, J.J.; Cano, A., & Hermenegildo, C. (2007). Estradiol counteracts oxidized LDL-induced asymmetric dimethylarginine production by cultured human endothelial cells. *Cardiovasc Res*, 73, 66-72.

Moon, S.K.; Thompson, L.J.; Madamanchi, N.; Ballinger, S.; Papaconstantinou, J.; Horaist, C.; Runge, M.S., & Patterson, C. (2001). Aging, oxidative responses, and proliferative capacity in cultured mouse aortic smooth muscle cells. *Am J Physiol Heart Circ Physiol*, 280, H2779-H2788.

Moreau, K.L.; Donato, A.J.; Seals, D.R.; DeSouza, C.A., & Tanaka, H. (2003). Regular exercise, hormone replacement therapy and the age-related decline in carotid arterial compliance in healthy women. *Cardiovasc Res*, 57, 861-868.

Mugge, A.; Riedel, M.; Barton, M.; Kuhn, M., & Lichtlen, P.R. (1993). Endothelium independent relaxation of human coronary arteries by 17β-oestradiol in vitro. *Cardiovasc Res*, 27, 1939-1942.

Murphy, J.G., & Khalil, R.A. (1999). Decreased $[Ca^{2+}]_i$ during inhibition of coronary smooth muscle contraction by 17β-estradiol, progesterone, and testosterone. *J Pharmacol Exp Ther*, 291, 44-52.

Murphy, J.G., & Khalil, R.A. (2000). Gender-specific reduction in contractility and $[Ca^{2+}]_i$ in vascular smooth muscle cells of female rat. *Am J Physiol Cell Physiol*, 278, C834-C844.

Nakajima, T.; Kitazawa, T.; Hamada, E.; Hazama, H.; Omata, M., & Kurachi, Y. (1995). 17β-Estradiol inhibits the voltage-dependent L-type Ca^{2+} currents in aortic smooth muscle cells. *Eur J Pharmacol*, 294, 625-635.

Nakano-Kurimoto, R.; Ikeda, K.; Uraoka, M.; Nakagawa, Y.; Yutaka, K.; Koide, M.; Takahashi, T.; Matoba, S.; Yamada, H.; Okigaki, M., & Matsubara, H. (2009). Replicative senescence of vascular smooth muscle cells enhances the calcification through initiating the osteoblastic transition. *Am J Physiol Heart Circ Physiol*, 297, H1673-H1684.

Newby, A.C. (2006). Matrix metalloproteinases regulate migration, proliferation, and death of vascular smooth muscle cells by degrading matrix and non-matrix substrates. *Cardiovasc Res*, 69, 614-624.

Nickenig, G.; Strehlow, K.; Wassmann, S.; Baumer, A.T.; Albory, K.; Sauer, H., & Bohm, M. (2000). Differential effects of estrogen and progesterone on AT(1) receptor gene expression in vascular smooth muscle cells. *Circulation*, 102, 1828-1833.

Novella, S.; Dantas, A.P.; Segarra, G.; Novensa, L.; Bueno, C.; Heras, M.; Hermenegildo, C., & Medina, P. (2010). Gathering of aging and estrogen withdrawal in vascular dysfunction of senescent accelerated mice. *Exp Gerontol*, 45, 868-874.

O'Rourke, M.F., & Hashimoto, J. (2007). Mechanical factors in arterial aging: a clinical perspective. *J Am Coll Cardiol*, 50, 1-13.

O'Rourke, M.F., & Nichols, W.W. (2005). Aortic diameter, aortic stiffness, and wave reflection increase with age and isolated systolic hypertension. *Hypertension*, 45, 652-658.

Ospina, J.A.; Krause, D.N., & Duckles, S.P. (2002). 17β-estradiol increases rat cerebrovascular prostacyclin synthesis by elevating cyclooxygenase-1 and prostacyclin synthase. *Stroke*, 33, 600-605.

Ouchi, Y.; Share, L.; Crofton, J.T.; Iitake, K., & Brooks, D.P. (1987). Sex difference in the development of deoxycorticosterone-salt hypertension in the rat. *Hypertension*, 9, 172-177.

Pau, C.Y.; Pau, K.Y., & Spies, H.G. (1998). Putative estrogen receptor beta and alpha mRNA expression in male and female rhesus macaques. *Mol Cell Endocrinol*, 146, 59-68.

Pereira, T.M.; Nogueira, B.V.; Lima, L.C.; Porto, M.L.; Arruda, J.A.; Vasquez, E.C., & Meyrelles, S.S. (2010). Cardiac and vascular changes in elderly atherosclerotic mice: the influence of gender. *Lipids Health Dis*, 9, 87.

Prakash, Y.S.; Togaibayeva, A.A.; Kannan, M.S.; Miller, V.M.; Fitzpatrick, L.A., & Sieck, G.C. (1999). Estrogen increases Ca^{2+} efflux from female porcine coronary arterial smooth muscle. *Am J Physiol*, 276, H926-H934.

Price, J.M.; Hellermann, A.; Hellermann, G., & Sutton, E.T. (2004). Aging enhances vascular dysfunction induced by the Alzheimer's peptide beta-amyloid. *Neurol Res*, 26, 305-311.

Qiu, H.; Depre, C.; Ghosh, K.; Resuello, R.G.; Natividad, F.F.; Rossi, F.; Peppas, A.; Shen, Y.T.; Vatner, D.E., & Vatner, S.F. (2007). Mechanism of gender-specific differences in aortic stiffness with aging in nonhuman primates. *Circulation*, 116, 669-676.

Redheuil, A.; Yu, W.C.; Wu, C.O.; Mousseaux, E.; de Cesare A.; Yan, R.; Kachenoura, N.; Bluemke, D., & Lima, J.A. (2010). Reduced ascending aortic strain and distensibility: earliest manifestations of vascular aging in humans. *Hypertension*, 55, 319-326.

Reid, J.D., & Andersen, M.E. (1993). Medial calcification (whitlockite) in the aorta. *Atherosclerosis*, 101, 213-224.

Robb, E.L., & Stuart, J.A. (2011). Resveratrol interacts with estrogen receptor-beta to inhibit cell replicative growth and enhance stress resistance by upregulating mitochondrial superoxide dismutase. *Free Radic Biol Med*, 50, 821-831.

Rodriguez-Manas, L.; El-Assar, M.; Vallejo, S.; Lopez-Doriga, P.; Solis, J.; Petidier, R.; Montes, M.; Nevado, J.; Castro, M.; Gomez-Guerrero, C.; Peiro, C., & Sanchez-Ferrer, C.F. (2009). Endothelial dysfunction in aged humans is related with oxidative stress and vascular inflammation. *Aging Cell*, 8, 226-238.

Rosamond, W.; Flegal, K.; Furie, K.; Go, A.; Greenlund, K.; Haase, N.; Hailpern, S.M.; Ho, M.; Howard, V.; Kissela, B.; Kittner, S.; Lloyd-Jones, D.; McDermott, M.; Meigs, J.; Moy, C.; Nichol, G.; O'Donnell, C.; Roger, V.; Sorlie, P.; Steinberger, J.; Thom, T.; Wilson, M., & Hong, Y. (2008). Heart disease and stroke statistics--2008 update: a report from the American Heart Association Statistics Committee and Stroke Statistics Subcommittee. *Circulation*, 117, e25-146.

Ross, R. (1993). The pathogenesis of atherosclerosis: a perspective for the 1990s. *Nature*, 362, 801-809.

Rossouw, J.E.; Anderson, G.L.; Prentice, R.L.; LaCroix, A.Z.; Kooperberg, C.; Stefanick, M.L.; Jackson, R.D.; Beresford, S.A.; Howard, B.V.; Johnson, K.C.; Kotchen, J.M., & Ockene, J. (2002). Risks and benefits of estrogen plus progestin in healthy postmenopausal women: principal results From the Women's Health Initiative randomized controlled trial. *JAMA*, 288, 321-333.

Rubio-Gayosso, I.; Sierra-Ramirez, A.; Garcia-Vazquez, A.; Martinez-Martinez, A.; Munoz-Garcia, O.; Morato, T., & Ceballos-Reyes, G. (2000). 17β-estradiol increases intracellular calcium concentration through a short-term and nongenomic mechanism in rat vascular endothelium in culture. *J Cardiovasc Pharmacol*, 36, 196-202.

Ruiz-Feria, C.A.; Yang, Y.; Thomason, D.B.; White, J.; Su, G., & Nishimura, H. (2009). Pulse wave velocity and age- and gender-dependent aortic wall hardening in fowl. *Comp Biochem Physiol A Mol Integr Physiol*, 154, 429-436.

Santhanam, L.; Christianson, D.W.; Nyhan, D., & Berkowitz, D.E. (2008). Arginase and vascular aging. *J Appl Physiol*, 105, 1632-1642.

Schmidt, R.J.; Beierwaltes, W.H., & Baylis, C. (2001). Effects of aging and alterations in dietary sodium intake on total nitric oxide production. *Am J Kidney Dis*, 37, 900-908.

Schwartz, S.M. (1997). Smooth muscle migration in atherosclerosis and restenosis. *J Clin Invest*, 100, S87-S89.

Seals, D.R.; Jablonski, K.L., & Donato, A.J. (2011). Aging and vascular endothelial function in humans. *Clin Sci (Lond)*, 120, 357-375.

Seely, E.W.; Brosnihan, K.B.; Jeunemaitre, X.; Okamura, K.; Williams, G.H.; Hollenberg, N.K., & Herrington, D.M. (2004). Effects of conjugated oestrogen and droloxifene on the renin-angiotensin system, blood pressure and renal blood flow in postmenopausal women. *Clin Endocrinol (Oxf)*, 60, 315-321.

Segers, P.; Rietzschel, E.R.; De Buyzere, M.L.; Vermeersch, S.J.; De Bacquer D.; Van Bortel, L.M.; De Backer G.; Gillebert, T.C., & Verdonck, P.R. (2007). Noninvasive (input) impedance, pulse wave velocity, and wave reflection in healthy middle-aged men and women. *Hypertension*, 49, 1248-1255.

Semba, R.D.; Najjar, S.S.; Sun, K.; Lakatta, E.G., & Ferrucci, L. (2009). Serum carboxymethyl-lysine, an advanced glycation end product, is associated with increased aortic pulse wave velocity in adults. *Am J Hypertens*, 22, 74-79.

Shaw, L.J.; Bairey Merz, C.N.; Pepine, C.J.; Reis, S.E.; Bittner, V.; Kelsey, S.F.; Olson, M.; Johnson, B.D.; Mankad, S.; Sharaf, B.L.; Rogers, W.J.; Wessel, T.R.; Arant, C.B.; Pohost, G.M.; Lerman, A.; Quyyumi, A.A., & Sopko, G. (2006). Insights from the NHLBI-Sponsored Women's Ischemia Syndrome Evaluation (WISE) Study: Part I: gender differences in traditional and novel risk factors, symptom evaluation, and gender-optimized diagnostic strategies. *J Am Coll Cardiol*, 47, S4-S20.

Sherwood, A.; Bower, J.K.; McFetridge-Durdle, J.; Blumenthal, J.A.; Newby, L.K., & Hinderliter, A.L. (2007). Age moderates the short-term effects of transdermal 17β-estradiol on endothelium-dependent vascular function in postmenopausal women. *Arterioscler Thromb Vasc Biol*, 27, 1782-1787.

Shwaery, G.T.; Vita, J.A., & Keaney, J.F., Jr. (1998). Antioxidant protection of LDL by physiologic concentrations of estrogens is specific for 17β-estradiol. *Atherosclerosis*, 138, 255-262.

Silva-Antonialli, M.M.; Fortes, Z.B.; Carvalho, M.H.; Scivoletto, R., & Nigro, D. (2000). Sexual dimorphism in the response of thoracic aorta from SHRs to losartan. *Gen Pharmacol*, 34, 329-335.

Sivritas, D.; Becher, M.U.; Ebrahimian, T.; Arfa, O.; Rapp, S.; Bohner, A.; Mueller, C.F.; Umemura, T.; Wassmann, S.; Nickenig, G., & Wassmann, K. (2011). Antiproliferative effect of estrogen in vascular smooth muscle cells is mediated by Kruppel-like factor-4 and manganese superoxide dismutase. *Basic Res Cardiol*, 106, 563-575.

Sobrino, A.; Mata, M.; Laguna-Fernandez, A.; Novella, S.; Oviedo, P.J.; Garcia-Perez, M.A.; Tarin, J.J.; Cano, A., & Hermenegildo, C. (2009). Estradiol stimulates vasodilatory and metabolic pathways in cultured human endothelial cells. *PLoS One*, 4, e8242.

Sobrino, A.; Oviedo, P.J.; Novella, S.; Laguna-Fernandez, A.; Bueno, C.; Garcia-Perez, M.A.; Tarin, J.J.; Cano, A., & Hermenegildo, C. (2010). Estradiol selectively stimulates endothelial prostacyclin production through estrogen receptor-α. *J Mol Endocrinol*, 44, 237-246.

Spina, M.; Garbisa, S.; Hinnie, J.; Hunter, J.C., & Serafini-Fracassini, A. (1983). Age-related changes in composition and mechanical properties of the tunica media of the upper thoracic human aorta. *Arteriosclerosis*, 3, 64-76.

Squadrito, G.L., & Pryor, W.A. (1998). Oxidative chemistry of nitric oxide: the roles of superoxide, peroxynitrite, and carbon dioxide. *Free Radic Biol Med*, 25, 392-403.

Staessen, J.; Bulpitt, C.J.; Fagard, R.; Lijnen, P., & Amery, A. (1989). The influence of menopause on blood pressure. *J Hum Hypertens*, 3, 427-433.

Stallone, J.N.; Crofton, J.T., & Share, L. (1991). Sexual dimorphism in vasopressin-induced contraction of rat aorta. *Am J Physiol*, 260, H453-H458.

Stice, J.P.; Eiserich, J.P., & Knowlton, A.A. (2009). Role of aging versus the loss of estrogens in the reduction in vascular function in female rats. *Endocrinology*, 150, 212-219.

Su, Y.; Kondrikov, D., & Block, E.R. (2005). Cytoskeletal regulation of nitric oxide synthase. *Cell Biochem Biophys*, 43, 439-449.

Su, Y.; Kondrikov, D., & Block, E.R. (2007). Beta-actin: a regulator of NOS-3. *Sci STKE*, 2007, e52.

Sumi, D., & Ignarro, L.J. (2003). Estrogen-related receptor alpha 1 up-regulates endothelial nitric oxide synthase expression. *Proc Natl Acad Sci U S A*, 100, 14451-14456.

Sumino, H.; Ichikawa, S.; Kasama, S.; Kumakura, H.; Takayama, Y.; Sakamaki, T., & Kurabayashi, M. (2005). Effect of transdermal hormone replacement therapy on carotid artery wall thickness and levels of vascular inflammatory markers in postmenopausal women. *Hypertens Res*, 28, 579-584.

Sumino, H.; Ichikawa, S.; Kasama, S.; Takahashi, T.; Kumakura, H.; Takayama, Y.; Kanda, T., & Kurabayashi, M. (2006). Different effects of oral conjugated estrogen and transdermal estradiol on arterial stiffness and vascular inflammatory markers in postmenopausal women. *Atherosclerosis*, 189, 436-442.

Taddei, S.; Virdis, A.; Ghiadoni, L.; Mattei, P.; Sudano, I.; Bernini, G.; Pinto, S., & Salvetti, A. (1996). Menopause is associated with endothelial dysfunction in women. *Hypertension*, 28, 576-582.

Takenouchi, Y.; Kobayashi, T.; Matsumoto, T., & Kamata, K. (2009). Gender differences in age-related endothelial function in the murine aorta. *Atherosclerosis*, 206, 397-404.

Tamaya, T.; Wada, K.; Nakagawa, M.; Misao, R.; Itoh, T.; Imai, A., & Mori, H. (1993). Sexual dimorphism of binding sites of testosterone and dihydrotestosterone in rabbit model. *Comp Biochem Physiol Comp Physiol*, 105, 745-749.

Thompson, G.R., & Partridge, J. (2004). Coronary calcification score: the coronary-risk impact factor. *Lancet*, 363, 557-559.

Thorin, E., & Thorin-Trescases, N. (2009). Vascular endothelial ageing, heartbeat after heartbeat. *Cardiovasc Res*, 84, 24-32.

Toda, T.; Tsuda, N.; Nishimori, I.; Leszczynski, D.E., & Kummerow, F.A. (1980). Morphometrical analysis of the aging process in human arteries and aorta. *Acta Anat (Basel)*, 106, 35-44.

Tostes, R.C.; David, F.L.; Carvalho, M.H.; Nigro, D.; Scivoletto, R., & Fortes, Z.B. (2000). Gender differences in vascular reactivity to endothelin-1 in deoxycorticosterone-salt hypertensive rats. *J Cardiovasc Pharmacol*, 36, S99-101.

Tostes, R.C.; Nigro, D.; Fortes, Z.B., & Carvalho, M.H. (2003). Effects of estrogen on the vascular system. *Braz J Med Biol Res*, 36, 1143-1158.

Touyz, R.M. (2003). Reactive oxygen species in vascular biology: role in arterial hypertension. *Expert Rev Cardiovasc Ther*, 1, 91-106.

Touyz, R.M.; Cruzado, M.; Tabet, F.; Yao, G.; Salomon, S., & Schiffrin, E.L. (2003). Redox-dependent MAP kinase signaling by Ang II in vascular smooth muscle cells: role of receptor tyrosine kinase transactivation. *Can J Physiol Pharmacol*, 81, 159-167.

Tracy, R.P. (2006). The five cardinal signs of inflammation: Calor, Dolor, Rubor, Tumor ... and Penuria (Apologies to Aulus Cornelius Celsus, De medicina, c. A.D. 25). *J Gerontol A Biol Sci Med Sci*, 61, 1051-1052.

Van Craenenbroeck, E.M., & Conraads, V.M. (2010). Endothelial progenitor cells in vascular health: focus on lifestyle. *Microvasc Res*, 79, 184-192.

Vasa, M.; Breitschopf, K.; Zeiher, A.M., & Dimmeler, S. (2000). Nitric oxide activates telomerase and delays endothelial cell senescence. *Circ Res*, 87, 540-542.

Virdis, A.; Ghiadoni, L.; Giannarelli, C., & Taddei, S. (2010). Endothelial dysfunction and vascular disease in later life. *Maturitas*, 67, 20-24.

Wallace, D.C. (2005). A mitochondrial paradigm of metabolic and degenerative diseases, aging, and cancer: a dawn for evolutionary medicine. *Annu Rev Genet*, 39, 359-407.

Wang, M.; Takagi, G.; Asai, K.; Resuello, R.G.; Natividad, F.F.; Vatner, D.E.; Vatner, S.F., & Lakatta, E.G. (2003). Aging increases aortic MMP-2 activity and angiotensin II in nonhuman primates. *Hypertension*, 41, 1308-1316.

Wassmann, S.; Baumer, A.T.; Strehlow, K.; van Eickels M.; Grohe, C.; Ahlbory, K.; Rosen, R.; Bohm, M., & Nickenig, G. (2001). Endothelial dysfunction and oxidative stress during estrogen deficiency in spontaneously hypertensive rats. *Circulation*, 103, 435-441.

Wassmann, S.; Wassmann, K., & Nickenig, G. (2004). Modulation of oxidant and antioxidant enzyme expression and function in vascular cells. *Hypertension*, 44, 381-386.

Watanabe, M.; Sawai, T.; Nagura, H., & Suyama, K. (1996). Age-related alteration of cross-linking amino acids of elastin in human aorta. *Tohoku J Exp Med*, 180, 115-130.

Wellman, G.C.; Bonev, A.D.; Nelson, M.T., & Brayden, J.E. (1996). Gender differences in coronary artery diameter involve estrogen, nitric oxide, and Ca^{2+}-dependent K^+ channels. *Circ Res*, 79, 1024-1030.

White, R.E.; Darkow, D.J., & Lang, J.L. (1995). Estrogen relaxes coronary arteries by opening BKCa channels through a cGMP-dependent mechanism. *Circ Res*, 77, 936-942.

Wong, A.J.; Pollard, T.D., & Herman, I.M. (1983). Actin filament stress fibers in vascular endothelial cells in vivo. *Science*, 219, 867-869.

Wu, Z.; Maric, C.; Roesch, D.M.; Zheng, W.; Verbalis, J.G., & Sandberg, K. (2003). Estrogen regulates adrenal angiotensin AT_1 receptors by modulating AT_1 receptor translation. *Endocrinology*, 144, 3251-3261.

Wynne, F.L.; Payne, J.A.; Cain, A.E.; Reckelhoff, J.F., & Khalil, R.A. (2004). Age-related reduction in estrogen receptor-mediated mechanisms of vascular relaxation in female spontaneously hypertensive rats. *Hypertension*, 43, 405-412.

Xiong, Y.; Yuan, L.W.; Deng, H.W.; Li, Y.J., & Chen, B.M. (2001). Elevated serum endogenous inhibitor of nitric oxide synthase and endothelial dysfunction in aged rats. *Clin Exp Pharmacol Physiol*, 28, 842-847.

Yoon, H.J.; Cho, S.W.; Ahn, B.W., & Yang, S.Y. (2010). Alterations in the activity and expression of endothelial NO synthase in aged human endothelial cells. *Mech Ageing Dev*, 131, 119-123.

Yoshida, Y.I.; Eda, S., & Masada, M. (2000). Alterations of tetrahydrobiopterin biosynthesis and pteridine levels in mouse tissues during growth and aging. *Brain Dev*, 22 Suppl 1, S45-S49.

Zhang, F.; Ram, J.L.; Standley, P.R., & Sowers, J.R. (1994). 17β-Estradiol attenuates voltage-dependent Ca^{2+} currents in A7r5 vascular smooth muscle cell line. *Am J Physiol*, 266, C975-C980.

Zhang, Y.; Stewart, K.G., & Davidge, S.T. (2000). Estrogen replacement reduces age-associated remodeling in rat mesenteric arteries. *Hypertension*, 36, 970-974.

30

Pharmacologic Inhibition of Cardiac Stem Cell Senescence

Daniela Cesselli[1], Angela Caragnano[1], Natascha Bergamin[1], Veronica Zanon[1], Nicoletta Finato[1], Ugolino Livi[2], Carlo Alberto Beltrami[1] and Antonio Paolo Beltrami[1]

[1]*Department of Medical and Biological Sciences, University of Udine, Udine,*
[2]*Department of Experimental and Clinical Medical Sciences, University of Udine, Udine, Italy*

1. Introduction

Mammalian aging may be viewed as a reduction in the capacity to adequately maintain tissue homeostasis or to repair tissues after injury(Sharpless and DePinho, 2007). When homeostatic control diminishes to the point at which tissue/organ integrity and function are no longer sufficiently maintained, physiological decline develops, and aging becomes apparent. Cells that express senescence markers accumulate at sites of chronic age-related pathology, such as osteoarthritis, atherosclerosis and chronic heart failure(Blasco, 2007; Campisi and d'Adda di Fagagna, 2007; Chimenti, et al., 2003; Deng, et al., 2008; Jeyapalan and Sedivy, 2008; Minamino and Komuro, 2008; Sharpless and DePinho, 2007; Shawi and Autexier, 2008; Torella, et al., 2004; Urbanek, et al., 2005). Thus, senescent cells are associated with aging and age-related diseases in vivo(Campisi, 2011).

The discovery of tissue-resident stem and progenitor cells has suggested that these cells are responsible for tissue homeostasis and regeneration(Hosoda, et al., 2009; Hsieh, et al., 2007; Li and Clevers, 2010). For this reason, pathological and patho-physiological conditions characterized by altered tissue homeostasis and impaired regenerative capacity can be viewed as a consequence of the reduction in stem cell number and/or function. Following the evolutionary theory of antagonistic pleiotropy, stem cell senescence can be considered a double edged-sword that exerts both a tumor-suppressor effect, by preventing the expansion of injured self-renewing cells, and detrimental effects, contributing to tumor invasiveness in a paracrine fashion or to aging by causing stem cell arrest or attrition (cancer-ageing hypothesis)(Campisi, 2005; Sharpless and DePinho, 2007). In line with this, stem cell aging has been demonstrated in hematopoietic stem cells, as well as in other self-renewing compartments(Beltrami, et al., 2011a).

The recognition that the heart possesses a pool of primitive, clonogenic, self-renewing, and multipotent cells responsible for tissue homeostasis has opened a new era of research aimed at harvesting, expanding and utilizing these cells for cardiac repair(Beltrami, et al., 2003).

However, experimental studies have demonstrated that, although the cardiac stem cell (CSC) pool is expanded acutely after myocardial infarction, this response is attenuated in chronic heart failure(Urbanek, et al., 2005). In addition, a significant accumulation of senescent CSC in cardiac tissue both in pathological settings and with aging has been described(Cesselli, et al., 2011; Chimenti, et al., 2003; Rota, et al., 2006). More recently, our group has demonstrated that both age and pathology exert detrimental effects on human CSC (hCSC). Specifically, they attenuate CSC telomerase activity, reduce telomeric length, determine telomere erosion, are associated with the presence of telomere induced dysfunction foci and impair CSC function(Cesselli, et al., 2011). Importantly, comparing the gene expression profile of CSC obtained from normal and pathological tissues we identified several possible molecular targets for pharmacological interventions aimed at reverting or attenuating the senescence processes.

Aims of this chapter will be to review the knowledge on the impact that CSC senescence exerts on cardiac function, to discuss interventions aimed at reverting it and to focus on original results investigating the effects of Rapamycin, Resveratrol and DETA/NO on CSC senescence.

2. Cellular senescence

In 1961 Hayflick applied the term *cellular senescence* to cells that ceased to divide in culture despite favorable growth conditions, based on the speculation that their behavior recapitulated organism aging(Hayflick and Moorhead, 1961). Since then, this phenomenon was proposed to be either a detrimental cause of aging or a beneficial tumor suppression mechanism. In fact, cell senescence plays both these roles, supporting the evolutionary theory of antagonistic pleiotropy that postulates that cellular processes, selected to benefit young organisms, may have unselected deleterious effects in older organisms(Campisi and d'Adda di Fagagna, 2007).

Cellular senescence is currently defined as a specialized form of growth arrest, confined to mitotic cells, induced by various stressful stimuli and characterized by several, although not specific, markers(Sharpless and DePinho, 2007). Specifically, senescent cells are characterized by a permanent growth arrest, resistance to apoptosis, an altered pattern of gene expression, and the expression of proteins that are characteristic of, although not exclusive to, the senescent state(Beltrami, et al., 2011a), such as the senescence-associated β-galactosidase (SA-βgal) (Dimri, et al., 1995).

Recently identified markers of cellular senescence are p16, DEC1, p15, and DCR2(Collado, et al., 2005), and the cytological markers: senescence-associated heterochromatin foci (SAHFs), and senescence associated DNA-damage foci (SDFs)(Di Micco, et al., 2008; Narita, et al., 2003). SDFs are present in senescent cells from mice and humans and contain proteins that are associated with DNA damage. When these foci result from dysfunctional telomeres they are defined as telomere-induced dysfunctional foci (TIFs) (Campisi and d'Adda di Fagagna, 2007; Jeyapalan and Sedivy, 2008; Sharpless and DePinho, 2007).

Regarding the molecular mechanisms responsible for cellular senescence, intrinsic and extrinsic pathways have been described. While the first one is initiated by intracellular damages/stimuli, the second one is related to extracellular molecules. Importantly, these two mechanisms are strictly interconnected since senescent cells are characterized by the production of molecules able to alter the microenvironment thus inducing senescence on the neighborhood cells through a paracrine mechanism(Campisi, 2005).

Intrinsic inductors of cellular senescence are either the progressive telomere erosion that is associated with cell proliferation (i.e. replicative senescence) (Deng, et al., 2008; Shawi and Autexier, 2008) or the formation of irreparable DNA lesions that induce a persistent DNA damage response (DDR) which keeps the cells alive, but arrests their proliferation (i.e. telomere independent, stress-induced premature senescence)(Beltrami, et al., 2011a). In this latter case, DDR is induced by activated oncogenes, and DNA double strand break-inducing agents, such as reactive oxygen species (ROS). Many proteins participate in the DDR, including protein kinases (e.g. ataxia telangiectasia mutated -ATM- and checkpoint-2 -CHK2-), adaptor proteins (e.g. 53BP1 and MDC1 -mediator of DNA damage checkpoint protein-1-) and chromatin modifiers (for example, γ-H2AX)(von Zglinicki, et al., 2005). Therefore, intrinsic inductors of cellular senescence initiate a DDR, consisting of the activation of ATM and ataxia telangiectasia- and Rad3-related (ATR), and downstream kinases CHK1 and CHK2, and phosphorylation of p53. Phosphorylated p53 transcriptionally up-regulates genes, such as p21, that mediate cellular senescence and/or apoptosis to inhibit tumorigenesis. Although less well-understood, telomere dysfunction could also activate the $p16^{INK4A}$–RB pathway and inhibit cellular proliferation(Campisi and d'Adda di Fagagna, 2007; Deng, et al., 2008; Sharpless and DePinho, 2007; Shawi and Autexier, 2008).

Recent reports have demonstrated that autophagy plays a crucial role in the induction of cellular senescence(Adams, 2009), either replicative (Young and Narita, 2010) or stress-induced premature senescence (Patschan and Goligorsky, 2008; Young and Narita, 2010). However, several interventions that extended lifespan in various species (e.g. caloric restriction, and negative regulation of insulin and mTOR pathways) are associated with the activation of autophagy(Vellai, 2009). To reconcile this observation with the observed accumulation of senescent cells in aged tissues and organs, Authors hypothesize that autophagy may play a beneficial role in mild but long-term stress conditions, counteracting the accumulated damage, while it contributes to senescence establishment in more severely damaged cells(Young and Narita, 2010). Until recently, the general notion was that once senescence was established, cells were locked into a senescent phenotype through a global induction of heterochromatin, which results in the formation of Senescence Associated Heterochromatin Foci (SAHF). In this process, the cyclin dependent kinase inhibitor p16INK4A seemed to play a primary role. However, recently it was shown that SAHF are induced mainly in response to activated oncogenes in a cell type- and insult- dependent manner(Kosar, et al., 2011).

Several *extrinsic inductors of cellular senescence* have also been described so far(Beltrami, et al., 2011a). Specifically, it has been demonstrated that: Advanced Glycation End-products (AGE) (Patschan and Goligorsky, 2008), Angiotensin II (Fukuda and Sata, 2008; Imanishi, et al., 2005; Kunieda, et al., 2006), IGFBP7, IL-6, IL-8(Kuilman, et al., 2008; Orjalo, et al., 2009), GROα, urokinase- or tissue-type plasminogen activators (uPA or tPA), the uPA receptor (uPAR), and inhibitors of these serine proteases (PAI-1 and -2) (Blasi and Carmeliet, 2002; Kortlever, et al., 2006), can induce cellular senescence in different cell types. In this regard, a special role is played by the altered secretome of senescent cells (e.g. Senescence Associated Secretory Phenotype - SASP-). In fact, it has been demonstrated that senescent cells may alter profoundly their microenvironment, by inducing cellular senescence in neighboring cells in a paracrine fashion, by remodeling the extracellular matrix and by stimulating inflammation(Acosta, et al., 2008; Coppe, et al., 2008; Wajapeyee, et al., 2008).

3. Cardiac stem cell senescence

The recognition that the human adult heart possesses a pool of resident cardiac progenitor cells (hCSC), which are self-renewing, clonogenic, and multipotent(Bearzi, et al., 2009; Bearzi, et al., 2007; Beltrami, et al., 2007; Castaldo, et al., 2008; Messina, et al., 2004; Smith, et al., 2007), changed the dogma of the heart as a terminally differentiated organ, offered new hints in the understanding of the pathophysiology of heart diseases and opened a new area of research focused on the use of stem cells for cardiac repair(Beltrami, et al., 2011b; Dimmeler and Leri, 2008). Several different hCSC populations have been identified and characterized on the basis of the expression of specific markers, i.e. c-Kit(Bearzi, et al., 2009; Bearzi, et al., 2007; Castaldo, et al., 2008), ABCG2(Meissner, et al., 2006) and Islet-1(Bu, et al., 2009), or utilizing selective culture conditions, i.e. cardio-spheres(Messina, et al., 2004; Smith, et al., 2007) and multipotent adult stem cells(Beltrami, et al., 2007). Whether these cells are distinct populations or whether they represent different stages of maturation of the same cell type is still a debated question (Beltrami, et al., 2011b; Laflamme and Murry, 2011). Nonetheless, moving from the robust evidence of the efficacy of cardiac stem cell therapy in animal models(Bearzi, et al., 2007; Smith, et al., 2007), the feasibility, safety and some hints on the efficacy of autologous CSC therapy in patients suffering from cardiac pathology is currently under investigation in several clinical trials (ClinicalTrials.gov identifier NCT00474461, NCT00893360, and NCT00981006). Autologous CSC represent a population of cells intrinsically committed to cardiac lineages and would offer the advantage to avoid immunological issues(Dimmeler and Leri, 2008). Nonetheless, it would be important to identify whether and at which extent cardiac diseases can affect this resident stem cell reservoir.

3.1 CSC senescence in cardiac pathologies

The first evidence that hCSC could undergo cellular senescence was given by Anversa's group showing that aged diseased hearts were characterized, at tissue level, by an accumulation of $p16^{INK4a}$-positive/c-Kit-positive CSC(Chimenti, et al., 2003). Later it was shown that chronic heart failure was associated, in human heart tissues, with an increase in the number of $p16^{INK4a}$-p53-positive senescent hCSC, further characterized by short telomeres(Urbanek, et al., 2005). More recently, our group provided a direct demonstration of the impact that both aging and pathology exert on hCSC function(Cesselli, et al., 2011). Specifically, we observed that age and pathological state are both associated with: a reduction in telomerase activity, telomeric shortening, and an increased frequency of CSC with telomere induced dysfunction foci, and eventually expressing $p16^{INK4a}$ and $p21^{CIP}$. These pathologic alterations were coupled with a reduced hCSC function; in fact, hCSC obtained from failing hearts showed, with respect to those obtained from healthy hearts, a significant reduction in clonogenic, proliferative, and migratory potential. Moreover, senescent hCSC displayed an altered gene expression profile, enriched in transcripts of proteins involved in the senescence associates secretory phenotype (SASP), such as IL6 and IGFBP7(Cesselli, et al., 2011). Of note, the underlying diseases of the patients enrolled in this study were different, ranging from ischemic cardiomyopathy to hypertrophic and dilated cardiomyopathy(Cesselli, et al., 2011), suggesting that, independently from the etiology, end stage heart failure is characterized by a progressive loss of the compartment of hCSC with high regenerative potential, paralleled by an increase in the pool of stem cells with minimal or no ability to divide and acquire cardiac cell lineages. Moreover, animal models showed an involvement of CSC senescence in other pathologies such as the diabetic cardiomyopathy (Rota, et al., 2006) and the antracyclin-induced cardiomyopathy(De Angelis, et al., 2010).

3.2 Pathways involved in hCSC senescence

Whith regard to the mechanisms responsible for the replication, differentiation, senescence, and death of hCSC, different growth-factor receptor systems have been shown to play a key role: IGF-1-IGF1R, IGF-2-IGF2R, HGF-c-Met and the renin angiotensin system (RAS)(Dimmeler and Leri, 2008). While IGF-1-IGF1R and HGF-c-Met seemed to exert a protective effect, IGF-2-IGF2R and the RAS up-regulation is associated with CSC senescence.

Specifically, the expression of IGF-1R and the production of IGF-1 are attenuated in aging CSC, and this negatively interferes with oxidative damage and telomere shortening(D'Amario, et al., 2011a; Torella, et al., 2004). In fact, IGF-1 - IGF-1R induces CSC division, upregulates telomerase activity, maintains telomere length, hinders replicative senescence, and preserves the population of functionally competent cardiac stem cells in animals(Torella, et al., 2004) and in humans(D'Amario, et al., 2011a).

Ageing is also associated with a reduction in HGF production, thus impairing the migratory ability of CSC in response to tissue damage(Gonzalez, et al., 2008; Khan, et al., 2011); importantly, CSC dysfunction was shown to be partially restored by HGF injection(Gonzalez, et al., 2008). Regarding IGF-2-IGF2R, it has been recently demonstrated that hCSC expressing IGF-2R are characterized, with respect to IGF-1R positive hCSC, by a more senescent phenotype and by a reduced in vivo regenerative capacity(Gonzalez, et al., 2008).

Similarly, it has been documented that a local RAS is present on hCSC and that the formation of Angiotensin II (Ang II), together with the expression of AT1R, increases with age in hCSC(D'Amario, et al., 2011a). Ang II generates ROS possibly contributing to the age-dependent accumulation of oxidative damage in the heart(Fiordaliso, et al., 2001; Smith, et al., 2007). In fact, the use of ACE-inhibitors positively interferes with heart failure and prolongs life in failing patients(McMurray and Pfeffer, 2005). Moreover, sustained oxidative stress can trigger telomere shortening and uncapping initiating a permanent DNA-damage response(von Zglinicki, et al., 2005). The importance of oxidative stress has been confirmed in a murine model of diabetes, where it has been shown the association of cardiomyopathy with the premature senescence and apoptosis of CSC; importantly, in this model the deletion of p66shc could prevent CSC senescence and was associated with the preservation of myocyte number and cardiac function(Rota, et al., 2006).

Despite these important data, it remains to be determined whether other pathways, that are involved in the senescence of other cell compartments, could contribute to hCSC senescence as well. For example, data on the role played by autophagy, mitochondrial dysfunction, nucleolar dysfunction and epigenetic changes are still missing(Beltrami, et al., 2011a). However, comparing the gene expression profile of hCSC isolated from end-stage failing hearts with that of hCSC isolated from normal hearts, it was possible to demonstrate changes in the expression of genes strictly related to these senescence associated pathways(Cesselli, et al., 2011). Importantly, the analysis identified several possible molecular targets for pharmacological interventions aimed at reverting or attenuating the senescence processes. Interestingly, some of them were very well known target of drugs commonly used in clinical practice, such as beta-blockers and ACE-inhibitors(Cesselli, et al., 2011).

4. How to interfere with cardiac stem cell senescence

Cell therapy is a promising option for treating ischemic disease and heart failure(Dimmeler and Leri, 2008). In fact, various experimental studies documented that tissue-resident primitive cells improve recovery after ischemia(Beltrami, et al., 2011b). Moreover, different groups have demonstrated the feasibility of isolating and expanding hCSC even from end-stage failing hearts(Bearzi, et al., 2007; Beltrami, et al., 2007; Itzhaki-Alfia, et al., 2009; Smith, et al., 2007). However, accumulated evidences indicate that both ageing and pathology are associated with hCSC senescence and functional impairment (Cesselli, et al., 2011; D'Amario, et al., 2011a; D'Amario, et al., 2011b; Itzhaki-Alfia, et al., 2009). In fact, hCSC obtained from failing hearts present reduced migration, proliferation and differentiation(Cesselli, et al., 2011), features considered to be crucial for the regenerative potential of this autologous cell source. Moreover, these cells are characterized by a gene expression profile enriched in elements that are part of the senescence associated secretory phenotype (SASP). Therefore, senescent hCSC can contribute to create a microenvironment favoring, through a paracrine mechanism, senescence on neighbor cells, inflammation and extracellular matrix remodeling, thus creating a vicious circle hampering regenerative purposes.

For this reason, it would be extremely intriguing any attempt aimed at "improving" the quality of the expanded cells, selecting the fraction of cells with the highest regenerative potential or devoid of senescent cells. Conversely, we can hypothesize an intervention aimed at attenuating/reverting the molecular pathways characterizing senescent cells. In this regard, three main strategies can be envisioned: a sorting-based strategy, a function-based strategy and a drug-based strategy.

4.1 Sorting-based strategy to enrich in non-senescent cells

The sorting-based strategy would consist in the physical selection of the cells of interest. Sorting can be achieved, for example, utilizing a fluorescence-activated cell sorting (FACS) or a magnetic activated cell sorting (MACS). The selection strategy can be either positive (we choose and sort "young" cells on the basis of specific surface antigens) or negative (we enrich in non-senescent cells removing from the un-fractioned population those cells we believe to be senescent). Both approaches require the knowledge of specific surface antigens able to recognize the right population to sort. D'Amario et al have recently given examples of positive selection, utilizing antibodies recognizing insulin-like growth factor (IGF)-1 receptors to select, within hCSC isolated from end-stage failing patients, a population of young cells characterized by high telomerase activity, intact telomere length and endowed with a high regenerative ability, being able to restore a large quantity of infarcted myocardium, thus representing a potent cell population for cardiac repair(D'Amario, et al.,

2011a). Although not yet utilized for a negative selection, AT-2(D'Amario, et al., 2011a), IGF-2R and CD49a(Cesselli, et al., 2011) are surface markers that, being more expressed in senescent cells, could be utilized to deplete hCSC culture of the most senescent cells.

The major drawback of the sorting-based approach is the fact that it adds a further grade of complexity to the procedure aimed at producing clinical grade hCSC, since it requires Good Manufacturing Practice-compliant cell sorting and large-scale expansion starting from a reduced number of cells.

4.2 Function-based strategy to enrich in non-senescent cells

It is possible to take advantage of the fact that non-senescent cells are functionally impaired to select cells whose stem cell properties are still preserved. For example, we showed that single-cell derived clones, obtained from hCSC isolated from end-stage failing patients, are less senescent than the overall population(Cesselli, et al., 2011). Again, this approach would be hard to transfer to clinical practice, since it requires Good Manufacturing Practice-compliant cell sorting and large-scale expansion starting from very few cells. In fact, we have recently shown that only 0.7% of the hCSC obtained from end stage failing hearts gives rise to highly proliferating clones(Cesselli, et al., 2011) and, since hCSC are finite cell lines(Beltrami, et al., 2007; Cesselli, et al., 2011), hCSC-derived clones could undergo replicative senescence as a consequence of the high number of population doublings that are required to obtain a number of cells suitable for clinical purposes.

Whether selecting cells on the basis of the ability to actively extrude Hoechst 33342 (side population) could enrich in less senescent cells is still unknown(Hierlihy, et al., 2002; Martin, et al., 2004). However, also in this case a Good Manufacturing Practice-compliant cell sorting would be required.

4.3 Drug-based strategy to enrich in non-senescent cells

Several molecular pathways have been either associated with the development of cell senescence or, on the contrary, with organism longevity (Beltrami, et al., 2011a). Interestingly, the key elements of these two are common and the possibility to act on them can be explored to interfere with stem cell senescence and dysfunction, ameliorating stem cell regenerative approaches and organ pathology.

Briefly, as shown in Figure 1, the pathways main involved are: Insulin/Insulin-like Growth Factor Signaling (IIS), mTOR, AMPK/Autophagy, Nitric Oxide/Estrogen/Telomerase, Sirtuins, and p38MAPK(Beltrami, et al., 2011a).

Although the *Insulin/Insulin-like Growth Factor Signaling (IIS)* is critical for nutrient homeostasis, growth and survival, experimental evidences show that reduced IIS signaling in animals is associated with life extension(Beltrami, et al., 2011a). Insulin like Growth Factors and insulin inhibit the FoxO family of transcription factors through a pathway involving Insulin Receptor Substrate (IRS), PI3K and Akt. FoxO transcription factors promote a variety of cellular responses that include apoptosis, cell cycle arrest, differentiation, resistance to oxidative stress, and autophagy(Ronnebaum and Patterson, 2010; Salih and Brunet, 2008). The transcriptional activities and biological effects of FoxO depend on post-translational modifications and, in this regard, Sirt1 is believed to increase the ability of FoxO to respond to stress through cell cycle arrest and other adaptations but inhibits FoxO transcription of apoptotic genes. Last, FoxO is required for preventing Akt-mediated cardiac hypertrophy(Ronnebaum and Patterson, 2010). Regarding the possibility to interfere with this pathway, we have previously reported that hCSC expressing IGF1-R represent a subset of young and fully functional cells(D'Amario, et al., 2011a), and that IGF1 was able to support proliferation and differentiation of IGF-1R-positive hCSC.

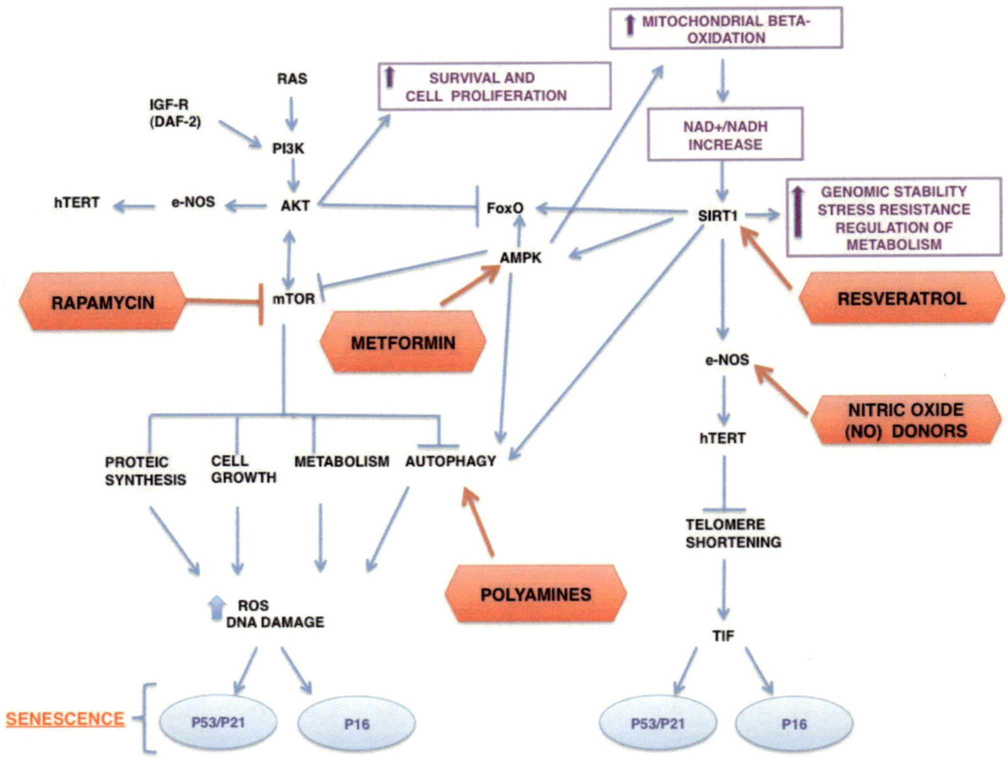

Fig. 1. Senescence pathways and possible pharmacological targets.

In aging, the *mammalian Target Of Rapamycin (mTOR)* plays a prominent role, which is, at least in part, mediated through IIS (Bhaskar and Hay, 2007). In fact, mTOR is activated by insulin, growth factors, nutrients and, indirectly, by Akt. mTOR forms two protein complexes; the Rapamycin-sensitive mTORC1, when bound to Raptor, and the Rapamycin insensitive mTORC2, when bound to Rictor. mTORC1 phosphorylates S6 kinase (S6K), eukariotic translation initiation factor 4E (eIF4E), and other factors involved in protein synthesis and hypertrophy. S6K, in turn, inhibits IRS by phosphorylation, while mTORC2 has a positive feedback on Akt. Nutrients and energy balance can regulate mTORC1, where aminoacids can activate it through the Rag family of GTPases, while AMPK, which is activated by ATP depletion, inhibits it (Bhaskar and Hay, 2007). Because of the central role of mTOR in ageing, Rapamycin has emerged as a very promising drug able to interfere with aging and, possibly, cell senescence(Blagosklonny, 2010). Importantly, Rapamycin is already used in clinical practice for its immunosuppressant and antiproliferative effects. Moreover, accumulated evidences display a possible role of Rapamycin in ageing and cell senescence. In fact, Rapamycin can extend the maximum lifespan of mice, when given late in life, restore self-renewal of hematopoietic stem cells of aged mice, and prevent epidermal stem cell exhaustion induced by Wnt-1 in mouse skin(Blagosklonny, 2010). Last, it has recently been shown that Rapamycin, the mTOR inhibitor PP242 or the IGF1R inhibitor PQ401, are able to increase the efficiency of iPS generation(Chen, et al., 2011). Despite the fact that rapamyicin is utilized in heart transplanted patients to avoid immunrejection, the effects of Rapamycin on hCSC senescence are still unexplored.

Nitric Oxide (NO) and estrogen signaling have been shown to counteract endothelial progenitor cell senescence through the catalytic subunit of human telomerase (hTERT)(Farsetti, et al., 2009). Estrogens' action is mediated either via genomic or nongenomic signaling pathways. The first ones follow the binding of estrogens to nuclear hormone receptors, which are capable of regulating transcription of a number of genes involved in development, metabolism, and differentiation following interaction with a hormone molecule. Therefore, estrogen receptors are ligand-dependent transcription factors. In addition, estrogens can trigger nongenomic signaling pathways through membrane associated estrogen receptors (mER) that activate both the PI3K and the Mitogen Activated Protein Kinase (MAPK) pathways. Estrogens can also activate Adenylate Cyclase and c-Src through the G-protein coupled estrogen receptor (GPER)(Meyer, et al., 2009). NO, on the other hand, is a free radical and an ancestral regulator of biological functions that include endothelial function, vasodilation, inflammation, and heart and muscle organogenesis(Farsetti, et al., 2009). NO is produced by a family of NO synthases (NOS) starting from L-arginine: neuronal NOS (n-NOS), endothelial NOS (e-NOS), and inducible NOS (i-NOS). Despite their names, the distribution of these enzymes is ubiquitous, but, while e-NOS and n-NOS are activated following an increase of intracellular calcium levels, i-NOS is calcium insensitive and is activated by inflammatory cytokines(Farsetti, et al., 2009). Importantly, it has been shown that VEGF-induced angiogenesis is mediated by NO and relies on hTERT activity. Estrogens, on the other hand, exert a beneficial role on the cardiovascular system which is, at least in part, mediated through the induction of e-NOS and hTERT(Farsetti, et al., 2009). Last, it has been recently shown that e-NOS and estrogen receptor (ERα) physically interact and cooperate in regulating hTERT and possibly other genes, thus delaying vascular senescence. Although NO production and endothelial nitric oxide synthase have been shown to be greater in longer living rodents, NO donors do not seem to influence animal maximum lifespan(Csiszar, et al., 2007). However, it has been shown both that NO can regulate telomerase activity(Farsetti, et al., 2009) and that it has a profound impact on mouse embryonic stem cell differentiation towards a cardiovascular fate(Spallotta, et al., 2010). Data on the effects of NO on hCSC are still missing.

Mammalian Sirtuins (Sirt) are yeast Sir2 orthologs possessing both NAD+ dependent- protein deacetylase and ADP-ribosyltransferase activity(Beltrami, et al., 2011a). Although Sir proteins are key regulators of *S. Cerevisiae, Drosophila,* and *C. Elegans* lifespan, the effect of Sirtuins on mammalian lifespan is less dramatic. Nonetheless, in mice lacking Sirt1, caloric restriction is unable to extend lifespan. Mammalians, in fact, possess at least 7 sirtuins, that act as metabolic sensors directly linking environmental signals to metabolic homeostasis and stress response. Sirt1, the most studied mammalian Sirtuin, controls gene expression, metabolism and aging, through a continuously growing list of substrates, that include: p53, members of the FoxO family, HES1 (hairy and enhancer of split 1), HEY2 (hairy/enhancer-of-split related with YRPW motif 2), PPARγ (peroxisome proliferator-activated receptor gamma), p300, PGC-1α (PPARγ coactivator), and NF- κB (nuclear factor kappaB)(Rahman and Islam, 2011). Although aging has been associated with stem cell senescence and dysfunction, the molecular mechanisms through which Sirt1 could protect primitive cells have not been completely delineated yet. However, the most prominent ones are: the positive regulation of telomeric length(Palacios, et al., 2010), the reduction of ROS production, the inhibition of p53(Rahman and Islam, 2011) and the induction of autophagy(Lee, et al., 2008). In this regard, Resveratrol is emerging as a potent drug able to delay age-related deteriorations and in mediating cardio-protection, conceivably by activating Sirt1(Petrovski, et al., 2011). In fact this polyphenolic compound has the ability to mimic the effects of caloric restriction by activating sirtuins and therefore acting modulating cell cycle, inhibiting apoptosis, increasing resistance to stress, and, finally, interfering with mTOR (Petrovski, et al., 2011). Accordingly, Resveratrol has shown beneficial effects against most degenerative and cardiovascular diseases from atherosclerosis, hypertension, ischemia/reperfusion, and heart failure to diabetes, obesity, and aging (Petrovski, et al., 2011). Importantly, pretreatment of either the infarcted heart or of cardiac stem cells with Resveratrol prior to cell injection results in an improvement of the regenerative capacities of the injected cells that eventually leads to improved heart function(Gorbunov, et al., 2011). However, in this specific case it was only evaluated the ability of Resveratrol to increase the engraftment of "normal" donor cells. In fact, up to now, the effects of Resveratrol on hCSC senescence remain to be elucidated. In addition, Resveratrol has been shown to be the most potent drug able to enhance iPS generation(Petrovski, et al., 2011).

p38MAPK is rapidly and transiently activated, by phosphorylation, following acute cellular stress. It is involved in senescence growth arrest by activating both p53 and pRb/p16INK4A pathways. Additionally, p38MAPK activity is required for the oncogene-induced premature senescence caused by oncogenic RAS, while its inhibition is able to delay replicative senescence, and to reverse the accelerated aging phenotype of fibroblasts obtained from Werner syndrome patients(Freund, et al., 2011). Further, p38MAPK is necessary and sufficient for the development of SASP in cells undergoing cellular senescence as a result of direct DNA damage or by oncogenic RAS(Freund, et al., 2011). Last, it was recently shown that p38MAPK inhibits Sirt1 by inducing its proteasomal degradation(Hong, et al., 2010). Although P38MAPK inhibitors have been successfully used to counteract in vitro the accelerated senescence phenotype seen in Werner syndrome progeria, it is still unclear whether this effect could be generalized to more physiological aging conditions. Importantly, it has been shown that p38MAPK inhibition can maintain hematopoietic stem cell quiescence, inhibiting the exhaustion of the hematopoietic stem cell pool(Ito, et al., 2006). In addition, p38MAPK inhibition can reduce cellular senescence in EPC exposed to doxorubicin (Spallarossa, et al., 2010). No data are available regarding hCSC. However, a role played by p38MAPK inhibition in inducing myocyte differentiation of embryonic stem cells has been reported(Gaur, et al., 2010).

Altogether, we can conclude that, although extremely interesting, the possibility to pharmacologically interfere with hCSC senescence has not yet been exploited.

5. Experimental data

In order to establish whether drugs known to interfere with the ageing processes could positively interfere with hCSC senescence and rescue their functional competence, hCSC obtained from failing hearts were cultured in the presence of increasing concentration of Rapamycin (1nM, 10nM, 100nM), Resveratrol (0.2μM, 0.5μM, 1μM) and DETA/NO (5μM, 10μM, 50μM). To reduce cell line variability, we selected hCSC obtained from ≈60 year old, male patients affected by end stage ischemic cardiomyopathy. After a 3-day treatment, cell lines (n=8) were analyzed both in terms of stem cell marker expression and cell proliferation, death and senescence. The ability of hCSC to differentiate and migrate was further assessed.

5.1 Methods

5.1.1 hCSC isolation and culture

Human atrial specimens, weighing 3-6 g, were collected over a period of five years from explanted hearts of patients in NHYA class 4 undergoing cardiac transplantation at the Cardiac Surgery Unit of the University Hospital of Udine, Italy. Informed consent was obtained in accordance with the Declaration of Helsinki and with approval by the Independent Ethics Committee of the University of Udine. Samples were employed for the isolation and expansion of c-kit-positive human cardiac stem cells (hCSC), as previously described (Bearzi, et al., 2009; Bearzi, et al., 2007; Beltrami, et al., 2007; Cesselli, et al., 2011). Specifically, two protocols were employed for the isolation of hCSC: enzymatic dissociation of the samples with collagenase and primary explant technique(Cesselli, et al., 2011). These two methodologies yielded comparable results up to 20-25 population doublings; efficiency and viability of hCSC were superimposable. Collagenase treatment was not found to affect these variables.

5.1.2 Pharmacological treatment of hCSC

After about 20 population doublings, growing cultures of hCSC were exposed to Rapamycin (1-100 nM, Sigma-Aldrich), 1-[N-(2-Aminoethyl)-N-(2-ammonioethyl)amino]diazen-1-ium-1,2-diolate or DETA/NO (5-50 μM, Sigma-Aldrich) and Resveratrol (0.2-1 μM, Sigma-Aldrich) for three days. At the end of the treatment, part of the cells was analyzed in terms of immunophenotype and to quantify cellular senescence, cell proliferation, and cell death. Part of the vehicle-treated and drug-treated cells was switched for n=2 days to a drug-free medium and subsequently assayed in terms of growth kinetic, differentiation and migration ability (see below).

5.1.3 Cell growth kinetic

Cells were seeded at a density of 2,000 cells/cm^2 in expansion medium. Cells were detached and counted at 1-2-5-9-12 and 14 days.

5.1.4 Cell differentiation assay

Muscle cell differentiation was achieved plating 0.5 to 1x10^4/cm^2 cells in expansion medium containing 5% FCS (Sigma-Aldrich, st. Louis, MO, USA), 10 ng/mL bFGF, 10 ng/mL VEGF, and 10 ng/mL IGF-1 (all from Peprotech EC, London, UK), but not EGF. Cells were allowed to become confluent and cultured for up to 4 weeks with medium exchanges every 4 days(Beltrami, et al., 2007; Cesselli, et al., 2011). Endothelial cell differentiation was obtained plating 0.5 to $1x10^4/cm^2$ hCSC in *EGM®-2* Endothelial Cell Growth Medium-*2* (Lonza, Switzerland) for 2 weeks.

5.1.5 Migration assay

In order to evaluate in vitro cell migration of drug treated or untreated hCSC, a scratch assay was performed(Liang, et al., 2007). In 33mm-plates at high confluence, scratches were created utilizing 200µl tips. Phase contrast images of the scratches were acquired at 3-hour intervals, until their complete closure, utilizing Leica DMI6000B. Images were then compared and quantified by ImageJ in order to calculate the rate of cell migration. The mean scratch width did not differ significantly in the different culture conditions ($p>0.05$).

5.1.6 Flow cytometry

Proliferating cells were detached with 0.25% trypsin-EDTA (Sigma-Aldrich) and, after a 20 minutes recovery phase, were incubated with either properly conjugated primary antibodies: CD13, CD29, CD49a, CD49b, CD49d, CD90, CD73, CD44, CD59, CD45, HLA-DR, CD117, CD271, CD34, (BD Biosciences), CD105, CD66e (Serotech), CD133 (Miltenyi Biotec), E-cadherin (Santa Cruz Biotechnology), ABCG-2 (Chemicon International), or with an unconjugated primary antibody: N-cadherin (Sigma-Aldrich). Unconjugated antibody was revealed using PE or FITC conjugated secondary antibodies (DakoCytomation). Properly conjugated isotype matched antibodies were used as a negative control.

Apoptosis and necrosis were evaluated utilizing the Annexin V-FITC Apoptosis Detection Kit (Bender MedSystem), following manufacturer's instructions.

The analysis was performed either by FACS-Calibur (BD Biosciences) or by CyAn (Dako Cytomation).

5.1.7 Immunofluorescence and fluorescence microscopy

Cells cultured either in expansion or in differentiation medium were fixed in 4% buffered paraformaldehyde for 20 minutes at room temperature (R.T.). For intracellular stainings, fixed cells were permeabilized for 8 minutes at R.T. with 0.1% Triton X-100 (Sigma-Aldrich) before exposing them to primary antibodies. Primary antibody incubation was performed over-night at 4°C using following dilutions: Oct-4 (Abcam, 1:150); Sox-2 (Chemicon, 1:150); Nanog (Abcam, 1:150), cKit (R&D; 1:100), p21 (Santa Cruz; 1:40), $p16^{INK4A}$ (CIN-TEK, pre-diluted), γH2A.X (Upstate, 1:500), Ki67 (Novocastra, 1:1000); α-Sarcomeric Actin (Sigma, 1:100) and CD31 (Dako, 1:50). To detect primary antibodies, A488 and A555 dyes labeled secondary antibodies, diluted 1:800, were employed (Molecular Probe, Invitrogen). Finally, 0.1 µg/ml DAPI (Sigma) was used to identify nuclei. Vectashield (Vector) was used as mounting medium. Confocal image acquisition was carried out by a Confocal Laser Microscope (Leica TCS-SP2, Leica Microsystems) utilizing either a 63x oil immersion objective (numerical aperture: 1.40) or a 40x oil immersion objective (numerical aperture: 1.25). Epifluorescence and phase contrast images were obtained utilizing a live cell imaging dedicated system consisting of a Leica DMI 6000B microscope connected to a Leica

DFC350FX camera (Leica Microsystems, Wetzlar, Germany). 10X (numerical aperture: 0.25), 40X oil immersion (numerical aperture: 1.25), and 63X oil immersion (numerical aperture: 1.40) objectives were employed for this purpose. Bright field images were captured utilizing a Leica DMD108 microscope (Leica Microsystems). 10X (numerical aperture: 0.40), 20X (numerical aperture: 0.70), and 40x (numerical aperture: 0.95) objectives were employed. Adobe Photoshop software was utilized to compose, overlay the images and adjust the contrast (Adobe, USA).

5.1.8 Statistics

Two-tailed unpaired- Student t- test and one-way Anova followed by Bonferroni post-test were utilized to compare means between two or more groups, respectively (Prism, version 4.0c). Results are expressed as mean±standard deviation. *P* values less than 0.05 were considered significant.

5.2 Results

We evaluated the effects of Rapamycin, Resveratrol and DETA/NO on hCSC stem cell marker expression, proliferation, senescence, death and function.

5.2.1 Effects of drugs on hCSC stem cell marker expression

As previously mentioned, hCSC obtained from failing hearts presented a mesenchymal immunophenotype and largely expressed the pluripotent state specific transcription factors Oct-4, Nanog and Sox-2. Drug treatment did not alter the mesenchymal immunophenotype and left unchanged the faction of cells expressing the pluripotent state specific transcription factors (data not shown).

5.2.2 Effects of drugs on hCSC proliferation, senescence and death

The effects exerted by Rapamyicin, Resveratrol and DETA/NO on hCSC proliferation, senescence and death resulted to be drug- and concentration- dependent; therefore, the effects exerted by each drug will be presented separately.

Rapamycin

As shown in Figure 1, Rapamycin mainly acts inhibiting mTOR-related pathway, thus inhibiting cell growth, autophagy and reducing oxidative stress. However, the anti-proliferative effect of the drugs is partially counteracted by a positive effect on Akt.

Accordingly, after a 3-day treatment hCSC, with respect to vehicle-treated cells, did not display changes in proliferation, as testified both by Ki67 expression and nuclear density (Figure 2).

Rapamycin was instead effective in reducing the fraction of senescent cells acting primarily on the fraction of cells expressing p16 that, at a 10nM concentration, resulted to be halved. No changes in the fraction of cells with DNA-damage foci were observed (Figure 2). DNA-damage foci positive cells were identified by the presence of the histonic protein γH2AX in the absence of Ki67 expression (Lawless, et al., 2010).

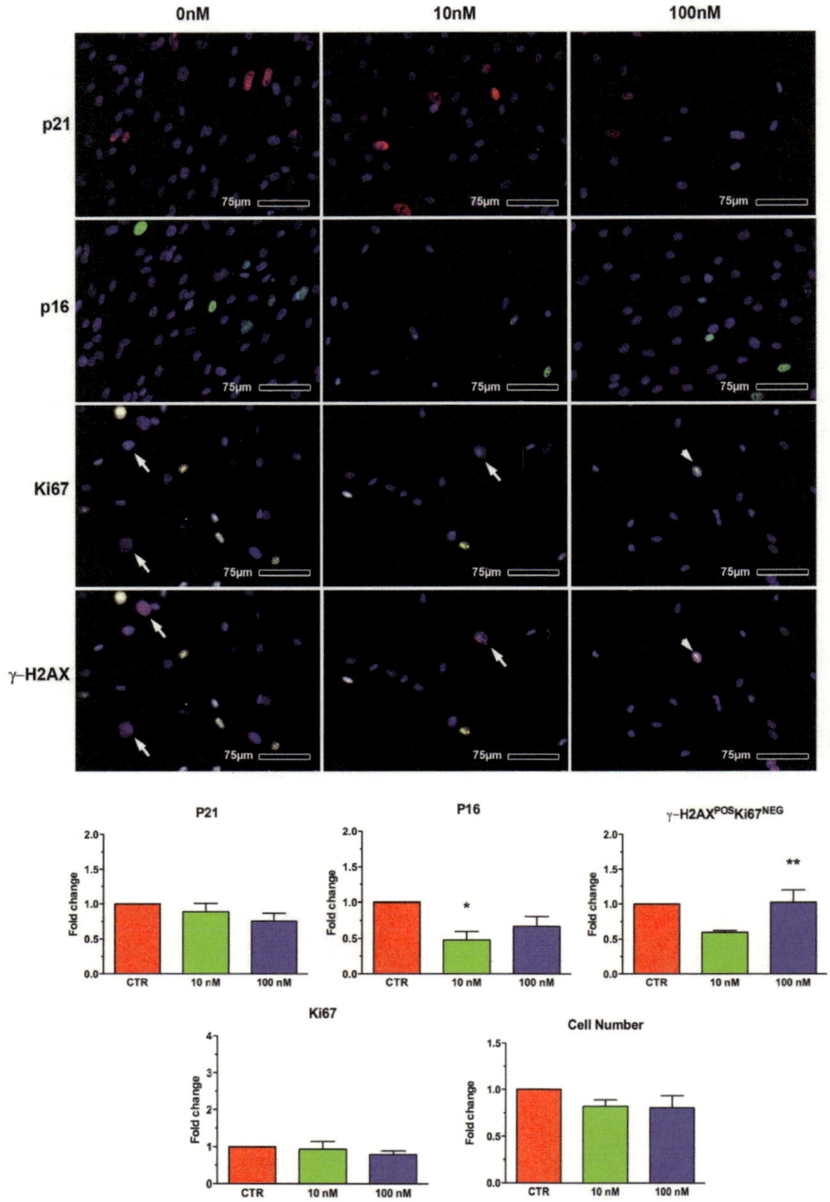

Fig. 2. **Effects of Rapamycin on hCSC.** hCSC were exposed for 3 days to 0nM (left panels), 1nM (central panels) and 10nM (right panels) Rapamyicin. Cells were then stained for p21 (red fluorescence), p16 (green fluorescence), Ki67 (yellow fluorescence) and γH2AX (magenta fluorescence). DNA-damage foci positive cells (arrows) were recognized as cells positive for γH2AX (magenta fluorescence) but negative for Ki67 (yellow fluorescence). Cells positive for both Ki67 and γH2AX (arrowheads) were excluded from the count. Histograms represent the fold changes in the fraction of cells expressing senescence (p21, p16, $\gamma H2AX^{+}Ki67^{-}$) and proliferation markers (Ki67) and in hCSC number of treated cells with respect to vehicle-treated cells (CTR). *, **, $p<0.05$ with respect to CTR and 10nM treated cells, respectively.

Interestingly, Rapamyicin at both concentrations tested increased the fraction of cells undergoing cell death through apoptosis (Figure 3).

In conclusion, Rapamyicin seemed to act reducing the fraction of p16-positive senescent cells, without affecting cell proliferation.

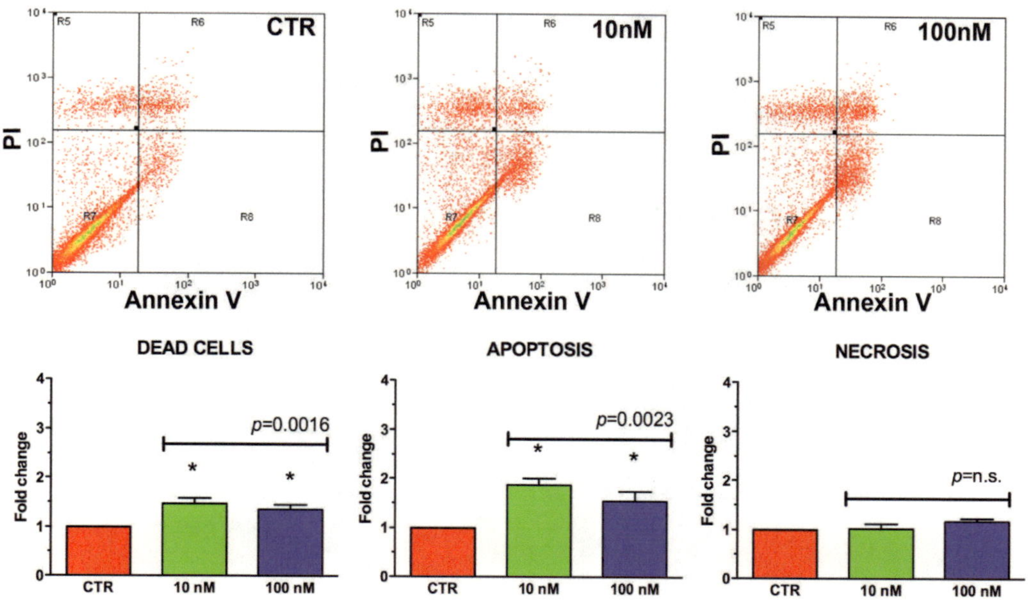

Fig. 3. **Effects of Rapamycin on hCSC death.** In the upper panel dot-plots graphically represent hCSC cultured in the presence of different concentrations of Rapamycin, stained for PI and AnnexinV and analyzed by FACS. Apoptotic cells were defined as AnnexinV^{+}PI$^{+/-}$ cells, necrotic cells as AnnexinV^{-}PI^{+}cells. In the lower panels, histograms represent the quantitative analysis of the fold change in the fraction of dead cells. *, $p<0.05$ with respect to vehicle-treated cells (CTR).

Resveratrol

As displayed in figure 1, Resveratrol has the ability to mimic the effects of caloric restriction by activating sirtuins and therefore acting modulating cell cycle, inhibiting apoptosis, increasing resistance to stress, and, finally, interfering with mTOR (Petrovski, et al., 2011).

Accordingly, Resveratrol-treated cells presented a larger fraction of Ki67-positive cells and an increased nuclear density (Figure 4). Importantly, the fraction of senescent cells resulted to be significantly reduced at both drug concentration used. Differently from Rapamyicin, acting on p16-positive cells, Resveratrol was effective in reducing the fraction of cells presenting DNA-damage foci and expressing p21 (Figure 4).

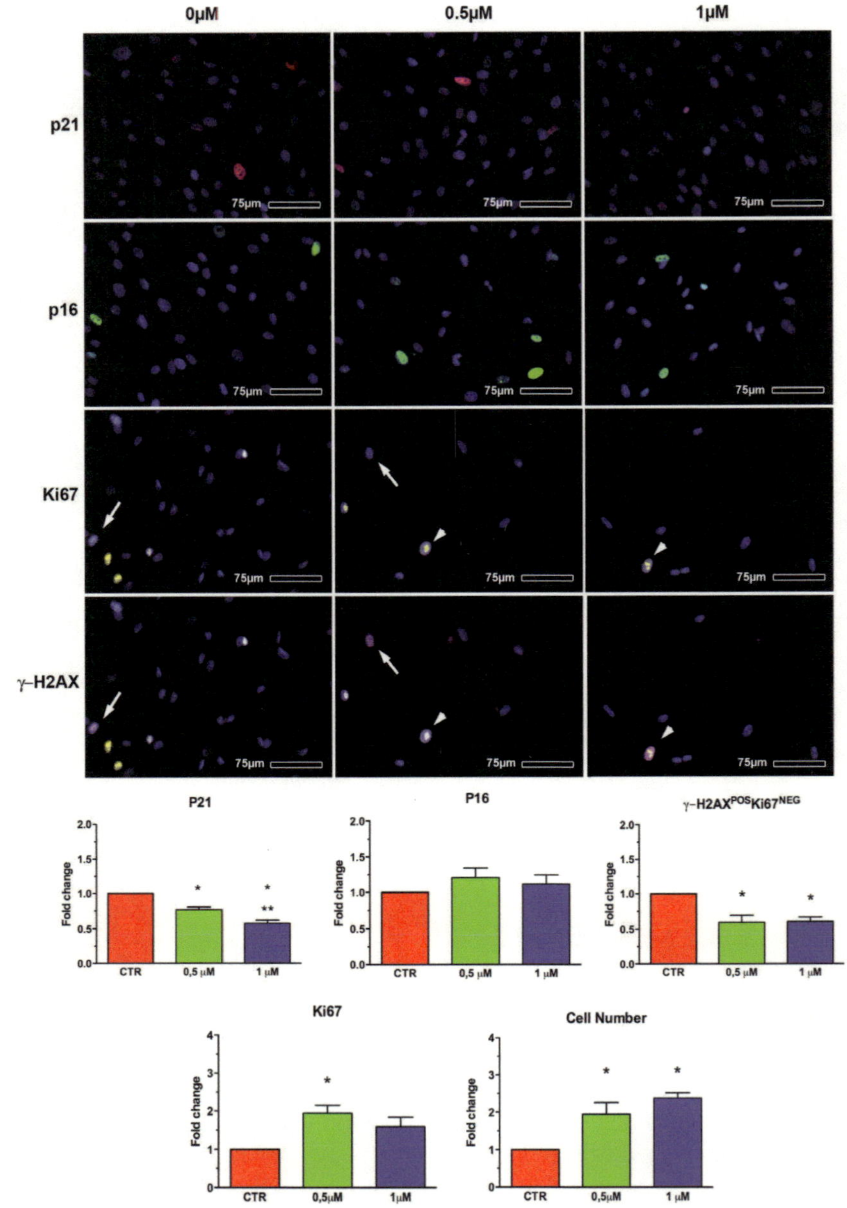

Fig. 4. **Effects of Resveratrol on hCSC.** hCSC were exposed for 3 days to 0µM (left panels), 0,5µM (central panels) and 1µM (right panels) Resveratrol. Cells were then stained for p21 (red fluorescence), p16 (green fluorescence), Ki67 (yellow fluorescence) and γH2AX (magenta fluorescence). DNA-damage foci positive cells (arrows) were recognized as cells positive for γH2AX (magenta fluorescence) but negative for Ki67 (yellow fluorescence). Cells positive for both Ki67 and γH2AX (arrowheads) were excluded from the count. Histograms represent the fold changes in the fraction of cells expressing senescence (p21, p16, $\gamma H2AX^{+}Ki67^{-}$) and proliferation markers (Ki67) and in hCSC number of treated cells with respect to vehicle-treated cells (CTR). *, $p<0.05$ with respect to CTR.

Moreover, Resveratrol significantly reduced the fraction of cells dying by necrosis (Figure 5).

Altogether these results indicate that Resveratrol presented beneficial effects on hCSC stimulating cell proliferation, reducing DNA-damage induced senescence and cell death.

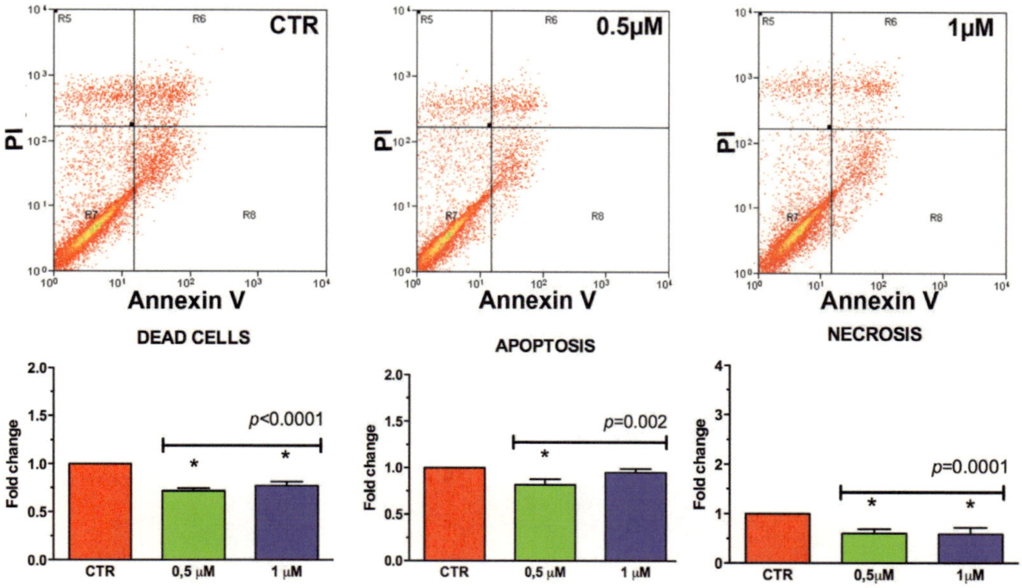

Fig. 5. **Effects of Resveratrol on hCSC death.** In the upper panel dot-plots graphically represent hCSC cultured in the presence of different concentrations of drug, stained for PI and AnnexinV and analyzed by FACS. Apoptotic cells were defined as $AnnexinV^{+}PI^{+/-}$ cells, necrotic cells as $AnnexinV^{-}PI^{+}$cells. In the lower panels, histograms represent the quantitative analysis of the fold change in the fraction of dead cells. *, p<0.05 with respect to vehicle-treated cells (CTR).

DETA/NO

As displayed in Figure 1, NO donors regulate telomerase activity. Moreover, it has been shown that it has a profound impact on stem cell differentiation towards a cardiovascular fate (Farsetti, et al., 2009).

After a 3-day treatment, DETA/NO-treated cells did not differ, with respect to vehicle-treated cells, in terms of nuclear density, while Ki67 resulted to be increased only in 10μM-treated cells (Figure 6). Importantly, all DETA/NO used concentrations significantly decreased the fraction of γH2AX-positive cells, with a trend to reduce the fraction of p21 positive cells only at 10 μM (Figure 6).

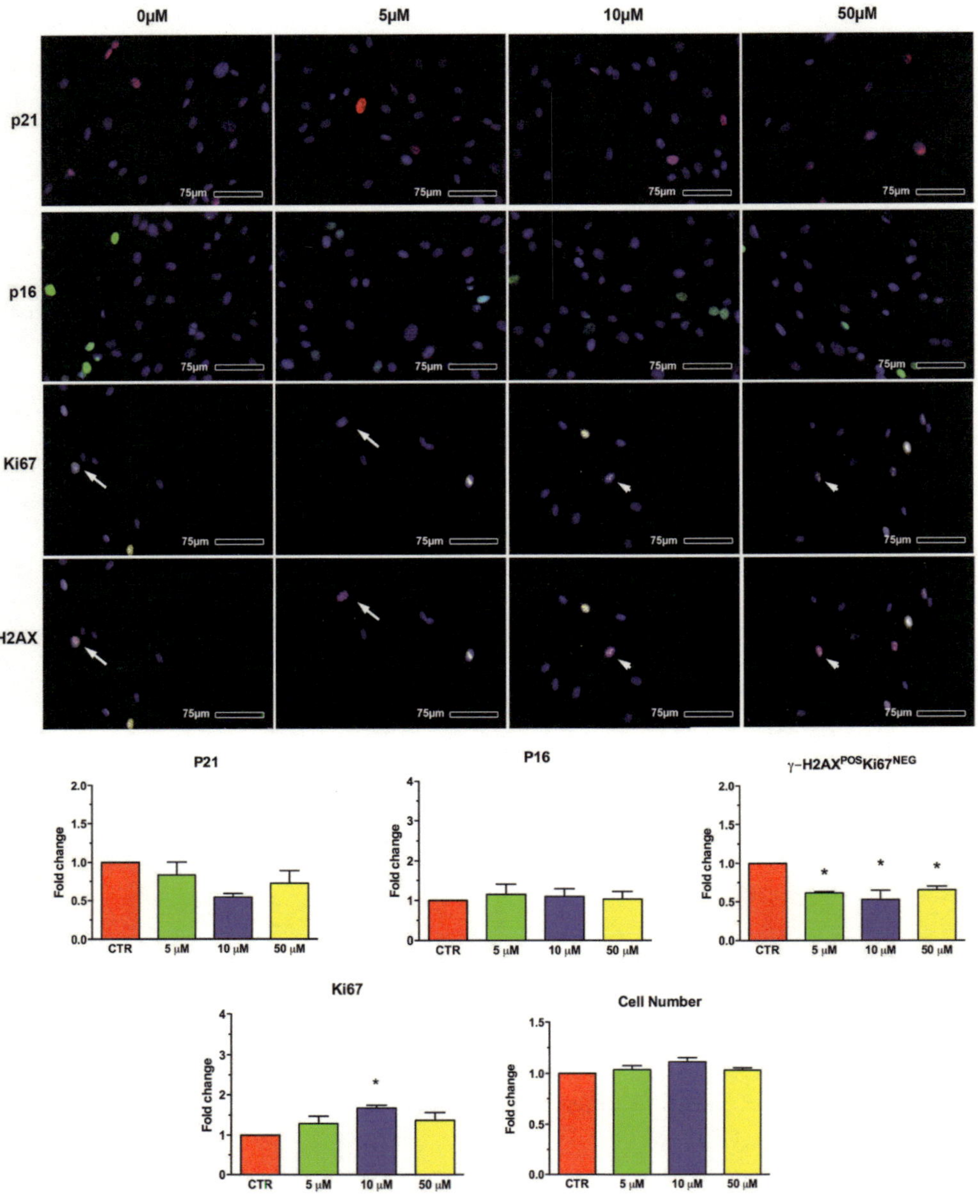

Fig. 6. **Effects of DETA/NO on hCSC.** hCSC were exposed for 3 days to DETA/NO 0μM, 5μM, 10μM and 50μM. Cells were then stained for p21 (red fluorescence), p16 (green fluorescence), Ki67 (yellow fluorescence) and γH2AX (magenta fluorescence). DNA-damage foci positive cells (arrows) were recognized as cells positive for γH2AX (magenta fluorescence) but negative for Ki67 (yellow fluorescence). Cells positive for both Ki67 and γH2AX (arrowheads) were excluded from the count. Histograms represent the fold changes in the fraction of cells expressing senescence (p21, p16, $\gamma H2AX^{+}Ki67^{-}$) and proliferation markers (Ki67) and in hCSC number of treated cells with respect to vehicle-treated cells (CTR). *, $p<0.05$ with respect to CTR.

No significantly changes in the fraction of dying cells was assessed (Figure 7).

In conclusion, DETA/NO seemed to act specifically by reducing the fraction of cells with DNA-damage foci eliciting a DNA-damage response. This is in line with its ability to activate telomerase activity.

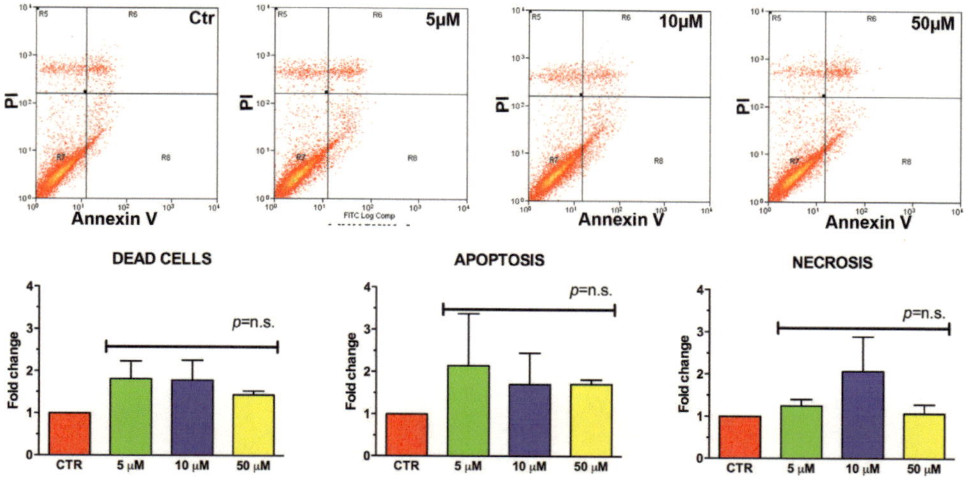

Fig. 7. **Effects of DETA/NO on hCSC death.** In the upper panel dot-plots graphically represent hCSC cultured in the presence of different concentrations of drug, stained for PI and AnnexinV and analyzed by FACS. Apoptotic cells were defined as AnnexinV^{+}PI$^{+/-}$ cells, necrotic cells as AnnexinV^{-}PI^{+}cells. In the lower panels, histograms represent the quantitative analysis of the fold change in the fraction of dead cells.

Altogether, the analysis of the effects of a three-day drug treatment of senescent hCSC, showed that, although all the utilized drugs exerted a beneficial effect in reducing the fraction of senescent cells, they differed not only in the pathway of cell senescence specifically targeted (p16 vs γH2AX/p21), but also in their ability to interfere with other key-processes such as cell proliferation and cell death. Table 1 summarizes the effects of the drugs on the principal cell processes and indicates the identified optimal drug concentration.

	Variable	Rapamycin	Resveratrol	DETA/NO
Senescence	**P16**	↓		
	P21		↓	↓
	γH2AX		↓	↓
Proliferation	**Ki67**		↑	↑ (10 μM)
	Nuclear density		↑	
Cell Death	**Apoptosis**	↑		
	Necrosis		↓	
Optimal drug concentration		10 nM	0.5 μM	10 μM

Table 1. Summary of drug effects on hCSC senescence, proliferation and death.

5.2.3 Effects of drugs on hCSC function

In order to verify whether the beneficial effects exerted by drugs on hCSC senescence were paralleled by an improvement in hCSC function, hCSC treated for three days with the optimal drug concentration were assayed, after two days of recovery, for: growth kinetic, differentiation capacity and migration abilities.

Growth kinetic

Despite the fact that during the three-day treatment only Resveratrol-treated cells resulted to increase their number (Figure 3, 5 and 7), all the drugs resulted to be effective in significantly reduce the population doubling time (Figure 8, p=0.002), suggesting that the reduction in the fraction of senescent cells was afterward associated with an increased proliferation rate.

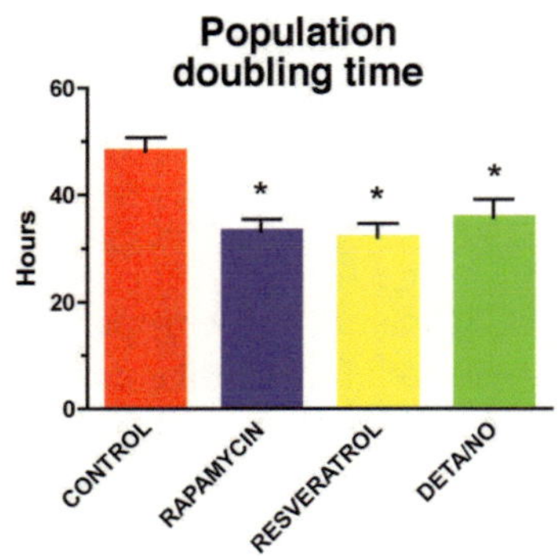

Fig. 8. Effects of drugs on hCSC population doubling time. *, $p<0.05$ with respect to vehicle-treated cells (CONTROL).

Differentiation ability

We investigated the ability of drug-treated hCSC to differentiate along the endothelial and myogenic fate. CD31 was utilized as endothelial marker, while alpha-sarcomeric actin as myogenic markers.

Interestingly, we have seen that cells treated for three days with drugs and then exposed to endothelial-differentiation inducing conditions displayed different behaviour. Specifically, while Rapamycin-treated cells significantly improved their ability to differentiate into endothelial cells expressing CD31, Resveratrol and DETA/NO did not (Figure 9).

Regarding, myocyte differentiation capacity, we noticed that cell cultures differed not only in the percentage of alpha-sarcomeric actin (ASA) positive cells, but also in the level of organization of the filaments. Therefore, we decided to use a score able to taking into account these two factors and defined as the product of the fraction of ASA-positive cells and an index expressing ASA organization, which ranged from 1 (not-organized) to 3 (well defined filaments)(Cesselli, et al., 2011). Applying these criteria, we established that Rapamycin did not interfere with the differentiation ability of hCSC, while the other two, especially DETA/NO, improved the myogenic potential of hCSC (Figure 10).

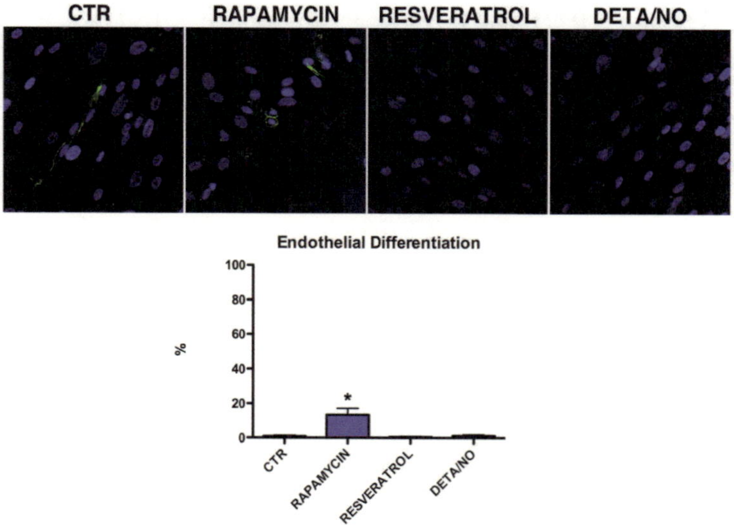

Fig. 9. **Effects of drugs on hCSC endothelial differentiation ability.** Green fluorescence represent CD31 expression on hCSC exposed to endothelial differentiation medium. Nuclei are depicted by the blue fluorescence of DAPI staining. Histograms represent the quantitative analysis of the fraction of CD31-positive cells in the cells treated with different drugs. *, p<0.05 vs vehicle-treated cells (CTR).

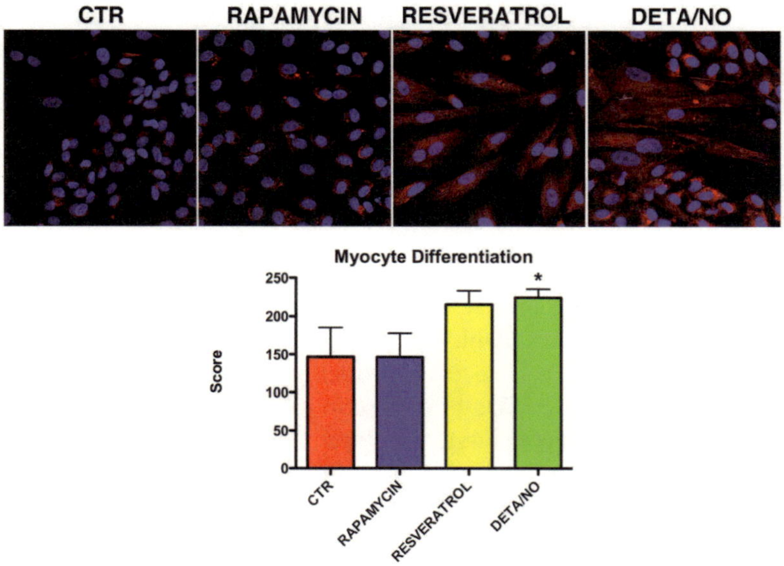

Fig. 10. **Effects of drugs on hCSC myocyte differentiation ability.** Red fluorescence represent alpha-sarcomeric actin expression on hCSC exposed to myocyte differentiation medium. Nuclei are depicted by the blue fluorescence of DAPI staining. Histograms represent the quantitative analysis of the level of myocyte differentiation of the cells treated with different drugs. See text for score meaning. *, p<0.05 vs vehicle-treated cells (CTR).

It remains to be demonstrated whether the improved differentiation ability of drug-treated cells is a consequence of the benefical effects of the drug on senescence or if it is due to a direct effect of the drug on differentiation pathways. In fact, the ability of DETA/NO to favor stem cell differentiation towards a cardiovascular fate has already been demonstrated in mouse embryonic stem cells (Farsetti, et al., 2009). Moreover, oxytocin, a hormone present also in the heart, induces embryonic and cardiac somatic stem cells to differentiate into cardiomyocytes, possibly through nitric oxide(Danalache, et al., 2007).

Migration capacity

In order to establish the migration speed of hCSC, a scratch assay was performed. With respect to vehicle treated cells, only DETA/NO-treated cells showed a trend to increase their migration ability (Figure 11), while Rapamycin and Resveratrol treated cells did not. Even in this case, it is difficult to establish whether DETA/NO would act directly on the migration ability of the cells, since it has already demonstrated a role of NO on SDF-1/CXCR4-mediated bone-marrow cell migration(Cui, et al., 2007).

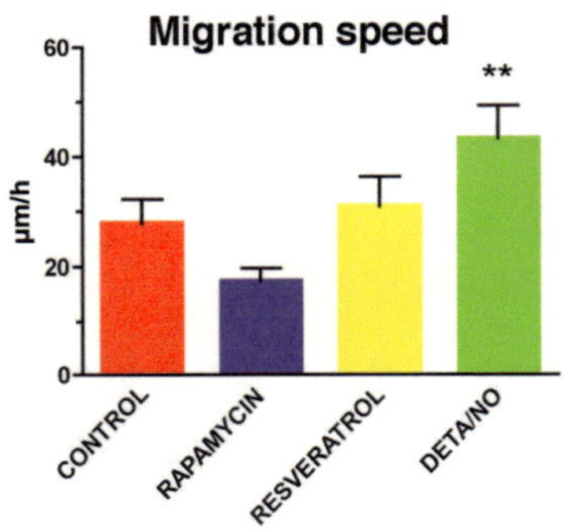

Fig. 11. **Effects of drugs on hCSC migration ability.** Histograms represent the quantitative analysis of migration speed of the cells treated with different drugs. **, $p<0.05$ vs Rapamycin-treated cells.

As a whole, drug treatment did not modify hCSC phenotype and stem cell marker expression. However, different effects were observed with respect to cell death, where Rapamycin increased of about 1.5 fold hCSC apoptosis ($p=0.002$), whereas Resveratrol showed a protective effect on cell necrosis, reducing it by 50% ($p=0.0001$). Although all drugs were associated with a significant decrease in the fraction of senescent cells, different pathways of cellular senescence were involved. Specifically, while Resveratrol and DETA/NO treatment were associated with a significant reduction by half of cells with DDR and p21 expression, Rapamycin treatment was mainly associated with a ≈60% reduction in p16 expression ($p<0.05$). Importantly, although all drug-treated cells showed, with respect to vehicle, an increase in cell proliferation, the effects on hCSC differentiation and migration ability were different. Specifically, Rapamycin treated cells displayed an improved endothelial differentiation capacity, while Resveratrol seemed to positively affect only the myogenic potential of hCSC. Finally, DETA/NO improved both the myocyte differentiation capacity and the migration ability of hCSC, without effects on endothelial differentiation capacity.

6. Conclusions

Severe heart failure is characterized by the loss of the growth reserve of the adult heart, dictated by a progressive decrease in the number of functionally-competent hCSC(Cesselli, et al., 2011). Despite these limitations, autologous CSC therapy is feasible and can be considered a therapeutic option for the large population of patients affected by severe heart failure(Beltrami, et al., 2011b; Segers and Lee, 2008). In fact, even in patients with advanced cardiomyopathies hCSC can be isolated from small myocardial biopsies and expanded in vitro(Cesselli, et al., 2011; D'Amario, et al., 2011b; Smith, et al., 2007). For this reason, it would be extremely intriguing any attempt aimed at "improving" the quality of the expanded cells, selecting the fraction of cells with the highest regenerative potential.

In this regard, Anversa's group showed that different membrane receptors influence the regenerative ability of hCSC and that IGF-1 receptor-positive hCSC are endowed with a high regenerative ability, representing a potent cell population for cardiac repair(D'Amario, et al., 2011a). However, this approach would require the sorting of cells expressing specific surface antigens, thus adding a further grade of complexity to the procedure aimed at producing clinical grade hCSC.

The strategy we wanted to undertake in this project was slightly different, since we decided to treat hCSC with drugs in culture. The results we obtained indicate that, although hCSC isolated from failing hearts are senescent and functionally impaired, it is possible to interfere pharmacologically, at least in vitro, with the senescence processes, rescuing the properties of the primitive cells. Specifically, we have shown that a three-day treatment with Rapamycin, Resveratrol or DETA/NO was able to reduce the fraction of senescent cells, improving their proliferative capacity. Importantly, the tested drugs seemed to exert their effects on different subpopulations of senescent cells; in fact, while Rapamycin mainly reduced the p16-positive fraction, DETA/NO and Resveratrol principally acted on the pool of cells characterized by DNA-damage foci and expressing p21. Similarly, different drugs showed different effects on hCSC function. In fact, while Rapamycin increased endothelial differentiation ability, DETA/NO improved hCSC myogenic and migration capacity.

These results represent the first demonstration that hCSC senescence can be attenuated in vitro, and that this is associated with an improved proliferative capacity.

Future research will be aimed: 1) at understanding more in depth the mechanism through which drugs exert their effects on cellular senescence, e.g. removal of senescent cells, modulation of SASP-mediated pathways; 2) establishing whether drug-treated cells possess an increased in vivo regenerative potential; 3) establishing criteria to define which is the best drug to use.

7. References

Acosta, J. C., O'Loghlen, A., Banito, A., Guijarro, M. V., Augert, A., Raguz, S., Fumagalli, M., Da Costa, M., Brown, C., Popov, N., Takatsu, Y., Melamed, J., d'Adda di Fagagna, F., Bernard, D., Hernando, E., & Gil, J. (2008). Chemokine signaling via the CXCR2 receptor reinforces senescence. Cell, 133(6), 1006-1018.

Adams, P. D. (2009). Healing and hurting: molecular mechanisms, functions, and pathologies of cellular senescence. Mol Cell, 36(1), 2-14.

Bearzi, C., Rota, M., Hosoda, T., Tillmanns, J., Nascimbene, A., De Angelis, A., Yasuzawa-Amano, S., Trofimova, I., Siggins, R. W., Lecapitaine, N., Cascapera, S., Beltrami, A. P., D'Alessandro, D. A., Zias, E., Quaini, F., Urbanek, K., Michler, R. E., Bolli, R., Kajstura, J., Leri, A., & Anversa, P. (2007). Human cardiac stem cells. Proc Natl Acad Sci U S A, 104(35), 14068-14073.

Bearzi, C., Leri, A., Lo Monaco, F., Rota, M., Gonzalez, A., Hosoda, T., Pepe, M., Qanud, K., Ojaimi, C., Bardelli, S., D'Amario, D., D'Alessandro, D. A., Michler, R. E., Dimmeler, S., Zeiher, A. M., Urbanek, K., Hintze, T. H., Kajstura, J., & Anversa, P. (2009). Identification of a coronary vascular progenitor cell in the human heart. Proc Natl Acad Sci U S A, 106(37), 15885-15890.

Beltrami, A. P., Barlucchi, L., Torella, D., Baker, M., Limana, F., Chimenti, S., Kasahara, H., Rota, M., Musso, E., Urbanek, K., Leri, A., Kajstura, J., Nadal-Ginard, B., & Anversa, P. (2003). Adult cardiac stem cells are multipotent and support myocardial regeneration. Cell, 114(6), 763-776.

Beltrami, A. P., Cesselli, D., Bergamin, N., Marcon, P., Rigo, S., Puppato, E., D'Aurizio, F., Verardo, R., Piazza, S., Pignatelli, A., Poz, A., Baccarani, U., Damiani, D., Fanin, R., Mariuzzi, L., Finato, N., Masolini, P., Burelli, S., Belluzzi, O., Schneider, C., & Beltrami, C. A. (2007). Multipotent cells can be generated in vitro from several adult human organs (heart, liver, and bone marrow). Blood, 110(9), 3438-3446.

Beltrami, A. P., Cesselli, D., & Beltrami, C. A. (2011a). At the stem of youth and health. Pharmacol Ther, 129(1), 3-20.

Beltrami, A. P., Cesselli, D., Beltrami, C. A., Cohen, I. S., & Gaudette, G. R. (2011b). Multiple Sources for Cardiac Stem Cells and Their Cardiogenic Potential, In: *Regenerating the Heart*, Cohen, I. S., & Gaudette, G. R., pp. 149-171, Humana Press.

Bhaskar, P. T., & Hay, N. (2007). The two TORCs and Akt. Dev Cell, 12(4), 487-502.

Blagosklonny, M. V. (2010). Rapamycin and quasi-programmed aging: Four years later. Cell Cycle, 9(10).

Blasco, M. A. (2007). Telomere length, stem cells and aging. Nat Chem Biol, 3(10), 640-649.

Blasi, F., & Carmeliet, P. (2002). uPAR: a versatile signalling orchestrator. Nat Rev Mol Cell Biol, 3(12), 932-943.

Bu, L., Jiang, X., Martin-Puig, S., Caron, L., Zhu, S., Shao, Y., Roberts, D. J., Huang, P. L., Domian, I. J., & Chien, K. R. (2009). Human ISL1 heart progenitors generate diverse multipotent cardiovascular cell lineages. Nature, 460(7251), 113-117.

Campisi, J. (2005). Senescent cells, tumor suppression, and organismal aging: good citizens, bad neighbors. Cell, 120(4), 513-522.

Campisi, J., & d'Adda di Fagagna, F. (2007). Cellular senescence: when bad things happen to good cells. Nat Rev Mol Cell Biol, 8(9), 729-740.

Campisi, J. (2011). Cellular senescence: putting the paradoxes in perspective. Curr Opin Genet Dev, 21(1), 107-112.

Castaldo, C., Di Meglio, F., Nurzynska, D., Romano, G., Maiello, C., Bancone, C., Muller, P., Bohm, M., Cotrufo, M., & Montagnani, S. (2008). CD117-positive cells in adult human heart are localized in the subepicardium, and their activation is associated with laminin-1 and alpha6 integrin expression. Stem Cells, 26(7), 1723-1731.

Cesselli, D., Beltrami, A. P., D'Aurizio, F., Marcon, P., Bergamin, N., Toffoletto, B., Pandolfi, M., Puppato, E., Marino, L., Signore, S., Livi, U., Verardo, R., Piazza, S., Marchionni, L., Fiorini, C., Schneider, C., Hosoda, T., Rota, M., Kajstura, J., Anversa, P., Beltrami, C. A., & Leri, A. (2011). Effects of age and heart failure on human cardiac stem cell function. Am J Pathol, 179(1), 349-366.

Chen, T., Shen, L., Yu, J., Wan, H., Guo, A., Chen, J., Long, Y., Zhao, J., & Pei, G. (2011). Rapamycin and other longevity-promoting compounds enhance the generation of mouse induced pluripotent stem cells. Aging Cell, 10(5), 908-911.

Chimenti, C., Kajstura, J., Torella, D., Urbanek, K., Heleniak, H., Colussi, C., Di Meglio, F., Nadal-Ginard, B., Frustaci, A., Leri, A., Maseri, A., & Anversa, P. (2003). Senescence and death of primitive cells and myocytes lead to premature cardiac aging and heart failure. Circ Res, 93(7), 604-613.

Collado, M., Gil, J., Efeyan, A., Guerra, C., Schuhmacher, A. J., Barradas, M., Benguria, A., Zaballos, A., Flores, J. M., Barbacid, M., Beach, D., & Serrano, M. (2005). Tumour biology: senescence in premalignant tumours. Nature, 436(7051), 642.

Coppe, J. P., Patil, C. K., Rodier, F., Sun, Y., Munoz, D. P., Goldstein, J., Nelson, P. S., Desprez, P. Y., & Campisi, J. (2008). Senescence-associated secretory phenotypes reveal cell-nonautonomous functions of oncogenic RAS and the p53 tumor suppressor. PLoS Biol, 6(12), 2853-2868.

Csiszar, A., Labinskyy, N., Zhao, X., Hu, F., Serpillon, S., Huang, Z., Ballabh, P., Levy, R. J., Hintze, T. H., Wolin, M. S., Austad, S. N., Podlutsky, A., & Ungvari, Z. (2007). Vascular superoxide and hydrogen peroxide production and oxidative stress resistance in two closely related rodent species with disparate longevity. Aging Cell, 6(6), 783-797.

Cui, X., Chen, J., Zacharek, A., Li, Y., Roberts, C., Kapke, A., Savant-Bhonsale, S., & Chopp, M. (2007). Nitric oxide donor upregulation of stromal cell-derived factor-1/chemokine (CXC motif) receptor 4 enhances bone marrow stromal cell migration into ischemic brain after stroke. Stem Cells, 25(11), 2777-2785.

D'Amario, D., Cabral-Da-Silva, M. C., Zheng, H., Fiorini, C., Goichberg, P., Steadman, E., Ferreira-Martins, J., Sanada, F., Piccoli, M., Cappetta, D., D'Alessandro, D. A., Michler, R. E., Hosoda, T., Anastasia, L., Rota, M., Leri, A., Anversa, P., & Kajstura, J. (2011a). Insulin-like growth factor-1 receptor identifies a pool of human cardiac stem cells with superior therapeutic potential for myocardial regeneration. Circ Res, 108(12), 1467-1481.

D'Amario, D., Fiorini, C., Campbell, P. M., Goichberg, P., Sanada, F., Zheng, H., Hosoda, T., Rota, M., Connell, J. M., Gallegos, R. P., Welt, F. G., Givertz, M. M., Mitchell, R. N., Leri, A., Kajstura, J., Pfeffer, M. A., & Anversa, P. (2011b). Functionally competent cardiac stem cells can be isolated from endomyocardial biopsies of patients with advanced cardiomyopathies. Circ Res, 108(7), 857-861.

Danalache, B. A., Paquin, J., Donghao, W., Grygorczyk, R., Moore, J. C., Mummery, C. L., Gutkowska, J., & Jankowski, M. (2007). Nitric oxide signaling in oxytocin-mediated cardiomyogenesis. Stem Cells, 25(3), 679-688.

De Angelis, A., Piegari, E., Cappetta, D., Marino, L., Filippelli, A., Berrino, L., Ferreira-Martins, J., Zheng, H., Hosoda, T., Rota, M., Urbanek, K., Kajstura, J., Leri, A., Rossi, F., & Anversa, P. (2010). Anthracycline cardiomyopathy is mediated by depletion of the cardiac stem cell pool and is rescued by restoration of progenitor cell function. Circulation, 121(2), 276-292.

Deng, Y., Chan, S. S., & Chang, S. (2008). Telomere dysfunction and tumour suppression: the senescence connection. Nat Rev Cancer, 8(6), 450-458.

Di Micco, R., Cicalese, A., Fumagalli, M., Dobreva, M., Verrecchia, A., Pelicci, P. G., & di Fagagna, F. (2008). DNA damage response activation in mouse embryonic fibroblasts undergoing replicative senescence and following spontaneous immortalization. Cell Cycle, 7(22), 3601-3606.

Dimmeler, S., & Leri, A. (2008). Aging and disease as modifiers of efficacy of cell therapy. Circ Res, 102(11), 1319-1330.

Dimri, G. P., Lee, X., Basile, G., Acosta, M., Scott, G., Roskelley, C., Medrano, E. E., Linskens, M., Rubelj, I., Pereira-Smith, O., & et al. (1995). A biomarker that identifies senescent human cells in culture and in aging skin in vivo. Proc Natl Acad Sci U S A, 92(20), 9363-9367.

Farsetti, A., Grasselli, A., Bacchetti, S., Gaetano, C., & Capogrossi, M. C. (2009). The telomerase tale in vascular aging: regulation by estrogens and nitric oxide signaling. J Appl Physiol, 106(1), 333-337.

Fiordaliso, F., Leri, A., Cesselli, D., Limana, F., Safai, B., Nadal-Ginard, B., Anversa, P., & Kajstura, J. (2001). Hyperglycemia activates p53 and p53-regulated genes leading to myocyte cell death. Diabetes, 50(10), 2363-2375.

Freund, A., Patil, C. K., & Campisi, J. (2011). p38MAPK is a novel DNA damage response-independent regulator of the senescence-associated secretory phenotype. EMBO J, 30(8), 1536-1548.

Fukuda, D., & Sata, M. (2008). Role of bone marrow renin-angiotensin system in the pathogenesis of atherosclerosis. Pharmacol Ther, 118(2), 268-276.

Gaur, M., Ritner, C., Sievers, R., Pedersen, A., Prasad, M., Bernstein, H. S., & Yeghiazarians, Y. (2010). Timed inhibition of p38MAPK directs accelerated differentiation of human embryonic stem cells into cardiomyocytes. Cytotherapy, 12(6), 807-817.

Gonzalez, A., Rota, M., Nurzynska, D., Misao, Y., Tillmanns, J., Ojaimi, C., Padin-Iruegas, M. E., Muller, P., Esposito, G., Bearzi, C., Vitale, S., Dawn, B., Sanganalmath, S. K., Baker, M., Hintze, T. H., Bolli, R., Urbanek, K., Hosoda, T., Anversa, P., Kajstura, J., & Leri, A. (2008). Activation of cardiac progenitor cells reverses the failing heart senescent phenotype and prolongs lifespan. Circ Res, 102(5), 597-606.

Gorbunov, N., Petrovski, G., Gurusamy, N., Ray, D., Kim, D. H., & Das, D. K. (2011). Regeneration of Infarcted Myocardium with Resveratrol-Modified Cardiac Stem Cells. J Cell Mol Med.

Hayflick, L., & Moorhead, P. S. (1961). The serial cultivation of human diploid cell strains. Exp Cell Res, 25, 585-621.

Hierlihy, A. M., Seale, P., Lobe, C. G., Rudnicki, M. A., & Megeney, L. A. (2002). The post-natal heart contains a myocardial stem cell population. FEBS Lett, 530(1-3), 239-243.

Hong, E. H., Lee, S. J., Kim, J. S., Lee, K. H., Um, H. D., Kim, J. H., Kim, S. J., Kim, J. I., & Hwang, S. G. (2010). Ionizing radiation induces cellular senescence of articular chondrocytes via negative regulation of SIRT1 by p38 kinase. J Biol Chem, 285(2), 1283-1295.

Hosoda, T., D'Amario, D., Cabral-Da-Silva, M. C., Zheng, H., Padin-Iruegas, M. E., Ogorek, B., Ferreira-Martins, J., Yasuzawa-Amano, S., Amano, K., Ide-Iwata, N., Cheng, W., Rota, M., Urbanek, K., Kajstura, J., Anversa, P., & Leri, A. (2009). Clonality of mouse and human cardiomyogenesis in vivo. Proc Natl Acad Sci U S A, 106(40), 17169-17174.

Hsieh, P. C., Segers, V. F., Davis, M. E., MacGillivray, C., Gannon, J., Molkentin, J. D., Robbins, J., & Lee, R. T. (2007). Evidence from a genetic fate-mapping study that stem cells refresh adult mammalian cardiomyocytes after injury. Nat Med, 13(8), 970-974.

Imanishi, T., Hano, T., & Nishio, I. (2005). Angiotensin II accelerates endothelial progenitor cell senescence through induction of oxidative stress. J Hypertens, 23(1), 97-104.

Ito, K., Hirao, A., Arai, F., Takubo, K., Matsuoka, S., Miyamoto, K., Ohmura, M., Naka, K., Hosokawa, K., Ikeda, Y., & Suda, T. (2006). Reactive oxygen species act through p38 MAPK to limit the lifespan of hematopoietic stem cells. Nat Med, 12(4), 446-451.

Itzhaki-Alfia, A., Leor, J., Raanani, E., Sternik, L., Spiegelstein, D., Netser, S., Holbova, R., Pevsner-Fischer, M., Lavee, J., & Barbash, I. M. (2009). Patient characteristics and cell source determine the number of isolated human cardiac progenitor cells. Circulation, 120(25), 2559-2566.

Jeyapalan, J. C., & Sedivy, J. M. (2008). Cellular senescence and organismal aging. Mech Ageing Dev, 129(7-8), 467-474.

Khan, M., Mohsin, S., Khan, S. N., & Riazuddin, S. (2011). Repair of senescent myocardium by mesenchymal stem cells is dependent on the age of donor mice. J Cell Mol Med, 15(7), 1515-1527.

Kortlever, R. M., Higgins, P. J., & Bernards, R. (2006). Plasminogen activator inhibitor-1 is a critical downstream target of p53 in the induction of replicative senescence. Nat Cell Biol, 8(8), 877-884.

Kosar, M., Bartkova, J., Hubackova, S., Hodny, Z., Lukas, J., & Bartek, J. (2011). Senescence-associated heterochromatin foci are dispensable for cellular senescence, occur in a cell type- and insult-dependent manner and follow expression of p16(ink4a). Cell Cycle, 10(3), 457-468.

Kuilman, T., Michaloglou, C., Vredeveld, L. C., Douma, S., van Doorn, R., Desmet, C. J., Aarden, L. A., Mooi, W. J., & Peeper, D. S. (2008). Oncogene-induced senescence relayed by an interleukin-dependent inflammatory network. Cell, 133(6), 1019-1031.

Kunieda, T., Minamino, T., Nishi, J., Tateno, K., Oyama, T., Katsuno, T., Miyauchi, H., Orimo, M., Okada, S., Takamura, M., Nagai, T., Kaneko, S., & Komuro, I. (2006). Angiotensin II induces premature senescence of vascular smooth muscle cells and accelerates the development of atherosclerosis via a p21-dependent pathway. Circulation, 114(9), 953-960.

Laflamme, M. A., & Murry, C. E. (2011). Heart regeneration. Nature, 473(7347), 326-335.

Lawless, C., Wang, C., Jurk, D., Merz, A., Zglinicki, T., & Passos, J. F. (2010). Quantitative assessment of markers for cell senescence. Exp Gerontol, 45(10), 772-778.

Lee, I. H., Cao, L., Mostoslavsky, R., Lombard, D. B., Liu, J., Bruns, N. E., Tsokos, M., Alt, F. W., & Finkel, T. (2008). A role for the NAD-dependent deacetylase Sirt1 in the regulation of autophagy. Proc Natl Acad Sci U S A, 105(9), 3374-3379.

Li, L., & Clevers, H. (2010). Coexistence of quiescent and active adult stem cells in mammals. Science, 327(5965), 542-545.

Liang, C. C., Park, A. Y., & Guan, J. L. (2007). In vitro scratch assay: a convenient and inexpensive method for analysis of cell migration in vitro. Nat Protoc, 2(2), 329-333.

Martin, C. M., Meeson, A. P., Robertson, S. M., Hawke, T. J., Richardson, J. A., Bates, S., Goetsch, S. C., Gallardo, T. D., & Garry, D. J. (2004). Persistent expression of the ATP-binding cassette transporter, Abcg2, identifies cardiac SP cells in the developing and adult heart. Dev Biol, 265(1), 262-275.

McMurray, J. J., & Pfeffer, M. A. (2005). Heart failure. Lancet, 365(9474), 1877-1889.

Meissner, K., Heydrich, B., Jedlitschky, G., Meyer Zu Schwabedissen, H., Mosyagin, I., Dazert, P., Eckel, L., Vogelgesang, S., Warzok, R. W., Bohm, M., Lehmann, C., Wendt, M., Cascorbi, I., & Kroemer, H. K. (2006). The ATP-binding cassette transporter ABCG2 (BCRP), a marker for side population stem cells, is expressed in human heart. J Histochem Cytochem, 54(2), 215-221.

Messina, E., De Angelis, L., Frati, G., Morrone, S., Chimenti, S., Fiordaliso, F., Salio, M., Battaglia, M., Latronico, M. V., Coletta, M., Vivarelli, E., Frati, L., Cossu, G., & Giacomello, A. (2004). Isolation and expansion of adult cardiac stem cells from human and murine heart. Circ Res, 95(9), 911-921.

Meyer, M. R., Haas, E., Prossnitz, E. R., & Barton, M. (2009). Non-genomic regulation of vascular cell function and growth by estrogen. Mol Cell Endocrinol, 308(1-2), 9-16.

Minamino, T., & Komuro, I. (2008). Vascular aging: insights from studies on cellular senescence, stem cell aging, and progeroid syndromes. Nat Clin Pract Cardiovasc Med, 5(10), 637-648.

Narita, M., Nunez, S., Heard, E., Lin, A. W., Hearn, S. A., Spector, D. L., Hannon, G. J., & Lowe, S. W. (2003). Rb-mediated heterochromatin formation and silencing of E2F target genes during cellular senescence. Cell, 113(6), 703-716.

Orjalo, A. V., Bhaumik, D., Gengler, B. K., Scott, G. K., & Campisi, J. (2009). Cell surface-bound IL-1alpha is an upstream regulator of the senescence-associated IL-6/IL-8 cytokine network. Proc Natl Acad Sci U S A, 106(40), 17031-17036.

Palacios, J. A., Herranz, D., De Bonis, M. L., Velasco, S., Serrano, M., & Blasco, M. A. (2010). SIRT1 contributes to telomere maintenance and augments global homologous recombination. J Cell Biol, 191(7), 1299-1313.

Patschan, S., & Goligorsky, M. S. (2008). Autophagy: The missing link between non-enzymatically glycated proteins inducing apoptosis and premature senescence of endothelial cells? Autophagy, 4(4), 521-523.

Petrovski, G., Gurusamy, N., & Das, D. K. (2011). Resveratrol in cardiovascular health and disease. Ann N Y Acad Sci, 1215, 22-33.

Rahman, S., & Islam, R. (2011). Mammalian Sirt1: insights on its biological functions. Cell Commun Signal, 9, 11.

Ronnebaum, S. M., & Patterson, C. (2010). The FoxO family in cardiac function and dysfunction. Annu Rev Physiol, 72, 81-94.

Rota, M., LeCapitaine, N., Hosoda, T., Boni, A., De Angelis, A., Padin-Iruegas, M. E., Esposito, G., Vitale, S., Urbanek, K., Casarsa, C., Giorgio, M., Luscher, T. F., Pelicci, P. G., Anversa, P., Leri, A., & Kajstura, J. (2006). Diabetes promotes cardiac stem cell aging and heart failure, which are prevented by deletion of the p66shc gene. Circ Res, 99(1), 42-52.

Salih, D. A., & Brunet, A. (2008). FoxO transcription factors in the maintenance of cellular homeostasis during aging. Curr Opin Cell Biol, 20(2), 126-136.

Sharpless, N. E., & DePinho, R. A. (2007). How stem cells age and why this makes us grow old. Nat Rev Mol Cell Biol, 8(9), 703-713.

Shawi, M., & Autexier, C. (2008). Telomerase, senescence and ageing. Mech Ageing Dev, 129(1-2), 3-10.

Smith, R. R., Barile, L., Cho, H. C., Leppo, M. K., Hare, J. M., Messina, E., Giacomello, A., Abraham, M. R., & Marban, E. (2007). Regenerative potential of cardiosphere-derived cells expanded from percutaneous endomyocardial biopsy specimens. Circulation, 115(7), 896-908.

Spallarossa, P., Altieri, P., Barisione, C., Passalacqua, M., Aloi, C., Fugazza, G., Frassoni, F., Podesta, M., Canepa, M., Ghigliotti, G., & Brunelli, C. (2010). p38 MAPK and JNK antagonistically control senescence and cytoplasmic p16INK4A expression in doxorubicin-treated endothelial progenitor cells. PLoS One, 5(12), e15583.

Spallotta, F., Rosati, J., Straino, S., Nanni, S., Grasselli, A., Ambrosino, V., Rotili, D., Valente, S., Farsetti, A., Mai, A., Capogrossi, M. C., Gaetano, C., & Illi, B. (2010). Nitric oxide determines mesodermic differentiation of mouse embryonic stem cells by activating class IIa histone deacetylases: potential therapeutic implications in a mouse model of hindlimb ischemia. Stem Cells, 28(3), 431-442.

Torella, D., Rota, M., Nurzynska, D., Musso, E., Monsen, A., Shiraishi, I., Zias, E., Walsh, K., Rosenzweig, A., Sussman, M. A., Urbanek, K., Nadal-Ginard, B., Kajstura, J., Anversa, P., & Leri, A. (2004). Cardiac stem cell and myocyte aging, heart failure, and insulin-like growth factor-1 overexpression. Circ Res, 94(4), 514-524.

Urbanek, K., Torella, D., Sheikh, F., De Angelis, A., Nurzynska, D., Silvestri, F., Beltrami, C. A., Bussani, R., Beltrami, A. P., Quaini, F., Bolli, R., Leri, A., Kajstura, J., & Anversa, P. (2005). Myocardial regeneration by activation of multipotent cardiac stem cells in ischemic heart failure. Proc Natl Acad Sci U S A, 102(24), 8692-8697.

Vellai, T. (2009). Autophagy genes and ageing. Cell Death Differ, 16(1), 94-102.
von Zglinicki, T., Saretzki, G., Ladhoff, J., d'Adda di Fagagna, F., & Jackson, S. P. (2005). Human cell senescence as a DNA damage response. Mech Ageing Dev, 126(1), 111-117.
Wajapeyee, N., Serra, R. W., Zhu, X., Mahalingam, M., & Green, M. R. (2008). Oncogenic BRAF induces senescence and apoptosis through pathways mediated by the secreted protein IGFBP7. Cell, 132(3), 363-374.
Young, A. R., & Narita, M. (2010). Connecting autophagy to senescence in pathophysiology. Curr Opin Cell Biol, 22(2), 234-240.

31

Central Immune Senescence, Reversal Potentials

Krisztian Kvell and Judit E. Pongracz
Department of Medical Biotechnology, University of Pecs, Hungary

1. Introduction

1.1 Ageing in focus

Ageing is a complex process that affects all living organisms. Senescence is not only conceivable in multicellular organisms, but also in unicellulars. Unlike certain diseases that have specific morbidity rates, ageing is a physiological process that affects all individuals that live long enough (unaffected by i.e. predation or famine) to experience senescence.

A pioneer of ageing research, August Weismann has established two rather opposing concepts for aging and even today both gather numerous followers. One is the adaptive concept, according to which ageing has evolved to cleanse the population from old, non-reproductive consumers. The other, non-adaptive concept suggests that ageing is due to greater weight on early survival / reproduction rather than vigour at later ages. This latter has been reshaped by the theory of antagonistic pleiotropy (Ljubuncic et al. 2009).

Due to advances in biomedical research and care, currently an average 55-aged person is expected to live up to 85 years of age at death on average in the Western societies. This number is expected to increase if biomedical research continues to develop at the current rate and by the year 2030 an average 55-aged person is expected to live up to 115 years of age at death (according to SENS plans) (de Grey 2007). If such forecasts prove to be true, it is of extraordinary significance and will likely trigger immense social and economical conflicts.

1.1.1 Ageing and society

Ageing of the population is one of the most important challenges for the developed world to face over the next decades. The current demographic trends and consequent shrinkage of the active workforce will put enormous pressure on the financing of social protection and health systems, likely to reduce living standards. Taken together with increased migration and emergence of novel infectious diseases, broad-scale provision of immunological protection constitutes a strategic aim for longer and healthier lifespan.

At present life-span is still significantly increasing in the Western civilisations, however, this increase is not accompanied by proportional increase in life spent in overall good health referred to as 'health-span'. There are current efforts to prolong health-span within expanding life-span. This would not only extend life spent in appropriate quality of life, but also has the potential to alleviate pressure on current public health systems. This chapter focuses on central immune senescence and therefore will enumerate potential mechanisms of extending human central immune fitness in the elderly.

1.1.2 Ageing of the immune system

Impaired immunological responsiveness in the elderly poses a major difficulty. The immunological competence of an individual is determined by the presence of mature lymphocytes formed in primary lymphoid organs, and specialized secondary lymphoid tissues performing diverse immune responses. Thus at systems level the maintenance of immunological equilibrium requires steady lymphocyte output, and controlled expansion. Lymphostromal interactions in both primary and secondary lymphoid tissues play essential roles in the development and function of lymphocyte subsets in adaptive immune responses. The thymic and lymph-node stromal microenvironments thus represent key elements in the development of the adaptive immune system. Consequently, impairment of the lymphoid microenvironment will ultimately lead to insufficient primary and secondary immune responses or to the decline of thymic selection, manifesting in immune senescence accompanied by late-onset autoimmune disorders, often observed in elderly. Self-tolerant cytotoxic and helper T-lymphocytes, the crucial regulator cells in adaptive immune responses, develop in the specialized epithelial network of the thymus. The thymus, however, gradually loses its capacity to support lymphopoiesis in an involution process that results in a decline of *de novo* T-cell production.

1.1.3 Significance of thymic involution studies

In contrast to the extensive studies addressing haemopoietic cells, the in-depth analysis of determinants for stromal competence during immunological ageing is far less detailed, despite its clear significance related to immunological responsiveness in the elderly. There is literature describing quantitative changes that occur during immunological senescence in peripheral immunologically competent tissues like the spleen or lymph nodes. Probably the best characterised, significant example is that of FDCs. Compared to young counterparts the aged follicular dendritic cells express significantly less CD21 ligand and FcγRII. As a consequence aged FDCs lose their ability to trap immune complexes and present antigens to B cells. This in turn leads to impaired germinal centre reactions and antibody production (Aydar et al. 2004). However, even these well characterised quantitative changes of the peripheral lymphoid tissues are less dramatic than the adipose involution of the thymus.

The manipulation of thymic immune senescence and the restoration of de-novo T-cell production should provide direct benefits for both adult and elderly patients. Such interventions shall increase health-span within life-span significantly reducing the healthcare costs alleviating the burden on healthcare systems.

1.2 T-cell development in the thymus

T-cell progenitors migrate to the thymus from the bone marrow where they undergo an extensive differentiation and selection process. After entering the thymus, thymocytes representing different stages of development occupy distinct regions of the thymus. The earliest $CD4^-CD8^-CD44^+CD25^-$ thymocyte progenitors, referred to as double negative 1

(DN1) cells are found near their site of entry at the cortico-medullary junction. The slightly more mature CD4-CD8-CD44+CD25+ (DN2) subset is found throughout the cortex, whereas CD4-CD8-CD44-CD25+ (DN3) subset is concentrated below the capsule. Following rearrangement of antigen receptor (TCR) genes (He et al. 2006) CD4+CD8+ (double positive or DP) thymocytes undergo positive (functional TCR) and negative (non self-reactive TCR) selection in the cortex and medulla, to finally leave the thymus for the periphery as CD4-CD8+ (cytotoxic) or CD4+CD8- (helper) single positive (SP), mature, naïve T-cells.

1.3 Thymic microenvironment in *de novo* T-cell production

Successful T-cell development requires the interaction of thymocytes with the thymic stroma, creating the special thymic microenvironment for T-cell differentiation and selection. A large proportion of the thymic stroma consists of epithelial cells that develop from the epithelial thymic anlage from the third pharyngeal pouch around embryonic day 10-11 in the mouse (Manley 2000). Following several differentiation steps, including expression of FoxN1 – a member of the forkhead transcription factor family (Mandinova et al. 2009) – that is essential for Mts24+ epithelial progenitors (Bennett et al. 2002; Gill et al. 2002) to develop into various epithelial subsets (Dooley et al. 2005) and to establish the special thymic epithelial cell phenotype (Manley 2000). FoxN1 expression in early stages of thymus organogenesis is regulated by secreted Wnt4 (Balciunaite et al. 2002) protein. The mature thymic epithelium consists of two major compartments, the cortex and the medulla, which apart from producing chemokines that attract haematopoietic stem cells to the thymus, also contribute the establishing the special thymic microenvironment. The thymic epithelial network regulates homing, intrathymic migration, and differentiation of developing T-lymphocytes through release of cytokines (e.g. interleukin-7 (Alves et al. 2009)), secretion of extracellular matrix components, and establishment of intercellular connections (Crisa L et al. 1996) (Schluns et al. 1997). Thymocytes bearing diverse TCR repertoire are selected by MHC (major-histocompatibility-complex) molecules and MHC bound-antigens presented by the thymic stroma, including epithelial cells. During T-cell development, characterised by progression through phenotypically distinct stages (Lind et al. 2001), thymocytes reside in spatially restricted domains of the mature thymus. T-cell precursors enter the thymus at the cortico-medullary junction (Blackburn et al. 2004), then migrate to the subcapsular zone of the outer cortex, back through the cortex, then to the medulla, where they finally leave to the periphery (Blackburn et al. 2004). Functional studies have shown, that the cortex is important in producing chemokines, which attract pro-thymocytes (Bleul et al. 2000) and are also essential for mediating positive selection (Anderson et al. 1994). Meanwhile the medullary epithelium has been implicated in driving the final stages of thymocyte maturation (Ge et al. 2000) and has a crucial role in tolerance induction (Farr et al. 1998; Derbinski et al. 2001). Additionally, the thymic epithelium is also the source of other secreted and cell surface proteins that regulate T-cell development. These proteins include bone morphogenic protein (BMP) (Bleul et al. 2005), Notch (Valsecchi 1997), and Wnt (Pongracz et al. 2003) family members.

1.4 Thymic involution during ageing

In comparison to other organs, ageing of the thymus is an accelerated process in all mammals. In humans, thymic senescence begins early, around late puberty and by 50 years of age 80% of the thymic stroma is converted into adipose tissue (Dixit 2010). As the thymic epithelium is replaced by adipose tissue, the whole process is called adipose involution (Marinova 2005). Due to decrease in functional thymic epithelial tissue mass, the thymus can no longer support the same output of naïve T-cell production (Ribeiro et al. 2007). T-lymphocyte composition in the periphery therefore exhibits the dominance of memory T-lymphocytes resulting in impaired responses towards novel, particularly viral infections (Chidgey et al. 2007; Gui et al. 2007; Grubeck-Loebenstein 2009). Since the thymic epithelium has also a key role in deleting auto-reactive T-cell clones, functional impairment increases the chances of developing auto-immune disease (Hsu et al. 2003). The transcription factor FoxN1, characteristic in thymus development is also affected by age. FoxN1 (Mandinova et al. 2009) is not only essential for progenitor epithelial cells of the thymic rudiment to develop into various epithelial subsets (Dooley et al. 2005) but also to maintain TEC identity in the differentiated, adult thymus. Decreased level of FoxN1 expression in adult TECs results in accelerated thymic involution (Chen et al. 2009; Cheng et al. 2010).

1.5 Thymic involution: developmental programme or senescence?

It has long been known that the thymus begins adipose involution and senescence rather early, but how early is that exactly? Recent studies have analysed the kinetics of thymic function and thymic mass versus age. It has been confirmed in both mouse and human thymic samples that the functional peek of thymic activity significantly precedes the peek of thymic mass and the first signs of adipose involution. In the mouse thymic activity is largely decreased by the age of one month compared to the newborn age (thymocyte precursor immigration at 6% and mature T cell emigration at 7% where 100% is measured at newborn age), yet the thymus reaches its largest size at one month of age (Shiraishi et al. 2003). Similar tendency has been described in humans where thymic function reaches its peak around the age of one year followed by the first signs of adipose infiltration by the age of approx. five years (Shiraishi et al. 2003). However, most studies describe significant thymic adipose involution starting around puberty / young adulthood. Therefore there is apparently significant detachment of thymic activity peak and thymic mass peak, and surprisingly activity peak significantly precedes mass peak.

The above described phenomenon raises the issue whether the early appearance of thymic involution belongs to senescence or developmental programme and how strictly these two may be separated? Similar questions are raised by the detection of miniature atherosclerotic lesions detected already at foetal age, a currently fashionable topic (Leduc et al. 2010).

1.6 Trans-differentiation of fibroblasts into adipocytes

The nuclear lamina consists of a matrix of proteins located next to the inner nuclear membrane. The lamina family of proteins makes up the matrix and that is highly conserved in evolution. The family of lamina associated polypeptides (LAP) has several members with similar functions. Studies with fibroblast cells have revealed that fibroblast to pre-adipocyte transformation is strongly connected to LAP2α, the member of the LAP2α protein family (Dorner et al. 2006). While most splice variants associate with the nuclear envelope, LAP2α is involved in several nucleoplasmic activities including cell-cycle control and differentiation (Berger et al. 1996; Hutchison et al. 2001). LAP2α is synthesized in the cytoplasm and is then transported into the nucleus by a PKC-dependent mechanism (Dreger et al. 1999). The mere over-expression of LAP2α in fibroblasts is known to directly up-regulate PPARγ expression, an acknowledged marker and key transcription factor of pre-adipocyte differentiation (Dorner et al. 2006). In pre-adipocytes PPARγ expression is followed by an increase of ADRP expression (adipose differentiation-related protein) a known direct target gene of PPARγ. Although LAP2α over-expression alone initiates pre-adipocyte differentiation in fibroblasts, it is not sufficient to complete the adipocyte differentiation programme in the absence of additional stimuli (Dorner et al. 2006).

1.7 Wnt signalling

1.7.1 Wnt signalling

The Wnt family of 19 secreted glycoproteins controls a variety of developmental processes including cell fate specification, cell proliferation, cell polarity and cell migration. There are two main signalling pathways involved in the signal transduction process from the Wnt receptor (Frizzled) complex: the canonical or β-catenin dependent, and the non-canonical pathway, which splits into the polar cell polarity (PCP) or c-Jun-N-Terminal Kinase (JNK) / Activating Protein (AP1) dependent and the Ca^{2+} or Protein kinase C (PKC) / Calmodulin Kinase (CaMKII) / Nuclear Factor of Activating T-cells (NFAT) dependent signalling pathways.

Based on their ability to activate a particular Wnt pathway, Wnt molecules have been grouped as canonical (Wnt1, Wnt3, Wnt3a, Wnt7a, Wnt7b, Wnt8) (Torres et al. 1996) and non-canonical pathway activators (Wnt5a, Wnt4, Wnt11) (Torres et al. 1996), although promiscuity is a feature of both ligands and receptors.

1.7.2 Canonical Wnt-pathway

The canonical or β-catenin / Tcf dependent Wnt pathway is extensively investigated, and has been shown to be present in the thymus both in developing thymocytes (Ioannidis et al. 2001; Staal 2001; Xu et al. 2003) as well as in the thymic epithelium (Balciunate et al. 2001, Pongracz et al. 2003). Generally, in the absence of canonical Wnt-s, glycogen synthase kinase-3β (GSK-3β) is active and phosphorylates β-catenin in the scaffolding protein complex of adenomatous polyposis coli (APC) and axin (Ikeda 1998; Yamamoto 1999). The phosporylated β-catenin is targeted for ubiquitination and 26S proteasome-mediated degradation, thereby decreasing the cytosolic level of β-catenin (Aberle 1997; Akiyama 2000). In the presence of Wnt-s, signals from the Wnt-Fz-LRP6 complex lead to the phosphorylation of three domains of Dishevelled (Dvl), a family of cytosolic signal transducer molecules (Noordermeer 1994). Activation of Dvl ultimately leads to phosphorylation and consequent inhibition of GSK-3β. Inhibition of GSK-3β results in stabilisation and finally cytosolic accumulation of β-catenin, which then translocates to the nucleus where is required to form active transcription complexes with members of the T-Cell Factor (LEF1, TCF1, TCF3, TCF4) transcription factor family (Staal et al. 2003) and transcription initiator p300 (Labalette et al. 2004). Successful assembly of the transcription complex leads to the activation of various target genes including cyclin-D1 (Shtutman et al. 1999; Tetsu et al. 1999), c-myc (He et al. 1998), c-jun (Mann et al. 1999), Fra-1 (Mann et al. 1999), VEGFR (Zhang et al. 2001).

1.7.3 Non-canonical Wnt-pathways

Generally, the two non-canonical signalling pathways are considered as regulators of canonical Wnt signalling and gene transcription. The two non-canonical Wnt pathways, the JNK/AP1 dependent, PCP (Yamanaka et al. 2002) and the PKC/CAMKII/NFAT dependent Ca^{2+} pathway (Wang et al. 2003), become activated following the formation of Wnt-Fz-LRP6 complex just like the canonical Wnt pathway. Although the non-canonical pathways differ from the canonical pathway in their dependency on the type of G-proteins (Malbon et al. 2001), activation of Dvl, downstream of Frizzled, is critical for further signal transduction in both (Boutros et al. 1998; Sheldahl et al. 2003). In further contrast to canonical Wnt signalling, phosphorylation of all three domains of Dvl, is not a requirement for transduction of non-canonical Wnt signals (Wharton Jr. 2001). Downstream of the cytosolic Dvl, the two non-canonical pathways activate different signalling cascades, which involve JNK or PKC and CaMKII, and trigger the transcription of different target genes. It has been proposed for non-canonical Wnt-signalling receptors to be linked directly to heterotrimeric G-proteins that activate phospholipase-C (PLC) isoforms, which in turn stimulate inositol lipid (i.e. Ca^{++} /PKC) signalling. Growing evidence, however, indicates that G-proteins are functionally diverse and that many of their cellular actions are independent of inositol lipid signalling (Peavy et al. 2005), indicating high levels of complexity in both the PKC dependent and independent Wnt signalling cascades. The JNK dependent PCP pathway, partly shares target genes with the canonical pathway, including cyclin-D1 (Schwabe et al. 2003) and matrix metalloproteinases (Nateri et al. 2005). Certainly, canonical Wnt signals can be rechanneled into the JNK pathway through naturally occurring, intracellular molecular switches, like the Dvl inhibitors, Naked-s (Nkd-1, Nkd-2) (Yan et al. 2001) leading to AP1 rather than TCF activation. AP1 is not a single protein, but a complex of various smaller proteins (cJun, JunB, JunD, cFos, FosB, Fra1, Fra2, ATF2, and CREB), which can form homo- and heterodimers. The composition of the AP1 complex is a decisive factor in the activation of target genes, therefore the regulation of AP1 composition is important. Two prominent members of the AP1 complex cJun and Fra1 are both targets of the canonical Wnt pathway (Mann et al. 1999), indicating strong cross-regulation between the canonical and the non-canonical JNK dependent Wnt signalling cascades (Nateri et al. 2005).

While there are shared ligands (Rosso et al. 2005; Wang et al. 2005) and target genes (Shtutman et al. 1999; Schwabe et al. 2003) in the canonical and JNK dependent Wnt pathways, Ca^{2+}/PKC dependent non-canonical signalling appears to be more independent of the other two pathways although cross-talk with both the β-catenin and the JNK pathways have been proposed (Kuhl et al. 2001). Generally, Ca^{2+} and PKC-dependent signals are frequently linked to AP1, NFkB and NFAT activation.

1.7.4 Inhibitory Wnt pathway

Besides the canonical and non-canonical Wnt pathways, inhibitory Fz pathways have also been described. Fz1 and Fz6 are, for example, able to transmit inhibitory Wnt signals. While Fz1 inhibits Wnt signal transduction via a G-protein dependent manner (Roman-Roman et al. 2004) (Zilberberg et al. 2004), Fz6 (Golan et al. 2004) inhibits Wnt dependent gene transcription by activating the transforming growth factor β–activated kinase 1 (TAK1), a member of the MAPKKK family, and nemo-like kinase (NLK) (Ishitani et al. 2003; Smit et al. 2004) via a Ca^{++} dependent signalling cascade. NLK phosphorylates TCF that consequently cannot bind to β-catenin, and the formation of active transcription complex becomes inhibited (Smit et al. 2004) .

1.7.5 Wnt-s in ageing

As Wnt-s are important regulators of stem cell survival and differentiation, recent studies have started to investigate the role of Wnt family members in ageing. Most studies confirmed that drastically reduced Wnt levels can trigger ageing as tissue specific stem cells fail to replenish mesenchymal tissues as a result of low Wnt signals. In contrast, the KLOTHO mouse, that carries a single gene mutation in KLOTHO, an endogenous Wnt antagonist also shows signs of accelerated ageing (Liu et al. 2007). It has been proposed that increased Wnt signalling leads to continuous stem cell proliferation which finally results in depletion of the stem cell pool (Brack et al. 2007).

1.7.6 Wnt-s in the thymus

The main source of Wnt glycoproteins in the thymus is the thymic epithelium, where 14 members of the Wnt family together with all 10 known Wnt receptors of the seven-loop transmembrane receptor family, Frizzleds (Fz) have been identified (Pongracz et al. 2003). That is a striking difference compared with thymocytes where developmentally regulated receptor expression is limited to Fz-5 and Fz-6 (Pongracz et al. 2003). The assembly of an active Wnt-Fz receptor complex also requires the presence of a co-receptor, the low density lipoprotein related protein 5 and 6 (LRP5/6) (Pinson 2000; Tamai 2000; Wehrli 2000), which is expressed both in thymocytes and thymic epithelial cells, indicating full ability in both cell types to respond to Wnt signals.

Initial experiments, by manipulating the level of some Wnt-s and soluble Fz-s, have shown perturbation of T-cell development (Staal 2001; Mulroy 2002), highlighting the importance of Wnt dependent signalling for T-cell proliferation and differentiation. Recent data (Pongracz et al. 2003) revealed differential expression of Wnt ligands and receptors in thymic cell types raising that T-cell development may be influenced by indirect events triggered by Wnt signalling within the thymic epithelium.

The canonical pathway has been shown to have an important role in thymocyte development regulating survival and differentiation (Ioannidis et al. 2001; Staal 2001; Pongracz et al. 2003; Xu et al. 2003). In a thymic epithelial cell study, transgenic expression of cyclin-D1, one of the principal target genes of Wnt signalling, has lead to the expansion of the entire epithelial compartment (Klug et al. 2000) suggesting that canonical Wnt signalling is involved in thymic epithelial cell proliferation, strengthening the argument, that thymic epithelial development is regulated by Wnt-s. So far, signalling studies have revealed, that Wnt4 can activate both the canonical (Lyons et al. 2004) and the non-canonical (Torres et al. 1996) (Chang et al. 2007; Kim et al. 2009) Wnt-pathways.

1.8 Steroids and ageing

Physiological steroids are implicated in the regulation of thymic ageing. For example both surgical and chemical castration have been demonstrated to decrease the progression of thymic ageing (Qiao et al. 2008) indicating that high steroid levels would accelerate the ageing process of the thymus. Still, steroids used in therapy have not been fully investigated for their effects on immune senescence. Autoimmune diseases and haematological malignancies are often treated by steroids, as they effectively promote apoptosis of leukaemia cells and trigger complex anti-inflammatory actions (Stahn et al. 2007). Apart from triggering decreased expression of cytokines and MHC class II (MHC II) molecules, glucocorticoid (GC) analogues like dexamethasone (DX) also induce apoptotic death of peripheral (Wust et al. 2008) and developing T-cells. In mouse models, GCs cause massive thymocyte depletion, especially in the $CD4^{+}CD8^{+}$ (DP) thymocyte population, (Wiegers et al. 2001; Berki et al. 2002; Jondal et al. 2004) blocking *de novo* T-cell production. Experiments have also demonstrated that high-dose GCs induce a dramatic (Blomgren et al. 1970) and apoptosis-associated (Boersma et al. 1979) involution of the thymus, and not only thymocytes but also TECs are seriously affected (Dardenne et al. 1986). Recent reports (Fletcher et al. 2009) have highlighted that TEC depletion appears reversible, and thymic epithelial stem cells play an important role in this process.

2. Thymic senescence – Current opinion

2.1 Physiological thymic senescence

2.1.1 Disintegration of epithelial network, adipose involution

Senescence exhibits characteristic histological changes in both the human and mouse thymus (Oksanen 1971; Marinova 2005). In young adult mice (at 1 month of age), histology reveals strict segregation of epithelial cell compartments by staining for medullary ($EpCAM1^{++}$, $Ly51^{-}$) and cortical ($EpCAM1^{+}$, $Ly51^{++}$) epithelial cellular subsets (Kvell et al. 2010). Thymic morphology shows high level of integrity just preceding puberty/early adulthood. However, the highly organized structure disintegrates and becomes chaotic by the age of 1 year. By this age the strict cortico-medullary delineation becomes disintegrated, degenerative vacuoles appear surrounded by areas showing strong co-staining with both epithelial markers. Also significant cellular areas appear that lack staining with either epithelial markers, a pattern completely absent at the young adult age. Staining for extracellular matrix components of fibroblast origin ($ER\text{-}TR7^{++}$) identifies mesenchymal elements. The staining pattern with ER-TR7 and EpCAM1 is strikingly different at the two ages examined. In young adult thymic tissue sections, a-EpCAM1 and a-ER-TR7- show little tendency for co-localization. In stark contrast, already by the age of 9 months a-EpCAM1 and ER-TR7-staining show significant overlap within the thymic medulla. The disorganization of thymic epithelial network is followed by the emergence of adipocytes. If thymic sections of senescent mice are co-stained with neutral lipid deposit-specific stains then histology shows the presence of relatively large, inflated cells in which the cytoplasm is pushed to the periphery by red-staining neutral lipid deposits, a pattern characteristic of adipose cells (Kvell et al. 2010).

2.1.2 Gene expression changes in the thymic epithelium during ageing

To investigate the underlying molecular events of thymic epithelial senescence, the gene expression changes may be investigated in TECs purified from 1 month and 1 year old mice (Kvell et al. 2010). The expression of both Wnt4 and FoxN1 decreases in thymic epithelial cells. Highly decreased level (or total absence in some cases) of FoxN1 could be the consequence of strong Wnt4 down-regulation by the age of 1 year, indicating that TECs can down-regulate FoxN1 expression while maintaining that of epithelial cell surface markers like EpCAM1 (Balciunaite et al. 2002). At the same time, mRNA levels of pre-adipocyte differentiation markers PPARγ and ADRP rise with age. This finding is in harmony with histological data demonstrating the emergence of adipocytes in the thymic lobes of senescent mice. The expression of lamin1, a key component of the nuclear lamina remains unaffected during senescence in thymic epithelial cells; whereas, the expression of LAP2α increases significantly. This degree of dissociation between lamin1 and LAP2α expression is of note and suggests functional differences despite conventionally anticipated association of lamin1 and LAP2 molecular family members. LAP2α up-regulation associated with age-related adipose involution is, however, in perfect agreement with other literature data suggesting the pre-adipocyte differentiation-promoting effect of LAP2α in fibroblasts (Dorner et al. 2006) and the same is suggested by our reports performed, however, with epithelial cells (Kvell et al. 2010).

According to literature, EMT is associated with differential expression of E- (decrease) and N-cadherin (increase) (Seike et al. 2009). TECs were tested for these markers to investigate whether the first step towards pre-adipocyte differentiation is the EMT of epithelial cells. In purified TECs while E-cadherin mRNA levels significantly decreased, N-cadherin gene expression showed a slight increase during ageing, indicating that EMT might be the initial step in epithelial cell transition and trans-differentiation.

2.1.3 Studies of LAP2α and Wnt4 effects on TEC

The hypothesis that both LAP2α and Wnt4 play important though opposite roles in thymic senescence may be addressed using LAP2α over-expressing or Wnt4-secreting transgenic TEP1 (mouse primary-derived thymic epithelial) cell lines. The use of a primary-derived model cell line provides the advantage of absolute purity, the complete lack of other cell types that could potentially affect the gene expression profile of epithelial cells (Beardsley et al. 1983). Using such cells quantitative RT-PCR analysis revealed that LAP2α over-expression triggers an immense surge of PPARγ expression. Such an increase in mRNA level suggests that this is not a plain quantitative, but rather a qualitative change. ADRP a direct target gene of PPARγ also becomes up-regulated although to a lesser extent. On the other hand in Wnt4-secreting cells the mRNA level of both PPARγ and ADRP decreased (Kvell et al. 2010).

2.1.4 Fz-4 and Fz-6 expression and distribution are affected by age

Once the preventive role of Wnt4 was established in adipocyte-type trans-differentiation of TECs, receptor associated signalling studies have ensued to investigate what signal modifications can lead to Wnt4 effects. Initially, expression levels of the Wnt4 receptors, Fz-4 and Fz-6 were analysed in thymi of young adult and mature adult (1 month and 9 months old) mice (Varecza et al. 2011). Q-RT-PCR analysis of TECs showed increased expression of both Fz-4 and Fz-6 mRNA with age. Immune-histochemistry using Fz-4 and Fz-6 specific antibodies confirmed elevated levels of both receptor proteins. Additionally, differential expression pattern of Fz-4 and Fz-6 was also observed in the thymic medulla and cortex. While in the young thymus the medulla (EpCAM1^{++}/Ly51^{-}) was preferentially stained for

Fz4 and Fz6, the cortex (EpCAM1+/Ly51+) only faintly stained for these receptors. In contrast to the young tissue, the 9 month old thymus shows a different pattern as the whole section including the cortex has become increasingly positive for both receptors (Varecza et al. 2011).

2.1.5 PKCδ translocation and its relation with Wnt4 signalling

Since Wnt4 levels as well as its receptors are modulated during the ageing process, further studies were performed to investigate active receptor signalling that is invariably associated with modified level of phosphorylation of receptor associated signalling molecules. Since Fz-s associate with Dvls that are phosphorylated by the δ isoform of PKCs, PKCδ activity was in focus. To test the involvement of PKCδ in Wnt4 signal transduction, increased Wnt4 levels were achieved using the supernatant of Wnt4-transgenic cell line (Varecza et al. 2011). Wild type TEP1 cells were exposed to SNs of control and Wnt4-secreting cells for 1 hour, then cytosolic and membrane fractions were isolated from cell lysates. Similar to previous studies with Wnt-5a (Giorgione et al. 2003), Western blot analysis revealed that within one hour of Wnt4 exposure PKCδ translocated into the membrane fraction where the cleavage products (Kanthasamy et al, 2006) characteristic of PKCδ activation were detectable. Additionally, increased membrane localisation of PKCδ was also detected in the Wnt4-overexpressing cell line. As both Fz-4 and Fz-6 levels increased with age, it was assumed that active receptor signalling might require more PKCδ during ageing. Indeed, apart from localisation of PKCδ to the membrane fraction, up-regulation of PKCδ was also detected in the ageing thymi. To investigate the role of PKCδ involvement in Wnt4 signalling, PKCδ activity level was modified by either over-expressing wild type PKCδ or by silencing PKCδ translation using siRNA technology. CTGF was used as a read-out gene based on data of previous experiments (Varecza et al. 2011). Surprisingly, although over-expression of PKCδ had no radical effect on Wnt4 target gene transcription, even moderate down-regulation of PKCδ was able to significantly increase CTGF expression in the presence of Wnt4, indicating that PKCδ might be involved in a negative regulatory loop.

2.1.6 Negative regulatory loops of signalling during senescence

As Fz-6 has been implicated in previous studies as a negative regulator of β-catenin dependent signalling, it was important to determine whether PKCδ is preferentially associated with either Wnt4 receptors. Experiments demonstrated age dependent increase of both Fz-6 and PKCδ as well as co-localisation of Fz-6 and PKCδ (Varecza et al. 2011). While in the young thymus Fz-6 and PKCδ co-localisation is more pronounced in the thymic cortex, in the ageing thymus it is the medulla that exhibits stronger staining for both proteins. While increased expression and activity of the Fz-6 receptor, a suppressor of the canonical Wnt signalling pathway explains some aspects of uneven target gene transcription following manipulation of PKCδ activity, parallel changes like up-regulation of Fz-4 also occur during ageing that might add to the complexity of the signalling process. Increase in Fz-4 levels in ageing mice correlated with increased CTGF gene expression.

If Fz-6 that also increases during senescence is truly a suppressor of β-catenin signalling then CTGF expression should have decreased or remained unchanged as Fz-4 transmitted signals would have been quenched by Fz-6 signalling. To test the above hypothesis, we have considered the following: CTGF has recently been reported to negatively regulate canonical Wnt signalling by blocking β-catenin stabilisation via GSK3β activation leading to phosphorylation and consequent degradation of β-catenin (Luo et al. 2004), indicating that CTGF might be part of a negative feed-back loop. The expression of Fz-8 (Mercurio et al. 2004) a recently reported receptor for CTGF increased in ageing mice, while FoxN1 the direct target of β-catenin dependent Wnt4 signalling (Balciunaite et al. 2002) became undetectable (Kvell et al. 2010).

2.2 Thymic senescence model

2.2.1 Steroid induced accelerated thymic senescence

A commonly held view is that the thymus involutes at puberty, and this model is based primarily on studies showing that growth hormone (GH) and sex steroids can affect cell production in the thymus and that their concentrations decrease with age (Min et al. 2006). As steroids are frequently applied medications, investigations were extended to identify similarities in induced and physiological senescence and potential mechanisms that might be able to reduce adipose involution of the thymus.

Similar to physiological senescence, the level of FoxN1 transcription factor and its regulator Wnt4 decreased in TECs within 24 hours following a single dose DX injection and remained low for over 1 week (Talaber et al. 2011).

However, in clinical treatments GC analogues are widely used for extended periods of time, rather than single shots. To mimic this pattern of clinical application, mice were injected with DX repeatedly for a time course of 1 month. Both Wnt4 and FoxN1 levels were measured drastically down-regulated, while the adipocyte differentiation factor ADRP, down-stream target of PPARγ was significantly increased. The results indicate that adipocyte-type trans-differentiation is completed at the molecular level over a much shorter time period following exogenous steroid-induced senescence compared to physiological rate senescence (Talaber et al. 2011).

2.2.2 Wnt4 inhibits steroid-induced adipose trans-differentiation

To test whether Wnt4 can prevent adipocyte type trans-differentiation, Wnt4 over-expressing TEP1 cell line was exposed to DX for a week. While in the control cell line DX exposure induced up-regulation of adipose trans-differentiation markers, within the Wnt4 over-expressing cell line, none of the adipose trans-differentiation markers were up-regulated indicating that Wnt4 alone can efficiently protect TECs against exogenous steroid-induced adipose trans-differentiation (Talaber et al. 2011).

3. Conclusions

3.1 Physiological thymic epithelial senescence

There are characteristic changes in the gene expression profile of purified thymic epithelial cells during thymic epithelial senescence (Kvell et al. 2010). Of note, Wnt4 level decreases, while LAP2α level increases. Also, the expression of the transcription factor FoxN1 required for maintaining thymic epithelial identity diminishes with age. On the other hand, adipose differentiation is confirmed at the molecular level by the increased expression of PPARγ and ADRP. This process is accompanied by shift from E-cadherin to N-cadherin, typical for EMT (epithelial to mesenchymal transition). These pioneer experiments confirm in both a model cell line and purified primary cells rendered transgenic for either Wnt4 or LAP2α that their opposing effects antagonistically influence adipose trans-differentiation of thymic epithelial cells via EMT. This has lead to the establishment of a novel, confirmed theory for the source of adipose cells replacing functional thymic epithelial network during senescence (see **Figure 1**). Apparently, these cells do not differentiate from invading or resident mesenchymal cells, but rather trans-differentiate (via EMT) from thymic epithelial cells (Kvell et al. 2010).

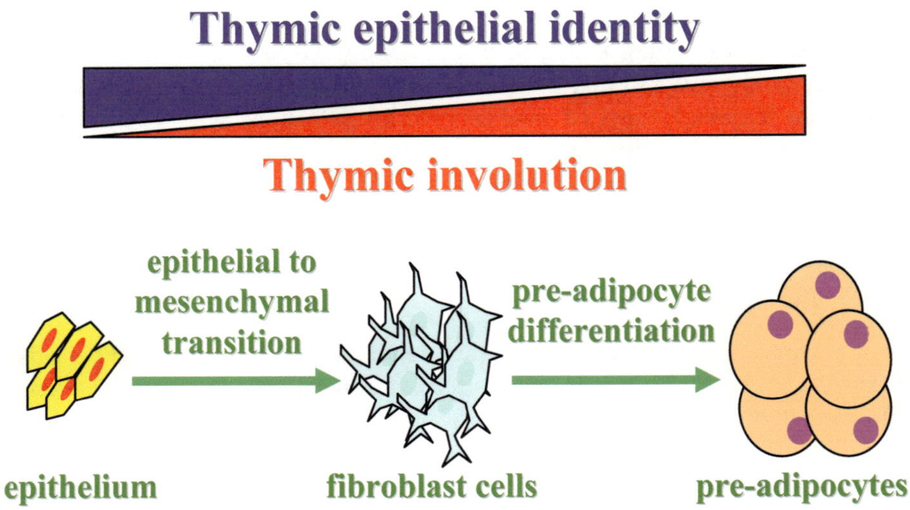

Fig. 1. Model of thymic involution process
Dedifferentiation of thymic epithelial cells triggers EMT (epithelial to mesenchymal transition) first, and then the resulting fibroblast cells undergo the conventional route of differentiation program towards adipocyte-lineage.

3.2 Signal transduction mechanisms involved in thymic epithelial senescence

While individual molecules, such as Wnt4 or LAP2α can serve as therapeutic targets to modify the ageing process, identification of complex interactions amongst signalling networks can provide further details. Investigation of Wnt signal transduction in the thymic epithelium has revealed that signalling pathways are activated or inhibited in an orderly fashion (Varecza et al. 2011). Initially, both Wnt4 receptors, Fz-4 and Fz-6 are up-regulated at young adult age. However, signals from Fz-4 and Fz-6 are different. While signals from Fz-4 initiate β-catenin dependent gene transcription, Fz-6 signals lead to suppression of β-catenin dependent signalling via increased activities of TGFβ-Activated Kinase (TAK) and Nemo-Like-Kinase (NLK). Fz-associated signals also require PKCδ to transmit Wnt signals. PKCδ associates with Fz-6 aiding suppression of β-catenin dependent signalling. Additional to Fz-6 signalling, connective tissue growth factor (CTGF, a β-catenin target gene) can also feedback on β-catenin dependent signal transduction. CTGF can interact with Fz-8 as well as LRP6, an important co-receptor of Wnt signalling and can trigger activation of GSK3β. This latter leads to accelerated proteasomal degradation of β-catenin and hence suppression of Wnt signals. Multiple signalling mechanisms that lead to suppression of Wnt signalling is summarized in **Figure 2** (Varecza et al. 2011).

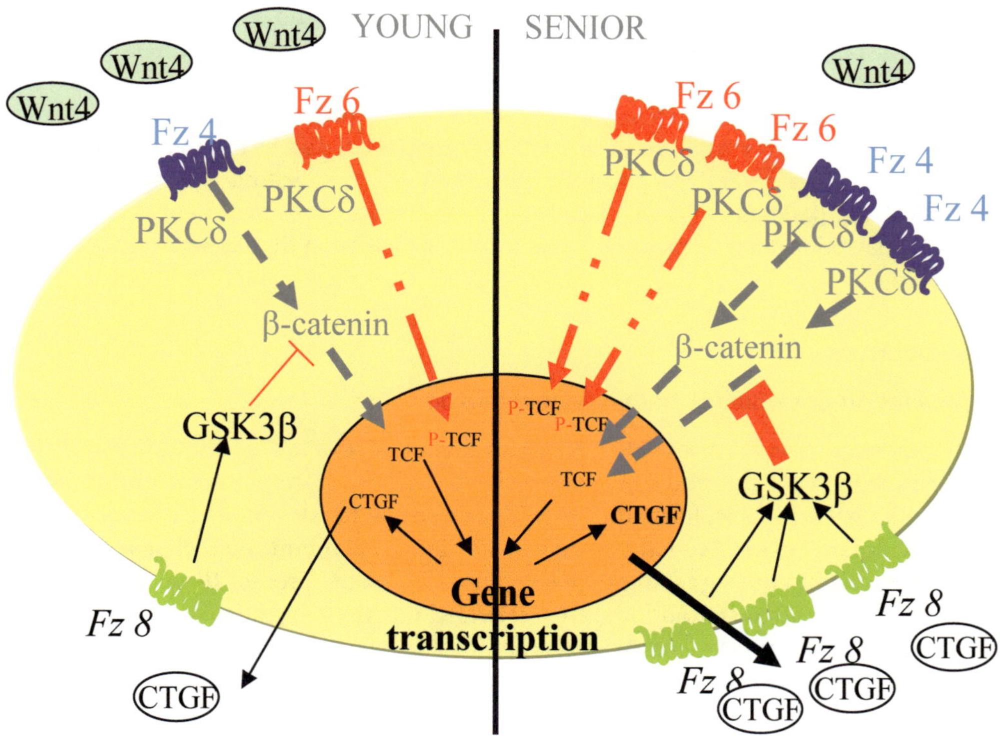

Fig. 2. Model of molecular mechanisms in thymic aging
At young age, Wnt4 levels are high and Wnt4 molecules compete for a moderate number of Fz receptors. While Fz-4 activates canonical Wnt signalling, signals from Fz-6 inhibit β-catenin dependent gene transcription keeping Wnt4 dependent signalling in balance. During the ageing process, Wnt4 levels decrease, while receptor expression increases with proportionally higher Fz-6. The β-catenin dependent Fz-4 signals lead to increased expression of CTGF. The CTGF receptor Fz8 is also up-regulated leading to enhanced activation of GSK3β. All these signalling events lead to loss of thymic epithelial cell characteristics and provide an opening for molecular events leading up to adipocyte type trans-differentiation.

3.3 Accelerated-rate, induced model of thymic epithelial senescence

Glucocorticoids are immunosuppressive drugs often used for treatment of autoimmune diseases and haematological malignancies. Although glucocorticoids can induce apoptotic cell death directly in developing thymocytes, how exogenous glucocorticoids affect the thymic epithelial network that provides the microenvironment for T cell development has been poorly characterised. The effect of DX (dexamethasone) on thymic epithelial cells has been tested both *in vitro* (model cell line) and *in vivo* (mouse model) (Talaber et al. 2011). *In vivo,* following single treatment with pharmacologically relevant dose of DX reversible changes in gene expression profile identical to physiological thymic epithelial senescence have been recorded, but occurring at a highly accelerated pace (see **Figure 1**). Specifically, the expression of Wnt4 and FoxN1 decreased, while LAP2α and PPARγ levels increased. Moreover, sustained DX treatment has induced the elevation of ADRP expression as well. The same changes of gene expression profile have been observed using the model TEP1 (thymic epithelial) cell line, however, *in vitro* studies have shown the molecular level rescue of thymic epithelial cells from adipose trans-differentiation due to the over-expression of Wnt4. These studies reveal the currently neglected effect of steroid therapy on thymic epithelial cells in patients receiving sustained or even single dose treatment and highlights novel potential side-effects appearing in the form of accelerated thymic senescence (Talaber et al. 2011).

4. Perspectives

4.1 Intervention possibilities of thymic rejuvenation

This chapter summarised current knowledge on thymic senescence, a central immune tissue that suffers significant morphological changes and functional impairment during ageing. The epithelial network is in focus that provides the niche for developing thymocytes until adipose involution begins. We have discussed physiological thymic epithelial senescence in detail with respect to the signalling pathways involved in the process (Kvell et al. 2010). It has also been shown that steroid induced accelerated rate thymic epithelial senescence quite resembles physiological rate senescence (except for its speed) at the molecular level (Talaber et al. 2011). The data presented confirm that Wnt4 can efficiently rescue thymic epithelial cells from steroid-induced adipose involution at the molecular level (Talaber et al. 2011). Since physiological and steroid-induced thymic epithelial senescence are identical at the molecular level, it is anticipated that sustained Wnt4 presence in the thymic context can efficiently prolong FoxN1 expression, maintain thymic epithelial identity and prevent trans-differentiation towards adipocyte lineage. The same works identify LAP2α as a pro-ageing molecular factor promoting the trans-differentiation of thymic epithelial cells into pre-adipocytes via EMT. The thymus selective decrease of LAP2α activity through small molecule compounds could theoretically shift the delicate molecular balance towards the same direction as increased Wnt4 presence.

However, there are also other methods that can efficiently support major functions of the thymus: T cell maturation and selection. An example is the thymus-specific enrichment of transgenic IL7 proteins using IL7-CCR9 fusion proteins that selectively home and accumulate in the thymic context to reinforce thymocyte development and maturation (Henson et al. 2005). This method has been characterised in detail and is currently being geared up towards potential human application in the form of inhalation products selectively delivering IL7 to the thymus (Aspinall et al. 2008).

The thymus-specific ablation of sex steroids also offers a target point for such interventions. Major involution in thymus mass occurs in parallel with the advance of puberty and correlation has been drawn with sex steroid levels. The use of thymus selective 11β-HSD1 inhibitor compounds could also theoretically decrease thymocyte sensitivity to steroid-induced apoptosis and steroid-induced epithelial molecular senescence, providing synergistic mechanism of action. Such artificial compounds (like the PF-00915275) have already been tested in healthy volunteers and were approved for safety (Courtney et al. 2008). However, these compounds do not specifically accumulate in the thymus and have not been tested in the thymic context.

Alternative methods for thymic rejuvenation include those targeting KGF, ghrelin and GH signal transduction pathways (Aspinall et al 2008). The ideal future thymus rejuvenation system that works selectively in the thymus at high efficiency and low side-effect ratio would likely constitute a combination of the above outlined methods and would efficiently aid restoration of immune competence.

4.2 Social and economic impact

By targeting and specifically inhibiting the molecular pathways that drive thymic adipose involution / immune senescence, it is possible to extend immune health-span within life-span, and improve health and quality of life, and also significantly decrease healthcare costs. This effect is expected to be very significant as - opposed to certain diseases - the physiological process of immune senescence affects all individuals, including currently healthy people.

It is to be evaluated whether an immune-fitness extending treatment would be predominantly useful as preventive treatment applied in younger individuals or would rather be useful as a reversal treatment in elderly individuals with various stages of thymic adipose degeneration. Both scenarios would affect vast segments of the population and would yield similarly significant economic and social benefit.

5. Acknowledgement

The authors are grateful to Prof. S. Amos (Institute of Haematology, Chaim Sheba Medical Centre, Tel-Hashomer, Israel) for providing the wild type murine LAP2α construct.

Experimental work performed by authors was funded by the following grants: OTKA PD 78310 to KK, Wellcome Trust 079415 and SROP-4.2.2/08/1/2008-0011 to JEP.

6. References

Aberle, H., Bauer, A., Stappert, J., Kispert, A., and Kemler, R. (1997). "b-Catenin is a target for the ubiquitin-proteosome pathway." EMBO J. 16: 3797-3804.

Akiyama, T. (2000). "Wnt/b-catenin signaling." Cytokine&Growth Factor Rev. 11: 273-282.

Alves NL, Richard-Le Goff O, Huntington ND, Sousa AP, Ribeiro VS, Bordack A, Vives FL, Peduto L, Chidgey A, Cumano A, Boyd R, Eberl G, Di Santo JP. (2009). "Characterization of the thymic IL-7 niche in vivo." Proc Natl Acad Sci U S A 106(5): 1512-7.

Anderson G, Owen JJ, Moore NC, Jenkinson EJ. "Thymic epithelial cells provide unique signals for positive selection of CD4+CD8+ thymocytes *in vitro*." J. Exp. Med. 179: 2027-2031.

Aspinall R, Mitchell W. Reversal of age-associated thymic atrophy: treatments, delivery, and side effects. Exp Gerontol. 2008 Jul;43(7):700-5.

Aydar Y, Balogh P, Tew JG, Szakal AK. Follicular dendritic cells in aging, a "bottle-neck" in the humoral immune response. Ageing Res Rev. 2004 Jan;3(1):15-29.

Balciunaite G, Keller MP, Balciunaite E, Piali L, Zuklys S, Mathieu YD, Gill J, Boyd R, Sussman DJ, Holländer GA. (2002). "Wnt glycoproteins regulate the expression of FoxN1, the gene defective in nude mice." Nat. Immunol. 3(11): 1102-1108.

Beardsley TR, Pierschbacher M, Wetzel GD, Hays EF. (1983). "Induction of T-Cell Maturation by a Cloned Line of Thymic Epithelium (TEPI) 10.1073/pnas.80.19.6005." Proceedings of the National Academy of Sciences 80(19): 6005-6009.

Bennett AR, Farley A, Blair NF, Gordon J, Sharp L, Blackburn CC. (2002). "Identification and characterization of thymic epithelial progenitor cells." Immunity 16(6): 803-814.

Berger R, Theodor L, Shoham J, Gokkel E, Brok-Simoni F, Avraham KB, Copeland NG, Jenkins NA, Rechavi G, Simon AJ. (1996). "The characterization and localization of the mouse thymopoietin/lamina-associated polypeptide 2 gene and its alternatively spliced products." Genome Res 6(5): 361-70.

Berki T, Pálinkás L, Boldizsár F, Németh P. (2002). "Glucocorticoid (GC) sensitivity and GC receptor expression differ in thymocyte subpopulations." Int Immunol 14(5): 463-9.

Blackburn, C. and N. Manley (2004). "Developing a new paradigm for thymus organogenesis." Nat Rev Immunol 4(4): 278-289.

Bleul, C. and T. Boehm (2000). "Chemokines define distinct microenvironments in the developing thymus." Eur. J. Immunol. 30: 3371-3379.

Bleul, C. and T. Boehm (2005). "BMP signaling is required for normal thymus development." J Immunol 175: 5213-5221.

Blomgren, H. and B. Andersson (1970). "Characteristics of the immunocompetent cells in the mouse thymus: cell population changes during cortisone-induced atrophy and subsequent regeneration." Cell Immunol 1(5): 545-60.

Boersma W, Betel I, van der Westen G. (1979). "Thymic regeneration after dexamethasone treatment as a model for subpopulation development." Eur J Immunol 9(1): 45-52.

Boutros M, Paricio N, Strutt DI, Mlodzik M. (1998). "Dishevelled activates JNK and discriminates between JNK pathways in planar polarity and wingless signaling." Cell 94: 109-118.

Brack AS, Conboy MJ, Roy S, Lee M, Kuo CJ, Keller C, Rando TA. (2007). "Increased Wnt Signaling During Aging Alters Muscle Stem Cell Fate and Increases Fibrosis." Science 317(5839): 807-810.

Chang J, Sonoyama W, Wang Z, Jin Q, Zhang C, Krebsbach PH, Giannobile W, Shi S, Wang CY. (2007). "Noncanonical Wnt-4 signaling enhances bone regeneration of mesenchymal stem cells in craniofacial defects through activation of p38 MAPK." Journal of Biological Chemistry 282(42): 30938-30948.

Chen L, Xiao S, Manley NR. (2009). "Foxn1 is required to maintain the postnatal thymic microenvironment in a dosage-sensitive manner." Blood 113(3): 567-574.

Cheng L, Guo J, Sun L, Fu J, Barnes PF, Metzger D, Chambon P, Oshima RG, Amagai T, Su DM. (2010). "Postnatal Tissue-specific Disruption of Transcription Factor FoxN1 Triggers Acute Thymic Atrophy." Journal of Biological Chemistry 285(8): 5836-5847.

Chidgey A, Dudakov J, Seach N, Boyd R.(2007). "Impact of niche aging on thymic regeneration and immune reconstitution." Semin Immunol 19(5): 331-40.

Courtney R, Stewart PM, Toh M, Ndongo MN, Calle RA, Hirshberg B. Modulation of 11beta-hydroxysteroid dehydrogenase (11betaHSD) activity biomarkers and pharmacokinetics of PF-00915275, a selective 11betaHSD1 inhibitor. J Clin Endocrinol Metab. 2008 Feb;93(2):550-6.

Crisa L, Cirulli V, Ellisman MH, Ishii JK, Elices MJ, Salomon DR. (1996). "Cell adhesion and migration are regulated at distinct stages of thymic T cell development: the roles of fibronectin, VLA4, and VLA5." J Exp Med 184(1): 21-28.

Dardenne M, Itoh T, Homo-Delarche F. (1986). "Presence of glucocorticoid receptors in cultured thymic epithelial cells." Cell Immunol 100(1): 112-8.

de Grey AD. “The natural biogerontology portfolio: "defeating aging" as a multi-stage ultra-grand challenge.” Ann N Y Acad Sci. 2007 Apr;1100:409-23.

Derbinski J, Schulte A, Kyewski B, Klein L. (2001). "Promiscuous gene expression in medullary thymic epithelial cells mirrors the peripheral self." Nat. Immunol. 2(11): 1032-1039.

Dixit, V. D. (2010). "Thymic fatness and approaches to enhance thymopoietic fitness in aging." Curr Opin Immunol 22(4): 521-8.

Dooley J, Erickson M, Roelink H, Farr AG. (2005). "Nude thymic rudiment lacking functional foxn1 resembles respiratory epithelium." Dev Dyn. 233(4): 1605-1612.

Dorner D, Vlcek S, Foeger N, Gajewski A, Makolm C, Gotzmann J, Hutchison CJ, Foisner R. (2006). "Lamina-associated polypeptide 2alpha regulates cell cycle progression and differentiation via the retinoblastoma-E2F pathway." J Cell Biol 173(1): 83-93.

Dreger M, Otto H, Neubauer G, Mann M, Hucho F. (1999). "Identification of phosphorylation sites in native lamina-associated polypeptide 2 beta." Biochemistry 38(29): 9426-34.

Farr, A. and A. Rudensky (1998). "Medullary thymic epithelium: a mosaic of epithelial "self"?" J. Exp. Med. 188(1): 1-4.

Fletcher AL, Lowen TE, Sakkal S, Reiseger JJ, Hammett MV, Seach N, Scott HS, Boyd RL, Chidgey AP. (2009). "Ablation and regeneration of tolerance-inducing medullary thymic epithelial cells after cyclosporine, cyclophosphamide, and dexamethasone treatment." J Immunol 183(2): 823-31.

Ge, Q. and W. Chen (2000). "Effect of murine thymic epithelial cell line (MTEC1) on the functional expression of CD4(+)CD8(-) thymocyte subgroups." Int. Immunol. 12(8): 1127-1133.

Gill J, Malin M, Holländer GA, Boyd R. (2002). "Generation of a complete thymic microenvironment by MTS24(+) thymic epithelial cells." Nat. Immunol. 3(7): 635-642.

Giorgione J, Hysell M, Harvey DF, Newton AC. (2003). "Contribution of the C1A and C1B domains to the membrane interaction of protein kinase C." Biochemistry 42(38): 11194-11202.

Golan T, Yaniv A, Bafico A, Liu G, Gazit A. (2004). "The human frizzled 6 (HFz6) acts as a negative regulator of the canonical Wnt b-catenin signaling cascade." J. Biol. Chem. 279(15): 14879-14888.

Grubeck-Loebenstein, B. (2009). "Fading Immune Protection in Old Age: Vaccination in the Elderly." J Comp Pathol.

Gui J, Zhu X, Dohkan J, Cheng L, Barnes PF, Su DM. (2007). "The aged thymus shows normal recruitment of lymphohematopoietic progenitors but has defects in thymic epithelial cells." Int Immunol 19(10): 1201-11.

He TC, Sparks AB, Rago C, Hermeking H, Zawel L, da Costa LT, Morin PJ, Vogelstein B, Kinzler KW. (1998). "Identification of c-MYC as a target of the APC pathway." Science 281(5382): 1509-1512.

He, X. and D. J. Kappes (2006). "CD4/CD8 lineage commitment: light at the end of the tunnel?" Curr Opin Immunol 18(2): 135-42.

Henson SM, Snelgrove R, Hussell T, Wells DJ, Aspinall R. An IL-7 fusion protein that shows increased thymopoietic ability. J Immunol. 2005 Sep 15;175(6):4112-8.

Hsu, H. C. and J. D. Mountz (2003). "Origin of late-onset autoimmune disease." Immunol Allergy Clin North Am 23(1): 65-82, vi.

Hutchison CJ, Alvarez-Reyes M, Vaughan OA. (2001). "Lamins in disease: why do ubiquitously expressed nuclear envelope proteins give rise to tissue-specific disease phenotypes?" J Cell Sci 114(Pt 1): 9-19.

Ikeda, S., Kishida, S., Yamamoto, H., Murai, H., Koyama, S., Kikuchi, A. (1998). "Axin, a negative regulator of the Wnt signaling pathway, forms a complex with GSK3b and b-catenin and promotes GSK-3b-dependent phosphorylation of b-catenin." The EMBO J. 17: 1371-1384.

Ioannidis V, Beermann F, Clevers H, Held W. (2001). "The b-catenin-TCF1 pathway ensures CD4+CD8+ thymocyte survival." Nature Immunology 2: 691-697.

Ishitani T, Kishida S, Hyodo-Miura J, Ueno N, Yasuda J, Waterman M, Shibuya H, Moon RT, Ninomiya-Tsuji J, Matsumoto K. (2003). "The TAK1-NLK Mitogen-activated protein kinase cascade functions in the Wnt-5a/Ca2+ pathway to antagonize Wnt/b-catenin signaling." Mol. Cell Biol. 23(1): 131-139.

Jin EJ, Park JH, Lee SY, Chun JS, Bang OS, Kang SS. (2006). "Wnt-5a is involved in TGF-beta3-stimulated chondrogenic differentiation of chick wing bud mesenchymal cells." Int J Biochem Cell Biol 38(2): 183-95.

Jondal M, Pazirandeh A, Okret S. (2004). "Different roles for glucocorticoids in thymocyte homeostasis?" Trends Immunol 25(11): 595-600.

Kanthasamy AG, Anantharam V, Zhang D, Latchoumycandane C, Jin H, Kaul S, Kanthasamy A. A novel peptide inhibitor targeted to caspase-3 cleavage site of a proapoptotic kinase protein kinase C delta (PKCdelta) protects against dopaminergic neuronal degeneration in Parkinson's disease models. Free Radic Biol Med. 2006 Nov 15;41(10):1578-89.

Kim YC, Clark RJ, Pelegri F, Alexander CM. (2009). "Wnt4 is not sufficient to induce lobuloalveolar mammary development." BMC Dev Biol 9: 55.

Klug DB, Crouch E, Carter C, Coghlan L, Conti CJ, Richie ER. (2000). "Transgenic expression of cyclin D1 in thymic epithelial precursors promotes epithelial and T cell development." J. Immunol. 164: 1881-1888.

Kühl M, Geis K, Sheldahl LC, Pukrop T, Moon RT, Wedlich D.(2001). "Antagonistic regulation of convergent extension movements in Xenopus by Wnt/beta-catenin and Wnt/Ca2+ signalling." Mech. Dev. 106: 61-76.

Kvell K, Varecza Z, Bartis D, Hesse S, Parnell S, Anderson G, Jenkinson EJ, Pongracz JE. Wnt4 and LAP2alpha as pacemakers of thymic epithelial senescence. PLoS One. 2010 May 18;5(5):e10701.

Labalette C, Renard CA, Neuveut C, Buendia MA, Wei Y. (2004). "Interaction and functional cooperation between the LIM protein FHL2, CBP/p300, and beta-catenin." Mol. Cell Biol. 24(24): 10689-10702.

Leduc L, Levy E, Bouity-Voubou M, Delvin E. Fetal programming of atherosclerosis: possible role of the mitochondria. Eur J Obstet Gynecol Reprod Biol. 2010 Apr;149(2):127-30.

Lind EF, Prockop SE, Porritt HE, Petrie HT.(2001). "Mapping precursor movement through the postnatal thymus reveals specific microenvironments supporting defined stages of early lymphoid development." J. Exp. Med. 194(2): 127-134.

Liu H, Fergusson MM, Castilho RM, Liu J, Cao L, Chen J, Malide D, Rovira II, Schimel D, Kuo CJ, Gutkind JS, Hwang PM, Finkel T. (2007). "Augmented Wnt Signaling in a Mammalian Model of Accelerated Aging." Science 317(5839): 803-806.

Ljubuncic P, Reznick AZ. "The evolutionary theories of aging revisited—a mini-review." Gerontology. 2009;55(2):205-16.

Luo Q, Kang Q, Si W, Jiang W, Park JK, Peng Y, Li X, Luu HH, Luo J, Montag AG, Haydon RC, He TC. (2004). "Connective tissue growth factor (CTGF) is regulated by Wnt and bone morphogenetic proteins signaling in osteoblast differentiation of mesenchymal stem cells." J Biol Chem 279(53): 55958-68.

Lyons JP, Mueller UW, Ji H, Everett C, Fang X, Hsieh JC, Barth AM, McCrea PD. (2004). "Wnt-4 activates the canonical beta-catenin-mediated Wnt pathway and binds Frizzled-6 CRD: functional implications of Wnt/beta-catenin activity in kidney epithelial cells." Exp Cell Res 298(2): 369-87.

Malbon CC, Wang H, Moon RT. (2001). "Wnt signaling and heterotrimeric G-proteins: strange bedfellows or a classic romance?" Biochem. Biophys. Res. Commun. 287(3): 589-93.

Mandinova A, Kolev V, Neel V, Hu B, Stonely W, Lieb J, Wu X, Colli C, Han R, Pazin MJ, Ostano P, Dummer R, Brissette JL, Dotto GP. (2009). "A positive FGFR3/FOXN1 feedback loop underlies benign skin keratosis versus squamous cell carcinoma formation in humans." J Clin Invest 119(10): 3127-37.

Manley, N. R. (2000). "Thymus organogenesis and molecular mechanisms of thymic epithelial cell differentiation." Sem. Immunol. 12: 421-428.

Mann B, Gelos M, Siedow A, Hanski ML, Gratchev A, Ilyas M, Bodmer WF, Moyer MP, Riecken EO, Buhr HJ, Hanski C. (1999). "Target genes of beta-catenin-T cell-factor/lymphoid-enhancer-factor signaling in human colorectal carcinomas." Proc. Natl. Acad. Sci U.S.A. 96(4): 1603-1608.

Marinova, T. T. (2005). "Epithelial framework reorganization during human thymus involution." Gerontology 51(1): 14-8.

Mercurio S, Latinkic B, Itasaki N, Krumlauf R, Smith JC. (2004). "Connective-tissue growth factor modulates WNT signalling and interacts with the WNT receptor complex." Development 131(9): 2137-47.

Michie AM, Soh JW, Hawley RG, Weinstein IB, Zuniga-Pflucker JC. (2001). "Allelic exclusion and differentiation by protein kinase C-mediated signals in immature thymocytes." Proc. Natl. Acad. Sci U.S.A. 98(2): 609-614.

Min H, Montecino-Rodriguez E, Dorshkind K. (2006). "Reassessing the role of growth hormone and sex steroids in thymic involution." Clinical Immunology 118(1): 117-123.

Mulroy, T., McMahon, J.A., Burakoff, S.J., McMahon, A.P., and Sen, J. (2002). "Wnt-1 and Wnt-4 regulated thymic cellularity." Eur. J. Immunol. 32: 967-971.

Nateri AS, Spencer-Dene B, Behrens A. (2005). "Interaction of phosphorylated c-Jun with TCF4 regulates intestinal cancer development." Nature July, Epub.

Newton, A. (2001). "Protein kinase C: structural and spatial regulation by phosphorylation, cofactors, and macromolecular interactions." Chem. Rev. 101: 2353-2364.

Noordermeer, J. K., J., Perrimon, N., and Nusse, R. (1994). "Dishevelled and armadillo act in the wingless signalling pathway in Drosophila." Nature 367: 80-83.

Oksanen, A. (1971). "Multilocular fat in thymuses of rats and mice associated with thymus involution: a light- and electron-microscope and histochemical study." J Pathol 105(3): 223-6.

Peavy RD, Hubbard KB, Lau A, Fields RB, Xu K, Lee CJ, Lee TT, Gernert K, Murphy TJ, Hepler JR. (2005). "Differential effects of Gq alpha, G14 alpha, and G15 alpha on vascular smooth muscle cell survival and gene expression profiles." Mol Pharmacol. 67(6): 2102-21014.

Pinson, K. I., Brennan, J., Monkley, S., Avery, B.J., Skarnes, W.C. (2000). "An LDL-receptor-related protein mediates Wnt signalling in mice." Nature 407(6803): 535-538.

Pongracz J, Hare K, Harman B, Anderson G, Jenkinson EJ. (2003). "Thymic epithelial cells provide Wnt signals to developing thymocytes." Eur. J. Immunol. 33: 1949-1956.

Qiao S, Chen L, Okret S, Jondal M. (2008). "Age-related synthesis of glucocorticoids in thymocytes." Exp Cell Res 314(16): 3027-35.

Ribeiro, R. M. and A. S. Perelson (2007). "Determining thymic output quantitatively: using models to interpret experimental T-cell receptor excision circle (TREC) data." Immunol Rev 216: 21-34.

Roman-Roman S, Shi DL, Stiot V, Haÿ E, Vayssière B, Garcia T, Baron R, Rawadi G. (2004). "Murine Frizzled-1 behaves as an antagonist of the canonical Wnt/beta-catenin signaling." J Biol Chem. 279: 5725-5733.

Rosso, S., D. Sussman, et al. (2005). "Wnt signaling through Dishevelled, Rac and JNK regulates dendritic development." Nat. Neuroscience 8: 34-42.

Schluns KS, Cook JE, Le PT. (1997). "TGF-beta differentially modulates epidermal growth factor-mediated increases in leukemia-inhibitory factor, IL-6, IL-1 alpha, and IL-1 beta in human thymic epithelial cells." J Immunol 158(6): 2704-12.

Schwabe RF, Bradham CA, Uehara T, Hatano E, Bennett BL, Schoonhoven R, Brenner DA. (2003). "c-Jun-N-terminal kinase drives cyclin D1 expression and proliferation during liver regeneration." Hepatology 37(4): 824-832.

Seike M, Mizutani H, Sudoh J, Gemma A. (2009). "Epithelial to mesenchymal transition of lung cancer cells." J Nippon Med Sch 76(4): 181.

Sheldahl LC, Slusarski DC, Pandur P, Miller JR, Kühl M, Moon RT. (2003). "Dishevelled activates Ca2+ flux, PKC, and CamKII in vertebrate embryos." J. Cell Biol. 161(4): 767-777.

Shiraishi J, Utsuyama M, Seki S, Akamatsu H, Sunamori M, Kasai M, Hirokawa K. Essential microenvironment for thymopoiesis is preserved in human adult and aged thymus. Clin Dev Immunol. 2003 Mar;10(1):53-9.

Shtutman M, Zhurinsky J, Simcha I, Albanese C, D'Amico M, Pestell R, Ben-Ze'ev A. (1999). "The cyclin D1 gene is a target of the beta-catenin/LEF-1 pathway." Proc. Natl. Acad. Sci U.S.A. 96(10): 5522-5527.

Smit L, Baas A, Kuipers J, Korswagen H, van de Wetering M, Clevers H. (2004). "Wnt activates the Tak1/Nemo-like kinase pathway." J Biol Chem 279(17): 17232-40.

Staal, F. J. and H. Clevers (2003). "Wnt signaling in the thymus." Curr. Opin. Immunol. 15(2): 204-208.

Staal, F. J. T., Meeldijk, J., Moerer, P., Jay, P., van de Weerdt, B.C.M., Vainio, S., Nolan, G.P., Clevers, H. (2001). "Wnt signaling is required for thymocyte development and activates Tcf-1 mediated transcription." Eur. J. Immunol. 31.: 285-293.

Stahn C, Löwenberg M, Hommes DW, Buttgereit F. (2007). "Molecular mechanisms of glucocorticoid action and selective glucocorticoid receptor agonists." Mol Cell Endocrinol 275(1-2): 71-8.

Talaber G, Kvell K, Varecza Z, Boldizsar F, Parnell SM, Jenkinson EJ, Anderson G, Berki T, Pongracz JE. Wnt-4 protects thymic epithelial cells against dexamethasone-induced enescence. Rejuvenation Res. 2011 Jun;14(3):241-8.

Tamai, K., Semenov, M., Kato, Y., Spkony, r., Chumming, L., Katsuyama, Y., Hess, F., Saint-jeannet, J.-P., He, X. (2000). "LDL-receptor-related proteins in Wnt signal transduction." Nature 407: 530-535.

Tanaka Y, Mamalaki C, Stockinger B, Kioussis D. (1993). "In vitro negative selection of alpha beta T cell receptor transgenic thymocytes by conditionally immortalized thymic cortical epithelial cell lines and dendritic cells." Eur. J. Immunol. 23(10): 2614-2621.

Tetsu, O. and F. McCormick (1999). "Beta-catenin regulates expression of cyclin D1 in colon carcinoma cells." Nature 398(6726): 422-426.

Torres MA, Yang-Snyder JA, Purcell SM, DeMarais AA, McGrew LL, Moon RT. (1996). "Activities of the Wnt-1 class of secreted signaling factors are antagonized by the Wnt-5A class and by a dominant negative cadherin in early Xenopus development." J. Cell Biol. 133(5): 1123-1137.

Valsecchi C, G. C., Ballabio A, Rugarli EI. (1997). "JAGGED2: a putative Notch ligand expressed in the apical ectodermal ridge and in sites of epithelial-mesenchymal interactions." Mech. Dev. 69(1-2): 203-207.

Varecza Z, Kvell K, Talabér G, Miskei G, Csongei V, Bartis D, Anderson G, Jenkinson EJ, Pongracz JE. Multiple suppression pathways of canonical Wnt signalling control thymic epithelial senescence. Mech Ageing Dev. 2011 May;132(5):249-56.

Wang, H. and C. Malbon (2003). "Wnt signaling, Ca2+, and cyclic GMP: visualizing frizzled functions." Science 300: 1529-1530.

Wang Z, Shu W, Lu MM, Morrisey EE.(2005). "Wnt7b activates canonical signaling in epithelial and vascular smooth muscle cells through interactions with Fzd1, Fzd10, and LRP5." Mol. Cell Biol. 25: 5022-5030.

Wehrli, M., Dougan, S.T., Caldwell, K., O'Keefe, L., Schwartz, S., Vaizel-Ohayon, D., Schejter, E., Tomlinson, A., DiNardo, S. (2000). "Arrow encodes an LDL-receptor-related protein essential for Wingless signalling." Nature 407(6803): 527-530.

Wharton Jr., K. A., Zimmermann, G., Rousset, R., Scott, M.P. (2001). "Vertebrate proteins related to Drosophila naked cuticle bind dishevelled and antagonize Wnt signaling." Developmental Biology 234: 93-106.

Wiegers GJ, Knoflach M, Böck G, Niederegger H, Dietrich H, Falus A, Boyd R, Wick G. (2001). "CD4(+)CD8(+)TCR(low) thymocytes express low levels of glucocorticoid receptors while being sensitive to glucocorticoid-induced apoptosis." Eur J Immunol 31(8): 2293-301.

Wüst S, van den Brandt J, Tischner D, Kleiman A, Tuckermann JP, Gold R, Lühder F, Reichardt HM. (2008). "Peripheral T cells are the therapeutic targets of glucocorticoids in experimental autoimmune encephalomyelitis." J Immunol 180(12): 8434-43.

Xu Y, Banerjee D, Huelsken J, Birchmeier W, Sen JM. (2003). "Deletion of b-catenin impairs T cell development." Nature Immunol. 4: 1177-1182.

Yamamoto, H., Kishida, S., Kishida, M., Ikeda, S., Takada, S., and Kikuchi, A. (1999). "Phosphorylation of axin, a Wnt signal negative regulator, by glycogen synthase kinase-3beta regulates its stability." EMBO J. 274: 10681-10684.

Yamanaka H, Moriguchi T, Masuyama N, Kusakabe M, Hanafusa H, Takada R, Takada S, Nishida E. (2002). "JNK functions in the non-canonical Wnt pathway to regulate convergent extension movements in vertebrates." EMBO Rep. 3(1): 69-75.

Yan D, Wallingford JB, Sun TQ, Nelson AM, Sakanaka C, Reinhard C, Harland RM, Fantl WJ, Williams LT. (2001). "Cell autonomous regulation of multiple Dishevelled-dependent pathways by mammalian Nkd." Proc. Natl. Acad. Sci U.S.A. 98(7): 3802-3807.

Zhang X, Gaspard JP, Chung DC. (2001). "Regulation of vascular endothelial growth factor by the Wnt and K-ras pathways in colonic neoplasia." Cancer Res. 61(16): 6050-6054.

Zilberberg A, Yaniv A, Gazit A. (2004). "The low density lipoprotein receptor-1, LRP1, iteracts with the human Frizzled-1 (HFz1) and down-regulates the canonical Wnt signaling pathway." J Biol Chem. 279: 17535-17542.

32

Age-Related Changes in Human Skin by Confocal Laser Scanning Microscope

Karine Cucumel, Jean Marie Botto, Nouha Domloge and Claude Dal Farra
Ashland Specialty Ingredients – Vincience
France

1. Introduction

Cutaneous aging is a complex biological phenomenon affecting the different constituents of the skin. Two independent processes, clinical and biological, affect the skin during aging. The first is called "chronological aging" and the second one, "extrinsic aging" or "photoaging", which is the result of out-door exposure (such as solar irradiation). In this study, we mainly investigated the features of "chronological aging".

With the advancement of skin research, and the more and more important requests from the cosmetic consumers to have access to technical information on the product efficacy, many non-invasive methods have recently been developed to evaluate and quantify skin-aging parameters. Indeed, numerous available tools allow studying skin-aging as defined by key clinically observed aging parameters such as surface texture, fine lines and wrinkles, skin pigmentation (age spots), firmness, and loss of skin tonicity and elasticity.

In the past decade, laser-scanning confocal microscopy was developed, providing images from *in vivo* human skin without tissue alteration. At the same time, numerous studies comparing and identifying structures imaged by conventional histological sectioning and confocal laser scanning microscope were performed especially by Rajadhyaksha et al., 1995 and Gonzales et al., 2004. Today, the commercially available tool is VivaScope® (Lucid® Inc.), which allows to observe the cellular structure in the whole epidermis, from the *stratum corneum* to the fibrous tissue of superficial dermis, not invasively (without alteration of the tissue), and in real time (without any fixatives). Thanks to the *in vivo* confocal microscopy, a new way to study the signs of age through the epidermis is born. The aim of this chapter was to investigate histometric parameters on several volunteers of different ages in order to better understand the aging process.

2. Focus on VivaScope®

2.1 Parameters of VivaScope® 1500

Confocal laser scanning microscopy opens a "window into your skin" without damaging the skin. Confocal laser scanning microscopy was performed by using the VivaScope® 1500 (Lucid® Inc.). This method allows the observation of the cutaneous micromorphology *in vivo*; thus, for the first time, a real time optical biopsy is possible.

The principle of *in vivo* confocal laser scanning microscopy consists of a laser that emits, with a wavelength of 830 nm, an illumination power inferior to 35 mW and a water immersion objective. The images obtained using this method have a similar resolution to that of classic microscopy: the lateral resolution is 1.25 μm and the vertical one, about 2 μm. The images are black and white, and parallel to the surface of the skin (Curiel-Lewandrowski et al., 2004; Gerger et al., 2006). In this method, the skin imaging is based on different reflection indices of the micro anatomical structures. Melanin offers the strongest contrast; therefore, the cytoplasm of melanocytes appears very bright. Keratin reflects less intensely, so that the cytoplasm of keratinocytes appears darker. Cell nuclei also appear dark, and collagen very bright (Rajadhyaksha et al., 1995).

This skin imaging technique represents a non-invasive and not painful method, and is not tissue-destructive. All these parameters allow imaging the epidermis up to the papillary dermis at a cellular level without any tissue damage. The skin is unaffected during the preparing procedures, thus minimizing visual artifacts. The data collected in real time are rapidly acquired and processed, and the segment of analyzed skin can be re-examined in order to evaluate the dynamic changes. Image stacks can be obtained by compiling images taken every 2 μm, from the horny layer to the dermis.

Confocal laser scanning microscopy can be used for numerous applications and research areas. The images it produces are especially well suited to assist physicians in performing screening examinations, diagnosing skin cancers, etc. This technology can also be applied in cases of burns, dermatitis, and in the cosmetics research industry (Pierard, 1993; Corcuff et al., 1996; Abramovits et al., 2003; Branzan et al., 2007; Ardigo M. & Gill M., 2008).

2.2 VivaScope® 1500 technical performance

Different images, from the *stratum corneum* to the upper part of the dermis, were collected, analyzed, and consecutively transformed into a digital image with different levels of gray. Different measurements can be performed, such as thickness of the *stratum corneum*, of the epidermis, and the number and height of dermal papillae. This paragraph will summarize the methodology to acquire different measurements.

2.2.1 Measurement of objective parameters: *Stratum corneum* and epidermis thicknesses

2.2.1.1 *Stratum corneum* thickness

The *stratum corneum* thickness was calculated measuring the intensity variation on vertical reconstruction of the epidermis with the software ImageJ IJ 43 (Abramoff et al., 2004) giving a plot profile. The process is explained in Figure 1. The plot profile gives the intensity of the luminosity at different depths at the place of the yellow line in the vertical reconstruction. (The yellow line is placed by the operating expert). The *stratum corneum* thickness can then be obtained from the graph but can be more precisely obtained by calculating the derivative of the plot profile using finite differences. The depth separation between the maximum and the minimum of the derivative measures the *stratum corneum* thickness. Five measurements were made on one stack per volunteer.

2.2.1.2 Epidermal thickness

The distance between the surface *(stratum corneum)* and the level showing the dermal tissue measures the thickness of the epidermis. In Figure 2, **A** represents the *stratum corneum* (beginning of the measurement area), **B**, the beginning of the dermal tissue (end of the measurement), and **C**, the measurement done with VivaScope® on H&E. For the epidermis thickness, we performed one measurement per stack, on eight stacks per volunteer. In our experiment, we decided to measure the thickness between interdigitations where the thickness is smaller, i.e. minimal thickness (called Emin).

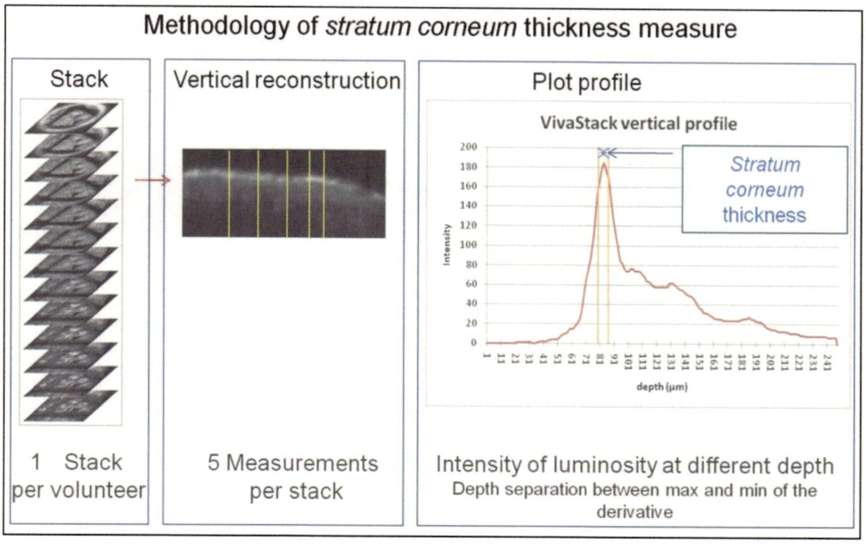

Fig. 1. Methodology of *stratum corneum* thickness measurement: From one volunteer, we collected series of images (stack), then the software provided from the stack a vertical section of the skin, the yellow line was placed by the expert to obtain the measure. The plot profile that gives the intensity at different depth is finally performed with ImageJ software and the calculation of the derivative measurement gave the precise thickness of the *stratum corneum*. Five measurements were made on one stack per volunteer.

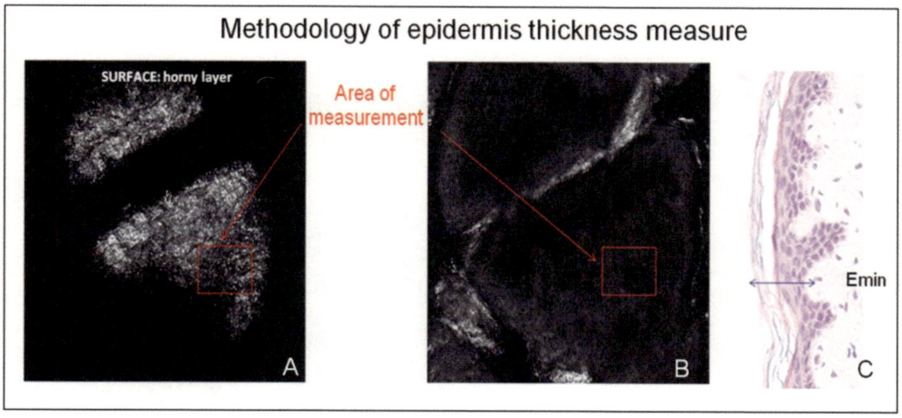

Fig. 2. Methodology of epidermis thickness measurement: The distance between the surface (*stratum corneum*) A and the level showing the first dermal tissue B measures the thickness of the epidermis. C represents the measurement done with the VivaScope® on a H&E biopsy section. For epidermis thickness, we made one measurement per stack, on eight stacks per volunteer.

2.2.2 Measurement of objective parameters: Dermal papillae

2.2.2.1 Measurement of the number of dermal papillae

The number of dermal papillae was evaluated by counting each active/functional papillae showing a lumen. Figure 3 explains how to recognize active/functional papillae from non-active dermal papillae. We made one measurement per stack, on eight stacks per volunteer.

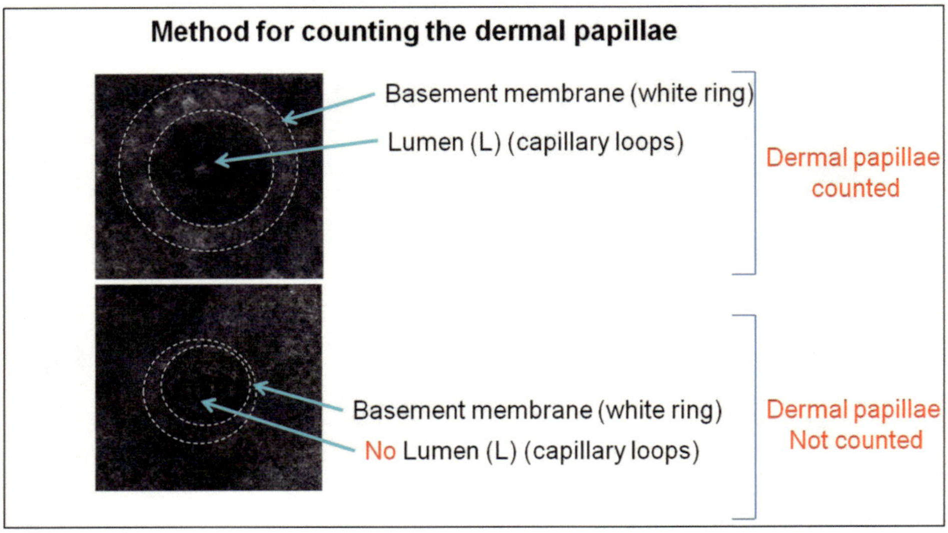

Fig. 3. The number of dermal papillae was evaluated by counting each active/functional papilla showing a lumen. The measurements were performed on eight stacks per volunteer and one measurement per stack.

To determine the height of dermal papillae, we measured the distance between the top of dermal papillae and the level showing no dermal papillae structure at all (Figure 4). We made the measurement on eight stacks per volunteer, and realized one measurement on two dermal papillae per stack. In total, we measured the height of 16 dermal papillae per volunteer.

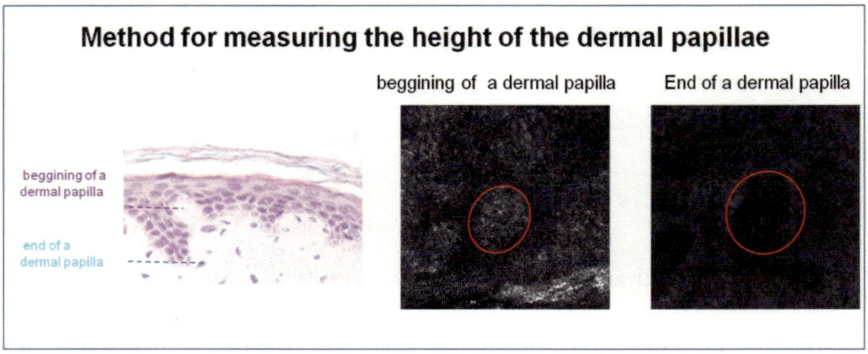

Fig. 4. The height of dermal papillae was measured as the distance between the top of dermal papillae and the level showing no dermal papillae structure at all. The measurements were performed on eight stacks per volunteer, and performed one measurement on two dermal papillae per stack. In total, we measured the height of 16 dermal papillae per volunteer.

2.2.2.2 Observations of reticular collagen

In some cases, we could also observe the reticular dermis, but we must note that we reached the detection limit at this point.

The clinical observations and measurements obtained by VivaScope® microscopy offer the cosmetic industry a great opportunity to trace the changes at different age-stages of the skin; and that will be presented in the second part of this chapter.

3. Skin changes at different age stages by *in vivo* confocal microscopy

3.1 Methodology of the clinical study

To investigate age-related changes, we studied five groups of five healthy volunteers each with Caucasian type of skin:

- The 20-30 group was composed of volunteers aged between 24 and 27 years (mean age: 25.2, 4 females, 1 male)
- The 30-40 group was composed of volunteers aged between 29 and 37 years (mean age: 33.8, 5 females),
- The 40-50 group was composed of volunteers aged between 41 and 46 years (mean age: 44.4, 5 females),
- The 50-60 group was composed of volunteers aged between 51 and 57 (mean age: 54.5, 3 females, 3 males),
- The 60-70 group, the older group, was composed of volunteers aged between 60 and 68 years (mean age: 63.6, 5 females).

Measurements were performed on their volar forearm, over two weeks in May.

For each group, we measured the epidermis and the horny layer thicknesses, the number and height of dermal papillae, and also carefully observed the granular cells, the morphology of dermal papillae, and when possible, the collagen fibers structure.

We compared these results with Hematoxylin-Eosin (H&E) stains on skin biopsies obtained from abdomen plastic surgery of females aged 20 to 79 years. In this part of the study, skin biopsies were fixed in successive baths of formol, alcohol, and xylene, then embedded in paraffin (Excelsior ES, Shandon, UK), and sectioned into 4 µm sections to be used for routine hematoxylin-eosin staining.

In this study, we observed very carefully the morphological features of the skin in the different volunteer groups; for each group, several biopsies were obtained, and for each of them, several skin cross-sections were studied and compared.

3.2 H&E staining observations

The following results are illustrated in Figure 5. In the different age groups, we observed:

- **Group 20-30:** The H&E skin coloration showed lots of dermal papillae as well as numerous invaginations, commonly called "rete pegs". The dermoepidermal junction was highly convoluted, and the basal cells appeared well organized without any damage. The papillary dermis appeared very dense.

- **Group 30-40:** At these ages, the structure of the epidermis was similar to that observed for 20-30 year-old donors. The interface between the epidermis and the dermis appeared highly convoluted due to the presence of rete pegs.
- **Group 40-50:** In this group, we observed a retraction of the rete pegs resulting in a flattened interface between epidermis and dermis. The dermal papillae were less apparent. The basal cells became less organized and the papillary dermis was less dense. It was in this group that we noticed the first morphological signs of age in the skin biopsies.
- **Group 50-60:** Here, the dermoepidermal junction was completely flat with a total absence of dermal papillae and so of rete pegs. The basal cells presented several damage and were disorganized. The papillary dermis decreased in density compared to the group 20-30.
- **Group 60-70:** The skin structure was similar to the one observed in the group 50-60. We found the same flattening of the dermoepidermal junction and the same damage of basal cells and papillary dermis.

observations	Comments
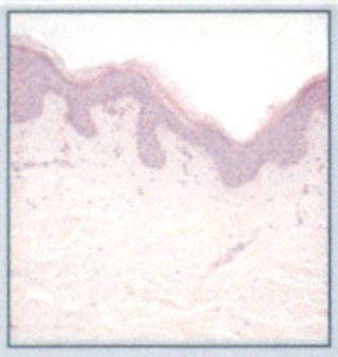	**Group 20-30:** The H&E skin staining showed lots of dermal papillae as well as numerous invaginations, commonly called "rete pegs". The dermoepidermal junction was highly convoluted, and the basal cells appeared well organized without any damage. The papillary dermis appeared very dense
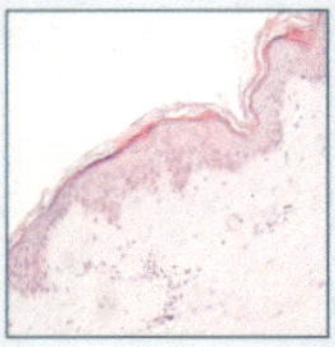	**Group 30-40** At these ages, the structure of the epidermis was similar to that observed for 20 years old donors. The interface between the epidermis and the dermis appeared highly convoluted due to the presence of rete pegs.
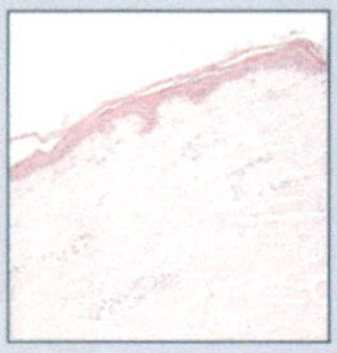	**Group 40-50:** In this group, we observed a retraction of the rete pegs resulting in a flattened interface between epidermis and dermis. The dermal papillae were less apparent. The basal cells became less organized and the papillary dermis was less dense. It was in this group that we noticed the first morphological signs of age in the skin biopsies.
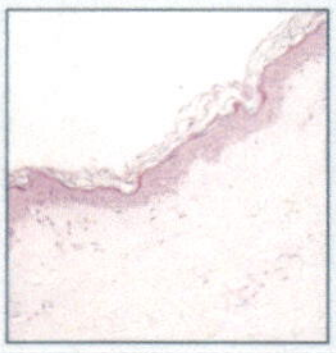	**Group 50-60:** Here, the dermoepidermal junction was completely flat with a total absence of dermal papillae and so of rete pegs. The basal cells presented several damage and were disorganized. The papillary dermis decreased in density compared to the group 20-30.
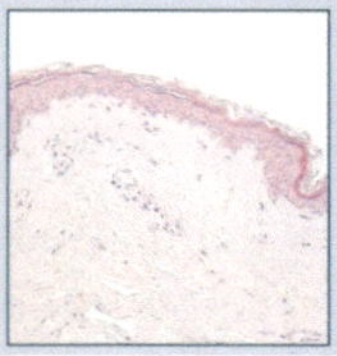	**Group 60-70:** the skin structure was similar to the one observed for the group 50-60. We found the same flattening of the dermoepidermal junction and the same damage of basal cells and papillary dermis.

Fig. 5. H&E staining biopsy observations and comments.

3.2.1 Results of H&E staining

In our light microscopy study, as largely described in the literature, we showed that aged skin revealed a thinner epidermis than young skin. This was primarily due to the retraction of rete pegs resulting in a flattened interface between epidermis and dermis and consequently to a flattened dermoepidermal junction. One of the consequences of this flattening is that aged epidermis becomes less resistant to shearing force, and less vascularized, leading to a bad nutrition of the basal cells. The observation of the *stratum corneum* in light microscopy study, as in other studies, showed that the number of horny cells did not seem to diminish with age, and thus the *stratum corneum* retained its normal thickness (Hull & Warfel, 1983).

In light microscopy, all the studies of the literature are in accordance regarding the evolution of skin thickness with age. However, conflicting results were found in the VivaScope® study and were challenging to interpret, as mentioned and discussed later on.

3.3 Confocal laser scanning microscope (VivaScope® 1500)

3.3.1 Horny layer and epidermis thicknesses

We measured and plotted the mean of horny layer and epidermal thicknesses as a function of age (Figure 6). The mean of horny layer and the epidermal thicknesses became thicker with age. The correlation between the thickening and age was statistically very significant for the *stratum corneum* and highly significant for the epidermal thickness. Table 1 gives the calculated correlation coefficient (r), which measures the correlation between the two variables: X for age and Y for the thickness.

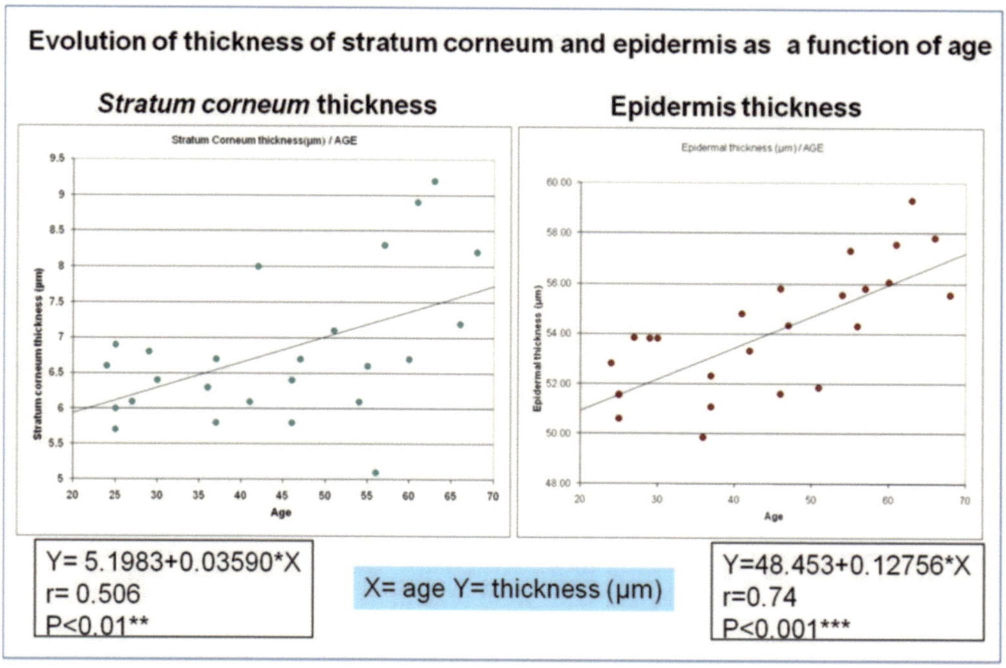

Fig. 6. Measurement and plot of horny layer and epidermis thicknesses as a function of age.

This correlation coefficient was positive, which implied that when age (X) increases, thickness (Y) also increases. The regression line can be used to predict the *stratum corneum* or epidermis thickness by entering the age of an individual.

Correlation test	p<	r=	Regression line	Mean		SD	
				X (age)	Y (thickness)	X	Y
***Stratum corneum* thickness / age**	0.01**	0.506	Y= 5.1983+0.03590*X	44.28	6.788	14.38	1.0199
Epidermal thickness / age	0.001***	0.74	Y=48.453+0.12756*X	44.28	54.102	14.38	2.479

: very significant *: highly significant

Table 1. Parameters of the graph representing the thicknesses of both horny layer and epidermis.

Furthermore, the correlation coefficient of the number and height of dermal papillae being close to 1 suggests that the number and the shape of dermal papillae could be considered as a very good aging indicator. According to the literature, we observed similar results with this technique to the ones that others obtained (Fenske and Lober, 1986; Zaghi et al., 2009).

3.4 Granular cell observation

For each group, we compared the organization and size of the granular cells. For each parameter observed, we assigned a category to each volunteer. Thus, for the granular cell morphology we used four categories: excellent, good, moderate and poor (the data are summarized in Table 2).

Age	excellent	good	moderate	poor
20-30	1	4		
30-40		3	2	
40-50			5	
50-60			2	3
60-70			1	4

Table 2. Granular cell observations: Excellent: very good organization, small and polygonal cells; Good: good organization, small and polygonal cells; Moderate: small cell disorganization and cell spreading, presence of no polygonal cells, vacuoles and dyskeratotic cells; Poor: cell disorganization and cell spreading, lots of cells with irregular shape, vacuoles, and condensed DNA.

- **Group 20-30 and group 30-40:** In these two groups, the granular layer displayed very well organized granular cells. The cells were regular in shape and size and had a good cohesion. We did not notice any cell damage (vacuole, dyskeratotic cells…). The granular layer had a honeycomb pattern as expected in young skin (discussed later in the next paragraph).

- **Group 40-50:** At this age, we observed the beginning of a disorganization of granular cells. The cells lost their polygonal shape and became bigger compared to young granular cells. Dyskeratotic cells appeared in this layer whereas the honeycomb pattern was less apparent.
- **Group 50-60 and group 60-70:** With age, the granular cell organization was completely lost. The cells had no longer a polygonal shape and their size was smaller. Numerous dyskeratotic cells appeared and the granular layer displayed cell spreading with a loss of cohesion.

3.5 Epidermal thickness assessment with VivaScope®

The effect of age on the thickness of the skin is one of the most controversial topics among dermatological researches. Indeed, in our study we observed a statistical correlation between thickening and age in both the horny layer and the epidermis. Focusing on the results of Table 1, we were able to observe a better correlation between epidermal thickness and age than horny layer thickness and age. Actually, this correlation difference pointed out that the *stratum corneum* is more influenced by the environment stress and volunteer's lifetime. Moreover, in the *stratum corneum* we observed that the correlation was not really linear but could look like a curve. This last finding suggested that the horny layer thickness could be constant during the first 50 years of life followed by a thickening in older individuals. More investigations have to be made to confirm these findings.

Controversially with others, we observed with the VivaScope® 1500 that the younger the skin is (and presumably healthier), the thinner the epidermis and the horny layer are. To our opinion, the relative thinness in younger skin (observed by this technique) correlated with what was seen in the granular cells in younger groups; the granular cells were more cohesive, often smaller than in the older groups, and better stacked, thus better organized. Hence, this relative thinness of the epidermis is not correlated with what was seen with light microscopy (i.e. the flattening of dermal junction) but correlated to a better internal organization of the granular cells. Besides, concerning the *stratum corneum*, with age, the cohesion between the corneocytes is lost (Fenske et al., 1986); therefore, they are not well organized and there is more space between each of them, which can explain the relative increase of the thickness.

3.6 Controversial results

Comparing measurements of the skin layer thickness between studies (and also from one individual to another, as well as between assessments) is especially challenging, due to the significant variations in measurements between individuals, between sites within each individual, between seasons, and hormonal differences between individuals.

Indeed, a study using confocal microscopy found that the thickness of living epidermis on the back of the arm decreased with age (Zaghi et al., 1986; Sandly-Møller et al., 2003). Another study using ultrasounds (Gniadecka et al., 1994) found an increase of facial skin thickness between 25 and 90 year-old people. In another study with 61 women with ages ranging from 18 to 94, authors found that the skin thickness increased on the forehead and buttock with age (Pellacani & Seidenari, 1999). In accordance with our results, in another study, Sauermann et al. (2002) considered a relatively old group with a mean age of 72.5 years and reported a significantly larger epidermal thickness in elderly volunteers. In the controversial study of Neerken et al. (2004), the thickness of the *stratum corneum* was found not to change with age, but in the older volunteer group, the minimum thickness of viable epidermis was somewhat larger (but no statistical difference between the investigated groups) and that the maximum thickness of the epidermis statistically significantly decreased with age. In our study, we chose to measure the minimum thickness of epidermis (see Figure 2 for reminder), and this can explain certain discrepancy compared with others.

When we focused on the methodology, we observed that Sauermann et al. measured the epidermal thickness on volar forearm with VivaScope® using the same method as we do, and found an increase in epidermal thickness with age.

Authors (Leveque et al., 1984) measured the total skin thickness on the dorsal and ventral forearm (epidermis + dermis) with Holtain Skinfold Caliper and found that the skin thickness decreased with age.

Takema et al. (1994) measured the skin thickness on the face and the ventral forearm by Dermascan A. They found that, with age, the skin thickness decreased in the area slightly sun-exposed (ventral forearm) whereas it increased in the area markedly sun-exposed.

Gambichler et al. (2006) measured the thickness of the epidermis on the forehead, pectoral area, forearm, buttock, upper back, and calf. They observed no inter-regional variation and a thinner epidermis in their older group.

Finally, Rigal & Leveque (1989) measured the skin thickness with ultrasound images for each decade of life (until 80-90 years) on the volar and dorsal forearms and observed an inter-regional difference. On the volar forearm, skin thickness did not vary significantly between the first and the seventh decade of life, but skin atrophy appeared after the eighth decade. On the dorsal forearm, they observed a phase of maturation (thickness increase) up to 15 years of age, and that atrophy signs began after the seventh decade.

Despite all these disagreements observed in bibliographic data, we can affirm that the keratinocyte turnover slows-down with age, leading to the accumulation and the increase in size of corneocytes in the *stratum corneum* (Leveque et al., 1984; Grove & Kligman; Marks, 1981). In our study, we observed that, with age, the granular cells increased in size, the shape changed, and the honeycomb pattern disappeared (correlating with an observed disorganization). According to Sauermann et al., the correlation between size of cells in the granular layer and age is consistent with a documented increase in corneocytes with age. Moreover, others (Fenske & Lober, 1986), who observed that in supra-basal cell layers the keratinocytes tend to display a decreased vertical height and an increased overall surface area, also reported this effect. Other authors suggested that this decrease in height and increase in irregularity could reflect the decrease in proliferation of the basal cell in aged skin (Sauermann et al., 2002). These changes, coupled with poor corneocytes adhesion, could lead to the increase of the thickness observed in our study.

3.7 Number and height of dermal papillae

Throughout different decades, we observed a statistically highly significant decrease in the number of dermal papillae ($p<0.001$). Therefore, mathematically, we could determine a negative correlation with r = -0.699 between the number of dermal papillae and age. The measured height of the dermal papillae also statistically highly significantly decreased ($p<0.001$), with a negative correlation of r = -0.854 (Figure 7).

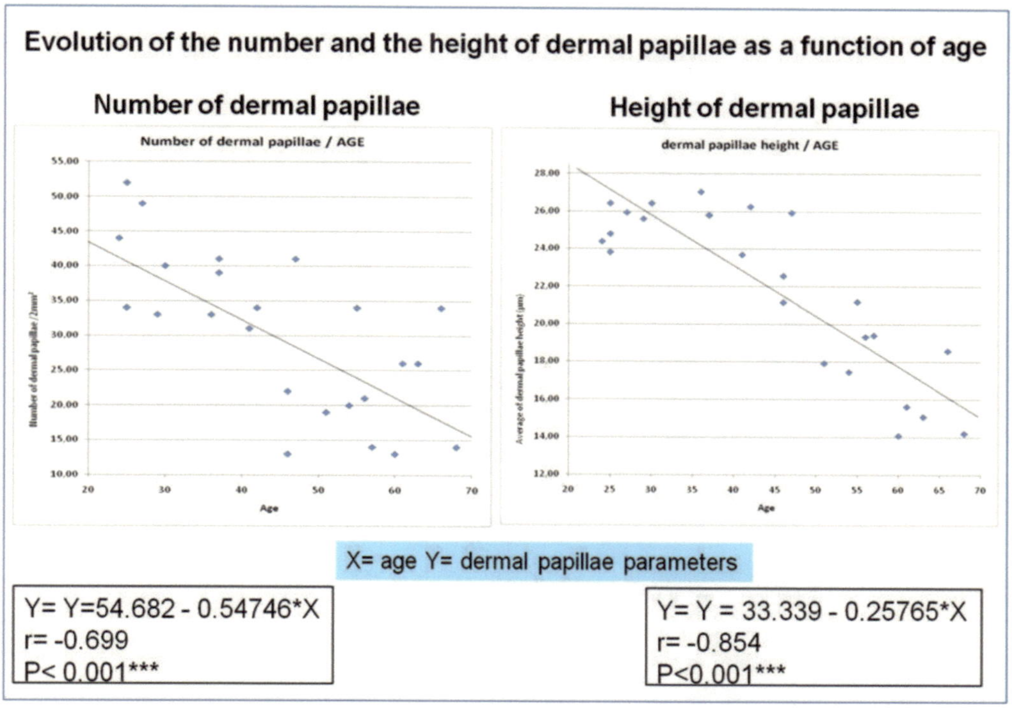

Fig. 7. Measurement and plot of the dermal papilla parameters (Number and height) as a function of age.

Furthermore, the correlation coefficient of the number and height of dermal papillae is close to 1, indicating that the number and shape of dermal papillae could be considered as very good aging indicators. According to the literature, we observed similar results with this technique as the ones that others obtained (Fenske and Lober, 1986; Zaghi et al., 2009).

3.8 Dermal papillae observations

The results of the observations are summarized in Figure 8.

- **Group 20-30:** At these ages, dermal papillae were numerous, round and very well delimited by a "white ring" (intense melanin content), which was constituted by the basal cells. Inside some papillae, we could observe capillary loops. All these observations demonstrated a good vascularization of the epidermis.
- **Group 30-40:** Dermal papillae were still round and pretty well defined although in that case we observed less melanin that interfered in the observation of dermal papillae. Nonetheless, the lumen of capillary loops is still observed, sign of a healthy skin.
- **Group 40-50:** The observed number of dermal papillae decreased in size. The shape was irregular and the dermal papillae were less defined. In this group of age, the capillary loops were hardly observable.

- **Group 50-60 and group 60-70:** The VivaScope® pictures did not display any dermal papillae. In the same manner, cells were disorganized, and the dermoepidermal junction was not observable. Moreover, vascularization was absent suggesting a poor epidermal nutritional status.

Dermal papillae	Comments
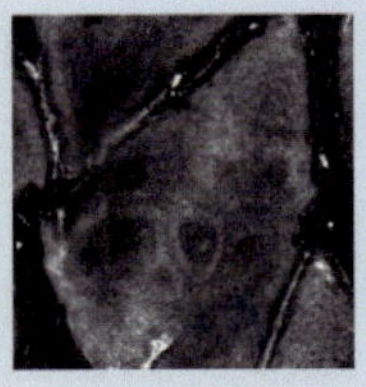	**Group 20-30:** At these ages, dermal papillae were numerous, round, and very well delimited by a "white ring", which was constituted by the basal cells. Inside some papillae, we could observe capillary loops. All these observations demonstrated a good vascularization of the epidermis.
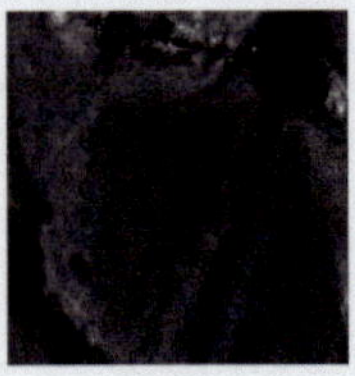	**Group 30-40:** Dermal papillae were still round and pretty well defined although, in that case, we only observed a few. Nonetheless, we could still see the lumen of capillary loops, a sign of healthy skin.
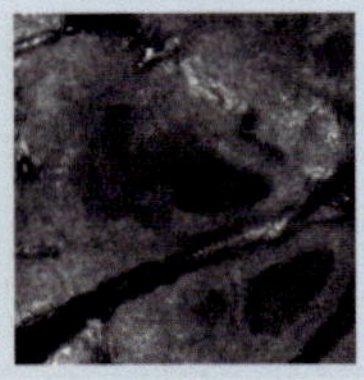	**Group 40-50:** The dermal papillae were less defined, and their shape irregular. In this group of age, capillary loops were hardly observable.
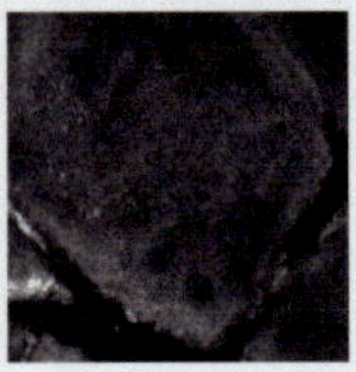	**Group 50-60:** The VivaScope® pictures did not display any dermal papillae. In the same manner, cells were disorganized and the dermoepidermal junction was not observable. Moreover, vascularization was absent, suggesting a poor epidermal nutritional status.
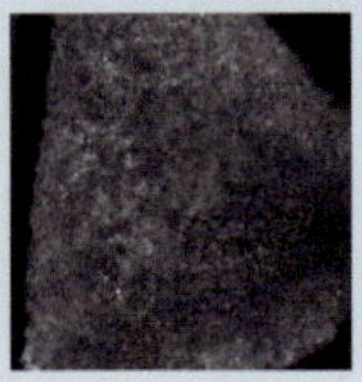	**group 60-70 (same as group 50-60)**

Fig. 8. Dermal papillae observations and comments.

3.9 Results on dermal papillae

Today, it is well accepted that the number of dermal papillae decreases with age, according to several studies (Fenske and Lober, 1986; Sauermann et al., 2002; Neerken et al., 2004) and we observed the same downward trend. The decrease in the number of dermal papillae with age reflects the flattening of the epidermal-dermal junction (Sauermann et al., 2002). In particular, this flattening demonstrates that not only the height of the dermal papillae decreases with age, but the number of interdigitations also drops with aging. The dermal papillae in the oldest groups were found irregular in shape; this feature could be explained by the reduction of the number of basal cells participating in the cellular cycle. This finding can be supported by the disappearance with age of the white ring surrounding dermal papillae that corresponded to basal cells.

After conducting this study, we conclude that the change in the number and morphology of dermal papillae are the parameters the most correlated with age. These parameters were closely linked to the dermal papilla function in supplying the epidermis with water and nutrients *via* dermal vasculature, and directly to the health of the epidermis. The morphology, number, and shape of dermal papillae could be great indicators of the epidermis health and age.

3.10 Collagen observations

The images obtained by the VivaScope® and the observations are compiled in Figure 9.

Collagen observations	Comments
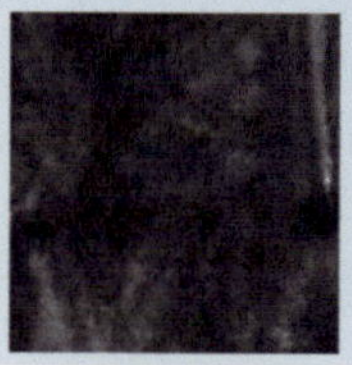	**Group 20-30 :** the younger group presented a very dense pattern and it was difficult to distinguish the fibers from each other. The collagen bundles were organized in tightly packed bundles.
	**group 30-40 : same as group 20-30**
	**Group 40-50:** at this rate of age we can see two different collagen aspects. We found dense collagen like in the younger groups and we found straight and filiform fibers that we can distinguish from the others material.
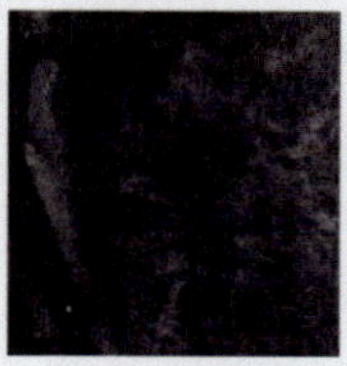	**Group 50-60** in older groups collagen fibers were judged filiform. We can easily see them as well as spaces between the fibers. The fibers looked like there were unraveling.
	**group 60-70: same as group 50-60**

Fig. 9. Collagen observations and comments.

- **Group 20-30 and group 30-40:** The younger group presented a very dense pattern of collagen and it was difficult to distinguish the collagen fibers from one another. The collagen bundles appeared organized in tightly packed bundles as discussed in the next paragraph.
- **Group 40-50:** At these ages, we could see two different collagen distribution patterns. We found dense collagen as in the younger groups, and straight and filiform fibers.
- **Group 50-60 and group 60-70:** In this group, collagen fibers were filiform. We could easily observe them, as well as spaces between the fibers, thus the fibers appeared individualized, isolated from one to another; therefore the fibers looked unraveled.

3.11 Results on collagen observations

With a confocal laser scanning microscope, also called VivaScope®, the collagen appearance of young skin was characterized by an organization in tightly packed bundles. At this age range, the collagen is the major dermal matrix component; collagen fiber bundles are compact and dense, which explains why we were not able to distinguish any structure in our observation. In contrast, in older groups, we managed to very well discern some collagen fibers from ground substance. This could be due to the decrease in the rate of collagen synthesis and the thickness of collagen fiber bundles (Fenske and Lober, 1986; Koehler et al., 2008). With age, the matrix becomes thinner, with straight collagen bundle fibers, giving an unraveled appearance to the bundles (Lavker et al., 1987; Zaghi et al., 2009).

4. Conclusion

To analyze the aging process, we investigated histometric parameters on biopsies from several donors of different ages, and performed a clinical study to observe the cutaneous micromorphology *in vivo*, using a confocal laser scanning microscope -VivaScope®1500- on groups of volunteers from 20 to 70 years of age.

The thickness of the epidermis and the horny layer seemed to be still controversial. However, regarding the effect of cosmetic ingredients contributing to an improvement of the skin's parameters, we observed that the healthier is the skin (a better-hydrated appearance), the thinner is the epidermis. The thinness parameter always correlates with an increase in the skin turnover and a decrease in size of granular cells.

As in the bibliographic data, we found that the number and height of dermal papillae decreased with age, and that these effects correlated with the flattening of epidermal-dermal junction seen in H&E staining biopsies. Therefore, after conducting this study, we came to the conclusion that the changes in the number and morphology of dermal papillae are the parameters the most correlated with age.

Finally, *in vivo* confocal laser scanning microscope can undoubtedly be considered as a sensitive and non-invasive tool allowing an easy study of the changes of different parameters of the whole epidermis, at all ages.

5. References

Abramoff, MD., Magalhaes, PJ., & Ram, SJ. (2004). Image Processing with ImageJ. *Biophotonics International*, Vol.11, No.7, pp.36-42.

Abramovits, W., & Stevenson, LC. (2003). Changing paradigms in dermatology: New ways to examine the skin using non-invasive imaging methods. *Clinics in Dermatology*, Vol.21, pp. 353-358.

Ardigo, M., & Gill, M. (2008). Blue nevus. In: *Reflectance confocal microscopy of cutaneous tumors*, Gonzalez S, Gill M, Halpern, AC, (EDs), 146–150, Informa Healthcare, USA.

Branzan, AL., Landthaler, M., & Szeimies, RM. (2007). *In vivo* confocal scanning laser microscopy in dermatology. *Laser in Medical Science*, Vol.22, pp. 73-82.

Corcuff, P., Gonnord, G., Pierard, GE., & Leveque, JL. (1996). *In vivo* confocal microscopy of human skin: a new design for cosmetology and dermatology. *Scanning*, vol.18, pp. 351-355.

Curiel-Lewandrowski, C., Williams, CM., Swindells, KJ,. Tahan, SR., Aster, S., Frankenthaler, RA., & González, S. (2004). Use of *In Vivo* Confocal Microscopy in Malignant Melanoma: an Aid in Diagnosis and Assessment of Surgical and Nonsurgical Therapeutic Approaches. *Archives of Dermatology*, vol.140, No.9, pp. 1127-32.

Fenske, NA., & Lober, CW. (1986). Structural and functional changes of normal aging skin. *Journal of American Academy of Dermatology*, vol.15, pp. 571-585.

Gambichler, T., Matip, R., Moussa, G., Altmeyer, P., & Hoffmann, K. (2006). *In vivo* data of epidermal thickness evaluated by optical coherence tomography: effects of age, gender, skin type, and anatomic site. *Journal of Dermatological Science*, vol.44, No.3, pp. 145-52.

Gerger, A., Koller, S., Weger, W., Richtig, E., Kerl, H., Samonigg, H., Krippl, P., & Smolle, J. (2006). Sensitivity and Specificity of Confocal Laser-Scanning Microscopy for *In Vivo* Diagnosis of Malignant Skin Tumors. *Cancer*, vol. 107, No.1, pp. 193-200.

Gniadecka, M., Gniadecki, R., Serup, J., & Sondergaard, J. (1994). Ultrasound structure and digital image analysis of the subepidermal low echogenic band in aged human skin: diurnal changes and inter individual variability. *Journal of Investigative Dermatology*, vol.102, No.3, pp. 362-365.

Gonzalez, S., Gilaberte-Calzada, Y., Gonzalez-Rodriguez, A., Torres, A., & Mihm, MC. (2004). *In vivo* reflectance-mode confocal scanning laser microscopy in dermatology. *Advances in Dermatology*, vol.20, pp. 371-387.

Grove, GL., & Kligman, AM. (1983). Age-associated changes in human epidermal cell renewal. *Journal of Gerontology*, vol.38, pp. 137-142.

Hull, MT., & Warfel, KA. (1983). Age-related changes in the cutaneous basal lamina: scanning electron microscopic study. *Journal of Investigative Dermatology*, vol.81, pp. 378–380.

Koehler, MJ., Hahn, S., Preller, A., Elsner, P., Ziemer, M., Bauer, A., König, K., Bückle, R., Fluhr, JW., & Kaatz, M. (2008). Morphological skin aging criteria by multiphoton laser scanning tomography: non-invasive *in vivo* scoring of the dermal fiber network. *Experimental Dermatology*, vol.17, pp. 519-523.

Lavker, RM., Zheng, PS., & Dong, G. (1987). Aged skin: A study by light, transmission electron, and scanning electron microscopy. *Journal of Investigative Dermatology*, vol.88, pp. 44s-51s.

Leveque, JL., Corcuff, P., De Rigal, J., & Agache, P. (1984). *In vivo* studies of the evolution of physical properties of human skin with age. *International Journal of Dermatology*, 23: 322-329.

Marks, R. (1981). Measurement of biological aging in human epidermis. *British Journal of Dermatology*, vol.104, pp. 627-633.

Neerken, S., Lucassen, GW., Bisschop, MA., Lenderink, E., & Nuijs, TA. (2004). Characterization of age-related effects in human skin: a comparative study that applies confocal laser scanning microscopy and optical coherence tomography. *Journal of Biomedical Optics*, vol.9, pp. 274-281.

Pellacani, G., & Seidenari, S. (1999). Variation in facial skin thickness and echogenicity with site and age. *Acta Dermato-Venereologica*, vol.79, pp. 366-369

Pierard, GE. (1993) *In vivo* confocal microscopy: a new paradigm in dermatology. *Dermatology*, vol.186, pp. 4-5

Rajadhyaksha, M., Grossman, M., Esterowitz, D., Webb, RH., & Anderson, RR. (1995). *In vivo* confocal scanning laser microscopy of human skin: melanin provides strong contrast. *Journal of Investigative Dermatology*, vol.104, pp. 946–52.

Rigal, J., & Lévêque, JL. (1989). Assessment of aging of the human skin *in vivo* ultrasonic imaging. *Journal of Investigative Dermatology*, Vol.93, pp. 621-625.

Sandby-Møller, J., Poulsen, T., & Wulf, HC. (2003). Epidermal thickness at different bodysites: relationship to age, gender, pigmentation, blood content, skin type and smoking habits. *Acta Dermato-Venereologica*, vol.83, No.6, pp. 410-3.

Sauermann, K., Clemann, S., Jaspers, S., Gambichler, T., Altmeyer, P., Hoffmann, K., & Ennen, J. (2002). Age related changes of human skin investigated with histometric measurements by confocal laser scanning microscopy *in vivo*. *Skin Research and Technology*, vol.8, pp. 52-56.

Takema, Y., Yorimoto, Y., Kawai, M., & Imokawa, G. (1994). Age-related changes in the elastic properties and thickness of human facial skin. *British Journal of Dermatology*. Vol.131, No.5, pp. 641-8.

Zaghi, D., Waller, JM., & Maibach, HI. (2009). The effects of aging on skin. *Nutritional Cosmetics*, pp. 63-77.

33

Imagistic Noninvasive Assessment of Skin Ageing and Anti-Ageing Therapies

Maria Crisan[1], Radu Badea[1], Carlo Cattani[2] and Diana Crisan[1]
[1]*University of Medicine and Pharmacy "Iuliu Hatieganu",*
[2]*University of Salerno,*
[1]*Romania*
[2]*Italy*

1. Introduction

The significant increase in life expectancy and the process of population ageing are aspects that generate important social and economic changes and influence the health and research policies throughout the world. The ageing phenomenon represents a natural, slow and irreversible process, which affects all body tissues, being determined by a multitude of factors that contribute in different proportions to the characteristic molecular, cellular, tissular and clinical changes. (Kohl et al, 2011)

The skin is a bio-membrane situated at the interface with the external environment. It reflects the state of health of the body, the human personality and has numerous psycho-social implications. Ageing is a complex process that implies external and internal factors. Chronological skin ageing comprises those changes in the skin that occur as a result of passage of time alone. Photo-ageing comprises those changes in the skin that are result of chronic sun exposure superimposed on chronological skin ageing. Several scientific theories on the ageing regulation at molecular, cellular and systemic levels have been postulated in order to define and control this process.

1.1 Ageing theories

For decades, researchers concluded that ageing comes as a consequence of both genetic and environmental influences. Among the environmental factors, solar UV radiation is the most important cause of premature aging.

1.1.1 The genetic theory

The theory of error accumulation, described by Orgel in 1963, interferes with the DNA replication, RNA transcription and translation into proteins. The risk for errors increases with age, determining at a certain moment a critical change in the genome that triggers senescence, apoptosis and cellular death.

1.1.2 The free radical theory

Postulated by Harman in 1956, this theory prooved that the reactive oxygen species interfere with the cellular and subcellular systems, inducing molecular degradations.

1.1.3 The mitochondrial theory

It is based on the fact that the mitochondria are the main source of free radicals within the cell. Skin exposure to sun determines the accumulation of mutations in the mitochondrial DNA, with implications in senescence (Shy et al, 2010).

1.1.4 The telomerase theory

Telomeres are sequences of nucleic acids extending from the ends of chromosomes. Every time our cells divide, telomeres are shortened, leading to cellular damage and cellular death associated with ageing. Telomerase, the "immortalizing" enzyme, appears to repair telomeres, manipulating the "clock" mechanism that controls the life span of dividing cells. The telomerase controls the telomere length and could be involved in the prevention of the ageing process. Recent studies have shown that specific molecules, applied topically or generally can activate the telomerase, preventing thus the shortening of the telomeres. (Han et al , 2009)

1.1.5 The theory of glycation

Maillard's theory is widely recognized as a general intrinsic ageing mechanism, focused on another potentially destructive agent, glucose. Glycation is the non-enzimatic reaction of a sugar and a protein forming multiple chemicals called advanced glycation end products (AGEs) (Pageon et al, 2010). The reaction products accumulate during the ageing process, and seem to also be involved in different pathologies associated with diabetes, atherosclerosis, Altzheimers disease, arthrytis (Bos et al, 2011). Proteins with a long biological half-life (collagen, elastin) are more affected. Glycation has different side effects on extracellular matrix fibers, leading to stiffer and more brittle collagen. In addition, elastin is easily glycated. Denaturated elastin is associated with slackened skin. It is important to mention that AGEs have cellular receptors that initiate inflammatory reactions when they are activated by an AGE complex. These reactions are associated with metabolic disorders, arterial diseases, the premature ageing process and the whole associated pathology. It has been reported that glycation affects the precise aggregation of collagen monomers into fibers, aspect that may be correlated with the different amplitude of the pixels when performing high-frequency ultrasound. Literature data as well as our own studies show that the echogenicity of the pixels and their density, correlated with the classical histological aspect of the integument, offer important information regarding age, cutaneous phototype, anti-ageing therapies, cutaneous pathologies etc. The extension of glycation in the skin can be measured with an instrument that measures a fluorometric chemical named pentosidine. Pentosidine is a fluorescent crosslinker that accumulates in a linear fashion in the collagen of all tissues. The fluorescence degree is correlated with the amount of accumulated pentosidine, age, risc of developing a certain pathology etc.

According to literature, collagen may be considered the key protein that allows the noninvasive assessment (fluorimetry, ultrasonography) of the cutaneous senescence process as well as the efficacy of various anti-ageing therapies. The non-invasive assessment of the cutaneous structure opens a new era of skin care and anti-ageing treatment.

Photoaging occurs as a result of cumulative damage from ultraviolet (UV) radiation. The UV rays induce and accelerate the glycation process, interact with cells and extracellular matrix, induce the synthesis and release of cytokines, stimulate the metalloproteinase synthesis, especially collagenase and elastase, and represent the major aggression factor on the cellular DNA. In photoaged skin collagen fibrils are disorganized, and abnormal elastin accumulates.

Despite the progress in aging research, these have yet to be an unanimous vote on one specific theory of ageing. Most of these theories have been disputed by researchers over and over again and many of them, as Dr.Hans Kugler editor of the Journal of Longevity Research, said, "...are dying of old age." Age-related changes do not occur uniformly in individuals because they are under genetic and environmental control. What is certain is that we are all involved in a global-ageing phenomenon.

1.2 Signs of skin ageing

The skin is the only organ completely displayed at the body surface and represents the ideal system for the study of both the intrinsic and extrinsic ageing process. Changes of the skin structure, such as wrinkles, irregularities of pigmentation, in contrast to ageing of other organs are visible and provide social clues to estimate the individual age.

1.2.1 Intrinsic aged skin occurs as a result of passage of time alone

Clinical manifestations include xerosis, laxity, wrinkles, slackness, benign tumors (cherry angiomas, seborrheic keratoses). Chronological ageing is affected by the changes of hormones and growth factors that appear with age. **Histological features** involve the epidermis, dermis and appendages. The hallmarks of intrinsic ageing are the thinning of the epidermis, flattening of the dermo-epidermal junction and reduction of extracellular matrix components.

1.2.2 Photoaged skin occurs as a result of cumulative damage from UV radiation

Clinical manifestations include roughness, irregular pigmentation, wrinkles, pseudo-scars, fine nodularity (elastotic material), telangiectasia, sebaceous hyperplasia,etc. **Histological manifestations** involve irregular epidermal thickness, nodular aggregations of elastotic material in the papillary dermis. The most obvious histological aspect is solar elastosis along with an increased amount of ground substance consisting of glycozaminoglycans and proteoglycans, and a decreased number of collagen fibers. Solar elastosis may correspond to the subepidermal low echogenicity band (SLEB) a specific imagistic parameter that appears on photoagressed areas. See Figure 3

In the reticular dermis collagen fibers appear degraded, clumped and fragmented. In addition, an inflammatory infiltrate can be identified. The elastosis process, collagen degenerescence, inflammatory infiltrates (histological aspects identified in usual or special stains) represent the morphological substrate of the sonograms. The amplitude and density of the pixels, correlated with the histological aspect, quantify different mollecular, cellular, biochemical and structural reactions that govern the ageing process.

The response to UV- induced damage is correlated with the individuals' skin type. Thus, subjects with skin type II show an atrophic and dysplastic response to UV rays, present fewer wrinkles, smoother skin, actinic keratoses, and epidermal malignancies (carcinoma, melanoma). The individuals with skin type III or IV show hyperplastic responses, present thick skin with coarse wrinkles. Our observations on 140 subjects have shown that individuals belonging to phototype class II (70 subjects) have a different imagistic pattern on photoexposed and photoprotected sites, in comparison to subjects belonging to phototype class III (70 subjects). The dynamics of the pixels on the studied areas indicate significant variations according to the phototype class and are correlated to different clinical aspects of the ageing process. The specific ageing features of phototype class II and III are shown in Table I.

	Phototype classs II	**Phototype class III**
Clinical aspects	Smooth skin, less superficial wrinkles, numerous pre-malignant lesions and cutanous carcinomas	Thick, pigmented, deeply wrinkled skin
Imagistic aspect: Photoexposed area (zigomatic area)	Thicker epidermis Thicker dermis Increased number of LEP, MEP, HEP	Thinner epidermis Thinner dermis Lower number of LEP, MEP, HEP
Imagistic aspect: Photoprotected area (medial arm)	Thiner epidermis Thicker dermis Higher amount of LEP Lower amount of MEP, MEP, LEPs/LEPi higher	Thicker epidermis Thinner dermis Lower amount of LEP Higher amount of MEP and HEP LEPs/LEPi lower

Table 1. Clinical and imagistic characteristics of skin phototype II and III.

It is well known that phenotypical and functional skin differences of individuals belonging to different ethnic backrounds are related to genetic factors, pigmentary system, life-time UV exposure, life-time style. In contrast to the studies on the pigmentary system, we can appreciate that there are other histological, biochemical differences, which govern the different shades of color. Despite the interest in finding objective markers for phototype classification, more complex studies comparing ageing and phototype between different ethnic groups remain to be published. Our observations suggest a complex interrelationship between the histological structure and the individual pigmentary system. The identification of certain measurable objective markers for every phototype will allow an optimisation of the phototherapy protocols and will reduce the photoinduced side-effects.

1.3 Histology of the skin

From histological point of view, skin consists of two layers of different origin, structure and function.

The epidermis (0,07 to 0,12 mm) is the outermost structure, derived from ectoderm, consisting of cells organized into five layeres. Stratum basale (germinativum), suported by a basement membrane consists of a single layer of mitotically active cells. Stratum spinosum, the thickest layer of the epidermis consists of polyhedral to flattened cells, attached to each other by unstable desmosomes, confering it a prickly appearance. Stratum granulosum consists of cells that contain lipid-rich granules that act as a waterproof barrier. Stratum lucidum is present only in thick skin. Stratum corneum is the most superficial layer, composed of numerous layers of flattened, keratinized cells.

The dermis (corium), lying directly beneath the epidermis is derived from the mesoderm and is subdivided into two layers: the superficial, loosely woven papillary layer and the deeper, much denser reticular layer.The dermis ranges in thickness from 0,6mm to 3mm. Histologically, the dermis is a dense, irregular collagenous connective tissue, containing mostly type I collagen fibers and networks of elastic fibers, which support the epidermis and bind the skin to the underlying hypodermis.

The papillary dermis is a loose connective tissue consisting of: type III collagen fibers, elastic fibers, fibroblasts, mast cells etc. The reticular layer is composed of dense, irregular collagenous connective tissue, displaying thick type I collagen fibers, closely packed into large bundles lying mostly parallel to the skin surface. Thick elastic fibers form networks that are more abundant around sebaceous and sweat glands. Proteoglycans fill the interstices of the reticular dermis. Cells are sparser and include fibroblasts, mast cells, macrophages, lymphocytes and fat cells. The hypodermis (subcutaneous adipose tissue) is considered a diffuse organ, normally well represented. From structural and functional point of view it is well integrated with the dermis and epidermis thru vessels and nerve structures. It lies underneath the reticulary dermis, being composed of adipose cells, disposed in adipose lobules, separated by conjunctive septa that contain blood vessels, lymphatics, nerve fibres and numerous mastocytes. The architecture of the adipose tissue differs for men and women. The subcutis is not part of the cutaneous structure, but is studied together with it, due to the associated pathology.

1.3.1 Epidermis

Epidermis is a stratified squamous nonkeratinized epithelium that covers the body on its surface. It consists of cells organized into five rows. Among keratinocytes that represent the most important cellular population, other cells, such as melanocytes, Langerhans cells and Merkel cells are found.

Imagistically, the epidermis appears as a hyperechogenic band, displayed parallel to the cutanous surface, having a thickness that can be assessed in mm. The thickness of the epidermis changes in relationship to the ageing process, applied therapy, associated pathology.

1.3.2 Dermo-epidermal junction

The junction between epidermis and dermis is a special ondulated basement membrane rich in collagen type IV filaments, collagen type III, collagen type VII, glycoproteins. The morphofunctional integrity of this barrier is essential for the skin protection function.

Imagistically, it is visualised as an extremly thin band situated at the limit of the hyperechogenic epidermis and the underlying dermis.

1.3.3 Dermis

Is a dense connective tissue, situated between the epidermis and hypodermis. The dermis consists of cells and extracellular matrix, composed of collagen and elastic fibres, proteoglycans, glycoproteins, tissular fluid. The limit with the hypodermis is a straight or sometimes ondulated line, because of the underlying adipose lobules, that are prominent in the lower dermis (visible aspect in „orange skin appearance" cellulitis). (Crisan, 2007)

Imagistically, we can assess the thickness of the dermis in mm as well as the number of pixels with different amplitudes, each codifying different structural, physiological or pathological aspects.

1.3.3.1 Extracellular matrix

Collagen is an important protein for the skin as it is essential for the structure and function of the extracellular matrix in the dermis. Thinner and wrinkled skin are typical signs of normal ageing and are consequences of reduced collagen. Collagen may be considered a "gold protein"for the assessment of the ageing process (fluorometrical, imagistical, clinical) and risc prediction of associated pathology. Collagen type I and II are the main types of collagen in the skin. In young subjects, there is a prominence of collagen type III or reticular fibres that are organised in fibrills and disposed at the level of papillary demis. In adults there is a prominence of type I collagen, organised in fibres disposed in parallel bands in the reticular or profound dermis. Collagen type IV forms filaments and is situated at the dermo-epidermal junction. In elderly subjects all types of collagen are diminuished. Collagen type I is the most common form (80%) in the dermis and is responsable for the cutaneous resistance. It is continuously produced and recycled throughout lifetime. In young subjects the synthesis process is prominent whereas in subjects over the age of 40, degradation processess are more common. (Uitto et al, 2008)

The key cell that forms and maintains the extracellular matrix is the fibroblast. The synthesis of the connective tissue fibres is initiated intracellularly, whereas the formation of filaments, fibrills or fibres are extracellular processes, controlled by several factors of the extracellular matrix. The main source of dermal echogenicity is represented by collagen fibres, disposed in an organized manner. Collagen and elastin are important proteins in maintaining the cutaneous architecture and ensuring the biostructural qualities of the integumentary system.

Proteoglycans beside glycoproteins and fibers are important components of the extracellular matrix. They consist of a protein core to which different glycozaminoglycans are linked. Hyaluronic acid binds uncovalently the proteoglycans, forming macromolecules that attract water, resulting in a true hydrating capsule with great importance for the hydration of the skin. With age, the amount of proteoglycans decreases and consequently the cutaneous hydration degree as well. The degree of hydration can be asssessed ultrasonographically by establishing the amount of low echogenic pixels in the skin.

1.4 Ultrasonography in dermatology

The imaging techniques have imposed themselves as usefull non-invasive methods for skin examination and diagnostic tools for skin conditions. During the past years conventional and high resolution ultrasonography (US) have extended their utility in the field of clinical dermatology (Schmid-Wendtner& Burgdorf W, 2005). The procedure involving ultrasound is a non invasive method allowing "in vivo" and "in real time" histological assessment of the cutaneous structure as well as its specific conditions. Several studies have prooven the similarities between sonograms and histological sections. (Jasaitiene et al, 2011)

The inclusion of this method among the procedures used for the diagnosis of skin diseases is an attempt to replace as much as possible the invasive procedures, especially biopsy, with non invasive ones. The motivation for the extensive use of US derives from its ability to reveal in detail the skin components, up to 1.5 cm in depth, to assess the axial and lateral tumoral extension, the inflammatory and degenerative processes, as well as the efficacy of different topical and general therapies.

1.4.1 High-frequency ultrasound

High-frequency ultrasound is a new, noninvasive method that allows an "in vivo assessment" of the physiological and pathological aspects of the integumentary system. It represents a more desirable and less emotionally-involving alternative to skin biopsy that is routinely used in the dermatological field. It also represents an important research tool for the characterization of skin properties on different intervals of age, allowing the establishment of an imagistic ageing model of the integumentary system. (Badea et al, 2010)

The use of high-frequency ultrasound in dermatology allows a clear identification of the skin layers and thus tissue assessment. At frequencies above 10 MHz, it was prooven that the technology provides enough resolution to characterize microstructures. High-frequency ultrasound allows, as the senescence process progresses, the identification of variations both in skin thickness and echogenicity, offering specific, ultrasonographic markers that allow an objective assessment of the skin ageing process. The changes of the extracellular matrix, consisting in variations of the dermal density and echogenicity throughout the physiological senescence process can be easily identified with the use of high-frequency ultrasound.

The ultrasonographic assessment of the integument can be performed with a 20 MHz high-frequency Dermascan device (Dermascan C, Cortex Technology, Denmark), as seen in Figure 1, that allows the "in vivo" acquirement of cross-sectional images of the skin (B mode) up to 2.5 cm in depth.

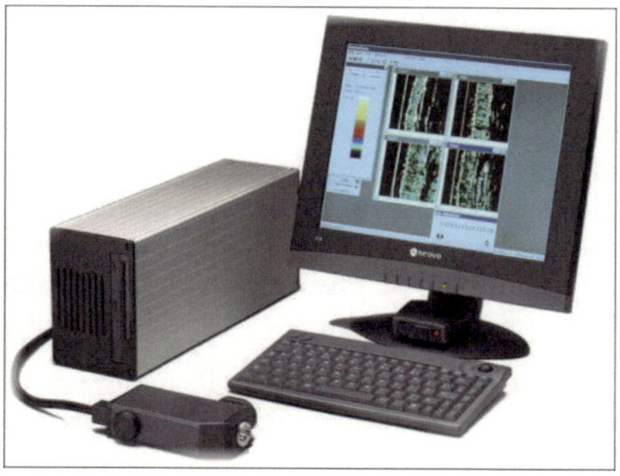

Fig. 1. Ultrasonographic equipment (Dermascan C, Cortex Technology, Dennmark).

The device consists of three major parts: a transducer, an elaboration system and a data storing system. The ultrasonic wave is partially reflected at the boundary between adjacent structures and generates echoes of different amplitudes. The intensity of the reflected echoes is evaluated by a microprocessor and visualized as a colored two-dimensional image. The color scale of echogenicity is: white- yellow - red - green - blue - black. On a normal cutaneous image, the epidermal echogenicity appears as a white band, the dermis is expressed as a 2 color composition: yellow and/or red, and the subcutaneous layer appears either green or black, as displayed in Figure 2.

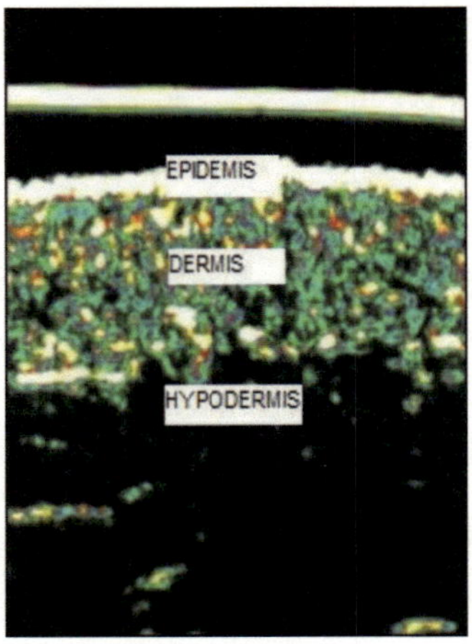

Fig. 2. Ultrasound image of the skin: epidermis, dermis, hypodermis

The ultrasonographic images are saved and processed with a specific image analysis software (Dermavision, Cortex Technology), that has a certain property: the amplitudes of the echoes of the pixels are given as a value on a numerical scale that ranges from 0-255. On this scale, the low echogenity pixel area corresponds to the 0-30 interval, the medium echogenity pixels to 50-150, and the high echogenity pixels to the 200-255 interval.

During the study, we can adjust the gain curve as well as the speed of ultrasound at tissular level. Ultrasonographic gel is applied on the aperture of the ring of the transducer, which is then placed perpendicularly to the skin surface for the acquirement of the cross-sectional image. There are several parameters that can be assessed by using Dermascan device and Dermavision analysis software as illustrated in Table 2

The thickness of the epidermis can be obtained by establishing the mean of three measurements performed in A-mode at three different sites of each image (the 2 extremities and the center of the analyzed image). The thickness of the dermis is obtained in B-mode, by measuring the distance between the dermo-epidermal and the dermo-hypodermic junction at the same three different sites and by establishing the mean of the three values. By selecting a certain interval from the 0-255 pixel scale, we obtain values corresponding to the low, medium and high echogenic pixels, present in the analyzed image.

Additionally, the LEP can be quantified separately in the upper (LEPs) and lower (LEPi) dermis. To separate the 2 areas, we draw a parallel line to the epidermal entrance echo, dividing the dermis into 2 equally thick parts. The ratio of LEP number in the upper and lower dermis (LEPs/LEPi) can be calculated.

PARAMETER	Description
Thickness of the epidermis **Thickness of dermis**	Given in mm
The number of LEP **(low echogenic pixels):**	Quantifiy the degree of cutaneous hydration, inflammatory processes, solar elastosis, collagen degeneration
The number of MEP **(medium echogenic pixels)**	Quantify the protein structures, the collagen and ellastin precursors (different assembly degrees)
The number of HEP **(high echogenic pixels):**	Quantify mature collagen assembled in fibres and disposed in parallel bands - marker of intrinsic ageing
SLEB - subepidermal low echogenicity band	A well delimited, subepidermal low echogenicity band (0-30), situated in the upper dermis, mainly present on photoexposed sites - marker of extrinsic ageing, shown in Figure 3
LEPs / LEPi ratio: number of low echogenic pixels in the upper dermis/number of low echogenic pixels in the lower dermis	Allows an appreciation of the density and integrity of the extracellular matrix, both from the upper and lower dermis, which varies according to age, UV-rays exposures, therapy - photoageing marker

Table 2. Ultrasonographic parameters

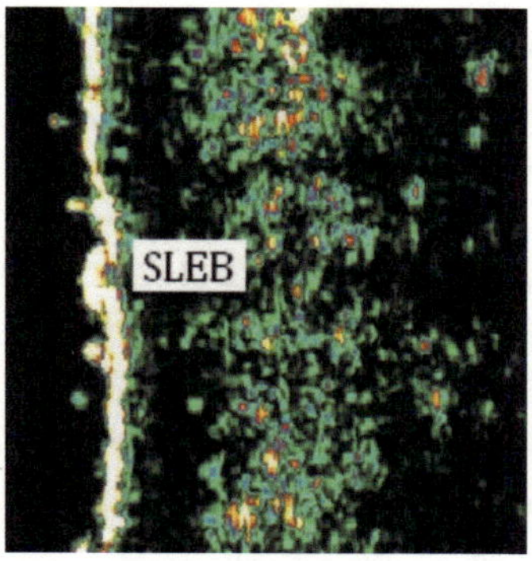

Fig. 3. Subepidermal low echogenicity band (SLEB)

The ultrasonographic skin examination with a high frequency transducer offers a 80 micrometer axial resolution, a 200 micrometer lateral resolution and a 1-2,5 cm depth [8,9]. According to the literature data and our experience, high frequency US is a non invasive instrument for skin examination having multiple applications both in the clinical and the research setting. We mention some of the most important contributions of the method in Table 3:

	Applications of high-frequency ultrasound
1.	Histologic skin evaluation and identification of each skin component (epidermis, dermis, dermo-epidermic and dermo-hypodermic junction, hypodermis); it is worth mentioning that the skin thickness is measured in"mm", while the density of the dermis is measured in number of pixels of different amplitude.
2.	Assessment and description of pigmentary and non-pigmentary tumoral structures: pigmented nevi, melanomas, carcinomas, dermoid cysts, sclerodermia, etc.
3.	Non invasive monitoring, both qualitative and quantitative, of the cutaneous alterations induced by senescence
4.	Monitoring of chronic inflammatory conditions
5.	Monitoring the efficacy of various therapies
6.	Objective markers for determining the phototype

Table 3. Applications of high-frequency ultrasonography in Dermatology

1.4.2 Conventional ultrasound

The use of conventional US has gained greatly in importance in clinical dermatology starting with the 70's. It proved to be a valuable diagnostic method and to have several indications, such as: a. identification and description of visible and palpable tumors, including melanoma; b. preoperative and postoperative assessment of periferal lymph nodes in all patients with malignant skin tumors; c. monitoring of metastases, especially during chemotherapy. (Wortsman et al, 2010) The main applications of US in dermatology in the present times are conventional cutaneous US and examination with the high frequency transducer.

2. High-frequency ultrasound study of the skin

2.1 High frequency ultrasound study of the skin aging process

High frequency ultrasound allows the "in vivo" appreciation of certain histological parameters and offers new characteristic markers, which may quantify the severity of the cutaneous senescence process. Moreover, it may differentiate between the chronological aging process and photoaging. It evaluates the physio-chemical properties of the integument, epidermis, dermis and subcutis that induce acoustical variations, expressed through certain changes of tissue echogenicity. Our study focused on measuring the changes in skin thickness and dermis echogenicity, as part of the complex ageing process, on different intervals of age.

The study was performed on 40 Caucasian patients, 12 men, 28 women, aged 4 -75 years and divided into four age categories: 4-20, 21-40, 41-60, >60. For each subject, cutaneous ultrasound images were taken from 3 different sites: dorsal forearm (DF), medial arm (MA) and zygomatic area (ZA). The data we obtained was statistically assessed, based on the ANOVA and Student T test, using the EPIINFO program. We evaluated the differences between values referring to different intervals of age at the 3 examined sites. A p value <0.05 was considered significant.

The **thickness of the epidermis** remains at approximately similar values on all examined sites, for all age intervals, with no statistically significant differences. The **thickness of the**

dermis shows certain variations. A growth of the dermal thickness at facial level can be noticed with aging. From a mean of approximately 1,320 mm on the 4-20 age interval, the dermis reached a value of 1,614 mm for the subjects taking part of the >60 age interval.

At dorsal forearm and medial arm level, we noticed that the dermis thickness varied in the same way: a decrease of the dermis thickness for the 20-40 age interval, followed by an increase for the 41-60 age interval. The 20-40 age interval, corresponding to the maturity period, is characterized by active synthesis processes, which lead to the thickening of the extracellular matrix.The degenerative processes that lead to the thinning of the dermis appear slowly after the age of 60. The variation pattern of the dermal and epidermal thickness with age can be observed in Table 4.

	Interval of age			
Area	**4-20**	**21-40**	**41-60**	**>60**
Epidermis DF (mm)	0,19675	0,182333	0,182667	0,186444
Epidermis MA (mm)	0,165375	0,163778	0,184889	0,169333
Epidermis ZA(mm)	0,175875	0,173333	0,155222	0,162333
Dermis DF (mm)	1,211875	1,191222	1,311556	1,168889
Dermis MA (mm)	0,856375	0,772889	0,838333	0,861
Dermis ZA (mm)	1,320375	1,45	1,448289	1,614

Table 4. Mean of dermis and epidermis thickness on 4 age intervals, at dorsal forearm (DF), medium arm (MA) and zygomatic area (ZA) level

Generally, considering the **total thickness of the integument** (dermis and epidermis), a significant increase may be noticed especially at the facial site, which prooves that the integument thickness increase is dependant on the severity of UV photoexposure. Also, comparing young subjects (aged 4-20) with elderly ones (>60), it is noticeable that the integument is thinner in the second group at dorsal forearm level, has similar values on the medial arm and increases at facial level.

The number of hypoechogenic pixels shows a significant variation in case of the dorsal forearm and medial arm of the patients taken into study, as follows: hypoechogenic pixels significantly decrease on the dorsal forearm in the 20-40 age interval compared to the 4-20 interval ($p= 0.038018$, $p<0.05$) and increase significantly in the >60 age interval in comparison to the 41-60 interval ($p= 0.00777$, $p<0.05$); on the medial arm, hypoechogenic pixels increase significantly in the 41-60 age interval, compared to 20-40 interval ($p= 0.018056$, $p<0.05$). The significant increase of hypoechogenic pixels after the age of 40, both on photoexposed and photoprotected sites, is correlated with the degenerative changes which are typical for the ageing process in general. Initially, elastic and reticular fibres from the papillary dermis are altered. Generally, we noticed that hypoechigenic pixels are more numerous in the upper dermis in elderly subjects on all studied areas, being correlated with the elastosis and cutaneous degenerescence processes.

Intermediate echogenic (50-100, 100-150) pixels increase significantly ($p<0.05$) on photoexposed sites in the 20-40 age interval (synthesis processes; assembly to filaments, microfibrils) and decrease after the age of 40 (decreased synthesis and degenerative processes). The repartition dynamics of the intermediate echogenic pixels in case of the 20-40 age interval indicates the presence of intense metabolic processes that continue on to the next intervals of age, but in a much slower rhythm. We consider this interval as a"critical age interval" that represents the optimal timing to inititate the prophylaxis of the senescence process and associated pathology.

Hyperechogenic pixels also display statistically significant variations on the three analyzed regions: on the dorsal forearm, high echogenic pixels increase significantly in the 20-40 interval of age, compared to the 4-20 interval ($p=0.025154$, $p<0.05$, and slightly decrease after the age of 40; on the medial arm, they decrease in the 40-60 age interval compared to the 20-40 age interval ($p= 0.038523$, $p<0.05$) and at facial site, high echogenic pixels increase in the 21-40 interval ($p= 0.025405$, $p< 0.05$) and decrease between 41-60 ($p= 0.048694$, $p<0.05$). The highest amount of hypoechogenic pixels was identified at facial level, an intensely photoagressed site, whereas the highest amount of hyperechogenic pixels was found at the medial arm site, a less photoexposed area. High echogenic pixels (200-255) are poorly expressed in patients belonging to the 4-20 age interval, and much better expressed in the 20-40 age interval on all studied areas. According to Table 5, the mean of hyperechogenic pixels is higher on photoprotected areas compared to the photoagressed ones for all intervals of age. Thus, we may consider hyperechogenic pixels as ultrasonographic markers of the chronological ageing process.

	0-30	**50-100**	**100-150**	**200-255**
DF				
0-20	11656.50	2184.12	627.62	470.50
20-40	7657.00	3581.55	1314.11	1221.55
40-60	12613.11	2413.44	740.555	701.33
>60	11007.44	2093.00	708.444	737.55
MA				
0-20	4792.50	2407.25	1036.50	1960.00
20-40	3371.55	2187.22	981.55	2687.22
40-60	5716.33	2225.88	916.11	1644.88
>60	5584.88	2204.66	822.22	1450.66
ZA				
0-20	15263.63	1568.87	348.25	120.75
20-40	13979.89	2670.00	821.77	602.22
40-60	17047.11	1561.88	394.77	213.22
>60	19055.56	1823.44	504.77	301.22

Table 5. Mean of 0-30, 50-100, 100-150, 200-255 pixels measured on subjects divided into 4 age intervals, at the examined sites: dorsal forearm (DF), medial arm (MA) and face level (ZA)

Subepidermal low echogenic band (SLEB) was identified in case of the subjects part of the 41-60 and >60 age intervals, and appeared especially on photoexposed sites (dorsal forearm, face) [10]. In some patients though, especially the younger ones, we were able to identify SLEB at medial arm level as well. On photo-aggressed sites, it may be noticed that the echogenicity of the upper dermis decreases with age.

SLEB may be considered a specific ultrasonographic parameter that allows a noninvasive quantification of the elastosis degree and actinic collagen degeneration. (Lacarrubba et al, 2008) SLEB varies in thickness and localization according to age and UV exposure. In young subjects, SLEB is present in the lower dermis and quantifies the degree of cutaneous hydration, since the extracellular matrix is rich in proteoglycans and hyaluronic acid.

Hyaluronic acid binds uncovalently the proteoglycans, forming macromolecules that attract water, forming a true hydrating capsule. In elderly subjects, SLEB quantifies the elastosis process and basophilic degenerescence of collagen, common aspects of the senescence process, but increased by UV. Thus, we may consider SLEB as a qualitative marker of the photoagression process.

The ultrasound study shows different echogenicity degrees for the **upper (LEPs) and lower (LEPi) dermis**. For the upper dermis, the study revealed an increase of hypoechogenic pixels (0-30), in comparison to the lower dermis, for all 4 age intervals studied. According to Figure 4, the hypoechogenicity degree is higher on photoexposed sites, both for the upper and the lower dermis. **LEPs/LEPi ratio** showed a statistically significant increase ($p<0.05$) for the 20-40 and 40-60 age intervals on photoexposed sites, especially at facial level ($p= 0.000999$, $p<0.05$).

On the medial arm , a progressive decrease was noticed till the age of 60, followed by a light increase in people >60 years. This aspect may be explained by the increase of hypoechogenic pixels in the upper dermis. Unlike the upper dermis, in the lower dermis, an increase of echogenicity may be noticed with ageing as visible in Figure 4. The ratio between the echogenicity of the upper and lower dermis represents an objective marker of the photoageing process.

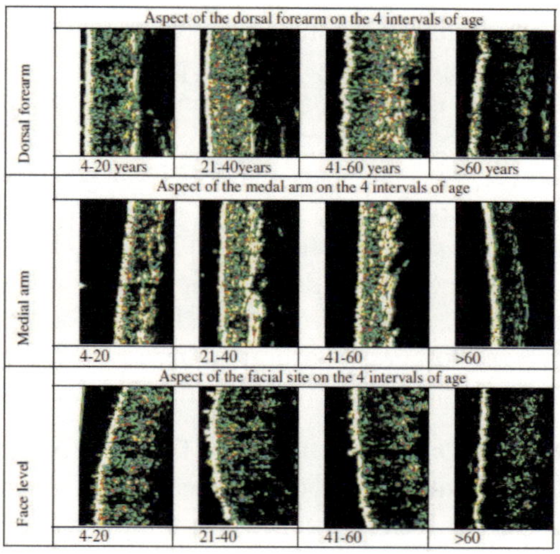

Fig. 4. Ultrasonographic aspect of the dorsal arm, medial arm and facial site on the 4 studied age intervals

The thickness of the integument, SLEB, as well as the dermal echogenicity are parameters that evaluate, with high accuracy the cutaneous senescence process at a microscopical level. The ratio between the echogenicity of the upper and lower dermis represents an objective marker of the photoaging process. SLEB is an ultrasonographic marker of the collagen degenerescence process and photoinduced cutaneous elastosis.

2.2 Non-invasive imagistic assessment by "in vivo" histological sections, of the efficacy of anti-ageing therapies

Taking into consideration that nowadays we assist a general ageing tendency of the world population, the antiaging therapy is a priority and a continuous challenge for researchers. The identification of the mechanisms involved in the cutaneous aging process and their impact on certain age categories, correlated with the hormonal and neurogenetic constellation of the subject would be highly desirable since it is estimated that about 31% of the population is over the age of 60 (US Census Bureau, online database.www.census.gov).

The increase of life expectancy, the psychosocial impact of the cutaneous aspect justifies the high amount of research studies of the ageing mechanisms as well as of the efficacy of certain anti-aging therapies. (Vaupel, 2010) The purpose of the 2 studies to be presented was the assessment with the help of high-frequency ultrasound of the cutaneous changes induced by topical use of Viniferol-containing products as well as by topical anti-ageing product (Interactive P63).

2.2.1 Efficacy of Viniferol as anti-ageing therapy

The first study assessed, with the help of high-frequency ultrasound, the cutaneous changes induced by topical use of products containing Viniferol. As far as the anti-ageing therapy is concerned, Viniferol ® (Resveratrol), an extract from Bordeaux vine stalks is one of the newest and more efficient anti-wrinkle and anti-ageing agents. Having a direct action upon the protein expression of the genes involved in the proliferation and differentiation of integumentary cells, Viniferol profoundly restructures and regenerates the skin. Due to its antioxidant properties, it reestablishes the metabolic balance of the cutaneous cells, slowing down the tissular degeneration and disorganization process (Vranesic-Bender, 2010). Even though the general anti-ageing effects of the flavonoids are well known, until now no scientific studies investigated the action of Viniferol at cutaneous level by using high-frequency ultrasound. Eighty female subjects, aged 22-75, who presented themselves to the practice for prophylaxis and anti-ageing therapy with flavonoids, were prospectively included in the study. 50% of the subjects belonged to Fitzpatrick phototype class II and 50% to phototype class III. The study excluded patients with known allergies to topical flavonoids, cutaneous facial lesions, resurfacing or other anti-ageing therapies in the last 2 months, or those who used phototherapy or oral contraception. The subjects taken into the study were divided into 2 categories: a study group and a control group.

The study group followed the proposed antiaging therapy for 12 weeks, according to a standard protocol. In the morning, a hydrating emollient cream, based on occlusive hydrating agents, was applied at facial level (including zygomatic area), lightly massaging the area for 2 minutes. In the evening, an anti-ageing product containing Viniferol, extracted from grapevine, was applied in the same manner. No other cosmetic products were used by the subjects during the 12 weeks of the study. The control group followed a placebo therapy for 12 weeks, using only moisturising cream in the morning and evening, applied at facial level. For every subject, ultrasonographic images were taken from zygomatic level initially and 12 weeks after local application of the emollient, hydrating product and anti-ageing, Viniferol-based cream. The data we obtained was analyzed, calculating the mean and standard deviation for the quantitative variables of every group and the proportions for the qualitative variables. The difference of means before and after treatment was tested using T-test for paired samples and the relationship between different parameters was assessed thru Spearmann correlation coefficients. A p-value <0.05 was considered significant.

All subjects involved in the study tolerated well the therapy, without evoking adverse effects (erythema, pruritus, ocular disturbance). Subjectively, post flavonoid-therapy a significant hydration of the skin throughout the day and an increase of the cutaneous tonicity was noticed.

After therapy, an increase of the mean **thickness of the epidermis** (0.129 ± 0.237 mm vs 0.150 ± 0.323 mm, p<0.000), and of the dermis (1.434 ± 0.241 mm vs 1.569 ± 0.219 mm, p<0.0001) was observed. (fig 3, 4)The **thickness of the dermis** increased mainly in the 40-60 age interval (1.413±0.280 mm vs 1.569±0.279 mm, p=0.001), and less, but still significantly < 40 years (1.416±0.266 mm vs 1.585±0.150 mm, p=0.015), while >60 years the increase was not statistically significant (1.480±0.157 mm vs 1.554±0.204 mm, p=0.097). At the same time, at dermal level, the **number of low echogenic pixels** decreased (15153.53 ± 3589.86 vs. 12958.48 ± 3628.35, p<0.0001), but this aspect was only noticed in the lower dermis (6949.75 ± 1966.93 vs 6257.62 ± 2224.88, p=0.016), not in the upper dermis (7290.55 ± 1794.60 vs 6940.65 ± 2150.30, p=0.168). Overall, the **LEPs/LEPi ratio** increased significantly after flavonoid therapy (1.092 ± 0.330 vs 1.259 ± 0.631, p=0.011). We also noticed an increase of **medium echogenic pixels** (3359.72 ± 1457.36 vs 3983.47 ± 1401.24, p=0.013) and **high echogenic pixels** (460.27 ± 323.93 vs 750.90 ± 493.82, p<0.0001) after therapy.The general variation pattern of the quantifiable ultrasonographic parameters after flavonoid therapy is illustrated in Table 6.

	Before treatment	**After treatment**	***P***
Thickness of epidermis (mm)	0.129 ± 0.237	0.150 ± 0.323	<0.0001
Thickness of dermis (mm)	1.434 ± 0.241	1.569 ± 0.219	<0.0001
LEP	15153.53 ± 3589.86	12958.48 ± 3628.35	<0.0001
MEP	3359.72 ± 1457.36	3983.47 ± 1401.24	0.013
HEP	460.27 ± 323.93	750.90 ± 493.82	<0.0001
LEPs	7290.55 ± 1794.60	6940.65 ± 2150.30	0.168
LEPi	6949.75 ± 1966.93	6257.62 ± 2224.88	0.016
LEPs/LEPi	1.092 ± 0.330	1.259 ± 0.631	0.011

Table 6. Cutaneous parameters quantified by high-frequency ultrasound before and after treatment

If we consider the variation of the ultrasonographic parameters after topical flavonoid therapy according to the phototype class of the subjects, it can be noticed that after therapy, there is a significant increase of the LEPs/LEPi ratio in the subjects belonging to phototype class II, not III, as shown in Table 7.

	Phototype 3			Phototype 2		
	Before treatment	After treatment	P	Before treatment	After treatment	P
Epidermis (mm)	0.1288±.026	0.151±0.027	<0.0001	0.129±0.021	0.148±0.037	0.020
Dermis (mm)	1.441±0.270	1.570±0.263	0.001	1.427±0.214	1.568±0.172	0.003
LEP	15059.25±4063.97	13864.75±3824.33	0.015	15247.8±3162.14	12052.2±730.34	<0.0001
MEP	3120.10±1725.95	3850.95±1487.32	0.046	3599.35±1122.42	4116.0±1334.62	0.151
HEP	379.35±280.94	645.50±373.59	<0.0001	541.20±350.25	856.3±581.03	0.004
LEPs	7071.65±1754.22	6961.1±2236.66	0.725	7509.45±1852.70	6920.20±2118.53	0.148
LEPi	7007.65±2150.80	6737.15±2205.91	0.480	6891.85±1818.86	5778.10±2193.29	0.010
LEPs/LEPi	1.035±0.262	1.096±0.300	0.200	1.1499±0.384	1.4227±0.820	**0.026**

Table 7. Variation of the cutaneous parameters quantified by high-frequency ultrasound before and after treatment, according to phototype

In the placebo group, we noticed no significant increase of the epidermis and a slight increase of the dermis after therapy (1.433 ± 0.34 mm vs. 1.486 ± 0.14 mm). The number of low echogenic pixels at dermal level also show a slight increase (13213 ± 1284 vs. 15374 ±2318 , p=0.1) due to an optimal hydration of the skin and a discrete decrease of high echogenity pixels (421,8 ± 121.18 vs 368. 3 ±104.03, p=0.07). The LEPs/LEPi ratio showed no particular display according to the age or phototype of the subjects.

Previous studies have shown that the thickness of the epidermis and dermis, as well as the dermal density are important parameters that assess the cutaneous regeneration process (Crisan M et al, 2009). The neosynthesis of the proteic structures induces an increase of the dermal echogenicity and density, local cell architecture changes and implicitly there is an increase of the dermis and epidermis thickness. It has been prooved that certain ultrasonographic markers, such as SLEB (subepidermal low echogenity band) or the LEPs/LEPi ratio can quantify the cutaneous senescence process, as well as the efficacy of various antiaging therapies.

The obtained results are in accordance with the data published in literature. Thus, locally applied flavonoids induce the neosynthesis of the fibrillary structures, but also of glicosaminoglycans, intense hydrophil molecules, favouring the cutaneous hydration. It is well known that flavonoids have important antiaging properties not only at cutaneous level, but at the level of the entire organism. Viniferol, a molecule with proven anti-ageing and antioxidant properties, exhibits a complex action at cutaneous level: it interacts with fibroblastic receptors, amplifies the interrelation fibrocyte-extracellular matrix, modulates the adhesivity molecules and interferes with the oxidative stress process and non-enzymatic glycation, with regenerative effect at cutaneous level.

After therapy, a significant increase of the mean thickness of the epidermis and dermis was noticed, fact that once again confirms the presence of a complex, regenerative dermal process, induced by flavonoids. The dermal thickness increased the most in the 40-60 age interval, to a lesser extent, but still significant under the age of 40, and insignificantly over 60 years. We can affirm that topical flavonoid products have the best efficacy on mature integument, with specific structural and hormonal characteristics. In young subjects (<40) the thickness of the dermis increases discretely as the dermis is a young connective tissue, rich in glicosaminoglycans and thus, properly hydrated. After the age of 60, interval characterized by the presence of degenerative changes of the extracellular matrix the flavonoid-based anti-ageing therapy induces less intense regenerative changes that could be amplified by the association of products able to interfere the characteristic age-related aging mechanisms. At the same time, concomitantly with the change in dermal thickness, the number of low echogenic pixels (LEP) decreased in the lower dermis, not in the upper part. The LEPs/LEPi ratio also increased significantly after therapy. The decrease of the number of low echogenic pixels in the lower dermis is proportionate with the significant increase of medium and high echogenic pixels that quantify proteic neosynthesis, as well as cytoarchitectural reorganizations of the extracellular matrix.

Our data shows important ultrasonographic changes at cutaneous level after anti-ageing therapy, as visible in Figure 5. Flavonoids have a complex action at the dermal level, interfering with several mechanisms involved in the senescence process. They act at the level of fibrocytes, on specific receptors, turning inactive mature cells into young, metabolically active ones.

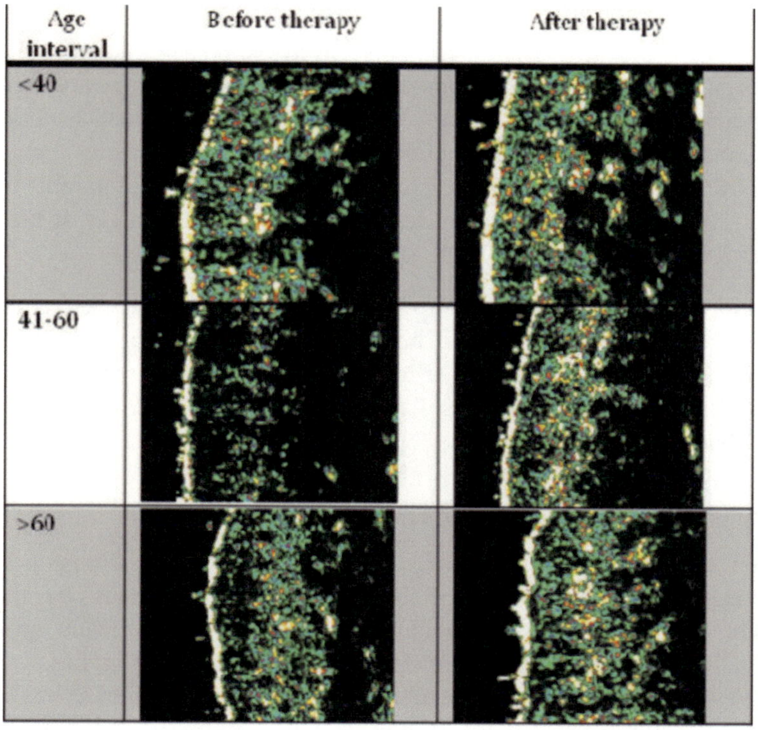

Fig. 5. Ultrasonographic skin aspect before and after topical therapy, on different age intervals

The synthesis of the proteic structures is initiated at intracellular level. The trophocollagen molecules, ellastin, the glicosaminoglycans are extracellularly assembled into microfibrills, fibers or proteoglycans. Depending on the biochemical structure, the level of organisation, architectural orientation and quantity, the proteins show a certain cutaneous echogenity degree. The low echogenity pixels that quantify the hydration degree of the extracellular matrix especially in the lower dermis are replaced by medium and high echogenity pixels, quantifying proteic synthesis. We can consider that MEP codify elastic and collagen precursors that are to be assembled into mature connective tissue fibers, codified by HEP.

The increase of the LEPs/LEPi ratio quantifies the replacement of the hypoechogenic pixels from the lower dermis with medium and high echogenic pixels as a result of protein neosynthesis. Type I collagen, that is prominant at the dermal level (punctiform hyperechogenic pixels) is organised in fibers, visible as hyperechogenic bands, having a parallel display in the lower dermis. These hyperechogenic bands, visible especially on photoprotected sites represent an ultrasonographic marker of the intrinsic aging process.

If we consider the significant changes of the ultrasonographic parameters after anti-ageing therapy depending on the phototype of the subject, a significant increase of the LEPs/LEPi ratio is present in the subjects in phototype II class, but not class III. This observation would justify the correlation of the anti-ageing therapy with the cutaneous phototype. Further studies are necessary to confirm the different reactivity of the phototype classes to local therapies.

Flavonoids, through complex mechanisms, interfere with the reactions involved in the senescence process, and induce the synthesis of the extracellular matrix. According to our data, Viniferol-based products are more efficient in the 40-60 age interval, characterized by complex biological changes at cutaneous level. Viniferol shows real and important anti-ageing properties, since it interferes concomitantly with the genetic, oxidative, immunologic, metabolic mechanisms that are involved in the cutaneous aging process. The prophylaxis of the ageing process should start before the age of 40, preferable in the "critical age interval" (20-40 years), that is characterized by important changes at tissular, cellular and molecular levels, (Crisan et al, 2010)

The optimization of the anti-ageing therapy, according to special studies requires targeted, personalized therapies, adapted to the hormonal, genetic, oxidative, immunologic and metabolic status of the subject, capable of interfering with deficient mechanisms on certain age intervals. Viniferol-based products have a higher efficacy in phototype II subjects compared to phototype III ones.

2.2.2 Efficacy of INTERACTIVE PEEL P63 as anti-ageing therapy

Interactive P63 is a metabolical dynamiser, capable of interacting simultaneously at different cutaneous levels, both on anabolic and catabolic mechanisms. It contains 8 active principles, among which: alfahidroxiacids, retinoids, a complex derived from growth factors, gluconolactone incapsulated in liposomes etc. This anti-ageing complex has a simulataneous action on three levels, epidermis, dermis and dermoepidermic junction. It has been tested in vitro on human fibroblasts cell cultures (Line Hs27) for cytotoxicity, apoptosis, proliferation index, collagen synthesys, matrix metaloproteinases activity.

This study included fifty female subjects aged 40-75, who addressed themselves to the practice for anti-ageing therapy. The subjects were divided into 2 groups of 30 and 20 patients. From the study group (30 subjects), 16 subjects belonged to Phototype class II, 14 subjects to phototype class III, wheareas from the placebo goup, 10 subjects were phototype II and the rest of 10 phototype III. The subjects were divided into 3 age categories: 40-50, 51-60, >60. The subjects from the study group underwent topical therapy with Interactive P63 product, whereas the rest of 20 subjects from the control group used a placebo product. The subjects taken into the study followed the proposed antiaging therapy for 12 weeks, according to a standard protocol. The Interactive P63 and placebo product were applied twice a week for 30 minutes at facial level for 12 weeks. During this period, no other treatments apart from moisturising cream were applied. For every subject, ultrasonographic images were taken from zygomatic area, initially and after 12 weeks of treatment. The data we obtained was analyzed, calculating the mean and standard deviation for all quantitative variables. The difference of means before and after treatment was tested using T test for paired samples. A p-value <0.05 was considered significant.

All subjects involved in the study tollerated well the therapy, without evoking adverse effects (erithema, pruritus, ocular disturbance) after 30 minutes of contact. In the Interactive P63 group, after therapy, an increase of the mean thickness of the epidermis (0.117 ± 0.021 mm vs 0.135 ± 0.023 mm, p=0.0024), and of the dermis (1.537 ± 0.23 mm vs 1.710 ± 0.244 mm, p=0.0076) was observed. At dermal level, the number of low echogenity pixels decreased in a significant manner after topical therapy (18484.4 ± 4666.5 mm vs. 14138.97 ± 3779.5 mm, p=0.00021) whereas the number of the medium (3118.63 ± 974.4 mm vs. 4608.93 ± 1105.6 mm, p=0.001) and high echogenic pixels (379.6 ± 274.17 mm vs. 1004.9 ± 458.78 mm, p<0.0001) increased significantly as displayed in Figure 6.

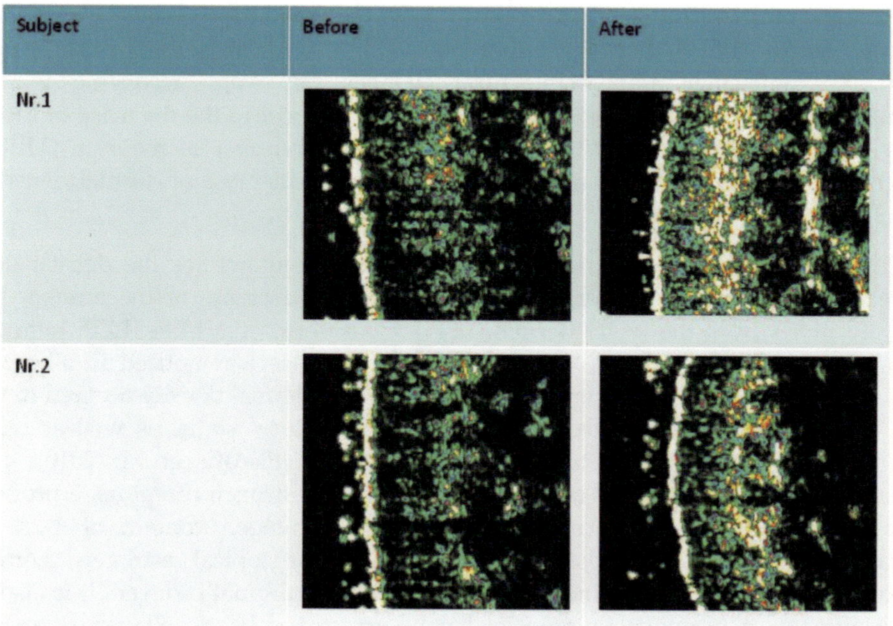

Fig. 6. Ultrasonographic evaluation of the zygomatic area, before and after topical P63 therapy

The LEPs/LEPi ratio increased significantly after therapy (1.149 ± 0.251 mm vs 1.574 ± 0.317 mm) especially due to the significant decrease of the number of low echogenic pixels (LEPi) in the lower dermis (8740.4±2711.01 vs 4921±2373.6, p=0.016).

If we consider the variation of the ultrasonographic parameters after topical therapy according to the phototype class of the subjects, it can be noticed in Figure 7 that after therapy, there is a significant increase of the LEPs/LEPi ratio in the subjects belonging to phototype class III, not II.

Considering the LEPs/LEPi parameter, we noticed a significant increase of the ratio in all subjects part of the study, especially in the 51-60 age interval (40-50 age interval: p=0.01, 51-60 age interval: p=0.0009, >60 age interval: p=0.02) as visible in Figure 8:

In the placebo group, we noticed a slight increase of the dermis (1.496 ± 0.14 mm vs. 1.571 ± 0.174, p=0.07) and of the dermal low echogenic pixels (13812 ± 2070 vs. 14787 ±2218 , p=0.08) due to an optimal hydration of the skin and a discret tendency of the high echogenity pixels to decrease (379,8 ± 137.18 vs 316.3 ±163.43, p=0.11). The LEPs/LEPi ratio showed no particular display according to the age or phototype of the subjects

INTERACTIVE P63 complex interacts concomitantly different mechanisms involved in the cutaneous aging process, conferring from imagistical point of view, a characteristic display of the pixels at cutaneous level. (Rouabhia et al, 2002) The increase of the epidermal/dermal thickness represents the morphological exppression of the changes induced by INTERACTIVE P63 complex at fibroblastic and extracellular matrix level. The activation of the fibroblasts as well as the inductive effect upon stem cells, associated with the inhibition of the mechanisms responsible for the distruction of the fibrillary structures, induce an increase of the dermal density. Thus, we noticed a general, significant decrease of the mean number of low echogenic pixels (LEP) at dermal level, more pronounced in the lower dermis (LEPi) than the upper one (LEPs), suggesting important structural, biochemical, mollecular and architectural changes that vary according to certain particular properties of the upper and lower dermis. Parallel to the decrease of LEP after therapy, a statistically significant increase of the mean number of medium (MEP) and high ecogenic pixels (HEP) was noticed, quantifying the increase of dermal density and thus, collagen neosynthesis.

The LEPs/ LEPi ratio, an essential imagistic marker that quantifies the dermal density, increased in a significant manner, due to the important decrease of the number of low echogenity pixels from the lower dermis (LEPi). Considering the LEPs/LEPi ratio on the three age categories: 40-50,51-60, >60 , a significant increase was noticed in all three age intervals. The fact that the most significant increase of the dermal density occured in **the 51-60 age** interval, may be correlated with the post-menopausal status as well as with the estrogen-like activity of INTERACTIVE P63 complex (El-Alfy et al, 2010). During menopause, due to a decrease of estrogen and cutaneous estrogen receptors, a progressive decrease of dermal collagen occurs, with a loss of collagen content of 1-2% every menopausal year. Several studies certify the fact that topical estrogen therapy in menopausal women induces an increase of almost 5.1% of dermal collagen. It is also a fact that the efficacy of hormone therapy is dependant on the basal collagen status at the beginning of the therapy. The initiation of a precoucious therapy in menopause has a prophylactic role, while a delayed therapy has a therapeutic purpose.

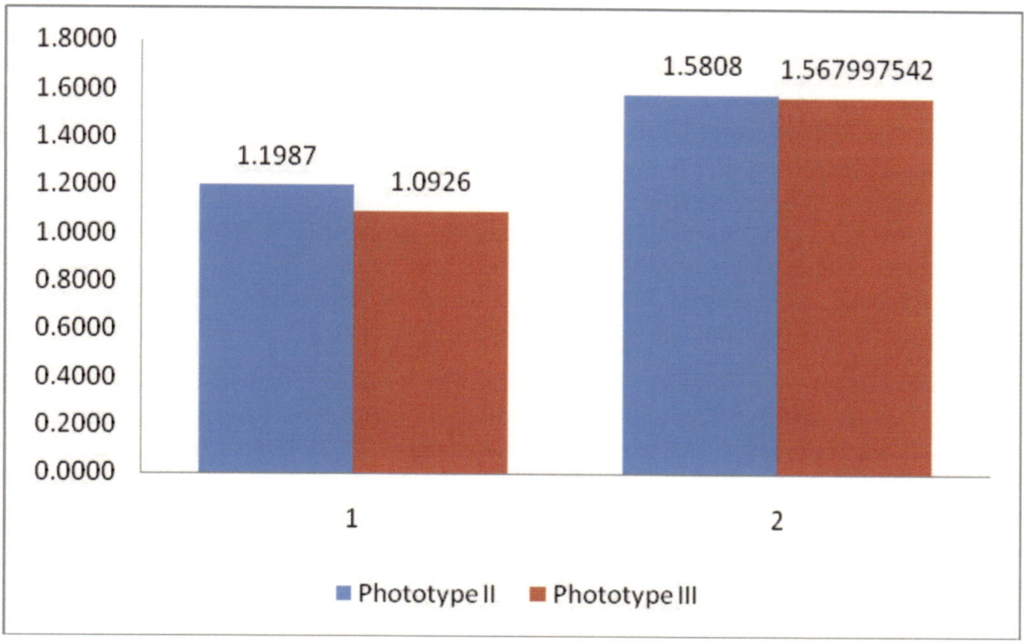

Fig. 7. Variation of the LEPs/LEPi ratio before and after topical therapy, according to phototype.

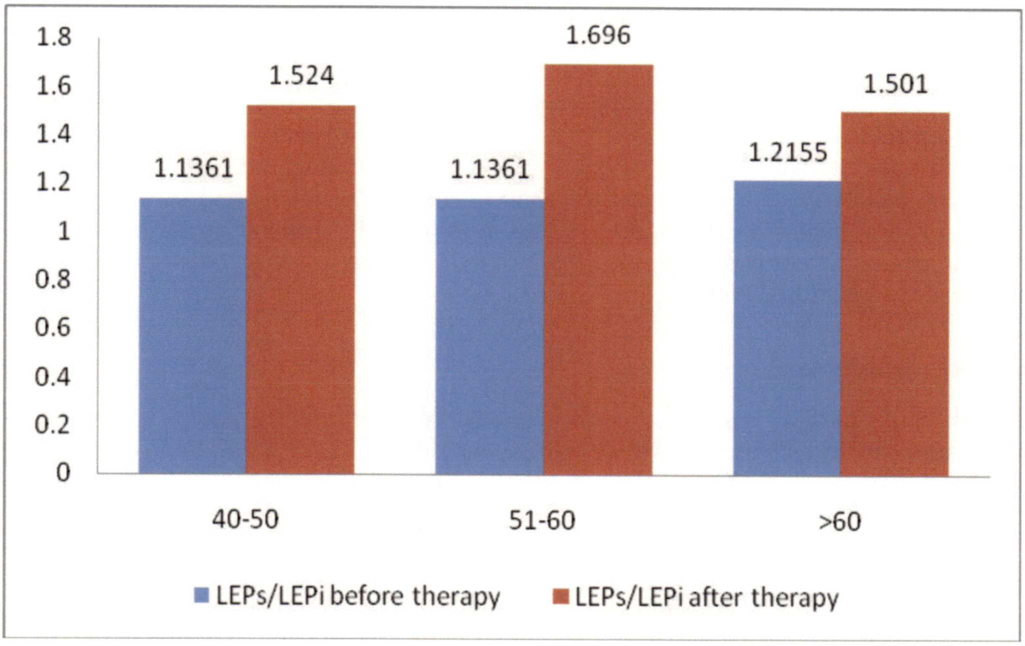

Fig. 8. The variation of the mean of the LEPs/LEPi ratio on different age interval before and after therapy

INTERACTIVE P63 complex acts at cellular level, interffering the cutaneous estrogenic receptors (α and β) that, even though with structural and functional similarities, have different expression conditions and act differently in menopause, explaining the changes regarding dermal density on age categories. Regarding the phototype of the subjects, a certain, particular reactivity is to be mentioned: a more significant growth of the dermal density in subjects belonging to phototype class III, compared to phototype class II. The LEPs/LEPi ratio showed no significant variation neither with the age or the phototype of the subjects. Interactive P 63 product acts on specific sensitive receptors may interfere with estrogen-like receptors, activating the fibroblast "key cell" and increases the synthesis of collagen. It has real and important anti-ageing properties on large age intervals, since it interferes concomitantly the oxidative, genetic, immunologic, hormonal and metabolic mechanisms. It is highly efficient especially in the 51-60 age interval and in phototype III patients.

In the past years, many advances in the diagnosis of skin ageing have become available for an earlier and more specific diagnosis. Our studies show the importance of high-frequency ultrasound as a noninvasive method for the assessment of the cutaneous senescence process. The correlations between the histological and imagistic parameters allow the establishment of noninvasive diagnosis and treatment protocols. Our observations require further development and review to determine the diagnostic accuracy. Some show great promise in assessing, with less invasive methodes, histological features required for an earlier diagnosis, or for establishing the efficacy of various therapies. The need to develop new strategies on how to prevent and how to accommodate the ageing society requires the elaboration of mathematical models in order to predict the evolution of the ageing phenomenon. (Crisan et al, 2010) The anti-ageing medicine may discover there is no limit to human life span.

3. Conclusions

High-frequency ultrasound is a non-invasive histological tool that allows the visualisation of "in vivo" histological sections, offering information with microscopical correspondence and also characteristic ultrasonographic markers. The efficacy of anti-ageing therapies varies with the age interval, according both to the applied product but also the cutaneous reactivity, phototype, hormonal and metabolical status. The prevention of the cutaneous ageing process should begin in the "critical age interval" and the improvement of the clinical aspect requires precocious, personalized therapies, using efficient substances, previously tested on cell-cultures.

4. Acknowledgment

Special thanks to all of my colleagues who contributed with usefull advice and pertinent observations to the elaboration of this chapter. I would also like to thank Cortex Technology for allowing us to use the Dermascan equipment, whitout which our study would not have been possible. This study is part of CNCSIS national research grant nr. 2624.

5. References

Badea R, Crişan M, Lupşor M, Fodor L.(2010). Diagnosis and characterization of cutaneous tumors using combined ultrasonographic procedures (conventional and high resolution ultrasonography). *Med Ultrason*. (4):317-22.

Bos DC, de Ranitz-Greven WL, de Valk HW. (2011) Advanced glycation end products, measured as skin autofluorescence and diabetes complications: a systematic review.*Diabetes Technol Ther.* Jul;13(7):773-9.

Crisan M, Cattani C, Badea R, Mitrea P et al. (2010) Modelling Cutaneous Senescence Process. *Lecture Notes in Computer Science,* (6017): 215-224

Crisan M, Cattani C, Badea R, Cosgarea R, Dudea S, Mitrea P, Lupsor M. (2009). Complex histological, genetical, ultrasonography and clinical studies in early noninvasive diagnosis of the photoinduced cutaneous senescence and in the photoinduced skin cancers, using computerized imaging, modern biotechnology and mathematical modelling methods." *Automatic computers applied mathematics,* vol.18.No.2, pg. 231-255 Scientific Journal ISSN 1221- 437X MEDIAMIRA SCIENCE PUBLISHER - ACAM CNCSIS - B +

Crisan M. (2007) Histology of the integumentary system with practical aplications. *Casa Cartii de Stiinta.* ISBN 973-686-935-0

El-Alfy, M., Deloche, C., Azzi, L., Bernard, B., Bernerd, F., Coutet, J., Chaussade, V., Martel, C., Leclaire, J. and Labrie, F. (2010). Skin responses to topical dehydroepiandrosterone: implications in antiageing treatment.. *British Journal of Dermatology,* 163: 968–976.

Han J, Quresh AA, Prescott J et al.(2009). Prospective study of telomere length and the risk of skin cancer. *J Invest Dermatol,* 129, 415-421

Jasaitiene D, Valiukeviciene S, Linkeviciute G, Raisutis R, Jasiuniene E, Kazys R. (2011) Principles of high-frequency ultrasonography for investigation of skin pathology.*J Eur Acad Dermatol Venereol;* 25(4): 375-382.

Kohl, E., Steinbauer, J., Landthaler, M. and Szeimies, R.-M. (2011), Skin ageing. *Journal of the European Academy of Dermatology and Venereology,* 25: no. doi: 10.1111/j.1468-3083.2010.03963.x

Lacarrubba F, Tedeschi A, Nardone B, Micali G. (2008) Mesotherapy for skin rejuvenation: assessment of the subepidermal low-echogenic band by ultrasound evaluation with cross-sectional B-mode scanning.. *Dermatol Ther. Suppl* 3:S1-5.

Pageon H. 2010. Reaction of glycation and human skin: the effects on the skin and its components, reconstructed skin as a model. (2009) *Pathol Biol (Paris).* Jun;58(3):226-31. Epub . Review.

Rouabhia and al. (2002). G factor P63 increases P63 protein and activates the differentiation of stem cells. (2009) *Arch Dermatol Res* ; 301(4):301-6.

Schmid-Wendtner MH, Burgdorf W (2005). Ultrasound scanning in dermatology. *Arch Dermatol.* Feb; 141(2):217-24.

Shi Y, Buffenstein R, Pulliam DA, Van Remmen H. (2010). Comparative studies of oxidative stress and mitochondrial function in aging. *Integr Comp Biol.* (5):869-79. Epub 2010 Jul2.

Uitto J. The role of elastin and collagen in cutaneous aging: intrinsic aging versus photoexposure. (2008). *J Drugs Dermatol.* (2 Suppl):s12-6

Vaupel JW. (2010). Biodemography of human ageing *Nature;* 464: 536-542.

Vranesić-Bender D. (2010) The role of nutraceuticals in anti-aging medicine. .*Acta Clin Croat.*;49(4):537-44.

Wortsman X, Wortsman J. (2010) Clinical usefulness of variable-frequency ultrasound in localized lesions of the skin. *J Am Acad Dermatol*; 62(2): 247-256.

34

The Level of ROS and DNA Damage Mediate with the Type of Cell Death, Senescence or Apoptosis

Takafumi Inoue and Norio Wake
Department of Obstetrics and Gynecology, Kyushu University, Fukuoka, Japan

1. Introduction

Cell senescence, originally defined as the proliferative arrest that occurs in normal cells after a limited number of cell divisions, is now more broadly regarded as a general biological program of terminal growth arrest. Replicative senescence of cells due to telomeric changes exhibits similar features with those seen in DNA damage (Vaziri et al., 1997; von Zglinicki, 2001). Therefore, DNA damage is expected to induce rapid cell growth arrest, which would be phenotypically indistinguishable from replicative senescence (Di Leonardo et al., 1994). This type of accelerated senescence that does not involve telomere shortening is triggered in normal cells by the expression of supraphysiological mitogenic signals (Orr et al., 1994). Not only normal cells, but also cancer cells can be induced readily to undergo senescence by genetic manipulation or by treatment with chemotherapeutic agents, radiation, or differentiating agents.

Reactive oxygen species (ROS), which are byproducts of normal cellular oxidative processes, are involved in senescence (Chen et al., 1998). Senescent cells have higher levels of ROS than normal cells (Hagen et al., 1997), and oxidative stress caused by sublethal doses of H_2O_2 or hyperoxia can force human fibroblasts to arrest in a manner similar to senescence (Dumount et al., 2000). Additionally, both oncogenic Ras and p53 induce senescence in association with increased intracellular ROS (Lee et al., 1999; Macip et al., 2003). p53 induces the accumulation of ROS presumably through a transcriptional influence on pro-oxidant genes (Polyak et al., 1997). Up-regulation of p21 also causes increased ROS levels in both normal and cancer cells (Macip et al., 2002), although the molecular mechanism remains unknown.

Recent evidence has suggested that p21 mediates apoptosis in a p53-independent manner (Roninson, 2003; Hsu et al., 1999), although its role in this apoptotic pathway remains controversial. In view of the possible roles played by ROS in both senescence and apoptosis, and the capacity of p21 to elevate ROS levels, we investigated the involvement of ROS in p21-induced cell death. Additionally, we studied how the status of p21 expression modulated ROS levels to achieve alternative cell fates.

2. Exogenous p21 protein induces senescence and apoptosis induced by p21 mediated through p53

We generated the recombinant adenovirus vector contained either the full-length p21 (Ad-p21). An adenovirus containing an empty vector (mock) was used as a control. We transferred these constructs into two cancer cell lines (LoVo, and HCT116) using an adenovirus infection system. The cell lines were initially selected based on their susceptibility (>80%) to adenovirus. The expression of p21 protein corresponding to the transfected vector was demonstrated by immunoblots (data not shown).

Infection of these cancer cell lines with 20MOI Ad-p21 resulted in growth arrest, which became irreversible after four days. This permanent growth arrest was accompanied by the presence of a senescence-specific marker, SA-β-gal positivity, as well as morphological changes such as a dramatic increase in cell size, and enlarged and prominent nuclei.

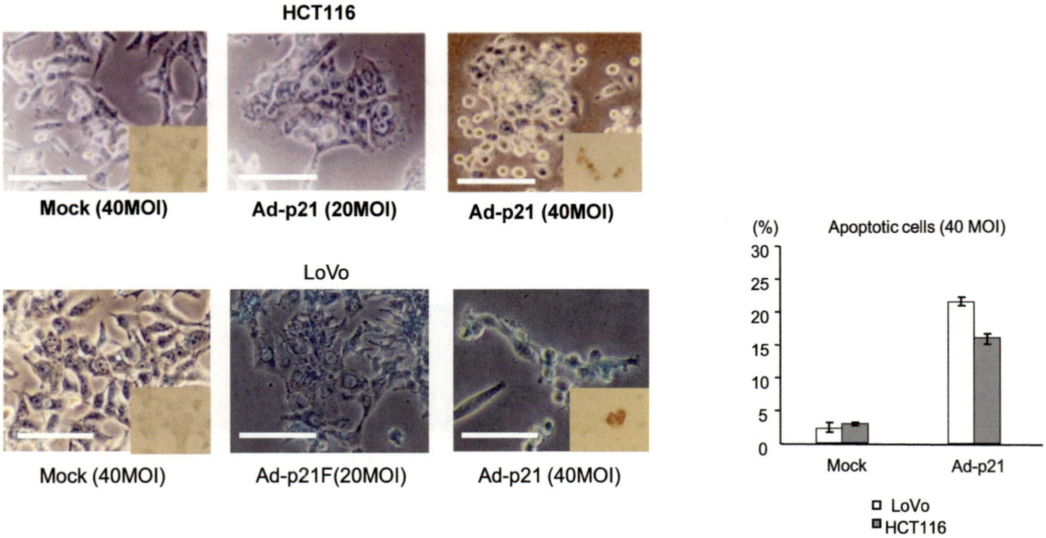

Fig. 1. Induction of senescence and apoptosis by p21 overexpression.
When LoVo and HCT116 cells were transfected with 20 MOI Ad-p21, cells were enlarged, flattened and had increased SA-β-gal positivity. At 40 MOI (LoVo and HCT116), cells were detached from the plate and floating. The small panel on the lower right for 40 MOI shows positive cells with the TUNEL assay. Mock transfected cells showed no change in morphology and were not positive for the TUNEL assays. The populations of apoptotic cells in LoVo and HCT116 infected with 40 MOI Ad-p21 after infection of 48 hrs are shown in right graph as indicated by the significant increased of sub G1 fraction. Data represent the average of three independent experiments and standards deviations are indicated by error bars. Bar=10μm

The apoptosis of cancer cells following DNA damage is p53-dependent and yet p21-independent (Waldman et al., 1996; Deng et al., 1995). However, due to differences in the experimental conditions for investigation the effects, contradictory conclusions have been drawn regarding the relationship between p21 and the induction of apoptosis (Tsao et al., 1999; Kagawa et al., 1999). In order to investigate the basis for the striking differences in the biologic responses to p21 expression, we measured the kinetics of p21 protein increase, as well as its expression levels following Ad-p21 infection by increasing MOI of the viral vector. Whereas 20 MOI Ad-p21 infection resulted in elongated, growth-arrested cells showing the morphological features of senescence, cells infected with 40 MOI Ad-p21 became rounded, contracted, and lost their ability to adhere to the plate with Apo-taq positive staining (Fig. 1). We used flow cytometry to measure the DNA contents of cancer cell lines following treatment Ad-p21. In LoVo and HCT116 cells, a hypoploid peak corresponding to a subG1 population had increased following infection with Ad-p21 (40 MOI) (data not shown). These results are characteristic of apoptosis.

3. The fate of cancer cells as a result of ROS generated by overexpressed p21 from adenoviral transfection

To investigate the roles of ROS in the senescent or apoptotic cell fates triggered by p21 expression in LoVo and HCT116 cells, we measured ROS levels with the fluorescent probe APF (Setsukinai et al., 2003), a marker of changes in the general accumulation of cellular oxidants. FACS analysis of APF-stained LoVo and HCT116 cells revealed a progressive increase in ROS levels following 20 MOI Ad-p21 infection. After three days of infection, when senescent morphological changes were first observed, the ROS levels in the cells were increased more than 2-fold. We next examined whether ROS levels were involved in the decision between senescence and apoptosis in LoVo and HTC116 cells. Both cells infected with 40 MOI Ad-p21 exhibited much higher ROS levels (4-fold) than did the cells infected with 20 MOI Ad-p21 (2-2.5 fold) (Fig. 2a).

We then established whether different cell fate outcomes were due to the levels of induced ROS and p21 protein. We investigated whether the antioxidant N-acetyl-L-cysteine (NAC), could protect cells from senescent phenotypes induced by 20 MOI Ad-p21 infection or the apoptotic phenotype by 40 MOI Ad-p21 infection. Both LoVo and HCT116 cells that harbored the wild type p53 gene were infected with 20MOI Ad-p21 were cultured in the presence of 10mM NAC for three days. Ad-p21 markedly induced SA-β-gal positive cells in the absence of NAC, and cultivation in the presence of NAC significantly suppressed the appearance of SA-β-gal-positive cells (Fig. 2b). Similarly, cultivation of LoVo and HCT116 cells in the presence of NAC for 3 days markedly inhibited apoptosis in response to 40 MOI Ad-p21 infection (Fig. 2c), thus suggesting that the induction of both senescence and apoptosis by p21 occurs via the generation of ROS.

4. Endogenous p21 protein up-regulation by sodium butyrate (NaB) induces cell death in a colon cancer cell line, HCT116

Next, we investigated whether up-regulation of endogenous p21 protein has an effect similar to that of Ad-p21 infection. We have previously demonstrated that NaB induced p21 expression, resulting in growth arrest and cell death in gynecologic cancer cells. [8]

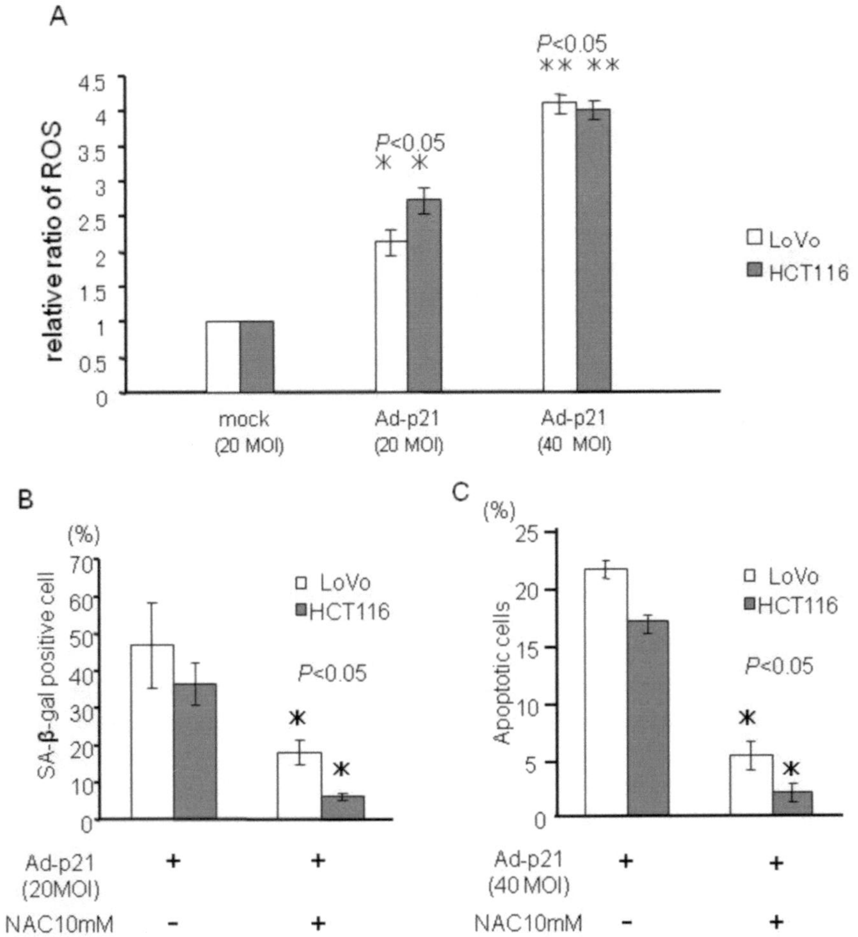

Fig. 2. ROS levels in cancer cell lines in response to p21 expression levels.

(a) ROS levels were evaluated by FACS analysis after staining LoVo and HCT116 cells with the fluorescent probe APF. Relative ratio of the geometric mean that is the average of the logarithm of the linear value for events expressed as the anti log in Ad-p21 (20 MOI or 40 MOI) infected cells as compared to the control (20MOI). Generated ROS levels were significantly higher in the cancer cells infected with 20 MOI Ad-p21 than those in control infected cells. *$P < 0.05$ In LoVo and HCT116 cells, generated ROS levels were significantly higher in the cancer cells infected with 40 MOI Ad-p21 than those in 20 MOI. **$P < 0.05$ Apoptosis was induced in the former and senescence in the latter.

(b) Senescence induced by p21-overexpression was inhibited by NAC (ROS scavenger). LoVo and HCT116 cells were cultured in 10 mM NAC and were infected with 20 MOI Ad-p21. The ratio of SA-β-gal positive cells after 74 hrs of the infection was significantly decreased in the presence of NAC. Results represent mean values of three experiments, and error bar shows the standard deviation.

(c) Induction of apoptosis with 40 MOI Ad-p21 was also inhibited by the addition of NAC in LoVo and HCT116 cells, as indicated by the significant decrease of sub G1 fraction. Results represent mean values of three experiments, and error bars shows the standard deviation.

To evaluate the induction of senescence in HCT116 cells, we analyzed the cell cycle alteration and SA-β gal staining in response to NaB. We measured the DNA contents of cancer cell lines treated with varying concentrations of NaB by flow cytometry. In HCT116, treatment with 0.5 to 1.0 mM NaB resulted in a decrease in the fraction of S phase (21%→4%) and G1 phase cells (57%→22%). Most cells accumulated in G2/M, suggesting arrest at the G2/M checkpoint. A hypoploid peak corresponding to the subG1 population was evident by flow cytometry following treatment with greater than 2.0mM NaB (Fig. 3a). This population corresponded to cells undergoing apoptotic cell death.

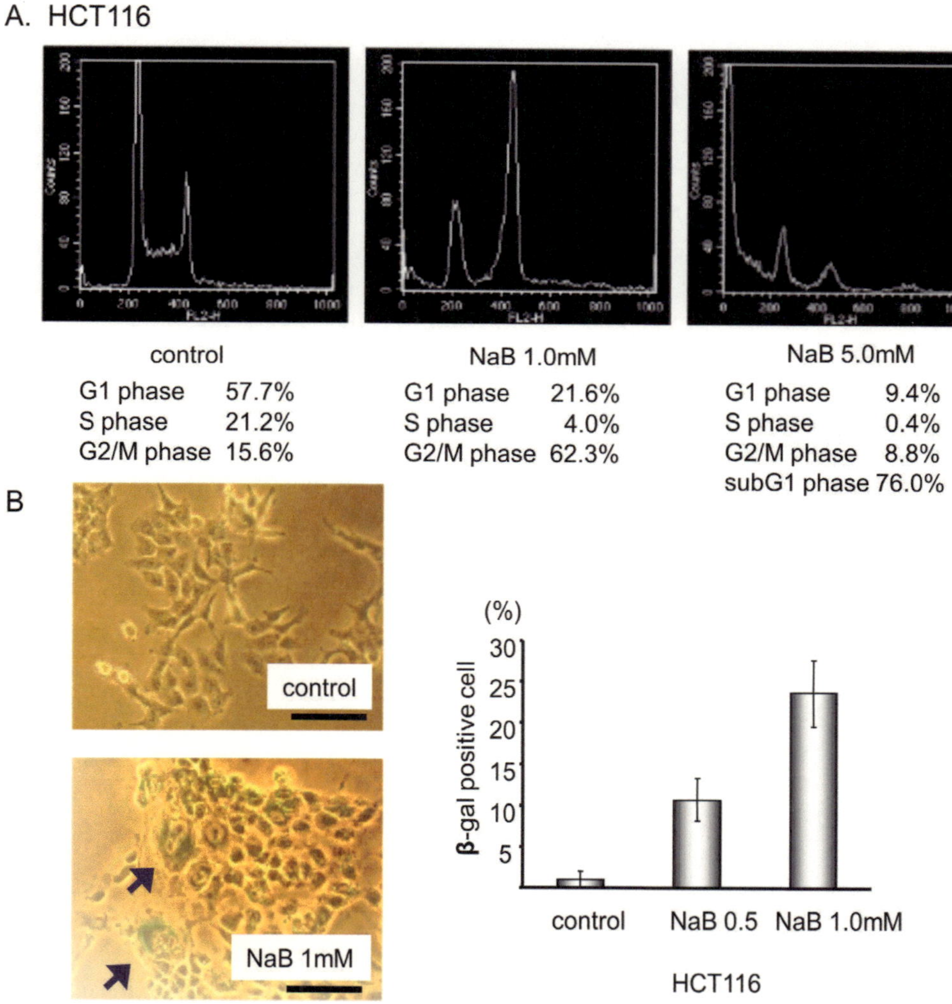

Fig. 3. (a) Effect of NaB on cell cycle analysis and the induction of cell death. DNA contents of HeLa and HCT116 cells with or without NaB for 24 hrs were analyzed by flow cytometry. NaB treatment reduced the percentage of cells in S phase and triggered the accumulation of cells in G2/M phase in HCT116 treated with of 1.0 mM NaB.
(b) Treatment with 1.0 mM NaB induced morphological change in HCT116 cells that included enlargement and flattening as well as an increase in the number of SA-β-gal positive cells (arrows). Bar=10μm

Incubation of HCT116 cells with 1.0 mM NaB for five days resulted in morphologic changes. These changes included an enlarged, flattened shape, increased cytoplasmic to nuclear ratio and decreased cell density accompanied by SA-β-gal staining (Fig. 3b).

5. Increased ROS levels in NaB-induced senescence and apoptosis of cancer cells

To investigate the contribution of ROS to senescence or apoptosis of HCT116 cells triggered by the treatment with different concentrations of NaB, we measured ROS levels as described above. FACS analysis of APF-stained cancer cell lines revealed a progressive increase in ROS levels following NaB treatment. The levels of ROS were increased following treatment both with 1 mM of NaB (2-3 fold) that induced senescence in HCT116 cells and with 5 mM of NaB (5-fold) that induced apoptosis compared with no treatment in HCT116 cells (Fig. 4a). The ROS level in apoptotic cells induced by NaB was markedly higher than that in senescent cells.

To further establish whether different cell fate outcomes were due to the induced ROS level, we investigated the effect of the antioxidant N-acetyl-L-cysteine (NAC) on the senescent phenotype. HCT116 cells were treated with 0.5 mM NaB in the presence or absence of 5mM NAC for 5 days. The increase of cell numbers in the G2/M fraction following treatment with 0.5 mM NaB was abrogated by co-treatment with 5mM NAC (Fig. 4b). As shown in Fig. 4c, culture in the presence of NAC significantly suppressed the number of SA-β-gal-positive HCT116 cells (23%→10%). This was accompanied by a decrease in ROS level, which suggested that the induction of senescence by NaB occurred via the generation of ROS. The treatment with NAC, however, could not prevent the apoptotic induction by higher concentrations of NaB in and HCT116 cells (data not shown), though the reason remained unknown.

6. DNA damage response (DDR) signals mediate NaB-induced cancer cell death

To clarify the association of NaB-induced cancer cell death with the DNA damage response, we next assayed for DDR signals including ATM and its downstream signals. One of the first processes initiated by DSB (double strand break) is massive phosphorylation of the tail of the histone variant H2AX (Redon et al., 2002). Foci of phosphorylated H2AX (γH2AX) are rapidly formed at the DSB sites and are thought to be essential for further recruitment of damage response proteins. γH2AX is dependent on the ATM protein and other members of the ATM family. (31) To examine the effect of NaB on DDR signals-related proteins, we analyzed the changes of DSB-related proteins expression levels in response to NaB by immunoblotting. Incubation with 1-5 mM NaB for 48 hrs resulted in the accumulation of γH2AX and ATM in HCT116 cells. The downstream proteins such as p53, phosphorylated p38 MAPK, and p21 were up-regulated by 1-5mM NaB after 48 hrs of incubation (Fig. 5a). In HCT116 cells, the levels of the DSB marker γH2AX were enhanced about 20 times when apoptosis was induced by incubating with 2 mM NaB and about 3.6 times when senescence was induced by 0.5 to 1.0 mM NaB for 24 hrs compared with the control (Fig. 5b).

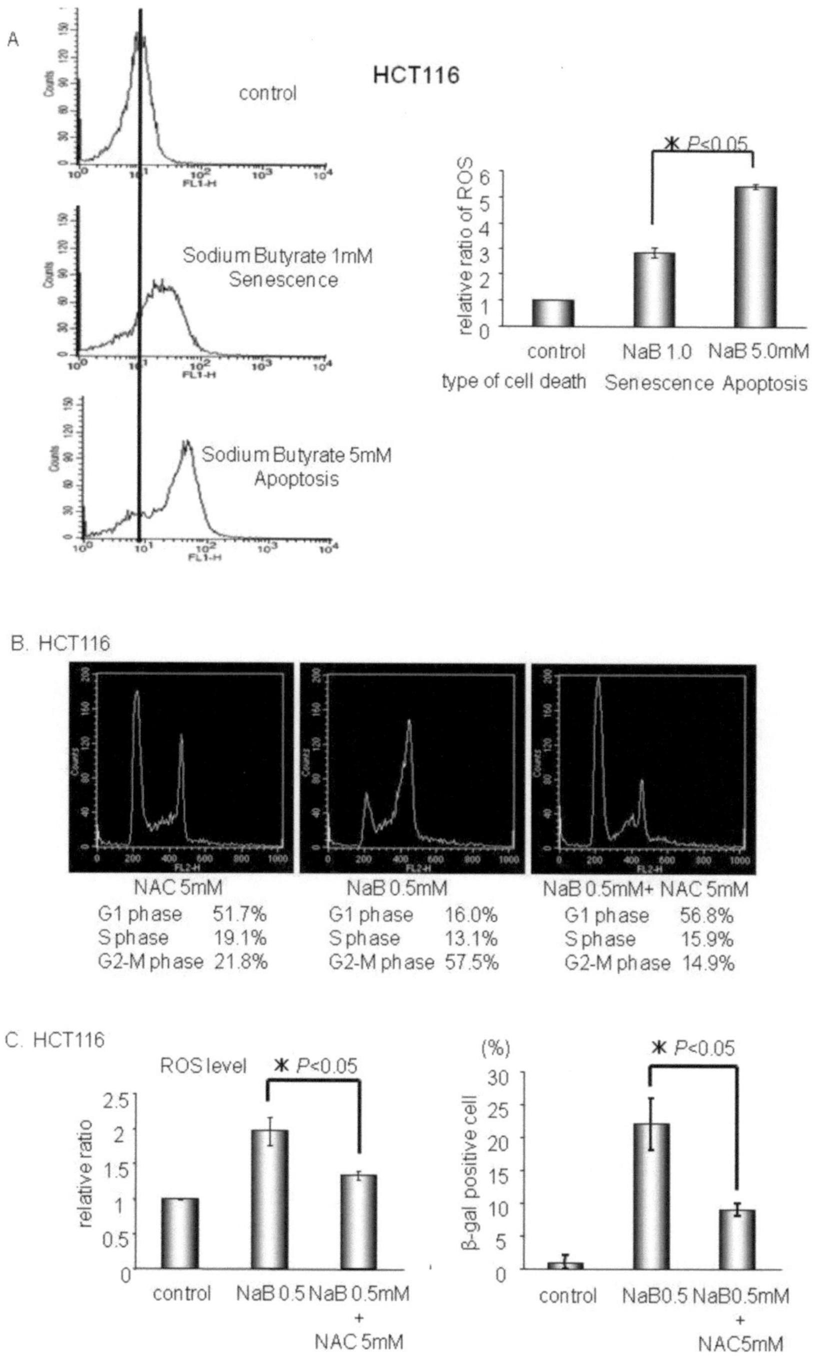

Fig. 4. Enhancement of ROS levels in cancer cell lines in response to NaB.
(a) ROS levels were evaluated by FACS analysis after staining HCT116 cells with the fluorescent probe APF. The ROS levels in apoptotic cells treated with 1.0 mM NaB are significantly higher than those in senescent cells induced by 5.0 mM NaB ($P<0.05$).

Data represent the average of three independent experiments and standards deviations are indicated by error bars.
(b) Treatment of NAC reduced the proportion of cells accumulating in G2/M phase and the ratio of senescent cells following NaB treatment. HCT116 cells were cultured with 0.5 mM NaB in the presence or absence of 0.5 mM NAC for 24 hrs.
(c) ROS level (left graph) and the ratio of senescent cells (right graph) after 96 hrs of treatment significantly decreased in the presence of NAC ($P<0.05$) compared to when NAC was absent. Results represent the mean values of three experiments, and error bars shows the standard deviation.

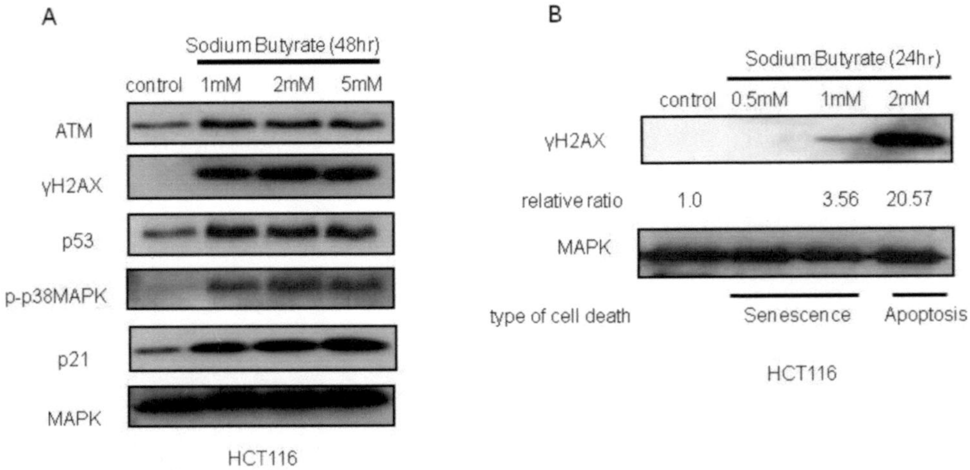

Fig. 5. NaB induced the expression of proteins associated with DSB.
(a) Western blot of ATM, phosphorylated H2AX (γH2AX), p53, phosphorylated p38 MAPK, p21 and MAPK after treatment with NaB treatment for 48hrs.
(b) The level of γH2AX protein in cells treated with 2.0 mM NaB for 24 hrs, was higher than that in cells treated with 1.0 mM NaB, a level which induced senescence. Levels of γH2AX associated with the type determination of cell death.

7. Conclusion

In this study, we obtained the following evidence. Exogenous and endogenous p21 up-regulation (Ad-p21 infection and NaB treatment) are able to induce senescence or apoptosis in cancer cell lines. The magnitude of ROS induced by p21 was critical for the p21-mediated cell fate decision. These findings help account for the differences in the p21-mediated cell fate decisions observed in various studies.

8. References

Chen QM, Bartholomew JC, Campisi J, Acosta M, Reagan JD, and Ames BN. Molecular analysis of H2O2-induced senescent-like growth arrest in normal human fibroblasts: p53 and Rb control G1 arrest but not cell replication. *Biochem J* 1998; 332: 43-50

Di Leonardo A, Linke SP, Clarkin K, and Wahl GM. DNA damage triggers a prolonged p53-dependent G1 arrest and long-term induction of Cip1 in normal fibroblasts. *Genes Dev* 1994; 8: 2540-51

Dumont P. Burton M, Chen QM, Gonos ES, Frippiat C, Mazarati J, Eliaers F, Remacle J, and Toussaint O. Induction of replicative senescence biomarkers by sublethal oxidative stress in normal human fibroblast. *Free Radical Biol Med* 2000; 28: 361-73

Deng C, Zhang P, Harper JW, Elledge SJ, and Leder P. Mice lacking p21CIP1/WAF1 undergoes normal development, but is defective in G1 checkpoint control. *Cell* 1995; 82: 675-84

Hsu SL, Chen MC, Chou YH, Hwang GY, and Yin SC. Induction of p21(CIP1/Waf1) and activation of p34(cdc2) involved in retinoic acid-induced apoptosis in human hepatoma Hep3B cells. *Exp Cell Res* 1999; 248: 87-96

Hagen TM, Yowe DL, Bartholomew JC, Wehr CM, Do KL, Park JY, and Ames BN. Mitochondria decay in hepatocytes from old rats: membrane potential declines, heterogeneity and oxidants increase. *Proc Natl Acad Sci U S A* 1997; 94: 3064-69

Kagawa S, Fujiwara T, Kadowaki Y, Fukazawa T, Sok-Joo R, Jack A, Roth JA, and Tanaka N. Overexpression of the $p21^{sdi1}$ gene induces senescence-like state in human cancer cells: implication for senescence-directed molecular therapy for cancer. *Cell Death and Differentiation* 1999; 6: 765-772

Lee AC, Fenster BE, Ito H, Takeda K, Bae NS, Hirai T, Yu ZX, Ferrans VJ, Howard BH, and Finkel T. Ras protein induce senescence by altering the intracellular levels of reactive oxygen spiecies. *J Biol Chem* 1999; 274: 7936-40

Macip S, Igarshi M, Berggren P, Yu J, Lee SW, and Aaroson SA. Influence of induced reactive oxygen species in p53-mediated cell gate decisions. *Mol Cell Biol* 2003; 23: 8576-85

Macip S, Igarshi M, Fang L, Chen A, Pan ZO, Lee SW, and Aaroson S. Inhibirion of p21-mediated ROS accumulation can rescue p21-induced senescence. *EMBO J* 2002; 21: 2180-88

Orr WC, and Sohal RS. Extension of life-span by overexpression of superoxide dismutase and catalase in Drosophila melanogaster. *Science* 1994; 263: 1128-30

Polyak K, Xia Y, Zweier JL, Kinzler KW, and Vogelstein B. A model for p53-induced apoptosis. *Nature* 1997; 389: 300-305

Roninson I. Tumor Cell Senescence in Cancer Treatment. Cancer Research 2003;63:2705-15

Redon C, Pilch D, Rogakou E, Sedelnikova O, Newrock K, Bonner W. Histone H2A variants H2AX and H2AZ. *Curr Opin Genet Dev* 2002; 12: 162-9

Setsukinai K, Urano Y, Kakinuma K, Majima HJ, Nagano T. Development of novel fluorescence probes that can reliably detect reactive oxygen species and distinguish specific species. *J Biol Chem* 2003; 278: 3170-75

Tsao Y, Huang S, Chang J, Hsieh J, Pong R, and Chen S. Adenovirus-mediated $p21^{(WAF1/SDII/CIP1)}$ gene transfer induces apoptosis of human cervical cancer cell lines. *Journal of Virology* 1999; 6: 4849-90

Vaziri H, West MD, Allsopp RC, Davison TS, Wu YS, Arrowsmith CH, Poirier GG., and Benchimol S. ATM-depenent telomere loss in aging human diploid fibroblasts and DNA damage lead to the posttranslational activation of p53 protein involving poly (ADP-ribose) polymerase. *EMBO J* 1997; 16: 6018-33 von Zglinicki, T. Telomeres and replicative senescence: Is it only length that counts? *Cancer Lett* 2001; 168: 111-6

Waldman T, Lengauer C, Kinzlar KW, and Vogelstein B. Uncoupling of S phase and mitosis induced by anticancer agent in cells lacking p21. Nature 1996;381:713-6

35

Reviewing the Life Cycle: Women's Lives in the Light of Social Changes

Anna Freixas, Bárbara Luque and Amalia Reina
Department of Psychology, Faculty of Educational Sciences
University of Cordova, Cordova
Spain

1. Introduction

Our chapter involves both a theoretical revision and a set of reflections that aim to analyse and redefine the significance of the final stages of the female life cycle, which has been revolutionised by two major set of circumstances: the increase in life expectation and the social changes that have taken place in the western world during the second half of the 20th century. In this regard, our reflections deal with the consequences that this spectacular prolongation of life has had for women. We also discuss the new significance that living into old age may have for women who will reach old age during the early decades of this century and who are the beneficiaries of the important social changes of the second half of the past century.

These important social changes have facilitated the virtually universal access of women to basic education, and of a very large proportion of women to higher education, as well as the generalisation and utilisation of new information and communication technologies. The incorporation of women into the labour market and the cash economy has altered relationships and the position of women in the world and has enabled them to renegotiate their intimate relationships, their sexuality and rates of birth-giving, and thus to modify to a great extent their future lives as elderly women during the first half of the 21th century.

2. Feminist critical gerontology

Our theoretical framework is based on critical gerontology, which analyses the extent to which political and socioeconomic factors interact to shape the experience of ageing, and treats age, gender, ethnic background and social class as variables on which the life course of the individual pivots, insofar as it predetermines their position in the social order. Critical gerontology shows a desire to explore the social construction of ageing within a broad sociopolitical and humanitarian context. The field also studies the disparate ways in which individuals grow old, and the social and political disempowerment than often accompany ageing (Minkler & Holstein, 2008: 196).

Feminist gerontology may be regarded as part of a project of development of those epistemologies which, from the perspective of the social sciences, question dominant perceptions of the lives of certain marginalized segments of the population. Feminist gerontological research attempts to document the experiences of elderly women and to promote new interpretations of female ageing, "asking questions about what 'everyone knows', and to examine ideas, positions, theories, and policies from the perspective of the least advantaged" (Minkler & Holstein, 2008: 199).

Critical feminist gerontology has documented the experience of elderly women, encouraging the development of more complete and more complex interpretations of their lives, and has discussed the necessity of studying and understanding their life trajectories in greater detail, revising the lacunae and inconsistencies that a large proportion of current gerontological studies offers, as a victim of the 'ideology of age'. Taking as its point of departure the notion that feminism is "a form of politics which aims to intervene in, and transform, the unequal power relations between men and women" (Hollows, 2001: 3), critical feminist gerontology emerges as a form of study via which we claim to alter the power relationships which, in this case, are mediated via age and gender (Ray, 2006; Freixas, 2008).

3. The new life course

One of the most significant processes of the 20th century has been the gradual ageing of the global population, particularly in the developed world, where life expectation has risen spectacularly. There are two immediate causes of this process in our society; the decline in birth-rates and the increase in life expectancy, which is due to the fall in the death rate at advanced ages. This faces us with a social fact that lacks precedents in human history. We have thus been witnesses to a structural change that has led to *the ageing of old people*, which is to say that the number of nonagerians and centenarians is growing, bringing social, cultural and health-care challenges as well as a duty to study the phenomenon. At this point in time, we can claim that as we approach old age, we still have many 'productive' years ahead of us, time that represents an unprecedented resource in terms of number and potential (Minkler & Holstein, 2008). Today's elderly women were the promoters of one of the most important demographic transformations in history, in that the reduction in their rates of giving birth led to a true demographic transition.

Ageing is not a process that can be viewed solely through the prism of age; it possesses other nuances of great importance, both collective and individual. Growing old for women is not the same as for men, nor does it have the same meaning for members of advanced and developing societies. It is not the same to grow old, having enjoyed a good education, with access to culture and to a health-care system, accompanied by professional activity and emotional and interpersonal relationships, as it is to do so outwith the limits of the system. The fundamental challenge is thus not to live longer, but how to live our extra years in terms of health, financial security, wellbeing, social insertion, and personal, cultural and social significance. Ageing is an achievement, a triumph, not a cataclysmic event (Freixas, 2002). The old vision of age as an inevitable process of loss, illness and decrepitude is no longer valid, as a significant proportion of women and men play important roles as active members of society and enjoy a degree of autonomy and satisfaction to very advanced ages.

The spectacular increase in life expectancy has changed people's psychological position in the life cycle. The old clichés regarding ageing and death once the barrier of the fifties had been passed, have been largely dispelled, and today, we can look forward to a long phase of life to which we must give meaning. Middle age (50 – 65), regarded as a cultural category, has acquired a recognised status as a stage of life distinct from the third age (65 - 80) and the fourth (older than 80). Studies of age need to add a description of each aspect of our state of mind that deals with the life cycle, revealing the fears and assumptions that invade it.

4. Gender and ageing

The characteristics of the lives of women, and their wide individual variations, make it difficult to analyse their experience in terms of the classical stages of development, which are adapted to the masculine model, which is still regarded as the norm. In such studies, theories of adult development have traditionally been based on largely male sample populations, whose experience and perspectives have ignored those of women, while the results obtained on the basis of such samples have been generalised to apply also to women, treating these as deficient when their experience and performance do not correspond to masculine standards. Virtually no studies have attempted to consider the significance and consequences of the differences in socialisation and the life options of women and men in old age.

It is several years since certain female authors first pointed out the necessity for the psychological study of the development of males and females to be separated. In spite of the fact that studies of the psychosocial development of women are still few and far between, we now possess a number of works that illustrate the lives of middle-aged and elderly women from other perspectives (Arber & Ginn, 1995; Bernard et al., 2000; Freixas, 1993; Friedan, 1993; Gannon, 1999; Greer, 1991; Pearsall, 1997). A large proportion of the available studies of the second part of the lives of women have been carried out on sample populations drawn from the middle class; white, heterosexual and with average levels of education, thus leaving in the shade knowledge of the experiences and lives of an important segment of the female population that is the process of becoming old.

A number of female writers (Barnett & Baruch, 1978; Freixas, 1997; Gilligan, 1982) have argued that the words of Erikson and Levinson —who proposed the development of the adult personality through unidirectional, irreversible, hierarchical and universal stages that do not take into account individual differences— does not represent the reality of the situation for women (Erikson, 1950; Levinson, 1978). The life experiences of men are intimately related to their chronological age, as a variable in which the events of their lives are framed, belonging as much to the family as to the occupational sphere. However, this type of model does not function in the life of women, for whom adulthood involves a wide variety of role models that are not based on chronological age, since their lives may offer a large number of combinations in which their occupation, partnership and child-rearing involve several levels of use of their time and commitment that mean that the roles of wife, mother and worker may possess different degrees of importance at different points of their life cycle. This tends not to occur in the lives of men, in whom the unidirectionality of events has usually been clearer. The differences in involvement in the public and private spheres is the cause of completely divergent paths of life, which means that in the development of women, the evolution of relationships frequently exerts greater pressure than does that of chronological age as such (Luque, 2008).

Viewed from a feminine perspective, ageing can be a wide-ranging challenge, insofar as they need to face their personal and social situation which, in many cases has left them in poverty and dependence. Furthermore, they need to uncover certain of the most deeply-rooted sociocultural demands that have anchored them to profoundly restrictive models, related to concepts of beauty and youth that have no respect for the natural processes of human development.

5. Social changes

The important social changes that have taken place in the West in the course of the 20th century have involved new social, political, cultural, sexual, family and financial organisations of such importance that they have transformed the social and private lives of both men and women. A good proportion of the successes achieved by the end of the 20th century originated in the feminist movement and its thinking.

5.1 The new social organisation

In the case of women, the new social organisation has produced such a degree of structural change that their lives will never again be marked by the social conditions that previously constrained them and in which they lived, deprived of education, liberty, financial resources, voting rights, and control of their own bodies and sexuality. Their lives remained at the mercy of men —fathers, husbands, brothers, priests— who were the sole possessors of all rights. These social changes have given them access to education, paid work, social and political participation, as well as to the use of their own property and to their bodies and sexuality, as mentioned above.

In the case of the 'new' elderly women of the 21st century, one of the principal effects of their longevity has been the lack of models of elderly women with meaningful lives. With the aim of filling this blank screen of some 30 years of extra life with content, and in the lack of social models to which we can look, the new elderly women of the first half of the 21st century will need to look to each other if they are to trace out a new route-map. We may assume that this new generation of elderly women will be happier than their grandmothers, given that they have succeeded in dismantling some of the social requirements that previously restricted their lives. Nevertheless, social change never takes place without pain, puzzlement and uncertainty. It is probable that the new life situations that we analyse in this chapter will noticeably improve their sense of satisfaction with life.

This, in the sense of a subjective perception of wellbeing beyond what the objective data might suggest, lies along two axes: that of 'control' of one's own life, and that of 'happiness'. The gender-based division of work that has ruled in industrialised societies has assigned to men the pole of 'control' (access to education, money, work outside the home, power, status) while limiting women to the pole of 'happiness' (relationships, emotions, care). This model of social organisation places men and women in different life spaces; the world of affect, relationships, care-giving, raising children, are all part of the feminine specialisation, while men are assigned the biblical tasks of earning the family's bread, going to war and defending their wives and their flocks, which in practice involves the total management of money and of political and private power. This model has led to the devaluation of all the activities and practices supplied by women, which has meant that the 'feminine space' has come to be regarded as inferior, and thus something to be avoided in the process of masculine identity, which has traditionally been constructed on the basis of denying its feminine side.

However, this division of social roles generated a lack of satisfaction among both parties, distancing men from the life of the emotions and women from power and from control of their own lives. The voices that demanded a more equitable division of these two spaces came from women, as they were more aware than men that this way of locating themselves in the world resulted in deficiencies which had lasting and irremediable consequences, especially in old age. For this reason, from the 1960s onwards, a good number of women progressively and definitively joined the world of paid labour, thus availing themselves of the use and management of their own money and possessions; meanwhile, they were also struggling to access education and the universities, and to have legislation passed that would give them better control of their lives, their bodies and their sexuality, giving them a radical transformation of their everyday life —although they might not have realised that at the time— above all, of the conditions of ageing, assuming the responsibility for their own well-being, not only physically, but also mentally and spiritually. All the above changes modified the relationships and the position of women in the world and enabled them to renegotiate their intimate relationships, their sexuality, birth-giving and, as a result, to modify to a great extent what will be their lives as elderly women during the first half of the 21st century.

We do not know whether these elderly women will be happier than their predecessors, because it is not age as such that is the cause of a lessening of pleasure in growing old, but rather the circumstances associated with life in old age that can determine a greater or lesser feeling of happiness. In this synthesis between the pole of control and the pole of happiness that marks the life of individuals, the old values of the popular song —'there are three things in life: health, money and love'— continue to be basic aims. Family, social and friendship networks, a higher level of education, good health and financial resources are the indicators that sustain us in adequate comfort in our old age.

5.2 Feminism and the life of older women

The great social changes that have marked the second half of the 20th century doubtless affect the pattern of life of men and women of all ages, in such a way that these important social changes will have important consequences for the old age experienced by women. Feminist movement has provided the foundations of the transformation of the public and private life of women —and thus of men— by overcoming the many social and cultural limitations that restricted their lives to the fields of reproduction and the private world.

The 60s and 70s of the previous century produced major social changes in favour of the civil rights of discriminated minorities —particularly those of black people and of women. The activities of the women's liberation movement encouraged the passing of laws that eliminated many of the social barriers that limited the lives of women in fields such as education, civil rights, reproductive and sexual rights, and of rights to work and to hold property, and so on.

Feminism, as a theoretical perspective and a social movement, has illuminated our understanding of power relationships within the family and emotional life, and has unveiled the system of maintenance and reproduction of such concepts. The feminist slogan 'the personal is political' led to a structural change. By claiming that the relationships that rule our private lives are power relationships, it suggests that many of the problems that we regard as 'personal' originate in society and, as such, can only be resolved by social and political change. On this basis, the creation of a collective consciousness mobilised women in their search for objectives and changes in their situation, although the emphasis on equality hid reflections on gender-based differences. Moreover, social recognition of rights has in many cases not been accompanied by true equality and the transformation of social, political, economic or personal life practices, in which women remain at a disadvantage, and which become significantly worse in old age.

The new elderly women of the 21st century to whom we refer in this chapter(1), born in the final third of the 20th century —heiresses of the benefits and discourses of the second wave of feminism, daughters of May'68 and the great social movements propelled by faith in change—, convinced that 'the personal is political' will revise each and every one of the elements of the social contract and of love: they will examine through a magnifying glass the received prescriptions regarding daily life and will denounce the patriarchal agreements that dominate both the personal and political spheres. They will insist on the deconstruction of identity inherited from the feminine 'mystique' (heterosexuality, femininity, passivity, obedience, maternity) across a continuum of crises of identity throughout their lives, until old age which, in the lack of a recognised legacy, offers itself as a blank space, without models and accompanied by many fears and ghosts; with a single strength derived from their links and the bank of arguments of feminist thinking and epistemology.

A good number of these women, who will make up an important fraction of the elderly population of the 21st century, have been characterised as refusing to passively accept the life models left to them by previous generations, have renegotiated the meaning of many received prescriptions and have modified the sense of ageing, taking as their point of departure vital and intellectual positions that are very different from those of their mothers and grandmothers. They have challenged cultural images of the 'little old lady'; asexual, self-sacrificing, lacking opinions, desires and necessities, always available, undervalued and weak, giving way to the model of an elderly woman who is active and sexual, attractive, who utilises her power and her new position in society, in her family, her network and her relationships (Kingsberg, 2002). These women will face old age with experiences of work, finance, family, status and power that are very different from those of their predecessors, and as such, enjoy greater financial, social and intellectual resources. All this has required the redefinition of many of the social roles that they have played up to the present day in terms of partnerships, family, paid employment, money and sexuality, etc. Theories of the life cycle have yet to develop a set of arguments that value the significance of these factors in individual and psychosocial terms.

On the other hand, the reflections produced by feminism at the end of the previous century regarding sexual differences have helped to give value to 'the feminine', and to recover the values that women have historically brought to relationships and the sustainability of life, recognising their civilising efforts (Libreria delle Donne di Milano, 1987). Thanks to these contributions, the elderly women of the 21st century find themselves occupying new fields of

[1] The new elderly women to whom we refer represent minor cultural, social, political, economic and personal avant garde. The elderly women of the 21st century also include women who remain rooted in the models of the previous century, for whom social change has not led to any real transformation of their lives, although it may do so for thair daughters, as a result of their efforts.

meaning and presence in which they do not feel a necessity to deny their femininity in occupying spaces that used to be dedicated to men and for which models were in short supply.

6. Elderly women of the 20th century / elderly women of the 21st century

In their youth, a large proportion of the women who are elderly today lived in social, economic and political situations characterised by poverty, deprivation and submission; they laboured within the family unit, in the fields, and in activities that accorded them neither social nor economic recognition. Nevertheless, many of these women were the promoters, whether voluntarily or involuntarily, of many of the social transformations enjoyed by the elderly women of the 21st century. Their role as pioneers in many areas has yet to be recognised. In reality, as Brody (2010) claims, they made up a 'new frontier' for themselves and for new generations. Also, to the extent to which they needed to overcome the many difficulties and deficiencies from which they emerged more than successfully, we may feel that they have demonstrated an admirable resilience. They have understood how to adapt to losses, to the new environments of life and work, to social and familial change, in a society that is profoundly changing and in which changes they have participated through their questioning. In this too, they were pioneers.

The demographic aspects are the basis of some of the great changes in the lives of elderly women. Thus, the increase in life expectancy will produce one of the most important transformations: while at the age of 60, or even earlier, life for both men and women had more or less come to an end during the first half of the 20th century, for the new elderly, the same age involves launching new initiatives; experiences and lives unlived until the moment at which they emerge as new expectations. To a great extent, this is because the increase in life expectancy is taking place in an epoch in which potent social changes have given the female population a wide range of new resources, both economic and intellectual as well as in the sphere of health. Furthermore, the revision carried out by women who were socialised under the model of submission to the patriarchy —feminists *avant la lettre*— will provide future generations with the ability to choose and to make decisions regarding their own lives that hitherto have been unthinkable.

On the other hand, the social and personal advances encouraged by feminism and the social movements will be concretised in a re-evaluation of age, and thus of the visibility and occupation of public space on the part of elderly people. Elderly women and men will enjoy a social and vital space and recognition that they have lacked until now.

6.1 Education, culture, freedom

One of the most important tasks in the process of ageing consists of 'assigning meaning to life itself', a task that demands a conjunction between reminiscence —giving meaning to one's own past life— and premonition —planning the future. To be able to identify a personal pathway to graceful ageing, accepting one's past and designing one's future, the new elderly women possess highly valuable elements, of which education is probably the most important. This group, born around the middle of the 20th century, does not include illiterate persons. The virtual universal access of women to basic general education and of an important fraction of the female population to higher education, as well as to the spread in the use and knowledge of the new information and communication technologies will offer them an extremely interesting panorama.

The new elderly women will communicate with their daughters, grandchildren and friends by email, and buy their airline and theatre tickets via the Internet, on which they will also check the weather and read the papers in their own homes.

Education allows access to information, and that in turn to liberty. The elderly women of the 21st century, given that they will have had an education, will be able to take up paid work (their own money) and will have had their own experiences of management and access to various forms of power and control. In no way do they resemble their grandmothers who, to the extent that they came from a society in which women were regarded as being less intellectually gifted than men, had very restricted access to education, which was reduced to a rudimentary level. This limited them to the role of housewife (wives, mothers, grandmothers) as the only possible occupation, leaving them in old age without money of their own and with very limited access to cultural and intellectual resources.

6.2 The work cycle of women

The most obvious consequence of the access of women to education is their incorporation into the labour market, which has markedly changed —although still with important limitations— domestic life, financial relationships within the family and, in consequence, the power relationships within the family and in social life. The model of social organisation of our culture is profoundly androcentric and not only ignores the peculiarities of the life cycle of women, but even punishes them for not running with the same rhythm as their male companions and being 'distracted' from their professional career by their child-care duties, performing tasks of care-giving and emotional support that are 'not the concern' of their male companions. All in all, the years dedicated to these tasks of sustaining life do not count in their curricula, thus giving men an advantage through their lack of solidarity in the tasks involved in civilising the world. A similar problem arise in the area of pensions, which are calculated according to a model of working life derived from the division of labour between the sexes, as a result of which the typical variability in the trajectory of the feminine career obviously operates to the disadvantage of the financial level of women in old age.

The financial insecurity which women in previous generations faced in old age is related to the fact that in many cases they entered and left the labour market as a function of the financial requirements of the family and the demands for care of their husbands and children. These are women who have abandoned interesting jobs in order to follow their husbands in his work, who have been unable to rise in their professional career for fear of injuring masculine honour, and who have left the house to work 'at anything' when their male's wage has not come in. All in all, the heterosexual definition currently defines the age of women who invested their capital in marriage, with the idea that this would supply their financial necessities in their old age, but when the hour of truth arrives find themselves in misery. Moreover, in a society in which women's most important value lies in their reproductive capacity, having an intellectual occupation was often seen in a negative and suspicious light, since intellectual work for women was considered to have a negative impact on childbirth (Hirdman, 1994).

We may think that some of the new elderly women —insofar as they have had a history of work that is more continuous and of higher status than that of their predecessors— will enjoy old-age pensions that will permit them to live the long later years of their life in a better financial situation than their mothers who, in accordance with the model of gender-based division of labour, put their efforts into unpaid domestic work, and thus found themselves consigned to poverty and financial dependence in their old age.

The fact that feminism has emphasised the necessity for women to have a 'purse of one's own' (Woolf, 1938) —a financially independent life, a career— should not be interpreted as a desire to adopt the masculine model of work. In fact, this is not the case, although some women are obliged to assimilate themselves to this model if they wish to advance in their professional careers. Many women of recent generations, in spite of their definitive incorporation into the world of work, continue to structure their working life around the requirements of the family and their duties of care. The flexibility in work demonstrated by women is not usually a matter of choice. They need flexible working conditions in order to be able to reconcile this aspect of life with the demands of the family.

Women want an equilibrium between paid work and their other activities, including leisure, care and voluntary work. One of the challenges of contemporary life will be to bear in mind the new, creative forms of life that women are putting into practice —most of them as solitary adventurers— given the difficult conditions that the traditional forms of relationship, derived from heterosexual romantic love, place on them.

6.3 Rethinking the model of retirement

The androcentric model of retirement, in which one changes from paid work to 'not working' from one day to the next, is probably in need of revision, attributing value to the work cycle of women who pursue extremely diverse career paths which, besides paid work *sensu strictu*, include care-giving, providing emotional support, voluntary work and a range of community and social activities of great importance and enormous social value, such as the irreplaceable tasks of making life more supportable and humane.

Just as diversity is the norm when we speak of the family types of the 21st century, so is it too when we observe the wide range of situations that have defined the social life of women since the late 20th century. The reflections aroused by a number of studies suggest a pre-retirement model of work that takes the form of a transition between working and retirement that could bring about an improvement in the experience of retirement, ameliorating the crisis of meaning and identity that can result from a single life-model, such as we often find among men (Everingham et al., 2007). In fact, some companies already ease the transition to retirement of both men and women by allowing them to reduce the number of hours worked and the range of tasks they undertake. For example, some universities reduce teaching hours, while maintaining the amount of time available for research, thus making best use of the intellectual capacity of their academic staff. Such a reduction in hours worked as retirement approaches could be adapted to a great extent to the range of women's careers.

It might be useful on financial grounds, given the erratic work-life histories of many women, with their serious consequences for retirement pensions, to lengthen their working lives, albeit in a partial fashion, allowing them to include periods of paid work alongside periods of other activities of interest, even if unpaid. This is not to forget the structural changes that are a result of our present longevity: for earlier generations, retirement coincided with the beginning of 'old age', the loss of one's faculties, senescence. Today, at 65, most of us enjoy an enviable state of health and can boast of knowledge and skills that make us useful in many spheres of work, social and community life. All of this favours the idea of creating *à la carte* retirement policies that would allow those who wish to do so, to compensate for some of the difficulties that they are liable to meet at the moment of compulsory retirement.

A unitary model of retirement does not correspond to the different implications of the work and family world of women. In fact, the new forms of retirement that society ought to be organising emerge from this plural reality and also, in these times of crisis, from that of the new generations of women and men for whom work will be no more than a matter of security, as it has long been for men, both historically and up until the present day. We might say that we find ourselves facing a society in which work insecurity is drawing both women and men down to the same level, and that the time has come to revise the forms of retirement, in order to be able to take new situations into account. This demand has been made time and time again by women. Although the different way in which women have interacted with the labour market has historically been regarded as 'second-best', the current crisis appears to be minimising gender differences in the world of work (Everingham et al., 2007).

The fear of financial insecurity will continue to be a prevalent feeling in the women of the coming generations who have worked intermittently, particularly for those who lack a partner but have family obligations. Such insecurity is based on the practice of part-time working, in the need to combine a number of obligations, and in the culture of flexible working that has left women in a financially vulnerable situation by denying them a secure income and a continuity of employment that would guarantee them a successful retirement. Thanks to a number of ideas derived from feminist thinking, the new generation of elderly women will probably take more seriously the topic of continuity of employment and pensions, which ought to reduce the numbers of elderly women in poverty.

6.4 Health and paid work

The health of elderly women in the 21st century is benefitting from the thinking derived from women's health-oriented networks which, since the end of the nineties, have produced interesting studies of differences in morbidity between men and women and have questioned diagnoses, treatments and medical practices regarding women's health (Valls et al., 2008). To date, little research has been done on the topic of the benefits of paid work on women's health, while the few studies that do exist suggest that social and relationships resulting from work outside the home protect women from mental and physical illness, by enabling them to raise their self-esteem and sense of security in decision-making, while offering them social support as well as a greater feeling of satisfaction with life (Sorensen & Verbrugge, 1987).

Paid work also offers other health advantages; it enables people to structure their own time and provides financial benefits, social contacts and professional identity. Where women are concerned, participation in the world of work improves their health insofar as it offers social status and power in addition to financial independence and self-esteem. The social support provided by paid work is valued by women as the most important element in keeping them there, quite apart from the potential financial necessity. The participants in Forssén and Carlstedt's study of health and paid work emphasised that this enabled them to control and relieve their illnesses and that it offered a number of health benefits, of which they mentioned the importance of enjoying a meaningful life, feeling competent and needed, and being recognised and enjoy a good mood, and that it helped to structure their days (Forssén & Carlstedt, 2007).

A topic of great importance in the lives of elderly females in the future will be the relationship that emerges between the massive incorporation of women into paid employment and their experiences of health. To what extent has the participation in the labour market been a source of physical and psychological health —even when such work has been hard, poorly paid and little recognised— in comparison with that of their predecessors as housewives or unpaid labour? Future studies ought to take into account the new relationships between women, their bodies, health and attractiveness, topics of great importance in the ageing process, while bearing in mind the double standard of ageing denounced by Susan Sontag (1972).

6.5 Body and beauty

Growing old is not easy in a society such as ours, in which the concept beauty is based on two elements that are difficult to maintain as we grow older: youth and slimness. Staying young when we have passed 60 is an oxymoron: we cannot be both old and young, while the need to remain slim, which is derived from an inadequate history of nutrition and an upbringing under an aesthetic model which itself is static, is no easy task in old age. The cultural change concerning the image of the female body has basically taken place since the early 20th century. Naomi Wolf located the start of our preoccupation with diet and slimness in the 1920s, when western women started to obtain the vote and legal emancipation, with certain swings that were functions of the greater or lesser exaltation of maternity as the destiny of women. However, it was most clearly after 1965, with the emergence of the skeletal model Twiggy, that women began to slim seriously and to suffer for the weight that they always regard as excessive. In spite of the fact that women have made advances in terms of rights, status and power, which ought to have brought them a greater sense of self-esteem and of competence and value, their obsession with weight has led them as a rule to feel unhappy, in spite of the advances that ought to have been concretised in the very opposite perception (Fredrickson & Roberts, 1997; Wolf, 1991).

Some of the sociocultural requirements regarding attractiveness that have such a great effect on the life of women while they are still young continue to place limits on their feeling of satisfaction with life and of wellbeing in their old age. Cultural requirements have historically impelled women to involve themselves in 'disciplinary practices' at a high physical, financial and psychological cost in order to maintain their appearance; practices that imply global strategies of control; in this case a biopolitics of control of the female body that leads women into a continual 'must do it', because otherwise they would not exist. Naomi Wolf put it succinctly as follows: "The real problem is the lack of choice." (Wolf, 1991: 354). Faced with this situation, the old women of the future will start to make decisions regarding how they wish to dress, make up and display themselves. They will develop a standard of personal care that is no longer a matter of pain or obligation, an imperative that makes them suffer because if they do not live up to it they will be excluded, but rather as an element of pleasure or enjoyment, of personal identity and acceptance of what nature has given to each of them, of liberty, of beauty, in order to feel good.

The new elderly women have managed to reflect individually and collectively about the messages and mandates they have received regarding attractiveness, and have been able to construct their own modes of thinking on this topic. Today, ideas of beauty have changed, and we can look to a new concept of beauty that integrates and fulfils them as individuals, that does not demand a particular external appearance, but rather looks into the interior of each individual being, taking self-esteem as its point of departure. Given that the conventional images of women older than 60 with which we have grown up no longer have anything to do with current reality, we will have to construct new patterns for them. The crucial topic here as far as new elderly women are concerned lies in the search for a model of beauty that moves them from the image of a wrinkled little old lady, dressed all in black, whose involvement in her own body image shines by its very absence, to a typology in which there is room for diversity and enjoyment rather than merely the obligation to wear mascara in the process of hiding one's age. All in all, it is a matter of questioning how far elderly women are prepared to go in identifying themselves with what is regarded as attractive in our society: how far they are willing to conform to a model in order to achieve a 'correct' image of growing old.

6.6 New family life

The demographic fact of greater longevity, allied to the lowering of the birth-rate, has altered the structure of the family; this has changed from that of the extended family with many children and few generations to one made up of few children and several generations. This situation has led to a change in the pattern of relationships, which are no longer horizontal (between brothers and sisters), to vertical links (between generations). However, new forms of social organisation have encouraged the appearance of new modes of family life that have already become the norm in the 21st century. Diversity characterises emotional life and the relationships of women who are currently in the process of becoming old, though not without some pain. In spite of everything, the family is, and will probably continue to be, an important aspect of the life of women for all time.

If anything does define the life of the old women of the 21st century, it is the fragmentation of their emotional and work careers. The concept of 'definitive' or 'for ever' under which their grandmothers were socialised, has disappeared at the stroke of a pen. We now live in what Ulrich Beck has called the "risk society", in which we have to be prepared for change, for the ephemeral, for breaks in long-term family and professional careers (Beck, 1992). The normal 'chaos of love' that has characterised our society since May'68 has fragmented our emotional lives (Beck & Beck-Gernsheim, 1995). No longer is anything 'for ever', while to introduce this concept into our emotional programme would not be a simple matter, particularly after having put so much effort into the creation of spaces of relationships and connections that were believed to be lasting.

The ideology of the traditional family has permeated the lives of women of all ages, in spite of the fact that for almost half a century new forms of family life have been emerging. The traditional family model (regarded as a universal model, in spite of the fact that it is basically the result of the gender-determined division of labour dating from the 19th century), which is characterised by the financial dependence of the woman and the lack of male involvement in care-giving and domestic tasks, has been followed by other family models derived from the incorporation of women into the labour market and feminist demands for fairness in the division of responsibilities. These new models have deconstructed the familiar myth, revealing a wide variety of models that have achieved similar degrees of legal, social and personal validity, among which we find the egalitarian heterosexual family, the female single-parent family as well as the male ditto, the homosexual family —both lesbian and gay—, and the recent concept of 'families of choice'. All of these models are derived from the social changes of the 20th century and from the theoretical thinking of the feminist movement (Fortin, 2005).

Heterosexual marriage continues to be a goal in the life of the new generation of elderly women, albeit to a lesser extent than before. What is certain is that in their time, many of these women married for love, rather than to obtain financial security as had previous generations, marrying men who, while they supported the discourse of equality in theory, continued in practice to behave like their fathers. Cohabitation with these husbands whose theoretical discourses displayed a social sensitivity and democratic framework, but who refused to renounce the privileges of their sex, which they assumed to be something 'natural', often generated relational conflicts which in turn raised the rates of separation and divorce (Coria, 2001). Women of recent generations who have wanted to maintain relationships with their partners on a basis of equality have had to deploy a range of strategic discourses and take part in various practices in order to control the context of daily life (Elizabeth, 2003). The inequalities in intimate relationships are not only a product of interpersonal relationships, but also the result of the limiting effects of cultural norms and other socially significant spaces, such as the family of origin.

6.7 New life-styles

Today, more and more people are adopting life-styles that combine intimacy, physical contact, emotional relationships and company, even though they live apart. Sharing interests, intimacy and social and personal activities need not involve sharing a home or a residence, which resolves some of the problems of cohabitation in later life with persons with whom one has not earlier come to agreement concerning everyday life together. It is thus clear that the structural changes of recent times involve a wide range of intimate relationships which, for the new generation of elderly women, involve moving on from a monogamous matrimonial relationship —which essentially means emotional and financial dependence— to a relationship that Anthony Giddens (1992) called a 'pure relationship' which is kept up only as far as both parties find that it gives them sufficient satisfaction to remain in it. Couples involved in such relationships lack models to follow, and in theory are more egalitarian, autonomous and happy than those in the classical model, preferring to replace marriage with some form of mutual commitment (Gross & Simmons, 2002).

In the new generation of elderly women we already find different 'trials' of relationships in which various alternatives to cohabitation within the framework of classical heterosexual marriage are practised. Some of these go in for cohabitation —i.e. living together with another person outwith a marriage contract— as an alternative to marriage as such. This mode tends to involve a more egalitarian relationship and may be more satisfactory for women. Another formula that has been tried out with some success is to be a couple, each of whose members live in their own house (LAT; living apart together), a formula that involves commitment, sexual relations and social recognition while satisfying the necessities for intimacy and autonomy, company and independence desired by many people in later life —particularly women. This formula, which is very similar to the 'pure relationship' described by Giddens (1992), is less institutionalised and requires a high level of negotiation. Meanwhile, a relationship with another person of the same sex is an option chosen by some mature women, who find areas of mutual understanding with their equals that they had not enjoyed in their heterosexual relationships. Recent legislation that recognises homosexual marriage has offered a certificate of legitimacy to this option, and has contributed to the elimination of social, cultural and family homophobia (Connidis, 2006).

6.8 Links and networks

Enjoying relationships in old age —whatever their configuration— has positive domestic, psychological, social and even financial benefits, insofar as they offer social and emotional support and physical and sexual contact, while also enabling care-giving and domestic tasks to be shared. Furthermore, networks allow different strategies for life in old age to be shared. This would appear to be a positive programme, but to make a success of it demands a good dose of internal freedom that no-one has ever said cannot be exploited, although women may not allow themselves to do so.

Women have always been creative experts in relationships of friendship which, as they grow older, display their inestimable value in the maintenance of wellbeing and a positive ageing process. For many reasons, the depositories of these links of friendship tend to be other women, whether younger, older or of similar ages, shading out differences in age, and giving and receiving, as appropriate, in rich intergenerational exchanges. Carolyn Heilbrun put it thus: "[since the 50s]...after a lifetime of solitude and few close and constant companions, women friends and colleagues, themselves now mature adults, whose intimacy helped to make the sixties my happiest decade" (Heilbrun, 1997: 4).

Too often is age associated with isolation; however, women of all ages form powerful networks of social and emotional support and set up instrumental and emotional links at time when life seems to be losing its balance, and these turn out to be extremely solid structures. Women have ample experience of this; since it is they who establish and maintain relationships within and beyond the family they are very well prepared to develop and maintain new social links when they find themselves facing the vicissitudes of old age.

Social networks are closely related to the quality of life, to the ability to deal with the stresses of everyday life, and to health and longevity. The greater life expectancy of women, their solid social networks and personal capacity for dealing successfully with the changing circumstances of life, ought to be recognised as closely interrelated feminine strengths.

6.9 Finally alone

Solitude is one of the great discoveries of maturity, at least for those who possess sufficient health and emotional support networks to enjoy it. Dreaded when we are young as a symbol of abandonment and lack of social participation, with the passing of the years it turns into a challenge, a personal space of liberty and happiness. In the first stage of adulthood, women are often so caught up in various central aspects of their own and others' lives that there comes a point in their later lives when solitude ceases to be something feared and turns into a happy meeting with oneself. Solitude is a temptation for persons who have lived with too much company and thus have scarcely enjoyed time and space to themselves. Heilbrun (1997) describes it as a pleasure for those who have managed to give meaning to their lives, as an opportunity to live in the present, as a gift that they do not wish to allow to escape. Solitude enables us to hold the reins of our daily lives, to organise our time.

Living alone is not usually a problem for most women. Used as they are to organising their own and others' lives, they suddenly find themselves on their own stage. Living alone brings a meeting with long-postponed desires that had become unrecognisable. Now they have all the time and space they need to organise their environment as they wish. All in all, they can embrace personal freedom and make room for their own desires.

The trends in gerontology that emphasise activity as a tool in successful ageing assign a value to 'doing' over to 'being', leaving little room for more quiet life choices, and obliging elderly persons to maintain family, leisure and care-giving activities and responsibilities that they have not chosen themselves. In the lives of elderly women, active ageing frequently implies yet other obligations: to remain active, to go out, participate, provide care, to show that one is bursting with life and activity. In reality, so-called productive and successful ageing imposes totalising ideals about the meaning of a 'good old age' (Minkler & Holstein, 2008).

6.10 The 'single'culture

If their predecessors were wives, mothers, daughters and neighbors, the new elderly women of the 21st century are partners, lovers, mothers and step-mothers, sisters, colleagues, cyber-girlfriends and, above all, divorcees. The elderly women of the future, i.e. women who are currently in their fifties, are twice as likely to be divorced as the elderly of today (Thomas & Fogg, 2000), to the extent that the current generation of the 'emerging elderly' has launched the practice of the 'single' life. On the one hand, they divorce and separate when the contradictions of equality in daily life become too obvious, while on the other, many of them opt much earlier to live a life that does not have room for heterosexual marriage.

It was this generation that deconstructed the old concept of 'spinster' that tormented and influenced the options of its mothers and grandmothers. The old women of the 21st century have continued to live with the specter of spinsterhood, although now only half-voiced, within a society that no believed in it. They do not wish to burden themselves with conventional marriage, while the convent is no longer an interesting option, so they have launched themselves on the paths of a profession and the control of their emotional life under new parameters. Whatever the reason, they have learned to live alone much earlier than their mothers, who only did so with the blessing of society when they had become widows, although the group of divorcees who had not made provision for the state of separation tends to find themselves in a poorer financial position in old age. In this way they can control all the threads of their life (economics, sexuality, independence), albeit not without difficulty, given the lack of models by which to view themselves.

In the face of the transitoriness of emotional relationships and the fragility of the ties of love, the new generations of elderly women have begun to practise forms of relationship and support that we might call 'families of choice': usually networks of women, spiced up with a few men, that make up a powerful support organisation and offer an antidote to solitude and isolation. Sources of cultural knowledge, of social support, of exchange of knowledge, of connections and emotional security, these new forms of family life enable elderly women to enjoy life alone in the security of knowing that nothing bad can happen to them, thanks to the efficient functioning of the structural networks of such 'families of choice'.

6.11 Habitat

One of the important conquests in the lives of elderly women is the possibility of deciding where and how to live, as much in terms of space as in forms of living and relationships. Present-day elderly women often find themselves living in old people's homes or in the homes of their children; perhaps even subjected to a peripatetic life, moving from the house of one child to the next, deprived of all intimacy, memories and mementos. The new generation of elderly women have considered how they are to be lodged in old age, about the design and features of the space in which they want to live, looking at it from their own perspective, and including in the balance the necessities that they may have in the future.

One's own house is the space that we have in which to live, to relate to the persons with whom we live, to receive our friends. It is also one's own personal and intimate space, in which we can enjoy freedom, but it is also the physical space in the city that enables us to participate in the community, maintain relationships and connections beyond the domestic circle, as active participants in the neighbourhood. The new generation of elderly women thus realise that they need a sufficiently intimate and private space that also provides for contact with the community and allows for relationships, avoiding dependence on the goodwill of other people.

In old age, we have to live in proximity with women and men of all ages; young people must not be deprived of the experience of relationships with elderly people, but nor can we grow old without participating in the interests and projects of younger generations. We are part of a community of care, with obvious mutual benefits (Tronto, 2000). If old people could maintain good connections with younger generations through participation in community life, they would retain an idea of themselves that was not fragmented by age and would contribute to a stimulating intergenerational continuity, in which reciprocity and interdependence would create a mutually enriching style of exchange. There would be fewer complaints, fewer aggravations, fewer misunderstandings. We would function as tribal chiefs, standing up for the interests of the future and preserve the valuable continuity between generations (Woodward, 1999).

6.12 A community of care

Caring is a crucial activity in human development; it configures us as emotional, empathetic beings, sensitive to the needs of our congeners. Caring activities comprise everything that we do to preserve life and wellbeing; our bodies, our souls and the environment, i.e. everything that enables us to sustain life on earth and makes us complete human beings. Caring is not a simple task. It produces internal satisfaction and peace of mind, but it costs us effort, and requires us to renounce alternatives. It generates internal contradictions and with them, feelings of guilt and frustration; it can also make us angry.

The ethics of care, as discussed by Carol Gilligan, assumes a moral virtue that goes beyond the simple assumption of responsibility like an obligation or a routine (Gilligan, 1982). It involves a personal commitment, internal and freely assumed, regarding the wellbeing of other persons. And precisely there lies one of its fundamental problems, whose crux is rooted in the differential traditional socialisation that has exempted men from this moral responsibility, to such an extent that, as Tronto (2000) claims, they have enjoyed the 'privilege of irresponsibility' in the care both of themselves and of others.

The unrewarded efforts of women on behalf of their children, partners and/or older members of the family is a public and social good that permits the economic development of society, thanks to the savings made by the state and the practical and emotional benefits that fall to individuals. Women find it difficult to set limits on the care they provide, just like the historical problems that they have experienced in offering their time gratis; in spite of this it is still the subject of contradictory feelings.

We live in a society in which the fall in the number of children per family reduces the proportion of the members of the group available to look after old people. Furthermore, caring for an old, dependent person does not offer the same pleasure as the care of a baby, whose day-by-day progress is obvious and stimulating. Care of the elderly is not a highly regarded activity, because the persons who receive such care are little valued by society (Calasanti, 2006). On the other hand, the realisation of dependence and the loss of capacities of a loved one force us to confront our own existence, precisely at the moment of our life cycle at which we are performing our own personal evaluation. This leads to clear physical and emotional wear and tear and generates many personal, partnership and intergenerational conflicts.

The new generation of elderly women may regard care-giving as an ethical and emotional opportunity that many of them assume, beyond the stress involved and the call of duty, which mixes feelings such as the need to protect the dignity of the loved one, company, and the desire to help the person involved to maintain a sense of self that protects their integrity. On the other hand, the experience of caring for a loved one offers an opportunity for emotional exchanges, for pardon, compassion, and is accompanied by an interesting and necessary reflection on dependence relationships. These also include those who perceive the necessity to liberate themselves from the oppression of care as a social demand that falls upon women, maintaining the right not to care for others and not to receive care themselves in the future, thus liberating the family from this responsibility and delegating it to the social services.

6.13 A social movement toward visibility

Finally, after so many years of playing an externally dictated role, the new generation of elderly women feel that they are entering a period of authenticity. In the second half of their lives, they may become what they have been building up in the course of time and they possess a full repertoire of knowhow that they can validate via participation social, neighbourly, political, cultural and leisure activities. The wisdom that accompanies the process of ageing enables them to distance from many of the preoccupations that in other periods had dominated their lives, and now they can create a space for the development of other persons; they have more time available, they enjoy collective activities as though they were a personal project and in this context can offer their experience, knowhow, and tricks and strategies learned in the course of their previous everyday lives.

The participation of middle-aged and elderly women in cultural, political and social organisations, in NGOs and women's associations has become a transformating element of great importance, for the psychological wellbeing of both the women themselves and for community, which benefits from the free, disinterested and wise richness of resources that the voluntary efforts bring to it.

Social participation and an active lifestyle are important elements of personal satisfaction throughout our lives. They generate pleasure, raise our self-esteem, and help to blunt the stressful and traumatic events that occur in the course of our lives. Nevertheless, not everyone feels the same necessity for interaction and social and community participation and, now and again, silence and solitude are essential, beyond the well-meaning prescriptions that would bring the elderly out on the streets at all times. Many women wish to combine activity with enjoyment of serenity and silence. To live occasionally parked by the wayside may also be a source of happiness; a necessity.

6.14 Citizens and pioneers

The passage from a fundamentally private life to the participation of this generation of women in public life is one of the key changes in the configuration of the ageing process in the women of the 21st century. Their personal position as 'citizens' with the experiences resulting from this concept and their refusal to be excluded from the practices of citizenship for which they have sacrificed so much as a generation demands a serious discussion. Citizens, women who participate in public life which, in the case of our future old women, does not usually begin in old age. Frequently, in earlier time, they were involved in other fields of neighbourhood, social and/or political activity. Some of them came from careers of social involvement in the public sphere and it is impossible to say whether their participation derives from their new situation as retirees or because they now have more free time. They are activist women who have grown old. In fact, such continuity in social involvement and participation is linked to high levels of education, independent of age or sex (Milan, 2005). We can say that we are faced with a 'culture of militancy' or of participation in its various forms, in elderly women.

Elderly women are active in many sectors of social life, as well as playing important roles in family care and voluntary work and in democratic and political life (Magarian, 2003). In their eagerness to combine different worlds; family, work, community, they have maintained a delicate balance between these public spheres and their family life, in which negotiations in terms of time and desires have often not been easy (Charpentier et al., 2008). The family and the needs of their loved ones have shaped the social commitments of these women, who have demonstrated a sustained willingness to reconcile their social, political and neighborhood connections with the needs of their families. This generation has left the house for the city; it has ventured to occupy new spaces, assumed new social roles and created new models of women in the public world, of committed citizens, beyond the frontiers of age. In the course of their lives, they have gained civil rights (the vote), personal and social rights (education, paid work, money of their own), and are convinced that 'the personal is political' (abortion, divorce, birth control, control of their bodies and of their sexuality).

They have been pioneers in many fields: in politics, in the universities, in trade unionism. They have fought for coeducational schools; they were the precursors of all the legislative changes that permit the access of women to the control of their sexuality, have gained contraception and the depenalisation of abortion. They were the first university women, the first lawyers, doctors, architects, scientists, philosophers, educators, the first female politicians to achieve power. Their valour has helped to ensure that women of subsequent generations enjoy better and easier access to civil rights, to their own bodies, to culture and the labour market, thanks to their participation in the tasks of political representation, the defence of their rights and in social activities and voluntary work. Although many of them do not define themselves as feminists, their lives and the personal and social victories for which they have struggled have clearly contributed to the improvements in women's lives.

All of the above they have done in the conviction that there has been a path not all of whose turnings they knew, and which lacked images that would show them alternative futures. There has been a debate regarding the necessity to build models of elderly women on which to base themselves at a distance of 15, 20 or 30 years, versus the wide range of possibilities that precisely the lack of such models open up for them, with the liberty that this situation offers to devise new forms; diverse, plural, contradictory, which would destroy the homogeneity of the images of the older person that has been available to social and family settings, and in which most of them do not recognise.

The new generation of elderly women requires personal models to live up to. Just now, they are the protagonists in a historical and demographic situation that lacks precedents. Never before so many women have lived for so long, in possession of so much freedom, knowledge, culture, financial independence and good health. The result is that life presents itself as an adventure in which it is possible to discover new territories that guide one's own path and that of coming generations, who will be able to feel that to grow old is not so bad after all. The new generation of elderly women now enjoys a consciousness that enables them to design their own future.

6.15 Useful or exploited?

The work done by women through all the ages, for low or zero remuneration and in many cases, as an obligation resulting from personal or family circumstances, must not be confused with civic commitment or citizen participation performed on a voluntary basis. The participation of elderly women in the life of the community can be regarded as a voluntary effort, although in many cases it has not been chosen by the women themselves. Often, civic commitments are "targeted at the privileged few who have the time, good health, resources and prior experience that allow them to engage in significant volunteer activities" (Minkler & Holstein, 2008: 199).

Too often do we regard elderly people in terms of their potential for voluntary work, taking care of a series of social necessities that no-one would otherwise cover. Elderly women have been trained in renouncing their own free time and their own desires, which makes it difficult for them to say 'no' and to set limits. They wish to be involved in the community and in society, but they occasionally feel that they are being exploited. Through their participation, they want to ensure continuity of the causes that they had earlier adopted (feminism, citizenship, society, family, etc.), and are proud of having paved the way for new generations. They are generative (Erikson, 1950), and wish to pass on their knowledge and their efforts to younger generations. They like to be regarded as active persons, forever learning, open to new trends and trying to change the world for the better (Charpentier et al., 2008).

However, the growing tendency to discuss elderly people in utilitarian terms also implies a form of ageism that is beginning to be questioned by the elderly themselves, as some of the traps that lie within the culture of participation are uncovered. Many societies have regarded old people as a vast and largely underutilized resource for meeting the needs of the community. On the other hand, certain feminist thinkers also demand the right of women to be 'non-productive' in their old age, to use their time for pure enjoyment or leisure activities (Minkler & Holstein, 2008).

7. Old women of today and tomorrow

Many of the vital, professional and relational transformations that women have achieved in the course of the 20th century were noted by the visionary writers of the late 19th and early 20th century; Edith Wharton, Charlotte Perkins Gilman, Kate Chopin, Willa Cather, Virginia Woolf, Katherine Mansfield, etc., who had the historical acuity to write stories and novels in which they advocated a new epoch of relationships and traced the paths of these great changes, proposing models of women who would be professionally, politically and emotionally independent. These are authors whose works have been a lighthouse that has illuminated the life of women, orienting the new life cycle of the women of the future.

If gerontological feminist research wishes to encourage interpretations of ageing that display the variety and complexity of lives and realities, if it wishes to suggest and invent new ways of ageing, overcoming the traditional ideas that restrict, limit and circumscribe the lives of old women, that is, if it wishes to alter the reality facing elderly women, it will need to be capable of generating an idea that, used as a motor, will result in an adequate explanatory framework. An idea that will enable old age to imagine and create and, what is more important, an idea that will help to destroy other beliefs that are currently being involuntarily sustained. For this, it will be necessary to recognise and name the changing contexts in which the women of today live their lives, which will in no way resemble those of their mothers and probably not those of their daughters either. The fact is that everything is simpler when it enjoys the support of a close community of empathetic beings that will allow the resolution of the dissonance that can be perceived between the manner in which old women perceive themselves and their image in society

The social changes that have transformed the lives of women and men in the course of the 20th century will require us to implement highly creative strategies aimed at living happily and peacefully during the last years of a long life. Although the tide of social change will carry the new generation of elderly women to different beaches than those which hosted their predecessors, they have not been brought there by circumstances alone. For the first time in history, these mature women have chosen their own route and navigated by their own charts. Obviously this will not eliminate shipwrecks, but it will make the voyage more interesting and more significant.

8. Conclusion

Although it is clear that the coming generations of old women are not going to resemble their grandmothers in almost anyway, they are not there yet. Growing old is a good time for evaluating the past, of successes achieved and of tasks still to be tackled. The difference between successes and the hopes that were their starting point may be a source of dissatisfaction and uneasiness from which the new elderly may have liberated themselves, insofar as they have managed to reject the model by which their grandmothers had been socialised. It is not a simple task to identify one's own desires, validate them and put them into practice, without feeling a certain dissonance.

Change is a characteristic of individuals of all ages, including the oldest of us. The characteristics of the elderly are also in constant flux due to changes in sociocultural, economic and health factors, new ideas, beliefs and social trends. Nothing is static, which means that gerontological research possesses an unending source of renovation and a huge field ahead of itself. New ideas that need to be studied in depth are constantly emerging, and to do so we need to listen to what older people are really saying… nor only to the words but to cries, whispers and silences (Brody, 1985). Although old people are more visible than ever, much research remains to be done in this respect. Evolutionary psychology and critical gerontology face an important task of explaining and understanding these new ages, beyond the catastrophic vision that dominates the theory in current use.

Topics still to be dealt with that are of decisive importance in the configuration of lives and professional careers include the essential redefinition of the central role played by the family in women's lives, in that life options appear to be less marked by the concept of romantic love. A new evaluation of the roles of men and women in the constitution and harmonious functioning of the family unit could ease the integration of women into the labour market, as well as a fairer share of the tasks of sustaining life, placing care-giving at the centre of the organisation of society and sharing responsibility for this task between both sexes (Carrasco, 2003; Luque & Freixas, 2008). All this can be made concrete in the course of time in a healthier and more comfortable old age for women.

Socialised as they are as 'beings in the service of others' it is difficult for them to identify the path of individuality, achievement of individual identity, and balancing the value of relationships with the necessity for silence and autonomy. There are still a number of extremely important topics that wear out the lives of women of all ages, and these topics have still to be dealt with through research and reflection: the definition of beauty on the part of women themselves; beauty at all ages; the redefinition of personal identity, beyond that given by domestic tasks; balancing the weight of love in the course of life; not being perennially available, trying to respect our way of thinking and our pathways; relationships beyond gender-related violence.

9. References

Arber, S. & Ginn, J. (Eds.) (1995). *Connecting gender and ageing: a sociological approach,* Open University Press, ISBN 0-335-19471-0, Maidenhead, Berkshire, UK

Barnett, R.C. & Baruch, G.K. (1978). Women in the middle years: A critique of research and theory. *Psychology of Women Quarterly*, No.3, pp.187-197, *ISSN* 0192-513X

Beck, U. (1992). *Risk Society: Towards a New Modernity*, Sage, ISBN 0-8039-8345-X, London, UK

Beck, U. & Beck-Gernsheim, E. (1995). *The Normal Chaos of Love*, Polity Press, ISBN 0-7456-1071-4, Cambridge, UK

Bernard, M.; Phillips, J.; Machin, L. & Davies, V.H. (Eds.) (2000). *Women Ageing. Changing Identities, Challenging Myths*, Routledge, ISBN 0-415-18944-6, London, UK

Brody, E.M. (1985). *Mental and physical health practices of older people*, Springer, ISBN 0-8261-4870-0, New York, USA

Brody, E.M. (2010). On being very, very old: An insider's perspective. *The Gerontologist*, Vol.50, No.1, pp. 2-10, *ISSN* 0016-9013

Calasanti, T.M. (2006). Gender and Old Age. Lessons from Spousal Care Work, In: *Age Matters. Realigning Feminist Thinking*, T.M. Calasanti & K.F. Slevin, (Eds.), 269-294, Routledge, ISBN 978-0415952248, New York, USA

Carrasco, C. (2003). *Tiempos, trabajos y flexibilidad: una cuestión de género*, Instituto de la Mujer, ISBN 207-03-074-X, Madrid, Spain

Charpentier, M.; Quéniart, A. & Jacques, J. (2008). Activism among older women in Quebec, Canada: Changing the world after age 65. *Journal of Women & Aging*, Vol.20, No. 3-4, pp. 343-360, ISSN 0895-2841

Connidis, I.A. (2006). Intimate relationships. Learning from later life experience, In: *Age Matters. Realigning Feminist Thinking*, T.M. Calasanti & K.F. Slevin, (Eds.), 123-153, Routledge, ISBN 978-0415952248, New York, USA

Coria, C. (2001). *El amor no es como nos contaron... ni como lo inventamos*, Paidós, ISBN 978-950-12-2683-6, Buenos Aires, Argentina

Elizabeth, V. (2003). To Marry, or Not to Marry: That is the Question. *Feminism & Psychology*, Vol.13, No.4, pp. 426-431, ISSN 0959-3535

Erikson, E.H. (1950). *Childhood and Society*, Norton, ISBN 0-393-31068-X, New York, USA

Everingham, C.; Warner-Smith, P. & Byles, J. (2007). Transforming retirement: Re-thinking models of retirement to accommodate the experiences of women. *Women's Studies International Forum*, Vol.30, No.6, pp. 512-522, ISSN 0277-5395

Forssén, A.S.K. & Carlstedt, G. (2007). Health-Promoting Aspects of a Paid Job: Findings in a Qualitative Interview Study With Elderly Women in Sweden. *Health Care for Women International*, Vol.28, pp. 909-929, ISSN 0739-9332

Fortin, P. (2005). Un regard féministe sur les modèles de famille. *Atlantis*, Vol.30, No.1, pp. 80-91, ISSN 0210-6124

Fredrickson, B.L. & Roberts, T.A. (1997). Objectification theory: Toward understanding women's lived experiences and mental health risks. *Psychology of Women Quarterly*, Vol.21, No.2, pp. 173-206, ISSN 0361-6843

Freixas, A. (1993). *Mujer y envejecimiento. Aspectos psicosociales*, laCaixa, ISBN 84-7664-399-3, Barcelona, Spain

Freixas, A. (1997). Envejecimiento y género: otras perspectivas necesarias. *Anuario de Psicología*, No.75, pp. 31-42, ISSN 0066-5126

Freixas, A. (2002). Dones i envelliment. Apunts per a una agenda. *DCIDOB*, No.82, pp. 36-39, ISSN 1133-6595

Freixas, A. (2008). La vida de las mujeres mayores a la luz de la investigación gerontológica feminista. *Anuario de Psicología,* Vol.39, No.1, pp. 41-57, ISSN 0066-5126

Friedan, B. (1993). *The fountain of age,* Simon & Schuster, ISBN 9780743299879, N. York, USA

Gannon, L. (1999). *Women and Aging. Transcending the Myths,* Routledge, ISBN 978-0415169103, London, UK

Giddens, A. (1992). *The transformation of intimacy. Sexuality, love and eroticism in modern societies,* Polity Press, ISBN 978-0804722148, Cambridge, UK

Gilligan, C. (1982). *In a Different Voice: Psychological Theory and Women's Development,* Harvard University Press, ISBN 0674445449, Cambridge, Ma, USA

Greer, G. (1991). *The Change. Women, Ageing and the Menopause,* Hamish Hamilton, ISBN 978-0449908532, London, UK

Gross , N. & Simmons, S. (2002). Intimacy as a double-edged phenomenon? An empirical test of Giddens. *Social Forces,* Vol. 81, No 2, pp. 531-555, ISSN 0037-7732

Heilbrun, C.G. (1997). *The last gift of time. Life beyond sixty,* Ballantine, ISBN 0-345-42295-3, New York, USA

Hirdman, Y. (1994). *Women from possibility to problem?,* Arbetsliuscentrum, ISBN 0-415-15350-6, Stockholm, Sweden

Hollows, J. (2001). *Feminism, Feminity and Popular Culture,* Manchester University Press, ISBN 9780719043956, Manchester, UK

Kingsberg, S.A. (2002). The impact of aging on sexual function in women and their partners. *Archives of Sexual Behavior,* Vol.31, No.5, pp. 431-437, ISSN 00040002

Libreria delle Donne di Milano (1987). *Non credere di avere diritti,* Rosenberg & Sellier, ISBN 8870112756, Turin, Italy

Levinson, D.J. (1978). *The seasons of a man's life,* Knopf, *ISBN 0345339010, New York, USA*

Luque, B. (2008). El itinerario profesional de las mujeres jóvenes: una carrera de obstáculos. *Anuario de Psicología,* Vol.39, No.1, 101-107, *ISSN* 0066-5126.

Luque, B. & Freixas, A. (2008). Itinerarios vitales y profesionales de mujeres y hombres y su relación con los proyectos iniciales. *Estudios de Psicología,* Vol.29, No2, pp. 197-207, ISSN 0210-9395

Magarian, A. (2003). Les mouvements associatifs. *Gérontologie et Societé,* No.106, pp. 249-261, ISSN 0151-0193

Milan, A. (2005). Volonté de participer. L'engagement politique chez les jeunes adultes. *Tendances sociales canadiennes,* (Statistique Canada, 1-008), pp. 2-7, ISSN 0831-5701

Minkler, M. & Holstein, M.B. (2008). From civil rights to… civic engagement? Concerns of two older critical gerontologist about a 'new social movement' and what it portends. *Journal of Aging Studies,* Vol.22, pp.196-204, ISSN 08904065

Moreno, H. (2011). Una buena encarnación. *Debate Feminista,*Vol.21, No.42, pp. 111-135, ISSN: 0188-9478

Pearsall, M. (Ed.). (1997). *The other within us. Feminist explorations of women and aging.* Westview Press, ISBN 978-0813381633, Boulder, Co, USA

Ray, R. E. (2006). The personal as political. The legacy of Betty Friedan. In: *Age Matters. Realigning Feminist Thinking,*T.M. Calsanti & K.F. Slevin, (Eds), 21-45, Routledge, ISBN 978-0415952248, New York, USA

Sontag, S. (1972, 23 sept.). The double standard of aging. *Saturday Review,* pp. 29-38

Sorensen, G. & Verbrugge, L.M. (1987). Women, work, and health. *Annual Review of Public Health,* Vol.8, pp. 235-251, ISSN 01637525

Thomas, G. & Fogg, S. (2000). *The best times, the worst of times. Older woman's retirement experience. Messages for future older women (Report)*, Older Women's Network, ISBN 1-900578-16-6, Sydney, Australia

Tronto, J. C. (2000). Age-Segregated Housing As a Moral Problem: An Exercise in Rethinking Ethics. In: *Mother Time. Women, Aging and Ethics,* M.U. Walker, (Ed.), 261-277, Rowman & Littlefield, ISBN 978-0847692606, Lanham, UK

Valls, C.; Banqué, M.; Fuentes, M. & Ojuel, J. (2008). Morbilidad diferencial entre mujeres y hombres. *Anuario de Psicología,* Vol. 39, No.1, pp. 9-22, ISSN 0066-5126

Wolf, N. (1991). *The Beauty Myth*e, Morrow, ISBN 978-0060512187, New York, USA

Woodward, K. (Ed.). (1999). *Figuring Age. Women, Bodies, Generations,* Indiana University Press, ISBN 0-253-21236-7, Bloomington, In, USA

Woolf, V. (1938). *Three Guineas,* ISBN 0-7012-0949-6, Hogarth Press, London, UK

36

Multi-Purpose Activities in Ergotherapy

Hulya Yucel
*Department of Physiotherapy and Rehabilitation,
Faculty of Health Sciences, Bezmi Alem University, Istanbul,
Turkey*

1. Introduction

The elderly population, both in terms of number and relative percentage in society, is increasing throughout the world. Society, relative to previous generations, will be older with a greater burden on health system resources due to chronic ongoing disease and illness management requirements. The demand for services of geriatrics and gerontology in turn increases. Health planners, who define funding levels within government, are required to consider this increasing life expectancy. Long-term care of the unhealthy elderly is a much-debated medical and political issue in developing countries. As the experiences of successful aging increases within society today, attention focusses on what defines successful aging and the factors that promote a healthy aged community (Bowling & Iliffe, 2006). For this reason, World Health Organisation (WHO) described active ageing as improving life expectancy, productivity and quality of life by promoting and maintaining the highest functional capacity of social well-being and physical and mental functioning (WHO, 1998).

Loneliness, a condition relatively common in the elderly, is being increasingly linked to negative quality of life predictors such as chronic diseases, depression and reduced social participation (Alpass&Neville, 2003; Jylha, 2004; Routasalo, 2007). Thoughts of being closer to death, loss of mobility and family bereavement reduce the sense of taking pleasure in life, affecting the extent of community involvement and levels of independence (Alpass&Neville, 2003). This greater isolation from society inhibits effective social behaviour and facilitates passive roles in interactions involving the elderly (Vitkus& Horowitz, 1987). The resulting loneliness and social isolation negatively impacts the psychosocial situation of well-being, the quality of life and cognitive skills (Routasalo et al., 2007).

Researches suggest the interest in and skills associated with activities of daily living are reduced with aging, because of changes in health and social issues commonly experienced in the elderly (Clark&Siebens, 2005; Routasalo et al., 2007; WHO, 1998). Remaining physically, mentally and socially active, things like "doing work", has great importance in maintaining functioning as does the need to avoid excessive levels of the more passive recreations, such as watching television. Indeed, many problems derive from having more unstructured free time. Meaningful leisure time in the elderly is essential to a good quality of life. In Yucel's thesis, the majority of elderly people stated that in their free time, they like to be involved in tasks such as reading and walking. The respondents would prefer not to participate regularly in physical activities. They could not give a concrete reason for this behaviour. One plausable explanation is the elderly may not be conscious enough about the benefits of regular activity programs and the consequences of their relative withdrawal from these (Yucel, 2008).

In a study in Brazil, the lack of adequate financial resources (40.3%) along with fatigue (38.1%) were identified as obstacles to the participation of the elderly in leisure activities (Reichert et al., 2007). Motivation is critical to the success of activity programs designed for the elderly. Many elderly have concerns about participating in activity programs, because they have developed negative behaviors and beliefs throughout their lives associated with activity. Barriers to activity programmes, such as having to park their cars long distances away, along with other factors such as snow and ice, inhibit involvement. Reducing these barriers to exercise is necessary for a more independent and "strong" elderly community (Resnick, 1991; Yoshimoto & Kawata, 1996).

Participating in activities and social integration is one of the important approaches to rehabilitation in the elderly. Ergotherapy programs are created to help to protect life roles in geriatrics. They promote active aging and overall quality of life through participation in activities designed and prescribed to the needs of the individuals (Boswell et al., 1997; Rosalie, 2003). Activity training, which facilitates an active aging process, is an important part of a comprehensive ergotherapy program in the elderly. It aims to care about health, to increase cognitive, emotional and physical capabilities, and ensure the independence of social functions through the choice of different activities in accordance with the individual requirements and needs of the elderly (Donohue et al., 1995; Lachenmayr&Mackenzie, 2004; Nelson, 1997; Vass et al., 2005).

In a survey of 815 elderly participants in Australia, the most desired activities overall were golf, walking, tennis and swimming. The underlying objectives of these activities were to stay healthy, that they were interested in that activity, they wanted to improve their physical capacity and maintain their overall joint mobility (Kolt et al., 2004). The quality of life of older people engaged in activities of their own choice were higher (Duncan-Myers&Huebner, 2000). Conversely, over 80% of elderly people in America spent their free time by visiting friends, watching television and listening to the radio (Lee&King, 2003). The type of activity is less important, because the differences reflect variables such as the individual's health, associated abilities and socio-economic status, than the actual participation itself. Participation is a stronger predictor of quality of life than the type of activity (Ward, 1979).

The maintenance of health and quality of life in older clientele is promoted through the participation in meaningful and purposeful activities (Csikszentmihaly, 1993; Glantz, 1996). The study of Inal et al. showed that life satisfaction scores are significantly higher in elderly people who are interested in a variety of crafts and regular walking (Inal, 2003). In people with life-long activity goals, such as participating in regular physical activity, the normal physiological changes that occur with aging were seen to be delayed or less severe. Elderly people who have defined leisure time activities have a higher quality of life.

Furthermore, Routasalo et al. (2007) showed increased psychological well-being and improved cognitive skills in the elderly by the implementation of activity training. The type of activity prescribed needs to be based on the individual. Studies have showed that leisure / hobbies / social activities are preferred for elderly that have mental health problems rather than physical problems (Mountain, 2005a). Cognitive tests increased significantly in patients with vascular dementia by applied activity treatment (Nagaya et al., 2005). These results suggest that activity training may be protective against the formation of a new dementia. Further investigation into the capacity of multi-purpose activity to inhibit the development of conditions such as depression and dementia in the elderly is necessary.

Whether activity prescribed to the elderly is given on an individual basis or should constitute a group format is open to debate. Researchers following the second world war investigated group behaviour. They concluded people need each other, not just to maintain themselves, but also to feel fulfilled in their lives. The most basic group is family with the members sharing responsibilities and performing required specific tasks. Families expanded roles includes activity such as plays, school activities and the involvement in religious and recreational organizations. All which enhance the integration of life goals and promote the individual's overall quality of life (Matsuo et al., 2003; Royeen & Reistetter, 1996; Yucel et al, 2006a). Some people are social, enjoy spending time with others, while others would prefer to be alone. Some still enjoy making new discoveries, while others want to continue with long-standing interests. Whether the activities are completed as an individual or in a group, whether they are novel or long standing, best reflects the needs and wants of the individual. The elderly should be encouraged to participate in activities appropriate for, and which interest, them. The regular continuity of activities is an important factor in enhancing quality of life.

Future research exploring concepts such as the reintroduction of extinct roles to the elderly, or increasing the diversity of the types of activity undertaken within a specific role, and the implications on quality of life and life satisfaction are necessary. Studies in different ethnic or cultural groups should be encouraged (Ross, 1990). Elderly people need increased diversity of activities to maximize the process of an active older age. Future education and training of health workers in geriatrics is necessary to promote a conciousness of the importance of roles in health outcomes and to provide the skills that facilitate the prescription of optimal activity; activity that best reflects the needs and wants of the individual older person. Activities are as necessary as eating or drinking and to have life; each individual should have regular activity within and outside the home based on their roles and physical and mental health.

This chapter will be issued as below:

Ergoterapy Approaches in Geriatrics, Importance of Leisure Time Activities, Multi-purpose Activities, Activity Training Models, Activity Training, Group Activities.

2. Ergotherapy aproaches

In geriatric rehabilitation, it is important to improve functional capacity and daily living skills of elderly, personal care about areas such as hygiene, rest and nutrition, and to ensure social-emotional support (Lewis&Bottomley, 2002). The goal should be to maintain the independence on functionality of the elderly or to restore if it is decreased.

Considering the following points facilitates to plan appropriate rehabilitation program in geriatrics:

1. There can be the capacity differences among elderly. In training programs which is planned within the scope of rehabilitation for the elderly, the capacity of individuals has to be known. Chosen approach is not important for any activity training for strengthening, but there are some circumstances to be considered peculiar to elderly. For example, late pupil dilation and thickening of the lens with aging mean

environmental clarity and projection can not be tolerated. Therefore three times much light are needed for function of the aged eyes. Additionally, the elderly can not detect the color differentiation which is necessary for driving, Activities of Daily Living (ADL) and ambulation. Such physiological changes affect the functionality of the elderly.

2. The level of activity differs from one aged to the other. For example, a 80 year old can fulfill the physical and cognitive functions whilst the other of the same age may not success.
3. Maximal health is directly associated with the maximal functional ability. Activities that give energy to the elderly to be alive and aim to provide independence in an active life and maintain health should be given to the elderly (Larson et al., 1986; Mountain, 2005a).

Day-care services in geriatric rehabilitation include observation of the elderly by caretakers, caregiver training, daily regular controls of drug intake etc., implementation of treatment services and social / recreational activities. General social services allow older people to maintain their lives in an appropriate environment. And also, they undertake transfer to the hospital and home from the hospital, prevention of diseases and preventive treatment. On the other hand, ergotherapy approaches come into prominence in determining the needs of the elderly, planning/implementation/monitoring of nursing program and revealing of changing needs over time (Mountain, 2005b).

Ergotherapy in geriatric rehabilitation mainly includes the following goals (Yucel, 2006b):

- To maintain basic and enstrumental ADL successfully by increasing physical and/or mental activity performance,
- To restore decreased ability and to improve or maintain quality of life,
- To help to continue on social habits in a society and provide psychosocial support and
- To provide educational support for caregivers.

There are some important cases to be considered in therapy sessions (Lewis&Bottomley, 2002):

1. An therapist who is more patient, relevant, knowledgeable and trustable, reduces the tension of the environment. During therapy session, the most important cause of high anxiety in the elderly is being fumble in front of family members and their own therapists, and fear of humiliation. Therefore, characteristics of therapists are important for the elderly to learn, in terms of providing psychological comfort.
2. Making frequent changes in the curriculum and environment of the elderly should be avoided as much as possible. Since unknown environment will bother elderly, training in their natural ambient is recommended. Once ability is gained, to adapt it to different environments later on will be more suitable.
3. The opportunity of visits to friends and relationships should be given to elderly to be social.
4. It should be put emphasis on family / caregiver training/ support. Family / caregiver training in assessment and treatment of the elderly is important. Because family members and caregivers provide actual physical and emotional support for the elderly. Therefore, their role in the solution of problems should be noted (Larson et al., 1986).
5. Physical and psychological comfort is essential. Ergonomic factors such as noise level, colors, lighting, ventilation, room temperature, comfortance of chair, table height and slipperiness of the floor should be considered. For example, the sounds of water or a computer come from behind should be eliminated.

6. To cope with a feeling of loneliness in the elderly:
   - meaningful relationships are developed,
   - recognizing the names of the people is encouraged to say
   - they are asked to remember the dates of birthdays accurately
   - communicating with plants, animals and children are provided
   - motivation for having something belong to them is provided and
   - alternative occupations are generated.
7. To strengthen the memory in the elderly;
   - audio-visual signals are used to introduce an object to be named permanently
   - principles of vocal motivation are applied to emphasize what is important in their lives
   - they are encouraged to tell their past experiences and to explain and discuss previous achievements
   - they are given sufficient time to remember the events
   - strategical games like chess take part of the programmes.

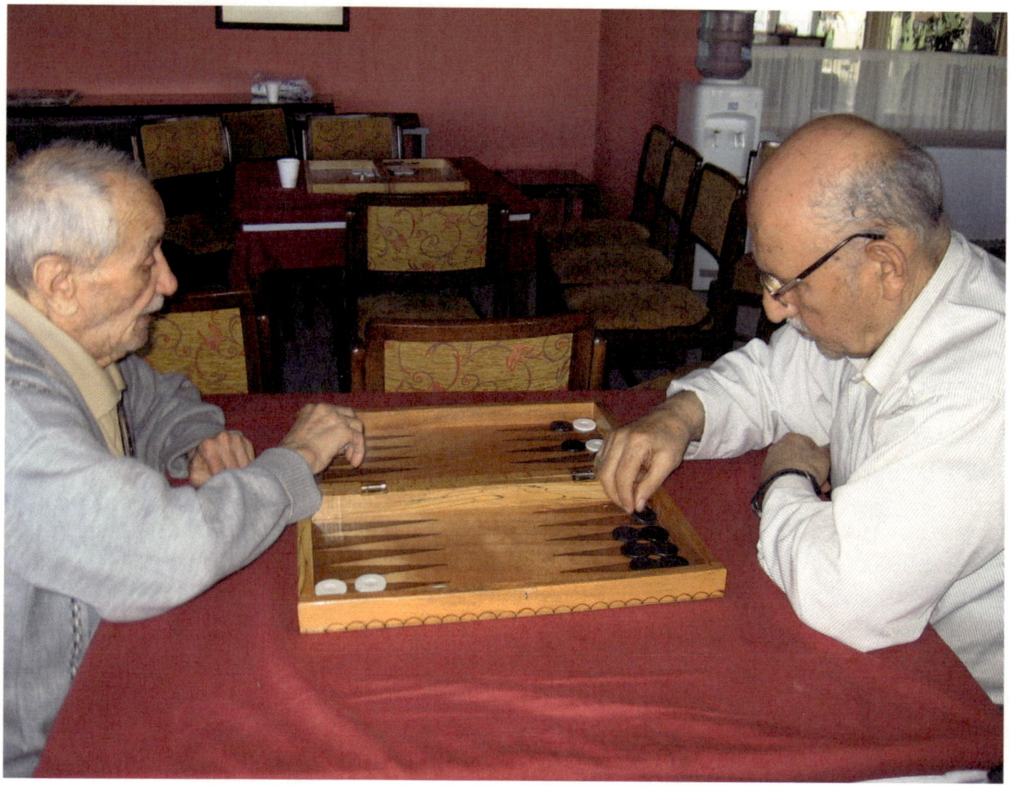

Fig. 1. Backgammon as a cognitive activity for memory strengthening

In ergotherapy, it is possible to increase skills such as spatial orientation, inductive thinking, fluid intelligence, problem solving and memory flexibility by using different methods. The advanced methods of testing and training are expected to contribute more higher-quality, productive and happy aging by reducing the decline in cognitive skills or by emphasizing cognitive characteristics during this period (Glantz, 1996). Reaching up and bending forward exercises or imagery exercises created from picking up apple from the tree, getting money from ground are effective in the elderly. Imagery exercises develops coordination and cognitive functions. They allow interactive training, because of facilitating a person to format an object mentally (Clark & Siebens, 2005; Nelson, 1997).

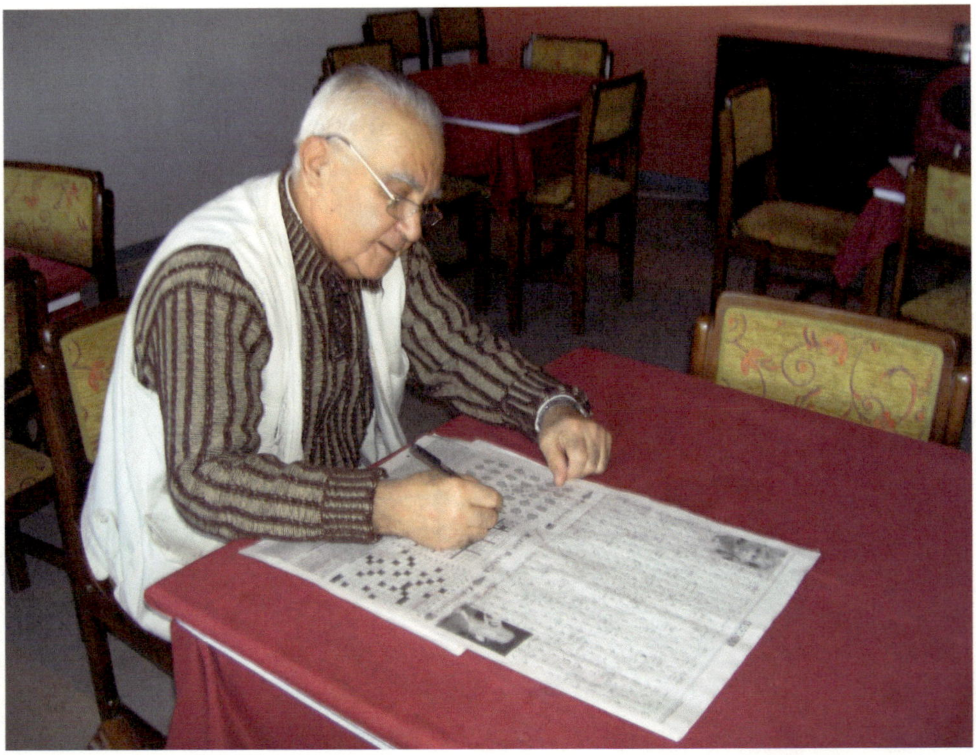

Fig. 2. Making puzzle and crosswords contributes to the cognitive health

Ergotherapy programs promote active aging and overall quality of life through participation in activities designed and prescribed to the needs of the individuals. The culture, satisfaction, motivation, interests and role in society of a person are taken into account. Elderly are encouraged to continue their habits and activities such as; gardening, non-strenuous sports, painting, handicrafts, building up a collection, simple repair work, singing and movie watching, which they used to enjoy participation. With some suggestions like "go on vacation, make hobbies and sports" elderly are removed from inactivity and negative psychology.

Old age is generally a period of limited environment. In fact, not only aging, but also an un-well organised environment for elderly restricts their power to live alone (Larson et al., 1986; Yucel et al., 2006a). Many elderly are not aware of being at risk of falling. 85% of falls happens especially on the stairs at home in the bathroom and bedroom. Therefore, this situation reveals that environmental changes and adaptations are needed for elderly to survive independently and self-sufficiently (Yucel et al., 2006a).

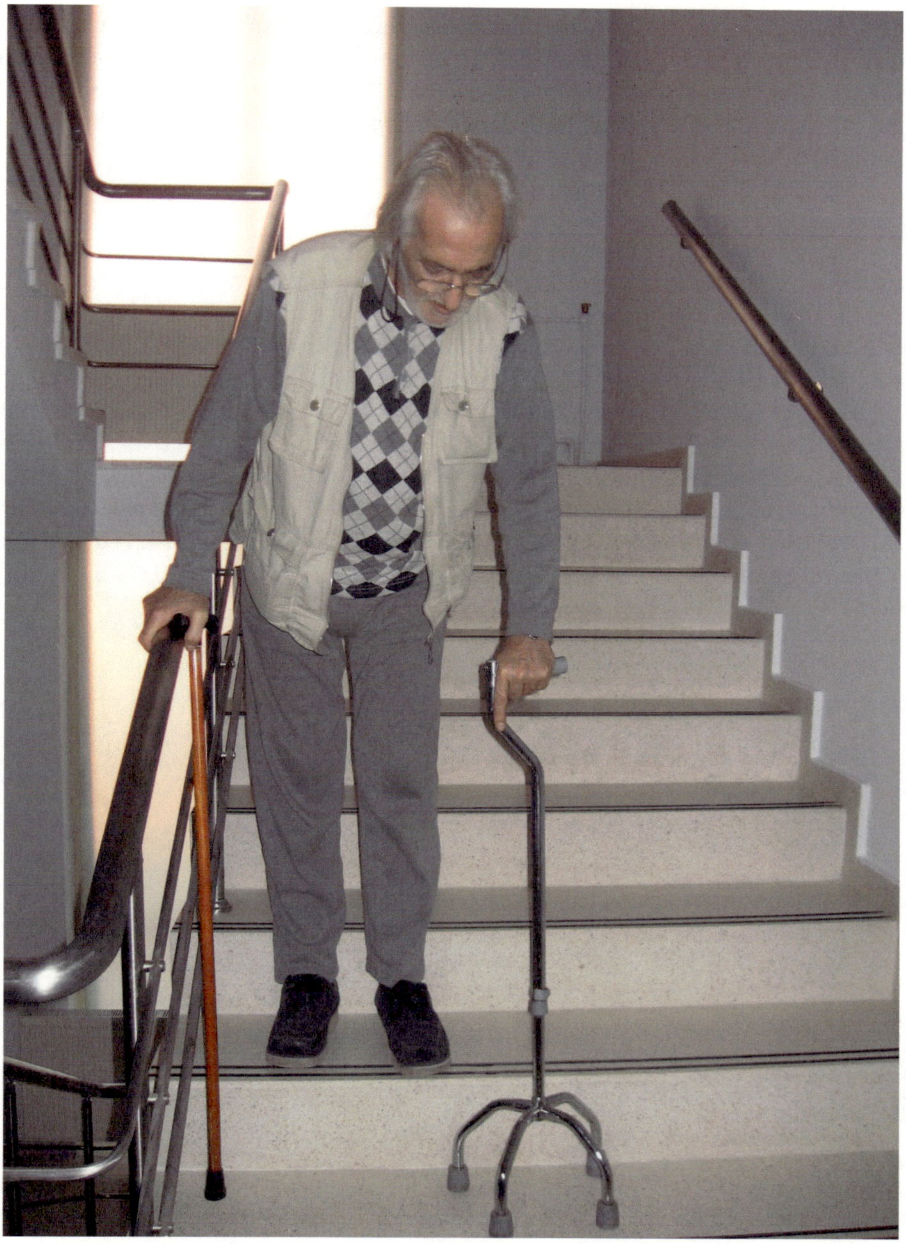

Fig. 3. Ergonomic accessibility with proper devices

Assistive aids such as walker should be suggested to increase stability during walking and to relieve stress in painful joints. An ergotherapist is needed to teach the use of assistive aids and joint protection techniques. Safety modifications and family / caregiver / elderly training reduce dangers. And providing adaptive tools which are necessary for age-related changes, positioning, teaching transfers and ambulation, training about health and prevention techniques and home exercise programs to increase the independence are the major topics of work field of a geriatric ergotherapist (Pu&Nelson, 2004).

As a result, service of the targeted rehabilitation to a person is the cornerstone of ergotherapy. Ergotherapy includes ADL, instrumental ADL, psychosocial well being, caregiver training, vocational rehabilitation, social / recreational leisure activities, lifestyle redesign, public health and environmental regulations for performing the roles successfully (Mountain, 2005a).

3. Leisure time activities

During lifelong, towards from young adulthood to middle age, interests and desires increase. Having more free time gives a person the opportunity to involve in an activity. But, leisure time activities in the elderly are more passive and home based. The time spent in outside cultural activities is quite less (Crombie et al., 2004). Older people often spend their times by visiting friends, listening to the radio, watching television and reading at their homes (Lee&King, 2003). Outdoor activities such as; sports, going to the theatre and cinema are activities with less continuity. There are some studies showing that this condition and low levels of recreational activity in the elderly are associated with changes in their body function (e.g. excess body mass index), marital status, low education level, male gender, genetic and metabolic factors (Mc Pherson&Kozlik, 1987; Mouton et al.,2000; Strain et al., 2002; Ross,1990).

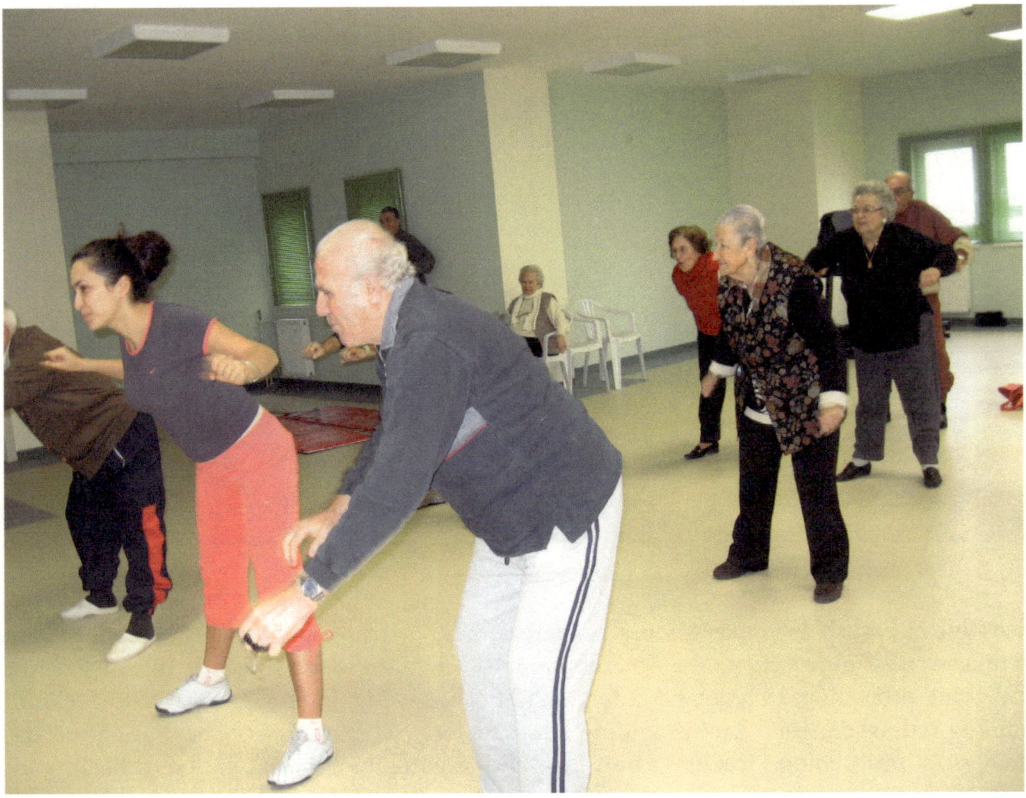

Fig. 4. Older people should participate in physical recreational activities

The habits of regular participation in physical activities among the elderly are decreased physiologically (Dipietro, 2001). Activities such as cycling are non-preferred activities, because they may often cause injuries (Gerson& Stevens, 2004). In literature there are some studies showing that male elderly are more active, but the role of women in recreational activities are more than men. Conversely, some studies show that women have less leisure time activity (Bruce & Devine, 2002).

Activity restriction in the elderly may be due to functional limitations in areas, such as vision, hearing and mobility (Cambois et al., 2005; Donohue et al., 1995). In a study in the United States, it has been shown that approximately 10% of the elderly have visual impairments cause depression, social dysfunction and lack of activity (Donohue et al., 1995). In the elderly with severe cognitive problems, some failures in memory, expression, orientation, visual perception and other complex abilities are obstacles that elderly require higher cortical functions to participate in some activities (Adler, 1997).

Elderly's interests and skills to leisure time activities may also be reduced due to changes in health and other social areas with ageing (Clark&Siebens, 2005; Routasalo et al., 2007; World Health Organisation (WHO)). Motivation is critical to the success of activity programs designed for the elderly. Many elderly have concerns about participating in activity programs, because they have developed negative behaviors and beliefs throughout their lives associated with activity. Barriers to activity programmes, such as having to park their cars long distances away, along with other factors such as snow and ice, inhibit involvement. Reducing these barriers to exercise is necessary for a more independent and "robust" elderly community (Resnick, 1991; Yoshimoto & Kawata, 1996).

4. Multi-purpose activities

Multi-purpose activities in ergotherapy programs have a positive impact on the independence of the elderly rather than delays of motor aging process. Scientists in twenty first century, specialized in therapeutic recreational activities, have begun to work to find significant and meaningful activities for the elderly (Cottrell, 1996; Heuvelen et al., 1998).

Snoezelen sensory training spreads over a wide area in clinical practice from learning disorders to dementia in the past decade. In this method, primary visual, hearing, touch, taste and smell senses are stimulated with the effect of light, soothing music, touch and relaxation oils (Chung et al., 2002; Lynch& Aspnes, 2004). Besides that vision and hearing are basic requirements of communication, touch is also an important physical sensation component. These sensory inputs should be taken into account in planning a major activity program for the elderly (Lewis& Bottomley, 2002).

Recreational rehabilitation in occupations such as; board games, handicrafts, playing a musical instrument, playing volleyball with balloon and dancing performs cognitive function activation by increasing the blood flow rate of the prefrontal region. There are some studies showed that having been in a leisure time activity like purposeful cognitive activities, such as reading at least two times a week significantly reduces the risk of dementia (Nagaya et al., 2005; Scarmeas et al., 2001; Yucel et al., 2006b, 2010).

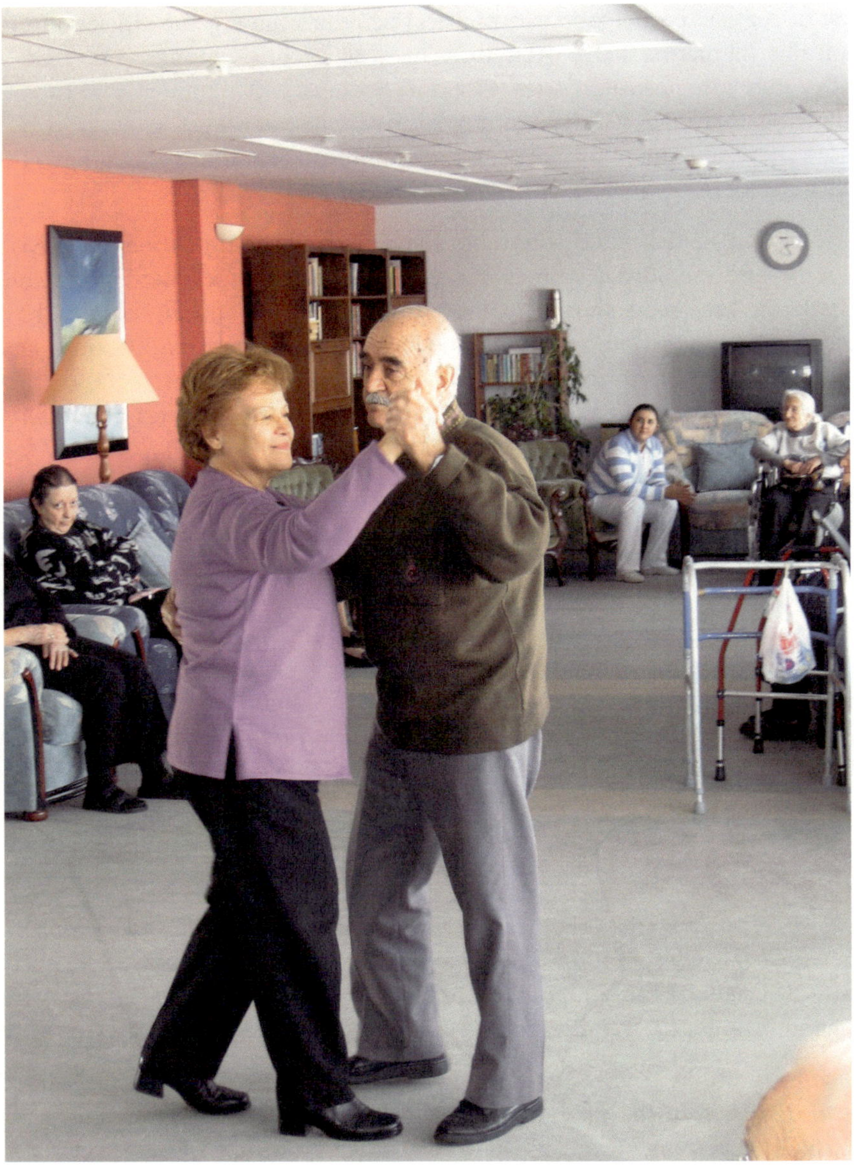

Fig. 5. Dancing performs cognitive function activation

Elderly are the people who are at risk for anxiety and depression. Social participations in activities such as painting, making music and religious meetings protect elderly from these risks (Lynch&Aspnes, 2004). In a study in the UK, it is stated that many activities are not effective as much as participating in religious gatherings that have a significant impact on well-being and quality of life in aged 50-74 (Routasalo et al.; 2007; Warr et al., 2004). Visiting friends and participating in social groups have positive effects on being healthy, having regular physical activities and carrying out ADL independently (Yoshimoto& Kawata, 1996). Reading is recommended in order to organize the behavior of depressive people and remove negative thoughts (Lynch& Aspnes, 2004). Baklien and Carlsson said that visiting a library and borrowing books keep people intellectually active (Baklien & Carlsson, 2000, as cited in Wikstrom, 2004).

One of the primary modalities used to treat depression in the elderly is medicine. However, taking anti-depressants without knowing the underlying reason can cause serious side effects. Therefore, alternative therapies are needed. There are many non-pharmacological treatment methods, such as the real orientation, behavioral therapy, sensory stimulation, music therapy and ergotherapy. Reminiscence therapy is also one of them. It is an effective method to gain self-confidence, socialization, well-being, expression and cognitive function. Reminiscence means discussion with a person or a group about activities, events and experiences done in the past, with the help of photos and / or music archive. The elderly indicate that they feel relaxed when they remember nice memories while looking at photo albums. This method reminds all the elderly of having lived a whole life and it still continues (Royeen & Reistetter, 1996; Stinson & Kirk, 2006; Woods et al., 2005).

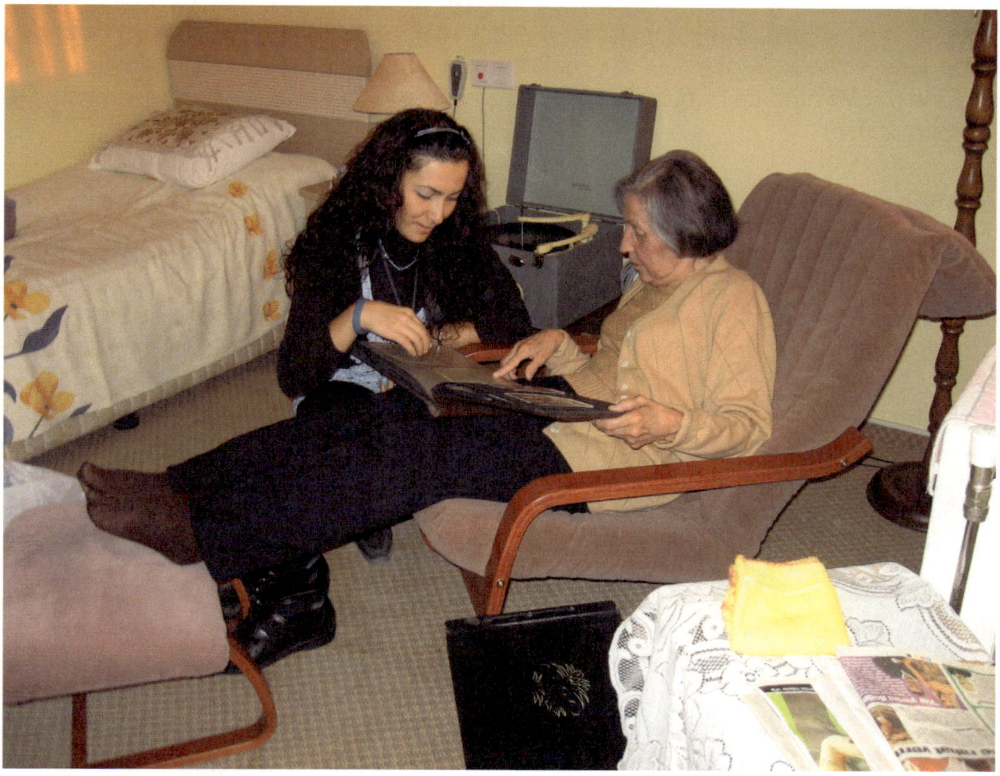

Fig. 6. Reminiscence therapy

Activities like looking at photo gallery and dancing are important for successful aging and perform daily activities independently. This kind of activities help the elderly to know that they are prepared for changing conditions, express themselves, change their perspectives about the life. Painting or deal with a music are a visual and auditory experience for them (Wikstrom, 2004). That the music takes place in activities becomes a positive influence on well-being of the elderly, especially who has depression and cognitive problems. Music therapy is a proven, easily accessible and useful method to be able to cope with behavior problems such as stress and anxiety. Activities with musics which old people's own choices are both suitable for the control of agitated behavior and cheap. Carefully selected music tone, type and rythm are important to make activities fun. Light and mid-rythmical music is preferred. Music therapy in different categories, such as orchestral music, piano and jazz, decreases the heart rate and respiratory rate, increases body temperature and also the body relaxation (Hsu& Lai, 2004; Lai, 1999, 2004; Lou, 2001; Sherratt et al., 2004; Sung& Chang, 2005; Hanser & Thompson, 1994). Nevertheless, another study has indicated that music does not have any effect on pain perception in stroke patients having upper extremity exercises (Kim&Koh, 2005). Playing a musical instrument is an effective activity to avoid the elderly from isolation and increase their socialization, and make their free time full (Zelazny, 2001).

Creative activities reduce depression and isolation, and increases the power of decision-making of the elderly. Art is a way of opening people's emotional windows and sensory capacity. This kind of activities allow the elderly to express themselves, permit positive effects of well-being, enable physical, sensory-motor and cognitive therapy and teach appropriate ways to respond to the challenges of passing years. For the aforementioned reasons activities hold an important role in ergotherapy (Callanan, 1994; Hannemann, 2006; Mountain, 2005b).

5. Activity training models

There are some basic models that activity training based on the elderly. According to the activity treatment model developed by Mosey in 1977 in the U.S., people's capabilities which are necessary to survive in a wide range of the community are enhanced. This model has been developed to understand why therapists should make assessment and treatment and they suggest specific activities or plan activities in a specific approach to a person. This activity model lost their validity today, because it could not provide an improvement due to focus on personal development. Other models have been developed based on roles. They allow short-term applications. The Canadian Model of Occupational Performance (CMOP) and The Model of Human Occupation (MOHO) are two of them. In these new models, cognitive and behavioral approaches took part in place of psychodynamic perspectives (Chacksfield, 2006; Forsyth & Kielhofner, 2006; Sumsion & Blank, 2006).

CMOP is focused on how a person is successful in self-care and productivity and how he/she performs the roles in leisure time activities and how much satisfaction gives this to him/her. MOHO emphasized on the personal preferences, habits, roles and performance capacity. For example, an elderly person with dementia has to carry out the activity of making a cup of tea. Talking, willingness, motor / physical / cognitive / mental abilities are required for this activity. Social and physical environment, routine work, past experiences and expectations, etc. are questioned by ergotherapist. Both models are not only in activity training, but nowadays also used frequently in all ergotherapy interventions for all the health problems that can be seen throughout the life.

6. Activity training

Activity training, which began to be more popular in the 1940's, is a part of a comprehensive rehabilitation program in the elderly who want to have active aging. It aimes to keep life healthy, increase cognitive, emotional and physical capabilities, ensure the independence of social functions through purposeful and appropriate activities designed to the desires and needs of the elderly (Donohue et al., 1995; Lachenmayr & Mackenzie, 2004; Maestre Castelblanque & Albert Cunat, 2005; Nelson, 1997; Vass et al., 1995). Older people find an opportunity to apply activities through their own choice for the expectations, that make them have more higher quality of life (Duncan-Myers & Huebner, 2000).

Ergotherapy plays a significant role to develop the skills in leisure time activities (Glantz, 1996). Ergotherapist explaines the meaning of one's activity by revealing age, gender, role performances, cultural values, wishes and preferences of a person. Evaluation of the special functional activity skills is one of the duty of ergotherapist (Mountain, 2005b). Ergotherapist recommends the elderly activities and social relationships to carry out daily activities, continue existing skills for social integration and gain new skills. Advices to continue a quiet and relax life, listening to the songs of the past, talking to tell, watching the beautiful scenery, being sufficient on maintaining self care, go for shopping, cooking and house cleaning, do sports/water exercises and acquisition of new hobbies are effective for the elderly. Accordingly, these activities help elderly to gain and protect abilities in fields such as communication, cognitive functions or hand motor control. Multi-purpose activity approaches aim to improve special functionality, reintegration activities supported by lifestyle / behavioral and family education, sensory stimulation, encourage the elderly to express themselves and ADL training (Wikstrom, 2004; Yucel et al., 2010).

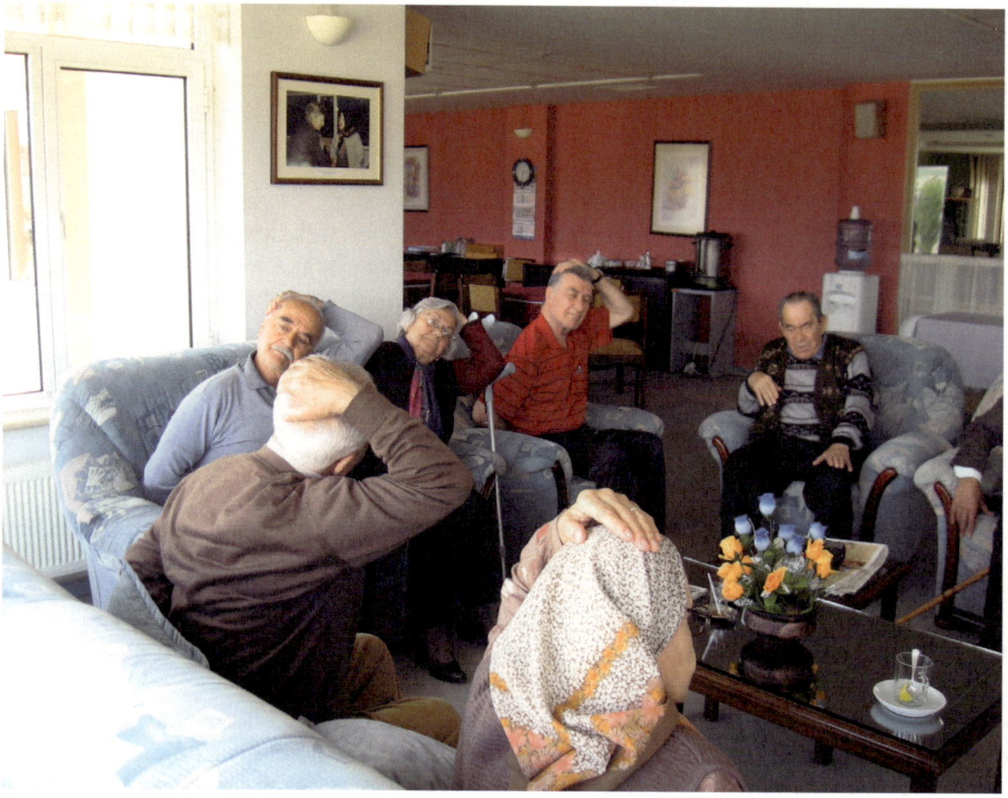

Fig. 7. Group exercise as multi-purpose activities

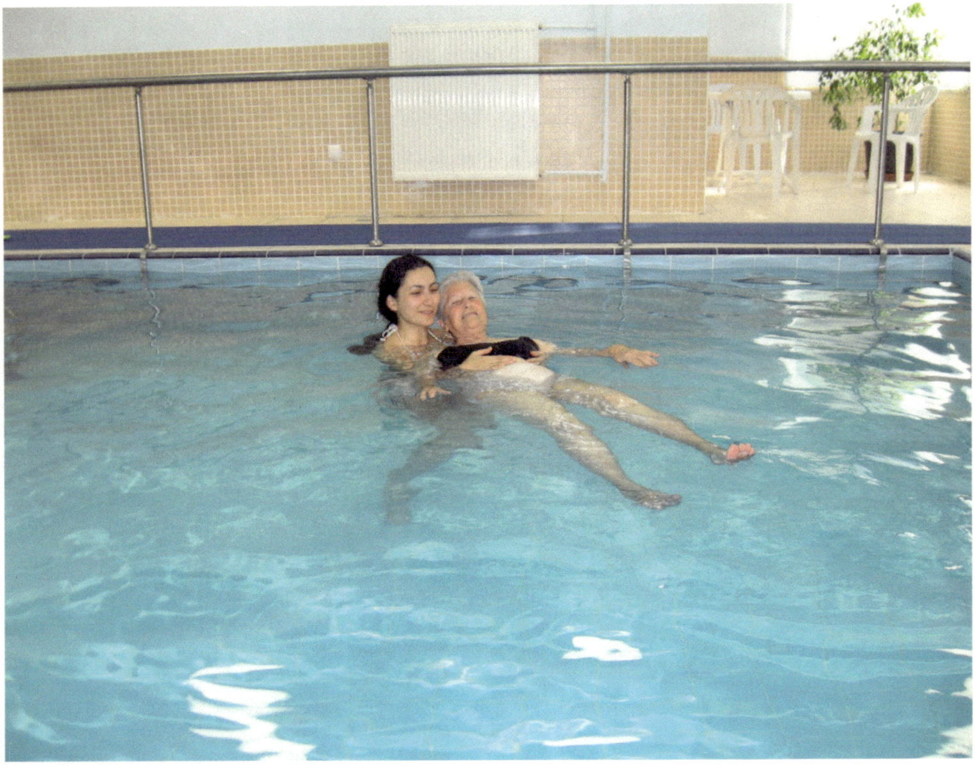

Fig. 8. Water exercises as an activity training method

The effects of multi-purpose activity training in the elderly:

1. It improves physical/psychosocial health and well-being.
2. It reduces the feeling of loneliness and establishes a close relationship with environment and increases the verbal interaction. Therefore, the elderly in a society peel off a thought of seeing themselves as redundant individuals. It is provided that the society accepts older people as unique individuals.
3. It provides environmental awareness, increases attention and problem-solving ability; reduces orientation distortion, and improves memory.
4. It decreases secondary complications such as decubitus ulcer, urinary tract infection, and it is protective against hypertension, diabetes mellitus, some cancers, osteporosis and depression (Crespo & Keteyian, 1996; Pang et al., 2005).
5. It reduces vital risk factors and contributes to the long-term protection of health status.

7. Group activities

There are many studies in the literature given activities to the elderly as individual or set in groups. However, general opinion is on behalf of effectiveness of group activity sessions. Because it is protective against feeling of loneleness and a lack of hope (Hannemann, 2006). Group activities develop self confidence, cognitive skills and ability of planning. Making a decision becomes easier. The elderly see their own prodecutivity, feel more comfortable and happy, and become more social in group (Landi et al., 1997).

Group activity is a modality which people, selected carefully, need emotional or physical support, are involved into a group by a trained therapist to help each other. Objectives of group activities are to increase awareness and to develop interpersonal and social skills by interaction with the other group members who provide feedback through behaviors. Compared to individual activities, the two main strong points of group activities are that the person can receive immediate feedback from their peers and there is an opportunity for therapist to observe the psychological, emotional and behavioral responses of each person.

Mills offers six different approaches to work with small group of models (Royeen & Reistetter, 1996):

1. Mechanical model: It is a model of mutual interaction with being independent from emotion, norms and believes. Each member controls the behaviors of other members of the group.
2. Organism model: In this model, group looks like a biological organism. Each member of the group has different role and responsibility due to his/her nature.
3. Complex model: This model advocates that independence in the changing needs of people and their obtained resources are limited.
4. Balance model: This model ensures a balance between internal needs and external requirements of the group.
5. Structural functional model: It is a model not only increases its resources, but it is also willing to change the structure and function of the group.
6. Growth model: This model develops depending on the capacity of members of the group and processes information.

Duncombe and Howe have formed ten different ergotherapy groups (Duncombe & Howe, 1985, as cited in Royeen& Reistetter, 1996):

1. Exercise group: Groups are generally formed in such exercises as volleyball, bowling and ping pong in rehabilitation centers and schools.
2. Dining group: This kind of groups are generally being in psychology and rehabilitation programs. Activities in these groups have menu planning, shopping, cooking and eating sections.
3. ADL Group: In these groups, people are prepared to live independently in the community by increasing the required self-care skills.
4. Handicraft group: In this group, art and craft skills are used for psychosocial evaluation and treatment of disabilities.
5. Task group: This group gives social, recreational and educational activities in tasks such as organizing a picnic and publishing newspaper to facilitate communication and socialization.
6. Self-expression group: In this group, interactive work among members is provided to the elderly with pictures, music and self-awareness exercises.
7. Reality orientation discussion group: Role simulation is provided to improve socialization and communication skills in this group.
8. Sensory-motor and sensory integration groups: Thorough these groups, integration of physical skills and sensory development are aimed to increase in the individuals with a wide range of problems like learning disabilities, hearing and visual problems and lack of sense of integrity.

9. Oriented sensation groups: Performing some roles in the style of the game and discussing in poetry and fantasy groups are performed in these groups.
10. Education group: There are groups, individuals and their families receive and discuss information on issues such as drugs.

There are some important factors to consider to determine the suitability of a person in a group (Ozmenler, 2005):

1. The possibility of a high level of a peer anxiety in a person, who has a negative reaction to be in a group, should be considered. Elderly who have destructive relationships with their peers do not want to be in a group, but that will be useful, if they can come to deal with being in a group. On the other hand, those who worry about authority too much, usually with fear of a therapist criticism, may be reluctant to express their thoughts and feelings in a seperate media. So that, they may accept the group as a nice treat and generally prefer group activities. Group media is more comfortable, because of being usually bilateral (one to one) environment (Landi et al., 1997).
2. Determining of impairments of the elderly is important to choose the best activity approach and assess their motivations, capacities and the strengths and weaknesses in their personality. For example, antisocial people do not find a heterogeneous group good and do not accept group standards.
3. It is needed that the therapist gives a detailed depiction of the process to the elderly as possible and to responds every question of the elderly.
4. Group activities are successful in three to fifteen members. Mostly groups with eight to ten members are preferred. The sufficient interactions may not be received in small groups with fewer members. With more than 10 members, the members or the therapist can not follow what is going on. Small groups are the smallest representatives of large communities. It may be difficult to work with large group. So, small groups are preferred (Royeen& Reistetter, 1996).
5. Groups are collected two times per week. One is with therapist and the other one is without therapist. It is important to maintain continuity of sessions. Usually group sessions take 1-2 hours. The time limit should be fixed.
6. Educational planning for the elderly often takes place in ergotherapy training programs. Visual aids and adaptations are used, such as timing and the number used for each person in the group.

The effectiveness of group activities are measured as follows:

How much did the group members reach the objectives?
What is satisfaction level in each individual?
What are quality and quantity of the product?

As a conclusion, good planning should be done in order to encourage the elderly to participate in the activity regularly and continuity. National campaigns are expected to be necessary and effective for the elderly to change perceptions about their levels of physical activity.

8. References

Adler, G. (1997). Driving and dementia: dilemmas and decisions. *Geriatrics,* 52, pp. 26-29, ISSN 0016-867X

Alpass, F.M. & Neville, S. (2003). Loneliness, health and depression in older males. *Aging and Mental Health,* 7 (3), pp. 212-216, ISSN1360-7863

Boswell, R.B.; Dawson, M. & Heininger, R. (1997). Quality of life defined by adults with spinal cord injuries. *Perceptual Motor Skills,* 84 (3), pp. 1140-1149, ISSN 0031-5125

Bowling, A. & Iliffe, S. (2006). Which model of successful aging should be used? Baseline findings from a British longitudinal survey of ageing. *Age Ageing,* 35 (6), pp. 607-14, ISSN 0002-0729

Bruce, D.G. & Devine, A. (2002). Recreational physical activity levels in healthy older women: The importance of fear of falling. *Journal of American Geriatric Society,* 50, pp. 84-89.

Callanan, B.O. (1994). Art therapy with the frail elderly. The *Journal of Long Term Home Health Care. The PRIDE Institute Journal,* 3 (2), pp. 20-23, ISSN 1072-4281

Cambois, E.; Robine, J.M. & Romieu, I. (2005). The influence of functional limitations and various demographic factors on self reported activity restriction at older ages. *Disability and Rehabilitation,* 5; 27 (15), pp. 871- 883, ISSN 0963-8288

Chacksfield, J. (2006). Activities therapy. In: *Foundations for practice in occupational therapy,* E.A. Duncan (Ed.), pp. 143-259, Elsevier Churchill Livingstone, London.

Chung, J.C.; Lai, C.K.; Chung, P.M. & French, H.P. (2002). Snoezelen for dementia. *Cochrane Database of Systematic Reviews*, (4): CD003152.

Clark, G.S. & Siebens, H.C. (2005). Geriatric Rehabilitation, In: *Physical Medicine and Rehabilitation,* J. Lisa (Ed.). pp.1531-1560, Lippincott Williams Wilkins, Philadelphia.

Cottrell, F.R.P. (1996). *Perspectives on purposeful activity: Foundation and future of occupational therapy.* The American Occupational Therapy Assosiation, Inc., USA.

Crespo, C. J. & Keteyian, S. J. (1996). Leisure-time physical activity among US Adults. Results from the third national health nutrition examination survey. *Arcieves of Internal Medicine,* 156, pp. 93-98, ISSN 0003-9926

Crombie, I.K.; Irvine, L. & Williams, B. (2004). Why older people do not participate in leisure time physical activity: asurvey activity levels, beliefs and deterrents. *Age Aging,* 33 (3), pp. 287-292, ISSN 0002-0729.

Csikszentmihaly, M. (1993). Activities and happiness: towards a science of occupation. *Journal of Occupational Science.* 1 (1), pp. 38-42.

Dipietro, L. (2001). Physical activity in aging: Changes in patterns and their relationship to health and function. *Journal of Gerontology,* 56A, pp. 13-22.

Donohue, B.; Acierno, R.; Hersen, M. & van Hasselt, V.B. (1995). Social skills training for depressed, visually impaired older adults. A treatment manual. *Behavioral Medicine.* 19 (4), pp. 379-424, ISSN 0896-4289

Duncan-Myers, A.M. & Huebner, R.A. (2000). Relationship between choice and quality of life among residents in long-term-care facilities. *American Journal of Occupational Therapy,* 54 (5), pp. 504-508, ISSN 0272-9490

Forsyth, K. & Kielhofner, G. (2006). The model of human occupation integrating theory into practice and practice into theory. In: *Foundations for practice in occupational therapy,* E.A. Duncan (Ed.), pp. 80-108, Elsevier Churchill Livingstone, London.

Gerson, L.W. & Stevens, J.A. (2004). Recreational injuries among older Americans. *Injury Prevention,* 10 (3), pp. 134-138, ISSN 1353-8047

Glantz, C.H. (1996). Evaluation and intervention for leisure activities. K.O. Larson (Ed.). *The role of occupational therapy with elderly (ROTE).* (s. 729-741). The American Occupational Therapy Association,USA.

Hannemann, B.T. (2006). Creativity with dementia patients. Can creativity and art stimulate dementia patients positively? *Gerontology,* 52 (1), pp. 59-65.

Hanser, S.B. & Thompson, L.W. (1994). Effects of a music therapy strategy on depressed older adults. *Journal of Gerontology,* 49 (6), pp. 265-269.

Heuvelen, M.G.; Kempen, G.M.; Ormel, J. & Rispens, P. (1998). Physical fitness related to age physical activity in older persons. *Medicine and Science in Sports Exercise,* 30 (3), pp. 434-441, ISSN 0195-9131

Hsu, W.C. & Lai, H.L. (2004). Effects of music on major depression in psychiatric inpatients. *Archives of Psychiatric Nursing,* 18 (5), pp. 193-199, ISSN 0883-9417

Inal, S.; Subaşı, F.; Ay Mungan, S.; Uzun, S.; Alpkaya, U.; Hayan, O. & Akarçay, V. (2003). Yaşlıların Fiziksel Kapasitelerinin ve Yaşam Kalitelerinin Değerlendirilmesi, *Geriatri* 6 (3), pp. 95-99.

Jylha, M. (2004). Old age and loneliness: cross-sectional and longitudinal analyses in Tampere longitudinal study on aging. *Canadian Journal of Aging,* 23 (2), pp. 157-168, ISSN 0714-9808

Kim, S.J.& Koh, I. (2005). The effects of music on pain perception of stroke patients during upper extremity joint exercises. *Journal of Music Therapy,* 42 (1), pp. 81-92, ISSN 0022-2917

Kolt, G.S; Driver, R.P. & Gilles, L.C. (2004). Why older Australians participate in exercise and sport.. *Journal of Aging and Physical Activity,* 12(2), pp. 185-198, ISSN 1063-8652

Lachenmayr, S. & Mackenzie, G. (2004). Building a foundation systems change: increasing access to physical activity programs for older adults. *Health Promotion and Practice,* 5 (4), pp. 451-458, ISSN 1524-8399

Lai, Y.M. (1999). Effects of music listening on depressed women in Taiwan. *Issues in Mental Health Nursing,* 20 (3), pp. 229-246, ISSN 0161-2840

Lai, H.L. (2004). Music preference and relaxation in Taiwanese elderly people. *Geriatric Nursing,* 25 (5), pp. 286-291, ISSN 0950-0448

Landi, F.; Zuccala, G. & Bernabei, R. (1997). Physiotherapy and occupational therapy, A geriatric experience in the acute care hospital. *American Journal of Physical Medicine and Rehabilitation,* 76, pp. 38-42, ISSN 0894-9115

Larson, R.; Mannell, R. & Zuzanek, J. (1986). Daily well being of older adults with friends and family. *Psychology and Aging,* 1(2), pp. 117-126, ISSN 0882-7974

Lee, R.E & King, A.C. (2003). Discretionary time among older adults: how do physical activity promotion interventions affect sedentary and active behaviors? *Annals of Behavioral Medicine,* 25 (2), pp. 112-119, ISSN 0883-6612

Lewis, C.B. & Bottomley, J.M. (2002). Principles and practice in geriatric rehabilitation, *In: Geriatric Physical Therapy. A Clinical Approach, pp.* 249-287, Prentice Hall, USA.

Lou, M.F. (2001). The use of music to decrease agitated behaviour of the demented elderly: the state of the science. *Scandinavian Journal of Caring Sciences,* 15 (2), pp. 165-173, ISSN 0283-9318

Lynch, T.R &Aspnes, A.K. (2004). Individual and group psychotherapy. In: *Textbook of Geriatric Psyciatry,* D.G. Blazer, D.C. Steffens & E.W. Busse. (Ed.). pp. 443-458, London.

Mac Pherson, B. & Kozlik, C. (1987). Age patterns in leisure participation, In: *Aging in Canada: Social perspectives,* V. Marshall (Ed.), pp. 89-95, Toronto: Fitzhenry and Whiteside.

Maestre Castelblanque, E. & Albert Cunat, V. (2005). Life style activities in older people without intellectual impairment: a population-based study. *Rural and Remote Health,* 5 (1), p. 344, ISSN1445-6354

Matsuo, M.; Nagasawa, J.; Yoshino A.; et.al. (2003). Effects of activity participation of the elderly on quality of life. *Yonago Acta Medica,* 46, pp. 17-24, ISSN 0513-5710

Mountain, G. (2005). Occupational Therapy Interventions, In: *Occupational therapy with older people.* (pp. 160-191). Whurr Publishers, London.

Mountain, G. (2005). Services to meet needs, In: *Occupational therapy with older people.* (pp. 102-135). Whurr Publishers, London.

Mouton, C.P.; Calmbach, W.L; Dhanda, R.; Espino, D.V & Hazuda, H. (2000). Barriers and benefits to leisure time physical activity among older Mexican Americans. *Archives of Family Medicine,* 9 (9), pp. 892-897, ISSN 1063-3987

Nagaya, M.; Endo, H.; Kachi, T. & Ota, T. (2005). Recreational rehabilitation improved cognitive function in vascular dementia. *Journal of American Geriatric Society,* 53 (5), pp. 911-912.

Nelson, D.L. (1997). Why the profession of occupational therapy will flourish in the 21 th century. *American Journal of Occupational Therapy,* 51 (1), pp. 13-24.

Ozmenler, N. (2005). Geriyatrik Psikiyatri, In: *Klinik Psikiatri,* H. Aydın, A. Bozkurt (Ed.), pp. 599-601, Ankara: Kaplan& Benjamin Sadock, Virginia Sadock.

Pang, M.Y.; Eng, J.J.; Dawson, A.S.; Mc Kay, H.A. & Harris, J.E. (2005). A community base fitness and mobility exercise program for older adults with chronic stroke: a randomized, controlled trial. *Journal of American Geriatric Society,* 53 (10), pp. 166-174.

Pu, C.T. & Nelson, M.E. Aging, function and exercise, In: *Exercise in Rehabilitation Medicine,* W.R. Frontera, D.M. Dawson ve D.M. Slovik (Eds.), pp. 391-424, USA: Human Kinetics.

Reichert, F.F.; Barros, A.J.; Domingues, M.R. & Hallal, P.C. (2007). The role of perceived personal barriers to engagement in leisure-time physical activity. *American Journal of Public Health,* 97 (3), pp. 515-519.

Resnick, B.M. (1991). Geriatric motivation: Clinically helping the elderly to comply. *Journal of Gerontological Nursing,* 17 (6), pp. 4-8, ISSN 0098-9134

Rosalie, A.K. (2003). Social assessment of geriatric patients. In: *Brocklehurst's Text book of Geriatric Medicine and Gerontology,* R.C. Tallis & H.M. Fillit (Eds.), p. 187, Churchill Livingstone, Spain.

Ross, R.R. (1990). Time-use in later life. *Journal of Advanced Nursing,* 15, pp. 394-399, ISSN 0309-2402

Routasalo, P.E.; Savikko, N. & Tivils, R.S. (2007). Effectiveness of psychosocial group rehabilitation in relieving loneliness of older people. *Advances in Gerontology,* 20 (3), pp. 24-32, ISSN 1561-9125

Royeen, M. & Reistetter, T.A. (1996). K.O. Larson (Ed.). *The role of occupational therapy with elderly (ROTE).* pp. 774-804. The American Occupational Therapy Association, USA.

Scarmeas, N.; Levy, G.; Tang, M.; Manly, J. & Stern, Y. (2001). Influence of leisure activity on the incidence of Alzheimer's disease. *Neurology,* 26; 57(12), pp. 2236-2242, ISSN:2090-5513

Sherratt, K.; Thornton, A. & Hatton, C. (2004). Emotional and behavioural responses to music in people with dementia: an observational study. *Aging and Mental Health,* 8 (3), pp. 233-241, ISSN 1360-7863

Stinson, C.K. & Kirk, E. (2006). Structured reminiscence: an intervention to decrease and increade depression and increase self-transcendence in older women. *Journal of Clinical Nursing,* 15 (2), pp. 208-218, ISSN 0962-1067

Strain, L.A.; Grabusic, C.C.; Searle, M.S. & Dunn, N.J. (2002). Continuing and ceasing leisure activities in later life: a longitudinal study. *The Gerontologist,* 42 (2), pp. 217-223, ISSN 0016-9013

Sumsion, T. & Blank, A. (2006). The canadian model of occupational performance (CMOP), *Foundations for practice in occupational therapy,* E.A. Duncan (Ed.), pp. 109-124, Elsevier Churchill Livingstone, London.

Sung, H.C. & Chang, A.M. (2005). Use of preferred music to decrease agitated behaviours in older people with dementia: a review of the literature. *Journal of Clinical Nursing,* 14 (9), pp. 1133-1140, ISSN 0962-1067

Vass, M.; Avlund, K. & Lauridsen, J. (2005). Feasible model for prevention of functional decline in older people: municipality-randomized, controlled trial. *Journal of American Geriatric Society.* 53 (4), pp. 563-568.

Vitkus, J. & Horowitz, L.M. (1987). Poor social performance of lonely people: lacking a skill or adopting a role? *Journal of Perceptual Social Psychology,* 52 (6), pp. 1266-1273.

Ward, R.A. (1979). The meaning of voluntary association participation to older people, *Journal of Gerontology,* 34 (3), pp. 438-445.

Warr, P.; Butcher, V. & Robertson, I. (2004). Activity and psychological well-being in older people. *Aging and Mental Health,* 8 (2), pp. 172-183, ISSN 1360-7863

WHO rapport (1998). A population aged 65 and above, 1997 in An Aging World, 30.10.2007, http://www.who.org/whr/1998/age-97-e.gif.

Wikstrom, B.M. (2004). Older adults and the arts: the importance of aesthetic forms of expression in later life. *Journal of Gerontological Nursing,* 30 (9), pp. 30-36, ISSN 0098-9134

Woods, B.; Spector, A.; Jones, C.; Orrell, M. & Davies, S. (2005). Reminiscence therapy for dementia. *Cochrane Database of Systematic Reviews,* 18 (2): CD001120.

Yoshimoto, T. & Kawata, C. (1996). Negative effect of perceived transportation problems on social activities of elderly people in a small town far from the nearest train station. *Japanese Journal of Geriatrics,* 33 (12), pp. 928-934, ISSN 0300-9173

Yucel, H.; Yıldırım, S.A. & Kayıhan, H. (2006). Assessments in Geriatric Rehabilitation. In: *Geriatri ve Gerontoloji,* S.Arıoğul (Ed.), pp. 183-197, Medikal&Nobel, Ankara.

Yucel, H.; Düger, T.; Uyanık, M. & Kayıhan, H. (2006). Occupational Therapy in Geriatric Rehabilitation, In: *Geriatri ve Gerontoloji,* S. Arıoğul (Ed.), pp. 205-221, Medikal & Nobel, Ankara.

Yucel, H. PhD Thesis, Hacettepe University, Institute of Health Sciences, Ankara, 2008

Yucel, H. & Kayıhan, H. (2010). Effects of multi-purpose activities on cognitive functions in the elderly who reside at home and the nursing home, *Turkish Clinics Medicine Sciences,* 30 (1): pp. 227-232.

Zelazny, C.M. (2001). Therapeutic instrumental music playing in hand rehabilitation for older adults with osteoarthritis: four case studies. *Journal of Music Therapy,* 38 (2), pp. 97-113, ISSN 0022-2917